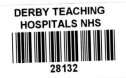

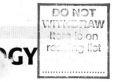
HISTOLOGY AND CELL BIOLOGY

An Introduction t

Fo

HISTOLOGY AND CELL BIOLOGY
An Introduction to Pathology

Fourth Edition

Abraham L. Kierszenbaum, M.D., Ph.D.
Emeritus Medical (Clinical) Professor
The Sophie Davis School of Biomedical Education
The City University of New York
New York, New York

Laura L. Tres, M.D., Ph.D.
Emeritus Medical (Clinical) Professor
The Sophie Davis School of Biomedical Education
The City University of New York
New York, New York

ELSEVIER

ELSEVIER
SAUNDERS

1600 John F. Kennedy Blvd.
Ste 1800
Philadelphia, PA 19103-2899

HISTOLOGY AND CELL BIOLOGY: AN INTRODUCTION TO PATHOLOGY   ISBN: 978-0-323-31330-8
Copyright © 2016, 2012, 2007, 2002 by Saunders, an imprint of Elsevier Inc.

Notices

Knowledge and best practice in this field are constantly changing. As new research and experience broaden our understanding, changes in research methods, professional practices, or medical treatment may become necessary.

Practitioners and researchers must always rely on their own experience and knowledge in evaluating and using any information, methods, compounds, or experiments described herein. In using such information or methods they should be mindful of their own safety and the safety of others, including parties for whom they have a professional responsibility.

With respect to any drug or pharmaceutical products identified, readers are advised to check the most current information provided (i) on procedures featured or (ii) by the manufacturer of each product to be administered, to verify the recommended dose or formula, the method and duration of administration, and contraindications. It is the responsibility of practitioners, relying on their own experience and knowledge of their patients, to make diagnoses, to determine dosages and the best treatment for each individual patient, and to take all appropriate safety precautions.

To the fullest extent of the law, neither the Publisher nor the authors, contributors, or editors assume any liability for any injury and/or damage to persons or property as a matter of products liability, negligence or otherwise, or from any use or operation of any methods, products, instructions, or ideas contained in the material herein.

Library of Congress Cataloging-in-Publication Data
Kierszenbaum, Abraham L., author.
   Histology and cell biology : an introduction to pathology / Abraham L. Kierszenbaum, Laura L. Tres. -- Fourth edition.
      p. ; cm.

   ISBN 978-0-323-31330-8 (hardcover : alk. paper)
   I. Tres, Laura L., author. II. Title.
      [DNLM: 1. Histology. 2. Pathologic Processes. 3. Cell Biology. 4. Pathology. QZ 4]
   RB25
   616.07--dc23

                                                                                            2014038010

Content Strategist: Meghan Ziegler
Content Development Specialist: Joanie Milnes
Publishing Services Manager: Anne Altepeter
Project Manager: Ted Rodgers
Cover designer: Xiaopei Chen

Printed in Canada
Last digit is the print number: 9 8 7 6 5 4 3 2 1

To our daughters Adriana and Silvia
To our grandchildren Ryan, Trevor, Kyle, and Marielle
To the beloved memory of our parents

PREFACE

The fourth edition of *Histology and Cell Biology: An Introduction to Pathology* contains revisions and additions that strengthen the visual approach to learning histology within the context of cell biology and pathology introduced in the previous editions. New in the fourth edition are a greater emphasis on pathology topics and the online audiovisual version of the histology-oriented Concept Mappings. The combined histology–cell biology–pathology approach intends to prepare medical students for the forthcoming learning of pathophysiology and clinical medicine. The practice of medicine changes relentlessly as new knowledge becomes known. Future physicians can find in this book the basis for continuing education to better help their patients by constantly integrating basic and clinical sciences.

The visual approach presented in this book emerged from many years of practicing pathology and teaching cell biology, histology, and pathology to medical students. Through the years, it became clear the need to communicate and reinforce relevant concepts of histology and pathology to be mastered under increasing time constraints resulting from changes in the basic science curriculum in most medical schools. The focal point of the teaching approach is to provide medical students with an integrated method wherein the learning of normal structure and pathologic conditions can reinforce each other. The cell biology and pathology components, although not complete, provide the necessary foundation for further learning and integration with medical sciences. Pathology students and residents may find this book useful for refreshing basic concepts of histology and cell biology. Histology and pathology are visually oriented sciences, and the visual cues included in this book can facilitate interpretation opportunities in clinical practice.

Similar to the previous editions, the fourth edition consists of six parts. Part I brings together histology, cell biology, and general pathology within the context of the basic tissues. Chapter 3, Cell Signaling, is an uncommon section in a histology book. It serves to unify the concept that the study of tissues and organs cannot be separated from molecular biology and general pathology. Parts II through VI present several organ systems grouped by their most relevant function for the purpose of integration. Instructors and students may find the grouping of organs useful for teaching and learning. Teachers may find the material beneficial for delivering a lecture using the same or a different presentation sequence. In Part VI, Organ Systems: The Reproductive System, the chapter headings depart from the traditional designation to emphasize prominent functions. All the information is presented in a clear, concise, and student-friendly manner using color graphics and photographs that are meant to be studied. In some cases the graphics reiterate the concise text; in others they add new information complementing or extending the text. Several boxes dispersed in most of the chapters introduce students to clinical and pathologic conditions based on recent and evolving molecular and biochemical knowledge.

Most chapters include one or more *Concept Mappings*. Each Concept Mapping provides a basic framework of interconnected concepts arranged in a hierarchical form leading to integration and critical thinking. Concept Mapping and Essential Concepts highlight key issues to remember, correlate, and extend in forthcoming courses during medical education. Students may find the new online audiovisual version of Concept Mappings convenient for reviewing and integrating the material when the time of in-course and board examinations arrives.

There are many people to be acknowledged and thanked. We are grateful for the numerous suggestions, comments, and encouragements from faculty and students. All of them provided valuable feedback to make the message clearer and more consistent. We also thank publishers who made available to students the Chinese, French, Greek, Japanese, Portuguese, Spanish, and Turkish editions. Our special appreciation goes to the production team of Elsevier in the Philadelphia and St. Louis offices for their magnificent effort in making sure that the fourth edition met high publishing standards.

Abraham L. Kierszenbaum and Laura L. Tres

New in the fourth edition are a greater emphasis on pathology topics and the online audiovisual version of the histology-oriented *Concept Mappings*.

The focal point of the teaching approach is to provide medical students with an integrated method wherein the learning of normal structure and pathologic conditions can reinforce each other.

Each *Concept Mapping* provides a basic framework of interconnected concepts arranged in a hierarchical form leading to integration and critical thinking.

HISTOLOGY AND CELL BIOLOGY
An Introduction to Pathology

Fourth Edition

1. Epithelium

Epithelia separate the internal environment from the external environment by forming sheets of polarized cells held together by specialized junctional complexes and cell adhesion molecules. Epithelial cells participate in embryo morphogenesis and organ development in response to intrinsic and extrinsic signaling by tailoring cell proliferation, differentiation and cell death. We address the structural characteristics of epithelial cells within a biochemical and molecular framework as an introduction to the transition from a normal to a pathologic status.

General classification of epithelia

The epithelium is a tightly cohesive sheet of cells that covers or lines body surfaces (for example, skin, intestine, secretory ducts) and forms the functional units of secretory glands (for example, salivary glands, liver). The main characteristics of epithelia are summarized in Box 1-A.

The traditional classification and nomenclature of different types of epithelia are based on two parameters:

1. The **shapes of individual cells.**

2. **The arrangement of the cells in one or more layers** (Figure 1-1).

Individual epithelial cells can be flattened (**squamous cells**), have equal dimensions (**cuboidal cells**), and be taller than wider (**columnar cells**).

According to the number of cell layers, an epithelium consisting of a **single cell layer** is classified as **simple epithelium.**

Simple epithelia, in turn, are subdivided into **simple squamous epithelium, simple cuboidal epithelium**, and **simple columnar epithelium**, according to the shape of their cell components. The specific name **endothelium** is used for the simple squamous epithelium lining the blood and lymphatic vessels. **Mesothelium** is the simple squamous epithelium lining all body cavities (peritoneum, pericardium, and pleura). Figure 1-2 provides examples of simple epithelia.

Stratified epithelia are composed of **more than one cell layer.** Stratified epithelia are subclassified according to the shapes of the cells at the superficial or outer layer into **stratified squamous epithelium, stratified cuboidal epithelium**, and **stratified columnar epithelium.**

Stratified squamous is the epithelium most frequently found and can be subdivided into **moderately keratinized** (also known as nonkeratinizing) or **highly keratinized** types (Figure 1-3). The cells of the outer layer of a nonkeratinizing squamous epithelium **retain**

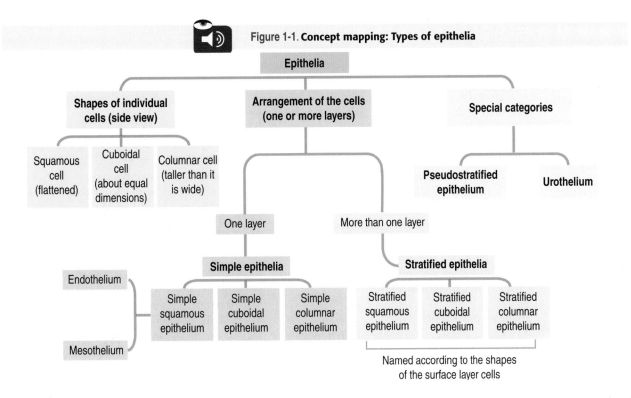

Figure 1-1. **Concept mapping: Types of epithelia**

Epithelia

Shapes of individual cells (side view) — Squamous cell (flattened), Cuboidal cell (about equal dimensions), Columnar cell (taller than it is wide)

Arrangement of the cells (one or more layers)

One layer — Simple epithelia — Endothelium, Mesothelium, Simple squamous epithelium, Simple cuboidal epithelium, Simple columnar epithelium

More than one layer — Stratified epithelia — Stratified squamous epithelium, Stratified cuboidal epithelium, Stratified columnar epithelium

Named according to the shapes of the surface layer cells

Special categories — Pseudostratified epithelium, Urothelium

Box 1-A | **Main characteristics of epithelia**

- Epithelia derive from the ectoderm, mesoderm, and endoderm.
- Epithelia line and cover all body surfaces except the articular cartilage, the enamel of the tooth, and the anterior surface of the iris.
- The basic functions of epithelia are **protection** (skin), **absorption** (small and large intestine), **transport of material** at the surface (mediated by cilia), **secretion** (glands), **excretion** (tubules of the kidneys), **gas exchange** (lung alveolus), and **gliding between surfaces** (mesothelium).
- Most epithelial cells renew continuously by mitosis.
- Epithelia lack a direct blood and lymphatic supply. Nutrients are delivered by diffusion.
- Epithelial cells have almost no free intercellular substances (in contrast to connective tissue).
- The cohesive nature of an epithelium is maintained by **cell adhesion molecules** and **junctional complexes**.
- Epithelia are anchored to a **basal lamina**. The basal lamina and connective tissue components cooperate to form the **basement membrane**.
- Epithelia have structural and functional **polarity**.

nuclei (for example, esophagus and vagina). **Nuclei are absent in the outer layer of the highly keratinized stratified squamous epithelium** (for example, the epidermis of the skin). Stratified epithelia have **basal cells** aligned along the basal lamina. Basal cells are mitotically active and continuously replace the differentiating cells of the upper layers.

Although rare, there are also **stratified cuboidal epithelia** (for example, in the ovarian follicles) and **stratified cuboidal epithelia** (for example, lining the intralobular ducts of salivary glands).

Two special categories are the **pseudostratified epithelium** and the **urothelium**. The pseudostratified epithelium consists of basal and columnar cells resting on the basal lamina. Only the columnar cells reach the luminal surface. Because the nuclei of the basal and columnar cells are seen at different levels, one has the impression of a stratified epithelial organization.

Within this category are the **pseudostratified columnar ciliated epithelium** of the trachea and the **pseudostratified columnar epithelium with stereocilia** of the epididymis (Figure 1-4).

The epithelium of the human urinary passages, also referred to as **urothelium**, has the characteristics of a pseudostratified epithelium: it consists of basal cells, intermediate cells and columnar dome-shaped cells, each extending thin cytoplasmic processes reaching the basal lamina (Figure 1-4). An important feature of this epithelium is its transitional height that varies with distention and contraction of the organ (see Chapter 14, Urinary System).

Epithelial cell polarity

An important aspect of an epithelium is its **polarity**. Polarity is essential to carry out specific functions of the various organ systems. Polarity is determined by

the distribution of proteins and lipids and the rearrangement of the cytoskeleton.

Most epithelial cells lining surfaces and cavities and have three **geometric** domains (Figure 1-5):

1. The **apical (uppermost) domain** is exposed to the lumen or external environment and displays **apical differentiations**.

2. The **lateral domain** faces neighboring epithelial cells linked to each other by **cell adhesion molecules** and **junctional complexes**.

3. The **basal domain** is associated with a **basal lamina** that separates the epithelium from underlying connective tissue, representing the internal environment. The basal lamina, of epithelial cell origin, is reinforced by components of the connective tissue. The basal lamina–connective tissue complex is designated the **basement membrane**.

From the **functional** perspective, sealing junctions segregate the plasma membrane of an epithelial cell into an **apical domain** and a **basolateral domain**. This segregation is supported by the asymmetric distribution of transporting molecules ensuring polarized secretory and absorptive functions of an epithelium.

For example, the apical domain has structures important for the **protection** of the epithelial surface (such as **cilia** in the respiratory tract) or for the **absorption** of substances (such as **microvilli** in the intestinal epithelium). In contrast, the basolateral domain facilitates directional or vectorial transport functions prevented from trespassing the sealing junctions.

Apical differentiations

The **apical domain** of some epithelial cells can display three types of differentiation:

1. **Cilia.**
2. **Microvilli.**
3. **Stereocilia.**

Cilia

There are two types of **cilia** (singular, **cilium**; Figure 1-6): **multiple motile cilia** and a **single** or a **primary non-motile cilium**.

Ciliogenesis, the assembly process of both types of cilia, is initiated by the **basal body**, a structure originated from a **basal body precursor** located in the **centrosome**. The basal body precursor multiplies and undergoes differentiation under control of six small, non-protein coding microRNAs that inhibit the translation of the mRNA encoding the **centrosomal protein CP110**. If the expression of CP110 protein increases by deletion of the regulatory microRNAs, basal bodies fail to dock to the apical plasma membrane, disrupting ciliogenesis and giving rise to **human respiratory disease** and **primary ciliary dyskinesia**.

Figure 1-2. **Simple epithelium**

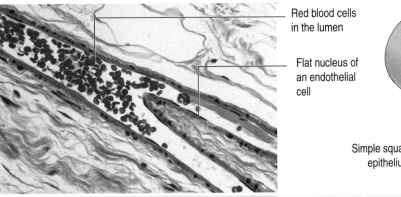

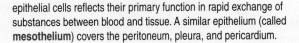

Red blood cells
in the lumen

Flat nucleus of
an endothelial
cell

Basal lamina

Lumen

Simple squamous
epithelium

Simple squamous epithelium (endothelium)

The inner lining of all blood vessels consists of a single layer of squamous endothelial cells. The thinness of the simple squamous epithelial cells reflects their primary function in rapid exchange of substances between blood and tissue. A similar epithelium (called **mesothelium**) covers the peritoneum, pleura, and pericardium.

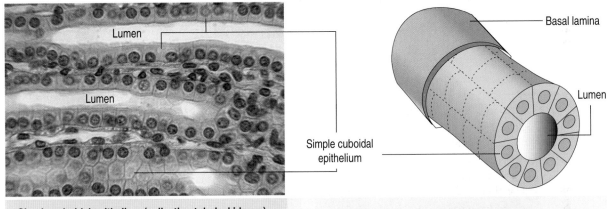

Lumen

Lumen

Basal lamina

Lumen

Simple cuboidal
epithelium

Simple cuboidal epithelium (collecting tubule, kidneys)

The inner lining of kidney tubules and thyroid follicles consists of a single layer of cuboidal cells. Cuboidal cells are highly polarized and participate in absorption, secretion (thyroid gland), and active ion transport (kidneys). Similar to the endothelium, a basal lamina attaches the cell to the subjacent connective tissue.

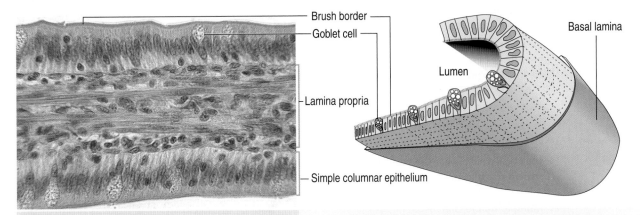

Brush border
Goblet cell

Lamina propria

Simple columnar epithelium

Basal lamina

Lumen

Simple columnar epithelium (small intestine)

The small intestine is lined by columnar epithelial cells with the nucleus in the medial portion of the cell. The apical domain contains finger-like projections called **microvilli** forming a **brush border**. Microvilli participate in the absorption of proteins, sugar, and lipids, which are released at the basolateral domain into the blood circulation for transport to the liver.

Goblet cells are present among the columnar epithelial cells. They can be distinguished by a dilated, goblet-like apical cytoplasm containing a light-stained mucus material. Mucus is released into the lumen and coats the epithelial cell surface. The **lamina propria** consists of loose connective tissue located beneath the epithelium.

Figure 1-3. Stratified epithelium

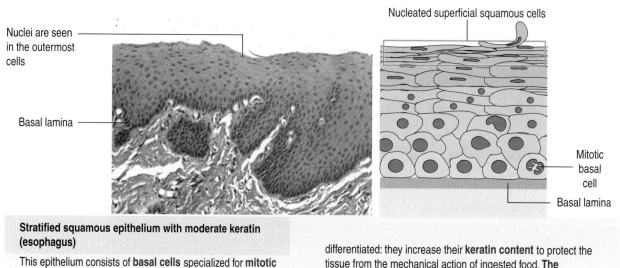

Nuclei are seen in the outermost cells

Basal lamina

Nucleated superficial squamous cells

Mitotic basal cell

Basal lamina

Stratified squamous epithelium with moderate keratin (esophagus)

This epithelium consists of **basal cells** specialized for **mitotic division**. Stratified cells covering the basal layer are differentiating cells. Cells of the outer layer are highly differentiated: they increase their **keratin content** to protect the tissue from the mechanical action of ingested food. **The outermost cells retain their nuclei.** This epithelium is also known as **nonkeratinizing**.

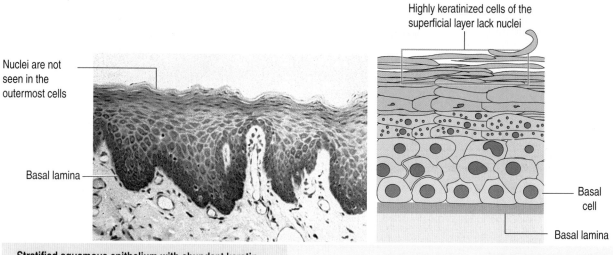

Nuclei are not seen in the outermost cells

Basal lamina

Highly keratinized cells of the superficial layer lack nuclei

Basal cell

Basal lamina

Stratified squamous epithelium with abundant keratin (epidermis)

This highly keratinized epithelium also consists of **basal cells** specialized for **mitotic division**. Stratified cells covering the basal layer are differentiating cells. Cells of the outer layer contain abundant **keratin** to prevent water loss and penetration of chemical and physical insults. **The outermost cells lack nuclei.** This epithelium is also known as **keratinizing**.

Under normal conditions, basal bodies migrate to the apical plasma membrane and extend into the extracellular space the **axoneme**, a microtubular structure that forms the basic structure of the cilium.

Multiple motile cilia

Multiple motile cilia function to **coordinate fluid or cargo flow on the surface of an epithelium.** They are cell projections originating from **basal bodies** anchored by **rootlets** to the apical portion of the cytoplasm (Figure 1-6).

A basal body contains nine **triplet** microtubules in a **helicoid array** without a central microtubular component. By contrast, a cilium consists of an **axoneme formed by a central pair of microtubules surrounded by nine concentrically arranged microtubular pairs. This assembly is known as the 9 + 2 microtubular doublet arrangement.** The axoneme is also a component of the sperm tail, or **flagellum**.

The trachea and the oviduct are lined by **ciliated epithelial cells**. In these epithelia, ciliary activity is important for the local defense of the respiratory system and for the transport of the fertilized egg to the uterine cavity.

Figure 1-4. **Pseudostratified epithelia**

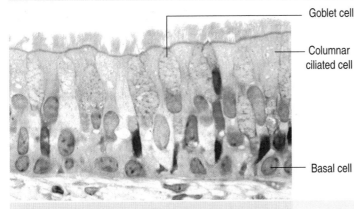

Goblet cell

Columnar ciliated cell

Basal cell

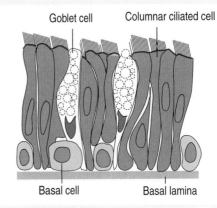

Goblet cell

Columnar ciliated cell

Basal cell

Basal lamina

Pseudostratified columnar ciliated epithelium (trachea)

This epithelium consists of three major cell types: (1) **Columnar cells** with **cilia** on their apical domain. (2) **Basal cells** anchored

to the basal lamina. (3) **Goblet cells**, mucus-secreting epithelial cells. Columnar ciliated and goblet cells attach to the basal lamina and reach the lumen. Basal cells do not reach the lumen.

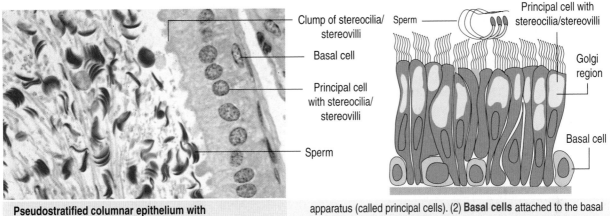

Clump of stereocilia/ stereovilli

Basal cell

Principal cell with stereocilia/ stereovilli

Sperm

Sperm

Principal cell with stereocilia/stereovilli

Golgi region

Basal cell

Pseudostratified columnar epithelium with stereocilia/stereovilli (epididymis)

The epididymal epithelium contains two major cell types. (1) **Columnar cells** with stereocilia and highly developed Golgi

apparatus (called principal cells). (2) **Basal cells** attached to the basal lamina. Basal and principal cells are associated with the basal lamina. Only principal cells reach the lumen. Sperm can be visualized in the lumen. Stereocilia is an early misnomer as they lack microtubules. An appropriate name is **stereovilli**.

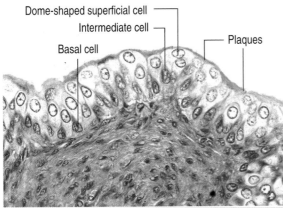

Dome-shaped superficial cell

Intermediate cell

Basal cell

Plaques

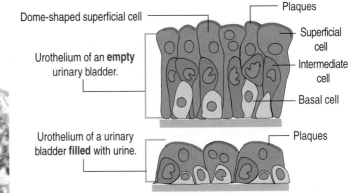

Dome-shaped superficial cell

Urothelium of an **empty** urinary bladder.

Plaques

Superficial cell

Intermediate cell

Basal cell

Urothelium of a urinary bladder **filled** with urine.

Plaques

Urothelium (urinary bladder)

The epithelium lining the urinary passages (also called **urothelium**), consists of three cell types. (1) **dome-shaped superficial cells** (often binucleated); (3) **pyriform-shaped intermediate cells**; and (2) **polyhedral-shaped basal cells**, all of them extending cytoplasmic processes anchored to the basal

lamina. In humans, the urothelium is a pseudostratified epithelium. A characteristic of the urothelium is its **transitional configuration** in response to distension and contraction tensional forces caused by urine. **Plaques** of aggregated proteins (**uroplakins**) are found on the apical plasma membrane of the dome-shaped superficial cells.

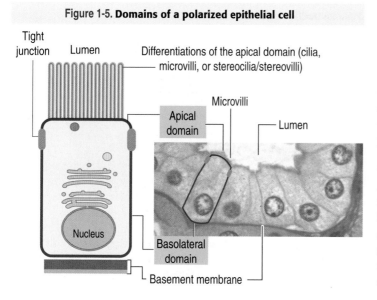

Figure 1-5. Domains of a polarized epithelial cell

Tight junction

Lumen

Differentiations of the apical domain (cilia, microvilli, or stereocilia/stereovilli)

Apical domain

Microvilli

Lumen

Nucleus

Basolateral domain

Basement membrane

Single or primary non-motile cilium

Some cells have a **single** or **primary non-motile cilium**. The importance of a single cilium emerges from rare recessive human disorders known as **ciliopathies** caused by structural or functional abnormalities of cilia. The structure and mechanism of assembly of a single cilium are shown in Figure 1-6.

The significant aspects of a primary cilium are:

1. It functions as a **sensor** that provides the cell with information about the surrounding external environment.

2. It participates in the early stages of embryonic patterning leading to organogenesis.

3. Many components of the **hedgehog signaling** pathway, essential at least in early development, are present in a single cilium.

4. The position of the single cilium, called **kinocilium**, of the hair cell of the organ of Corti in the inner ear determines the correct polarity of the adjacent actin-containing stereocilia, essential for maintaining body balance and for hearing (see Chapter 9, Sensory Organs: Vision and Hearing).

Microvilli

Microvilli (singular, **microvillus**; Figure 1-7) are finger-like cell projections of the apical epithelial cell surface containing a core of cross-linked microfilaments (a polymer of G-actin monomers).

At the cytoplasmic end of the microvillus, bundles of **actin** and other proteins extend into the **terminal web**, a filamentous network of cytoskeletal proteins running parallel to the apical domain of the epithelial cell.

The intestinal epithelium and portions of the nephron in the kidney are lined by epithelial cells with microvilli forming a **brush border**. In general, a brush border indicates the **absorptive** function of the cell.

Stereocilia (stereovilli)

Stereocilia (singular, **stereocilium**; see Figure 1-7) are long and **branching** finger-like projections of the apical epithelial cell surface. Similar to microvilli, stereocilia contain a core of cross-linked actin with other proteins. **Stereocilia (or stereovilli) do not have axonemes.** Stereocilia/stereovilli are typical of the epithelial lining of the epididymis and contribute to the process of sperm maturation occurring in this organ.

Cell adhesion molecules

A sheet of epithelial cells results from the tight attachment of similar cells to each other and to the **basal lamina**, a component of the extracellular matrix. **Cell adhesion molecules** enable interepithelial cell contact, and this contact is stabilized by specialized **cell junctions**. A consequence of this arrangement is the apical and basolateral domain polarity of an epithelial sheet.

Although cell adhesion molecules and cell junctions are considered here within the framework of epithelia, nonepithelial cells also can use cell adhesion molecules and junctions to establish contact with each other, enabling cell-cell communication. A typical example of nonepithelial cells connected by specialized junctions is the cardiac muscle (see Chapter 7, Muscle Tissue).

There are two major groups of cell adhesion molecules (see Box 1-B):

1. **Ca^{2+}-dependent molecules**, including **cadherins** and **selectins.**

2. **Ca^{2+}-independent molecules**, which compose the **immunoglobulin superfamily** and **integrins.**

Many cells can use different cell adhesion molecules to mediate cell-cell attachment. Integrins are mainly involved in cell–extracellular matrix interactions. Cadherins and integrins establish a link between the internal cytoskeleton of a cell and the exterior of another cell (cadherins) or the extracellular matrix (integrins).

Cadherins

Cadherins (Figure 1-8) are a family of Ca^{2+}-dependent molecules with a major role in cell adhesion and morphogenesis.

The importance of cadherins in human disease is indicated by the process known as epithelial-mesenchymal transition (EMT). EMT is the switching of polarized epithelial cells to a fibroblast-like or mesenchymal phenotype characterized by the loss of intercellular adhesion and increased cell migration.

During EMT, epithelial cadherins (E-cadherins), Crumbs (a group of apical polarity proteins) and cytokeratins (a cytoskeletal intermediate filament protein) are downregulated, whereas mesenchymal markers, such as vimentin (another intermediate filament protein), are upregulated.

A loss of E-cadherins is associated with the acquisi-

Figure 1-6. Apical differentiations of epithelial cells: Cilia and primary cilium

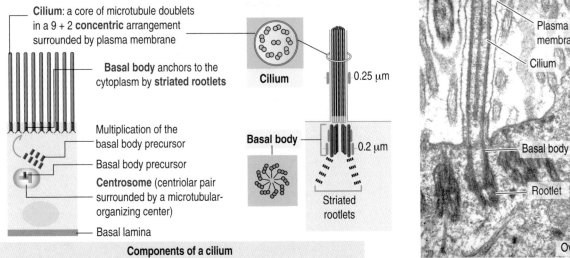

Cilium: a core of microtubule doublets in a 9 + 2 **concentric** arrangement surrounded by plasma membrane

Basal body anchors to the cytoplasm by **striated rootlets**

Multiplication of the basal body precursor

Basal body precursor

Centrosome (centriolar pair surrounded by a microtubular-organizing center)

Basal lamina

Cilium

0.25 μm

Basal body

0.2 μm

Striated rootlets

Plasma membrane

Cilium

Basal body

Rootlet

Oviduct

Basal body 9³ + 0

Cilium 9² + 2

Components of a cilium

Cilia develop from **basal bodies** located in the apical domain of the cytoplasm. **Basal body precursors** derive from the **centrosome**, multiply, mature and dock to the apical plasma membrane of the cell. A basal body, consisting of **nine peripheral microtubule triplets** (9^3 [triplets] + 0) in a **helicoidal** arrangement, extends into the extracellular space an **axoneme**, a microtubular structure surrounded by the plasma membrane. **Rootlets** anchor the basal body to the cytoplasm. Central microtubules are not present in basal bodies and centrioles. The **cilium** consists of a concentric array of nine microtubule doublets surrounding a central pair of microtubules (9^2 [doublets] + 2).

Assembly of the cilium

The cilium is formed and maintained by the transport of tubulins along the axoneme mediated by proteins of the intraflagellar transport (IFT) system. IFT trafficking from the base of the cilium to the tip (anterograde transport; to the microtubule plus end) is mediated by kinesin motor proteins mobilizing IFT protein complexes. Dynein motor participates in retrograde transport (to the microtubule minus end; base of the cilium). IFT proteins form a platform for transporting cargo between the base and tip of the cilium.

Disruption of the kinesin motor or IFT proteins blocks cilia formation. Basal body proteins influence ciliary trafficking. Among these are components of the BBSome, which are named after their association with **Bardet-Biedl syndrome** (BBS). BBSome proteins may help loading protein cargo to the ciliary axoneme.

Proteins of the **hedgehog signaling pathway** participate in intraciliary and intraflagellar transport.

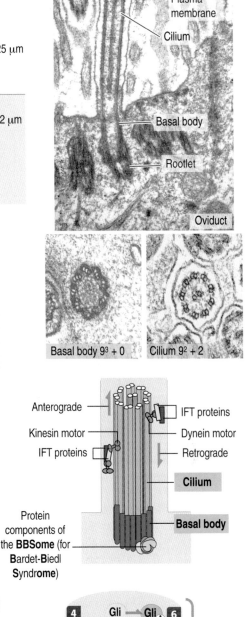

Anterograde

Kinesin motor

IFT proteins

IFT proteins

Dynein motor

Retrograde

Cilium

Protein components of the **BBSome** (for Bardet-Biedl **S**yndrome)

Basal body

Primary cilium and Hedgehog signaling

Hedgehog (Hh) signaling requires primary cilia for activation. The trafficking of Hh pathway proteins along primary cilia is a key factor in epithelial cell differentiation.
1 In the **absence** of Hh secretory protein, **Ptc** (for patched; the receptor of Hh), the transmembrane protein **Smo** (for Smoothened) is blocked from entering the cilium. Smo is stored in vesicles near the basal body.
2 Upon Hh binding, Ptc is internalized and Smo, free from blocking, moves to the plasma membrane **3** and activates the Hh pathway by **antagonizing** the function of **Sufu** (suppressor of fused) **4**.
5 The motor kinesin **KIF7** transports **Gli** (for glioma) transcription factors to the tip of the cilium. If Smo is not available to inactivate Sufu (because of the absence of Hh), Gli is degraded or processed to become a repressor. If the suppressive function of Sufu is antagonized, Gli is processed to an activator form (**GliA**) **6**.
7 Activated GliA is then transported out of the cilium into the nucleus (by **dynein motor** and **IFT proteins**) to activate epithelial differentiation genes.

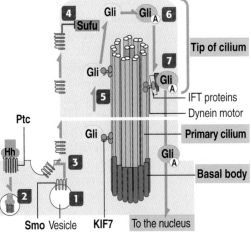

Tip of cilium

IFT proteins

Dynein motor

Primary cilium

Basal body

Ptc

Hh

Smo   Vesicle   KIF7   To the nucleus

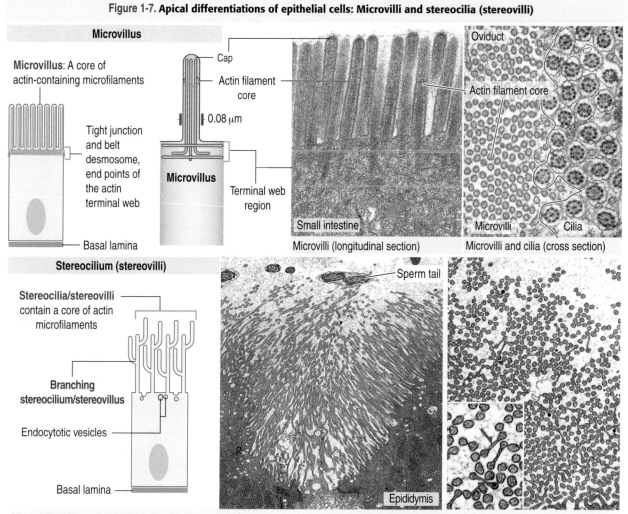

Figure 1-7. Apical differentiations of epithelial cells: Microvilli and stereocilia (stereovilli)

Microvillus

Microvillus: A core of actin-containing microfilaments

Tight junction and belt desmosome, end points of the actin terminal web

Basal lamina

Cap

Actin filament core

0.08 μm

Microvillus

Terminal web region

Oviduct

Actin filament core

Small intestine

Microvilli (longitudinal section)

Microvilli   Cilia

Microvilli and cilia (cross section)

Stereocilium (stereovilli)

Stereocilia/stereovilli contain a core of actin microfilaments

Branching stereocilium/stereovillus

Endocytotic vesicles

Basal lamina

Sperm tail

Epididymis

Microvilli and **stereocilia (stereovilli)** have the same substructure: Core of **actin microfilaments** and actin-associated proteins.

In the intestinal epithelium, actin extends into the **terminal web,** a network of cytoskeletal proteins in a collar-like arrangement at the apical domain of the cytoplasm. Although microvilli have comparable length, **stereocilia/stereovilli are longer and branch,** and the apical domain of the cell contains endocytotic vesicles. The bridges connecting adjacent stereocilia (blue arrows) are indicators of their branching.

tion of invasive behavior by tumor cells (**metastasis**) as we discuss in Chapter 4, Connective Tissue and Chapter 17, Digestive Glands.

There are more than 40 different cadherins. **E-cadherin** is found along the lateral cell surfaces and is responsible for the maintenance of most epithelial layers. The removal of calcium or the use of a blocking antibody to E-cadherin in epithelial cell cultures breaks down cell-cell attachment, and the formation of stabilizing junctions is disrupted. E-cadherin molecules form *cis*-homophilic dimers ("like-to-like"), which bind to dimers of the **same** or **different class of cadherins in the opposite cell membrane** (*trans*-homophilic or heterophilic ["like-to-unlike"] interaction). These forms of binding require the presence of calcium and result in a specialized zipper-like cell-cell adhesion pattern.

N-cadherin is found in the central nervous system,

the lens of the eye, and in skeletal and cardiac muscle. **P-cadherin** is observed in placenta (trophoblast).

The cytoplasmic domain of cadherins is linked to **actin** through intermediate proteins known collectively as the **catenin** (Latin *catena*, chain) **complex.** The complex includes **catenins** (α, β, and **p120**) and actin-binding proteins (α-actinin, vinculin, and formin-1, among others).

The catenin complex has at least three distinct roles in the function of cadherins:

1. Catenins mediate a direct link to filamentous actin.

2. They interact with regulatory molecules of the actin cytoskeleton.

3. They control the adhesive state of the extracellular domain of cadherins.

The association of actin to the cadherin-catenin complex is essential for cell morphogenesis, changes

Figure 1-8. Cadherins

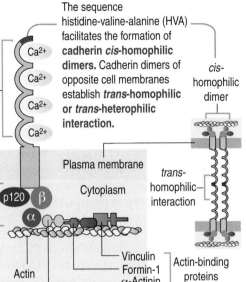

Four domains in the extracellular portion of cadherin bind to calcium. The function of cadherins is Ca²⁺-dependent.

β-catenin binds to the intracellular tail of cadherin and the β-catenin/cadherin complex recruits α-catenin, which binds directly to actin. p120 catenin is a regulator of cadherin function.

The sequence histidine-valine-alanine (HVA) facilitates the formation of **cadherin cis-homophilic dimers.** Cadherin dimers of opposite cell membranes establish *trans*-homophilic or *trans*-heterophilic interaction.

cis-homophilic dimer

Plasma membrane

trans-homophilic-interaction

Cytoplasm

p120 β

α

Actin

Vinculin
Formin-1
α-Actinin

Actin-binding proteins

Cadherins are the main adhesion proteins holding epithelial cells together in a sheet arrangement. The removal of calcium disrupts tissue cohesiveness. The cytoplasmic tail interacts with actin filaments through numerous intracellular attachment proteins, including three **catenin** proteins. β-catenin can also act as a transcriptional cofactor.

in cell shape, and the establishment of cell polarity.

Members of the cadherin family also are present **between cytoplasmic plaques** of the zonula and the macula adherens. β-catenin plays a significant role in **colorectal carcinogenesis** (see Chapter 16, Lower Digestive Segment).

Selectins

Selectins (Figure 1-9), similar to cadherins, are Ca²⁺-dependent cell adhesion molecules. In contrast to cadherins, selectins bind to carbohydrates and belong to the family of **C-type lectins** (Latin *lectum*, to select).

Each selectin has a carbohydrate-recognition domain (CRD) with binding affinity to a **specific oligosaccharide** attached to a protein (glycoprotein)

or a lipid (glycolipid). The molecular configuration of the CRD is controlled by **calcium**.

Selectins participate in the movement of **leukocytes** (Greek *leukos*, white, *kytos*, cell) circulating in blood (neutrophils, monocytes, B and T cells) toward tissues by **extravasation**. Extravasation is the essence of homing, a mechanism that enables leukocytes to escape from blood circulation and reach the sites of inflammation (see Figure 1-12). Homing also permits thymus-derived T cells to home in on peripheral lymph nodes (see Chapter 10, Immune-Lymphatic System).

The three major classes of cell surface selectins are as follows:

1. **P-selectin**, found in platelets and activated endothelial cells lining blood vessels.

2. **E-selectin**, found on activated endothelial cells.

3. **L-selectin**, found on leukocytes.

P-selectin is stored in cytoplasmic vesicles in endothelial cells. When endothelial cells are activated by inflammatory signaling, P-selectin appears on the cell surface.

On their surface, leukocytes contain **sialyl Lewis-x antigen**, a specific oligosaccharide ligand for P-selectin. P-selectin binding to the antigen slows down streaming leukocytes in blood, and they begin to roll along the endothelial cell surfaces. P-selectins get additional help from members of the immunoglobulin (Ig) superfamily and integrins to stabilize leukocyte attachment, leading to extravasation (see Figure 1-12).

Ig superfamily

N-CAM (for **neural cell adhesion molecule**) belongs to the Ig superfamily and mediates homophilic and heterophilic interactions.

In contrast to cadherins and selectins, members of the Ig superfamily are Ca²⁺-independent cell adhesion molecules and are encoded by a single gene. Members of the Ig superfamily are generated by the alternative messenger RNA (mRNA) splicing and have differences in glycosylation.

A conserved feature shared by all members of the Ig superfamily is an extracellular segment with one or more **folded domains characteristic of immunoglobulins** (Figure 1-10).

Of particular interest is **CD4**, a member of the Ig superfamily and the receptor for the **human immunodeficiency virus type 1** (**HIV-1**) in a subclass of lymphocytes known as T cells or helper cells. We discuss the significance of several members of the Ig superfamily in Chapter 10, Immune-Lymphatic System.

Other members of the Ig superfamily play important roles in the homing process during inflammation. Examples include **intercellular adhesion molecules 1 and 2** (**ICAM-1 and ICAM-2**) on endothelial cell

---

Box 1-B | Cell adhesion molecules: Highlights to remember

• Cell adhesion molecules can be classified as Ca²⁺-dependent and Ca²⁺-independent.

• Ca²⁺-dependent adhesion molecules include cadherins and selectins.

• Ca²⁺-independent adhesion molecules include cell adhesion molecules of the immunoglobulin superfamily (CAMs) and integrins.

• Cadherins and CAMs display *trans*-homophilic interaction across the intercellular space.

• Integrins are the only cell adhesion molecules consisting of two subunits: α and β.

• Cadherins and integrins interact with F-actin through adapters (catenins for cadherins, and vinculin, talin, and α-actinin for integrins).

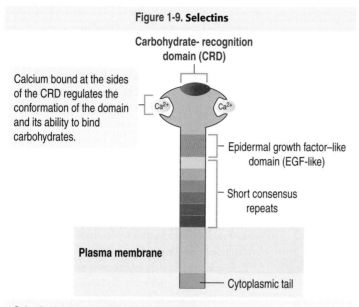

Figure 1-9. Selectins

Carbohydrate- recognition domain (CRD)

Calcium bound at the sides of the CRD regulates the conformation of the domain and its ability to bind carbohydrates.

Ca^{2+} Ca^{2+}

Epidermal growth factor–like domain (EGF-like)

Short consensus repeats

Plasma membrane

Cytoplasmic tail

Selectins have three extracellular domains:
1. A **carbohydrate-recognition domain** (CRD) specific for a particular sugar (galactose, mannose, *N*-acetylglucosamine, and others).
2. A domain homologous to a repeat found in epidermal growth factor (**EGF-like**).
3. Many **consensus repeats** found in complement regulatory proteins.
   There are three major types of selectins:
1. L-selectin, carried by lymphocytes and with binding affinity to sulfated carbohydrates.
2. E-selectin, expressed by activated endothelial cells.
3. P-selectin, expressed by platelets and activated endothelial cells.
   Selectins, together with integrins and intercellular cell adhesion molecules (ICAMs), play a significant role in inflammation and in the periodic migration of lymphocytes from the circulation into lymphoid organs (**homing**).

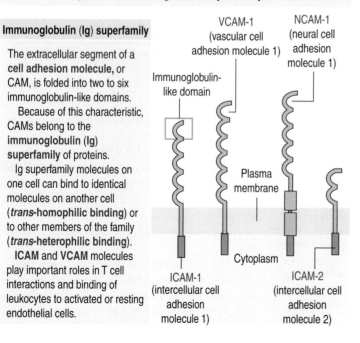

Figure 1-10. Immunoglobulin superfamily

Immunoglobulin (Ig) superfamily

The extracellular segment of a **cell adhesion molecule,** or CAM, is folded into two to six immunoglobulin-like domains.
   Because of this characteristic, CAMs belong to the **immunoglobulin (Ig) superfamily** of proteins.
   Ig superfamily molecules on one cell can bind to identical molecules on another cell (*trans*-homophilic binding) or to other members of the family (*trans*-heterophilic binding).
   ICAM and **VCAM** molecules play important roles in T cell interactions and binding of leukocytes to activated or resting endothelial cells.

VCAM-1 (vascular cell adhesion molecule 1)

NCAM-1 (neural cell adhesion molecule 1)

Immunoglobulin-like domain

Plasma membrane

Cytoplasm

ICAM-1 (intercellular cell adhesion molecule 1)

ICAM-2 (intercellular cell adhesion molecule 2)

surfaces. ICAM-1 is expressed when an inflammation is in progress to facilitate the transendothelial migration of leukocytes (see Chapter 6, Blood and Hematopoiesis).

Integrins

Integrins (Figure 1-11) differ from cadherins, selectins, and members of the Ig superfamily in that integrins are **heterodimers** formed by two associated α and β subunits encoded by different genes. There are about 22 integrin heterodimers consisting of 17 forms of α subunits and 8 forms of β subunits.

Almost every cell expresses one or several integrins. Similar to cadherins, the cytoplasmic domain of β integrin subunit is linked to **actin** filaments through **connecting proteins** (see **Figure 1-11**).

The extracellular domain of β integrin subunit binds to the **tripeptide RGD (Arg-Gly-Asp)** sequence present in **laminin** and **fibronectin**, two major components of the **basement membrane**, a specific type of extracellular matrix. Laminin and fibronectin interact with various collagen types (including **type IV collagen**), **heparan sulfate proteoglycan perlecan**, and **entactin** (also called **nidogen**).

The integrin–extracellular matrix relationship is critical for cell migration to precise sites during embryogenesis and can be regulated when cell motility is required. In addition to their role in cell-matrix interactions, integrins also mediate cell-cell interaction.

Integrins containing β_2 subunits are expressed on the surface of leukocytes and mediate cell-cell binding in preparation for extravasation. An example is $\alpha_1\beta_2$ integrin on non-adherent leukocytes that bind to ligands on endothelial cell surfaces following activation by extracellular stimulation, resulting in leukocyte extravasation during homing (the recruitment of leukocytes to extravascular spaces). We discuss the mechanism of cell homing in Figure 1-12 and expand it within the context of inflammation in Chapter 10, Immune-Lymphatic System.

Integrins are bidirectional signaling receptors. Integrins can be activated by proteins binding to their extracellular and intracellular domains. When integrins bind to extracellular matrix molecules, a protein complex binds to the cytoskeleton and several signaling pathways are activated.

Genetic mutations of integrins or integrin regulators have been associated with **Glanzmann's thrombo-asthenia** (mutations in β_3 integrin subunit), **leukocyte adhesion deficiency** (type I, caused by mutations in β_2 integrin subunit; type II, resulting from the absence of fucosyl-containing ligands for selectins due to a hereditary defect of endogenous fucose metabolism; and type III, determined by mutations in kindlin) and **skin diseases** (mutations in kindlin, α_2, α_6, and β_4 integrin subunits).

Figure 1-11. Integrins

Integrins differ from the other cell adhesion proteins:
1. They consist of **two subunits**.
2. They have a dual function: they bind to the extracellular matrix and the internal cytoskeleton.

The α subunit of an integrin has two chains linked by a disulfide linkage and a globular head with binding sites for divalent cations.

The β subunit has two significant characteristics: (1) The extracellular chain contains repeating cysteine-rich regions. (2) The intracellular portion interacts with actin filaments through connecting proteins: **talin** and **focal adhesion kinase**, the first proteins to be recruited.

In its active conformation, talin binds the β-integrin cytoplasmic domain. **Kindlin, an integrin coactivator,** binds to the β-integrin cytoplasmic domain and increases talin-induced integrin activation. The **IPP complex** (consisting of intergrin-linked kinase, PINCH [for Particularly Interesting New Cysteine-Histidine-rich protein] and parvin) recruits α-**actinin** and **paxillin** to the cell adhesion site.

In its active conformation state, β-integrin connects actin to the extracellular matrix proteins **fibronectin** and **laminin**, through their RGD-binding sites.

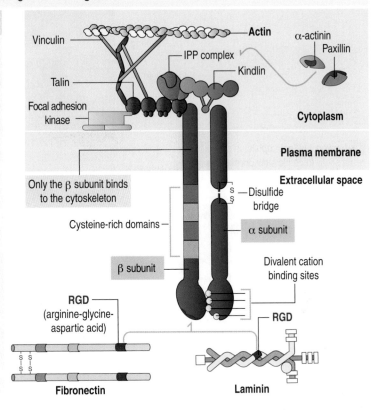

ADAM proteins

The reversal of integrin-mediated cell binding to the extracellular matrix can be disrupted by proteins called **ADAM** (for *a d*isintegrin *a*nd *m*etalloprotease). ADAMs have pivotal roles in fertilization, angiogenesis, neurogenesis, heart development, cancer and Alzheimer's disease (see Chapter 8, Nervous Tissue).

A typical ADAM protein (Figure 1-13) contains an **extracellular domain** and an **intracellular domain**. The extracellular domain consists of several portions including a **disintegrin domain** and a **metalloprotease domain**.

1. A disintegrin domain binds to integrins and competitively prevents integrin-mediated binding of cells to laminin, fibronectin, and other extracellular matrix proteins.

2. A metalloprotease domain degrades matrix components and enables cell migration.

A significant function of ADAMs is **protein ectodomain shedding**, consisting of the proteolytic release of the ectodomain of a membrane protein cleaved adjacent to the plasma membrane. ADAMs are members of the family of **sheddases**.

Ectodomain shedding targets for cleavage the **proinflammatory cytokine tumor necrosis factor ligand** (TNFL) and **all ligands of the epidermal growth factor receptor**. A released soluble ectodomain of a cytokine or growth factor can function at a distance from the site of cleavage (paracrine signaling). Ectodomain shedding of a receptor can inactivate

the receptor by functioning as a decoy sequestering soluble ligands away from the plasma membrane-bound unoccupied receptor.

A defect in **TNF receptor 1** (TNFR1) shedding, determined by a mutation in the receptor cleavage site, causes a **periodic febrile** because of continuous availability of TNFR1 for TNFL binding. Consequently, recurring fever occurs by increased inflammatory responses.

Cell junctions

Although cell adhesion molecules are responsible for cell-cell adhesion, cell junctions are necessary for providing stronger stability. In addition, the movement of solutes, ions, and water through an epithelial layer occurs **across** and **between** individual cell components.

The **transcellular pathway** is controlled by numerous channels and transporters.

The **paracellular pathway** is regulated by a continuous intercellular contact or **cell junctions**. A deficiency in the cell junctions accounts for acquired and inherited diseases caused by inefficient epithelial barriers.

Cell junctions are **symmetrical** structures formed between two adjacent cells. There are three major classes of **symmetrical** cell junctions (Figure 1-14; see Box 1-C):

1. **Tight junctions.**
2. **Anchoring junctions.**
3. **Gap** or **communicating junctions.**

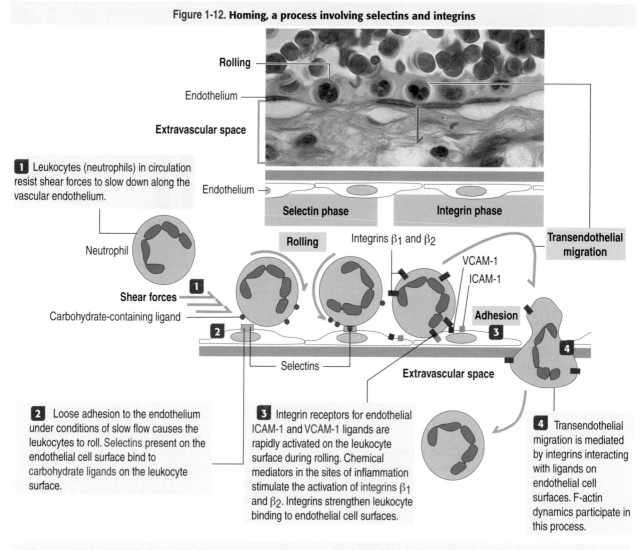

Figure 1-12. Homing, a process involving selectins and integrins

Rolling

Endothelium

Extravascular space

1 Leukocytes (neutrophils) in circulation resist shear forces to slow down along the vascular endothelium.

Endothelium →

Selectin phase

Integrin phase

Neutrophil

Rolling

Integrins β_1 and β_2

VCAM-1
ICAM-1

Transendothelial migration

Shear forces

Carbohydrate-containing ligand

1

2

Adhesion

3

4

Selectins

Extravascular space

2 Loose adhesion to the endothelium under conditions of slow flow causes the leukocytes to roll. Selectins present on the endothelial cell surface bind to carbohydrate ligands on the leukocyte surface.

3 Integrin receptors for endothelial ICAM-1 and VCAM-1 ligands are rapidly activated on the leukocyte surface during rolling. Chemical mediators in the sites of inflammation stimulate the activation of integrins β_1 and β_2. Integrins strengthen leukocyte binding to endothelial cell surfaces.

4 Transendothelial migration is mediated by integrins interacting with ligands on endothelial cell surfaces. F-actin dynamics participate in this process.

Most leukocytes circulate in blood without interacting with other blood cells or endothelial cells lining the blood vessels. However, a subset of **lymphocytes** participates in a continuous recirculation process through lymphoid tissues. This homing process involves many diverse adhesion molecules that help lymphocytes to home to various lymphoid compartments of the body.

The lymphocyte-endothelial cell interaction requires two types of cell adhesion proteins: **selectins** and **integrins**. **Neutrophils** use a similar mechanism to escape from blood vessels, primarily **postcapillary venules**, into inflammatory sites. The migration of leukocytes from the bloodstream to the tissue occurs in several steps as illustrated.

Tight junctions

Tight junctions (also called **occluding junctions**) (Figure 1-15) have two major functions:

1. They determine **epithelial cell polarity** by separating the apical domain from the basolateral domain and preventing the free diffusion of lipids and proteins between them.

2. They prevent the free passage of substances across an epithelial cell layer (**paracellular pathway barrier**).

Cell membranes of two adjacent cells come together at regular intervals to seal the apical intercellular space. These areas of close contact continue around the entire surface of the cell like a belt, forming anastomosing strips of the transmembrane

proteins **occludin** and **claudin**. Occludin and claudin belong to the family of **tetraspanins** with four transmembrane domains, two outer loops, and two short cytoplasmic tails.

Occludin interacts with four major **zonula occludin** (ZO) proteins: ZO-1, ZO-2, ZO-3, and **afadin**. **Claudin** (Latin *claudere*, to close), a family of 16 proteins forming linear fibrils in the tight junctions, confers barrier properties on the paracellular pathway. A mutation in the gene encoding **claudin 16** is the cause of a rare human **renal magnesium wasting syndrome** characterized by hypomagnesemia and seizures.

Two members of the Ig superfamily, **nectins** and **junctional adhesion molecules** (**JAMs**), are pres-

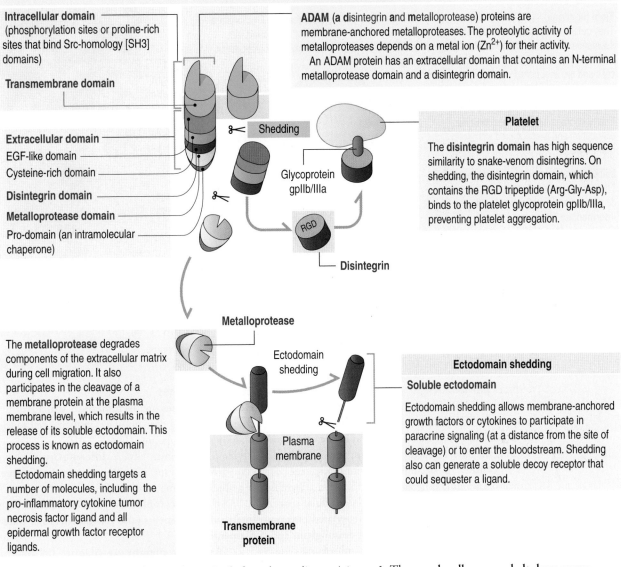

Figure 1-13. ADAM protein, a sheddase

Intracellular domain
(phosphorylation sites or proline-rich sites that bind Src-homology [SH3] domains)

Transmembrane domain

Extracellular domain
EGF-like domain
Cysteine-rich domain

Disintegrin domain

Metalloprotease domain

Pro-domain (an intramolecular chaperone)

ADAM (a **d**isintegrin **a**nd **m**etalloprotease) proteins are membrane-anchored metalloproteases. The proteolytic activity of metalloproteases depends on a metal ion (Zn^{2+}) for their activity.
An ADAM protein has an extracellular domain that contains an N-terminal metalloprotease domain and a disintegrin domain.

Shedding

Glycoprotein gpIIb/IIIa

RGD

Disintegrin

Platelet

The **disintegrin domain** has high sequence similarity to snake-venom disintegrins. On shedding, the disintegrin domain, which contains the RGD tripeptide (Arg-Gly-Asp), binds to the platelet glycoprotein gpIIb/IIIa, preventing platelet aggregation.

Metalloprotease

The **metalloprotease** degrades components of the extracellular matrix during cell migration. It also participates in the cleavage of a membrane protein at the plasma membrane level, which results in the release of its soluble ectodomain. This process is known as ectodomain shedding.
Ectodomain shedding targets a number of molecules, including the pro-inflammatory cytokine tumor necrosis factor ligand and all epidermal growth factor receptor ligands.

Ectodomain shedding

Plasma membrane

Transmembrane protein

Ectodomain shedding

Soluble ectodomain

Ectodomain shedding allows membrane-anchored growth factors or cytokines to participate in paracrine signaling (at a distance from the site of cleavage) or to enter the bloodstream. Shedding also can generate a soluble decoy receptor that could sequester a ligand.

---

ent in tight junctions. Both form homodimers (*cis* homodimers) and then *trans* homodimers across the intercellular space. Nectins are connected to actin filaments through the protein **afadin**. The targeted deletion of the *afadin* gene in mice results in embryonic lethality. A mutation in the *nectin-1* gene is responsible for **cleft lip/palate and ectodermal dysplasia** (CLEPD1) of skin, hairs, nails, and teeth in humans. Nectin-2–deficient male mice are sterile.

Tight junctions can be visualized by **freeze-fracturing** a network of **branching and anastomosing sealing strands**. We discuss in Chapter 2, Epithelial Glands, the procedure of freeze-fracturing for the study of cell membranes.

Anchoring junctions

Anchoring junctions are found below the tight junctions, usually near the apical surface of an epithelium. There are three classes of **anchoring junctions** (see Figures 1-14, 1-16, 1-18, and 1-19):

1. The **zonula adherens** or **belt desmosome**
2. The **macula adherens** or **spot desmosome**
3. The **hemidesmosome**

Zonula adherens or belt desmosome

Similar to the tight junctions, the **zonula adherens** is a **beltlike junction**. The zonula adherens (Figure 1-16) is associated with **actin microfilaments**. This association is mediated by the interaction of **cadherins** (**desmocollins** and **desmogleins**) with **catenins** (α, β, and p120). The main desmogleins expressed in the epidermis of the skin are desmoglein 1 and desmoglein 3 (Figure 1-17).

Macula adherens or spot desmosome

The **macula adherens** (also called **desmosome**) is a **spotlike** junction associated with **keratin intermediate filaments** (also known as **tonofilaments**) extending from one spot to another on the lateral and basal cell surfaces of epithelial cells (Figure 1-18). Spot desmo-

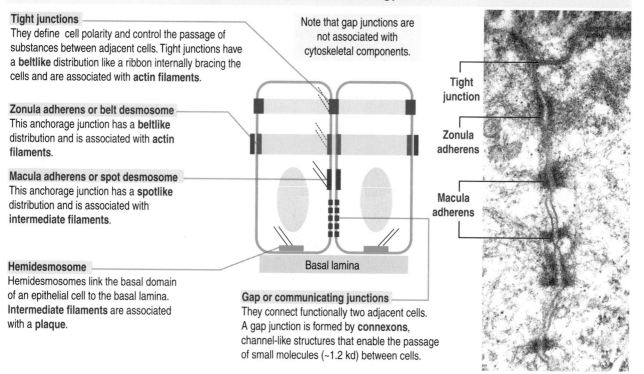

Figure 1-14. Anchoring and communicating junctions

Tight junctions
They define cell polarity and control the passage of substances between adjacent cells. Tight junctions have a **beltlike** distribution like a ribbon internally bracing the cells and are associated with **actin filaments**.

Zonula adherens or belt desmosome
This anchorage junction has a **beltlike** distribution and is associated with **actin filaments**.

Macula adherens or spot desmosome
This anchorage junction has a **spotlike** distribution and is associated with **intermediate filaments**.

Hemidesmosome
Hemidesmosomes link the basal domain of an epithelial cell to the basal lamina. **Intermediate filaments** are associated with a **plaque**.

Note that gap junctions are not associated with cytoskeletal components.

Basal lamina

Gap or communicating junctions
They connect functionally two adjacent cells. A gap junction is formed by **connexons**, channel-like structures that enable the passage of small molecules (~1.2 kd) between cells.

Tight junction

Zonula adherens

Macula adherens

---

somes provide strength and rigidity to an epithelial cell layer. Spot desmosomes are also present in the intercalated disks linking adjacent cardiocytes in heart (see Chapter 7, Muscle Tissue) and in the meninges lining the outer surfaces of the brain and spinal cord.

In contrast to occluding junctions, adjacent cell membranes linked by zonula and macula adherens are separated by a relatively wide intercellular space. This space is occupied by the glycosylated portion of proteins of the **cadherin** family, **desmogleins** and **desmocollins**, anchored to **cytoplasmic plaques** containing **desmoplakin, plakoglobin,** and **plakophilin.**

The cytoplasmic plaques are attached to the cytosolic face of the plasma membrane. The interlocking of similar cadherins binds two cells together by Ca^{2+}-dependent homophilic or heterophilic interaction, as we have already seen. Inherited disorders of some of the desmosomal components are indicated in Figure 1-18.

The human desmosomal cadherins genes include four desmogleins and three desmocollins. Their cytoplasmic regions interact with plakoglobin and plakophilin.

Desmoplakin interacts with the intermediate filaments keratin in epidermis, desmin in the intercalated disks, and vimentin in the meninges. **Desmoglein 1** and **desmoglein 3** maintain the cohesiveness of the epidermis, a stratified squamous epithelium. Autoantibodies to desmoglein 1 cause a blistering disease (disruption of cell adhesion) of the skin called **pemphigus foliaceus** (see Figure 1-17).

Hemidesmosomes

Hemidesmosomes are **asymmetrical** structures anchoring the basal domain of an epithelial cell to the underlying basal lamina (Figure 1-19).

Hemidesmosomes have a different organization compared with a macula adherens or a desmosome. A hemidesmosome consists of:

1. An **inner cytoplasmic plate** associated with intermediate filaments (also called **keratins** or **tonofilaments**)

2. An **outer membrane plaque** linking the hemidesmosome to the basal lamina by **anchoring filaments** (composed of **laminin 5**) and **integrin** $\alpha_6\beta_4$

Although hemidesmosomes look like half-desmosomes, none of the biochemical components present in the desmosome is found in hemidesmosomes. Hemidesmosomes increase the overall stability of epithelial tissues by linking intermediate filaments of the cytoskeleton with components of the basal lamina.

We consider additional details of the hemidesmosomes and their role in autoimmune diseases of the skin when we discuss the structure of intermediate filaments in the cytoskeleton section.

Gap junctions or communicating junctions

Gap junctions are symmetrical communicating junctions formed by integral membrane proteins called **connexins.**

Six connexin monomers associate to form a connexon, a hollow cylindrical structure that spans the plasma membrane. The end-to-end alignment of

Figure 1-15. Molecular organization of tight junctions

Tight junctions are circumferential belts at the apical domain of epithelial cells and linking adjacent endothelial cells. Tight junctions seal the space between epithelial cells and regulate the passage of water and flux of ions between adjacent epithelial cells (**paracellular pathway**). Molecules across the cell follow a **transcellular pathway**.

Afadin-nectin complex is anchored to ZO-1. Nectins form *cis*-homodimers, which interact with each other (*trans*-homo interaction) through the extracellular region.

Junctional adhesion molecules (JAMs) are associated to afadin and ZO-1. JAMs *cis*-homodimers interact with each other (*trans*-homo interaction) and determine the formation of cell polarity.

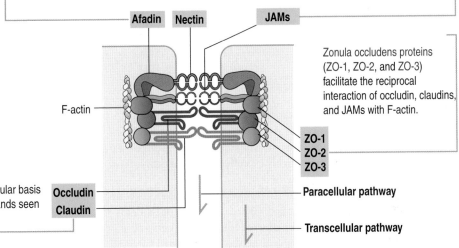

Afadin   Nectin   JAMs

F-actin

Zonula occludens proteins (ZO-1, ZO-2, and ZO-3) facilitate the reciprocal interaction of occludin, claudins, and JAMs with F-actin.

ZO-1
ZO-2
ZO-3

Occludin and claudins are the molecular basis for the formation of tight junction strands seen in freeze-fracture preparations.

Occludin
Claudin

Paracellular pathway

Transcellular pathway

Nectins and JAMs are members of the immunoglobulin subfamily. Their structure is characterized by immunoglobulin loops, each stabilized by disulfide bonds. Nectins and JAMs *cis*-homodimers mediate *trans*-homo cell-cell adhesion.

Occludin and claudins are members of the tetraspanin family of proteins, containing four transmembrane domains, two loops, and two cytoplasmic tails.

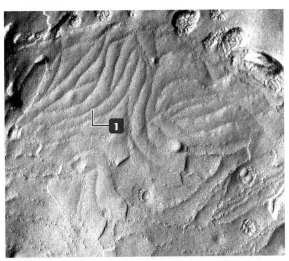

1 In **freeze-fracture preparations**, tight junctions appear as branching and **interconnected sealing ridges** forming a network near the apical domain of the cell. The ridges represent the transmembrane proteins **occludin** and **claudins** associated with the fractured protoplasmic face (PF).

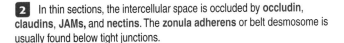

Lumen   Actin microfilaments   Zonula adherens   Plasma membrane

2 In thin sections, the intercellular space is occluded by **occludin**, **claudins, JAMs,** and **nectins.** The **zonula adherens** or belt desmosome is usually found below tight junctions.

connexons in adjacent cells provides a direct channel of communication (1.5 to 2 nm in diameter) between the cytoplasm of two adjacent cells (Figure 1-20). Connexons have a **clustering** tendency and can form patches about 0.3 mm in diameter.

These junctions facilitate the movement of molecules 1.2 nm in diameter (for example, Ca^{2+} and cyclic adenosine monophosphate [cAMP]) between cells). The connexon axial channels close when the concentration of Ca^{2+} is high. This junction is responsible for the chemical and electrical "**coupling**" between adjacent cells. A typical example is **cardiac muscle cells** connected by gap junctions to enable the transmission of electrical signals.

Figure 1-16. Zonula adherens (belt desmosome)

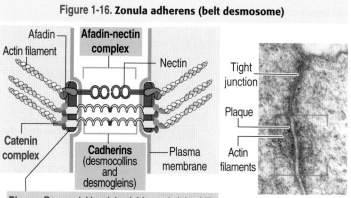

Afadin
Actin filament
Afadin-nectin complex
Nectin
Catenin complex
Cadherins (desmocollins and desmogleins)
Plasma membrane
Tight junction
Plaque
Actin filaments

Plaque: Desmoplakin, plakoglobin, and plakophilin

Clinical significance: Connexin mutations

Several diseases occur when genes encoding connexins are mutated. Mutations in the *connexin 26* (*Cx26*) **gene**, highly expressed in cells of the cochlea, are associated with **deafness**.

Mutations in the *connexin 32* (*Cx32*) gene are found in X-linked **Charcot-Marie-Tooth demyelinating neuropathy** resulting in progressive degeneration of peripheral nerves, characterized by distal muscle weakness and atrophy and impairment of deep tendon reflexes.

Connexin 32 (Cx32) protein is expressed in Schwann cells, which are involved in the production of rolled myelin tubes around the axons in the peripheral nervous system (see Chapter 8, Nervous Tissue). Gap junctions couple different parts of the rolled myelin tubes of the *same Schwann cell*, rather than different cells. A loss of the functional axial channels in myelin leads to the demyelinating disorder.

Mutations in the *connexin 50* (*Cx50*) gene are associated with **congenital cataracts**, leading to blindness.

Bone cells (osteoblasts/osteocytes) are connected by gap junctions and express connexin 43 (Cx43) and connexin 45 (Cx45) proteins. A deletion of the *Cx43* gene determines skeletal defects and delays in mineralization.

Basement membrane

The basement membrane consists of two components (Figure 1-21):

1. The **basal lamina**, a sheetlike extracellular matrix in direct contact with epithelial cell surfaces. The basal lamina results from the self-assembly of laminin molecules with type IV collagen, entactin, and proteoglycans.

2. A **reticular lamina**, formed by type III collagen fibers, supports the basal lamina and is continuous with the connective tissue.

The basal and reticular laminae can be distinguished by electron microscopy. Under the light microscope, the combined basal and reticular laminae receive the name of basement membrane, which can be recognized by the **periodic acid–Schiff** (**PAS**) stain (see Figure 1-21; see Box 1-D).

The PAS stain enables the pathologist to determine whether an epithelial malignant tumor has invaded the subjacent connective tissue by cancerous cells breaking through the basement membrane.

The basal lamina has specific functions in different tissues. The double basal lamina of the renal corpuscle constitutes the most important element of the **glomerular filtration barrier** during the initial step in the formation of urine (see Chapter 14, Urinary System).

In skeletal muscle, the basal lamina maintains the integrity of the tissue, and its disruption gives rise to **muscular dystrophies** (see Chapter 7, Muscle Tissue).

Laminin (Figure 1-22) is a cross-shaped protein consisting of three chains: the α **chain**, the β **chain**, and the γ **chain**. Laminin molecules can associate with each other to form a meshlike polymer. Laminin and **type IV collagen** are the major components of the basal lamina, and both are synthesized by epithelial cells resting on the lamina.

Laminin has binding sites for **nidogen** (also called entactin), **proteoglycans** (in particular, heparan sulfate **perlecan**), α-**dystroglycan** (see Chapter 7, Muscle Tissue), and **integrins**.

Figure 1-17. Desmogleins in skin disease: Pemphigus foliaceus

Desmoglein 1 predominates above the stratum spinosum.

Desmoglein 3 predominates in the strata basale and spinosum.

Layers of the epidermis

Stratum corneum
Stratum granulosum
Stratum spinosum
Stratum basale
Basal lamina
Dermis

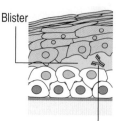

Blister

Pemphigus foliaceus is an autoantibody-mediated blistering disease in which antibodies against **desmoglein 1** cause a loss of adhesion of keratinocytes in the superficial layers of the epidermis.

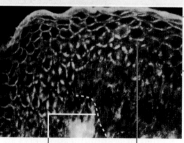

Superficial layers of the epidermis

Basal lamina

Intercellular deposits of immunoglobulins throughout the upper layers of the epidermis in contrast with the basal layers.

Immunofluorescence image from Weedon D: Skin Pathology. 2nd edition. London, Churchill Livingstone, 2002.

Figure 1-18. Macula adherens (spot desmosome)

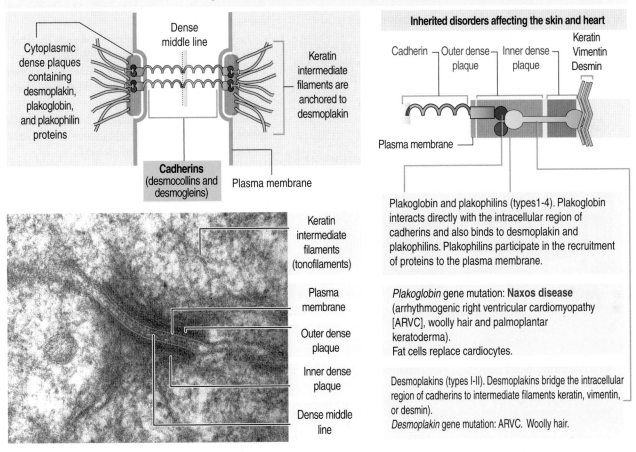

Cytoplasmic dense plaques containing desmoplakin, plakoglobin, and plakophilin proteins

Dense middle line

Keratin intermediate filaments are anchored to desmoplakin

Cadherins (desmocollins and desmogleins)

Plasma membrane

Inherited disorders affecting the skin and heart

Cadherin — Outer dense plaque — Inner dense plaque — Keratin Vimentin Desmin

Plasma membrane

Keratin intermediate filaments (tonofilaments)

Plasma membrane

Outer dense plaque

Inner dense plaque

Dense middle line

Plakoglobin and plakophilins (types1-4). Plakoglobin interacts directly with the intracellular region of cadherins and also binds to desmoplakin and plakophilins. Plakophilins participate in the recruitment of proteins to the plasma membrane.

Plakoglobin gene mutation: **Naxos disease** (arrhythmogenic right ventricular cardiomyopathy [ARVC], woolly hair and palmoplantar keratoderma).
Fat cells replace cardiocytes.

Desmoplakins (types I-II). Desmoplakins bridge the intracellular region of cadherins to intermediate filaments keratin, vimentin, or desmin).
Desmoplakin gene mutation: ARVC. Woolly hair.

Fibronectin (see Figure 1-22) consists of two protein chains cross-linked by disulfide bonds. Fibronectin is the main adhesion molecule of the extracellular matrix of the connective tissue and is produced by fibroblasts. Fibronectin has binding sites for **heparin** present in proteoglycans, several types of **collagens** (types I, II, III, and V), and **fibrin** (derived from fibrinogen during blood coagulation).

Fibronectin circulating in blood is synthesized in the liver by hepatocytes. It differs from fibronectin produced by fibroblasts in that it lacks one or two repeats (designated EDA and EDB for extra domain A and extra domain B) as a result of alternative mRNA splicing. Circulating fibronectin binds to fibrin, a component of the blood clot formed at the site of blood vessel damage. The RGD domain of immobilized fibronectin binds to integrin expressed on the surface of activated platelets, and the blood clot enlarges. We return to the topic of blood coagulation or hemostasis in Chapter 6, Blood and Hematopoiesis.

Figure 1-19. Hemidesmosome

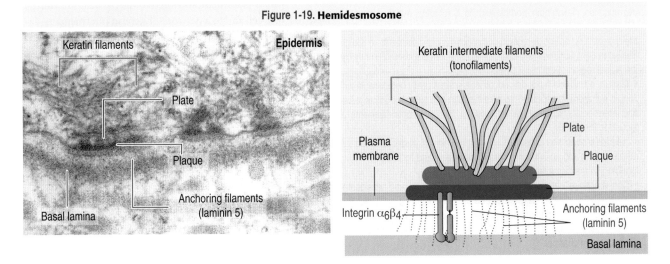

Keratin filaments

Epidermis

Plate

Plaque

Basal lamina

Anchoring filaments (laminin 5)

Keratin intermediate filaments (tonofilaments)

Plasma membrane

Plate

Plaque

Integrin α6β4

Anchoring filaments (laminin 5)

Basal lamina

Figure 1-20. **Gap junctions**

The intercellular channel is an axial channel that allows the direct passage of small signaling molecules between adjacent cells to coordinate cell responses.

Clusters of intercellular channels are known as gap junctions because of the narrow extracellular gap that separates the apposed plasma membranes.

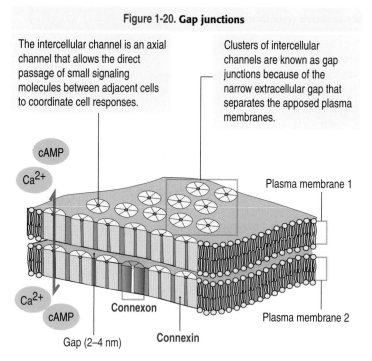

Six connexin monomers assemble to form a **hexameric connexon**, a cylinder with a central open channel. Connexons in the plasma membrane of one cell align with connexons of an adjacent cell, forming a **hydrophilic intercellular channel** connecting the cytoplasm of the apposed cells.

Box 1-C | Cell junctions: Highlights to remember

- Cell junctions can be classified as **symmetrical** and **asymmetrical**. Symmetrical junctions include tight junctions, belt desmosome (zonula adherens), desmosomes (macula adherens), and gap junctions. The hemidesmosome is an asymmetrical junction
- **Tight junctions** contain occludin and claudin, belonging to the protein family of tetraspanins because four segments of each protein span the plasma membrane. An additional component is the afadin-nectin protein complex.
   Junctional adhesion molecules (JAMs), zonula occludens (ZO) proteins ZO-1, ZO-2, and ZO-3 and F-actin are additional protein components. Tight junctions form a circumferential gasket that controls the paracellular pathway of molecules.
- **Zonula adherens** (belt desmosome) consists of a **plaque** that contains desmoplakin, plakoglobin, and plakophilin. Cadherins, mainly desmocollins and desmogleins dimers, and the afadin-nectin complex extend from the plaque to the extracellular space. A catenin complex links actin filaments to the plaque. Similar to tight junctions, the belt desmosome forms a circumferential gasket at the apical region of epithelial cells.
- **Macula adherens** (spot desmosome) are structurally comparable with the zonula adherens except that the afadin-nectin and catenin complexes are absent and intermediate filaments (tonofilaments), instead of actin filaments, are attached to the plaque.
- **Hemidesmosomes** consist of an inner membrane **plate**, to which tonofilaments attach, and an outer membrane **plaque**, linked by integrin $\alpha_6\beta_4$ and laminin 5 to the basal lamina.
- Tight junctions, belt desmosomes, spot desmosomes, and hemidesmosomes are anchoring junctions. **Gap junctions** are not anchoring junctions. Instead, gap junctions are communicating junctions connecting adjacent cells. The basic unit of a gap junction is the connexon, formed by 6 connexin molecules encircling a central channel.

Epithelium: Highlights to remember

Figure 1-23 presents the highlights of cell adhesion molecules and cell junctions.

1. An epithelium is a continuous sheet of polarized cells supported by a basement membrane.

2. The polarized nature of an epithelium depends on the tight junctions that separate the polarized cells into apical and basolateral regions.

3. Tight junctions control the paracellular pathway of solutes, ions, and water. Tight junctions form a belt around the circumference of each cell.

4. Endothelial cells, the constituents of a simple squamous epithelium, are linked by tight and spot desmosomes tightly regulated to maintain the integrity of the endothelium and protect the vessels from unregulated permeability, inflammation, and reactions leading to blood coagulation in the lumen (see Chapter 12, Cardiovascular System).

5. Leukocytes reach the site of infection by attaching to endothelial cell surfaces and migrate across the endothelium into the underlying tissues by a mechanism called **diapedesis**. Leukocytes find their way through endothelial cell-cell junctions after docking to activated or resting endothelial cells by the endothelial cell adhesion molecules ICAM-1 and VCAM-1 (see Figure 1-10). ICAM-1 and VCAM-1 bind to β_2 and β_1 integrin subunits in leukocytes (see Figure 1-12).

6. The cohesive nature of the epithelium depends on three factors: cell junctions, cell adhesive molecules and the interaction of integrins with the extracellular matrix, produced to a large extent by fibroblasts.

7. The basal lamina is essential for the differentiation of epithelial cells during embryogenesis.

Note in Figure 1-23 that:

1. The basal domain of epithelial cells interacts with the basal lamina through hemidesmosomes and integrins. Hemidesmosomes, so called because of their appearance as half-desmosomes in electron micrographs, are anchored to the basal lamina ouside the cell and to a network of keratin intermediate filaments inside the cell through a plate-plaque complex. Mutations in hemidesmosome components cause severe skin blistering as a result of a rupture of the anchoring molecular integrity.

2. Integrins interact directly with laminin and fibronectin, in particular the RGD domain to which integrins bind. Inside the cell, integrins interact with actin microfilaments. Integrins connect the extracellular environment to the intracellular space. We have seen that some ADAM proteins can use their disintegrin domain to prevent integrin binding to extracellular matrix ligands.

3. Collagens and proteoglycans do not interact directly with the basal domain of epithelial cells.

Figure 1-21. Basement membrane

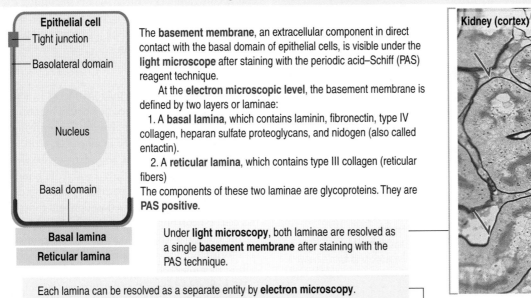

Epithelial cell
- Tight junction
- Basolateral domain
- Nucleus
- Basal domain

Basal lamina

Reticular lamina

The **basement membrane**, an extracellular component in direct contact with the basal domain of epithelial cells, is visible under the **light microscope** after staining with the periodic acid–Schiff (PAS) reagent technique.

At the **electron microscopic level**, the basement membrane is defined by two layers or laminae:

1. A **basal lamina**, which contains laminin, fibronectin, type IV collagen, heparan sulfate proteoglycans, and nidogen (also called entactin).

2. A **reticular lamina**, which contains type III collagen (reticular fibers)

The components of these two laminae are glycoproteins. They are **PAS positive**.

Under **light microscopy**, both laminae are resolved as a single **basement membrane** after staining with the PAS technique.

Kidney (cortex)

Each lamina can be resolved as a separate entity by **electron microscopy**.

Epithelial cell

Basal lamina   Reticular lamina   Nucleus of a fibroblast producing components of the reticular lamina

---

Instead, this interaction is mediated by laminin and fibronectin, which contain specific binding sites for collagens, the proteoglycan perlecan, and nidogen.

4. The lateral domains of adjacent epithelial cells communicate by gap junctions (not shown in Figure 1-23). In contrast to tight junctions and belt and spot desmosomes, gap junctions are not anchoring devices. They consist of intercellular channels connecting the cytoplasm of adjacent cells. They are communicating junctions.

5. Cadherins and the afadin-nectin complex are present in tight junctions and zonula adherens. Actin microfilaments are associated with these two junctions but there is a difference: catenins are present in zonula adherens but not in tight junctions.

Cytoskeleton

Cytoskeleton is a three-dimensional network of proteins distributed throughout the cytoplasm of eukaryotic cells.

The cytoskeleton has roles in:

1. **Cell movement** (crawling of blood cells along blood-vessel walls, migration of fibroblasts during wound healing, and movement of cells during embryonic development)

2. **Support and strength for the cell**

Box 1-D | Periodic acid–Schiff (PAS) reaction

- PAS is a widely used histochemical technique to show 1,2-glycol or 1,2-amino-alcohol groups, such as those present in glycogen, mucus, and glycoproteins.
- **Periodic acid**, an oxidant, converts these groups to **aldehydes**. The **Schiff reagent**, a colorless fuchsin, reacts with the aldehydes to form a characteristic **red-purple (magenta)** product.
- Some important PAS-positive structures are the **basement membrane**, **glycocalyx**, **mucus** produced by goblet cells, stored **glycoprotein hormones** in cells of the pituitary gland, and **collagens**.

Figure 1-22. Laminin and fibronectin

Laminin

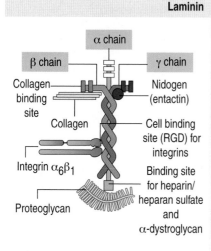

Laminin is the major component of the basal lamina. It consists of three disulfide-linked polypeptide chains designated α, β, and γ chains. Variants for each chain give rise to several laminin isoforms with different structure and function.

Laminins have binding sites for cell surface receptors (**integrins**), **type IV collagen**, and other adhesion proteins (e.g., **nidogen**, also known as **entactin**).

Laminin monomers self-associate to form a network that is part of the **basal lamina**.

Fibronectin

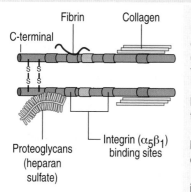

Fibronectin is a glycoprotein formed by two identical chains joined by disulfide linkages close to the C-terminal.

There are two forms of fibronectin:

1. **Plasma fibronectin**, produced by **hepatocytes** and secreted into the bloodstream.

2. **Cellular fibronectin**, produced by **fibroblasts**, forms part of the extracellular matrix.

Fibronectin has binding sites for **integrins, collagen, heparan sulfate,** and **fibrin**.

3. **Phagocytosis**
4. **Cytokinesis**
5. **Cell-cell and cell–extracellular matrix adherence**
6. **Changes in cell shape**

The components of the cytoskeleton were originally identified by **electron microscopy**. These early studies described a system of cytoplasmic "cables" that fell into three size groups, as follows:

1. **Microfilaments** (7 nm thick)
2. **Intermediate filaments** (10 nm thick)
3. **Microtubules** (25 nm in diameter)

Biochemical studies, involving the extraction of cytoskeletal proteins from cells with detergents and salts and in vitro translation of specific mRNA, showed that each class of filaments has a unique protein organization. When cytoskeletal proteins were purified, they were used as antigens for the production of antibodies. Antibodies are used as tools for the localization of the various cytoskeletal proteins in the cell. The **immunocytochemical localization**

of cytoskeletal proteins (Figure 1-24) and **cell treatment with various chemical agents** disrupting the normal organization of the cytoskeleton have been instrumental in understanding the organization and function of the cytoskeleton.

Microfilaments

The main component of microfilaments is **actin**. Actin filaments are composed of globular monomers (**G-actin**, 42 kd), which polymerize to form long helical filaments intertwined in a helix (**F-actin**).

Actin is a versatile and abundant cytoskeletal component forming static and contractile bundles and filamentous networks specified by actin-binding proteins and their distinctive location and function in a cell. F-actin bundles are present in the microvilli of the intestinal (Figure 1-25) and renal epithelial cells (brush border) and the stereocilia from the hair cells of the inner ear.

We have already seen that the intracellular portion of the cell adhesion molecules cadherins and integrin β_1 interacts with F-actin through linker proteins (see Figures 1-8 and 1-11). As discussed in Chapter 6, Blood and Hematopoiesis, actin, together with spectrin, forms a filamentous network on the inner face of the red blood cell membrane that is crucial for maintaining the shape and integrity of red blood cells. **Spectrin** is a tetramer consisting of two distinct polypeptide chains (α and β).

Actin filaments are polar. Growth of actin filaments may occur at both ends; however, one end (the "**barbed end**" or **plus end**) grows faster than the other end (the "**pointed end**" or **minus end**). The names correspond to the arrowhead appearance of myosin head bound at an angle to actin.

Actin filaments can branch in the **leading edge** (**lamellipodia**) of cells involved in either motility or interaction with other cell types. F-actin branching is initiated from the side of a preexisting actin filament by Arp2/3 (for **actin-related protein**), an actin nucleating complex of seven proteins (Figure 1-26). **Formin** regulates the assembly of unbranched actin in cell protrusions such as the intestinal microvilli (see Figure 1-25).

Actin monomers have a binding site for adenosine triphosphate (ATP), which is hydrolyzed to adenosine diphosphate (ADP) as polymerization proceeds. **Actin polymerization is ATP-dependent** (see Box 1-E).

The kinetics of actin polymerization involves a mechanism known as **treadmilling: G-actin monomers assembled at one end of the filament concurrently disassemble at the other end** (see Figure 1-26). Four types of proteins control treadmilling (see Figure 1-26), as follows:

1. **Thymosin** sequesters pools of G-actin monomers within cells.

Figure 1-23. Summary of cell junctions and cell adhesion molecules

Zonula adherens (belt desmosome)
It consists of a **dense plaque** associated with the **catenin complex** (α-catenin, β-catenin and p120), α-actinin, vinculin and formin-1. **Actin filaments** are attached to the catenin complex. The intercellular space is bridged by **cadherins** and the **afadin-nectin complex** connecting the opposite dense plaques.

Tight junctions (occluding junctions)
Consist of the transmembrane proteins **occludin** and **claudins**, associated with **ZO-1, ZO-2, ZO-3**, and the **afadin-nectin complex** at the intracellular side. Occludin and claudins seal the intercellular space.

Macula adherens (spot desmosome)
Desmosomes are symmetrical structures consisting of: (1) plaques containing **desmoplakins**, **plakoglobin** and **plakophilins** (2) linking **cadherins** (mainly **desmocollins and desmogleins**) and (3) keratin filaments attached to the plaques.

Immunoglobulin superfamily
Cell adhesion molecules belong to the immunoglobulin superfamily because they contain domains similar to immunoglobulins. CAMs do not require Ca^{2+} to maintain **homophilic** adhesive interactions.

Selectin
Selectins are Ca^{2+}-dependent molecules with binding affinity for **sugars**. Selectins have an important role in the **homing process**.

Hemidesmosomes
Hemidesmosomes consist of an **inner plate**, the anchoring site of the intermediate filament keratin and an **outer plaque**, attached to the basal lamina by two major components: anchoring filaments (laminin 5) and integrin $\alpha_6\beta_4$.

Integrins
On the **extracellular side**, integrins interact directly with fibronectin and laminin. On the **intracellular side**, the β subunits of integrin interact with actin through intermediate proteins (including α-**actinin**, **vinculin**, and **talin**).

Laminin
Laminin consists of three polypeptide chains (α, β, and γ) with binding sites for type IV collagen, proteoglycan perlecan, integrin, and nidogen.

Proteoglycans
Proteoglycans (mainly heparan sulfate perlecan) interact directly with fibronectin and laminin.

Labels in figure: Catenin complex · Actin · Claudin · Occludin · Afadin-nectin complex · ZO-1, ZO-2, and ZO-3 · Afadin-nectin complex · Cadherins · Perlecan · Fibronectin · Collagens · Type IV collagen · Nidogen (entactin)

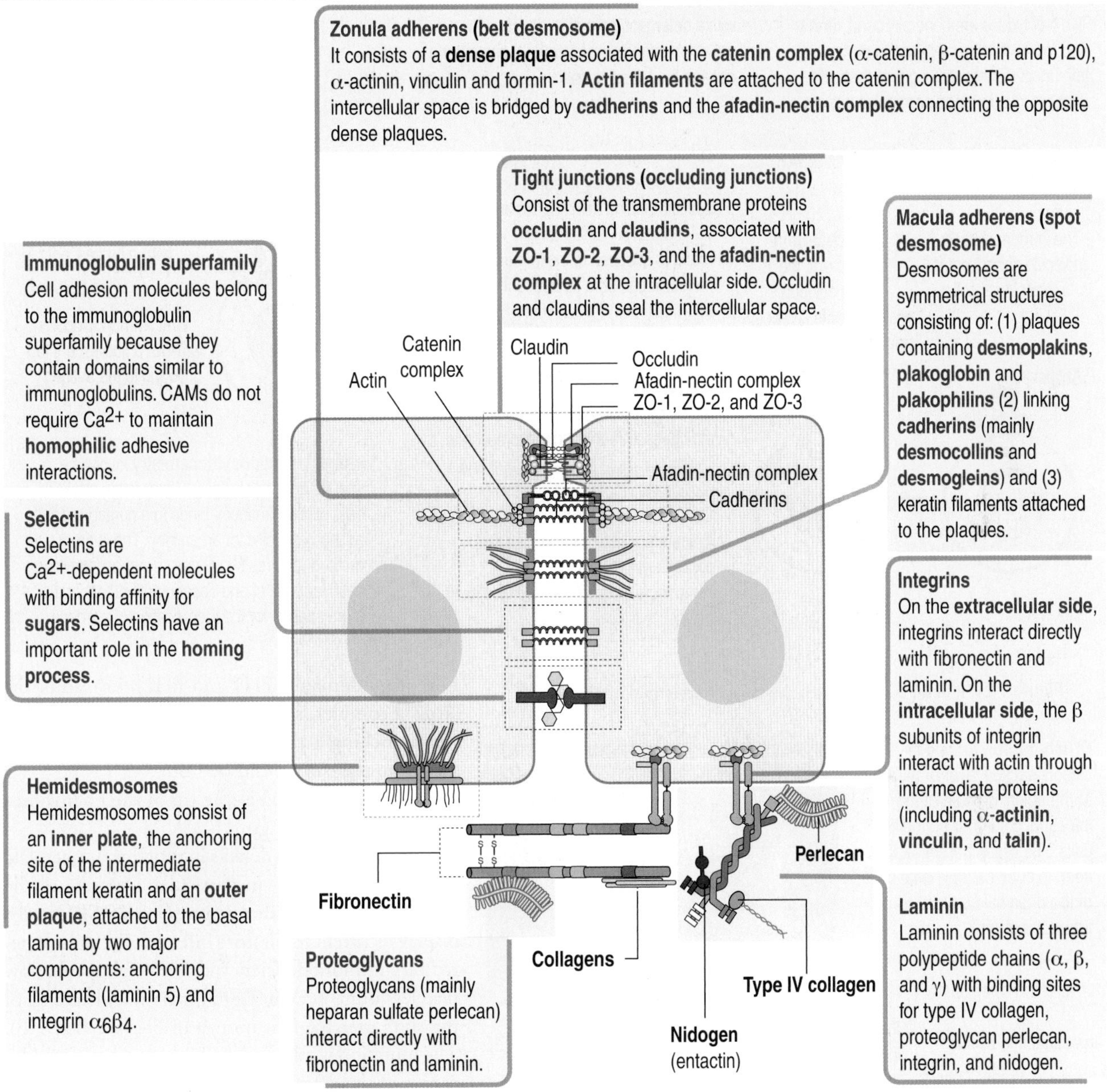

2. **Profilin** suppresses nucleation of G-actin and promotes F-actin growth at the barbed end. Profilin can favor the assembly of monomeric G-actin into filaments by facilitating the exchange of bound ADP for ATP. **Only ATP-actin monomers can be assembled into filaments.**

3. **Cofilin** (also known as actin depolymerizing factor) triggers depolymerization of ADP-bound actin at the pointed end. Similar to profilin and thymosin, cofilin forms a dimeric complex with G-actin.

4. **Gelsolin** has a dual role: it is a **capping protein** and prevents the loss and addition of actin monomers, and it is a **severing protein**. In the presence of Ca^{2+}, gelsolin fragments actin filaments and remains bound to the barbed end, forming a cap that prevents further filament growth.

In the core of the **intestinal microvilli**, the assembly of G-actin monomers into filaments and the organization of these filaments into thick bundles are controlled by various types of **actin-binding or actin-related proteins.** A bundle of parallel nonbranching actin filaments, forming the core of the **microvillus**, is held together by actin-linking proteins, **villin** and **fimbrin**. Side arms of **myosin-I** and the Ca^{2+}-binding protein **calmodulin** anchor the bundle to the plasma membrane (see Figure 1-25).

Arp2/3 and additional regulatory proteins form a nucleation complex for the assembly of **branching actin filaments**.

Branching actin filaments assemble at the leading edge of a cell during cell motility. In microvilli, **formins** (proteins with highly conserved formin-

Figure 1-24. Immunocytochemistry

Two techniques are generally used: **direct and indirect immunocytochemistry.** Immunocytochemistry requires that cells under study are made permeable, usually with a detergent, so that **antibody molecules (immunoglobulins)** can enter a cell and bind to an antigen.

Direct immunofluorescence

The immunoglobulin molecule cannot enter into an intact cell

After detergent treatment, the immunoglobulin molecule enters the cell and binds to the antigen

Antigen

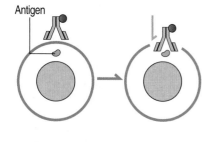

Direct immunocytochemistry involves a specific antibody or some agent with specific binding affinity to an antigen tagged with a visible marker. Visible markers attached to the immunoglobulin molecule can be a fluorescent dye such as **fluorescein** (green fluorescence) or **rhodamine** (red fluorescence). When examined with a fluorescence microscope, only labeled components are visible as bright, fluorescent structures. Direct immunofluorescence involves a single incubation step and provides a simple detection system. Gold particles (electron-dense) attached to immunoglobulin molecules are convenient markers for immunocytochemistry at the electron microscopic level.

Indirect immunofluorescence

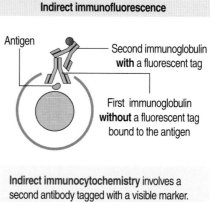

Antigen

Second immunoglobulin **with** a fluorescent tag

First immunoglobulin **without** a fluorescent tag bound to the antigen

Indirect immunocytochemistry involves a second antibody tagged with a visible marker. This second antibody binds to a nontagged first antibody specific for an antigen. The indirect method requires two separate incubations (one each for the first and second antibodies) and is more specific for the identification of antigens.

Figure 1-25. F-actin bundles form the core of intestinal microvilli

Brush border, formed by a closely packed layer of microvilli, at the apical domain of the intestinal columnar epithelial cells. The brush border is also seen in cuboidal epithelial cells of the proximal convoluted tubule (nephron).

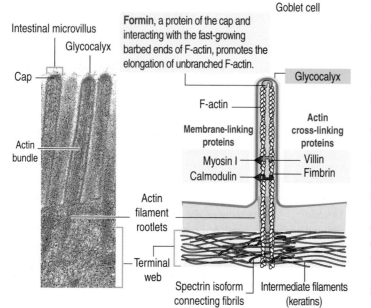

Goblet cell

Intestinal microvillus

Glycocalyx

Cap

Actin bundle

Formin, a protein of the cap and interacting with the fast-growing barbed ends of F-actin, promotes the elongation of unbranched F-actin.

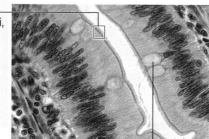

Glycocalyx

F-actin

Membrane-linking proteins

Myosin I

Calmodulin

Actin cross-linking proteins

Villin

Fimbrin

Actin filament rootlets

Terminal web

Spectrin isoform connecting fibrils

Intermediate filaments (keratins)

homology domains, FH1 and FH2), instead of the Arp2/3 complex, seem to regulate the elongation of **nonbranching actin filaments**, while remaining attached to the barbed end (see Box 1-E).

Formins are located at the tip of the microvillus, the **cap region** (see Figure 1-25).

Male patients with defects in proteins that activate the Arp2/3 complex, in particular a protein of the **Wiskott-Aldrich syndrome protein (WASP)** family, display recurrent respiratory infections because of hereditary immunodeficiency, thrombocytopenia (low platelet count) present from birth on and eczema of the skin after the first month of life (see Box 1-F). The mutation is inherited from the mother, a healthy carrier of the defective gene.

Microvilli and stereocilia are comparable structures, although they differ in length and the number of actin filaments:

1. **Intestinal microvilli** are 1 to 2 μm long, 0.1 μm wide, and consist of 20 to 30 bundled actin filaments.

2. **Stereocilia in hair cells of the inner ear** have a tapered shape at their base, the length range is 1.5 to 5.5 μm, and each actin bundle contains up to 900 actin filaments.

Hair cells are extremely sensitive to mechanical displacement, and a slight movement of the stereocilium is amplified into changes in electric potential transmitted to the brain.

We study hair cells of the inner ear in Chapter 9, Sensory Organs: Vision and Hearing.

Figure 1-26. Role of actin binding proteins in the assembly and disassembly of F-actin

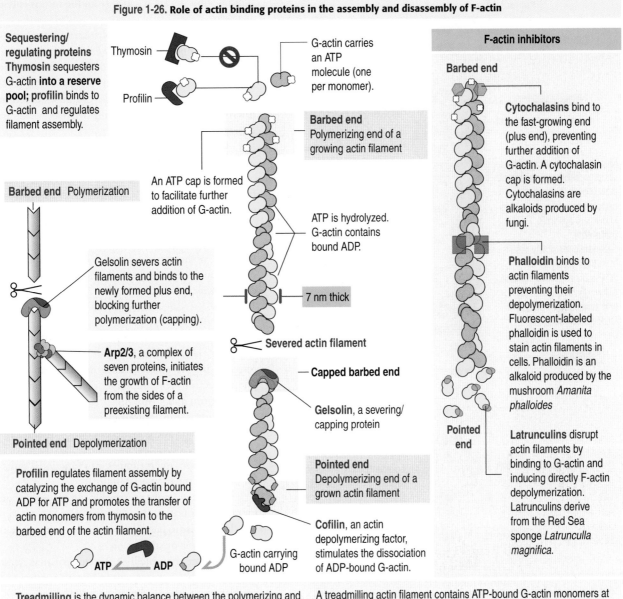

Sequestering/ regulating proteins Thymosin sequesters G-actin **into a reserve pool; profilin** binds to G-actin and regulates filament assembly.

Thymosin

Profilin

G-actin carries an ATP molecule (one per monomer).

Barbed end Polymerizing end of a growing actin filament

An ATP cap is formed to facilitate further addition of G-actin.

ATP is hydrolyzed. G-actin contains bound ADP.

7 nm thick

Barbed end Polymerization

Gelsolin severs actin filaments and binds to the newly formed plus end, blocking further polymerization (capping).

Arp2/3, a complex of seven proteins, initiates the growth of F-actin from the sides of a preexisting filament.

Severed actin filament

Capped barbed end

Gelsolin, a severing/ capping protein

Pointed end Depolymerization

Profilin regulates filament assembly by catalyzing the exchange of G-actin bound ADP for ATP and promotes the transfer of actin monomers from thymosin to the barbed end of the actin filament.

Pointed end Depolymerizing end of a grown actin filament

ATP — ADP

Cofilin, an actin depolymerizing factor, stimulates the dissociation of ADP-bound G-actin.

G-actin carrying bound ADP

F-actin inhibitors

Barbed end

Cytochalasins bind to the fast-growing end (plus end), preventing further addition of G-actin. A cytochalasin cap is formed. Cytochalasins are alkaloids produced by fungi.

Phalloidin binds to actin filaments preventing their depolymerization. Fluorescent-labeled phalloidin is used to stain actin filaments in cells. Phalloidin is an alkaloid produced by the mushroom *Amanita phalloides*

Pointed end

Latrunculins disrupt actin filaments by binding to G-actin and inducing directly F-actin depolymerization. Latrunculins derive from the Red Sea sponge *Latrunculla magnifica*.

Treadmilling is the dynamic balance between the polymerizing and depolymerizing ends to maintain the length of an actin filament.

A treadmilling actin filament contains ATP-bound G-actin monomers at the barbed end, whereas the ones at the pointed end are ADP-bound.

Microtubules

Microtubules are composed of **tubulin dimers** (Figure 1-27; see Box 1-G). Each tubulin dimer consists of two tightly bound tubulin molecules: α-**tubulin** and β-**tubulin**. Tubulin subunits are arranged in longitudinal rows called **protofilaments**. Thirteen protofilaments associate side by side with each other to form a cylinder of **microtubules** with a hollow core. The diameter of a microtubule is **25 nm**.

Similar to actin filaments, microtubules are structurally **polarized**. Microtubules have a **plus end**, which grows more rapidly than the **minus end** (see Figure 1-27).

In contrast to actin filaments, most individual microtubules seem to undergo **alternate phases of slow growth and rapid depolymerization**. This process, called **dynamic instability**, consists of three major steps:

1. A **polymerization phase**, in which GTP-tubulin

Box 1-E | Microfilaments: Highlights to remember

• **Microfilaments** consist of G-actin, globular monomers, which polymerize in the presence of **ATP** into a long intertwined in a helix filamentous polymer, F-actin, that is 7 nm thick.

• F-actin has a distinct polarity: a barbed or polymerization end, and a pointed or depolymerizing end. Profilin has two roles: it severs F-actin and regulates F-actin assembly by catalyzing the exchange of G-actin bound ADP for ATP. Cofilin is a depolymerizing factor. The Arp2/3 complex initiates the branching of F-actin.

• **Treadmilling** is the dynamic balance between the polymerizing and depoly-merizing ends of F-actin.

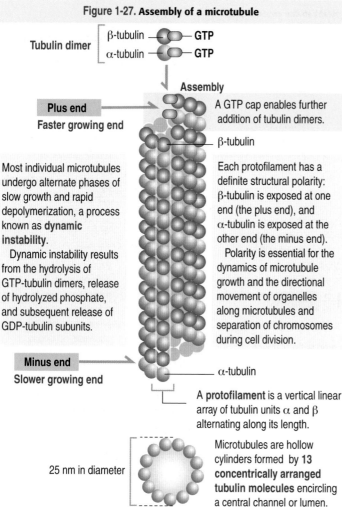

Figure 1-27. Assembly of a microtubule

Tubulin dimer

β-tubulin —— GTP
α-tubulin —— GTP

Assembly

A GTP cap enables further addition of tubulin dimers.

Plus end
Faster growing end

β-tubulin

Most individual microtubules undergo alternate phases of slow growth and rapid depolymerization, a process known as **dynamic instability**.

Dynamic instability results from the hydrolysis of GTP-tubulin dimers, release of hydrolyzed phosphate, and subsequent release of GDP-tubulin subunits.

Each protofilament has a definite structural polarity: β-tubulin is exposed at one end (the plus end), and α-tubulin is exposed at the other end (the minus end).

Polarity is essential for the dynamics of microtubule growth and the directional movement of organelles along microtubules and separation of chromosomes during cell division.

Minus end
Slower growing end

α-tubulin

A **protofilament** is a vertical linear array of tubulin units α and β alternating along its length.

25 nm in diameter

Microtubules are hollow cylinders formed by **13 concentrically arranged tubulin molecules** encircling a central channel or lumen.

subunits add to the plus end of the microtubule and a **GTP cap** is assembled to facilitate further growth.

2. The **release of hydrolyzed phosphate (Pi)** from tubulin-bound GTP.

3. A **depolymerization phase**, in which GDP-

Box 1-F | Wiskott-Aldrich syndrome

• The Arp2/3 complex is necessary for nucleating the assembly of branched networks of actin filaments. The function of phagocytic cells and platelets depends on a functional actin cytoskeleton.

• Numerous proteins activate the Arp2/3 complex. Without these proteins, the Arp2/3 complex is inactive.

• Two major proteins that bind and activate the Arp2/3 complex include the Wiskott-Aldrich syndrome protein (WASP) family, which consists of several members (WASP, neuronal WASP [N-WASP] and SCAR/WAVE1-3 [**s**uppressor of **cAM**P receptor/**WA**SP family **ve**rprolin-homologous protein 1-3]). Additional members belong to the cortactin family, which includes cortactin and hemato-poietic-specific protein.

• Mutations in the *WASP* gene, present in the X chromosome, are character-ized by recurrent respiratory infections (defective function of T and B cells), a reduction in the number of platelets (thrombocytopenia) leading to increased susceptibility to bleeding, and eczema of the skin. Males but not females are affected by the Wiskott-Aldrich syndrome.

---

tubulin subunits are released from the minus end at a fast rate.

The polymerization-to-depolymerization transition frequency is known as *catastrophe*; the depolymeriza-tion-to-polymerization transition frequency is known as *rescue*.

The stability of microtubules can be modified by **microtubule-associated proteins (MAPs)**. MAPs are classified into two groups:

1. Classical MAPs, such as MAP1A, MAP1B, MAP2, and tau.

2. Nonclassical MAPs, including Lis1 and DCX family members. MAPs stabilize microtubules by phosphorylation/dephosphorylation.

In Chapter 7, Nervous Tissue, we discuss the sig-nificance of tau phosphorylation and dephosphory-lation in **Alzheimer's disease**. A lack of expression of Lis1 causes a sever brain developmental disorder called **lissencephaly**.

Centrosome

The centrosome, the major microtubule-organizing center in cells, consist of a **pair of centrioles** sur-rounded by the **pericentriolar material**, an amor-phous, electron-dense substance rich in proteins such as pericentrin and γ-tubulin.

The centrosome has four major functions:

1. It nucleates the polymerization of tubulin sub-units into microtubules.

2. It organizes microtubules into functional units, for example, the mitotic spindle.

3. It duplicates once every cell cycle in preparation for cell division.

4. It gives rise to basal body precursors, the origina-tors of multiple or single cilia.

Centrosome abnormalities, in particular an increase in their number, are frequent in human tumors and correlate with advanced tumor grade and metastasis. Therefore, **centrosome amplification** has a lethal effect by preventing cells to assemble normal mi-totic spindles but also enhancing the potential of tumorigenesis.

Centrosomes are part of the **mitotic center,** which, together with the **mitotic spindle**, constitutes the **mitotic (or meiotic) apparatus** (Figure 1-28). A centriole is a small cylinder (0.2 μm wide and 0.4 μm long) composed of **nine microtubule triplets** in a helicoid array. In contrast to most cytoplasmic microtubules, which display dynamic instability, the centriolar microtubules are very stable.

During interphase, centrioles are oriented at right angles to each other. Before mitosis, centrioles repli-cate and form **two pairs**. During mitosis, each pair can be found at opposite poles of the cell, where they direct the formation of the **mitotic or meiotic spindle**.

There are three types of microtubules extending

Figure 1-28. Mitotic apparatus

The mitotic (or meiotic) apparatus consists of two components:
1. The **mitotic center**.
2. The **mitotic spindle**.

The three components of the mitotic center are the **microtubule organizing center** surrounding a pair of **centrioles** and **radiating microtubules** (also called astral microtubules) anchoring the mitotic center to the plasma membrane.

The mitotic spindle consists of two major classes of microtubules originating in the mitotic center: the **kinetochore microtubules**, anchored to the **centromeres** of the metaphase chromosomes, and the **polar microtubules**, which overlap with each other in the center of the cell and are not attached to chromosomes.

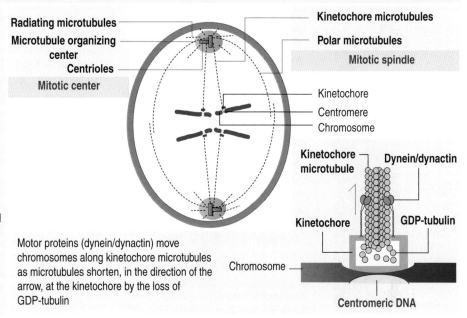

Radiating microtubules
Microtubule organizing center
Centrioles
Mitotic center

Kinetochore microtubules
Polar microtubules
Mitotic spindle

Kinetochore
Centromere
Chromosome

Kinetochore microtubule
Dynein/dynactin
Kinetochore
GDP-tubulin
Chromosome
Centromeric DNA

Motor proteins (dynein/dynactin) move chromosomes along kinetochore microtubules as microtubules shorten, in the direction of the arrow, at the kinetochore by the loss of GDP-tubulin

from the centrosomes:

1. **Radiating** or **astral microtubules**, anchoring each centrosome to the plasma membrane.

2. **Kinetochore microtubules**, attaching the chromosome-associated kinetochore to the centrosomes.

3. **Polar microtubules**, extending from the two poles of the spindle where opposite centrosomes are located (see Figure 1-28).

Kinetochores are formed by several proteins assembled on centromeric DNA during mitosis and meiosis. The centromere is the chromosomal site where the kinetochore assembles. If kinetochores fail to assemble, chromosomes cannot segregate properly (see Box 1-H).

The **pericentriolar material** contains the γ-**tubulin ring complex** and numerous proteins, including **peri-**

Figure 1-29. Axoneme

One of the principal functions of the **inner sheath** and **radial spokes** is the stabilization of axonemal bending. **Tektins** are filamentous proteins extending along the microtubules. Together with nexin links, tektins may provide a scaffold to microtubules or have a role in the assembly of axoneme-associated structures.

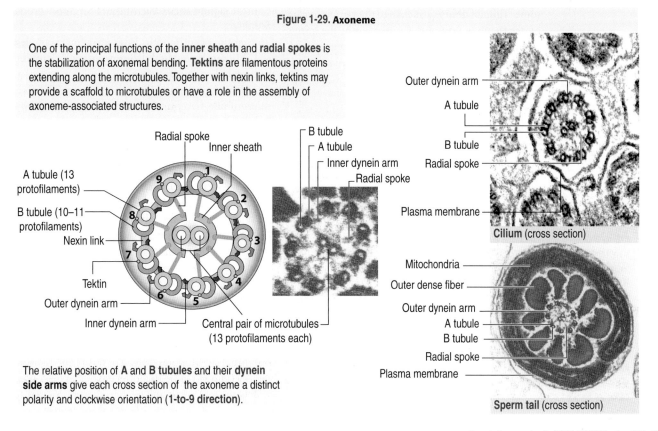

Radial spoke
Inner sheath
A tubule (13 protofilaments)
B tubule (10–11 protofilaments)
Nexin link
Tektin
Outer dynein arm
Inner dynein arm
Central pair of microtubules (13 protofilaments each)

B tubule
A tubule
Inner dynein arm
Radial spoke

Outer dynein arm
A tubule
B tubule
Radial spoke
Plasma membrane
Cilium (cross section)

Mitochondria
Outer dense fiber
Outer dynein arm
A tubule
B tubule
Radial spoke
Plasma membrane
Sperm tail (cross section)

The relative position of **A** and **B tubules** and their **dynein side arms** give each cross section of the axoneme a distinct polarity and clockwise orientation (**1-to-9 direction**).

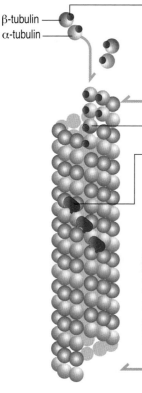

Figure 1-30. Agents that prevent microtubular function

β-tubulin
α-tubulin

Colchicine binding to tubulin dimers prevents their assembly into microtubules. **Vinblastine** and **vincristine**, used in antitumor therapy, also inhibit tubulin polymerization. **Nocodazole** is another protein inhibitor of tubulin polymerization.

Plus end

Tubulin-colchicine complex

Taxol binds to microtubules preventing their depolymerization. Taxol disrupts mitosis by affecting the dynamic assembly and disassembly of the mitotic spindle required for the separation of chromosomes into daughter cells.

Antimitotic drugs are potent inhibitors of the polymerization and depolymerization of microtubules of the mitotic spindle. Antimitotic drugs bind to diverse sites on tubulin, and their combination can be therapeutically more efficient.

Minus end

centrin. Each γ-tubulin ring complex is the nucleation site or template for the assembly and growth of one microtubule. The centrioles do not have a direct role in the nucleation of microtubules in the centrosome. Tubulin dimers associate to the γ-tubulin ring by the α-tubulin subunit. Consequently, the minus end of each microtubule points to the centrosome; the plus end, the growing end, is oriented outward, free in the cytoplasm.

The axoneme of cilia and flagella

Early in this chapter, we indicate that centrosomes give rise to **precursor basal bodies**, which are the outgrowth origin of cilia (see Figure 1-6) and flagella.

Motile cilia and flagella are cytoplasmic extensions

---

containing a core of microtubules, the **axoneme** (Figure 1-29). The axoneme consists of nine peripheral microtubule doublets surrounding a central pair of microtubules. This arrangement is known as the **9 + 2** configuration.

Each peripheral doublet consists of a complete microtubule (called an **A tubule**, with **13** protofilaments), sharing its wall with a second, partially completed microtubule (called a **B tubule**, with **10** to **11** protofilaments). Extending inward from the A tubule are **radial spokes** that insert into an amorphous **inner sheath** surrounding the central microtubule pair. Adjacent peripheral doublets are linked by the protein **nexin** (see Box 1-I).

Projecting from the sides of the A tubule are sets of protein arms: the **inner** and **outer arms of dynein**, a microtubule-associated adenosine triphosphatase (ATPase). In the presence of ATP, the sliding of peripheral doublets relative to each other bends cilia and flagella. Sliding and bending of microtubules are the basic events of their motility.

Ciliopathies can occur when defects occur during:

1. The multiplication and docking of the centrosome-derived precursor basal bodies. An example is the enhanced expression of the protein CP110 that prevents the attachment of basal bodies to the plasma membrane, leading to primary ciliary dyskinesia.

2. The transport of proteins during the assembly of cilia and flagella, resulting in the **Bardet-Biedl syndrome** (see Box 1-J; see Figure 1-6).

Clinical significance: Microtubule-targeted drugs. Sterility

Two groups of antimitotic drugs act on microtubules:

1. **Microtubule-destabilizing agents**, which inhibit microtubule polymerization.

2. **Microtubule-stabilizing agents**, which affect microtubule function by suppressing dynamic instability.

The **first group** includes **colchicine, colcemid, vincristine**, and **vinblastine**, which bind to tubulin and inhibit microtubule polymerization, blocking mitosis. Colchicine is used clinically in the treatment of gout. Vincristine and vinblastine, from *Vinca* alkaloids isolated from the leaves of the periwinkle plant, have been successfully used in childhood hematologic malignancies (leukemias). Neurotoxicity, resulting from the disruption of the microtubule-dependent axonal flow (loss of microtubules and binding of motor proteins to microtubules), and myelosuppression are two side effects of microtubule-targeted drugs.

The **second group** includes **taxol** (isolated from the bark of the yew tree) with an opposite effect: It stabilizes microtubules instead of inhibiting their assembly (Figure 1-30). Paclitaxel (taxol) has been used widely to treat breast and ovarian cancers. Similar to *Vinca* alkaloids, its main side effects are neurotoxicity

---

Box 1-G | Microtubules: Highlights to remember

- **Microtubules** are structures consisting of tubulin dimers, α and β, which polymerize in the presence of **GTP** into longitudinal rows of protofilaments. Each tubulin monomer binds one GTP molecule. Thirteen parallel protofilaments form a cylinder or microtubule 25 nm in diameter.
- Similar to F-actin, microtubules have a distinct polarity: a plus or polymerizing end and a minus or depolymerizing end.
- Microtubules undergo alternate phases of slow growth and rapid depolymerization, a process known as dynamic instability.
- Centrioles, basal bodies, and axonemes of cilia and flagella contain a precise array of microtubules.
- Kinesin and cytoplasmic dynein, two molecular motor proteins, use microtubules as tracks for the transport of vesicle and nonvesicle cargos.

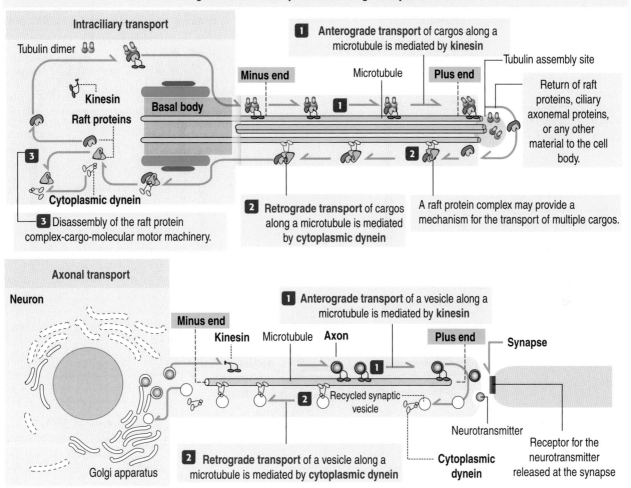

Figure 1-31. Intraciliary and axonal cargo transport

Intraciliary transport

Tubulin dimer

Kinesin

Raft proteins

3 Disassembly of the raft protein complex-cargo-molecular motor machinery.

Cytoplasmic dynein

Basal body

Minus end

Microtubule

Plus end

1 Anterograde transport of cargos along a microtubule is mediated by **kinesin**

1

2

Tubulin assembly site

Return of raft proteins, ciliary axonemal proteins, or any other material to the cell body.

2 Retrograde transport of cargos along a microtubule is mediated by **cytoplasmic dynein**

A raft protein complex may provide a mechanism for the transport of multiple cargos.

Axonal transport

Neuron

Minus end

Kinesin

Microtubule

Axon

Plus end

Synapse

1 Anterograde transport of a vesicle along a microtubule is mediated by **kinesin**

1

2

Recycled synaptic vesicle

Neurotransmitter

Cytoplasmic dynein

Receptor for the neurotransmitter released at the synapse

Golgi apparatus

2 Retrograde transport of a vesicle along a microtubule is mediated by **cytoplasmic dynein**

and suppression of hematopoiesis.

Kartagener's syndrome is an autosomal recessive **ciliary dyskinesia** frequently associated with **bronchiectasis** (permanent dilation of bronchi and bronchioles) and **sterility** in men.

Kartagener's syndrome is the result of structural abnormalities in the axoneme (**defective or absent dynein**) that prevent mucociliary clearance in the airways (leading to persistent infections) and reduce sperm motility and egg transport in the oviduct (leading to sterility).

Box 1-H | Differences between centromeres and kinetochores

- The terms **centromere** and **kinetochore** are often used synonymously, but do not mean the same thing.
- The **centromere** (not the centrosome) is the chromosomal site associated with microtubules of the spindle. Centromeres can be recognized cytologically as a narrow chromatin region on metaphase chromosomes known as **primary constriction** where centromeric DNA is present.
- The **kinetochore** consists of proteins assembled on the centromeric chromatin on sister chromatids. The assembly of the kinetochore depends exclusively on the presence of centromeric DNA sequences. The centromere and the kinetochore mediate attachment of the kinetochore microtubules of the spindle.

Microtubules: Cargo transport and motor proteins

The transport of vesicles and nonvesicle cargos occurs along microtubules and F-actin.

Specific molecular motors associate to microtubules and F-actin to mobilize cargos to specific intracellular sites.

Microtubule-based molecular motors include kinesin and cytoplasmic dynein for the **long-range** transport of cargos.

F-actin–based molecular motors include unconventional myosin Va and VIIa for the **short-range** transport of cargos. We discuss additional aspects of the F-actin–based cargo transport mechanism during the transport of **melanosomes** in Chapter 11, Integumentary System.

Three examples of microtubule-based cargo transport in mammalian systems are as follows (see Box 1-K):

1. Axonemal transport, including flagella (**intraflagellar transport**) and cilia (**intraciliary transport**) (Figure 1-31). During axonemal transport, particles are mobilized by kinesin and cytoplasmic dynein along the microtubule doublets of the axoneme.

Defective axonemal transport results in the abnor-

Figure 1-32. Classes of myosin molecules and how they work

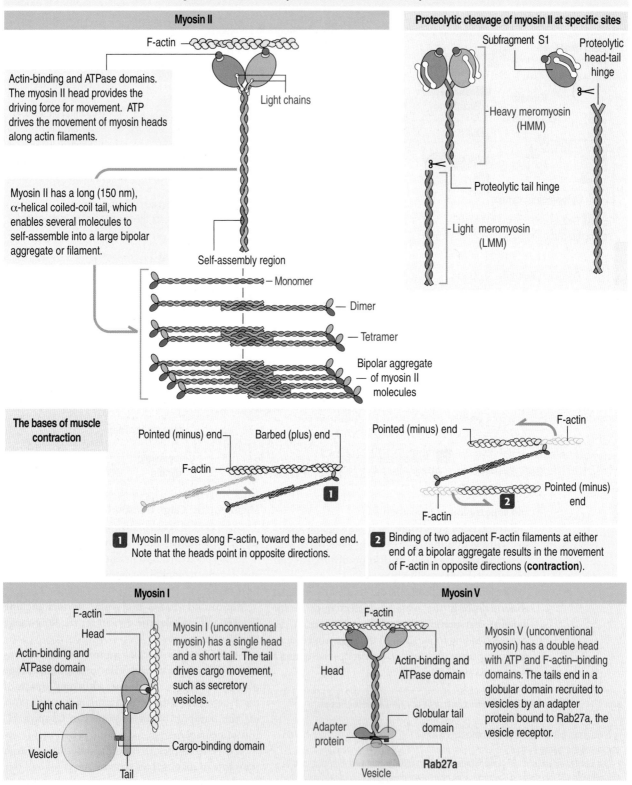

Myosin II

F-actin

Actin-binding and ATPase domains. The myosin II head provides the driving force for movement. ATP drives the movement of myosin heads along actin filaments.

Light chains

Myosin II has a long (150 nm), α-helical coiled-coil tail, which enables several molecules to self-assemble into a large bipolar aggregate or filament.

Self-assembly region

Monomer
Dimer
Tetramer
Bipolar aggregate of myosin II molecules

Proteolytic cleavage of myosin II at specific sites

Subfragment S1
Proteolytic head-tail hinge
Heavy meromyosin (HMM)
Proteolytic tail hinge
Light meromyosin (LMM)

The bases of muscle contraction

Pointed (minus) end — Barbed (plus) end
F-actin

Pointed (minus) end
F-actin
Pointed (minus) end
F-actin

1 Myosin II moves along F-actin, toward the barbed end. Note that the heads point in opposite directions.

2 Binding of two adjacent F-actin filaments at either end of a bipolar aggregate results in the movement of F-actin in opposite directions (**contraction**).

Myosin I

F-actin
Head
Actin-binding and ATPase domain
Light chain
Vesicle
Tail
Cargo-binding domain

Myosin I (unconventional myosin) has a single head and a short tail. The tail drives cargo movement, such as secretory vesicles.

Myosin V

F-actin
Head
Actin-binding and ATPase domain
Adapter protein
Globular tail domain
Rab27a
Vesicle

Myosin V (unconventional myosin) has a double head with ATP and F-actin–binding domains. The tails end in a globular domain recruited to vesicles by an adapter protein bound to Rab27a, the vesicle receptor.

mal assembly of cilia and flagella, including **polycystic kidney disease**, **retinal degeneration**, **respiratory ciliary dysfunction**, and **lack of sperm tail development**. As indicated before (see Box 1-J), the **Bardet-Biedl syndrome** is a disorder caused by basal body/ciliary

dysfunction secondary to a defective microtubule-based transport function.

2. **Axonal transport**, along the axon of neurons (see Figure 1-31).

3. **Intramanchette transport**, along microtubules

- **Microtubules**: Major component of the axoneme. Motor proteins use microtubules of the axoneme as tracks for intraciliary or intraflagellar cargo transport. Microtubule-based axonal transport also depends on motor proteins.
- **Tektins**: Intermediate filament-like proteins extending along the length of axonemal microtubules and, presumably, adding mechanical strength to the axoneme.
- **Dynein arms**: ATPase responsible for ciliary and flagellar movement. The heads are in contact with the adjacent outer microtubules at a periodic distance and move along them.
- **Nexin links**: A beltlike arrangement stabilizing the nine outer concentric pairs of microtubules.
- **Radial spokes**: Project from each of the nine outer microtubule doublets to the inner sheath surrounding the central pair.
- **Inner sheath**: A structure surrounding the central pair of microtubules, in contact with the globular end of the radial spokes.

of the manchette, a transient structure assembled during the elongation of the spermatid head (see Chapter 20, Spermatogenesis).

Microtubules: Axonal transport

Axons are cytoplasmic extensions of neurons responsible for the conduction of neuronal impulses. Membrane-bound vesicles containing **neurotransmitters** produced in the cell body of the neuron travel to the terminal portion of the axon, where the content of the vesicle is released at the **synapse**.

Bundles of microtubules form tracks within the axon to carry these vesicles. Vesicles are transported by two motor proteins (see Figure 1-31):

1. **Kinesin**
2. **Cytoplasmic dynein**

Kinesins and **cytoplasmic dyneins** participate in two types of intracellular transport movements:

1. **Saltatory movement**, defined by the continuous and random movement of mitochondria and vesicles.
2. **Axonal transport**, a more direct intracellular movement of membrane-bound structures.

Kinesins and cytoplasmic dyneins have two ATP-binding heads and a tail. Energy derives from continuous ATP hydrolysis by ATPases present in the heads. The head domains interact with microtubules, and the tail binds to specific receptor binding sites

- Bardet-Biedl syndrome (BBS) is a pleiotropic (multisystemic) disorder that includes age-related retinal dystrophy, obesity, polydactyly, renal dysplasia, reproductive tract abnormalities, and learning disabilities.
- BBS is a disorder of **basal bodies** and **cilia** resulting from a **defective microtubule-based transport function** (intraciliary transport) required for the assembly, maintenance, and function of basal bodies, cilia, and flagella (intraflagellar transport).
- Eight BBS genes (*BBS1-8*) have been identified. The degree of clinical variability in BBS is not fully explained.

on the surface of vesicles and organelles.

Kinesin uses energy from ATP hydrolysis to move vesicles from the cell body of the neuron toward the end portion of the axon (**anterograde transport**). Cytoplasmic dynein also uses ATP to move vesicles in the opposite direction (**retrograde transport**).

Myosin family of proteins

Members of the myosin family of proteins bind and hydrolyze ATP to provide energy for their movement along actin filaments from the pointed (minus) end to the barbed (plus) end. **Myosin I** and **myosin II** are the predominant members of the myosin family (Figure 1-32; see Box 1-L).

Myosin I, regarded as an **unconventional** myosin, is found in all cell types and has only one head domain and a tail. The head is associated with a single light chain. The head interacts with actin filaments and contains ATPase, which enables myosin I to move along the filaments by binding, detaching, and re-binding. The tail binds to vesicles or organelles. When myosin I moves along an actin filament, the vesicle or organelle is transported. Myosin I molecules are smaller than myosin II molecules, lack a long tail, and do not form dimers.

Myosin II, a **conventional** myosin, is present in muscle and nonmuscle cells. Myosin II consists of a pair of identical molecules. Each molecule consists of an ATPase-containing head domain and a long rodlike tail. The tails of the dimer link to each other along their entire length to form a two-stranded coiled rod. The tail of myosin II self-assembles into dimers, tetramers, and a bipolar filament with the heads pointing away from the midline.

The two heads, linked together but pointing in opposite directions, bind to adjacent actin filaments of opposite polarity. Each myosin head bound to F-actin moves toward the barbed (positive) end. Consequently, the two actin filaments are moved against each other, and contraction occurs (see Figure 1-32).

Heads and tails of myosin II can be cleaved by enzymes (trypsin or papain) into **light meromyosin** (**LMM**) and **heavy meromyosin** (**HMM**). LMM forms filaments, but lacks ATPase activity and does not bind to actin. HMM binds to actin, is capable of ATP hydrolysis, and does not form filaments. HMM is responsible for generating force during muscle contraction. HMM can be cleaved further into two subfragments called **S1**. Each S1 fragment contains ATPase and light chains and binds actin.

Myosin V, an **unconventional** myosin, is double-headed with a coiled double tail. The head region binds to F-actin; the distal globular ends of the tails bind to **Rab27a**, a receptor on vesicle membranes. Myosin Va mediates vesicular transport along F-actin tracks. A specific example is the transport of melanosomes from melanocytes to keratinocytes, first along microtubules and later along F-actin (see Chapter 11, Integumentary System).

Mutations in the *Rab27a* and *myosin Va* genes disrupt the F-actin transport of melanosomes. An example in humans is **Griscelli syndrome**, a rare autosomal recessive disorder characterized by pigment dilution of the hair caused by defects in melanosome transport and associated with disrupted T cell cytotoxic activity and neurologic complications.

Figure 1-33 summarizes the relevant structural and functional characteristics of motor proteins.

Myosin light-chain kinase

The self-assembly of myosin II and interaction with actin filaments in nonmuscle cells takes place in certain sites according to functional needs. These events are controlled by the enzyme **myosin light-chain kinase** (MLCK), which **phosphorylates one of the myosin light chains** (called the **regulatory light chain**) present on the myosin head. The activity of MLCK is regulated by the Ca^{2+}-binding protein **calmodulin** (Figure 1-34).

MLCK has a **catalytic domain** and a **regulatory domain**. When calmodulin and Ca^{2+} bind to the regulatory domain, the catalytic activity of the kinase is released. The MLCK–calmodulin–Ca^{2+} complex catalyzes the transfer of a phosphate group from ATP to the myosin light chain, and myosin cycles along F-actin to generate force and muscle contraction.

Phosphorylation of one of the myosin light chains results in two effects:

1. It exposes the actin-binding site on the myosin head. This step is essential for an interaction of the myosin head with the F-actin bundle.

2. It releases the myosin tail from its sticky attachment site near the myosin head. This step also is critical because only myosin II stretched tails can self-assemble and generate bipolar filaments, a requirement for muscle contraction (see Figure 1-33).

In smooth muscle cells, a **phosphatase** removes the phosphate group from myosin light chains. Skeletal muscle contraction does not require phosphorylation of the myosin light chains. We discuss additional details of muscle contraction when we study the muscle tissue (see Chapter 7, Muscle Tissue).

Intermediate filaments

Intermediate filaments (Figure 1-35) represent a heterogeneous group of structures so named because their diameter (10 nm) is intermediate between those of microtubules (25 nm) and microfilaments (7 nm). Intermediate filaments are the most stable cytoskeletal structures.

Detergent and salt treatments extract microfilament and microtubule components and leave intermediate filaments insoluble. The structure of the intermediate filament does not fluctuate between assembly and disassembly states similar to microtubules and microfilaments. Note that in contrast to microtubules and actin filaments, which are assembled from globular proteins with nucleotide-binding and hydrolyzing activity, intermediate filaments consists of filamentous monomers lacking enzymatic activity. In contrast to actin and tubulin, the assembly and disassembly of intermediate filament monomers are regulated by **phosphorylation** and **dephosphorylation**, respectively.

Intermediate filament protein monomers consist of

Figure 1-33. Comparison of motor proteins

	Myosin I	Myosin II	Kinesin	Cytoplasmic dynein
Number of heads	One	Two	Two	Two
Tail binds to	Cell membrane	Myosin II	Vesicle	Vesicle
Head binds to	Actin	Actin	Microtubule	Microtubule
Direction of head motion toward the	Barbed (plus) end	Barbed (plus) end	Plus end	Minus end

three domains (see Figure 1-35): A central α-helical **rod domain** is flanked by a nonhelical N-terminal **head domain** and a C-terminal **tail domain**.

The assembly of intermediate filaments occurs in four steps:

1. A pair of filamentous monomers of variable length and amino acid sequence of the head and tail domains, form a **parallel dimer** through their central rod domain coiled around each other.

2. A **tetrameric unit** is then assembled by two **antiparallel half staggered coiled dimers**. Therefore, in contrast to microtubules and actin filaments, the antiparallel alignment of the initial tetramers determines a lack of structural polarity of intermediate filament (absence of plus and minus ends). One end

of an intermediate filament cannot be distinguished from another. If molecular motors associate to an intermediate filament, they would find it difficult to identify one direction from another.

3. **Eight tetramers** associate laterally to form a 16 nm-thick **unit length filament** (ULF).

4. Individual ULFs join end-to-end to form a short filaments that continue growing longitudinally by annealing to other ULFs and existing intermediate filaments. The elongation of the filament is followed by internal compaction to achieve the 10 nm-thick intermediate filament.

The tight association of dimers, tetramers and ULFs provide intermediate filaments with high tensile strength and resistance to stretching, compression, twisting and bending forces.

Intermediate filaments **provide structural strength or scaffolding for the attachment of other structures**. Intermediate filaments form extensive cytoplasmic networks extending from cage-like perinuclear arrangements to the cell surface.

Intermediate filaments of different molecular classes are characteristic of particular tissues or states of differentiation (for example, in the epidermis of skin). Five major types of intermediate filament proteins have been identified on the basis of sequence similarities in the α-helical rod domain. They are referred to as **types I** through **V** (see Box 1-M). About 50 intermediate filament proteins have been reported so far.

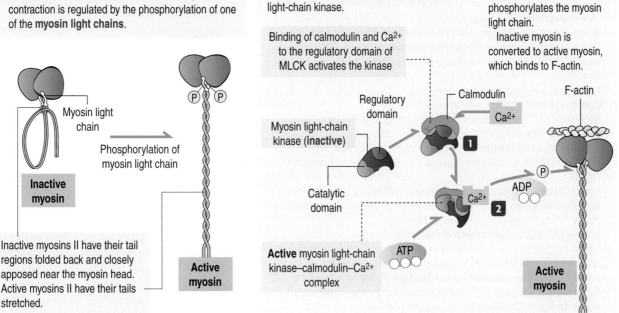

Figure 1-34. Light-chain phosphorylation of myosin II in nonmuscle cells

In **skeletal muscle**, the regulation of actin-myosin interaction is mediated by the binding of Ca²⁺ to troponin.

In **smooth muscle** and **nonmuscle cells**, contraction is regulated by the phosphorylation of one of the **myosin light chains**.

Myosin light chain

Phosphorylation of myosin light chain

Inactive myosin

Active myosin

Inactive myosins II have their tail regions folded back and closely apposed near the myosin head. Active myosins II have their tails stretched.

1 The activity of myosin light-chain kinase is regulated by the **calmodulin-Ca²⁺ complex**. An increase in cytosolic Ca²⁺ induces calmodulin binding to the regulatory domain of myosin light-chain kinase.

Binding of calmodulin and Ca²⁺ to the regulatory domain of MLCK activates the kinase

Regulatory domain

Myosin light-chain kinase (**inactive**)

Catalytic domain

Active myosin light-chain kinase–calmodulin–Ca²⁺ complex

ATP

2 The active myosin light-chain kinase–calmodulin–Ca²⁺ complex, in the presence of ATP, phosphorylates the myosin light chain.

Inactive myosin is converted to active myosin, which binds to F-actin.

Calmodulin

Ca²⁺

F-actin

ADP

Ca²⁺

Active myosin

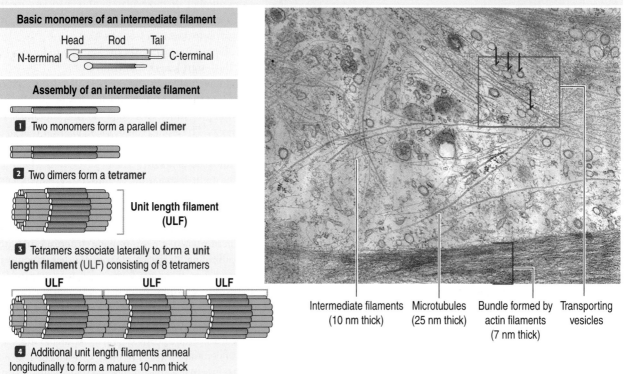

Basic monomers of an intermediate filament

Assembly of an intermediate filament

1 Two monomers form a parallel **dimer**

2 Two dimers form a **tetramer**

Unit length filament (ULF)

3 Tetramers associate laterally to form a **unit length filament** (ULF) consisting of 8 tetramers

4 Additional unit length filaments anneal longitudinally to form a mature 10-nm thick **intermediate filament**

Intermediate filaments (10 nm thick) Microtubules (25 nm thick) Bundle formed by actin filaments (7 nm thick) Transporting vesicles

Type I (acidic keratins) and type II (neutral to basic keratins). This class of proteins forms the intermediate filament cytoskeleton of **epithelial cells** (called **cytokeratins** to distinguish them from the keratins of hair and nails). Equal amounts of acidic (40 to 60 kd) and neutral-basic (50 to 70 kd) cytokeratins **combine** to form this type of intermediate filament protein. **Type I and type II intermediate filament keratins form tonofilaments associated with molecules present in the cytoplasmic plaques of desmosomes and hemidesmosomes** (see Figures 1-18 and 1-19). We come back to intermediate filament–binding proteins, such as **filaggrins**, when we discuss the differentiation of keratinocytes in the epidermis of the skin (Chapter 11, Integumentary System), and **plectin**, when we analyze the cytoskeletal protective network of skeletal muscle cells (Chapter 7, Muscle Tissue).

In the **epidermis**, the basal cells express keratins K5 and K14. The upper differentiating cells express keratins K1 and K10. In some regions of the epidermis, such as in the palmoplantar region, keratin K9 is found. Mutations in K5 and K14 cause hereditary blistering skin diseases belonging to the clinical type **epidermolysis bullosa simplex** (see later, Clinical significance: Intermediate filaments and skin blistering diseases).

Type III. This group includes the following intermediate filament proteins:

Vimentin (54 kd) is generally found in cells of **mesenchymal origin.**

Desmin (53 kd) is a component of **skeletal muscle cells** and is localized to the Z disk of the **sarcomere** (see Chapter 7, Muscle Tissue). This intermediate filament protein keeps individual contractile elements of the sarcomeres attached to the Z disk and plays a role in coordinating muscle cell contraction. Desmin

---

Box 1-M | Intermediate filament proteins: Highlights to remember

- **Type I (acidic) and type II (basic)**
  Keratins (40-70 kd): Keratins assemble as type I and type II heteropolymers. Different keratin types are coexpressed in epithelial cells, hair, and nails. Keratin gene mutations occur in several skin diseases (blistering and epidermolysis diseases).
- **Type III (can self-assemble as homopolymers)**
  Vimentin (54 kd): Present in mesenchymal-derived cells.
  Desmin (53 kd): A component of Z disks of striated muscle and smooth muscle cells.
  Glial fibrillary acidic protein (GFAP 51 kd): Present in astrocytes.
  Peripherin (57 kd): A component of axons in the peripheral nervous system.
- **Type IV**
  Neurofilaments (NF): Three forms coexpressed and forming heteropolymers in neurons: NF-L (light, 60 to 70 kd), NF-M (medium, 105 to 110 kd) and NF-H (heavy, 135 to 150 kd).
  α-Internexin (66 kd): A component of developing neurons.
- **Type V**
  Lamin A and lamin B (60 to 70 kd, 63-68 kd): Present in the nuclear lamina associated to the inner layer of the nuclear envelope. Maintain the integrity of the nuclear envelope. A group of human diseases, laminopathies, is associated with *lamin A* gene (*LMNA*) mutations (see Box 1-N).

is also found in **smooth muscle cells**.

Glial fibrillary acidic protein (GFAP) (51 kd) is observed in **astrocytes** and some Schwann cells (see Chapter 8, Nervous Tissue).

Peripherin (57 kd) is a component of neurons of the peripheral nervous system and is coexpressed with neurofilament proteins (see Chapter 8, Nervous Tissue).

Type IV. This group includes neurofilaments, nestin, syncoilin and α-internexin. Neurofilaments are the main components.

Neurofilaments (NFs) are found in axons and dendrites of **neurons**. Three types of proteins can be found in a neurofilament: **NF-L** (60 to 70 kd), **NF-M** (105 to 110 kd), and **NF-H** (135 to 150 kd), for low-molecular-weight, middle-molecular-weight, and high-molecular-weight neurofilaments. Abnormal accumulations of neurofilaments (neurofibrillary tangles) are a characteristic feature of a number of neuropathologic conditions.

α-Internexin (66 kd) is found predominantly in the central nervous system (particularly in the spinal cord and optic nerve).

Type V. Proteins of this group, the **nuclear lamins**, are encoded by three genes: *LMNA, LMNB1,* and *LMNB2*.

Lamin A and **lamin C** arise from the alternative splicing of transcripts encoded by the ***LMNA*** gene. The ***LMNB1*** gene encodes **lamin B1** expressed in all somatic cells. The ***LMNB2*** gene encodes **lamin B2**, expressed in all somatic cells, and **lamin B3**, that is specific for spermatogenic cells.

Nuclear lamins (60 to 75 kd) **differ from the other intermediate filament proteins in that they organize an orthogonal meshwork, the nuclear lamina**, in association with the inner membrane of the nuclear envelope.

Lamins provide mechanical support for the nuclear envelope and bind chromatin. Because of their clinical relevance, we come back to nuclear lamins and associated proteins when we discuss the organization of the nuclear envelope.

Figure 1-36. Structure and composition of a hemidesmosome

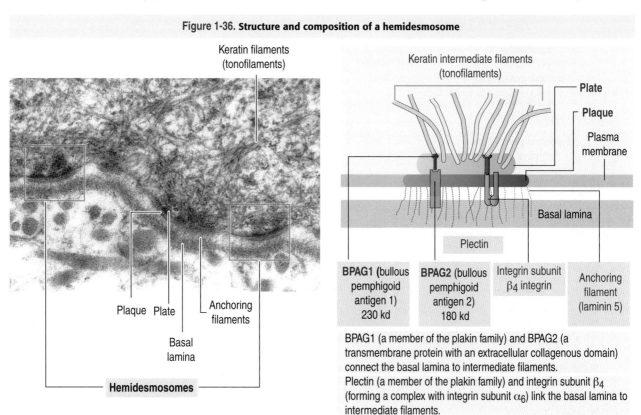

Keratin filaments (tonofilaments)

Keratin intermediate filaments (tonofilaments)

Plate
Plaque
Plasma membrane
Basal lamina

Plectin

Plaque Plate

Anchoring filaments

Basal lamina

Hemidesmosomes

| BPAG1 (bullous pemphigoid antigen 1) 230 kd | BPAG2 (bullous pemphigoid antigen 2) 180 kd | Integrin subunit β4 integrin | Anchoring filament (laminin 5) |

BPAG1 (a member of the plakin family) and BPAG2 (a transmembrane protein with an extracellular collagenous domain) connect the basal lamina to intermediate filaments.
Plectin (a member of the plakin family) and integrin subunit β4 (forming a complex with integrin subunit α6) link the basal lamina to intermediate filaments.

1 A circulating antibody to bullous pemphigoid antigen (BPAG1 or BPAG2) triggers a local response that induces mast cells to release **eosinophil chemotactic factor** (ECF) to attract eosinophils.

2 Eosinophils release proteases causing the breakdown of anchoring filaments linking the attachment plaque of the hemidesmosome to the basal lamina. A blister develops.

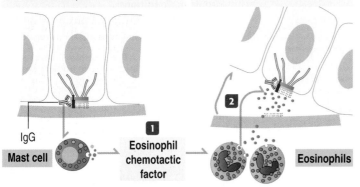

and lamin C as essential for the correct tissue-specific expression of certain genes.

2. The **mechanical stress hypothesis** proposes that a defect in lamin A and lamin C weakens the structural integrity of the nuclear envelope.

During mitosis, the **phosphorylation** of lamin **serine residues** causes a transient disassembly of the meshwork, followed by a breakdown of the nuclear envelope into small fragments. At the end of mitosis, lamins are **dephosphorylated**, and the lamin meshwork and the nuclear envelope reorganize. See the cell nucleus section concerning the mechanism of phosphorylation and dephosphorylation of lamins during the cell cycle.

Hemidesmosomes and intermediate filaments

Hemidesmosomes are specialized junctions observed in basal cells of the stratified squamous epithelium attaching to the basement membrane (Figure 1-36). **Inside the cell**, the proteins **BPAG1** (for **bullous pemphigoid antigen 1**) and **plectin** (members of the **plakin family** of cross-linker proteins) are associated to **intermediate filaments** (also called **tonofilaments**). Plectin connects intermediate filaments to the integrin subunit β_4.

On the extracellular side, integrin $\alpha_6\beta_4$, **BPAG2** (for **bullous pemphigoid antigen 2**) and **laminin 5**, a protein present in specialized structures called **anchoring filaments**, link hemidesmosomes to the basal lamina.

A group of human diseases, known as **laminopathies**, are linked to defects in proteins of the nuclear envelope, including lamins (see Box 1-N). Numerous laminopathies affect cardiac and skeletal muscle, adipose tissue (**lipodystrophies**), and motor and sensory peripheral nerves.

Two hypotheses concerning the pathogenic mechanism of laminopathies have been considered:

1. The **gene expression hypothesis** regards lamin A

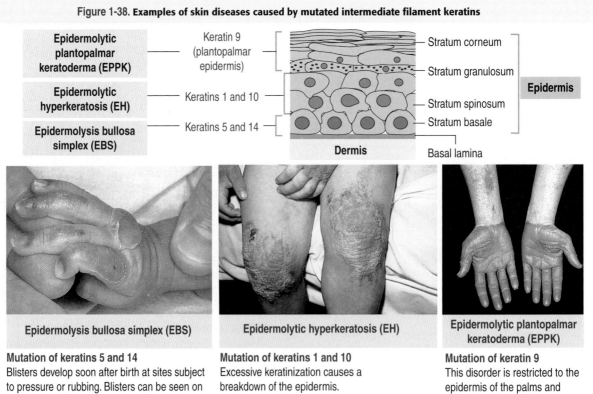

Figure 1-38. **Examples of skin diseases caused by mutated intermediate filament keratins**

Epidermolytic plantopalmar keratoderma (EPPK)	Keratin 9 (plantopalmar epidermis)
Epidermolytic hyperkeratosis (EH)	Keratins 1 and 10
Epidermolysis bullosa simplex (EBS)	Keratins 5 and 14

Stratum corneum
Stratum granulosum
Stratum spinosum
Stratum basale
Basal lamina
Epidermis
Dermis

Epidermolysis bullosa simplex (EBS)

Mutation of keratins 5 and 14
Blisters develop soon after birth at sites subject to pressure or rubbing. Blisters can be seen on the fingers of an infant.

Epidermolytic hyperkeratosis (EH)

Mutation of keratins 1 and 10
Excessive keratinization causes a breakdown of the epidermis.

Epidermolytic plantopalmar keratoderma (EPPK)

Mutation of keratin 9
This disorder is restricted to the epidermis of the palms and soles.

Photographs from Callen JP, et al.: Color Atlas of Dermatology. Philadelphia, WB Saunders, 1993.

Figure 1-39. Nuclear envelope and nuclear pore complex

Proteins of the nuclear pore complex are collectively designated **nucleoporins**

Filamentous **Phe-Gly nucleoporins** in the central channel contain docking sites for nuclear transport factor-cargo proteins entering the channel from either cytoplasmic or nuclear sites.

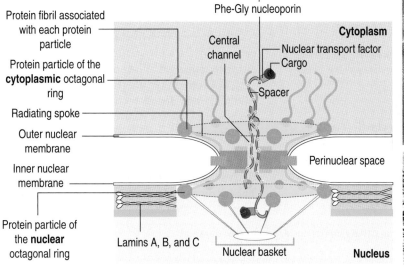

Phe-Gly nucleoporin

Protein fibril associated with each protein particle

Protein particle of the **cytoplasmic** octagonal ring

Radiating spoke

Outer nuclear membrane

Inner nuclear membrane

Protein particle of the **nuclear** octagonal ring

Central channel

Cytoplasm

Nuclear transport factor

Cargo

Spacer

Perinuclear space

Lamins A, B, and C

Nuclear basket

Nucleus

Nuclear pores

Freeze fracture | top view

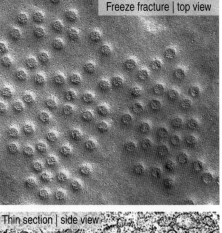

Thin section | side view

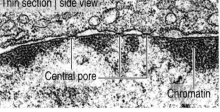

Central pore

Chromatin

F-actin

Intermediate filament protein

F-actin

Nesprin-1/2

Plectin

Nesprin-3 Nesprin-1/2

Outer nuclear membrane

Lamin B receptor (**LBR**)

Sun1 dimer

Perinuclear space

Emerin

Inner nuclear membrane

Lamin B1/B2

Lamin A/C

Chromatin

Lamina-associated polypeptide 1C (**LAP1C**)

Lamina-associated polypeptide 2β (**LAP2β**)

Lamins

Lamins bind to inner nuclear membrane proteins lamin B receptor (LBR), emerin, lamina-associated polypeptides 1C (LAP1C) and 2β (LAP2β). Sun 1 dimer protein links lamins to nesprins inserted in the outer nuclear membrane. Nesprin-1/2 associates with F-actin and nesprin-3 binds to plectin, which in turn associates with intermediate filament proteins.

Mutations of emerin, which binds to both lamins A and B, and lamin B receptor, which binds to lamin B, give rise to **Emery-Dreifuss muscular dystrophy** and **Pelger-Huet anomaly in blood granulocytes** (incomplete differentiation).

Homozygous mutation in lamin B receptor causes **Greenberg skeletal dysplasia**, an embryonic lethal chondrodystrophy.

The plakin-related protein BPAG1 associates to BPAG2, a transmembrane protein with an extracellular collagenous domain.

Putting all things together, BPAG1 constitutes a bridge between the transmembrane protein BPAG2 and intermediate filaments. If this bridge is disrupted, as in bullous pemphigoid, the epidermis becomes detached from the basal lamina anchoring sites. BPAG1 and BPAG2 were discovered in patients with bullous pemphigoid, an autoimmune disease.

Clinical significance: Skin blistering diseases
Bullous pemphigoid is an autoimmune blistering disease similar to **pemphigus vulgaris** (called "pemphigoid", similar to pemphigus). Blisters or bullae develop at the epidermis-dermis junction when circulating immunoglobulin G (IgG) cross-reacts with bullous pemphigoid antigen 1 or 2. IgG-antigen complexes lead to the formation of complement complexes (C3, C5b, and C9), which damage the attachment of hemidesmosomes and perturb the synthesis

• Lamins, type V intermediate filament proteins, are the main components of the nuclear lamina.
• Lamins bind to proteins of the inner nuclear membrane, including emerin (with eight transmembrane spans), lamin B receptor, lamina-associated polypeptides 1 and 2β, and nesprin-1α, a protein with several spectrin-like repeats that binds lamin A and emerin (see Figure 1-39).
• Lamins and their associated proteins have roles in chromatin organization, spacing of nuclear pore complexes, and reassembly of the nucleus after cell division.
• Mutations of lamins and lamin-binding proteins cause various diseases (called laminopathies) (see Box 1-N). Hutchinson-Gilford progeria syndrome (premature aging) is caused by a mutation in lamin A.

of anchoring proteins by basal cells (Figure 1-37).

The production of local toxins causes the degranulation of mast cells and release of chemotactic factors attracting eosinophils. Enzymes released by eosinophils cause blisters or bullae.

Intermediate filaments strengthen the cellular cytoskeleton. The expression of mutant keratin genes results in the **abnormal assembly of keratin filaments**, which **weakens the mechanical strength of cells** and causes inherited skin diseases, as shown in Figure 1-38:

1. **Epidermolysis bullosa simplex** (EBS), characterized by skin blisters after minor trauma. EBS is determined by **keratin 5** and **14** mutant genes.

2. **Epidermolytic hyperkeratosis** (EH), in which patients have excessive keratinization of the epidermis owing to mutations of **keratin 1** and **10** genes.

3. **Epidermolytic plantopalmar keratoderma** (EPPK), a skin disease producing fragmentation of the epidermis of the palms and soles, caused by a mutation of the **keratin 9** gene.

Cell nucleus
Nuclear envelope and nuclear pore complex
The cell nucleus consists of three major components:

Figure 1-40. Ran GTPase directs nucleocytoplasmic transport

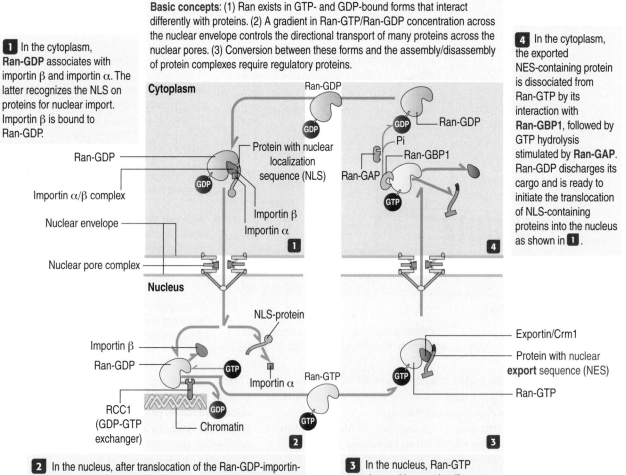

Basic concepts: (1) Ran exists in GTP- and GDP-bound forms that interact differently with proteins. (2) A gradient in Ran-GTP/Ran-GDP concentration across the nuclear envelope controls the directional transport of many proteins across the nuclear pores. (3) Conversion between these forms and the assembly/disassembly of protein complexes require regulatory proteins.

1 In the cytoplasm, **Ran-GDP** associates with importin β and importin α. The latter recognizes the NLS on proteins for nuclear import. Importin β is bound to Ran-GDP.

4 In the cytoplasm, the exported NES-containing protein is dissociated from Ran-GTP by its interaction with **Ran-GBP1**, followed by GTP hydrolysis stimulated by **Ran-GAP**. Ran-GDP discharges its cargo and is ready to initiate the translocation of NLS-containing proteins into the nucleus as shown in **1**.

2 In the nucleus, after translocation of the Ran-GDP-importin-αβ/NLS protein complex, **importin** β is released from Ran, and **importin** α detaches from the **NLS-containing protein**, which becomes free. **RCC1**, a guanine nucleotide exchanger bound to chromatin, generates **Ran-GTP**.

3 In the nucleus, Ran-GTP associates with exportins (for example, **exportin Crm1**) required for export into the cytoplasm of **NES-containing proteins**.

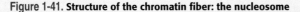

Figure 1-41. Structure of the chromatin fiber: the nucleosome

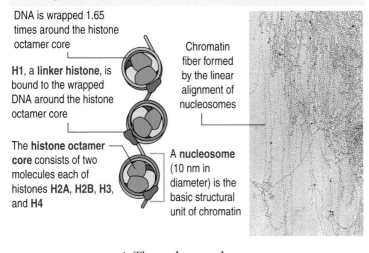

DNA is wrapped 1.65 times around the histone octamer core

H1, a **linker histone**, is bound to the wrapped DNA around the histone octamer core

The **histone octamer core** consists of two molecules each of histones **H2A, H2B, H3,** and **H4**

Chromatin fiber formed by the linear alignment of nucleosomes

A **nucleosome** (10 nm in diameter) is the basic structural unit of chromatin

1. The **nuclear envelope.**
2. **Chromatin.**
3. The **nucleolus.**

The **nuclear envelope** consists of two concentric membranes separated by a perinuclear space. The **inner nuclear membrane** is associated with the **nuclear lamina** (see Box 1-O), **chromatin,** and **ribonucleoproteins.** The **outer nuclear membrane** is continuous with the membranes of the endoplasmic reticulum and can be associated with ribosomes.

The **nuclear pore complex** has a **tripartite structure,** composed of a **central cylindrical body** placed between **inner** and **outer octagonal rings,** each consisting of eight protein particles. The central cylinder consists of a central plug and eight radiating **spokes** (Figure 1-39). The exact role of individual nuclear pore complex proteins in nucleocytoplasmic trafficking is unclear.

Figure 1-42. X chromosome inactivation

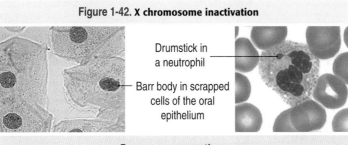

Drumstick in a neutrophil

Barr body in scrapped cells of the oral epithelium

Dosage compensation

The inactive X chromosome remains condensed during most of the interphase of the cell cycle.

It is visualized as a densely stained chromatin mass (**Barr body** or **X chromatin**) in a variable number of nuclei (about 30%-80%) of a normal female. A small **drumstick** is observed in 1% to 10% of neutrophils in the female.

The inactivation of one of the X chromosomes is **random** (paternal or maternal X chromosome).

If a cell has more than two X chromosomes, the extra ones are inactivated and the maximum number of Barr bodies per nucleus will be one less than the total number of X chromosomes in the karyotype.

Nuclear pore complexes embedded in the nuclear envelope establish bidirectional communication gates for the trafficking of macromolecules between the cytoplasm and the nucleus. Small molecules (less than 40 to 60 kd) can diffuse passively through the nuclear pore complex. Proteins of any size, containing a **nuclear localization amino acid sequence** (**NLS,** Pro-Lys-Lys-Lys-Arg-Lys-Val), can be imported into the nucleus, however, by an energy-dependent mechanism (requiring ATP and GTP).

Nucleocytoplasmic transport: Ran-GTPase

Protein nuclear import/export is controlled by **Ran** (for Ras-like nuclear GTPase), **a small GTPase of the Ras superfamily** that dictates the directionality of nucleocytoplasmic transport.

Ran shuttles across the nuclear pores and accumulates inside the nucleus by an active transport mechanism (Figure 1-40).

1. **In the nucleus,** a high concentration of Ran-GTP is achieved by **RCC1,** a GDP-GTP exchanger protein bound to chromatin. Ran-GTP determines the dissociation of imported proteins containing **NLS** by binding to **importin β,** the transporter receptor protein.

2. **In the opposite direction, from the nucleus to the cytoplasm,** binding of Ran-GTP to the carrier protein **exportin/Crm1** facilitates the assembly of complexes containing proteins with **nuclear export sequence** (**NES**).

3. **In the cytoplasm,** Ran-GTP is converted to Ran-GDP by Ran-GTPase, which is activated by two cooperating proteins: **Ran-GAP** (Ran-GTPase-activating protein) and **RanBP** (Ran-GTP binding protein). Consequently, the exported protein is dissociated from its transporter receptor protein exportin/Crm1 and Ran-GTP. Importin and exportins are recycled by transport back across the nuclear pore complex.

Chromatin

Chromatin is defined as particles or "beads" (called **nucleosomes**) on a double- stranded DNA string (Figure 1-41). Each nucleosome consists of a **histone octamer core** and about two turns of DNA wound around the histone core. The histone octamer contains two molecules each of H2A, H2B, H3, and H4 histones. H1 histone cross-links the DNA molecule wrapped around the octamer.

Chromatin is packed in separate chromosomes that can be visualized during mitosis (or meiosis). During interphase (phases G_1, S, and G_2 of the cell cycle), individual chromosomes cannot be identified as such, but are present in a diffuse or noncondensed state.

Diffuse chromatin, called **euchromatin** ("good chromatin"), is transcriptionally (RNA synthesis) active and represents about 10% of total chromatin.

Figure 1-43. Components of the nucleus and nucleolus

The nucleus of eukaryotic cells is separated from the cytoplasm by the **nuclear envelope**, a double concentric membrane derived from the endoplasmic reticulum. The nuclear envelope is interrupted at random intervals by **nuclear pore complexes**, nucleoporin-containing structures that regulate the passage of molecules between the nuclear and cytoplasmic compartments.

Nucleolar proteins **nucleolin** and **fibrillarin** are found in the dense fibrillar component. **Nucleostemin** is present in the granular component. **RNA polymerase I** occupies the fibrillar center.

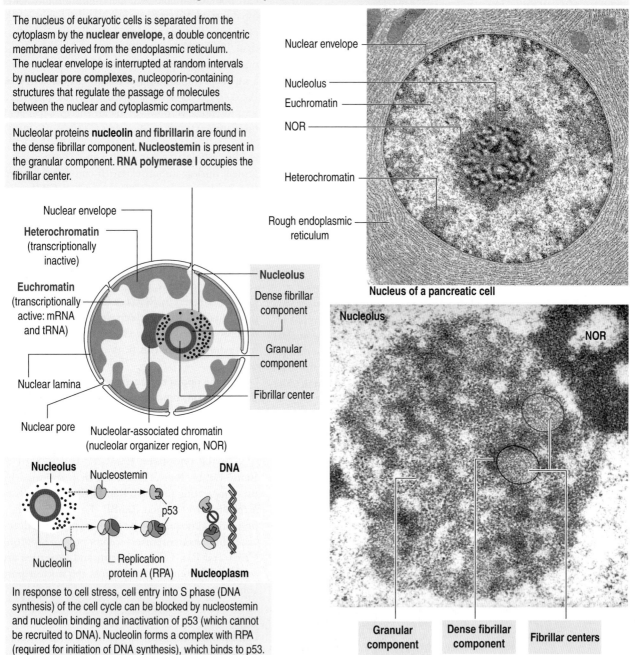

Nucleus of a pancreatic cell

In response to cell stress, cell entry into S phase (DNA synthesis) of the cell cycle can be blocked by nucleostemin and nucleolin binding and inactivation of p53 (which cannot be recruited to DNA). Nucleolin forms a complex with RPA (required for initiation of DNA synthesis), which binds to p53.

Euchromatin is the site of synthesis on **nonribosomal RNAs**, including **mRNA** and **transfer RNA (tRNA)** precursors.

Condensed chromatin, called **heterochromatin** ("different chromatin"), is transcriptionally inactive and represents about 90% of total chromatin (Figure 1-42).

Dosage compensation: X chromosome inactivation

X chromosome inactivation, known as **dosage compensation**, starts early in embryonic stem cell differentiation and is characterized by four features:

1. All but one of the X chromosomes undergoes inactivation.

2. The choice of the inactivated X chromosome is random. Either the paternal or the maternal X chromosome is inactivated.

3. The inactivation processes is heritable through subsequent rounds of cell division. The choice remains nonrandom for all subsequent cell descendants.

4. Both X chromosomes in oocytes remain active.

The transcriptional inactivation of one of the two X chromosomes is observed in the trophoblast on day 12 after fertilization and on day 16 in the embryo.

In humans, the inactivated X chromosome is recognized by the presence of the **Barr body**, a

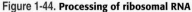

Figure 1-44. Processing of ribosomal RNA

Mature rRNA precursor molecule (45S)

RNA polymerase

RNA polymerase

Chromatin fiber

Direction of RNA synthesis (5' to 3' end)

Nascent rRNA precursor molecule

Chromatin fiber

Direction of RNA synthesis (5' to 3' end)

Nascent rRNA precursor molecule

Electron micrograph from Franke WW et al.: Morphology of transcriptional units of rDNA. Exp Cell Res 100:233-244, 1976.

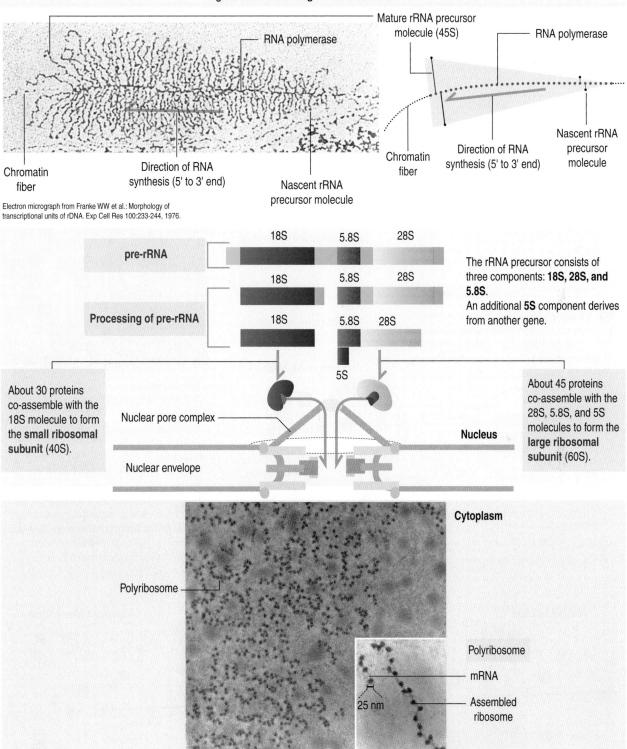

pre-rRNA

18S   5.8S   28S

Processing of pre-rRNA

18S   5.8S   28S

18S   5.8S   28S

5S

The rRNA precursor consists of three components: **18S, 28S, and 5.8S**.
An additional **5S** component derives from another gene.

About 30 proteins co-assemble with the 18S molecule to form the **small ribosomal subunit** (40S).

Nuclear pore complex

About 45 proteins co-assemble with the 28S, 5.8S, and 5S molecules to form the **large ribosomal subunit** (60S).

Nucleus

Nuclear envelope

Cytoplasm

Polyribosome

Polyribosome

mRNA

25 nm

Assembled ribosome

heterochromatin mass observed adjacent to the nuclear envelope or in the form of a **drumstick** in polymorphonuclear leukocytes (see Figure 1-42). If a cell has more than two X chromosomes, the extra X chromosomes are inactivated, and more than one Barr body is visualized.

The concept of dosage compensation is relevant to the understanding of tumor-suppressor inactivation and oncogene inactivation when a single active copy of an X-linked genes is affected. Some genes located on the inactivated X chromosome escape inactivation in normal cells and several of these genes, most of which encode growth factors, are implicated in human cancer. For example, the gene encoding

Figure 1-45. **Localization of nucleic acids using light microscopy**

Feulgen reaction

1 **Hydrolysis with hydrochloric acid** forms aldehyde groups on deoxyribose (DNA sugar) but not ribose (RNA sugar).

2 DNA-containing chromatin stains purple because aldehyde groups reacting with the colorless **Schiff's reagent** yield a **purple product**.

Cytoplasm
Nucleus
Nucleolus

HCl

The nucleolus is unstained (DNA-containing intranucleolar fibrillar centers are not resolved with the light microscope).

Basophilia

1 **Toluidine blue**, a basic dye, binds to the negatively charged phosphate groups on DNA and RNA. Chromatin (DNA), the nucleolus (RNA), and ribosomes attached to the endoplasmic reticulum (RNA) stain blue. These structures are **basophilic**.

Rough endoplasmic reticulum

Nucleolus

DNAse

2 Pretreatment with DNAse followed by toluidine blue staining identify RNA-containing sites.

RNAse

Rough endoplasmic reticulum

Nucleus

Nucleolus

Nucleus

3 Pretreatment with RNAse followed by toluidine blue staining identify DNA-containing sites.

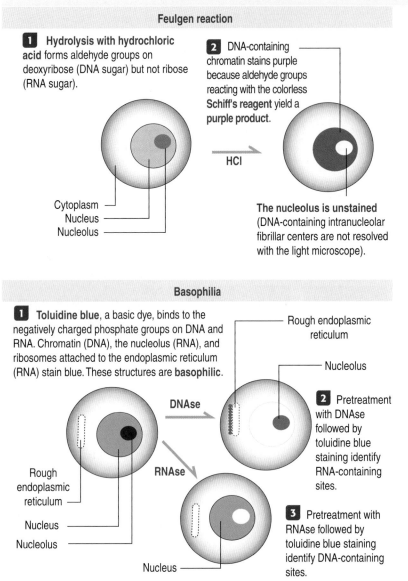

Autoradiography

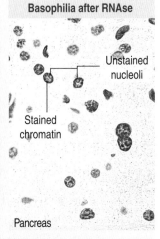

This autoradiogram illustrates the uptake of [^{3}H]thymidine by nuclei of intestinal epithelial cells (duodenum).

The radiolabeled precursor was injected into an experimental animal, which was sacrificed 24 hours later.

Histologic sections were coated with a photographic emulsion and exposed in the dark for 48 hours. Development of the photographic emulsion followed by staining of the section reveals the localization of silver grain (black dots) on some nuclei that were passing through the S phase (DNA synthesis) of their cell cycle.

Feulgen reaction	PAS reaction	Basophilia	Basophilia after RNAse

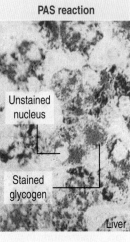

Feulgen positive chromatin

Feulgen negative nucleolus

Pancreas

DNA stains purple. Proteins in the nucleolus are stained green with a contrast dye.

Unstained nucleus

Stained glycogen

Liver

Glycogen in the cytoplasm of hepatocytes stains purple. The nucleus is unstained.

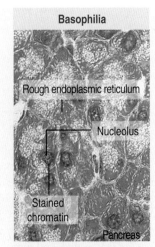

Rough endoplasmic reticulum

Nucleolus

Stained chromatin

Pancreas

Nucleic acids (DNA in chromatin and RNA in nucleolus and rough endoplasmic reticulum) are stained.

Unstained nucleoli

Stained chromatin

Pancreas

After RNAse treatment, only chromatin stains. Nucleoli and rough endoplasmic reticulum are not stained.

• The nucleolus is the site of synthesis, processing, and modification of pre-rRNA and initial preribosomal assembly. It also houses proteins unrelated to ribosome synthesis and shuttling between the nucleolus and the nucleoplasm to serve specific functions.
• The nucleolus consists of three components: (1) fibrillar centers; (2) a dense fibrillar component surrounding the fibrillar centers; and (3) a granular component. Pre-rRNA synthesis occurs at the interface between the fibrillar centers and the surrounding dense fibrillar component. Nascent pre-rRNA transcripts extend into the dense fibrillar component and migrate to the granular component where processing, modification, and preribosomal assembly occur.
• The fibrillar centers contain chromatin and transcription factors, including RNA polymerase I. The dense fibrillar component, the site of initial pre-rRNA processing, contains small ribonucleoproteins involved in RNA modification. The granular component accounts for about 75% of the nucleolar mass; the granules correspond to preribosomes.
• The nucleolus disappears during mitotic prophase and reassembles at the end of telophase at specific chromosomal regions named **nucleolar-organizer regions (NORs)**.

gastrin-releasing peptide receptor is associated with an increased risk in lung cancer in women. We come back to X-linked dominant and recessive inheritance at the end of this chapter.

Nucleolus

The **nucleolus** is the site of synthesis and processing of **ribosomal RNA (rRNA)** and **assembly of ribosomal subunits**. The *rRNA* genes are arranged in an array of multiple copies transcribed by RNA polymerase I.

The nucleolus houses several proteins, including **fibrillarin** and **nucleolin**, required for pre-rRNA processing. In addition, the nucleolus contains **nucleostemin**, a protein unrelated to ribosomal biogenesis. Nucleolin and nucleostemin are shuttling proteins;

• Both reactions use the **Schiff reagent**.
• In the **PAS reaction, periodic acid** forms aldehyde groups in sugars of glycoproteins by an **oxidation process.**
• In the Feulgen reaction, **hydrochloric acid** forms aldehyde groups in deoxyribose by **hydrolysis**.

Many cytologic stains use **acidic** and **basic** dyes.
• **Basic** or **cationic dyes** have positively charged color radicals forming electrostatic linkages with acidic groups (e.g., phosphate groups in nucleic acids). **Toluidine blue** is a cationic dye that binds to phosphate groups in DNA and RNA to give a blue color. DNA and RNA are considered to be **basophilic** (having binding affinity for a basic dye).
• **Acidic** or **anionic dyes** have negatively charged color radicals establishing electrostatic linkages with basic groups. **Eosin** is an anionic dye that stains many basic proteins. Basic proteins are considered to be **acidophilic** (having affinity for an acidic dye).

they relocalize from the nucleolus to the nucleoplasm where they interact with **protein p53**, a protector of DNA damage by preventing DNA replication in response to genomic stress. We come back to p53 later (see Figure 1-52).

Essentially, the nucleolus is a multifunctional nuclear structure consisting of stable proteins involved in ribosomal synthesis and molecules shuttling between the nucleolus and nucleoplasm to fulfill non-nucleolar functions.

Structurally, the nucleolus consists of three major components (Figure 1-43; see Box 1-P):

1. A **fibrillar center** (corresponding to chromatin containing repeated rRNA genes and the presence of **RNA polymerase I** and **signal recognition particle [SRP] RNA**).

2. A dense **fibrillar component** (where nascent rRNA is present and undergoing some of its processing). **Fibrillarin** and **nucleolin** are found in the fibrillar dense component.

3. A **granular component** (where the assembly of ribosomal subunits, containing **18S rRNA** [small subunit] and **28S rRNA** [large subunit], is completed). **Nucleostemin**, a protein unrelated to ribosomal biogenesis, coexists with the granular components.

Nucleoli are typically surrounded by a shell of heterochromatin, mostly from centromeric and pericentromeric chromosomal regions.

The nucleolus dissociates during mitosis, then reappears at the beginning of the G_1 phase. More than one nucleolar mass, each representing the product of a chromosome with a **nucleolar organizing region (NOR)**, can be observed in the nucleus. In some cells with an extended interphase, such as neurons, a single large nucleolus is organized by the fusion of several nucleolar masses.

The active process of rRNA synthesis can be visualized at the electron microscopic level (Figure 1-44) by spreading the contents of nuclei of cells with hundreds of nucleoli (e.g., amphibian oocytes). **rRNA genes** can be seen as repeating **gene units** along the chromatin axis, like "Christmas trees," pointing in the same direction and separated by nontranscribed **spacers**. The entire rRNA gene region is covered by more than 100 **RNA polymerase I** molecules synthesizing an equivalent number of **fibrils**, each with a terminal **granule**.

Each fibril represents an rRNA precursor (45S) ribonucleoprotein molecule oriented perpendicularly to the chromatin axis similar to the branches of a tree. The **45S** rRNA precursor is detached from the chromatin axis and cleaved into **28S, 18S,** and **5.8S rRNAs**.

The 18S rRNA and associated proteins form the **small ribosomal subunit**. The 28S and 5.8S, together with 5S rRNA made outside the nucleolus, and associated proteins form the **large ribosomal subunit.**

Acid fuchsin	Sulfonated red derivative of basic fuchsin which binds to collagen and to many cytoplasmic components
Alcian blue	A dye of uncertain chemical nature, often combined with PAS (see below) and used as a differential stain for acidic glycoproteins (mucins), which appear blue
Azure A	A basic dye, such as methylene blue and thionin, which stains nucleic acids. It is a component of many blood stains. It stains cartilage, mast cell granules metachromatically (purple to red)
Basic fuchsin	A mixture of closely related basic triphenylmethane dyes, each a propeller-shaped molecule with three nitrogen attached in *p*-position to each benzene ring
Cresyl violet	A basic dye which is used to stain nucleoproteins, Nissl bodies, and others. It has metachromatic properties for glycoproteins and mast cell granules
Feulgen reaction	Specific for the demonstration of DNA. Hydrolysis with HCl forms aldehyde groups on the DNA sugar (deoxyribose) but not on RNA sugar (ribose). Aldehydes react with reduced basic fuchsin (Schiff's reagent) to form a purple color. Robert Feulgen (German, 1884-1955).
Giemsa stain	Combined blood stain consisting of methylene blue, azure and eosin. The staining results are similar to those of Wright's stain. Gustav Giemsa (German, 1867-1948).
Gomori techniques	A group of different histochemical techniques named after George Gomori (Hungarian, 1904-1957). Used for: acid and alkaline phosphatases, a silver method for reticular fibers, a stain for pancreatic cells, elastic fibers and glycoproteins, and a reaction to demonstrate iron pigments.
Hematoxylin and eosin	A routine staining combination. Hematoxylin is used in combination with metal ions (aluminum or iron) to form colored chelate complexes. These act as cations and bind preferentially to acidic (anionic) groups. Hematoxylin stains nuclei blue; eosin stains the cytoplasm pink.
Mallory stain	Used for connective tissue. It contains aniline blue, orange G and azocarmine (or acid fuchsin). Connective tissue collagen bundles, in general, stain blue; muscle stains red; epithelium appears red due to red nuclei; red blood cells are orange-red. Frank Burr Mallory (American, 1862-1941).
Masson trichrome stain	A combination of acid fuchsin, orange G and light green. Nuclei appear black, cytoplasm red. Collagen fibers and glycoproteins are green; red blood cells are yellow to orange; muscle stains red. Claude Laurent Masson (French, 1880-1959).
Metachromasia	The property of certain biological compounds to change the color of such dyes as toluidine blue or thionine. For example, glycoproteins found in cartilage and mast cell granules will stain red or violet instead of blue with toluidine blue (Greek *meta*, after; *chroma*, color).
Orcein (resorcinol)	A natural dye obtained from lichens. Stains elastic fibers dark brown.
Periodic acid-Schiff reaction (PAS)	Used to demonstrate 1,2-aminoalcohol groups in glycogen and glycoproteins. Periodic acid converts these groups to aldehydes. Schiff's reagent (a leucofuchsin) reacts in turn with the aldehydes to form a characteristic red-purple product. Ugo Schiff (German, 1834-1915).
Sudan III, IV and Sudan black	Fat soluble substances used to stain fat in frozen sections. These azo dyes are soluble in non-aqueous, lipid phases and are preferentially concentrated by solution in fat droplets. Sudanophilia is the affinity for Sudan stain.
Toluidine blue	A basic stain which binds to nucleic acids. Also stains mast cell granules, glycoproteins and cartilage metachromatically (see Metachromasia).
van Gieson stain	It consists of picric acid and basic fuchsin. It is used to stain connective tissue. It stains collagen fibers red and elastic fibers and muscle yellow. Combined with hematoxylin, it stains nuclei blue brown. Ira van Gieson (American, 1865-1913).
Vital dyes	Non-toxic dyes administered to a living organism and taken up by phagocytosis. Trypan blue is used for vital staining. Carbon particles can also be used to demonstrate phagocytosis. Supravital dyes are added to the culture medium of cells.
Wright blood stain	It uses eosin and methylene blue to differentiate blood cell types and malarial parasites. James Homer Wright (American, 1869-1928).

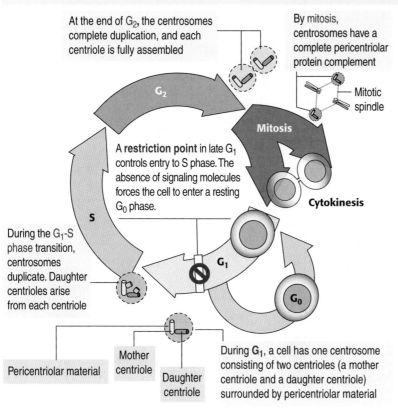

Figure 1-46. Phases of the cell cycle

At the end of G$_2$, the centrosomes complete duplication, and each centriole is fully assembled

By mitosis, centrosomes have a complete pericentriolar protein complement

Mitotic spindle

G$_2$

Mitosis

A **restriction point** in late G$_1$ controls entry to S phase. The absence of signaling molecules forces the cell to enter a resting G$_0$ phase.

Cytokinesis

S

During the G$_1$-S phase transition, centrosomes duplicate. Daughter centrioles arise from each centriole

G$_1$

G$_0$

Pericentriolar material

Mother centriole

Daughter centriole

During **G$_1$**, a cell has one centrosome consisting of two centrioles (a mother centriole and a daughter centriole) surrounded by pericentriolar material

Cell division in eukaryotic cells: the nuclear cycle and centrosome cycle

The cell cycle is divided into **four phases**: G$_1$ (gap 1), S, G$_2$ (gap 2), and mitosis. Mitosis is followed in most cases by cytokinesis. DNA replication occurs during the S phase and can be detected by **autoradiography** using [^{3}H]thymidine as a labeled precursor.

The **duration of the phases of the cell cycle** varies. The mitotic phase is the shortest (about 1 hour for a total cycle time of 24 hours). The G$_1$ phase is the longest (about 11 hours). The S phase is completed within 8 hours; G$_2$ in about 4 hours.

Some cells stop cell division or divide occasionally to replace cells lost by injury or cell death. These cells leave the G$_1$ phase of the cell cycle and become quiescent by entering the so-called **G$_0$ phase**. Although G$_0$ cells are metabolically active, they have lost their proliferation potential unless appropriate extracellular signals enable their reentry to the cell cycle.

The mRNA precursor is transcribed by RNA polymerase II, and the tRNA precursor is transcribed by RNA polymerase III.

Localization of nucleic acids

Cytochemistry and **autoradiography** (Figure 1-45) provide information about the cellular distribution and synthesis of nucleic acids. The **Feulgen reaction is specific for the localization of DNA** (see Box 1-Q).

Box 1-T | Cell cycle: Highlights to remember

• Cell division requires the coordination of three cycles: cytoplasmic cycle, nuclear cycle, and centrosome cycle. The centrosome cycle plays a role in regulating the cytoplasmic and nuclear cycles.
• The **cytoplasmic cycle** depends on the availability of cyclins activated and de-activated by cyclin-dependent kinases (Cdks). Cdk inhibitors inactivate Cdk-cyclin complexes. Cdk inhibitors are up-regulated at the transcriptional level to arrest, if necessary, the cytoplasmic and nuclear cycle.
• The **nuclear cycle** involves DNA duplication and chromosomal condensation. **Cdk2** phosphorylation of a protein complex bound to the origin of DNA replication recruits DNA polymerase to initiate and complete DNA synthesis in S-phase. **Cdk1** phosphorylation triggers chromosomal condensation (mediated by **histone H3** phosphorylation) and breakdown of the nuclear envelope (determined by nuclear lamin phosphorylation).
• During the **centrosome cycle**, the two centrioles of a centrosome duplicate during S-phase after phosphorylation of centrosome substrates by **Cdk2**. Daughter centrioles derive from each centriole.
• Cdks are involved in the coordination of the cytoplasmic, nuclear, and centrosome cycles.
• Cdk2 activity is required to initiate DNA replication and centriolar duplication.

Basic dyes, such as toluidine blue, stain DNA and RNA (**see** Box 1-R). Pretreatment with deoxyribonuclease (DNAse) and ribonuclease (RNAse) defines the distribution sites of DNA and RNA by selective removal of one of the nucleic acids.

Box 1-S provides basic information about the most frequently cytochemical techniques used in Histology and Pathology.

Autoradiography and **radiolabeled precursors** for one of the nucleic acids can determine the timing of their synthesis. In this technique, a radioactive precursor of DNA ([^{3}H]thymidine) or RNA ([^{3}H]uridine) is exposed to living cells. As a result of exposure to the radiolabel, any synthesized DNA or RNA contains the precursor. The radioactivity is detected by coating the cells with a thin layer of a photographic emulsion. Silver-containing crystals of the emulsion are exposed to structures of the cell containing radioactive DNA or RNA. After development of the emulsion, silver grains indicate the location of the labeled structures. This approach has been used extensively for determining the duration of several phases of the cell cycle.

Cell cycle

The cell cycle is defined as **the interval between two successive mitotic divisions resulting in the production of two daughter cells** (Figure 1-46).

The cell cycle is traditionally divided into two major phases:

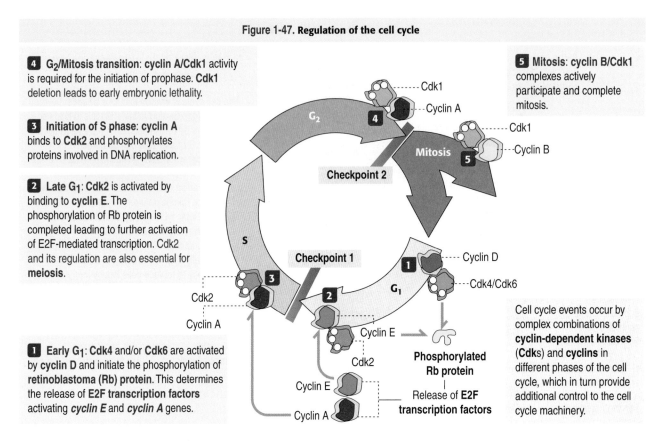

Figure 1-47. Regulation of the cell cycle

4 G₂/Mitosis transition: cyclin A/Cdk1 activity is required for the initiation of prophase. Cdk1 deletion leads to early embryonic lethality.

3 Initiation of S phase: cyclin A binds to **Cdk2** and phosphorylates proteins involved in DNA replication.

2 Late G₁: **Cdk2** is activated by binding to **cyclin E**. The phosphorylation of Rb protein is completed leading to further activation of E2F-mediated transcription. Cdk2 and its regulation are also essential for **meiosis**.

1 Early G₁: Cdk4 and/or Cdk6 are activated by **cyclin D** and initiate the phosphorylation of **retinoblastoma (Rb) protein**. This determines the release of **E2F transcription factors** activating *cyclin E* and *cyclin A* genes.

5 Mitosis: cyclin B/Cdk1 complexes actively participate and complete mitosis.

Cell cycle events occur by complex combinations of **cyclin-dependent kinases (Cdks)** and **cyclins** in different phases of the cell cycle, which in turn provide additional control to the cell cycle machinery.

1. **Interphase.**
2. **Mitosis** (also known as the **M phase**).

The most relevant event of interphase is the **S phase**, when the DNA in the nucleus is replicated. S phase is preceded by an interval or **gap** called the **G₁ phase**. The beginning of mitosis is preceded by the **G₂ phase**, a phase in which the cell ensures that DNA replication is completed before starting the M phase.

Essentially, G₁ and G₂ phases provide time for cell growth before and after DNA synthesis. Cell growth is required for doubling the cell mass in preparation for cell division.

Cells in G₁ can make a commitment to DNA replication and enter the S phase or stop their progression into the following S phase. If a cell does not enter the S phase, it remains in a **resting state** known as G₀, where it can remain for days, months, or years before reentering the cell cycle.

In a more contemporary view, the cycle is regarded as the coordinated progression and completion of three separate cycles:

1. A **cytoplasmic cycle**, consisting of the sequential activation of **cyclin-dependent protein kinases** in the presence of **cyclins**.

2. A **nuclear cycle**, in which DNA is replicated and chromosomes condense in preparation for cell division.

3. A **centrosome cycle**, consisting of the duplication of the two centrioles, called mother and daughter centrioles, and assembly of pericentriolar

proteins in preparation for the organization of the mitotic spindle curing mitosis or meiosis (see Figure 1-46). Recall from our previous discussion on the centrosome as a microtubule organizing center that γ-**tubulin ring** complexes are microtubule-nucleating complexes interacting with the protein **pericentrin** in the pericentriolar material. If this interaction is disrupted, the cell cycle is arrested during the G₂-M phase transition, and the cell undergoes programmed cell death or apoptosis. **Basal bodies**, the origin site of cilia and flagella, derive from centrosomes.

The activities of cyclin-dependent protein kinases–cyclin complexes coordinate the timed progression of the nuclear and centrosome cycles. Figure 1-47 provides additional details.

Autoradiography and FACS

The various phases of the cell cycle can be studied by autoradiography. Cells in the S phase can be recognized by detecting the synthesis of DNA using [³H]thymidine as a radiolabeled precursor. Cells can be stained through the developed emulsion layer to determine the precise localization sites of the overlapping silver grains.

The time progression of cells through the different phases of the cell cycle can be estimated using both brief and prolonged [³H]thymidine pulses. The number of cells radiolabeled during interphase (generally about 30%) represent the **labeling index** of the S phase. The fraction of radiolabeled cells seen in

Figure 1-48. Assembly and disassembly of the nuclear envelope

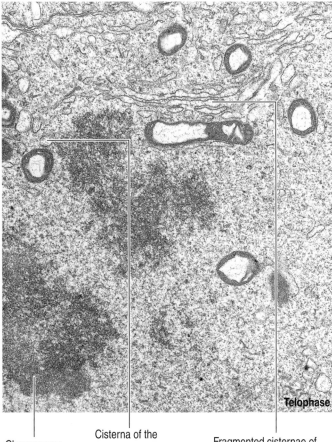

Chromosome

Cisterna of the endoplasmic reticulum associated to chromatin

Fragmented cisternae of the endoplasmic reticulum

Telophase

1 During interphase, the nuclear lamina, a network of lamins A, B, and C, associates with chromatin and the inner membrane of the nuclear envelope.

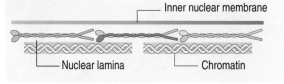

Inner nuclear membrane

Nuclear lamina

Chromatin

2 At mitosis, first protein kinase C and then cyclin A–activated Cdk1 kinase phosphorylate lamins, causing the filaments to dissociate into free lamin dimers.

Head Rod Tail

Lamin dimers

Phosphorylation site

3 As the nuclear lamina dissociates, the nuclear envelope undergoes breakdown. Lamin A, lamin B, and lamin C remain phosphorylated and dispersed. The components of the nuclear pore complex disassemble and disperse. Cisternae of the endoplasmic reticulum are a reservoir of the future nuclear envelope.

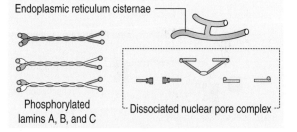

Endoplasmic reticulum cisternae

Phosphorylated lamins A, B, and C

Dissociated nuclear pore complex

Sequential events during the reassembly of the nuclear envelope

4 During anaphase, soluble proteins of the nuclear pore complex (nucleoporins) bind to the surface of chromatin.

5 During late anaphase, lamina-associated polypeptide 2β (LAP2β), lamin B receptor (LBR), and emerin, transmembrane proteins of the inner nuclear membrane, appear on the surface of chromatin.

6 During late telophase, cisternae of the endoplasmic reticulum anchor to LAP2β, LBR, and emerin, and the reconstitution of the nuclear envelope starts.

7 Before cytokinesis, lamin B becomes dephosphorylated by protein phosphatase 1 and, together with lamins C and A, initiates the formation of the nuclear lamina. The formation of the nuclear lamina starts on completion of the reconstruction of the nuclear envelope.

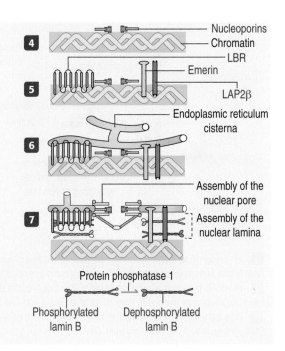

Nucleoporins
Chromatin
LBR
Emerin
LAP2β
Endoplasmic reticulum cisterna
Assembly of the nuclear pore
Assembly of the nuclear lamina

Protein phosphatase 1

Phosphorylated lamin B

Dephosphorylated lamin B

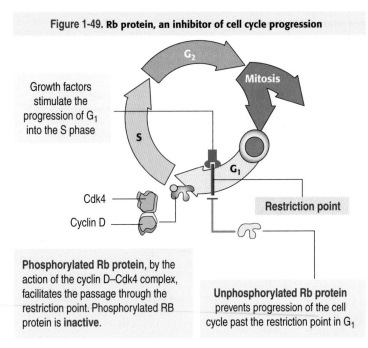

Figure 1-49. Rb protein, an inhibitor of cell cycle progression

Growth factors stimulate the progression of G_1 into the S phase

G2

Mitosis

S

G1

Cdk4

Cyclin D

Restriction point

Phosphorylated Rb protein, by the action of the cyclin D–Cdk4 complex, facilitates the passage through the restriction point. Phosphorylated RB protein is **inactive**.

Unphosphorylated Rb protein prevents progression of the cell cycle past the restriction point in G_1

mitosis (**mitotic index**) indicates that the radiolabeled precursor, which entered the cell during the S phase, progressed through the G_2 phase into M phase.

An alternative to autoradiography is the measurement of **DNA content** (**C value** 1.5 pg per haploid

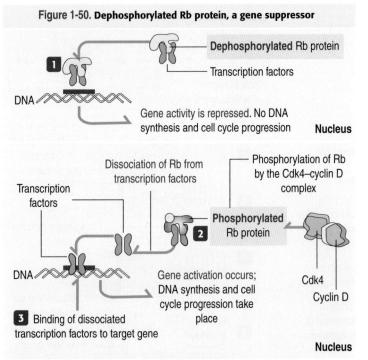

Figure 1-50. Dephosphorylated Rb protein, a gene suppressor

1

Dephosphorylated Rb protein

Transcription factors

DNA

Gene activity is repressed. No DNA synthesis and cell cycle progression

Nucleus

Dissociation of Rb from transcription factors

Phosphorylation of Rb by the Cdk4–cyclin D complex

Transcription factors

Phosphorylated Rb protein **2**

DNA

Gene activation occurs; DNA synthesis and cell cycle progression take place

Cdk4

Cyclin D

3 Binding of dissociated transcription factors to target gene

Nucleus

1 Rb protein in its **dephosphorylated form** binds to a group of transcription factors and represses gene transcription of normally activated target genes.
2 When Rb protein is **phosphorylated** by the Cdk4–cyclin D complex, transcription factors dissociate from Rb protein during late G_1.
3 Free transcription factors stimulate the expression of genes required for DNA synthesis and cell cycle progression.

cell) using a **fluorescence-activated cell sorter (FACS)**. Cells are stained with a fluorescent dye, which binds to DNA. The amount of fluorescence detected by the FACS is equivalent to the amount of DNA in each cell (for example, 2C in G_1; 4C at the end of S phase; 4C during G_2).

Breakdown and reassembly of the nuclear envelope

The disassembly of the nuclear envelope occurs at the end of the mitotic and meiotic prophase. It involves the fragmentation of the nuclear envelope, the dissociation of the nuclear pore complexes, and the depolymerization of the nuclear lamina (Figure 1-48).

The nuclear lamina is composed of type V intermediate filament proteins, **lamins A, B, and C**, which associate with each other to form the nuclear lamina.

Phosphorylation of lamins, catalyzed first by **protein kinase C** and later by **cyclin A–activated Cdk1 kinase**, results in the disassembly of the nuclear lamina. In addition, the components of the nuclear pore complex, the nucleoporins, and the membranous cisternae of the endoplasmic reticulum also disperse. The endoplasmic reticulum is the nuclear membrane reservoir for nuclear envelope reassembly.

During anaphase, nucleoporins and three transmembrane protein components of the inner nuclear membrane, **lamina-associated polypeptide 2β, lamin B receptor**, and **emerin**, attach to the surface of the chromosomes (chromatin). Then, cisternae of the endoplasmic reticulum are recruited by nucleoporins and inner nuclear membrane proteins, and the nuclear envelope is rebuilt by the end of telophase.

A final step in the reconstruction of the nuclear envelope is the dephosphorylation of lamin B by **protein phosphatase 1**. Dephosphorylated lamin B associates with lamins A and C to form the nuclear lamina before cytokinesis.

This sequence of events stresses the impact of gene mutations affecting the expression of lamin A or lamin-binding proteins (see Box 1-N) as causes of laminopathies.

Tumor-suppressor genes: The retinoblastoma model

Not only Cdk-cyclin complexes control the progression and completion of the cell cycle. Tissues use two strategies to restrict cell proliferation:

1. By limiting mitogenic factors, such as platelet-derived growth factor (PDGF) and fibroblast-growth factor (FGF), which **stimulate cell growth**.

2. By regulatory genes that actively **suppress proliferation**. These genes, called **suppressor genes**, control normal cell proliferation.

The **retinoblastoma model** provides important clues on how suppressor genes work (Figure 1-49). Each cell has duplicate copies of the **retinoblastoma**

Figure 1-51. The telomerase complex

Human telomeres consist of many kilobases of TTAGGG repeats, with a G-rich leading stand and a C-rich lagging strand. The G-strand extends into the 3' direction, forming the G-overhang.

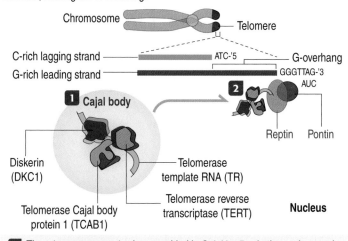

1 The telomerase complex is assembled in Cajal bodies in the nucleus and is shuttled to the telomeres by the accessory protein TCAB1.

2 The ATPases pontin and reptin activate the telomeric complex at the chromosome ends and initiate nucleotide addition. By this mechanism, the telomeric complex compensates for the shortening of telomeres, maintaining telomere length and stability. Telomere stability is essential for the highly proliferative stem cells. A complex of six proteins, called shelterin, regulates the length of the telomere (not shown).

(*Rb*) **gene** as a safety backup. When the **two copies** of the *Rb* gene are mutated, an abnormal **Rb protein** induces cancerous growth of retinal cells.

When a single copy of the *Rb* gene pair is mutated, the remaining *Rb* gene copy functions normally and suppresses unregulated cell proliferation unless a second mutation occurs. In children with only a single intact *Rb* gene copy, all cells of the developing embryo grow normally. Late in gestation, retinal cells may lose the normal copy of the *Rb* gene, and a retinoblastoma develops.

The *Rb* gene specifies a **nuclear protein** involved in regulating the activity of a group of proteins, **transcription factors**, involved in DNA synthesis and cell cycle progression. When Rb protein is **dephosphorylated**, it binds to transcription factors. Although the Rb protein–transcription factor complex can bind to target genes, the activity of the transcription factors is repressed.

When Rb protein is **phosphorylated** by the **Cdk4–cyclin D** complex, it dissociates from the transcription factor complex, which activates specific gene expression (Figure 1-50). Phosphorylated Rb protein switches transcription factors from suppression to activation required for DNA synthesis and progression of the cell cycle.

Figure 1-52. The p53 pathway

How p53 tumor suppression activity works — **E3 ubiquitin ligase MDM2 modulates the stability of p53**

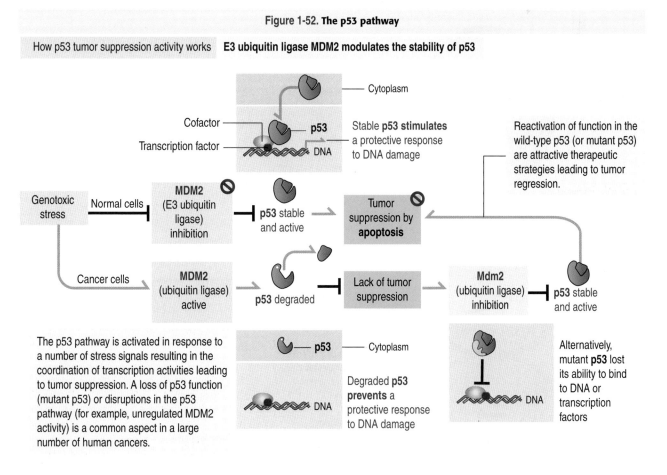

The p53 pathway is activated in response to a number of stress signals resulting in the coordination of transcription activities leading to tumor suppression. A loss of p53 function (mutant p53) or disruptions in the p53 pathway (for example, unregulated MDM2 activity) is a common aspect in a large number of human cancers.

Figure 1-53. **Phases of mitosis**

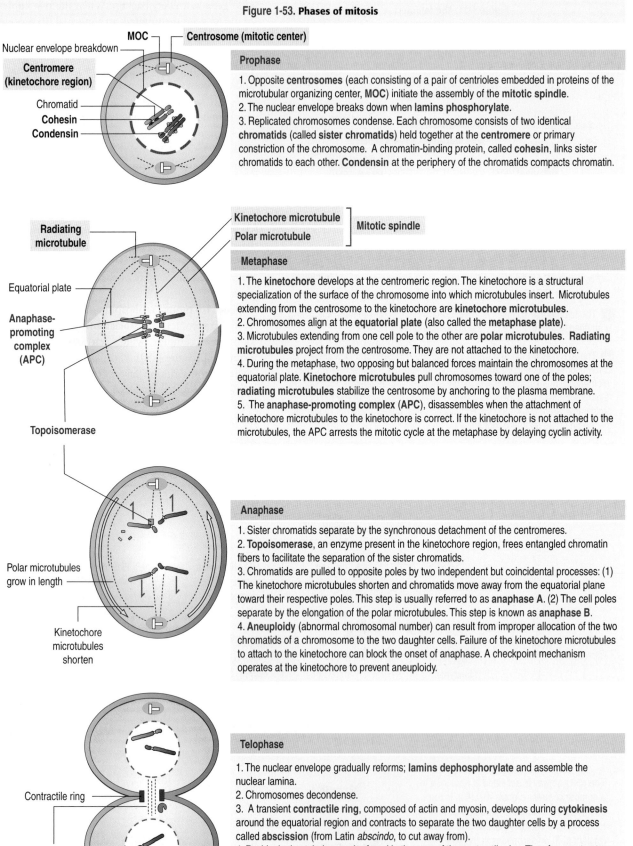

MOC — **Centrosome (mitotic center)**

Nuclear envelope breakdown

Centromere (kinetochore region)

Chromatid

Cohesin

Condensin

Prophase

1. Opposite **centrosomes** (each consisting of a pair of centrioles embedded in proteins of the microtubular organizing center, **MOC**) initiate the assembly of the **mitotic spindle**.
2. The nuclear envelope breaks down when **lamins phosphorylate**.
3. Replicated chromosomes condense. Each chromosome consists of two identical **chromatids** (called **sister chromatids**) held together at the **centromere** or primary constriction of the chromosome. A chromatin-binding protein, called **cohesin**, links sister chromatids to each other. **Condensin** at the periphery of the chromatids compacts chromatin.

Radiating microtubule

Kinetochore microtubule
Polar microtubule
Mitotic spindle

Equatorial plate

Anaphase-promoting complex (APC)

Topoisomerase

Metaphase

1. The **kinetochore** develops at the centromeric region. The kinetochore is a structural specialization of the surface of the chromosome into which microtubules insert. Microtubules extending from the centrosome to the kinetochore are **kinetochore microtubules**.
2. Chromosomes align at the **equatorial plate** (also called the **metaphase plate**).
3. Microtubules extending from one cell pole to the other are **polar microtubules**. **Radiating microtubules** project from the centrosome. They are not attached to the kinetochore.
4. During the metaphase, two opposing but balanced forces maintain the chromosomes at the equatorial plate. **Kinetochore microtubules** pull chromosomes toward one of the poles; **radiating microtubules** stabilize the centrosome by anchoring to the plasma membrane.
5. The **anaphase-promoting complex** (APC), disassembles when the attachment of kinetochore microtubules to the kinetochore is correct. If the kinetochore is not attached to the microtubules, the APC arrests the mitotic cycle at the metaphase by delaying cyclin activity.

Polar microtubules grow in length

Kinetochore microtubules shorten

Anaphase

1. Sister chromatids separate by the synchronous detachment of the centromeres.
2. **Topoisomerase**, an enzyme present in the kinetochore region, frees entangled chromatin fibers to facilitate the separation of the sister chromatids.
3. Chromatids are pulled to opposite poles by two independent but coincidental processes: (1) The kinetochore microtubules shorten and chromatids move away from the equatorial plane toward their respective poles. This step is usually referred to as **anaphase A**. (2) The cell poles separate by the elongation of the polar microtubules. This step is known as **anaphase B**.
4. **Aneuploidy** (abnormal chromosomal number) can result from improper allocation of the two chromatids of a chromosome to the two daughter cells. Failure of the kinetochore microtubules to attach to the kinetochore can block the onset of anaphase. A checkpoint mechanism operates at the kinetochore to prevent aneuploidy.

Contractile ring

Midbody

Telophase

1. The nuclear envelope gradually reforms; **lamins dephosphorylate** and assemble the nuclear lamina.
2. Chromosomes decondense.
3. A transient **contractile ring**, composed of actin and myosin, develops during **cytokinesis** around the equatorial region and contracts to separate the two daughter cells by a process called **abscission** (from Latin *abscindo*, to cut away from).
4. Residual microtubules can be found in the core of the contractile ring. They form a structure known as the **midbody**.
5. Radiating, kinetochore, and polar microtubules disappear.

Box 1-U | **p53: Highlights to remember**

- The tumor-suppressor protein p53 protects the integrity of DNA in response to harmful stress, called genotoxic stress.
- The protective function depends on the ability of p53 to induce programmed cell death or apoptosis or arrest cell cycle activities, when a cell undergoes genotoxic stress.
- How does p53 work? As a transcription factor, p53 controls the transcriptional activation of proapoptotic genes and the inactivation of antiapoptotic genes. By this mechanism, a cell affected by genotoxic stress is eliminated.
- What can go wrong? A loss of p53 function may occur by a mutation of the *TP53* gene, which encodes p53, or by an abnormal signaling pathway controlling p53 function (see Figure 1-52).
- Why is p53 important? Cancer cells are highly sensitive to apoptotic signals, but can survive if there is a loss of p53 function.

Clinical significance: Retinoblastoma tumors

Retinoblastoma, a tumor that occurs early in life, arises as a consequence of mutations in *Rb1* gene, which encodes the retinoblastoma tumour-suppressor protein Rb.

Children with the **familial form** of retinoblastoma usually have multiple tumor sites growing in both eyes.

A second type of retinoblastoma, the **sporadic form**, is seen in children whose parents have no history of the disease. Once cured, these patients, as adults, do not transmit the disease to the next generation. Children with the sporadic retinoblastoma are genetically normal at fertilization, but during embryonic development two somatic mutations occur in a cell lineage, giving rise to the **cone photoreceptor precursor** of the retina. The resulting **double-mutated *Rb*** genes induce cone photoreceptor precursor cells to proliferate into a retinoblastoma.

In **familial retinoblastoma**, the fertilized egg already carries a single mutant *Rb* gene, acquired from the sperm or egg. All cells derived from the zygote carry this mutation, including the cells of the retina. The remaining normal *Rb* gene must undergo a mutation to reach the double-mutated condition required for tumor formation.

Retinoblastoma is only one of several tumors that arise through loss or inactivation of critical genes. **Wilms' tumor** of the kidney is caused by the loss of a growth-regulating gene, called *WT-1*. Similar to the *Rb* gene, both copies must be mutated before a cell begins to grow out of control.

One suppressor gene that does not fit easily into this model is *p53*, the most frequently mutated gene in human tumors (leukemias, lymphomas, brain tumors, and breast cancer, among others). The *p53* gene encodes the **p53 protein**, a tetramer that binds to a specific sequence of DNA involved in the transcriptional control of certain genes.

A mutation that affects one of the four subunits of **p53** may compromise the function of the remaining three subunits. In contrast to the mutations that affect most other suppressor genes by knocking out gene function completely, the *p53* mutations can result in either mild or aggressive growth. We discuss below details of p53 functional regulation.

In Chapter 16, Lower Digestive Segment, we study the tumor-suppressor *adenomatous polyposis coli (APC)* gene responsible for a hereditary form of colon cancer (**familial adenomatous polyposis**) derived from the malignant transformation of some of the many **polyps** (benign tumors) observed in individuals affected by this condition.

Telomerase: Aging, senescence, and cancer

Somatic cells can undergo a limited number of cell divisions, after which they enter a state of **senescence**. In contrast, tumor cells have an unlimited life span required for the formation of a tumor. In vitro studies using cultured cells have provided a model for the study of the biological clock of normal somatic cells.

The **loss of telomeres** represent a sort of molecular clock that appears to drive aging. The **telomeres** are the ends of chromosomes formed by a stretch of repeated nucleotide sequences (see Figure 1-51). Telomeres are responsible for maintaining chromosomal integrity and represent the cellular biological clock. When DNA polymerases fail to copy the chromosomal ends, telomeres decrease in size with every cell division. Cellular senescence occurs when the telomeres shorten to a point at which the integrity of a chromosome cannot be maintained.

The length of the telomeres in male and female germinal cells and hematopoietic stem cells is protected by the enzyme **telomerase**, a ribonucleoprotein with reverse transcriptase activity that uses an RNA template to maintain the length of the telomeres. Telomerase is not present in somatic cells.

Most tumor cells express high levels of telomerase. The telomerase complex (see Figure 1-51) consists of the catalytic **telomerase reverse transcriptase (TERT)**, the RNA subunit telomerase **template RNA (TR)**, which provides the template for repeat synthesis of chromosome ends, and **dyskerin (DKC1)**, an auxiliary protein. This complex is assembled in **Cajal bodies** in the nucleus and is transported to

Box 1-V | **Li-Fraumeni syndrome**

- **Li-Fraumeni syndrome (LFS)** is an autosomal dominant condition characterized by a predisposition to cancer.
- Several types of cancer develop in a young individual (younger than 45 years old): brain tumors, breast tumors (40% of the tumors in females), acute leukemia, and soft tissue and bone sarcomas.
- LFS syndrome is caused by a mutation of the tumor-suppressor gene encoding **p53**, a transcription factor with a cell cycle regulatory function.
- The incidence of LFS is low. Although the initial cancer can be successfully treated in affected children, there is a significant risk in the subsequent development of a second primary malignant tumor.

the telomeres by an accessory protein, **telomerase Cajal protein 1** (**TCAB1**). Two ATPases, **pontin** and **reptin**, activate the telomerase complex at the chromosomal end and initiate nucleotide addition.

Telomere dysfunction has been directly implicated in two diseases: **dyskeratosis congenita** and **idiopathic pulmonary fibrosis**. Dyskeratosis congenita is characterized by bone marrow failure, abnormal skin pigmentation, nail dystrophy, and leukoplakia (patches of keratosis on the tongue and the inside of the cheeks). Idiopathic pulmonary fibrosis leads to the progressive destruction of the lung tissue with a fatal outcome. Short telomeres are observed in both diseases.

Senescence appears to be triggered by more than a single mechanism. The accumulation of damage and stress in cells is the consequence of additive factors derived from shorter telomeres, reactive oxygen species and mitochondrial dysfunction. The dysfunction of the tumor suppressive retinoblastoma pathway, that we have already discussed, and the tumor suppressive p53 signaling pathway, that we are describing below, added to an unstable telomerase pathway, may push cells towards senescence or malignancy.

Clinical significance: The p53 signaling pathway

p53 is a critical transcriptional activator of numerous target genes (see Box 1-U). Its role, as a **cellular stress sensor**, is to respond to DNA damage, oxidative stress and ischemia by controlling apoptosis through transcription-dependent and transcription independent (mitochondrial dysfunction) mechanisms leading to cell cycle arrest or limit cell damage.

Autophagy, necrosis and apoptosis are three distinct forms of cell death following acute cell injury (for example, ischemia/reperfusion injury and oxidative damage occurring in cerebral stroke and myocardial infarction).

Under low levels of genotoxic stress, p53 induces the expression of antioxidants, thereby supporting cell survival. Increasing levels of DNA damage stimulate the generation of increased reactive oxygen species (ROS) levels to eliminate cells that are not fit to survive or sustain too much damage.

Loss of p53 function by mutations in p53 or by a disruption of the p53 signaling pathway is frequently associated with human cancers. This observation underscores the significant importance of p53 in tumor suppression.

As tumor suppressor, the function of p53 is controlled by sequestration and inhibition of its negative regulator, the **E3 ubiquitin ligase MDM2** (Figure 1-52). **When MDM2 is inhibited, p53 remain stable and active** to operate within the context of DNA damage or tumor suppression leading to apoptosis or cell cycle arrest. **If MDM2 is active, p53 is degraded**

and the tumor suppression effect is lost.

Mutations of the *TP53* gene, which encodes the p53 protein, are observed in 50% of human cancers. The loss of *TP53* gene expression by an autosomal dominant mutation is responsible for a multicancer phenotype known as **Li-Fraumeni syndrome** (see Box 1-V).

The inactivation of p53 tumor suppression role has important therapeutic implications in cancer patients receiving chemotherapy with a potential genotoxic effect. A negative side effect of chemotherapy is the p53-driven apoptosis in sensitive tissues (for example, stem cells in bone marrow and intestinal epithelium) thus compromising effective tumor suppressor function. Efforts are directed towards understanding the molecular mechanisms by which p53 can discriminate between acute DNA damage (**genotoxic insult**) and tumor suppression (**oncogenic signaling**). The goal is to block p53-dependent side effects of chemotherapy without the risk of compromising p53 tumor suppression function.

Pharmacologic agents binding to MDM2 could stabilize and increase the levels of p53 in cancer cells to exert a tumor-suppressor activity through its death-inducing functions.

Mitosis

Mitosis is preceded by the duplication of a pair of **centrioles** during the S phase of the cell cycle to form two centrosomes. Centrioles are embedded in proteins of the **microtubule-organizing center** (**MOC**). Each centrosome moves toward opposite sites of the nucleus.

The primary function of the centrosome is the formation and maintenance of the **mitotic spindle** consisting of microtubules. About 1000 new microtubules can be generated per minute on each centrosome using a pool of tubulin dimers derived from disassembled cytoplasmic microtubules.

Mitosis is divided into four substages: **prophase**, **metaphase**, **anaphase**, and **telophase**. The highlights of mitosis are summarized in Figure 1-53.

Basic Concepts of Medical Genetics

Medical genetics studies human biological variations related to health and disease. Figure 1-54 provides a Concept Mapping to help you integrate the relevant aspects of human development and genetics diseases described below. Box 1-W illustrates the **standard genetic symbols** used for pedigree analysis.

Genetic diseases can be caused by:

1. **Chromosomal disorders**: chromosome numerical abnormalities and chromosome structural abnormalities.

2. **Mendelian inheritance: Single gene defects**

3. **Non-mendelian inheritance: Multifactorial**

disorders, somatic cell genetics disorders, and mitochondrial disorders.

We start this section by defining basic aspects of **human development**, with particular reference to teratogens, and by describing specific aspects of **congenital disease**, **congenital malformations** and **congenital deformations**.

Human development is divided into an **embryonic period** and a **fetal period**. The embryonic period starts at fertilization and ends 10 weeks later, when the age of the embryo is 8 weeks. At this time, all the precursor organs are formed. During the embryonic period, the embryo is susceptible to birth defects caused by **teratogens** (Greek *teras*, monster; *gen*, producing), including:

1. **Alcohol** (**fetal alcohol syndrome**).

2. **Maternal infections** (rubella, toxoplasmosis, cytomegalovirus or herpes simplex virus).

3. **Radiation** (x-ray exposure or radiation therapy).

4. **Nutritional deficiencies** (such as **spina bifida**, caused by a folate deficiency).

After 8 weeks, the developing organism is called **fetus** and continues its development, completed by week 40.

A **congenital disease** is present at birth but may not be apparent after a few years (for example, an abnormality in heart development such as an atrial or ventricular septum defect).

A **congenital malformation** occurs during embryonic development and is caused by a genetic defect. Congenital malformations include:

1. **Agenesis**: an organ fails to develop.

2. **Hypoplasia** (Greek *hypo*, under; *plasis*, y molding): an organ fails to achieve complete development.

3. **Dysplasia** (Prefix Greek *dys*, difficult; *plasis*, a molding): the organization of a tissue is abnormal.

4. **Dysraphism** (*dys*; *rhaphe*, **suture**): a failure during embryonic fusion (for example, a **myelomeningocele**, known as **spina bifida**).

5. **Atresia** (Prefix Greek *a*, not; *tresis*, a hole): the lumen of an organ is not formed.

6. **Ectopia** (Greek *ektopos*, out of place): an organ or tissue failing to reach a normal location (for example, testicular maldescent or crytorchid).

7. Lack of involution by apoptosis of a temporary embryological structure (for example, persistent thyroglossal duct).

A **congenital deformation**, such as hip dislocation or clubfoot, is the result of maternal mechanical factors affecting fetal development (for example, a distorted uterus due to leiomyomas, benign tumors of the smooth muscle cell wall).

Chromosomal disorders

Chromosomal disorders can be in the **number** of individual chromosomes or **structural abnormalities** of individual chromosome.

Regarding **chromosome numerical abnormalities**:

1. Normal human somatic cells contain 46 chromosomes, the **diploid number**.

2. Normal human gamete cells, sperm and egg, contain 22 autosome chromosomes and 1 sex chromosome (X or Y in males and X in females), the **haploid number**.

3. **Polyploidy** is the condition whereby the chromosome number exceeds the diploid number and this number is an exact multiple of the haploid number. **Tetraploidy** is four times the haploid number (92 chromosomes). Tetraploid hepatocytes are observed during liver regeneration. Megakaryocytes are normally polyploid cells (they have 8-16 times the haploid number).

4. **Aneuploidy** (Greek *an*, without; *eu*, good; *ploidy*, condition) arises from non-disjunction of paired sister chromatids (during first meiotic division) or chromosomes (during second meiotic division). An aneuploidy individual has fewer or more than the normal diploid number of chromosomes. This condition is usually deleterious, in particular when it affects the number of autosomes.

A lack of an X chromosome in female cells has severe effects; but females with supernumerary X chromosomes are usually normal or nearly normal because of X chromosome inactivation, a mechanism that balances the dosage of X-linked genes with that of XY males.

Chromosome structural abnormalities are the result of chromosomal breakage observed by exposure to ionizing radiations and in inherited conditions (such as in ataxia telangiectasia and Fanconi syndrome):

1. **Translocation** is the transfer of broken chromosomal material between chromosomes.

There are three forms of translocation: **reciprocal translocation**, when there is reciprocal breaking and rejoining of any pair of chromosomes without overall gain or loss of genetic material; **centric fusion (Robertsonian translocation)**, when two acrocentric chromosomes break close or at the centromere and rejoin into a single chromosome with two centromeres (dicentric chromosome) and a fragment with no centromere (acentric) that will be lost at the subsequent cell division; and **insertional translocation**, involving three breaks in one or two chromosomes, resulting in an interstitial deletion of a segment of one chromosome, that is inserted into the gap of the other.

2. **Deletion**: a chromosomal segment breaks and is lost.

3. **Inversion**: a broken chromosome segment is reinserted in the same chromosome but in an inverted orientation.

4. **Ring chromosome**: the terminal ends of the arms of a chromosome are lost and the two proximal ends rejoin to form a closed circle.

5. **Duplications**, when an additional copy of a chromosome is present. Duplications are more frequent than deletions and less harmful.

6. **Isochromosome**: a chromosome with a deletion of one arm with a duplication of the other.

Other **chromosomal variants** are:

1. **Mosaic**: an individual with two or more cell lines derived from a single zygote. For example, in female mammalian somatic tissues, one X chromosome is active and the other is transcriptionally inactive (an indication of dosage compensation, as you know). These tissues are regarded **mosaic** (whether the maternal or paternal X chromosome is active in cells of the somatic tissues).

2. **Chimera**: an individual with two or more cell lines derived from two separate zygotes.

Mendelian inheritance: Single gene disorders

In human, there are 44 autosomes consisting of 22 homologous pairs, with genes present in pairs (one of paternal origin and the other from maternal origin) and located in a specific site, or **locus**, within each chromosome. Alternative forms of a gene are called **alleles** (Greek *allelon*, reciprocally).

If both pairs of genes are identical, the individual is **homozygous**; if different, the individual is **heterozygous**.

Any gene determines a characteristic, or **trait**. A trait expressed in the heterozygote is **dominant**, and, if only expressed in the homozygote, it is **recessive**.

Genetic diseases can be caused by defects in a **single gene** or a **group of genes**. The defects are expressed as **dominant** or **recessive** (**mendelian inheritance**). or require a coexisting environmental factor before a disease is produced (**polygenic** or **multifactorial inheritance**), with partial contribution of genetic factors.

Single gene defect disorders can be:

1. **Autosomal chromosome-linked** or **sex chromosome-linked** (mainly X chromosome-linked, affecting males devoid of **dosage compensation** as in females).

As we have seen, one of the X chromosomes in XX female cells undergoes inactivation. A structural representation of X chromosome inactivation is a condense chromatin structure at the nuclear periphery of female cells, known as **Barr body**. X chromosome inactivation silences most of the genes encoded on this chromosome, a condition called **functional unisomy**.

Unisomy is the condition of an individual or cell carrying only one member of a pair of homologous chromosomes. For example, male cells have only one X chromosome, a situation known as **genetic unisomy**.

2. **Homozygous**, when the defective gene is present on **both members** of a chromosomal pair.

3. **Heterozygous**, when the defective gene is present on only **one member** of a chromosomal pair.

The **mendelian inheritance patterns** of a single gene defect **are the following**:

1. **Autosomal dominant inheritance: expressed in heterozygotes; on the average half of offspring is affected.**

For example, f**amilial hypercholesterolemia** is caused by a single mutant gene on the short arm of chromosome 19, encoding a receptor for low density lipoprotein (LDL). Defect in the receptor results in defective clearance of circulating LDL, including cholesterol. Males and females are affected, each is a heterozygote and can transmit the condition if each has married an affected person (a normal homozygote). The expected proportion of affected individuals is 50%.

2. **Autosomal recessive inheritance: expressed in homozygotes; low risk to offspring.**

For example, **sickle cell disease** is produced by sickled-shaped red blood cells that may occlude blood vessels, causing recurrent infarctions of the lung and spleen (see Chapter 6, Blood and Hematopoiesis).

The disease results from **defective hemoglobin S (HbS)** caused by a substitution of valine for glutamic acid. The predominant hemoglobin in normal individuals is HbA. A parent with sickle cell anemia that marries to a homozygous normal person (HbA/HbA) will produce unaffected heterozygous (HbA/HbS). If

---

Box 1-W | Pedigree analysis: Highlights to remember

- The pedigree is a common tool used in medical genetics. It is constructed like a tree using standard genetic symbols to show inheritance patterns for specific phenotypic characteristics. A human pedigree starts with a family member, called the propositus, that attracts the attention of the geneticist as a means to trace back the progression of the phenotype through the family.
- The following symbols are used:

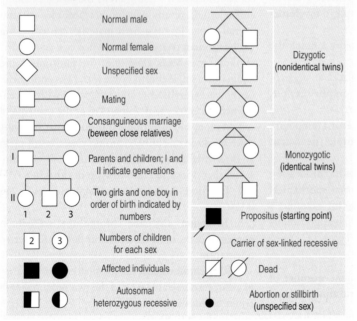

Normal male	
Normal female	
Unspecified sex	
Mating	Dizygotic (nonidentical twins)
Consanguineous marriage (beween close relatives)	
Parents and children; I and II indicate generations	Monozygotic (identical twins)
Two girls and one boy in order of birth indicated by numbers	
Numbers of children for each sex	Propositus (starting point)
Affected individuals	Carrier of sex-linked recessive
Autosomal heterozygous recessive	Dead
	Abortion or stillbirth (unspecified sex)

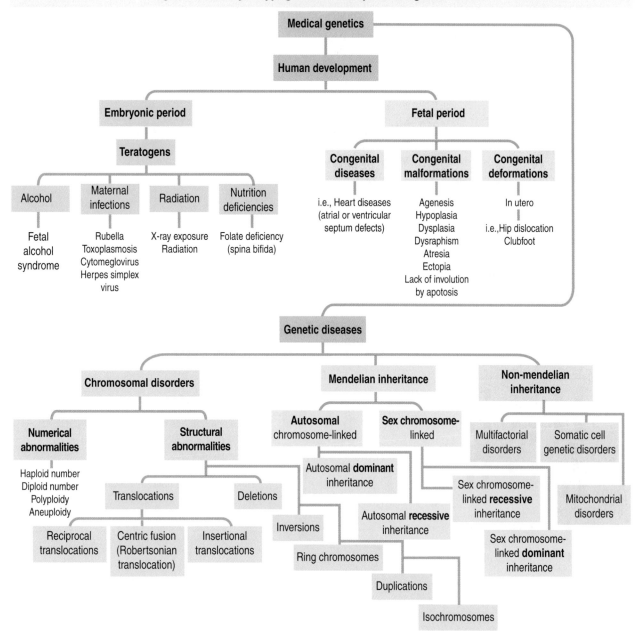

Figure 1-54. Concept Mapping: Human development and genetic diseases

a HbS/HbS individual marries a heterozygote, there is one in two chance on the average that each child may be affected. If both parents have sickle cell disease, all children will have sickle cell disease.

3. **Sex-linked recessive inheritance.** Male-to-female X chromosome trait transmission will result in all daughter carriers (female-to-female transmission, 50% of the daughters are carriers). There is no male-to-male transmission of a gene defect.

An example is **muscular dystrophy** (**Duchenne muscular dystrophy**), a condition that causes progressive muscular weakness with significant elevation of creatine kinase and other muscle enzymes in blood. Heterozygous females are carriers (clinically unaffected) but transmit the condition. When a carrier

female that marries a normal male, one-half of the daughters will be carriers and one-half of the sons will be affected.

4. **Sex-linked dominant inheritance.** X chromosome disorders are observed in the heterozygous female and in the heterozygous male (with a mutant allele on his single X chromosome). An affected male transmits the trait to all his daughters but none of his sons. Direct male-to male transmission cannot take place.

Vitamin D-resistant rickets (even the dietary intake of vitamin D is normal) and the X-linked form of Charcot-Marie-Tooth disease (hereditary motor and sensory neuropathy) are X chromosome-linked dominant conditions.

Figure 1-55. **Nomenclature of human chromosomes and abnormal karyotype**

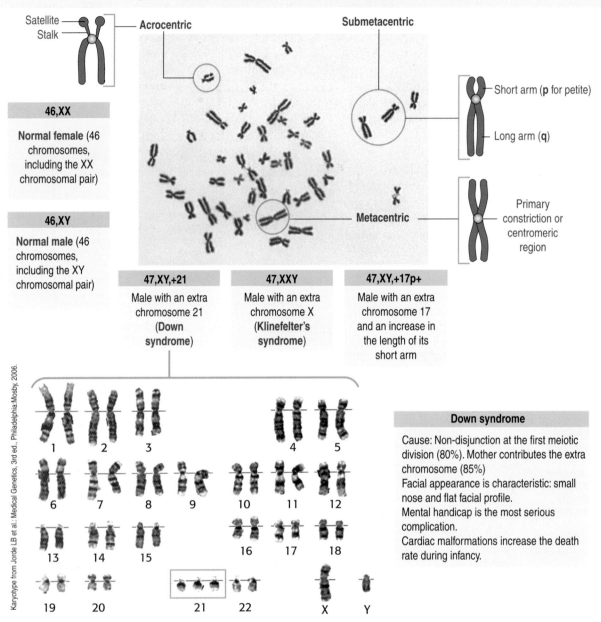

Karyotype from Jorde LB et al.: Medical Genetics, 3rd ed., Philadelphia:Mosby, 2006.

46,XX

Normal female (46 chromosomes, including the XX chromosomal pair)

46,XY

Normal male (46 chromosomes, including the XY chromosomal pair)

Acrocentric

Submetacentric

Short arm (**p** for petite)

Long arm (**q**)

Metacentric

Primary constriction or centromeric region

47,XY,+21

Male with an extra chromosome 21 (**Down syndrome**)

47,XXY

Male with an extra chromosome X (**Klinefelter's syndrome**)

47,XY,+17p+

Male with an extra chromosome 17 and an increase in the length of its short arm

Down syndrome

Cause: Non-disjunction at the first meiotic division (80%). Mother contributes the extra chromosome (85%)
Facial appearance is characteristic: small nose and flat facial profile.
Mental handicap is the most serious complication.
Cardiac malformations increase the death rate during infancy.

Similarly, in Y chromosome-linked dominant inheritance, only males are affected when the male transmits a Y-linked trait.

Non-mendelian Inheritance

Polygenic diseases arise from the participation of dispersed genes, each contributing to the characteristics of the disease lacking a distinct phenotype.

Multifactorial disorders arise on a conditioning genetic background (predisposition to a disease) that will only occur when triggering environmental factors are present.

Multifactorial traits may be **discontinuous** (distinct phenotypes) or **continuous** (a lack of distinct phenotypes). Cleft lip and palate, congenital heart disease, neural tube defect and pyloric stenosis are

congenital malformation inherited as a discontinuous multifactorial traits. Examples of continuous multifactorial traits are height, weight, skin color, and blood pressure..

In contrast to mendelian inheritance disorders, pedigree analysis is not applicable and **twin concordance** and family correlations studies are required.

Twins may be genetically identical (**monozygotic**) or non-identical (**dizygotic**). Monozygotic twins arise from a single zygote which splits into two embryos. Dizygotic twins result from two eggs each fertilized by a sperm, have two amniotic sacs and two placentas, each with separate circulation. Most monozygotic twins have a single placenta with common blood circulation.

Twins are **concordant** if they show a discontinuous trait (such as height) and **discordant** if only one shows the trait. Monozygotic twins have identical genotypes; dizygotic twins are like siblings (brothers and sisters). If there is a chromosomal disorder or a specific single gene trait, the monozygotic concordance rate will be 100%. For discontinuous multifactorial traits of genetic and environmental nature, the monozygotic concordance rate will be less than 100% but higher than in the dizygotic twins. This range tells us about the increasing importance of the genetic contribution and heritability to a chromosomal disorder or a specific single gene trait when monozygotic concordance is higher.

Relatives share a proportion of their genes and family correlations studies can provide support for multifactorial inheritance of a trait.

Most cancers are regarded as **somatic cell genetic disorders**. Some familial cancers have germline mutations; others display somatic cell mutations leading to malignancy. A mutation in a fertilized egg that occurs after the first cell division, may affect the gonadal cells (gonadal mosaic) or the somatic cells (somatic mosaic).

Mitochondrial disorders caused by mutations in DNA mitochondrial are transmitted to all children of an affected mother but not to the offspring of an affected father. We discuss further the patterns of maternal inheritance of mitochondrial disorders in Chapter 2, Epithelial Glands.

Karyotyping (chromosome analysis)

Cytogenetics is the analysis of the structure of normal and abnormal chromosomes (Greek *chromos*, colored; *soma*, body).

A **karyotype** (or **chromosome analysis**) is a description of the number and structure of the chromosomes. A standard karyotype is based on the use of metaphase cells from any population of dividing cells (Figure 1-55). Lymphocytes in peripheral blood are the most frequently used cells, but bone marrow cells, cultured fibroblasts or cells from amniotic fluid or chorionic villi can also be used.

Cells are cultured in the presence of a mitogen (for example, phytohemagglutinin) for 3-4 days and treated with colcemid to disrupt mitotic spindles to enrich the sample in metaphase cells. Cells are collected and treated with an hypotonic solution to swell the cells and disperse chromosomes on a microscope before fixation and staining. **Giemsa staining** is generally used to produce **G-banding**, alternate light and dark band patterns characteristic for each chromosome pair.

There are **22 pairs of autosomes** and **one pair of sex chromosomes (XX or XY) in the human**. Chromosomes can be classified according to the length and position of the centromere.

In the notation of human cytogenetics, the total number of chromosomes (46) is followed by the total number of sex chromosomes (see Figure 1-55). A **normal male** is identified as **46,XY** (46 chromosomes, including the XY chromosomal pair) and a female as **46,XX** (46 chromosomes, including the XX chromosomal pair).

Extra autosomes are indicated by placing the number of the extra chromosomes after the sex chromosomes with a plus (+) sign. 47,XY+21 is the karyotype of a male with trisomy 21 (Down syndrome, see Figure 1-55).

A male with an extra X chromosome is symbolized as **47,XXY**. A plus or minus sign is placed following a chromosome symbol to indicate the increase or decrease in arm length. The letter **p** symbolizes the **short arm** and **q** the **long arm**. **47,XY,+17p+ identifies a male with 47 chromosomes, including an additional chromosome 17, with an increase in the length of its short arm.**

Essential concepts	**Epithelium**

• Epithelium is one of the four basic tissues. The three additional basic tissues are connective tissue, muscle tissue, and nervous tissue.

Epithelia can be classified into three major groups based on:

(1) The number of cell layers (one layer: simple epithelium; more than one layer: stratified epithelium).

(2) The shape of the cells (squamous epithelium, cuboidal epithelium, and columnar epithelium).

(3) The shape of the cells at the outermost layer (stratified squamous epithelium, stratified cuboidal epithelium, and stratified columnar epithelium).

The stratified squamous epithelium can be subdivided into moderately keratinized (usually called nonkeratinized) and highly keratinized

types. The name endothelium identifies the simple squamous epithelium lining blood and lymphatic vessels. The name mesothelium is used to describe the simple squamous or cuboidal lining of serosa (peritoneum, pleura, and pericardium). Tumors originating in the mesothelium are called **mesotheliomas**.

• An important cytoskeletal component of epithelial cells are keratin proteins (cytokeratins). The pathologist looks for the presence of keratins to determine the epithelial origin of a tumor (called **carcinoma**, in contrast to connective tissue–derived tumors called **sarcomas**).

• An intermediate type is the pseudostratified epithelium, in which all the cells are in contact

with the basal lamina, but not all of them reach the lumen. The transitional epithelium, or urothelium, lining the urinary passages, can be regarded as a pseudostratified epithelium, although it has the appearance of a stratified squamous epithelium. The outermost cells of the urothelium of the urinary bladder have the property of changing their geometry and surface configuration in response to tensional forces exerted by urine.

• A refinement in the classification of selected epithelia relies on apical differentiations, such as cilia, microvilli, and stereocilia. A pseudostratified epithelium with cilia is seen along the respiratory tract and the oviduct. Simple cuboidal epithelium of specific segments of the nephron and the simple columnar epithelium of the small intestine contain microvilli forming a brush border along the apical domain. Stereocilia are seen in the epithelial lining of the epididymis and hair cells of the inner ear.

Epithelial cells organize layers of cells that are closely linked by specialized plasma membrane–associated structures, such as tight junctions, anchoring junctions (belt and spot desmosomes and hemidesmosomes), and gap junctions.

• Epithelial cells are highly polarized. They have an apical domain and a basolateral domain. The boundaries of the domains are defined by the distribution of junctions and their components, the polarized distribution of the actin cytoskeleton, and the presence of a basement membrane at the basal surface.

• The apical domain of some epithelial cells displays differentiations projecting into the lumen. The apical differentiations can be motile (multiple cilia) and nonmotile (primary cilium, microvilli and stereocilia/stereovilli).

There are multiple motile cilia, that coordinate fluid or cargo flow on the surface of an epithelium and a single or primary non-motile cilium, a mechanosensor that houses components of the hedgehog signaling system.

Cilia contain an axoneme, formed by a concentric array of nine microtubule doublets surrounding a central pair. Cilia originate from a basal body precursor—a centrosome derivative—inserted in the apical plasma membrane.

In contrast to the axoneme, the basal body and the centriole are formed by nine microtubule triplets in a helicoid arrangement. There are no central microtubules in basal bodies and centrioles. The nonmotile microvilli and stereocilia contain an actin microfilament core. Microvilli have a uniform length. Stereocilia are longer, their length is variable, and, in the epididymal epithelium, they have a tendency to branch.

• The position and stability of the epithelial

cell layer are maintained by cell adhesion molecules and cell junctions.

• Cell adhesion molecules can be classified as:
(1) Ca²⁺-dependent.
(2) Ca²⁺-independent.

Cadherins and selectins are Ca²⁺-dependent. Cell adhesion molecules (CAMs) of the immunoglobulin-like family and integrins are Ca²⁺-independent. In contrast to cadherins, selectins, and CAMs, integrins consist of two subunits, α and β, forming a heterodimer.

Cadherins constitute homophilic cis-homodimers (like-to-like), which interact through the extracellular domain with similar or different dimers present in the adjacent epithelial cell (forming trans-homodimers or trans-heterodimers [like to unlike]). The intracellular domain of cadherins interacts with the catenin complex consisting of catenins α and β and p120. The catenin complex interacts with filamentous actin through adapter proteins (α-actinin, formin-1, and vinculin).

Selectins bind carbohydrate ligands through their carbohydrate recognition domain. Selectins play an important role in homing, the transendothelial migration of neutrophils, lymphocytes, and macrophages during inflammation and the deposit of fatty streaks in the subendothelial space of blood vessels during early atherosclerotic lesions.

The extracellular immunoglobulin-like domain of CAMs binds to identical (homotypic binding) or different molecules (heterotypic binding) on another adjacent cell. The CAM CD4 is the receptor of HIV-1 in T cells (helper cells).

Integrins are heterodimers formed by two associated subunits, α and β. The extracellular domain of the integrin subunit β binds to laminin and fibronectin, two components of the basal lamina. Proteoglycans and collagens bind to laminin and fibronectin to form the reticular lamina. The intracellular domain of integrin subunit β binds to filamentous actin through the adapter proteins, including α-actinin, vinculin, kindlin, and talin. Integrins establish a

link between the extracellular matrix and the internal cytoskeleton.

• The basement membrane is a PAS-positive (periodic acid-Schiff staining) structure present at the basal domain of epithelial cells. It consists of a basal lamina and a reticular lamina, which can be defined by electron microscopy. The pathologist looks for the integrity of the basal lamina to determine if growing malignant epithelial cells are restricted to the epithelial layer (carcinoma in situ) or have invaded the underlying connective tissue where blood and lymphatic vessels are present.

• Related to the function of integrins are the ADAM proteins. The disintegrin domain of selected ADAMs can block integrin-binding affinities. The metalloprotease domain of ADAMs can participate in the shedding of the extracellular domain of plasma membrane–anchored growth factors, cytokines, and receptors. ADAMs have roles in angiogenesis, apoptosis, neurogenesis, and cancer.

• Cell junctions not only maintain the mechanical integrity of the epithelium but also can function as signaling structures reporting cell position and are able to modulate cell growth or programmed cell death (apoptosis). Intercellular junctions can be:
(1) Symmetrical, such as tight junctions, belt desmosomes (zonula adherens), spot desmosomes (macula adherens) and gap junctions.
(2) Asymmetrical, such as hemidesmosomes.

• Tight junctions consist of two transmembrane proteins—the tetraspanins occludin and claudin—and two immunoglobulin-like proteins—junctional adhesion molecules (JAMs) and nectins. Nectins are associated to the protein afadin forming the afadin-nectin complex. JAMs and nectins form dimers (called cis-dimers) and dimers inserted in the opposing plasma membrane interact with

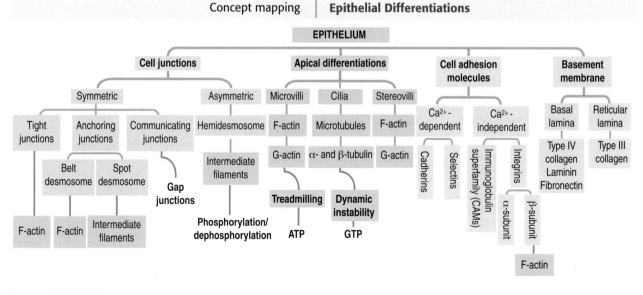

Concept mapping | **Epithelial Differentiations**

each other (*trans*-dimers).

The adapter proteins zonula occludens ZO-1, ZO-2, and ZO-3 link occludin, claudins, JAMs, and the afadin-nectin complex to actin microfilaments. Claudins constitute the backbone of tight junction strands visualized on freeze-fracture electron micrographs.

Tight junctions constitute a circumferential fence separating the apical domain from the basolateral domain. Materials can cross epithelial and endothelial cellular sheets by two distinct pathways: the transcellular pathway and the paracellular pathway. Tight junctions regulate the paracellular transport of ions and molecules in a charge-dependent and size-dependent fashion.

Similar to tight junctions, **zonula adherens (belt desmosome)** also have a circumferential distribution and interact with filamentous actin. A distinctive feature is the presence of a plaque containing desmoplakin, plakoglobins and plakophilins. Cadherins (desmocollins and desmogleins) and the afadin-nectin complex link the plasma membranes of adjacent epithelial cells. The intracellular region of cadherins interacts with actin through the catenin complex.

Macula adherens (spot desmosome) provides strength and rigidity to the epithelial cell layer, particularly in the stratified squamous epithelium, and links adjacent cardiocytes (fascia adherens and desmosome) as a component of the intercalated disk. In contrast to the belt desmosome, spot desmosomes are spotlike. The plaque—which contains desmoplakin, plakoglobins, and plakophilins—is the insertion site of intermediate filament keratins (called tonofilaments) or desmin (intercalated disk). The intermediate filament-binding protein in the plaque is desmoplakin. The catenin complex is not present. Desmocollins and desmogleins are the predominant cadherins.

Hemidesmosomes are asymmetrical anchoring junctions found at the basal region of epithelial cells. Hemidesmosomes consist of two components: an inner plate, associated to intermediate filaments, and an outer plaque anchoring the hemidesmosome to the basal lamina by anchoring filaments (laminin 5).

Gap junctions are symmetrical communicating junctions (instead of anchoring junctions). Gap junctions consist of clusters of intercellular channels connecting the cytoplasm of adjacent cells. There are more than 20 connexin monomers, each identified by the assigned molecular mass. Six connexin monomers form a connexon inserted into the plasma membrane. Connexons pair with their counterparts in the plasma membrane of an adjacent cell and form an axial intercellular channel allowing the cell-to-cell diffusion of ions and small molecules. A mutation in *connexin32* (*Cx32*) gene in the myelin-producing Schwann cell is the cause of the X-chromosome–linked **Charcot-Marie-Tooth disease**, a demyelinating disorder of the peripheral nervous system.

• The **basement membrane** consists of two components:

(1) A basal lamina, in direct contact with the epithelial basal cell surface.

(2) A reticular lamina, formed by fibronectin and collagen fibers and continuous with the connective tissue.

The basal lamina consists of laminin, type IV collagen, entactin, and proteoglycans. The basal lamina is an important component of the glomerular filtration barrier in the kidneys. A basal lamina covers the surface of muscle cells and contributes to maintaining the integrity of the skeletal muscle fiber during contraction. A disruption of the basal lamina–cell muscle relationship gives rise to **muscular dystrophies**. The basement membrane can be recognized by light microscopy by the PAS stain.

• The **cytoskeleton** consists of:

(1) Microfilaments (7 nm thick).

(2) Microtubules (25 nm in diameter).

(3) Intermediate filaments (10 nm in diameter).

The basic unit of a **microfilaments** is the G-actin monomer. The ATP-dependent polymerization of monomers forms a 7-nm-thick F-actin filament. Monomers added on the barbed end of the filament move, or treadmill, along the filament until they detach by depolymerization at the pointed end.

Motor proteins, such as myosin Va, transport vesicle cargos along F-actin. Defective myosin Va is the cause of **Griscelli syndrome**, a disorder in the transport of melanosomes from melanocytes to keratinocytes in the epidermis. Patients with Griscelli syndrome have silvery hair, partial albinism, occasional neurologic defects, and immunodeficiency.

F-actin associated with myosin II forms the contractile structures of skeletal and cardiac muscle cells. They represent the myofilament components of myofibrils. Myofibrils, consisting of a linear chain of sarcomeres, are the basic contractile unit found in the cytoplasm of striated muscle cells.

Microtubules are composed of α and β tubulin dimers. Tubulin dimers arranged longitudinally form protofilaments. Thirteen protofilaments associate side-by-side with each other to form a microtubule. Microtubules undergo alternate phases of slow growth and rapid depolymerization, a process called dynamic instability. The polymerization of tubulin subunits is GTP-dependent.

The **centrosome** consists of a pair of centrioles surrounded by a pericentriolar protein matrix. Each centriole consists of nine triplets of microtubules arranged in a helicoid manner. Centrioles duplicate during the cell cycle in preparation for the assembly of the mitotic spindle during cell division. A basal body precursor is produced inside the centrosome, multiplies, differentiates into basal a basal body and docks to the plasma membrane to develop a cilium.

The **mitotic apparatus** consists of two opposite mitotic centers bridged by the mitotic spindle. Each mitotic center is represented by the centrosome (a pair of centrioles embedded in a protein matrix, the microtubular organizing center, MOC) and radiating

microtubules. The mitotic spindle consists of kinetochore microtubules and polar microtubules. Kinetochore microtubules attach to the kinetochore, a cluster of proteins associated with the centromere, the primary constriction of a chromosome. Centrosome and centromere sound alike words but they represent two different structures.

Microtubules are a target of **cancer chemotherapy** with the purpose of blocking cell division of tumor cells by destabilizing or stabilizing dynamic instability. Derivatives of *Vinca* alkaloids and taxol have been widely used.

The **axoneme** consists of nine microtubule doublets in a concentric array, surrounding a central pair of microtubules. Each doublet consists of a tubule A, formed by 13 protofilaments and closely attached to tubule B, formed by 10 to 11 protofilaments. Axonemes are present in cilia and flagella of the sperm tail. Dynein arms, an ATPase, are linked to tubule A. ATPase hydrolyzes ATP to use energy for the sliding of microtubules, the basis for ciliary and flagellar movement.

Microtubules provide tracks for motor protein transporting vesicle and nonvesicle cargos within the cell. Molecular motors, such as kinesin and cytoplasmic dynein, mediate the transport of cargos.

There are three specific microtubule-based transport systems:

(1) Axonemal transport, which includes intraciliary and intraflagellar transport.

(2) Axonal transport.

(3) Intramanchette transport. Manchette is a transient microtubular structure involved in sperm development.

Bardet-Biedl syndrome, a disorder of basal bodies and cilia resulting from defective intraciliary transport, is characterized by retinal dystrophy, obesity, polydactyly, renal dysplasia, reproductive tract abnormalities, and learning disabilities.

Kartagener's syndrome, characterized by defective or absent dynein arms, is associated with bronchiectasis and infertility (reduced sperm motility and egg transport in the oviduct).

Intermediate filaments are formed by monomers displaying a central coiled-coil flanked by globular regions. A pair of monomers form a parallel dimer. A tetramer is assembled by two antiparallel half staggered dimers. Eight tetramers associate side-by-side to form a unit length filament (ULF). ULFs join end-to-end and continue extending longitudinally by adding ULFs to form 10 nm-thick intermediate filaments.

In contrast to F-actin and microtubules, the assembly of intermediate filaments is regulated by phosphorylation-dephosphorylation.

There are several types of intermediate filaments, including:

(1) Type I and Type II keratins (markers of epithelial cells).

(2) Type III: Vimentin (present in mesenchymal-derived cells), desmin (abundant in muscle cells), and glial fribrillary acidic protein (a marker of glial cells).

(3) Type IV: Neurofilaments (found in neurons).

(4) Type V: Lamins (forming the nuclear lamina associated to the inner layer of the nuclear envelope).

Disorders of keratins cause **blistering diseases** of the skin. Defective gene expression of lamins causes a group of diseases called **laminopathies** affecting muscle tissue (e.g., **Emery-Dreifuss muscular dystrophy**), nervous tissue (e.g., **Charcot-Marie-Tooth disease type 2B1**), and adipose tissue (e.g., **Dunnigan-type familial lipodystrophy**).

• The **cell nucleus** consists of the nuclear envelope, chromatin, and the nucleolus. The nuclear envelope has nuclear pores, a tripartite structure consisting of inner and outer octagonal rings and a central cylindrical body. Nuclear pores contain several proteins called nucleoporins. Ran-GTPase regulates nucleo-cytoplasmic transport across nuclear pores by enabling the passage of proteins with a nuclear import sequence bound to a protein complex of importins α and β and Ran-GDP. In the nucleus, Ran-GDP is converted to Ran-GTP by RCCI, a GDP-GTP exchanger and the importin-imported protein complex is dissociated. Ran-GTP associates with exportins, and proteins with a nuclear export sequence are transported to the cytoplasm. Ran-GTP interacts with Ran-GBP1, and is converted to Ran-GDP by hydrolysis stimulated by Ran-GAP. The cargo is discharged, and Ran-GDP is ready to initiate another transport cycle.

Two forms of **chromatin** exist: heterochromatin (transcriptionally inactive) and euchromatin (transcriptionally active). One of the two X chromosomes in every female somatic cell remains condensed, a process known as dosage compensation. The condensed X chromosome can be visualized as a mass of heterochromatin adjacent to the nuclear envelope (called **Barr body**) and in the form of a drumstick in polymorphonuclear leukocytes.

The **nucleolus** consists of a fibrillar center (chromatin containing repeat rRNA genes, RNA polymerase I, and SRP); a dense fibrillar component (containing the proteins fibrillarin and nucleolin); and a granular component (the assembly sites of ribosomal subunits).

• Staining techniques and autoradiography can determine the localization of nucleic acids in cells. The **Feulgen reaction** detects DNA. **Basic dyes** can localize DNA and RNA. RNAse and DNAse cell pretreatment can define the identity of the basophilic staining. Autoradiography is based on the administration of a radiolabeled precursor to living cells. Radioactive sites can be traced using a photographic emulsion, which after developing and fixation, produces silver grain in sites where the radiolabeled precursor is localized. This procedure enables the study of the cell cycle and the detection of sites involved in protein synthesis, glycosylation, and transport. Fluorescence-activated cell sorting enables the identification and separation of cell types using cell surface markers, and the study of the cell cycle based on the content of DNA.

• **Cell cycle** is defined as the interval between two successive cell divisions resulting in the production of two daughter cells. Traditionally, the cell cycle consists of two major phases:

(1) Interphase.

(2) Mitosis.

Interphase includes the S phase (DNA synthesis), preceded by the G1 phase and followed by the G2 phase. The phases of mitosis are:

(1) Prophase: the centrosomes organize the mitotic spindle; lamins phosphorylate and the nuclear envelope breaks down; each chromosome consists of sister chromatids held together at the centromere; the protein cohesin holds together the noncentromeric regions; condensin compacts the chromatin.

(2) Metaphase: kinetochore microtubules attach to the kinetochore present in each chromosome; chromosomes align at the equatorial plate; the anaphase-promoting complex disassembles if the attachment of the kinetochore microtubules is correct.

(3) Anaphase: topoisomerase frees entangled chromatin fibers; chromatids separate from each other and move closer to their respective poles—anaphase A—and cell poles separated by the action of polar microtubules—anaphase B.

(4) Telophase: lamins dephosphorylate and the nuclear envelope reassembles; chromosomes decondense; a contractile ring (actin-myosin) develops during cytokinesis; microtubules of the spindle disappear.

In a more contemporary view, the cell cycle consists of three distinct cycles:

(1) Cytoplasmic cycle (sequential activation of cyclin-dependent protein kinases.

(2) Nuclear cycle (DNA replication and chromosome condensation).

(3) Centrosome cycle (duplication of the two centrioles—mother and daughter centrioles—in preparation for assembly of the mitotic apparatus).

• Cyclin-dependent protein kinases control the progression and completion of the cell cycle. Tumor-suppressor proteins control cell cycle progression. Dephosphorylated Rb protein, a tumor-suppressor, binds to transcription factors and represses gene activity. Transcription factors dissociate from phosphorylated Rb protein and stimulate cell cycle progression. **Retinoblastoma**, a malignant tumor of the eye, is observed when the *Rb* gene is mutated.

Another tumor-suppressor protein is p53, a transcription factor with a cell cycle regulatory function. Mutations of the *p53* gene are seen in patients with leukemias, lymphomas, and brain tumors. **p53 has a protective cell function**: it can induce apoptosis or arrest the cell cycle when the cell undergoes harmful stress (called **genotoxic stress**). Mutations of the *p53* gene prevent this protective function.

Li-Fraumeni syndrome is caused by a mutation of the *p53* gene. Young patients have a predisposition to cancer (e.g., brain tumors, breast tumors, acute leukemia, and soft tissue and bone sarcomas).

• Breakdown of the nuclear envelope occurs at the end of prophase. It involves the fragmentation of the nuclear envelope, dissociation of nuclear pore complexes, and phosphorylation of lamins (depolymerization). Reassembly of the nuclear envelope involves the dephosphorylation of lamins by a protein phosphatase.

Telomeres at the end regions of chromosomes are formed by a stretch of repeated nucleotide sequences. When DNA polymerase fails to copy the chromosomal ends, telomeres decrease in length with every cell division until the integrity of the chromosome cannot be maintained. Male and female germinal cells can protect the telomeres by the enzyme telomerase, which is not present in somatic cells. Most tumor cells express telomerase.

• **Genetic diseases** can be caused by:

(1) Chromosomal disorders (numerical [polyploidy, tetraploidy and aneuploidy] and structural [translocation, deletion, inversion, ring chromosome, duplication and isochromosome] abnormalities).

(2) Mendelian inheritance (autosomal or sex chromosome-linked dominant and recessive single gene defects that can be homozygous or heterozygous).

(3) Non-mendelian inheritance (including multifactorial disorders [discontinuous or continuous], somatic cell genetic disorders [cancer] and mitochondrial disorders [determined by mutations in mitochondrial DNA transmitted to all children of an affected mother but not to the offspring of an affected father]).

Human development is divided into an embryonic period (from fertilization to the 8-week embryo) and a fetal period (after week 8 to week 40). Birth defects caused by teratogens predominate during the embryonic period. Teratogens include alcohol (fetal alcohol syndrome), maternal infections, exposure to radiations, nutritional deficiencies (spina bifida caused by a folate deficiency).

Congenital diseases are present at birth but not fully apparent after a few years. Congenital malformations (including agenesis, hypoplasia, dysplasia, dysraphism, atresia, ectopia and lack of involution by apoptosis) take place during embryonic development and are caused by genetic defects. Congenital deformations occur in utero by mechanical factors.

Karyotyping is the structural and numerical analysis of metaphase chromosomes. A normal male has a chromosomal complement 46,XY (46 chromosomes, including the XY chromosomal pair). A normal female has 46,XX (46 chromosomes, including the XX chromosomal pair). Depending on the position of the centromere or primary constriction, chromosomes are classified as metacentric, submetacentric, and acrocentric.

2. Epithelial Glands

There are two types of epithelial glands: exocrine glands and endocrine glands. Exocrine glands secrete their product onto body surfaces through a duct; endocrine glands are ductless and secrete their products, hormones, into the interstitial spaces before entering the blood circulation. Exocrine glands are classified as simple and branched or compound glands. Secretory cells of exocrine glands discharge their products in three different mechanisms: a merocrine mechanism, utilizing membrane-bound secretory vesicles; an apocrine mechanism, by releasing a secretory product surrounded by a rim of cytosol; and a holocrine mechanism, involving the release of a disintegrating cell that becomes the secretory product. This chapter integrates the structure and function of exocrine glands with basic concepts of cell and molecular biology.

Development of epithelial glands

Most glands develop as epithelial outgrowths into the underlying connective tissue (Figure 2-1). **Exocrine glands** remain connected to the surface of the epithelium by an excretory duct that transports the secretory product to the outside. **Endocrine glands lack an excretory duct**, and their product is released into the blood circulation.

Endocrine glands are surrounded by fenestrated capillaries and commonly store the secretions they synthesize and release after stimulation by chemical or electrical signals. Exocrine and endocrine glands can be found together (for example, in the pancreas), as separate structures in endocrine organs (thyroid and parathyroid glands), or as single cells (enteroendocrine cells). Endocrine glands will be studied later in Chapter 18, Neuroendocrine System, and Chapter 19, Endocrine System.

Classification of epithelial glands

Glands are classified according to the type of **excretory duct** into **simple** and **branched** (also called **compound**) glands. The gland can be **simple** (Figure 2-2) when the excretory duct is unbranched. The gland can be **branched** when the excretory duct subdivides (Figure 2-3).

Secretory portion: Unicellular and multicellular

An **exocrine gland** has two components: a **secretory portion** and an **excretory duct**. The **secretory portion** of a gland may be composed of one cell type (**unicellular**, for example, **goblet cells** in the respiratory epithelium and intestine) or many cells (**multicellular**).

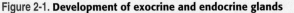

Figure 2-1. Development of exocrine and endocrine glands

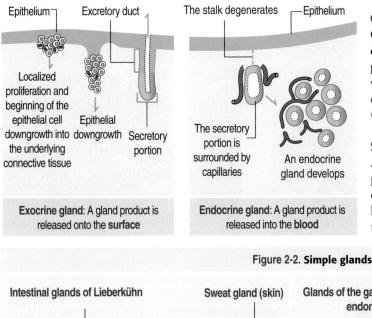

Exocrine gland: A gland product is released onto the **surface**

Endocrine gland: A gland product is released into the **blood**

Figure 2-2. Simple glands

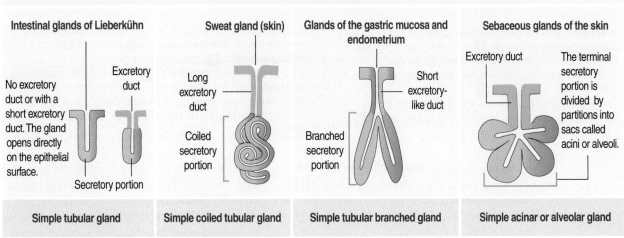

Intestinal glands of Lieberkühn

No excretory duct or with a short excretory duct. The gland opens directly on the epithelial surface.

Excretory duct

Secretory portion

Simple tubular gland

Sweat gland (skin)

Long excretory duct

Coiled secretory portion

Simple coiled tubular gland

Glands of the gastric mucosa and endometrium

Short excretory-like duct

Branched secretory portion

Simple tubular branched gland

Sebaceous glands of the skin

Excretory duct

The terminal secretory portion is divided by partitions into sacs called acini or alveoli.

Simple acinar or alveolar gland

Figure 2-3. Glands with branched ducts

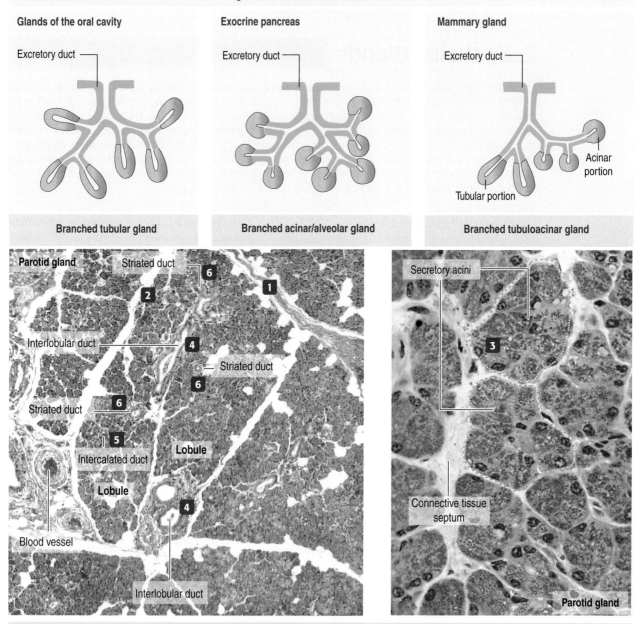

Glands of the oral cavity

Excretory duct

Branched tubular gland

Exocrine pancreas

Excretory duct

Branched acinar/alveolar gland

Mammary gland

Excretory duct

Acinar portion

Tubular portion

Branched tubuloacinar gland

Parotid gland

Striated duct — 6

2

1

Interlobular duct — 4

Striated duct
6

Striated duct — 6

5

Intercalated duct

Lobule

Lobule

4

Blood vessel

Interlobular duct

Secretory acini

3

Connective tissue septum

Parotid gland

General organization of a branched (compound) gland

A **branched gland** is surrounded by a connective tissue capsule that sends partitions or **septa** 1 inside the gland to organize large units called **lobes** (interlobar septa; not shown).

Lobes are subdivided by connective tissue **interlobular septa** into small subunits called **lobules** 2.

A branched gland consists of a varying number of secretory units classified according to their morphology as **tubular**, **acinar** 3, or **tubuloacinar**. The secretion drains into excretory ducts located between lobules (**interlobular ducts** 4). Within a lobule, **intercalated ducts** 5, smaller than the diameter of an acinus, connect acini with **striated ducts** (6). Striated ducts, present only in salivary glands but not in pancreas, drain into **interlobular ducts**. **Interlobular ducts** converge to form **lobar ducts** (not shown). See Figure 2-4, and Chapter 17, Digestive Glands, for additional information.

According to the **shape** of the secretory portion (see Figures 2-2 and 2-3), glands can be **tubular**, **coiled**, or **alveolar** (Latin *alveolus*, small hollow sac; plural *alveoli*), also called **acinar** (Latin *acinus*, grape; plural *acini*).

Simple tubular glands are found in the small and large intestine. The sweat glands of the skin are typical coiled glands. The sebaceous gland of the skin is an example of an alveolar gland. The gastric mucosa and endometrium have branched **secretory units**.

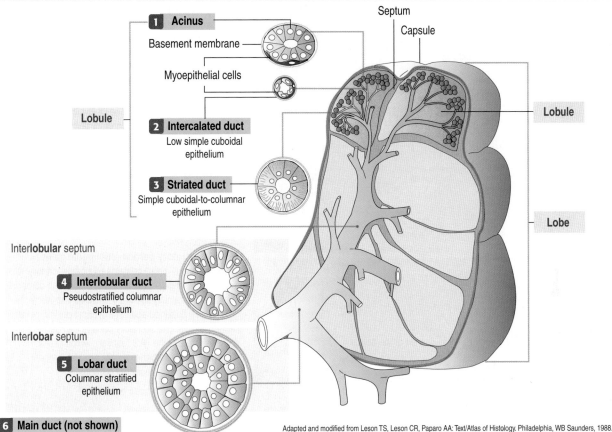

Figure 2-4. Histologic overview of a compound salivary gland

1 Acinus
- Basement membrane
- Myoepithelial cells

2 Intercalated duct
Low simple cuboidal epithelium

3 Striated duct
Simple cuboidal-to-columnar epithelium

Lobule

Interlobular septum

4 Interlobular duct
Pseudostratified columnar epithelium

Interlobar septum

5 Lobar duct
Columnar stratified epithelium

6 Main duct (not shown)

Septum
Capsule
Lobule
Lobe

Adapted and modified from Leson TS, Leson CR, Paparo AA: Text/Atlas of Histology. Philadelphia, WB Saunders, 1988.

All **branched exocrine glands** contain epithelial components (secretory acini and ducts) called **parenchyma**, and supporting connective tissue, including blood and lymphatic vessels and nerves, called the **stroma**.

The gland is enclosed by a connective tissue **capsule** that branches inside the gland forming **septa** (singular *septum*) that subdivide the **parenchyma**.

In large branched glands, the parenchyma is anatomically subdivided into **lobes**. Adjacent lobes are separated by **interlobar septa**. A lobe is formed by **lobules**, separated from each other by a thin **interlobular septa**.

Septa support the major branches of the **excretory duct, blood and lymphatic vessels**, and **nerves**. **Interlobular ducts** extend along **interlobular septa**; lobar ducts extend along **interlobar septa**. Intercalated and striated ducts lie within lobules and are surrounded by little connective tissue.

Intercalated and **striated ducts** are lined by a **simple cuboidal-to-simple columnar epithelium**, whereas the epithelial lining of **interlobular ducts** is pseudostratified columnar. **Lobar ducts** are lined by a **stratified columnar epithelium**.

Shape of the secretory portion

Glands can be classified as **simple tubular** or **simple alveolar** (or acinar) according to the **shape of the secretory portion**. In addition, tubular and alveolar secretory portions can coexist with branching excretory ducts; the gland is called **a branched (or compound) tubulo-alveolar** (or acinar) gland (for example, the salivary glands). The mammary gland is an example of a branched alveolar gland.

A branched gland (Figure 2-4) is surrounded by a connective tissue **capsule**. **Septa** or **trabeculae** extend from the capsule into the glandular tissue. Large **interlobar septa** divide the gland into a number of **lobes**. Branches from the interlobar septa, **interlobular septa**, subdivide the lobes into smaller compartments called **lobules**.

During development, a main excretory duct gives rise to branches that lie between lobes, inside the **interlobar** septa. Small branches derived from each of these ducts generate small subdivisions. These branches can be found first between lobules (in **interlobular septa**) and within lobules (**intercalated and striated ducts**). Additional details are presented in Chapter 17, Digestive Glands.

Types of secretion

Based on the type of secretion, exocrine glands can be classified as **mucous glands**, when their products are rich in **glycoproteins** and water; **serous glands**, with secretions enriched with **proteins** and water; and **mixed glands**, which contain both mucous and serous cells (Figure 2-5).

Figure 2-5. Histologic differences between submandibular, sublingual, and parotid glands

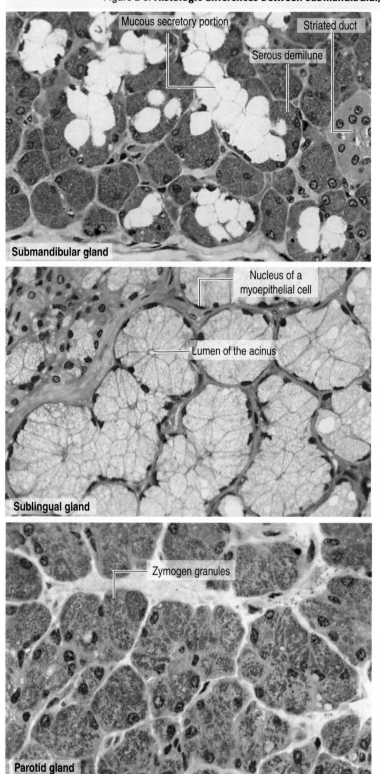

Submandibular gland

- Mucous secretory portion
- Serous demilune
- Striated duct

Sublingual gland

- Nucleus of a myoepithelial cell
- Lumen of the acinus

Parotid gland

- Zymogen granules

Mixed secretory portion
(submandibular or submaxillary gland)

The **submandibular gland** contains both serous and mucous secretory portions and they produce a seromucous secretion delivered into the same lumen. Mixed secretory units are made up of mucous cells and a small cap of serous cells on one side. The cap is called the **serous demilune** because of its crescent moon shape. Surrounding each secretory unit and the initial portion of the excretory duct are the **myoepithelial cells**. Myoepithelial cells are placed between the secretory cells and the basal lamina and their long and branched cytoplasmic processes form a loose basket. Their function is to contract and squeeze the secretion out of the secretory portion and along the duct system.

Mucous secretory portion (sublingual gland)

The **sublingual gland** contains mucous secretory portions that appear pale because of the high content of mucus-containing secretory vesicles. The nuclei generally lie flattened against the basal portion of the secretory cells. The secretory content can be demonstrated by the PAS reaction, which stains glycoproteins. Myoepithelial cells are also present around the mucous secretory portions.

Mucous acinar cell

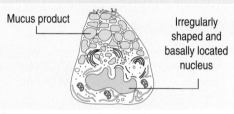

- Mucus product
- Irregularly shaped and basally located nucleus

Serous secretory portion (parotid gland)

The **parotid gland** contains serous secretory portions. The serous-secreting cells have a large spherical nucleus, a basal region in which the rough endoplasmic reticulum predominates, and an apical region with red-stained **zymogen granules**. Zymogen granules represent secretory vesicles containing enzyme precursors.

Serous acinar cell

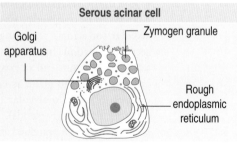

- Golgi apparatus
- Zymogen granule
- Rough endoplasmic reticulum

Mechanisms of secretion

Exocrine glands can also be classified on the basis of **how the secretory product is released** (Figure 2-6).

In **merocrine secretion** (Greek *meros*, part; *krinein*, to separate), the product is released by **exocytosis**. Secretory granules are enclosed by a membrane that fuses with the apical plasma membrane during discharge or exocytosis. An example is the secretion of zymogen granules by the pancreas.

In **apocrine secretion** (Greek *apoknino*, to separate), the release of the secretory product involves **partial loss of the apical portion of the cell**. An example is

Figure 2-6. Mechanisms of glandular secretion

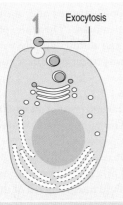
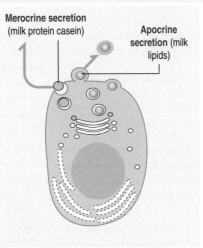
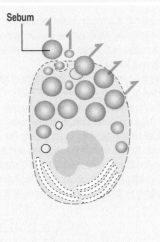

Exocytosis

Merocrine secretion
(milk protein casein)

Apocrine secretion (milk lipids)

Sebum

Merocrine secretion

The secretory vesicle approaches the apical domain of an epithelial cell. The vesicular membrane fuses with the plasma membrane to release its contents into the extracellular space.

The fused plasma membrane can be taken back into the cell by **endocytosis** and recycled for further use by secretory vesicles.

Apocrine secretion

Some of the apical cytoplasm is pinched off with the contained secretions.

Mammary glands secrete milk lipids by apocrine secretion and the milk protein casein by merocrine secretion.

Holocrine secretion

The cell produces and accumulates a secretory product in the cytoplasm, such as sebum in sebaceous glands, and then disintegrates to release the secretory material.

the secretion of **lipids** by epithelial cells of the mammary gland. **Proteins** secreted by epithelial cells of the mammary gland follow the merocrine pathway (exocytosis).

In **holocrine secretion** (Greek *holos*, all), the secretory product constitutes **the entire cell and its product**. An example is the sebaceous glands of the skin, which produce a secretion called **sebum**.

Plasma membrane and cytomembranes

A review of major concepts of cell membranes and organelles and their clinical relevance are presented in this chapter. Epithelial glands are a convenient topic for this integration. We initiate the review by addressing the structural and biochemical characteristics of the plasma membrane. Additional information related to plasma membrane–mediated cell signaling is presented in Chapter 3, Cell Signaling.

The **plasma membrane** determines the structural and functional boundaries of a cell. Intracellular membranes, called **cytomembranes**, separate diverse cellular processes into compartments known as **organelles**. The nucleus, mitochondria, peroxisomes, and lysosomes are membrane-bound organelles; lipids and glycogen are not membrane-bound and are known as **inclusions**.

Plasma membrane

The plasma membrane consists of **lipids** and **proteins**. The phospholipid bilayer is the fundamental structure of the membrane and forms a bilayer barrier between two aqueous compartments: the extracellular and intracellular compartments. Proteins are embedded within the phospholipid bilayer and carry out specific functions of the plasma membrane such as cell-cell recognition and selective transport of molecules (see Box 2-A).

Phospholipid bilayer

Membrane lipids have three general functions:

1. Cell membranes consist of **polar lipids** with a hydrophobic portion that self-associates, and a hydrophilic portion, that interacts with water–containing molecules. This **amphipathic property** enables cells and organelles to establish an internal setting separated from the external environment.

2. Lipids enable some intramembranous proteins to aggregate and others to disperse.

Phospholipids, ceramide and cholesterol are synthesized in the endoplasmic reticulum. Sphingolipids synthesis takes place in the Golgi apparatus.

3. Lipids can participate in cell signaling (for example, phosphatidylinositol and diacylglycerol).

The four major phospholipids of plasma membranes are **phosphatidylcholine, phosphatidylethanolamine, phosphatidylserine** and **sphingomyelin** (Figure 2-7). They represent more than one half the lipid of most membranes. A fifth phospholipid, **phosphatidylinositol**, is localized to the inner leaflet of the plasma membrane.

In addition to phospholipids, the plasma membrane of animal cells contains **glycolipids** and **cholesterol**. Glycolipids, a minor membrane component, are found in the outer leaflet, with the carbohydrate moieties exposed on the cell surface.

Cholesterol, a major membrane constituent, is

present in about the same amounts as are phospholipids. Cholesterol, a rigid ring structure, is inserted into the phospholipid bilayer to modulate membrane fluidity by restricting the movement of phospholipid fatty acid chains at high temperatures. Cholesterol is not present in bacteria.

Two general aspects of the phospholipid bilayer are important to remember:

1. **The structure of phospholipids accounts for the function of membranes as barriers between two aqueous compartments.** The hydrophobic fatty acid chains in the interior of the phospholipid bilayer are responsible for the membranes being impermeable to water-soluble molecules.

2. **The phospholipid bilayer is a viscous fluid.** The long hydrocarbon chains of the fatty acids of most phospholipids are loosely packed and can move in the interior of the membrane. Therefore, phospholipids and proteins can diffuse laterally within the membrane to perform critical membrane functions.

Membrane proteins

Most plasma membranes consist of about 50% lipid and 50% protein. The carbohydrate component of glycolipids and glycoproteins represents 5% to 10% of the membrane mass. The surface of a plasma membrane is coated by a **glycocalyx** (see Box 2-B).

According to the **fluid mosaic model** of the membrane structure, membranes are two-dimensional fluids in which proteins are inserted into lipid bilayers. It is difficult for membrane proteins and phospholipids to switch back and forth between the inner and outer leaflets of the membrane. However, because they exist in a fluid environment, both proteins and lipids are able to diffuse laterally through the plane of the membrane. However, not all proteins can diffuse freely; the mobility of membrane proteins is limited by their association with the cytoskeleton.

Restrictions in the mobility of membrane proteins are responsible for the polarized nature of epithelial cells, divided into distinct **apical** and **basolateral domains** that differ in protein composition and function. Tight junctions between adjacent epithelial cells

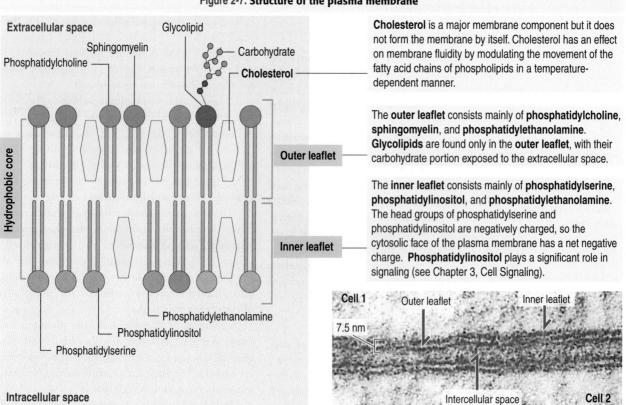

Figure 2-7. Structure of the plasma membrane

Extracellular space

Phosphatidylcholine
Sphingomyelin
Glycolipid
Carbohydrate
Cholesterol

Hydrophobic core

Outer leaflet

Inner leaflet

Phosphatidylethanolamine
Phosphatidylinositol
Phosphatidylserine

Intracellular space

Cholesterol is a major membrane component but it does not form the membrane by itself. Cholesterol has an effect on membrane fluidity by modulating the movement of the fatty acid chains of phospholipids in a temperature-dependent manner.

The **outer leaflet** consists mainly of **phosphatidylcholine**, **sphingomyelin**, and **phosphatidylethanolamine**. **Glycolipids** are found only in the **outer leaflet**, with their carbohydrate portion exposed to the extracellular space.

The **inner leaflet** consists mainly of **phosphatidylserine**, **phosphatidylinositol**, and **phosphatidylethanolamine**. The head groups of phosphatidylserine and phosphatidylinositol are negatively charged, so the cytosolic face of the plasma membrane has a net negative charge. **Phosphatidylinositol** plays a significant role in signaling (see Chapter 3, Cell Signaling).

Cell 1
Outer leaflet
Inner leaflet
7.5 nm
Intercellular space
Cell 2

• The extracellular domain of a plasma membrane is generally glycosylated by the carbohydrate portions of glycolipids and transmembrane glycoproteins. The surface of the cell is, therefore, covered by a carbohydrate coat, known as the **glycocalyx**.
• The glycocalyx protects the cell surface and facilitates cell-cell interactions. An appropriate example is the mechanism of **homing**, a process allowing leukocytes to leave blood vessels and mediate inflammatory responses. As you recall, the initial step in adhesion between endothelial cells and leukocytes is mediated by **selectins**, a family of transmembrane proteins which recognize specific sugars on the cell surface.

(discussed in Chapter 1, Epithelium) not only seal the space between cells but also serve as barriers to the diffusion of proteins and lipids between the apical and basolateral domains of the plasma membrane.

Two major classes of membrane-associated proteins are recognized (Figure 2-8):

 1. **Peripheral proteins**.
 2. **Integral membrane proteins**.

Peripheral membrane proteins are not inserted into the hydrophobic interior of the membrane but are, instead, indirectly associated with membranes through protein-protein ionic bond interactions, which are disrupted by solutions of **high salt concentration** or **extreme pH**.

Portions of integral membrane proteins are inserted into the lipid bilayer. They can only be released by solubilization using **detergents**. Detergents are chemical agents that contain both hydrophobic and hydrophilic groups. The **hydrophobic groups** of the detergent penetrate the membrane lipids and bind to the membrane-inserted hydrophobic portion of the

protein. The **hydrophilic groups** combine with the protein, forming aqueous-soluble detergent-protein complexes.

Numerous integral proteins are **transmembrane proteins**, spanning the lipid bilayer, with segments exposed on both sides of the membrane. Transmembrane proteins can be visualized by the **freeze-fracture technique**.

Freeze-fracture: Differences between a surface and a face

The **freeze-fracture technique** is valuable for the visualization of intramembranous proteins with the electron microscope. This technique provided the first evidence for the presence of transmembrane proteins in the plasma membrane and cytomembranes.

Specimens are frozen at liquid nitrogen temperature (–196°C) and "split" with a knife (under high vacuum) along the hydrophobic core of the membrane. As a result, two complementary halves, corresponding to each membrane bilayer, are produced. Each membrane half has a **surface** and a **face**. The face is artificially produced during membrane splitting.

A replica of the specimen is generated by evaporating a very thin layer of a heavy metal (generally platinum with a thickness of 1.0 to 1.5 nm) at a 45° angle to produce a contrasting shadowing effect. The platinum replica is then detached from the real specimen by floating it on a water surface, mounted on a metal grid, and examined under the electron microscope.

Figure 2-9 indicates the nomenclature for the

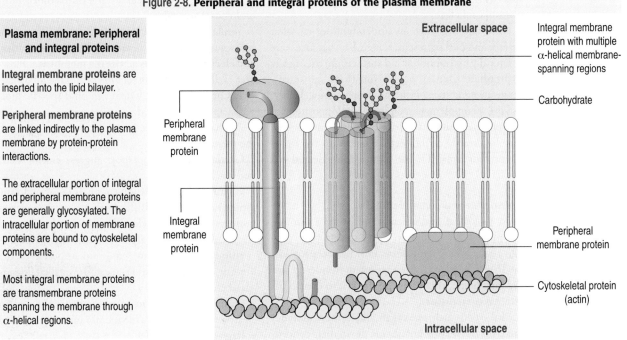

Figure 2-8. Peripheral and integral proteins of the plasma membrane

Plasma membrane: Peripheral and integral proteins

Integral membrane proteins are inserted into the lipid bilayer.

Peripheral membrane proteins are linked indirectly to the plasma membrane by protein-protein interactions.

The extracellular portion of integral and peripheral membrane proteins are generally glycosylated. The intracellular portion of membrane proteins are bound to cytoskeletal components.

Most integral membrane proteins are transmembrane proteins spanning the membrane through α-helical regions.

Extracellular space

Integral membrane protein with multiple α-helical membrane-spanning regions

Carbohydrate

Peripheral membrane protein

Integral membrane protein

Peripheral membrane protein

Cytoskeletal protein (actin)

Intracellular space

Figure 2-9. Freeze-fracture: Differences between surface and face

Freeze-fracture of a cell membrane splits the bilayer into two leaflets. **Each leaflet has a surface and a face.** The surface of each leaflet faces either the extracellular surface (**ES**) or intracellular or protoplasmic surface (**PS**). The extracellular and protoplasmic faces (**EF** and **PF**) are artificially produced by splitting the membrane bilayer along its hydrophobic core. After membrane fracture, membrane proteins remain associated to the protoplasmic membrane leaflet and appear as **particles in the PF replica.** The region once occupied by the protein shows **a complementary pit in the EF replica.**

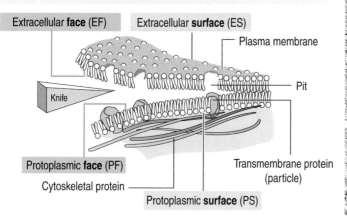

Extracellular **face (EF)**
Extracellular **surface (ES)**
Plasma membrane
Pit
Knife
Protoplasmic **face (PF)**
Cytoskeletal protein
Transmembrane protein (particle)
Protoplasmic **surface (PS)**

Secretory vesicles
Golgi apparatus
Outer membrane
Nuclear pores
Inner membrane
Nucleus

identification of surfaces and faces in electron micrographs of freeze-fracture preparations.

The **surface** of the plasma membrane exposed to the **extracellular space** is labeled **ES**, for **extracellular surface**. The **surface** of the plasma membrane exposed to the **cytoplasm** (also called protoplasm) is labeled **PS**, for **protoplasmic surface**.

The **face** of the membrane leaflet looking to the **extracellular space** (the exocytoplasmic leaflet in the illustration) is labeled **EF**, for **extracellular face**. Similarly, the face of the leaflet facing the **protoplasmic space** (identified as a protoplasmic leaflet) is **PF**, for **protoplasmic face**.

Now that we have an understanding of what surface and face represent, remember that **faces** are chemically **hydrophobic** and **surfaces** are chemically **hydrophilic**. One last point: Note that a transmembrane protein stays with the protoplasmic leaflet, leaving a complementary **pit** in the opposite exocytoplasmic leaflet. Why? Cytoskeletal components may be directly or indirectly attached to the tip of the protein exposed to the cytoplasmic side and will not let go.

Transporter and channel proteins
Most biological molecules cannot diffuse through the phospholipid bilayer. Specific transport proteins, such as **carrier proteins** and **channel proteins**, mediate the selective passage of molecules across the membrane, thus allowing the cell to control its internal composition.

Molecules (such as **oxygen** and **carbon dioxide**) can cross the plasma membrane down their concentration gradient by dissolving first in the phospholipid bilayer and then in the aqueous environment at the cytosolic or extracellular side of the membrane. This mechanism, known as **passive diffusion**, does not involve membrane proteins. Lipid substances can also cross the bilayer.

Other biological molecules (such as **glucose, charged molecules**, and **small ions** H^+, Na^+, K^+ and Cl^-) are unable to dissolve in the hydrophobic interior of the phospholipid bilayer. They require the help of specific **transport proteins** (Figure 2-10) and **channel proteins**, which facilitate the diffusion of most biological molecules.

Similar to passive diffusion, **facilitated diffusion** of biological molecules **is determined by concentration and electrical gradients across the membrane**. However, facilitated diffusion requires one of the following:

1. **Carrier proteins**, which can bind specific molecules to be transported.

2. **Channel proteins**, forming open gates through the membrane.

Carrier proteins transport sugars, amino acids and nucleosides.

Channel proteins are ion channels involved in the rapid transport of ions (faster transport than carrier proteins), are **highly selective of molecular size and electrical charge**, and **are not continuously open.**

Some channels open "gates" in response to the binding of a signaling molecule and are called **ligand-gated channels.**

Other channels open in response to changes in electric potential across the membrane and are called **voltage-gated channels.**

Figure 2-10. Transporters

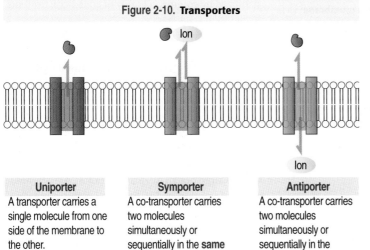

Uniporter
A transporter carries a single molecule from one side of the membrane to the other.

Symporter
A co-transporter carries two molecules simultaneously or sequentially in the **same direction.**

Antiporter
A co-transporter carries two molecules simultaneously or sequentially in the **opposite direction.**

Endoplasmic reticulum

The **endoplasmic reticulum** is an interconnected network of membrane-bound channels within the cytoplasm, part of the **cytomembrane** system and distinct from the **plasma membrane**.

The endoplasmic reticulum system, consisting of **cisternae** (flat sacs), **tubules**, and **vesicles**, divides the cytoplasm into two compartments:

1. The **luminal** or **endoplasmic compartment.**
2. The **cytoplasmic** or **cytosolic compartment.**

Smooth endoplasmic reticulum

The **smooth endoplasmic reticulum** lacks ribosomes and is generally in proximity to deposits of glycogen and lipids in the cytoplasm. The smooth endoplasmic reticulum has an important role in **detoxification reactions** required for the conversion of harmful

lipid-soluble or water-insoluble substances into water-soluble compounds more convenient for discharge by the kidneys. It also participates in **steroidogenesis** (see Chapter 19, Endocrine System).

Products released into the luminal compartment of the endoplasmic reticulum are transported to the Golgi apparatus by a transporting vesicle and eventually to the exterior of the cell by exocytosis.

One can visualize the sequence in which the lumen of the cytomembrane system is interconnected and remains as such in an imaginary stage; you can visualize that the **luminal compartment of a secretory cell is continuous with the exterior of the cell** (Figure 2-11). The surrounding space is the cytosolic compartment in which soluble proteins, cytoskeletal components, and organelles are present.

Now, let us visualize the membrane of each component of the cytomembrane system as consisting of two leaflets (Figure 2-12):

1. The **exocytoplasmic leaflet** (facing the extracellular space).

2. The **protoplasmic leaflet** (facing the cytosolic compartment).

Let us imagine that exocytoplasmic and protoplasmic leaflets form a continuum. During the **freeze-fracturing process**, the knife fractures the membrane as it jumps from one fracture plane to the other across the hydrophobic core and splits membranes into two leaflets. The knife cannot stay with a single membrane because cytomembrane-bound organelles occupy different levels and have random orientations within the cell. This randomness will be apparent during the examination of the replica.

The sample may contain a combination of exocytoplasmic and protoplasmic leaflets which, in turn, can expose surfaces and faces. As you already know, membrane proteins tend to remain associated with the protoplasmic leaflet and appear as **particles on the PF** (protoplasmic face). A shallow **complementary pit is visualized in the EF** (extracellular face).

Rough endoplasmic reticulum

The **rough endoplasmic reticulum** is recognized under the light microscope as a diffuse basophilic cytoplasmic structure called **ergastoplasm**.

The rough endoplasmic reticulum is involved in the synthesis of proteins, carried out by their attached **ribosomes** (Figure 2-13). In contrast, the membranes of the smooth endoplasmic reticulum lack attached ribosomes (see Figure 2-13). Most proteins exit the rough endoplasmic reticulum in vesicles transported to the *cis* portion of the Golgi apparatus (see Figures 2-16 and 2-17). Other proteins are retained by the rough endoplasmic reticulum to participate in the initial steps of protein synthesis (see Figure 2-15). The retained proteins contain the targeting sequence

Figure 2-11. Intracellular compartments

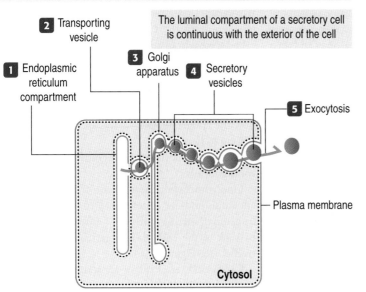

The luminal compartment of a secretory cell is continuous with the exterior of the cell

2 Transporting vesicle

1 Endoplasmic reticulum compartment

3 Golgi apparatus

4 Secretory vesicles

5 Exocytosis

Plasma membrane

Cytosol

Figure 2-12. **Leaflets of cytomembranes and plasma membrane**

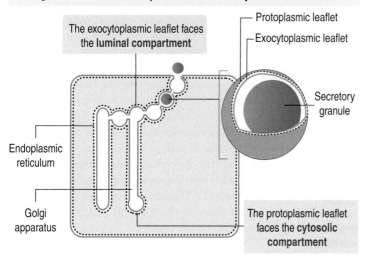

The exocytoplasmic leaflet faces the **luminal compartment**

Protoplasmic leaflet

Exocytoplasmic leaflet

Secretory granule

Endoplasmic reticulum

Golgi apparatus

The protoplasmic leaflet faces the **cytosolic compartment**

Lys-Asp-Glu-Leu (KDEL) at the C-terminal. A lack of the KDEL sequence marks proteins for transport to the Golgi apparatus.

Protein synthesis and sorting

The role of the endoplasmic reticulum in protein synthesis and sorting was demonstrated by incubating pancreatic acinar cells in a medium containing radiolabeled amino acids and localizing radiolabeled proteins by autoradiography.

The secretory pathway taken by secretory proteins includes the following sequence: rough endoplasmic reticulum, to Golgi apparatus, to secretory vesicles, to the extracellular space or lumen (Figure 2-14). Plasma membrane and lysosomal proteins also follow the sequence of rough endoplasmic reticulum to Golgi apparatus but are retained within the cell.

Proteins targeted to the nucleus, mitochondria, or peroxisomes are synthesized on free ribosomes and then released into the cytosol. In contrast, proteins for secretion or targeted to the endoplasmic reticulum, Golgi apparatus, lysosomes, or plasma membrane are synthesized by membrane-bound ribosomes and then transferred to the endoplasmic reticulum as protein synthesis progresses.

Ribosomes attach to the endoplasmic reticulum under the guidance of the amino acid sequence of the polypeptide chain being synthesized. Ribosomes synthesizing proteins for secretion are directed to the endoplasmic reticulum by a signal sequence at the growing end of the polypeptide chain.

The mechanism by which secretory proteins are directed to the endoplasmic reticulum is explained by the **signal hypothesis** (Figure 2-15).

Golgi apparatus

The Golgi apparatus consists of a cluster of flattened stacks of sacs called **cisternae** (Figures 2-16 and 2-17)

stabilized by **golgins**, a family of coiled-coil proteins. Each Golgi stack has:

1. An entry, or *cis*, face, adjacent to the endoplasmic reticulum.

2. An exit, or *trans*, face, continuous with the *trans*-Golgi network (**TGN**), pointing toward the plasma membrane or the nucleus.

Cisternae of the *medial*-Golgi are interposed between the *cis*-Golgi and the *trans*-Golgi.

Cargos derived from the endoplasmic reticulum transport soluble proteins and membrane to the *cis*-Golgi. **Cargo** designates newly synthesized membrane and proteins destined to be stored within a cell compartment or secreted to the cell exterior.

The material travels through the cisternae by means of **transport vesicles** that bud off from one cisterna and tether and fuse with the next in the presence of golgins. **Golgins** form an appendicular network on the *cis*-Golgi, around the rims of the sacs and on the *trans*-Golgi, with roles in Golgi structure stabilization and vesicle trafficking.

Finally, vesicle cargos translocate from the *trans*-Golgi to the TGN, the tubular-vesicular distribution center of cargos to the cell surface or to another cellular compartment (for example, lysosomes).

The Golgi apparatus undergoes a permanent turnover. It disassembles during mitosis/meiosis and reassembles in interphase.

Functions of the Golgi apparatus

Three specific functions are carried by the Golgi apparatus:

1. **Modification of carbohydrates attached to glycoproteins and proteoglycans received from the endoplasmic reticulum**. This process is called **glycosylation**. A characteristic glycosylation event within the Golgi is the modification of *N*-linked oligosaccharides on glycoproteins. More than 200 enzymes participate in the biosynthesis of glycoproteins and glycolipids in the Golgi apparatus. The enzymes called **glycosyltransferases** add specific sugar residues; the enzymes called **glycosidases** remove specific sugar residues.

2. **Sorting of cargos to several destinations within the cell**. We discuss in another section of this chapter how the Golgi apparatus marks specific proteins for sorting to lysosomes.

3. The **synthesis of sphingomyelin and glycosphingolipids**.

Once processed, cargos bud off from the Golgi apparatus and are either sorted to the **secretory of lysosomal sorting pathway** (anterograde traffic) or back to the **endoplasmic reticulum** (retrograde traffic) (see Figure 2-16).

Certain classes of cargos are stored into secretory granules for later release in response to an extracel-

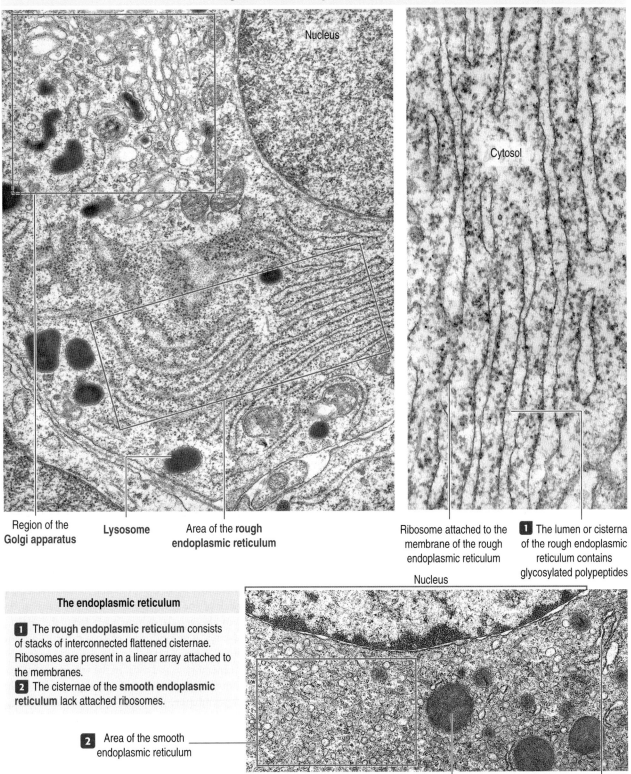

Figure 2-13. The endoplasmic reticulum

Nucleus

Cytosol

Region of the **Golgi apparatus**

Lysosome

Area of the **rough endoplasmic reticulum**

Ribosome attached to the membrane of the rough endoplasmic reticulum

1 The lumen or cisterna of the rough endoplasmic reticulum contains glycosylated polypeptides

Nucleus

The endoplasmic reticulum

1 The **rough endoplasmic reticulum** consists of stacks of interconnected flattened cisternae. Ribosomes are present in a linear array attached to the membranes.

2 The cisternae of the **smooth endoplasmic reticulum** lack attached ribosomes.

2 Area of the smooth endoplasmic reticulum

Mitochondrium

Rough endoplasmic reticulum

lular signal. This mechanism is called **facultative** or **regulated secretion**. Other cargos can be secreted continuously without a need of a stimulus. This mechanism is called **constitutive secretion**; it supplies newly synthesized lipids and proteins to the plasma membrane or proteins to be released outside the cell such as proteins of the extracellular matrix or immunoglobulins during immune reactions.

Cargo sorting occurs along **microtubules** or **actin filaments** with the help of motor proteins. The pres-

Figure 2-14. **Protein synthesis, transport, and secretion by exocrine pancreatic cells**

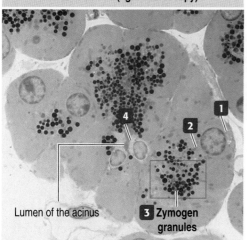

Pancreatic acinus (light microscopy)

Lumen of the acinus

3 **Zymogen granules**

Pancreatic acinar cells secrete newly synthesized proteins into the digestive tract.

When cells were labeled with a radioactive amino acid to trace the intracellular pathway of the secreted proteins, it was found by autoradiography that, after a 3-minute labeling, newly synthesized proteins were localized in the rough endoplasmic reticulum **1**.

Later on, the radiolabeled proteins were found to translocate to the Golgi apparatus **2** and then, within secretory vesicles as zymogen granules **3**, to the plasma membrane and the extracellular space **4**.

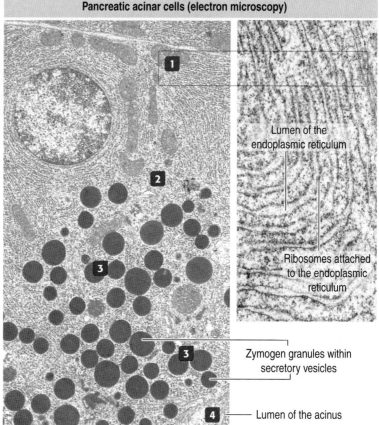

Pancreatic acinar cells (electron microscopy)

Lumen of the endoplasmic reticulum

Ribosomes attached to the endoplasmic reticulum

Zymogen granules within secretory vesicles

Lumen of the acinus

---

ence of **specific lipids domains** in the membrane of a vesicle cargo recruit **coating proteins** and **tethering golgins** to sort the cargo in the direction of an **acceptor membrane** site. Essentially, the sorting and transport of cargos depend on specialized coats preparing the cargo to be moved along the cytoskeleton by molecular motor proteins. **Tethering golgins** (coiled-coil proteins) attach the cargo to the cytoskeleton. When the vesicle cargo reaches an acceptor membrane, it fuses with the help of **fusion proteins**.

Vesicle transport

Vesicle transport involves the mobilization of proteins and membrane between cytomembrane compartments. The **exocytosis** or **secretory pathway** starts in the endoplasmic reticulum, continues through the Golgi apparatus, and ends on the cell surface. The **endocytic pathway** consists in the internalization and degradation of extracellular material from the plasma membrane, through endosomes to lysosomes.

These two events depend on distinctive proteins coating the cytosolic side of the membrane of the transport vesicle that becomes a **coated vesicle**. The coat helps the recruitment of molecules for transport. Before fusion with the acceptor membrane, the vesicle sheds its coat, allowing the membranes to interact directly and fuse.

Transport vesicles are coated by the protein **clathrin**. Clathrin-coated vesicles are seen in the exocytosis/secretory and endocytosis pathway.

In the endocytosis pathway (Figure 2-18), vesicles start at the plasma membrane as **clathrin-coated pits**. Clathrin molecules assemble in a basket-like arrangement on the cytosolic face of the plasma membrane and the pit shape changes into a vesicle.

Dynamin, a small GTP-binding protein, surrounds the neck of the invaginated coated pit, causing the neck of the vesicle to pinch off from the plasma membrane. A second class of coat proteins are the **adaptins**. Adaptins stabilize the clathrin coat to the vesicle membrane and assist in the selection of cargos for transport by binding to **cargo receptors** on the vesicle membrane. When the cargo reaches the target acceptor membrane, the coat proteins are shed and the membranes can fuse.

Sorting of clathrin-coated vesicles and COP-coated vesicles

A continual process of **budding** and **fusion** of **transport vesicles** mobilizes products from the endoplasmic reticulum to the Golgi apparatus (anterograde traffic), between membranous stacks of the Golgi apparatus, and from the Golgi apparatus to the endoplasmic reticulum (retrograde traffic) (see Figure 2-16).

Figure 2-15. Protein synthesis: Signal hypothesis

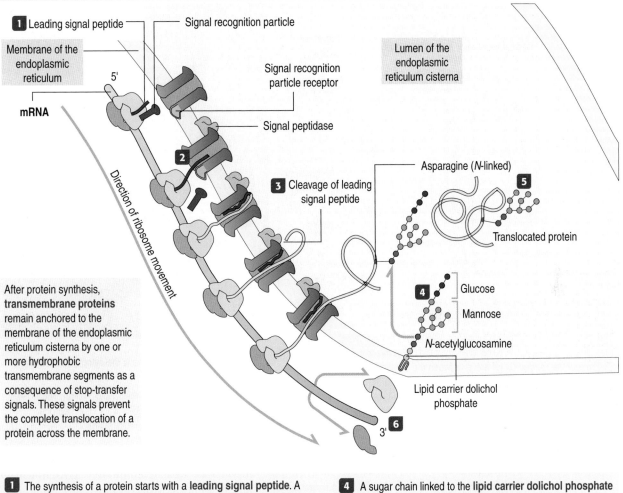

1 Leading signal peptide

Signal recognition particle

Membrane of the endoplasmic reticulum

Lumen of the endoplasmic reticulum cisterna

Signal recognition particle receptor

5'

mRNA

Signal peptidase

2

Direction of ribosome movement

3 Cleavage of leading signal peptide

Asparagine (*N*-linked)

5

Translocated protein

4 Glucose

Mannose

N-acetylglucosamine

Lipid carrier dolichol phosphate

After protein synthesis, **transmembrane proteins** remain anchored to the membrane of the endoplasmic reticulum cisterna by one or more hydrophobic transmembrane segments as a consequence of stop-transfer signals. These signals prevent the complete translocation of a protein across the membrane.

3' **6**

---

1 The synthesis of a protein starts with a **leading signal peptide**. A **signal recognition particle (SRP)** binds to the ribosome and stops further growth of the protein. The complex is anchored to the cytoplasmic side of the endoplasmic reticulum cisterna where SRP binds to the **SRP receptor**. After binding, SRP is removed from the complex.

2 The protein reinitiates its growth and the leading peptide crosses the lipid bilayer into the lumen of the rough endoplasmic reticulum.

3 **Signal peptidase** removes the leading peptide and protein elongation continues.

4 A sugar chain linked to the **lipid carrier dolichol phosphate** is attached to the asparagine residue (*N*-glycosylation).

5 The synthesized protein is released. **Glucose** and one **mannose** are removed from the previously attached oligosaccharide.

6 Ribosome subunits disassemble at the 3'-end of the mRNA.

The vesicular transport mechanism involves two types of coated vesicles (Figure 2-19):

1. **Clathrin-coated vesicles**, transporting products from the Golgi apparatus to lysosomes, and carrying products from the exterior of the cell to lysosomes (for example, cholesterol; see Figure 2-18).

2. **COP-coated vesicles** (COP stands for **co**at **p**rotein), transporting products between stacks of the Golgi apparatus (**COPI-coated vesicles**), and from the endoplasmic reticulum to the Golgi apparatus (**COPII-coated vesicles**).

We have already seen that **adaptins** mediate the binding of clathrin to the vesicular membrane as well as select specific molecules to be trapped in a vesicle.

What about COP-coated vesicles?

A guanosine triphosphate (GTP)-binding protein called **ARF** (for **a**denosine diphosphate [ADP]-**r**ibosylation **f**actor), is required for the assembly of COPI and COPII molecules to form a protein coat called a **coatomer** on the cytosolic side of a transporting vesicle.

When GTP is converted to guanosine diphosphate (GDP) by hydrolysis, the coatomer dissociates from the vesicle just before the vesicle fuses with a target membrane. ARF is related to **Ras proteins**, a group of oncogene proteins also regulated by the alternate binding of GTP and GDP (see the MAP kinase pathway in Chapter 3, Cell Signaling).

Figure 2-16. **Secretory and lysosomal sorting pathways**

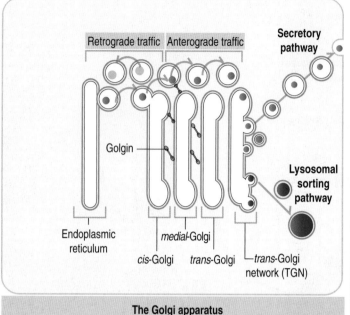

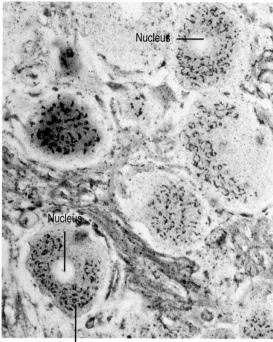

Multiple Golgi apparatus sites in the cytoplasm of neurons

First described in 1898 by Camillo Golgi (Italian, 1843–1926. Nobel Prize in Physiology-Medicine 1906) in neurons impregnated with silver salts (Golgi stain).

The Golgi apparatus

The cisterna closest to the endoplasmic reticulum is the **cis-Golgi**, whereas the cisterna closest to the apical domain of the cell is the **trans-Golgi**. Cisterna of the **medial-Golgi** are in between the **cis-Golgi** and the **trans-Golgi**. The **trans-Golgi network (TGN)** is the sorting site of vesicles or cargos. Transporting vesicles bud from one stack and fuse with the next in an **anterograde traffic** (endoplasmic reticulum to Golgi) or **retrograde traffic** (Golgi to endoplasmic reticulum). **Golgins** stabilize cisternae and vesicles.

Vesicle fusion to a target membrane: NSF and SNARE proteins

The fusion of a transporting vesicle to a target membrane (Figure 2-20) requires the **recognition of the specific target membrane** so the **vesicle and target membranes can fuse** to deliver the transported cargo.

Vesicle fusion is mediated by two interacting cytosolic proteins: **NSF** (for *N*-ethylmaleimide-sensitive fusion) and **SNAPs** (for **s**oluble **N**SF **a**ttachment **p**roteins). NSF and SNAP bind to specific membrane receptors called SNARE (for **SNAP** **re**ceptors). SNAREs are present on the transporting vesicle (v-SNARE) and target membranes (t-SNARE) and represent **docking proteins**. Following docking, the SNARE complex recruits NSF and SNAPs to produce the fusion of the vesicle and target membranes.

Lysosomal sorting pathway: M6P and its receptor

Lysosomal hydrolases are synthesized in the endoplasmic reticulum, transported to the *cis*-Golgi, and finally sorted to **lysosomes**. This sorting mechanism involves two important steps (Figure 2-21):

1. The insertion in the *cis*-Golgi of **mannose-6-phosphate** (**M6P**) into oligosaccharides attached to glycoproteins destined to lysosomes.

2. The presence in the TGN of the **transmembrane M6P receptor protein** in the sorting vesicle.

By this mechanism, M6P-containing lysosomal enzymes are separated from other glycoproteins in vesicles with the M6P receptor. After being transported to a clathrin-coated transporting vesicle, lysosomal enzymes dissociate from the M6P receptor and become surrounded by a membrane to form a **lysosome**. Membranes containing free M6P receptor are returned to the Golgi apparatus for **recycling**.

Receptor-mediated endocytosis: Cholesterol uptake

Receptor-mediated endocytosis increases the capacity of the cell to internalize specific macromolecules with great efficiency and in large amount. A classic example is the uptake of cholesterol used to make new cell membranes. As you recall from your biochemistry course, cholesterol is highly insoluble and is mobilized in the bloodstream bound to protein as low-density lipoprotein (LDL) particles. LDL carries about 75% of the cholesterol and circulates in blood for about 2 to 3 days. Approximately 70% of LDL is cleared from blood by cells containing **LDL receptors**; the remainder is removed by a scavenger pathway using a receptor-independent mechanism.

The internalization of a **ligand** (such as LDL, transferrin, polypeptide hormones, or growth factors) by a cell requires a specific **membrane receptor**. The LDL

Figure 2-17. **Compartments of the Golgi apparatus**

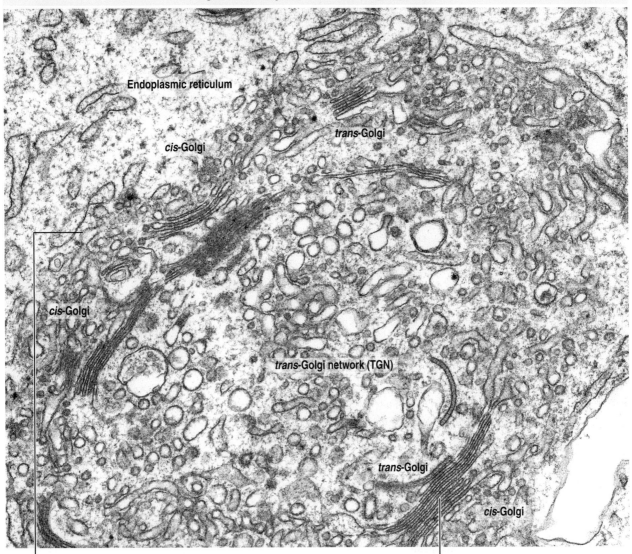

Endoplasmic reticulum

cis-Golgi

trans-Golgi

cis-Golgi

trans-Golgi network (TGN)

trans-Golgi

cis-Golgi

Endoplasmic reticulum export domain

***medial*-Golgi**

Golgi apparatus

The **Golgi apparatus** is visualized under the electron microscope as a series of curved flattened saccules or cisternae stacked upon one another. The ends of the saccules are dilated and can form spherical vesicles. The saccules and vesicles contain proteins being glycosylated for further secretion or sorting.

The Golgi apparatus consists of four major functionally distinct compartments:

1. The *cis*-Golgi is the entry site to the Golgi apparatus of products derived from the endoplasmic reticulum.
2. The *trans*-Golgi is the exit site of cargos.
3. The *medial*-Golgi is interposed between the *cis*-Golgi and the *trans*-Golgi.
4. The *trans*-Golgi network (TGN) is the sorting site of cargos for transport to lysosomes or secretion (exocytosis).

receptor–LDL complex is internalized by **receptor-mediated endocytosis**. We have seen that this process involves the assembly of the protein **clathrin** on the cytosolic side of the plasma membrane, which forms a **coated pit** (see Figure 2-18).

The function of clathrin, together with **adaptin**, is to concentrate receptor-ligand complexes in a small surface area of the plasma membrane. Receptors with their bound ligands move by lateral diffusion in the plane of the lipid bilayer. The coated pit invaginates to form a **coated vesicle**, which pinches off from the plasma membrane to transport receptor-ligand complexes to a specific intracellular pathway, usually an **endosome**. Recall that **dynamin** assembles around the neck of the budding coated vesicle to pinch off the vesicle from the plasma membrane with the help of other proteins recruited to the neck site.

After internalization, clathrin of the coated vesicle

Figure 2-18. Endocytosis pathway: Cholesterol uptake

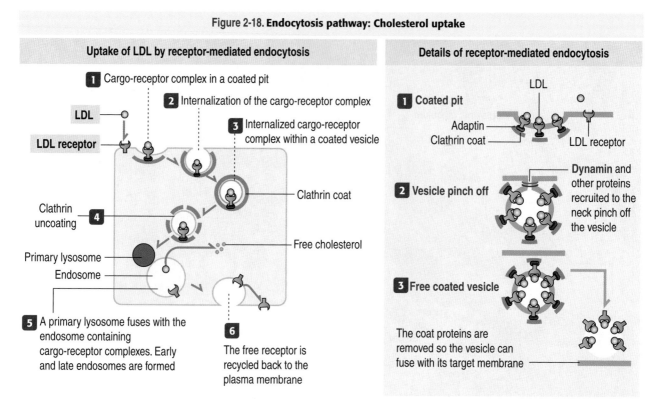

Uptake of LDL by receptor-mediated endocytosis

1 Cargo-receptor complex in a coated pit

2 Internalization of the cargo-receptor complex

LDL

LDL receptor

3 Internalized cargo-receptor complex within a coated vesicle

Clathrin coat

Clathrin uncoating

4

Free cholesterol

Primary lysosome

Endosome

5 A primary lysosome fuses with the endosome containing cargo-receptor complexes. Early and late endosomes are formed

6 The free receptor is recycled back to the plasma membrane

Details of receptor-mediated endocytosis

LDL

1 Coated pit

Adaptin

Clathrin coat

LDL receptor

2 Vesicle pinch off

Dynamin and other proteins recruited to the neck pinch off the vesicle

3 Free coated vesicle

The coat proteins are removed so the vesicle can fuse with its target membrane

---

is removed and the uncoated vesicle fuses with the endosome, with an internal low pH. In this acidic environment, LDL detaches from the receptor and is delivered to an inactive **primary lysosome**, which changes into a **secondary lysosome** engaged in substrate degradation. LDL is broken down by lysosomal hydrolytic enzymes and is released into the cytosol as free cholesterol, where it can be used for new membrane synthesis.

The LDL receptor, in turn, is continuously recycled back to the plasma membrane to be used again. The LDL receptor can recycle every 10 minutes and can make several hundred cycles in its 20-hour life span.

Cholesterol is required for the synthesis of steroid hormones, the production of bile acids in liver hepatocytes, and the synthesis of cell membranes.

Box 2-C | Macroautophagy and autophagy

• There are different types of autophagy. **Macroautophagy** (commonly referred to autophagy) is non-selective and consists in the random sequestration, degradation and recycling of intracellular components into double-membraned autophagosomes. **Autophagy** is a selective process defined by the type of material being delivered across the lysosomal membrane (chaperone-mediated autophagy).
• Non-selective macroautophagy and selective autophagy use proteins encoded by autophagy-related (*Atg*) genes to form autophagosomes that fuse with lysosomes to become degradative autolysosomes.
• Tumor cells induce autophagy in response to starvation or damaging stress to promote cell survival. This particular aspect suggests that inhibition of the mechanism of autophagy could be useful to improve cancer therapy. Alternatively, defective chronic autophagy may lead to a damaging tissue inflammatory state conducive to tumor development, an important aspect of cancer prevention.

Clinical significance: Familial hypercholesterolemia
The mechanism of cholesterol uptake is disrupted in **familial hypercholesterolemia**, characterized by an elevation of LDL, the predominant cholesterol transport protein in the plasma. The primary defect is a **mutation in the gene encoding the LDL receptor**, required for the internalization of dietary cholesterol by most cells. High levels of LDL cholesterol in blood plasma lead to the formation of **atherosclerotic plaques** in the coronary vessels, a common cause of **myocardial infarction**.

Patients with familial hypercholesterolemia have three types of defective receptors:

1. LDL receptors incapable of binding LDL.
2. LDL receptors that bind LDL but at a reduced capacity.
3. LDL receptors that can bind LDL normally but are incapable of internalization.

Lysosomes

Lysosomes are membrane-bound organelles of heterogeneous size and morphology that contain acid hydrolases. Lysosomes are regarded as the end degradation compartment of the endocytic pathway and also participate in the digestion of intracellular material during the non-selective process of **macroautophagy**, commonly referred to autophagy (see Box 2-C). In addition, lysosomes function as secretory organelles in response to external stimulation (see Box 2-D)

Two types of lysosomes are recognized:

1. **Primary lysosomes** (Figure 2-22), defined as the

Figure 2-19. Clathrin- and COP-mediated vesicle transport

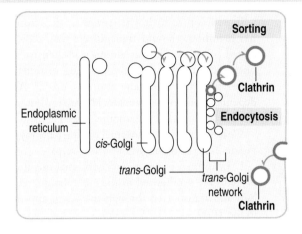

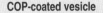

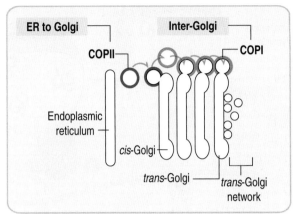

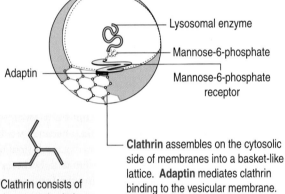

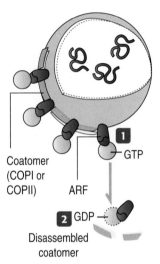

Clathrin consists of three protein chains

Clathrin assembles on the cytosolic side of membranes into a basket-like lattice. **Adaptin** mediates clathrin binding to the vesicular membrane.

1. **ARF** (ADP-ribosylation factor) bound to GTP associates with the membrane of the Golgi stacks to promote binding of COP coat protein (**coatomer**), leading to vesicle budding.

2. Hydrolysis of bound **GTP** changes ARF to **GDP**-bound, leading to the disassembly of the vesicle coat before the vesicle fuses with a target membrane.

Vesicular transport consists of:
1. The formation of a vesicle by budding from a membrane.
2. The assembly of a protein coat on the cytosolic surface of transport vesicles.

There are **two types of coated vesicles:**
1. **Clathrin-coated,** found in endocytic vesicles and vesicles sorted from the *trans*-Golgi network to a lysosome.
2. **COP-coated vesicles** (COP stands for coat protein), observed in transporting vesicles between stacks of the Golgi apparatus (**COPI-coated vesicles**) or from the endoplasmic reticulum to the Golgi apparatus (**COPII-coated vesicles**).

COP assembly is regulated by two different mechanisms:
1. Clathrin binding to a vesicle is mediated by **adaptins**.
2. COP binding to a vesicle is mediated by **GTP-bound ARF**. The coatomer sheds when GTP hydrolysis changes **ARF-GTP bound** to **ARF-GDP-bound**. Then, the vesicle fuses with the acceptor or target membrane.

ARF is a member of the **Ras protein family** (involved as oncogenes in cancer; see the MAP kinase pathway in Chapter 3, Cell Signaling).

Ras-related proteins (called **Rab proteins**) are also involved in vesicular transport.

primary storage site of lysosomal hydrolases.

2. **Secondary lysosomes** (corresponding to **phagolysosomes** and **autolysosomes**), regarded as lysosomes engaged in a substrate degradation process.

As discussed, the plasma membrane can internalize extracellular particles and fluids using vesicles resulting from the invagination of the membrane by a process called **endocytosis**. Endocytosis has two important goals: **to bring material into the cell**, and **to recycle the plasma membrane**. The reverse process,

called **exocytosis**, is the transport outside the cell of products processed or synthesized by the cell.

Endocytosis involves three major types of vesicles:

1. **Clathrin-free phagosomes,** used to internalize large particles (for example, virus, bacteria, or cell debris).

2. **Clathrin-coated vesicles,** to take in small macromolecules.

3. **Pinocytosis** (cellular drinking), to internalize fluids in a vesicle called **caveola** coated by **caveolin**.

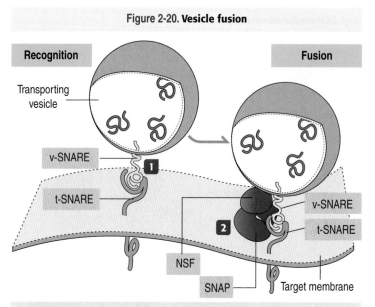

Figure 2-20. Vesicle fusion

Recognition		Fusion

Transporting vesicle

v-SNARE

t-SNARE

1

2

v-SNARE

t-SNARE

NSF

SNAP

Target membrane

Vesicle fusion involves two steps: Target membrane recognition and fusion

1 The **recognition** of the appropriate target membrane by a receptor on the **vesicle** (**v-SNARE**) and a receptor on the **target membrane** (**t-SNARE**).

2 The **fusion** of the vesicle and target membranes. Fusion involves two proteins:
1. **NSF** (for *N*-ethylmaleimide-**s**ensitive **f**usion);
2. **SNAP**s (for **s**oluble **N**SF **a**ttachment **p**roteins). NSF and SNAP are recruited by SNAREs (for **SNAP** **re**ceptors) to induce fusion of vesicle and target membranes.

Most cells take in fluid by pinocytosis but phagocytosis is the function of specialized cells, including **macrophages**. We study them in Chapter 4, Connective Tissue (macrophages), Chapter 6, Blood and Hematopoiesis (white blood cells), and Chapter

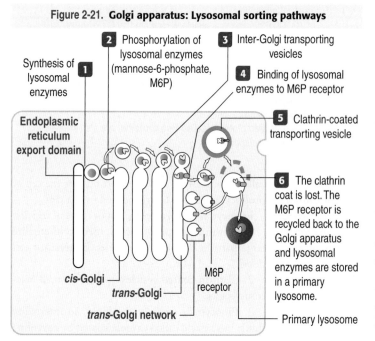

Figure 2-21. Golgi apparatus: Lysosomal sorting pathways

1 Synthesis of lysosomal enzymes

2 Phosphorylation of lysosomal enzymes (mannose-6-phosphate, M6P)

3 Inter-Golgi transporting vesicles

4 Binding of lysosomal enzymes to M6P receptor

5 Clathrin-coated transporting vesicle

Endoplasmic reticulum export domain

6 The clathrin coat is lost. The M6P receptor is recycled back to the Golgi apparatus and lysosomal enzymes are stored in a primary lysosome.

cis-Golgi

trans-Golgi

trans-Golgi network

M6P receptor

Primary lysosome

10, Immune-Lymphatic System (macrophages and antigen-presenting cells). Phagocytic cells scavenge cell remnants during apoptosis and aging blood cells in spleen.

In addition to hydrolytic enzymes, the lysosome has **membrane-bound transporters** that allow digested products, such as amino acids, sugars, and nucleotides, to reach the cytosol for reuse or excretion. The lysosomal membrane also contains an **ATP-dependent pump** that provides H$^+$ into the lysosome to maintain an acidic environment (see Figure 2-22).

We now review the **lysosomal sorting pathway** (see Figure 2-21) to highlight important steps:

1. Lysosomal enzymes and lysosomal membrane proteins are synthesized in the endoplasmic reticulum and transported through the Golgi apparatus to the TGN.

2. An important event in the *cis*-Golgi is the tagging of lysosomal enzymes with a specific phosphorylated sugar group, M6P, that is recognized in membranes of the *trans*-Golgi region by the corresponding receptor, M6P receptor.

3. The tagging enables enzymes to be sorted and packaged into transport vesicles that leave the TGN network toward the lysosomes.

There is a coordinated genetic control of lysosomal biogenesis. The transcription factor **TFEB** (for transcription factor EB) regulates the expression of several lysosomal genes and also coordinates the formation of autophagosomes and their fusion with lysosomes. Overexpression of TFEB increases the formation of new lysosomes during starvation and autophagy.

Phagocytosis, endocytosis, and macroautophagy

The different **endocytic pathways** of various materials to lysosomes are illustrated in Figure 2-22. Note some important events and corresponding terminology:

1. **Lysosomes can fuse with endosomes, autophagosomes and phagosomes** to form a hybrid organelle (a **secondary lysosome**) by mixing their contents so the bulk of the endocytic cargo can be degraded.

2. **Endocytic vesicles fuse with early endosomes and late endosomes** before cargo delivery to a lysosome. Endosomes lack M6P receptor, a distinction from lysosomes.

3. The fusion of late endosomes with lysosomes results in a depletion of lysosomes. Lysosomes are recovered from the hybrid organelle by the removal of late endosome constituents. Small vesicular structures with lysosomal protease content in the presence of proton-pumping ATPase and Ca^{2+} bud off from hybrid organelles.

4. Phagocytosis is essential for specialized cells to take up invading pathogens, fragments of apoptotic cells and other foreign material into the **phagosome**. Lysosomes fuse with phagosomes to form a hybrid

Figure 2-22. **Types of lysosomes**

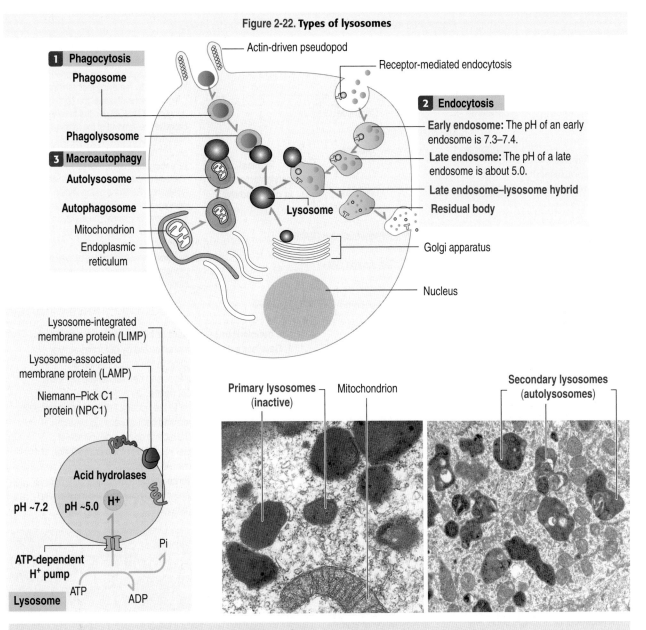

1 Phagocytosis
Phagosome

Actin-driven pseudopod

Receptor-mediated endocytosis

2 Endocytosis

Phagolysosome

3 Macroautophagy

Autolysosome

Autophagosome

Mitochondrion

Endoplasmic reticulum

Lysosome

Early endosome: The pH of an early endosome is 7.3–7.4.

Late endosome: The pH of a late endosome is about 5.0.

Late endosome–lysosome hybrid

Residual body

Golgi apparatus

Nucleus

Lysosome-integrated membrane protein (LIMP)

Lysosome-associated membrane protein (LAMP)

Niemann–Pick C1 protein (NPC1)

Acid hydrolases

pH ~7.2   pH ~5.0   H+

ATP-dependent H+ pump

Pi

Lysosome

ATP   ADP

Primary lysosomes (inactive) — Mitochondrion

Secondary lysosomes (autolysosomes)

Lysosomes

Lysosomes are organelles, which contain about 40 types of hydrolytic enzymes active in an acidic environment (pH ~5.0). Their function is to degrade proteins, nucleic acids, oligosaccharides, and phospholipids.

The surrounding membrane has three characteristics:
1. It separates hydrolytic enzymes from the cytosol.
2. It harbors transport proteins (**LIMPs, LAMPs,** and **NPC1**) that translocate hydrolases into the lysosome (LIMPs and LAMPs) and with a role in lysosomal cholesterol efflux (NPC1).
3. It contains an **ATP-dependent H+ pump** to maintain an acidic intralysosomal environment.

There are three major pathways for the intracellular degradation of materials. Extracellular particles can be taken up by phagocytosis and endocytosis. Aged intracellular components are degraded by macroautophagy, a non-selective process.

1 Phagocytosis: The material that is phagocytosed is enclosed within a phagosome, which then fuses with a lysosome to form a phagolysosome. Abundant phagosomes are observed in macrophages.
2 Endocytosis: The material that is endocytosed is delivered to an early endosome and then to a late endosome. The membrane of a late endosome contains the H+ pump, the early endosome does not. A lysosome fuses with the late endosome (hybrid organelle) to begin its catalytic function. Endocytosis is characteristic of receptor-mediated endocytosis of polypeptide hormones and growth factors. A residual body is a structure containing partially digested material.
3 Macroautophagy: Macroautophagy starts with the endoplasmic reticulum enclosing an aged cell component to form an autophagosome, which then fuses with a lysosome to form a hybrid autolysosome and its content is digested.

Figure 2-23. Lysosomal storage disorders: Tay-Sachs disease

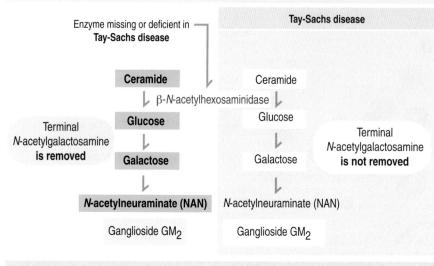

Tay-Sachs disease

Enzyme missing or deficient in
Tay-Sachs disease

Ceramide

Ceramide

β-*N*-acetylhexosaminidase

Glucose

Glucose

Terminal
N-acetylgalactosamine
is removed

Terminal
N-acetylgalactosamine
is not removed

Galactose

Galactose

N-acetylneuraminate (NAN)

N-acetylneuraminate (NAN)

Ganglioside GM$_2$

Ganglioside GM$_2$

Gangliosides are sphingolipids rich in carbohydrates predominant in the nervous system. Gangliosides are degraded inside lysosomes by removing their terminal sugars.

In **Tay-Sachs disease**, the content of ganglioside M$_2$ (GM$_2$) in the brain is high because the removal of the terminal *N*-acetylgalactosamine is slow or it does not occur. **The missing lysosomal enzyme is β-*N*-acetylhexosaminidase.**

Affected neurons contain lipids within lysosomes. Retarded psychomotor development and weakness are early symptoms. Dementia, blindness, and death usually occur within 3 years after birth. Amniocentesis to assay for β-*N*-acetylhexosaminidase activity during prenatal development can diagnose the inherited autosomal recessive disease.

Lysosomal storage disorders

The hydrolytic enzymes within lysosomes are involved in the breakdown of sphingolipids, glycoproteins, and glycoproteins into soluble products. These molecular complexes can derive from the turnover of intracellular organelles or enter the cell by phagocytosis.

A number of genetic diseases lacking lysosomal enzymes result in the progressive accumulation within the cell of partially degraded insoluble products. This condition leads to clinical conditions known as **lysosomal storage disorders** (LSDs).

These disorders include broad categories depending on the major accumulating insoluble product and the substrate for the defective lysosomal enzyme.

The **deficient breakdown of sphingolipids** is the cause of:
1. **Gaucher's disease**, characterized by defective activity of a **glucocerebrosidase**, resulting in the accumulation of glucocerebrosides in the spleen and central nervous system.
2. **Niemann-Pick disease**, defined by a defective **sphingomyelinase**, leading to the accumulation of sphingomyelin and cholesterol in the spleen and central nervous system.
3. **Tay-Sachs disease**, characterized by a deficiency of β-*N*-acetylhexosaminidase, resulting in the accumulation of gangliosides in the central nervous system.

The **diagnosis** of these three lysosomal storage disorders is based on the detection of enzymatic activity in leukocytes and cultured fibroblasts of the patients.

Gaucher's disease
(or glucosylceramide lipidosis) is characterized by three forms:

Type 1 does not have a neurologic component and occurs in late childhood or adolescence. It affects bone, liver, spleen (see histologic image) and lungs.

Type 2 occurs early one, at 2 to 3 months of age, is associated with neurologic symptoms and death usually occurs by 2 years of age.

Type 3 is seen in the adult, is associated with hepatosplenomegaly and has a neurologic component. Death occurs by the fourth decade.

One of the many macrophages (**Gaucher cells**) with cytoplasmic accumulation of lipid material and eccentric nucleus

Red pulp

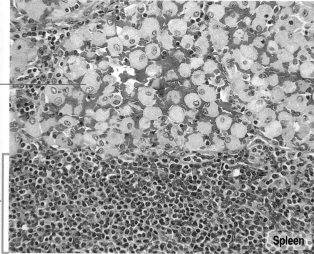

Spleen

phagolysosome where cargo degradation occurs.

5. **Macroautophagy** involves the degradation of cytoplasmic components of the cell itself enclosed in an **autophagosome** that fuses with a lysosome to form a hybrid **autolysosome**.

Note that autophagosomes are structures with a double membrane. The sequestered cytoplasmic material is degraded into small molecules transported across the lysosomal membrane to the cytosol for reuse (for example, the production of new proteins). Autophagy is essential for cell survival and cell homeostasis. We discuss molecular aspects of authophagy in Chapter 3, Cell Signaling.

6. Exocytosis of lysosomal contents can take place

by lysosomal membrane fusion with the plasma membrane in the presence of SNAREs. Some of the cells types with "secretory" lysosomes are included in Box 2-D.

Clinical significance: Lysosomal storage disorders
Lysosomal storage disorders or **diseases** (LSDs) are caused by the progressive accumulation of cell membrane components within cells because of a hereditary deficiency of enzymes required for their breakdown.

Loss of function mutations in proteins critical for lysosomal function (such as lysosomal enzymes, lysosomal integral membrane proteins, proteins involved in post-translational modifications and trafficking of lysosomal proteins) cause substrate accumulation and lysosomal storage defects.

Two-thirds of LSDs lead to neuronal dysfunction and neurodegeneration. Many affected individuals are clinically normal at birth, an indication that impaired lysosomal function does not affect neuronal function during early brain development.

You may like to focus again on Figure 2-21 and Figure 2-22 to review the pathway followed by hydrolytic enzymes to reach the lysosome and the highlights of the sequence steps of endocytosis, phagocytosis and macroautophagy. These cellular trafficking pathways are the bases for understanding the clinical value of **substrate reduction therapy** (**SRT**; using inhibitors to block substrate synthesis), and **enzyme replacement therapy** (**ERT**; utilizing the membrane-associated M6P receptor for the uptake of lysosomal enzymes into cells after intravenous administration).

An important pathologic concept to grasp is that **defective lysosomal enzyme carriers, rather than the lysosomal storage material itself, can account for the cellular pathologies in LSDs.** Essentially, not all lysosomal diseases are storage disorders.

For example, a deficiency in the lysosomal integral membrane protein type 2 (LIMP-2), with binding affinity to the lysosomal enzyme β-glucocerebrosidase (β-Glc) in the endoplasmic reticulum and involved in the transport of β-Glc to the lysosome, is deficient in **Gaucher disease**. Consequently, LIMP-2 mutations determine a reduction in lysosomal β-Glc activity.

Furthermore, the microscopic analysis of biopsied tissues and biochemical evaluation of accumulated cellular substrates can determine the underlying enzymatic defects of lysosomal storage material. For example, deficiencies in the proteins Niemann-Pick disease type C1 and C3 (NPC1 and NPC2), required for the release of cholesterol from the lysosome, causes cholesterol accumulation in **Niemann-Pick disease**. In other words, although the precise transport mechanism is sometimes not entirely clear, a cellular storage defect can often offer clues for SRT and ERT clinical strategies.

Additional details on the mechanism leading to **Tay-Sachs disease** (**GM2 gangliosidosis**), characterized by an increased in brain weight due to gliosis (proliferation of glial cells in response to damage of the central nervous system), neuronal atrophy (caused by abnormal whorled lysosomes displacing the nucleus) and axonal defects abnormalities in myelin), are presented in Figure 2-23.

Mitochondria

The mitochondrion (Greek *mito*, thread; *chondrion*, granule) is a highly compartmentalized organelle. The primary function of mitochondria is to house the enzymatic machinery for oxidative phosphorylation resulting in the production of adenosine triphosphate (**ATP**) and the release of energy from the metabolism of molecules.

A mitochondrion consists of an **outer mitochondrial membrane** and an **inner mitochondrial membrane** creating an **intermembrane space** between them (Figure 2-24). The inner mitochondrial membrane surrounds a large compartment called the **matrix**. The matrix is partitioned by infoldings of the inner mitochondrial membrane known as **cristae**. Cristae amplify the inner mitochondrial membrane on which ATP synthesis takes place.

Mitochondria contain DNA and RNA, including ribosomes to synthesize some of their own proteins in the matrix. Only 1% of mitochondrial proteins are encoded by mitochondrial DNA. Most of mitochondrial proteins are encoded by nuclear genes, synthesized in cytosol ribosomes and imported into mitochondria by targeting signals that are recognized by the **translocase of the outer mitochondrial membrane complex** (**TOM**) on the outer mitochondrial membrane. TOM is the most common entry route of imported mitochondrial proteins. **Targeting polypeptide signals** and **chaperones** (Hsp60 and Hsp70)

Box 2-D | Secretory lysosomes

- Some cell types can store and secrete lysosomal hydrolytic enzymes. An example is the **osteoclast**, a cell involved in bone resorption following the release of the enzyme **cathepsin K** from a lysosomal compartment into the acidic environment created by an H^+-ATPase pump within the Howship's lacuna (see Chapter 4, Connective Tissue).
- Secretory lysosomes are found in cells of the immune system. **CD8$^+$ cytolytic T cells** and **natural killer cells** secrete the pore-forming protein **perforin** by means of secretory lysosomes to destroy target cells (see Chapter 10, Immune-Lymphatic System).
- **Melanocytes** have **melanosomes**, lysosomal-related organelles transporting **melanin** to keratinocytes to produce skin and hair pigmentation (see Chapter 11, Integumentary System).
- A number of autosomal human genetic diseases give rise to immune dysfunction and defects in pigmentation (for example, **Chediak-Higashi syndrome** and **Griscelli syndrome 1** (see Chapter 11, Integumentary System).

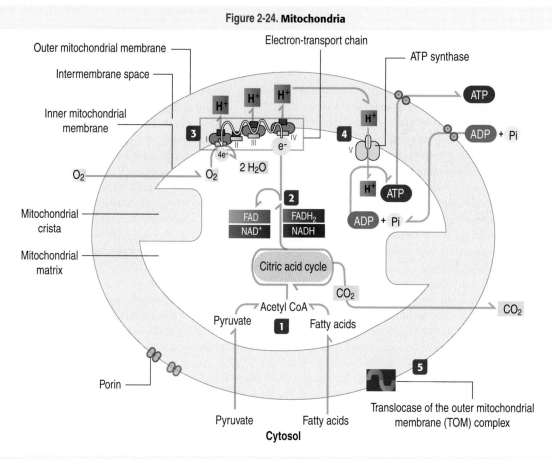

Figure 2-24. Mitochondria

Outer mitochondrial membrane

Intermembrane space

Inner mitochondrial membrane

Electron-transport chain

ATP synthase

Mitochondrial crista

Mitochondrial matrix

H^+ H^+ H^+

3 II III IV

$4e^-$ e^-

O_2 O_2 2 H_2O

H^+ **4** V

H^+ ATP

ADP + Pi

ATP

ADP + Pi

2

FAD	FADH$_2$
NAD$^+$	NADH

Citric acid cycle

CO_2 CO_2

Acetyl CoA

Pyruvate **1** Fatty acids

Porin

5

Pyruvate Fatty acids Translocase of the outer mitochondrial membrane (TOM) complex

Cytosol

1 **Pyruvate** and **fatty acids** are transported from the cytosol to the mitochondria across the outer mitochondrial membrane and converted in the mitochondrial matrix into **acetyl coenzyme A** (acetyl CoA) by enzymes of the **citric acid cycle**. CO_2 is released from the cell as waste metabolic product. **Porins** are permeable aqueous channels located along the outer mitochondrial membrane.

2 The citric acid cycle generates high-energy electrons carried by nicotinamide adenine dinucleotide (**NADH**) and flavin adenine dinucleotide (**FADH$_2$**). These carriers donate their high-energy electrons to the electron-transport chain located in the inner mitochondrial membrane. High-energy electrons produced during the **citric acid cycle** are utilized by the electron-transport chain complexes (I, II, III, and IV) to produce adenosine triphosphate (**ATP**).

3 The electrons pass along the chain to molecular oxygen (O_2) to form water (H_2O). Four electrons and four H$^+$ added to each molecule of O_2 for two molecules of H_2O.

4 As electrons travel through the chain, energy in the form of protons (H$^+$) is released across the inner membrane into the intermembrane space. The resulting H$^+$ gradient drives ATP synthesis by **ATP synthase** (V) utilizing adenosine diphosphate (ADP) and Pi coming from the cytosol. ATP produced in the mitochondrial matrix is released into the cytosol.

5 Translocase of the outer mitochondrial membrane (TOM) is the common entry gate of precursor proteins encoded by the cell nucleus. After passing through the TOM complex, the precursors use different mitochondrial pathways.

enable proteins to reach the matrix (Figure 2-25).

The outer mitochondrial membrane is permeable. It contains **porins**, proteins that form aqueous channels permeable to water-soluble molecules with a reduced molecular mass (less than 5 kd), such as sugars, amino acids and ions. The inner mitochondrial membrane is impermeable to the passage of ions and small molecules.

The inner mitochondrial membrane is the site of electron-transport and proton (H$^+$) pumping and contains the ATP synthase. Most of the proteins embedded in the inner mitochondrial membrane

are components of the **electron-transport chain**, involved in oxidative phosphorylation.

The mechanism of ATP synthesis is called **oxidative phosphorylation**. It consists in the addition of a phosphate group to adenosine diphosphate (ADP) to form ATP and the utilization of O_2. It is also called **chemiosmotic** because it involves a **chemical component** (the synthesis of ATP) and an **osmotic component** (the electron-transport and H$^+$ pumping process).

The mitochondrial matrix contains **pyruvate** (derived from carbohydrates) and **fatty acids** (derived

Figure 2-25. **Types of mitochondria and protein import**

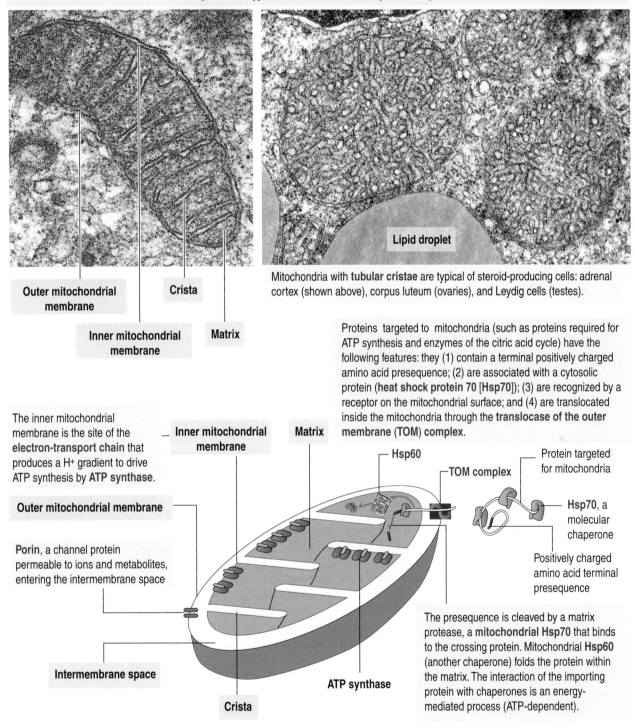

Outer mitochondrial membrane

Crista

Inner mitochondrial membrane

Matrix

Lipid droplet

Mitochondria with **tubular cristae** are typical of steroid-producing cells: adrenal cortex (shown above), corpus luteum (ovaries), and Leydig cells (testes).

Proteins targeted to mitochondria (such as proteins required for ATP synthesis and enzymes of the citric acid cycle) have the following features: they (1) contain a terminal positively charged amino acid presequence; (2) are associated with a cytosolic protein (**heat shock protein 70 [Hsp70]**); (3) are recognized by a receptor on the mitochondrial surface; and (4) are translocated inside the mitochondria through the **translocase of the outer membrane (TOM) complex.**

The inner mitochondrial membrane is the site of the **electron-transport chain** that produces a H+ gradient to drive ATP synthesis by **ATP synthase.**

Inner mitochondrial membrane

Matrix

Hsp60

TOM complex

Protein targeted for mitochondria

Outer mitochondrial membrane

Porin, a channel protein permeable to ions and metabolites, entering the intermembrane space

Hsp70, a molecular chaperone

Positively charged amino acid terminal presequence

The presequence is cleaved by a matrix protease, a **mitochondrial Hsp70** that binds to the crossing protein. Mitochondrial **Hsp60** (another chaperone) folds the protein within the matrix. The interaction of the importing protein with chaperones is an energy-mediated process (ATP-dependent).

Intermembrane space

ATP synthase

Crista

from fat). These two small molecules are selectively transported across the inner mitochondrial membrane and then converted to acetyl coenzyme A (**acetyl CoA**) in the matrix.

The citric acid cycle converts acetyl CoA to CO_2 (released from the cell as waste metabolic product) and high-energy electrons, carried by nicotinamide adenine dinucleotide (**NADH**)– and flavin adenine dinucleotide (**FADH$_2$**)–activated carrier molecules.

NADH and FADH$_2$ donate high-energy electrons to the electron-transport chain lodged in the inner mitochondrial membrane and become oxidized to NAD^+ and FAD. The electrons travel rapidly along the transport chain to O_2 to form water (H_2O).

As the high-energy electrons travel along the electron-transport chain, energy is released by proton pumps as H+ across the inner mitochondrial membrane into the intermembrane space. The H+

gradient then drives the synthesis of ATP.

Note that:

1. The inner mitochondrial membrane converts the energy derived from the high-energy electrons of NADH into a different type of energy: the high-energy phosphate bond of ATP.

2. The electron-transport chain (or **respiratory chain**) contributes to the consumption of O_2 as a phosphate group is added to ADP to form ATP.

The components of the **electron-transport chain** are present in many copies embedded in the lipid bilayer of the inner mitochondrial membrane. They are grouped into three large respiratory enzyme complexes in the receiving order of electrons:

1. The **NADH dehydrogenase complex**.
2. The **cytochrome b-c_1 complex**.
3. The **cytochrome oxidase complex**.

Each complex is a system that pumps H^+ across the inner mitochondrial membrane into the intermembrane space as electrons travel through the complex. If this mechanism did not exist, the energy released during electron transfer would produce heat.

Cyanide and **azide** are poisons that bind to cytochrome oxidase complexes to stop electron transport, thereby blocking ATP production.

Cytochrome c is a small protein that shuttles electrons between the cytochrome b-c_1 complex and the cytochrome oxidase complex.

When the cytochrome oxidase complex receives electrons from cytochrome c, it becomes oxidized and donates electrons to O_2 to form H_2O. Four electrons from cytochrome c and four H^+ from the aqueous environment are added to each molecule of O_2 to form $2H_2O$.

The H^+ gradient across the inner mitochondrial membrane is used to steer ATP synthesis. **ATP synthase** is a large enzyme embedded in the inner mitochondrial membrane involved in ATP synthesis.

H^+ flow back across the inner mitochondrial membrane down the electrochemical gradient through a hydrophilic route within ATP synthase to drive the reaction between ADP and Pi to produce ATP.

This reaction takes place in the enzymatic component of ATP synthase projecting into the mitochondrial matrix like a lollipop head. About 100 molecules of ATP are produced per second. About three H^+ cross the ATP synthase to form each molecule of ATP. ADP molecules produced by ATP hydrolysis in the cytosol are drawn back into mitochondria for recharging to ATP. ATP molecules produced in the mitochondrial matrix are released into the cytosol for their use.

Mitochondria participate in apoptosis, steroidogenesis, and thermogenesis

Mitochondria participate in three significant functions:

1. **Programmed cell death** or **apoptosis**.
2. **Steroidogenesis** (production of steroid hormones).
3. **Thermogenesis**.

Concerning apoptosis, mitochondria contain **procaspases-2, -3, and -9** (precursors of proteolytic enzymes), **apoptosis initiation factor** (AIF), and **cytochrome c**. The release of these proteins in the cytosol initiates apoptosis. We come back to mitochondria and apoptosis in Chapter 3, Cell Signaling.

With regard to steroidogenesis, mitochondrial membranes contain enzymes involved in the synthesis of the steroids aldosterone, cortisol, and androgens. We discuss the participation of mitochondria in steroid production in Chapter 19, Endocrine System, and Chapter 20, Spermatogenesis.

Concerning thermogenesis, most of the energy from oxidation is dissipated as heat rather than converted to ATP. **Uncoupling proteins** (UCPs), members of the superfamily of mitochondrial anion-carrier proteins present in the mitochondrial inner membrane, mediate the regulated discharge of H^+ (called **proton leak**), resulting in the release of heat. Proton leak across the mitochondrial inner membrane is mediated by **UCP-1**.

UCP-1 is present in the mitochondrial inner membrane of **brown adipocytes**. Its role is to mediate regulated **thermogenesis** in response to cold exposure (see section on adipose tissue in Chapter 4, Connective Tissue).

Clinical significance: Mitochondrial maternal inheritance

Mitochondrial DNA (mtDNA) is transmitted by the mother (maternal inheritance). Both males and females can be affected by mitochondrial diseases, but males seem unable to transmit the disorder to the offspring. Maternal inheritance of mtDNA is regarded as an evolutionary advantageous event because of the potential damage of mtDNA by reactive oxygen species (ROS) involved in fertilization.

Motile sperm reaching the oviduct for fertilization eliminate their mtDNA before fertilization, leaving vacuolar mitochondria. Yet, residual mtDNA in the fertilizing sperm can be unevenly distributed in the zygote during early embryo development. Consequently, paternal mtDNA inheritance effects cannot be disregarded.

Myoclonic epilepsy with ragged red fibers (MERRF) is characterized by generalized muscle weakness, loss of coordination (**ataxia**), and multiple seizures. The major complications are respiratory and cardiac failure because the respiratory and cardiac muscles are affected. Muscle cells and neurons are the most affected because of their need for significant amounts of ATP to function.

Figure 2-26. Peroxisome

1 Proteins for peroxisomes are synthesized by free cytosolic ribosomes and then transported into peroxisomes. Phospholipids and membrane proteins are also imported to peroxisomes from the endoplasmic reticulum.

2 Matrix proteins are targeted to the interior of the peroxisome by **peroxisome targeting signals (PTSs)** bound to **peroxin 5 (PEX5)**. **Peroxisomal membrane proteins** are targeted to the peroxisomal membrane by the shuttling receptor **PEX19** bound to the PTS. The complex docks to **PEX16** at the peroxisomal membrane.

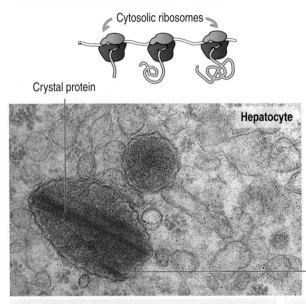

Cytosolic ribosomes

Crystal protein

Hepatocyte

Peroxisome

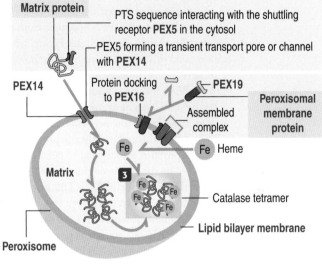

Matrix protein

PTS sequence interacting with the shuttling receptor **PEX5** in the cytosol

PEX5 forming a transient transport pore or channel with **PEX14**

PEX14

Protein docking to **PEX16**

PEX19

Peroxisomal membrane protein

Assembled complex

Fe — Fe Heme

Matrix

3

Fe Fe Fe Fe Fe

Catalase tetramer

Lipid bilayer membrane

4 **Zellweger syndrome**, one of the four diseases within the group of **peroxisome biogenesis disorders**, is a fatal condition caused by the defective assembly of peroxisomes due to mutations in genes encoding PEX1, PEX2, PEX3, PEX5, PEX6, and PEX12.

Newly synthesized peroxisomal enzymes remain in the cytosol and eventually are degraded. Cells in patients with Zellweger syndrome contain **empty peroxisomes**.

3 **Catalase**, the major protein of the peroxisome, decomposes H_2O_2 into H_2O.

Catalase is a tetramer of apocatalase molecules assembled within the peroxisome.

Heme is added to each monomer to prevent it from moving back into the cytosol across the peroxisomal membrane.

Peroxisomes are abundant in the liver (hepatocytes).

Histologic preparations of muscle biopsies of individuals with MERRF display a peripheral red-stained material corresponding to **aggregates of abnormal mitochondria**, giving a ragged appearance to red muscle fibers. **MERRF is caused by a point mutation in a mitochondrial DNA gene encoding tRNA for lysine**. An abnormal tRNA causes a deficiency in the synthesis of proteins required for electron transport and ATP production.

Three maternally inherited mitochondrial diseases affect males more severely than females:

1. About 85% of individuals affected by **Leber's hereditary optic neuropathy (LHON)** are male. The disease is confined to the eye. Individuals suffer a sudden loss of vision in the second and third decades of life.

2. **Pearson marrow-pancreas syndrome** (anemia and mitochondrial myopathy observed in childhood).

3. **Male infertility**. Almost all the energy for sperm motility derives from mitochondria.

Peroxisomes

Peroxisomes, organelles present in all mammalian cells except erythrocytes, contain at least one oxidase and one catalase for the β-oxidation of **very long chain fatty acids (VLCFA)** as well as to the α-oxidation of branched-chain fatty acids. In addition, several of the peroxisomal pathways are conducive to the production of hydrogen peroxide, and its subsequent breakdown by catalase.

Peroxisomes are bound by single membranes enclosing a dense matrix containing metabolic enzymes, substrates and cofactors forming **crystalloid cores** (Figure 2-26). The peroxisomal membrane is a lipid bilayer with embedded peroxisomal membrane proteins synthesized on free ribosomes in the cytosol and then imported into peroxisomes.

Peroxisome biogenesis can take place through two pathways:

1. *De novo* generation pathway: Peroxisomes can be formed from **pre-peroxisomal vesicles** budding off from the endoplasmic reticulum and fusing with each other to form **mature peroxisomes**.

2. **Fission generation pathway**: Pre-existing peroxisomes can generate new peroxisomes by growth

and fission (mediated by PEX11, dynamin-related proteins and a fission protein), using new proteins and lipids derived from vesicles originated in the endoplasmic reticulum.

Peroxisomes contain different peroxisomal proteins, including **peroxins (PEX)**, involved in peroxisomal biogenesis. PEX are receptor proteins shuttling between the cytosol and the peroxisome after binding to the **peroxisome targeting signal (PTS)** of the protein to be imported. PEX uncouple from the PTS before the protein is imported (see Figure 2-26). PEX are encoded by *PEX* genes, some of them associated with **peroxisome biogenesis disorders**. To date, 15 human *PEX* genes have been identified.

Peroxisome biogenesis involves the targeting and import into pre-existing peroxisomes of **matrix proteins** and **peroxisomal membrane proteins.**

Matrix proteins are targeted to peroxisomes from the cytosol by the PTS recognized in the cytosol by the shuttling receptor PEX5. The import process consists of three consecutive steps (see Figure 2-26):

1. PEX5 interacts with PEX14 at the peroxisomal membrane forming a **transport pore or channel.**

2. Matrix proteins dock and translocate inside the peroxisome across the transport pore.

3. The importing pore disassembles and PEX5 recycles back to the cytosol for another import round.

Peroxisomal membrane proteins are targeted to peroxisomal membranes through the interaction of the PTS with the shuttling receptor PEX19 in the cytosol and then the docking of this complex to PEX16 bound to the peroxisomal membrane. Peroxisomal membrane proteins can also be targeted to peroxisomes by insertion into the membrane of the sendoplasmic reticulum followed by vesicular transport to peroxisomes.

Catalase (peroxidase), a major peroxisome enzyme, decomposes hydrogen peroxide into water or is utilized to oxidize other organic compounds (uric acid, amino acids, and fatty acids). Peroxisomes, like mitochondria, degrade fatty acids. The oxidation of fatty acids by mitochondria and peroxisomes provides metabolic energy.

Peroxisomes participate in the biosynthesis of lipids. Cholesterol and dolichol are synthesized in both peroxisomes and endoplasmic reticulum. In the human liver, peroxisomes are involved in the synthesis of **bile acids** (derived from cholesterol).

Peroxisomes contain enzymes involved in the synthesis of **plasmalogens**, phospholipids in which one of the hydrocarbon chains is linked to glycerol by an ether bond (instead of an ester bond). **Plasmalogens contribute more than 80% of the phospholipid content of myelin in brain** and are involved in the protection of cells from ROS reduced damage.

Clinical significance: Peroxisomal disorders
The significant role that peroxisomes play in human metabolism is highlighted by devastating disorders attributed to defects in peroxisome biogenesis and function.

There are two types of peroxisomal disorders:

1. **Single peroxisomal enzyme deficiencies**, caused by mutations of genes encoding peroxisomal enzymes.

2. **Peroxisomal biogenesis disorders (PBDs)**, determined by mutations of *PEX* genes, involved in peroxisome biogenesis and function. Most PBDs consist of severe neurologic dysfunction due to central nervous system malformations, myelin abnormalities, and neuronal degeneration.

PBDs include four diseases: **infantile Refsum disease (IRD)**, **neonatal adrenoleukodystrophy (NALD)**, **rhizomelic chondrodysplasia**, and the cerebrohepatorenal **Zellweger syndrome (ZS)**.

All peroxisomal disorders, except X-linked NALD, are autosomal recessive. A defect in the transport of VLCFA across the peroxisomal membrane is the cause of NALD. Accumulation of VLCFA in the adrenal cortex causes adrenal atrophy. Incorporation of VLCFA in myelin disrupts its structure.

IRD, NALD and ZS are caused by mutations of *PEX* genes. Therefore, they share a common pathogenic feature: deficient peroxisomal assembly.

ZS (see Figure 2-26) is the most severe within the group of PBDs. It is fatal within the first year of life. The primary defect is the mutation of the *PEX1, PEX2, PEX3, PEX5, PEX6 AND PEX12* genes encoding proteins necessary for the import of membrane and matrix proteins.

The clinical characteristics of ZS include:

1. **Dysmorphic facial features** (prominent forehead, broad nasal bridge, large fontanelles and flat supraorbital ridges).

2. **Hepatomegalia** (enlargement of the liver; hepatic fibrosis and cirrhosis). Hepatocellular peroxisomes are absent or severely decreased.

3. **Neurologic abnormalities** (defective neuronal migration). Affected children may show at birth muscle hypotonicity, an inability to move, and a failure to suck or swallow.

We have seen than peroxisomes are the sites for oxidation of VLCFA. So increased level of this molecule in blood plasma is an indication of ZS. Prenatal analysis for VLCFA and plasmalogen are used from amniotic tests and absence of peroxisomes in liver biopsy is another indicator of ZS.

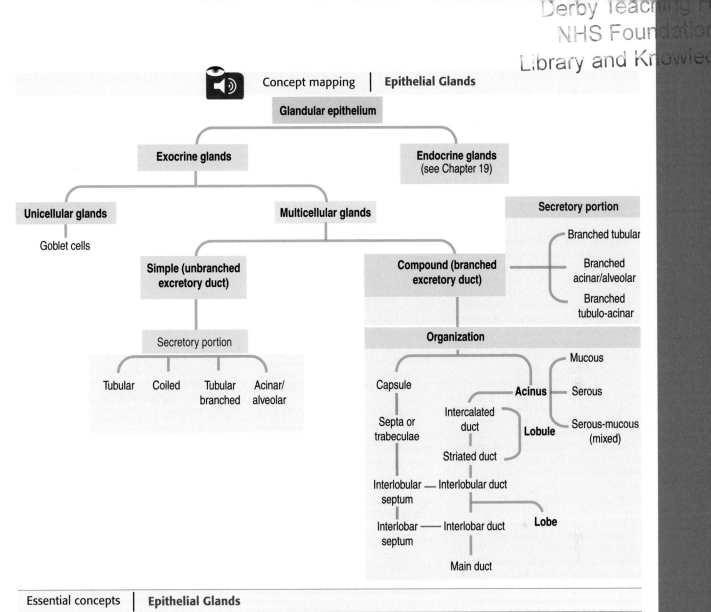

Concept mapping | **Epithelial Glands**

Essential concepts | **Epithelial Glands**

• There are two types of glands:
  (1) Exocrine glands, that secrete their products through ducts onto an internal or external space.
  (2) Endocrine glands, that lack ducts and secrete their products into the blood.

• There are different types of exocrine glands:
  (1) Unicellular (a single cell, for example, the goblet cell of the intestinal or respiratory epithelium).
  (2) Multicellular glands. Multicellular glands form the parenchyma of organs such as the pancreas and the prostate.

• Exocrine glands have two structural components:
  (1) The secretory units, whose cells synthesize and secrete a product called secretion.
  (2) The excretory ducts, that transport the secretion to an epithelial surface.

• Glands with a single unbranched duct are called simple glands. Larger glands have a branched duct system and are called branched or compound glands. Branched glands are surrounded by a connective tissue capsule that

sends partitions or septa (together with blood vessels and nerve fibers) into the mass of the gland, which becomes partitioned into lobes.
  Thinner septa divide lobes into smaller units called lobules. Duct branches are present in the interlobar, interlobular, and intralobular connective tissue septa as interlobar ducts, interlobular ducts, and intercalated/striated ducts connected to the secretory units (acini).

• A simple gland can be straight, coiled, or branched (the term "branched" refers to the secretory unit, but not to the excretory duct). The gland is called simple tubular, simple coiled, or simple branched tubular.
  A gland with a secretory unit with a rounded form is called simple acinar or alveolar gland. The secretory unit can be tubular and the gland is called simple tubular.

• In a branched acinar gland, the acini are lined by secretory cells surrounding a narrow lumen. The acini and alveoli of the salivary glands and the mammary glands contain contractile basket-like myoepithelial cells. The acinar cellular organization can be part of the wall of short tubular ducts and also form their endings. The

gland is then called branched tubuloacinar gland (for example, mammary gland).

• Glands can secrete:
  (1) Mucus (mucous glands).
  (2) Proteins (serous glands).
  (3) A combination of mucus and proteins (mixed glands). Mixed glands contain both mucous and serous cells, the latter forming a crescentic or half-moon–shaped region (serous demilunes) capping the acini.

• When a gland releases its product by exocytosis, it is called merocrine gland (such as the pancreas). A gland in which the apical region of a cell is pinched off and released into the lumen is called apocrine gland (an example is the mammary gland). When the whole cell is released and is part of the secretion, the gland is called holocrine gland (such as the sebaceous glands of the skin).

Cytomembranes and the plasma membrane. Intracellular membranes, called cytomembranes, separate diverse cellular processes into compartments. Cytomembranes are components of the endoplasmic reticulum and Golgi apparatus. The nucleus, mitochondria, lysosomes, and peroxisomes are bound by cytomembranes and are called organelles. The nucleus and mitochondria are surrounded by a double membrane; lysosomes and peroxisomes are surrounded by a single membrane. Lipids and glycogen are not membrane-bound and are called inclusions.

• The plasma membrane is the structural and functional boundary of a cell. It separates the intracellular environment from the extracellular space.

The plasma membrane consists of lipids and proteins. Phospholipids (phosphatidylcholine, phosphatidylethanolamine, phosphatidylserine and sphingomyelin) form a bilayer consisting of outer and inner leaflets. Phosphatidylinositol is another phospholipid, with an important role in cell signaling, localized to the inner leaflet of the plasma membrane. Cholesterol is inserted into the phospholipid bilayer and modulates membrane fluidity.

Integral membrane proteins are transmembrane proteins spanning the lipid bilayer through α-helical regions. Peripheral membrane proteins are indirectly linked to the plasma membrane by protein-protein interactions. Peripheral membrane proteins exposed to the cytosol interact with cytoskeletal components. The extracellular portion of integral and peripheral membrane proteins is generally glycosylated. A glycocalyx coats the surface of most epithelial cells.

• Freeze-fracture combined with electron microscopy enables the visualization of intramembranous proteins. A frozen and fractured specimen is used to produce a thin metal replica of the two surfaces of a membrane and its two artificial faces.

The lipid bilayer membranes are frozen at liquid nitrogen temperature (−196°C) and "split" along the middle of the hydrophobic core. As a result, two complementary halves of a membrane are produced and the hydrophobic face exposed.

Each half or monolayer of the membrane has a surface and a face. The original monolayer facing the extracellular environment exhibits a surface designated extracellular surface (ES); the corresponding area facing the hydrophobic core of the membrane becomes the extracellular face (EF) and was created artificially after "splitting" the membrane. The original monolayer facing the intracellular or protoplasmic environment has a surface called the protoplasmic surface (PS); the corresponding area facing the hydrophobic core is the protoplasmic face (PF).

Membrane proteins tend to remain associated to the cytoplasmic or protoplasmic leaflet and appear as particles on the P fracture face (PF). Pits complementary to the particles and representing the space once occupied by the protein, are present on the E fracture face (EF).

• **Transporters** include carrier proteins and channel proteins. They mediate the selective passage of molecules across the cell membrane. Gases (such as oxygen and carbon dioxide) can cross membranes by passive diffusion. Glucose, electrically charged molecules, and small ions require transport proteins and channel proteins for facilitated diffusion across a membrane.

Channel proteins can be ligand-gated channels (gates which open upon ligand binding) or voltage-gated channels (which open in response to changes in electrical potential across the membrane).

• Cytomembranes, represented in part by the endoplasmic reticulum and Golgi apparatus, establish a continuum between intracellular compartments and the extracellular space. The lumen of cisternae, tubules, and vesicles is continuous with the extracellular space. The membranous wall separates the luminal compartment from the cytosolic compartment. Products released into the lumen of the endoplasmic reticulum are transported to the Golgi apparatus by transporting vesicles and eventually to the cell exterior by exocytosis.

Imagine that there is a continuum in this secretory sequence and that all the luminal spaces are virtually interconnected and continuous with the cell exterior. The freeze-fracture technique takes advantage of this virtual arrangement if you consider that the membrane splitting knife can jump from the exocytoplasmic leaflet of a membrane-bound vesicle to the exocytoplasmic leaflet of the plasma membrane exposed to the environment.

• The cytomembranes of the endoplasmic reticulum can be associated with ribosomes (rough endoplasmic reticulum) or lack ribosomes (smooth endoplasmic reticulum). The rough endoplasmic reticulum participates in protein synthesis and transport to the Golgi apparatus.

The smooth endoplasmic reticulum has a significant role in cell detoxification reactions required for converting harmful lipid-soluble substances into water-insoluble material. The smooth endoplasmic reticulum is generally adjacent to glycogen deposits and lipid droplets (nonmembrane-bound inclusions).

Proteins targeted to the nucleus, mitochondria, or peroxisomes and cytoskeletal proteins are synthesized on free ribosomes (polyribosomes) and released in the cytosol.

• The **Golgi apparatus** is involved in the attachment of oligosaccharides to proteins and lipids involving glycosyltransferases. It consists of four compartments:
  (1) A *cis*-Golgi, the receiving site from the endoplasmic reticulum.
  (2) A *medial*-Golgi, interposed between the *cis*-Golgi and *trans*-Golgi.
  (3) A *trans*-Golgi, the exit site.
  (4) A *trans*-Golgi network (TGN), a sorting site.
  Golgins, a family of coiled-coil proteins,

stabilize the flattened stacks of sacs of the Golgi apparatus.

Clathrin-coated vesicles are observed during lysosomal sorting and endocytosis. COP- (for coat proteins) coated vesicles are seen trafficking between Golgi stacks (COPI) and from the endoplasmic reticulum to the Golgi (COPII).

Golgi-derived products can be released from the cell by exocytosis or sorted to lysosomes. Exocytosis can be continuous and does not require a triggering signal. This form of secretion is called constitutive secretion.

Certain classes of Golgi-derived cargos are stored into secretory granules and released by exocytosis under control of a chemical or electrical signal. This mechanism is called facultative or regulated secretion.

The sorting mechanism of lysosomes involves two steps:
  (1) The insertion of mannose-6-phosphate (M6P) into glycoproteins destined to lysosomes.
  (2) The presence of the transmembrane M6P receptor protein in the membrane of the transporting vesicle. This mechanism separates M6P-containing lysosomal enzymes from other glycoproteins.

• **Lysosomes** are organelles surrounded by a single membrane. Two types of **lysosomes** are recognized:
  (1) Primary lysosomes (inactive), the primary storage of lysosomal enzymes.
  (2) Secondary lysosomes (autolysosomes), engaged in a catalytic process.
  Lysosomes target internalized extracellular material for degradation through the activity of lysosomal hydrolytic enzymes operating at an acidic pH (5.0).
  There are three major pathways involved in intracellular degradation of materials:
  (1) **Phagocytosis** (the pagocytosed material is enclosed within a phagosome that fuses with a lysosome to form a phagolysosome).
  (2) **Endocytosis** (the endocytosed material is delivered to an early endosome and then to a late endosome that fuses with a lysosome).
  (3) **Macroautophagy** (the endoplasmic reticulum encloses an aged cell component to form an autophagosome that fuses with a lysosome to form an autolysosome).

Specific cells have secretory lysosomes (hydrolytic enzymes are secreted). Examples include:
  (1) The osteoclast, involved in bone resorption.
  (2) Cytolytic T cells and natural killer cells, engaged in the destruction of target cells.
  (3) Melanocytes, releasing melanin derived from melanosomes (lysosome-related organelles) to produce skin and hair pigmentation.

Lysosomal storage disorders occur when hereditary deficiency in lysosomal enzymes prevents the normal breakdown of cell components that accumulate progressively in cells.. Examples are **Tay-Sachs disease** (accumulation of ganglioside GM_2 in the brain), **Gaucher's disease** (accumulation of glucocerebrosides in the spleen and central nervous system), and **Niemann-Pick disease** (accumulation of sphingomyelin in the spleen and central nervous system).

Internalization of material occurs by the process of endocytosis. The reverse process is called exocytosis. Endocytosis involves the internalization of virus or bacteria by phagocytosis using clathrin-independent vesicles and the uptake of small macromolecules utilizing clathin-coated vesicles.

Receptor-mediated endocytosis of a ligand requires a plasma membrane receptor. The ligand-receptor complex is internalized by the process of receptor-mediated endocytosis.

This process involves:

(1) The formation of a clathrin-coated pit (to concentrate ligand-receptor complexes in a small surface area).

(2) The invagination of the coated pit to form a coated vesicle.

(3) The pinching off of the coated vesicle from the plasma membrane.

(4) Transport of the vesicle to an endosome.

(5) Removal of the clathrin coat before fusion of the vesicle with the endosome.

(6) Recycling back of the receptor-containing vesicle to the plasma membrane.

This transport mechanism is defective in **familial hypercholesterolemia** because of a mutation in the gene encoding the receptor for the ligand low-density lipoprotein (LDL).

High levels of cholesterol in blood plasma result in the formation of atheromas in the intima of blood vessels.

• The fusion of a vesicle to a target membrane requires:

(1) Recognition of a specific target membrane site.

(2) Vesicle-membrane fusion.

Vesicle-membrane fusion is mediated by two interacting cytosolic proteins:

(1) NSF (for *N*-ethylmaleimide–sensitive fusion).

(2) SNAP (for soluble NSF attachment protein).

NSF and SNAP bind to specific membrane receptors called SNARE (for SNAP receptors). SNARE ligands on the membrane of the transporting vesicle (vesicle-SNARE, v-SNARE) and the target membrane receptor (target-SNARE, t-SNARE) are responsible for docking the vesicle to the target membrane. Following docking, NSF and SNAP are recruited to produce fusion.

• **Mitochondria** are organelles surrounded by a double membrane. The outer mitochondrial membrane is separated by an intermembrane space from the inner mitochondrial membrane. The inner membrane folds into cristae extending into the mitochondrial matrix.

The inner mitochondrial membrane harbors the electron-transport chain and adenosine triphosphate (ATP) synthase.

The mitochondrial matrix contains most of the enzymes of the citric acid cycle. Mitochondria participate in apoptosis (programmed cell death), steroidogenesis, and thermogenesis in brown fat.

Mitochondria are transmitted by the mother (maternal inheritance). Males do not transmit mitochondria at fertilization. Both males and females can be affected by mitochondrial disease, but males never transmit the disorder.

Myoclonic epilepsy with ragged red fibers (MERRF) manifests with muscle weakness, loss of coordination (ataxia), and multiple sizures. MERRF is caused by a mutation in a mitochondrial DNA gene encoding lysine tRNA.

Maternally inherited mitochondrial diseases affecting males more severely than females are **Leber's hereditary optic neuropathy (LHON)**, **Pearson marrow-pancreas syndrome**, and **male infertility**.

• **Peroxisomes** are organelles surrounded by a single membrane. Peroxisomes contain crystaloid cores containing oxidases and catalases, enzymes that oxidize organic compounds and decompose hydrogen peroxide into water. Peroxisomes are involved in the synthesis of bile acids and biosynthesis of lipids.

Peroxisome biogenesis involve two pathways:

(1) De novo generation pathway, consisting in pre-peroxisomal vesicles budding off from the endoplasmic reticulum and fusing to form mature peroxisomes.

(2) The fission generation pathway, derived from the fission and growth of a pre-existing peroxisome.

Peroxisomes contain peroxins, receptor proteins shuttling between the cytosol and the peroxisome, matrix proteins, and peroxisomal membrane proteins.

How do peroxins work? Peroxins bind to the peroxisome targeting signal of the matrix proteins to be imported across transporting pores or channels.

In fact, peroxisomal membrane proteins build the pores serving as transporting gates for proteins that need to gain access inside the peroxisome.

Thus, mutations in the peroxin encoding genes (about 15 genes in human) determine peroxisome biogenesis disorders (PBDs).

There are two types of PBDs:

(1) Single peroxisomal enzyme deficiencies.

(2) PBDs caused by mutations of peroxin genes.

Neurologic dysfunction–caused by malformations of the central nervous system, myelinization abnormalities and neuronal defective migration–characterize PBDs.

Zellweger syndrome, a severe and fatal cerebrohepatorenal disorder, is determined by the failure of peroxisomal enzymes to be imported from the cytosol into the peroxisome. Deficient peroxisomal assembly in hepatocytes is associated with fibrosis and cirrhosis.

Additional PBDs include infantile Refsum disease, neonatal adrenoleukodystrophy and rhizomelic chondrodysplasia.

3. Cell Signaling

Cells respond to extracellular signals produced by other cells or by themselves. This mechanism, called cell signaling, allows cell-cell communication and is necessary for the functional regulation and integration of multicellular organisms. Our discussion in this chapter not only provides the basis for understanding cell signaling pathways but serves also as an introduction to General Pathology, including aging, cell senescence and neoplasia and the role of cell injury in human disease, including necrosis, apoptosis and necroptosis and the mechanisms of autophagy, ubiquitin-proteasome proteolysis and mitophagy.

Signaling molecules can transmit information by acting as **ligands** binding to **receptors** expressed by their target cells. Some signaling molecules can act on the cell surface after binding to cell surface receptors; others can cross the plasma membrane and bind to intracellular receptors in the cytoplasm and nucleus.

An understanding of the molecular aspects of cell signaling is clinically relevant to uncover potential targets of novel therapeutics for the treatment of metabolic dysfunctions and diseases.

Types of cell signaling and feedback action

Signaling molecules use different routes to reach their targets (Figure 3-1):

1. **Endocrine cell signaling** involves a signaling molecule, a **hormone**, secreted by an **endocrine cell and transported through the circulation to act on distant target cells**. An example is the steroid hormone testosterone produced in the testes, that stimulates the development and maintenance of the male reproductive tract using the vascular route. **Neuroendocrine cell signaling** is a specific form of endocrine signaling involving a product secreted by a nerve cell into the bloodstream and acting on distant cells.

2. **Paracrine cell signaling** is mediated by a molecule acting **locally** to regulate the behavior of a **nearby cell**. A paracrine molecule diffuses over small distances to reach a target cell.

Neurotransmitter or synaptic cell signaling is a specialized form of paracrine signaling. Neurons secrete neurotransmitters that diffuse short distances and bind to receptors on target cells.

Juxtacrine cell signaling is **contact-dependent signaling**. It requires the contact of proteins of adjacent plasma membranes for signaling to occur. An example is the **immunologic synapse**, a combination of cell-cell adhesion and signaling that takes place when the plasma membranes of an antigen-presenting cells and a T cell are in contact with each other.

3. **Autocrine cell signaling** is defined by **cells responding to signaling molecules that they themselves produce**. A classic example is the response of cells of the immune system to foreign antigens or growth factors that trigger their own proliferation and differentiation. Abnormal autocrine signaling leads to the unregulated growth of cancer cells.

Cell signaling mechanisms require a feedback action. In general, after a signaling molecule binds to its receptor, the target cells exerts either a **negative** or **positive feedback** action to regulate the release of the targeting hormone (Figure 3-2).

Hormones and ligands

Binding of a hormone or ligand to its receptor initiates a cascade of intracellular reactions (called s**ignal transduction**) to regulate critical functions such as **embryonic and fetal development, cell proliferation and differentiation, movement, metabolism, and behavior.**

Ligands include:
1. **Steroid hormones.**
2. **Peptide hormones, neuropeptides and growth factors.**
3. **Nitric oxide.**
4. **Neurotransmitters.**
5. **Eicosanoids.**

Steroid hormones

Steroid hormones (Box 3-A) are lipid-soluble molecules that diffuse across the phospholipid bilayer of the plasma membrane of target cells, bind to intracellular receptors in the cytoplasm, enter the nucleus as **steroid hormone-receptor complexes** and bind to specific receptor sites on chromatin (specifically **hormone-response elements** at the DNA) to activate or repress gene expression (Figure 3-3). Steroid receptors are members of the **steroid receptor superfamily.**

Steroid hormones are synthesized from **cholesterol** and include **testosterone, estrogen, progesterone and corticosteroids**. Steroid hormones are usually secreted as they are synthesized and are transported in the bloodstream bound to protein carriers.

Testosterone, estrogen, and progesterone are **sex steroids** and are produced predominantly by the gonads. In the **androgen insensitivity syndrome** (also

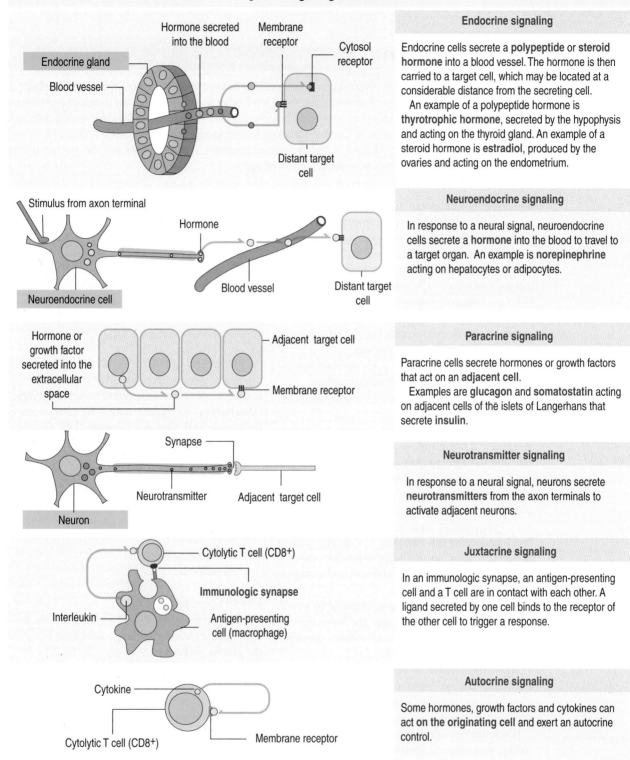

Figure 3-1. Signaling mechanisms

Endocrine signaling

Endocrine cells secrete a **polypeptide** or **steroid hormone** into a blood vessel. The hormone is then carried to a target cell, which may be located at a considerable distance from the secreting cell.

An example of a polypeptide hormone is **thyrotrophic hormone**, secreted by the hypophysis and acting on the thyroid gland. An example of a steroid hormone is **estradiol**, produced by the ovaries and acting on the endometrium.

Neuroendocrine signaling

In response to a neural signal, neuroendocrine cells secrete a **hormone** into the blood to travel to a target organ. An example is **norepinephrine** acting on hepatocytes or adipocytes.

Paracrine signaling

Paracrine cells secrete hormones or growth factors that act on an **adjacent cell**.

Examples are **glucagon** and **somatostatin** acting on adjacent cells of the islets of Langerhans that secrete **insulin**.

Neurotransmitter signaling

In response to a neural signal, neurons secrete **neurotransmitters** from the axon terminals to activate adjacent neurons.

Juxtacrine signaling

In an immunologic synapse, an antigen-presenting cell and a T cell are in contact with each other. A ligand secreted by one cell binds to the receptor of the other cell to trigger a response.

Autocrine signaling

Some hormones, growth factors and cytokines can act **on the originating cell** and exert an autocrine control.

known as the **testicular feminization syndrome, Tfm**), there is a mutation in the gene expressing the **testosterone receptor** such that the receptor cannot bind the hormone, and hence the cells do not respond to the hormone. Although genetically male, the individual develops the secondary sexual characteristics of a female. We discuss the androgen insensitivity syndrome in Chapter 21, Sperm Transport and Maturation. We discuss their functional roles in Chapter 20, Spermatogenesis, and Chapter 22, Follicle Development and The Menstrual Cycle.

Corticosteroids are synthesized in the cortex of the adrenal gland and include two major classes: **glucocorticoids**, which stimulate the production of

Figure 3-2. Positive and negative feedback

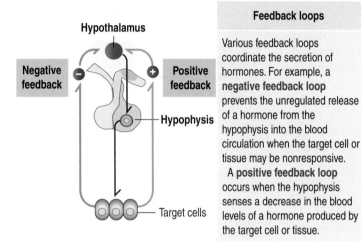

Feedback loops

Various feedback loops coordinate the secretion of hormones. For example, a **negative feedback loop** prevents the unregulated release of a hormone from the hypophysis into the blood circulation when the target cell or tissue may be nonresponsive.

A **positive feedback loop** occurs when the hypophysis senses a decrease in the blood levels of a hormone produced by the target cell or tissue.

glucose, and **mineralocorticoids**, which act on the kidneys to regulate water and salt balance. We address structural and functional aspects of corticosteroids in Chapter 19, Endocrine System.

There are types of cell signaling molecules structurally and functionally distinct from steroids but act on target cells by binding to intracellular receptors after entering the cell by diffusion across the plasma membrane. They include **thyroid hormones** (produced in the thyroid gland to regulate development

Figure 3-3. Mechanism of action of steroid hormones

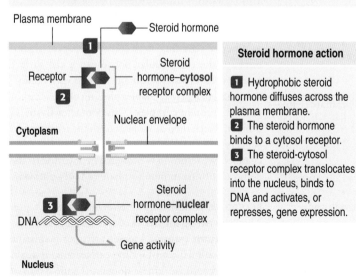

Steroid hormone action

1 Hydrophobic steroid hormone diffuses across the plasma membrane.
2 The steroid hormone binds to a cytosol receptor.
3 The steroid-cytosol receptor complex translocates into the nucleus, binds to DNA and activates, or represses, gene expression.

and metabolism), **vitamin D₃** (regulates calcium metabolism and bone growth; see Chapter 19, Endocrine System), and **retinoids** (synthesized from vitamin A to regulate development, wound healing and epidermal differentiation; see Chapter 11, Integumentary System). The synthetic pathway of thyroid hormones and some of their actions are presented in Chapter 19, Endocrine System.

Peptide hormones and growth factors

A large variety of signaling molecules bind to cell surface receptors. Unlike intracellular steroid receptors, membrane bound receptors of peptide/protein ligands affect cellular function by transduction signaling. Several groups are recognized:

1. **Peptide hormones** (see Box 3-B): This group includes insulin, glucagon and hormones secreted by the hypophysis and peptides secreted by neurons (**enkephalins** and **endorphins**), that decrease pain responses in the central nervous system. See Chapter 18, Neuroendocrine System, and Chapter 19, Endocrine System, for a detailed discussion of peptide hormones and neuropeptides.

2. **Growth factors**: This group of peptides controls cell growth and differentiation (**nerve growth factor**, NGF; **epidermal growth factor**, EGF; **platelet-derived growth factor**, PDGF).

NGF is a member of a family of peptides called **neurotrophins**, which regulate the development and viability of neurons. EGF stimulates cell proliferation and is essential during embryonic development and in the adult. PDGF is stored in blood platelets and released during clotting.

Nitric oxide

Nitric oxide is a simple gas synthesized from the amino acid **arginine** by the enzyme **nitric oxide synthase**. It acts as a paracrine signaling molecule in the nervous, immune, and circulatory systems. Like steroid hormones, nitric oxide can diffuse across the plasma membrane of its target cells. Unlike steroids, nitric oxide does not bind to an intracellular receptor to regulate transcription. Instead, **it regulates the activity of intracellular target enzymes**.

The following are relevant characteristics of nitric oxide:

1. It is an unstable molecule with a limited half-life (seconds).

2. It has local effects.

3. A well-defined function of nitric oxide signaling is the **dilation of blood vessels**. For example, the release of the neurotransmitter acetylcholine from nerve cell endings in the blood vessel muscle cell wall stimulates the release of nitric oxide from endothelial cells.

Nitric oxide increases the activity of the second

messenger cyclic guanosine monophosphate (cGMP) in smooth muscle cells, which then causes cell muscle relaxation and blood vessel dilation (see Chapter 21, Sperm Transport and Maturation).

Nitroglycerin, a pharmacologic agent used in the treatment of heart disease, is converted to nitric oxide, which increases heart blood flow by dilation of the coronary blood vessels.

Neurotransmitters

These cell signaling molecules are released by neurons and act on cell surface receptors present in neurons or other type of target cells (such as muscle cells).

This group includes **acetylcholine**, **dopamine**, **epinephrine** (adrenaline), **serotonin**, **histamine**, **glutamate**, and γ-**aminobutyric acid** (GABA). The release of neurotransmitters from neurons is triggered by an **action potential**. Released neurotransmitters diffuse across the **synaptic cleft** and bind to surface receptors on the target cells.

There are differences that distinguish the **mechanism of action of neurotransmitters**. For example, **acetylcholine is a ligand-gated ion channel**. It induces a change in conformation of ion channels to control ion flow across the plasma membrane in target cells.

Neurotransmitter receptors can be associated to G proteins (see below), a class of signaling molecules linking cell surface receptors to intracellular responses.

Some neurotransmitters have a **dual function**. For example, epinephrine (noradrenaline; produced in the medulla of the adrenal gland) can act as a neurotransmitter and as a hormone to induce the breakdown of glycogen in muscle cells.

Eicosanoids

Eicosanoids are lipid-containing **inflammatory mediators** produced in leukocytes and other cells of the

immune system that, **in contrast to steroids, bind to cell surface receptors** (Box 3-C).

Prostaglandins, prostacyclin, thromboxanes, and **leukotrienes** are members of this group of molecules. They stimulate blood platelet aggregation, inflammatory responses, and smooth muscle contraction.

Leukotrienes (Greek *leukos*, white; Chemistry *triene*, a compound containing three double bonds) are synthesized by the oxidation of **arachidonic acid** by the enzyme arachidonate lipoxygenase.

During the synthesis of prostaglandins, arachidonic acid is converted to **prostaglandin H$_2$** by the enzyme **prostaglandin synthase**. This enzyme is inhibited by **aspirin** and **anti-inflammatory drugs. Inhibition of prostaglandin synthase by aspirin reduces pain, inflammation, platelet aggregation, and blood clotting** (prevention of strokes).

Cell surface receptors

Most ligands responsible for cell signaling and signaling transduction bind to receptors on the surface of target cells.

Ligand binding to hormone and growth factor receptors activates a series of **intracellular targets located downstream of the receptor**, in particular the activity of intracellular proteins, or, like neurotransmitter receptors, controlling the flow of water (**aquaporins**) and electrolytes across ligand-gated ion channels located on the plasma membrane.

Several functional aspects of specific cell surface receptors are relevant:

1. G protein–coupled receptors.
2. Receptor and nonreceptor tyrosine kinases.
3. Cytokine receptors.
4. Tyrosine phosphatases and serine–threonine kinases.

G protein–coupled receptors

Members of a large family of **G proteins** (more than 1000 guanine nucleotide–binding proteins) are present at the inner leaflet of the plasma membrane (Figure 3-4).

When a signaling molecule or **receptor ligand** binds to the extracellular portion of a cell surface receptor, its cytosolic domain undergoes a conformational change that enables binding of the receptor to the G protein complex. This contact activates G protein, which then dissociates from the receptor and triggers an intracellular signal to an enzyme or ion channel. We return to G protein when we discuss the cyclic adenosine monophosphate (cAMP) pathway.

Receptor and nonreceptor tyrosine kinases

There are two main classes of tyrosine kinases:

1. **Receptor tyrosine kinases** are transmembrane proteins with a ligand-binding extracellular domain and an intracellular kinase domain (Figure 3-5).

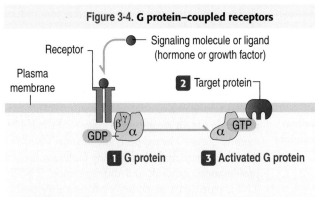

Figure 3-4. G protein–coupled receptors

Receptor

Signaling molecule or ligand (hormone or growth factor)

Plasma membrane

2 Target protein

β γ

α

GDP

α GTP

1 G protein

3 Activated G protein

Cytoplasm

G protein

1 G protein consists of three subunits (α, β, and γ). The α subunit regulates G protein activity.

In the resting state, guanosine diphosphate (GDP) is bound to the α subunit in a complex with β and γ subunits.

2 G protein transmits a cell surface signal to an adjacent **target molecule** (**adenylyl cyclase** or **ion channel**).

3 Hormone binding stimulates the release of GDP and its exchange for guanosine triphosphate (GTP).

The activated GTP-bound α subunit dissociates from β and γ and interacts with a target to induce a response.

---

2. **Nonreceptor tyrosine kinases are** located in the cytosol, nucleus and inner side of the plasma membrane.

Receptor tyrosine kinases (see Figure 3-5), in contrast with G protein–coupled receptors, are enzymes that phosphorylate substrate proteins on **tyrosine** residues. **EGF, NGF, PDGF, insulin and several growth factors are receptor tyrosine kinases.**

Most of the receptor tyrosine kinases consist of single polypeptides, although the insulin receptor

and other growth factors consist of a pair of polypeptide chains.

Binding of a ligand (such as a growth factor) to the extracellular domain of these receptors induces **receptor dimerization** that results in **receptor autophosphorylation** (the two polypeptide chains phosphorylate one another). The autophosphorylation of the receptors determines the binding of downstream signaling molecules to the tyrosine kinase domain.

Downstream signaling molecules bind to phosphotyrosine residues through **SH2 domains** (for Src homology 2). *Src* (for **sarcoma**) is a gene present in the tumor-producing Rous sarcoma virus and encodes a protein that functions as a tyrosine kinase.

The subfamily of **nonreceptor tyrosine kinases** includes the **Src family**, the **Fujinami poultry sarcoma/feline sarcoma** (Fps/Fes), and **Fes-related** (Fer) subfamily.

How do receptor and nonreceptor tyrosine kinases differ functionally from each other? In the absence of a ligand, receptor tyrosine kinases are unphosphorylated and monomeric, whereas nonreceptor tyrosine kinase is maintained in an inactive state by cellular inhibitor proteins. Activation occurs when the inhibitors are dissociated or by recruitment to transmembrane receptors that trigger autophosphorylation. Tyrosine kinase activity terminates when tyrosine phosphatases hydrolyze tyrosyl phosphates and by induction of inhibitory molecules.

The activity of tyrosine kinases in cancer cells can be affected by unregulated autophosphorylation in the absence of a ligand, by disrupting autoregulation of the tyrosine kinase, or by overexpression of receptor tyrosine kinase and/or its ligand. Abnormal activation of tyrosine kinases can stimulate the proliferation and anticancer drug resistance of malignant cells.

Tyrosine kinase activity can be inhibited by **ima-**

Figure 3-5. Tyrosine kinases

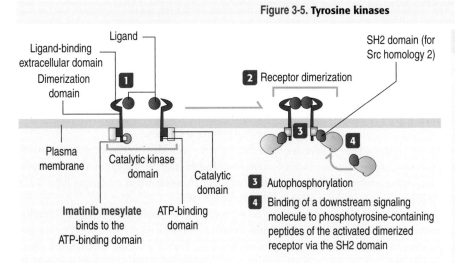

Ligand-binding extracellular domain

Ligand

Dimerization domain

1

Plasma membrane

Catalytic kinase domain

Catalytic domain

Imatinib mesylate binds to the ATP-binding domain

ATP-binding domain

2 Receptor dimerization

SH2 domain (for Src homology 2)

3

4

3 Autophosphorylation

4 Binding of a downstream signaling molecule to phosphotyrosine-containing peptides of the activated dimerized receptor via the SH2 domain

Cytoplasm

Tyrosine kinase receptor

Binding of a signaling molecule (for example, a growth factor) triggers **receptor dimerization** and **autophosphorylation** (the two polypeptide chains phosphorylate each other).

Downstream signaling molecules, with an **SH2 domain**, bind to phosphotyrosine-containing peptides of the activated receptor.

Imatinib mesylate binds to the adenosine triphosphate (ATP)-binding domain and prevents downstream signaling. Imatinib is used in the treatment of hematologic malignancies associated with tyrosine kinase dysregulation.

tinib mesylate, a molecule that binds to the adenosine triphosphate (ATP)–binding domain of the tyrosine kinase catalytic domain (see Figure 3-5). Imatinib can induce hematologic remission in patients with **chronic myeloid leukemia** and tumors caused by activated receptor tyrosine kinase PDGF receptor (**chronic myelomonocytic leukemia**) and c-kit (**systemic mastocytosis** and **mast cell leukemias**). Imatinib has been successfully used in the treatment of gastrointestinal solid tumors.

Cytokine receptors

This family of receptors consists of several subfamilies classified on their differing structure and activities. They include:

1. **Type I cytokine receptors** (to which interleukin ligands bind) and **type II cytokine receptors** (mainly for interferon ligands).

2. **Chemokine receptors and chemokine ligands** (CC, CXC, CX3C and CXCR1; the spacing between cysteins (C) determines the bound type of chemokine ligand).

3. **Tumor necrosis factor receptor superfamily.**

4. **Transforming growth factor-β (TGFβ) receptors.**

All cytokine receptors are associated with one or more members of the JAK-STAT pathway. Cytokines and cytokine receptors regulate hematopoiesis, immune responses, inflammation and tissue healing through the JAK-STAT pathway that, consequently, represents a potential therapeutic target. We discuss below details of the JAK-STAT pathway (see Figure 3-9).

Note that tyrosine kinases are not intrinsic components of the cytokine receptors but instead they are noncovalently linked. Upon ligand binding to the cytokine receptor, the activity of **intracellular tyrosine kinases** is stimulated. A ligand induces the dimerization and cross-phosphorylation of the associated JAK tyrosine kinases. Activated kinases phosphorylate tyrosine residues on the receptors, providing binding sites for downstream signaling molecules that contain the SH2 domain.

Hyperactivation mutations of the **type I cytokine receptor** signaling pathway are associated with **myeloproliferative diseases** and other hematologic defects. Abnormal activation of type I cytokine receptor correlates with **leukemias** and **lymphomas**. Defective **type II cytokine receptor** signaling are associated with immune deficiencies and inflammatory conditions.

The **chemokine receptor** consists of seven transmembrane domains with extracellular loops (determining ligand specificity) and G–coupled proteins at the intracellular domain (to enable downstream signaling). **Chemokine ligands** (CC, CXC, CX3C and CXCR1) are 8 kd to 14 kd in size. Binding of chemokine ligands to chemokine receptors induce chemotaxis (cell migration during homing) of target inflammatory cells. Migrating cells are attracted to sites with higher concentrations of chemokines (concentration gradient). We discuss homing and inflammation in Chapter 6, Blood and Hematopoiesis.

The **tumor necrosis factor receptor (TNFR) superfamily (death receptors)** belongs to the cytokine receptor group. The receptors and ligands (TNFL) of this family participate in signaling pathways for cell proliferation, survival, and differentiation. TNFR/TNFL participate in chronic inflammatory conditions such as rheumatoid arthritis (see Chapter 5, Osteogenesis) and inflammatory bowel disease (see Chapter 16, Lower Digestive Segment).

TNFR are active as self-assembling noncovalent trimers. The cytoplasmic domain of TNFR is the docking site of signaling molecules, such as the cytoplasmic adaptor protein TRAF (TNF receptor–associated factors) and Dead Domain (DD). From a functional perspective, adaptor proteins allow the regulatory flexibility of the dead receptors. As we discuss in the Apoptosis section of this chapter (see Figure 3-15), the Fas receptor has a DD domain that binds to the Fas-associated DD (FADD) protein adaptor that ultimately recruits and activates caspase 8 to cause cell death.

Finally, RANKL (for transmembrane receptor for activation of nuclear factor kappa B ligand), a member of the TNF superfamily with binding affinity to RANK receptor, has a significant tole in the development of osteoclasts from monocyte precursors (see Chapter 4, Connective Tissue). RANK/RANKL signaling regulates the differentiation of mammary gland alveolar buds into tubulo-alveolar structures in preparation for lactation.

Members of the **TGF-β** family are protein kinases that phosphorylate serine and threonine residues (rather than tyrosine). TGF-β inhibits the proliferation of their target cells. Like tyrosine kinase and cytokine receptors, binding of ligand to the TGF-β receptor induces receptor dimerization and the cytosolic serine or threonine kinase domain cross-phosphorylates the polypeptide chains of the receptor.

Receptors linked to tyrosine phosphatases and serine-threonine kinases

So far, we have seen that receptors with enzymatic activity stimulate protein phosphorylation at tyrosine residues. However other receptors have other enzymatic activities.

Some receptors associate with tyrosine phosphatases to remove phosphate groups from phosphotyrosine residues. Therefore, **they regulate the effect of tyrosine kinases by arresting signals initiated by tyrosine phosphorylation.**

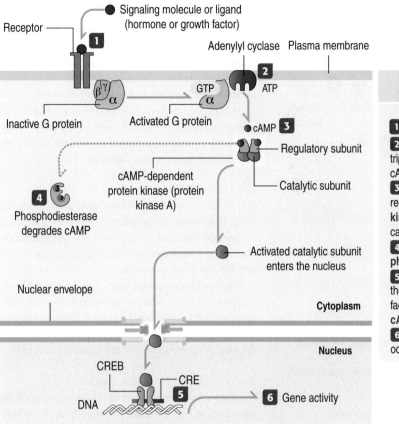

Figure 3-6. Cyclic adenosine monophosphate (cAMP) pathway

Signaling molecule or ligand (hormone or growth factor)

Receptor

Adenylyl cyclase   Plasma membrane

GTP   ATP

Inactive G protein   Activated G protein

cAMP

Regulatory subunit

cAMP-dependent protein kinase (protein kinase A)

Catalytic subunit

Phosphodiesterase degrades cAMP

Activated catalytic subunit enters the nucleus

Nuclear envelope

Cytoplasm

Nucleus

CREB

CRE

DNA

Gene activity

cAMP signaling pathway

1 A ligand binds to a cell receptor.
2 **Adenylyl cyclase**, activated by the guanosine triphosphate (GTP)–bound G protein subunit α, forms cAMP from ATP.
3 cAMP, the second messenger, binds to the regulatory subunits of **cAMP-dependent protein kinase (protein kinase A)** and releases the catalytic subunits.
4 cAMP is degraded by a **cAMP-dependent phosphodiesterase**.
5 The activated catalytic subunit translocates into the nucleus and phosphorylates the transcription factor **CREB (CRE-binding protein)** bound to the **cAMP response element (CRE)**.
6 Specific gene expression of inducible genes occurs.

Major signal transduction pathways

Upon ligand binding, most cell surface receptors stimulate intracellular target enzymes **to transmit and amplify a signal**. An amplified signal can be propagated to the nucleus to regulate gene expression in response to an external cell stimulus.

The major intracellular signaling pathways include:

1. The **cAMP pathway.**
2. The **cGMP pathway.**
3. The **phospholipid–Ca²⁺ pathway.**
4. The **Ca²⁺-calmodulin pathway.**
5. The **Ras** (for rat sarcoma virus), **Raf** (for rapidly accelerated fibrosarcoma) and **MAP** (for mitogen-activated protein) **kinase pathway.**
6. The **JAK-STAT** (for Janus kinase–signal transducers and activators of transcription) **pathway.**
7. The **NF-κB** (for nuclear factor involved in the transcription of the κ light chain gene in B lymphocytes) **transcription factor pathway.**
8. The **integrin-actin pathway.**

The cAMP pathway

The intracellular signaling pathway mediated by **cAMP** was discovered in 1958 by Earl Sutherland while studying the action of **epinephrine**, a hormone that breaks down glycogen into glucose before muscle contraction.

When epinephrine binds to its receptor, there is an increase in the intracellular concentration of cAMP. cAMP is formed from adenosine triphosphate (ATP) by the action of the enzyme **adenylyl cyclase** and degraded to adenosine monophosphate (AMP) by the enzyme **cAMP phosphodiesterase**. This mechanism led to the concept of a **first messenger** (epinephrine) mediating a cell-signaling effect by a **second messenger**, cAMP. The epinephrine receptor is linked to adenylyl cyclase by G protein, which stimulates cyclase activity upon epinephrine binding.

The intracellular signaling effects of cAMP (Figure 3-6) are mediated by the enzyme **cAMP-dependent protein kinase** (or **protein kinase A**). **In its inactive form, protein kinase A is a tetramer composed of two regulatory subunits** (to which cAMP binds) **and two catalytic subunits**. Binding of cAMP results in the **dissociation of the catalytic subunits**. Free catalytic subunits can phosphorylate **serine residues** on target proteins.

In the epinephrine-dependent regulation of glycogen metabolism, protein kinase A phosphorylates two enzymes:

1. **Phosphorylase kinase**, which in turn phosphorylates glycogen phosphorylase to break down glycogen into glucose-1-phosphate.

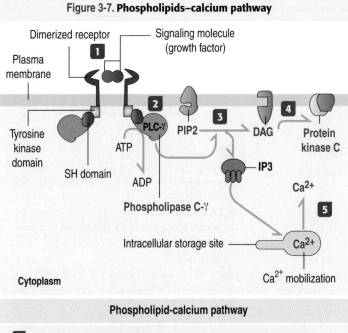

Figure 3-7. Phospholipids–calcium pathway

Phospholipid-calcium pathway

1 A signaling molecule binds and activates the protein kinase domains of a dimerized receptor.

2 Phospholipase C-γ (**PLC**-γ) contains an **SH domain** that mediates its association with activated receptor tyrosine kinases.

3 PLC-γ catalyzes the hydrolysis of **PIP2** to produce **diacylglycerol (DAG)** and **IP3**.

4 DAG activates **protein kinase C**.

5 IP$_3$ signals the **release of Ca^{2+}** from intracellular storage sites.

which activates cAMP-inducible genes.

Finally, cAMP effects can be direct, independent of protein phosphorylation. An example is the direct regulation of **ion channels in the olfactory epithelium. Odorant receptors** in sensory neurons of the olfactory epithelium are linked to G protein, which stimulates adenylyl cyclase to increase intracellular cAMP (see Chapter 13, Respiratory System).

cAMP does not stimulate protein kinase A in sensory neurons but acts directly to open Na$^+$ channels in the plasma membrane to initiate membrane depolarization and nerve impulses.

The cGMP pathway

cGMP is also a second messenger. It is produced from guanosine triphosphate (GTP) by guanylate cyclase and degraded to GMP by a phosphodiesterase. Guanylate cyclases are activated by nitric oxide and peptide signaling molecules.

The best characterized role of cGMP is in photoreceptor rod cells of the retina, where it converts light signals to nerve impulses. Chapter 9, Sensory Organs: Vision and Hearing, in the eye section, provides a detailed description of this cell signaling process.

The phospholipid–calcium pathway

Another second messenger involved in intracellular signaling derives from the phospholipid **phosphatidylinositol 4,5-bisphosphate** (PIP2) present in the inner leaflet of the plasma membrane (Figure 3-7).

The hydrolysis of PIP2 by the enzyme **phospholipase C (PLC)**, stimulated by a number of hormones and growth factors, produces two second messengers: **diacylglycerol** and **inositol 1,4,5-trisphosphate** (IP3). These two messengers stimulate two downstream signaling pathway cascades: **protein kinase C** and **Ca^{2+} mobilization**.

Two forms of PLC exist: **PLC-β** and **PLC-γ**. PLC-β is activated by G protein. PLC-γ contains SH2 domains that enable association with receptor tyrosine kinases. Tyrosine phosphorylation increases PLC-γ activity, which in turn stimulates the breakdown of PIP2.

Diacylglycerol, derived from PIP2 hydrolysis, activates members of the **protein kinase C** family (**protein serine and threonine kinases**).

Phorbol esters are tumor growth–promoting agents acting, like diacylglycerol, by stimulation of protein kinase C activities. Protein kinase C activates other intracellular targets such as protein kinases of the **MAP kinase pathway** to phosphorylate transcription factors leading to changes in gene expression and cell proliferation.

The calcium–calmodulin pathway

Although the second messenger diacylglycerol re-

2. **Glycogen synthase**, which is involved in the synthesis of glycogen. Phosphorylation of glycogen synthase prevents the synthesis of glycogen.

Note that an elevation of cAMP results in two distinct events: the breakdown of glycogen and, at the same time, a blockage of further glycogen synthesis. Also note that the binding of epinephrine to a single receptor leads to a signal amplification mechanism during intracellular signaling mediated by many molecules of cAMP. cAMP signal amplification is further enhanced by the phosphorylation of many molecules of phosphorylase kinase and glycogen synthase by the catalytic subunits dissociated from protein kinase A. It is important to realize that protein phosphorylation can be rapidly reversed by **protein phosphatases** present in the cytosol and as transmembrane proteins. These protein phosphatases can terminate responses initiated by the activation of kinases by removing phosphorylated residues.

cAMP also has an effect on the transcription of specific target genes that contain a regulatory sequence called the **cAMP response element (CRE)**. Catalytic subunits of protein kinase A enter the nucleus after dissociation from the regulatory subunits. Within the nucleus, catalytic subunits phosphorylate a transcription factor called **CRE-binding protein (CREB)**,

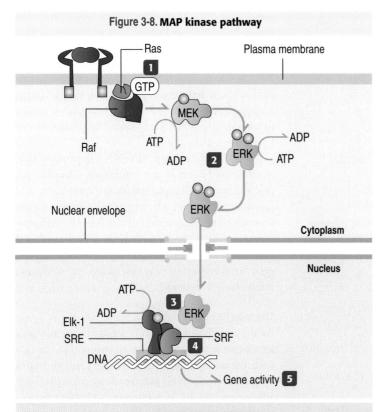

Figure 3-8. MAP kinase pathway

Plasma membrane

Ras

GTP

Raf

MEK

ATP

ADP

ERK

ADP

ATP

ERK

Nuclear envelope

Cytoplasm

Nucleus

ATP

ADP

Elk-1

SRE

ERK

SRF

DNA

Gene activity **5**

Activation of ERK-MAP kinase

1 Ligand binding to a growth factor receptor activates the small GTP-binding protein **Ras** (rat sarcoma virus), which interacts with **Raf** protein kinase.

2 Raf phosphorylates and activates **MEK** (MAP kinase or ERK kinase), which then activates **ERK** (extracellular signal–regulated kinase) by phosphorylation of tyrosine and threonine residues.

3 Activated ERK translocates into the nucleus where it phosphorylates the transcription factor **Elk-1**.

4 Activated Elk-1 binds to **SRE** (serum response element) forming a complex with **SRF** (serum response factor).

5 Gene induction occurs.

calcium-calmodulin pathway is described in Chapter 1, Epithelium.

The Ras, Raf, and MAP kinase pathway

This pathway involves evolutionarily conserved protein kinases (yeast to humans) with roles in cell growth and differentiation. **MAP kinases** are protein serine and threonine kinases activated by growth factors and other signaling molecules (Figure 3-8).

A well-characterized form of MAP kinase is the ERK family. Members of the **ERK** (for extracellular signal–regulated kinase) family act **through either protein tyrosine kinase or G protein–associated receptors**. Both cAMP and Ca^{2+}-dependent pathways can stimulate or inhibit the ERK pathway in different cell types.

The activation of ERK is mediated by two protein kinases: **Raf**, a protein serine or threonine kinase, which, in turn, activates a second kinase called **MEK** (for MAP kinase or ERK kinase). Stimulation of a growth factor receptor leads to the activation of the GTP-binding protein **Ras** (for rat sarcoma virus), which interacts with Raf. Raf phosphorylates and activates MEK, which then activates ERK by phosphorylation of serine and threonine residues. ERK then phosphorylates nuclear and cytosolic target proteins.

In the nucleus, activated ERK phosphorylates the transcription factors **Elk-1** (for E-26-like protein 1) and **serum response factor** (SRF), which recognize the regulatory sequence called **serum response element** (SRE).

In addition to ERK, mammalian cells contain two other MAP kinases called **JNK** and **p38 MAP kinases**. Cytokines, heat shock and ultraviolet irradiation stimulate JNK and p38 MAP kinase activation mediated by small GTP-binding proteins different from Ras. These kinases are not activated by MEK but by a distinct dual kinase called **MKK** (for MAP kinase kinase). JNK kinases have been associated with the development of insulin restistance.

A key element in the ERK pathway are the **Ras proteins**, a group of oncogenic proteins of tumor viruses that cause sarcomas in rats. Mutations in the Ras gene have been linked to human cancer. **Ras proteins are guanine nucleotide–binding protein with functional properties similar to the G protein α subunits** (activated by **GTP** and inactivated by guanosine diphosphate [**GDP**]).

A difference with G protein is that Ras proteins do not associate with βγ subunits. Ras is activated by **guanine nucleotide exchange factors** to facilitate the release of GDP in exchange for GTP. The activity of the Ras-GTP complex is terminated by GTP hydrolysis, which is stimulated by **GTPase-activating proteins**.

In human cancers, mutation of Ras genes results

mains associated with the plasma membrane, the other second messenger IP3, derived from PIP2, is released into the cytosol to activate ion pumps and free Ca^{2+} from intracellular storage sites. High cytosolic Ca^{2+} concentrations (from a basal level of 0.1 μM to an increased 1.0 μM concentration after cytosolic release) activate several Ca^{2+}-dependent protein kinases and phosphatases.

Calmodulin is a Ca^{2+}-dependent protein that is activated when the Ca^{2+} concentration increases to 0.5 μM. Ca^{2+}-calmodulin complexes bind to a number of cytosolic target proteins to regulate cell responses.

Note that Ca^{2+} **is an important second messenger** and that its intracellular concentration can be increased not only by its release from intracellular storage sites but also by increasing the entry of Ca^{2+} into the cell from the extracellular space. The regulation of myosin light chain kinase activity by the

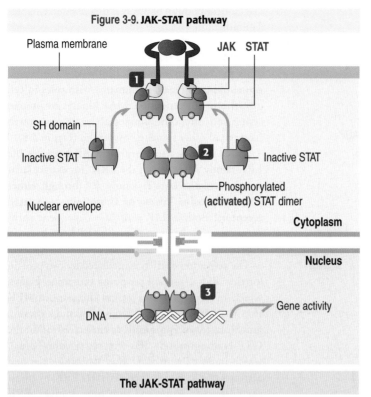

Figure 3-9. JAK-STAT pathway

Plasma membrane

JAK STAT

1

SH domain

Inactive STAT

2

Inactive STAT

Phosphorylated
(activated) STAT dimer

Nuclear envelope

Cytoplasm

Nucleus

3

DNA

Gene activity

The JAK-STAT pathway

1 Ligand binding to a cytokine receptor leads to the attachment of the inactive transcription factor STAT to the receptor-associated **JAK protein tyrosine kinase** via their **SH2 domains**.
2 Phosphorylated **STAT dimerizes**.
3 The phosphorylated STAT dimer translocates to the nucleus where it activates transcription of target genes.

in a breakdown failure of GTP and, therefore, the mutated Ras protein remains continuously in the active GTP-bound form.

The JAK-STAT pathway

The preceding MAP kinase pathway links the cell surface to the nucleus signaling mediated by a protein kinase cascade leading to the phosphorylation of transcription factors. The development of the erythroid lineage (red blood cell formation) in bone marrow stimulated by erythropoietin involves the JAK-STAT pathway (see Chapter 6, Blood and Hematopoiesis).

The JAK-STAT pathway provides a close connection between protein tyrosine kinases and transcription factors by directly affecting transcription factors (Figure 3-9).

STAT (for **signal transducers and activators of transcription**) **proteins** are transcription factors with an SH2 domain. STAT proteins are present in the **cytoplasm** in an inactive state. Stimulation of a receptor by ligand binding recruits STAT proteins, which bind to the cytoplasmic portion of receptor-associated **JAK protein tyrosine kinase** through their SH2 domain and become phosphorylated. Phosphorylated STAT proteins then dimerize and

translocate into the nucleus, where they activate the transcription of target genes.

NF-κB transcription factor pathway

NF-κB (for nuclear factor involved in the transcription of the κ light chain gene in B lymphocytes) is a transcription factor involved in immune responses in several cells. NF-κB is activated by protein kinase C (Figure 3-10).

In its **inactive state**, the NF-κB protein heterodimer is bound to the **inhibitory subunit** I-κB and the complex is retained in the cytoplasm. The phosphorylation of I-κB, triggered by protein kinase C, leads to the destruction of I-κB by the 26S proteasome and the release of NF-κB. The free NF-κB heterodimer translocates into the nucleus to activate gene transcription in response to immunologic and inflammatory signaling.

The integrin-actin pathway

As discussed in Chapter 1, Epithelium, integrin heterodimers are cell surface receptors that interact with the extracellular matrix (ECM) and the actin cytoskeleton through intermediary proteins. Cell adhesion to the ECM is essential for embryonic development, tissue stability, homing and homeostasis.

Actin relationship to integrins enables not only a mechanical role of F-actin in cell adhesion buy also the transmission of chemical signals inside the cell initiated at the ECM. Although integrin subunits α and β do not have an intrinsic kinase domain, they utilize associated proteins to transmit signals. Integrin-mediated interaction between the ECM and the actin cytoskeleton generally takes place at **focal adhesion** sites on the cell surface where integrins aggregate.

As shown in Figure 1-11 in Chapter 1, Epithelium, **talin** binds to the cytoplasmic domain of β subunit of integrin. Vinculin does not interact directly with β subunit tails, but interacts with talin and α-actinin; the latter interacts with F-actin. Focal adhesion kinase (FAK), which interacts with talin, phosphorylates their associated proteins, including paxillin. These interactions determine a conformational change that enables the extracellular domain of integrins to increase their binding affinity for extracellular ligands. As you recall, the β subunit of integrin binds to the RGD (arginine-glycine-aspartic acid) domain present in laminin and fibronectin, two ligands present in the ECM.

General Pathology: Specific signaling pathways

There are additional signaling pathways with important roles in embryonic and fetal development, body axis patterning, cell migration and cell proliferation. All of them contain numerous components subject to diverse regulatory steps and crosstalk mechanisms.

Figure 3-10. NF-κB transcription factor pathway

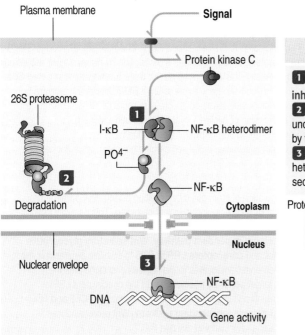

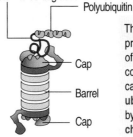

Activation of NF-κB

1 NF-κB is a protein heterodimer that, when associated with the **inhibitory subunit** I-κB, forms an **inactive complex** present in the cytoplasm.

2 When protein kinase C is stimulated, I-κB is phosphorylated and undergoes **phosphorylation-dependent degradation**, after ubiquitinization, by the 26S proteasome.

3 Removal of I-κB uncovers the nuclear localization sites of the NF-κB heterodimer that translocates into the nucleus, binds to specific DNA sequences, and regulates gene expression.

The **26S proteasome** is a giant multimeric protease found in the cytoplasm and nucleus of many cells. It consists of a barrel-shaped core, where proteins are degraded, and two caps that recognize proteins with attached **ubiquitin**. Ubiquitinized proteins are taken up by the 26S proteasome and degraded in the **chamber** of the barrel component.

Some of them use different downstream effectors activated by specific transcription factors.

Box 3-D presents the basic elements of:

1. **Hedgehog (HH) signaling.**
2. **Wingless (Wnt)/β-catenin signaling.**
3. **Notch signaling pathways.**

Box 3-E provides relevant features of:

4. **Transforming growth factor-β (TGF-β) signaling.**
5. **Bone morphogenetic protein (BMP) signaling,** a member of the TGF-β superfamily.
6. **Fibroblast growth factor (FGF) signaling.**

The clinical relevance and multifunctional nature of these pathways are represented by mutations leading to a number of diseases. We will refer to these pathways in several chapters.

General Pathology: Stem cell niches and stemness

Cells in the body show a remarkable range in ability to divide and grow. Some cells (for example, nerve cells and erythrocytes) reach a mature, differentiated state and usually do not divide. Such cells are referred to as **postmitotic cells.**

Other cells, called **stem cells**, show continuous division throughout life (for example, epithelial cells lining the intestine and stem cells that give rise to the various blood cell types). Many other cells are intermediate between these two extremes and remain quiescent most of the time but can be triggered to divide by appropriate signals. Liver cells are an example. If the liver is damaged, cell division can be triggered to compensate for the lost cells.

Stem cells have three properties (Figure 3-11):

1. **Self-renewal.**
2. **Proliferation.**
3. **Differentiation.**

These properties depend in part on the specific microenvironment where they reside, called **stem cell niche.** The stem cell niche provides stem cells the appropriate signals to remain into a quiescent state, preventing their progression towards final differentiation, or to become activated.

The interplay between the stem cell niche and the cellular state of a stem cell is governed by **stemness. Stemness is the characteristic gene expression profile of different stem cells not observed in ordinary, nonstem cells. Stemness genes** (enriched in stem cells) include *Nanog, Oct4, Myc, Sox2* and *Klf4* (Krüpel-like factor 4). The concept of stemness is relevant to the pursuit of reprogramming other cells into stem cells, the realm of regenerative medicine.

Stem cells have the potential to generate a large number of mature cells continuously throughout life. When stem cells divide by mitosis, some of the progeny differentiates into a specific cell type. Other progeny remains as stem cells within the stem cell niche.

The intestinal epithelium, the epidermis of the skin, the hematopoietic system, and spermatogenic cells of the seminiferous epithelium share this property. We discuss in detail the significance of stem cells in each of these tissues in the appropriate chapters.

Hedgehog (HH) signaling

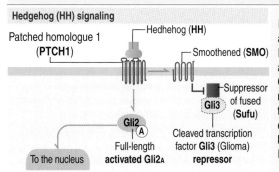

Key functions: Involved in switching Gli factors from transcriptional repressors into activators in the cytoplasm to allow HH-specific transcriptional events.

Pathway: HH proteins bind to the **receptor PTCH1** and then signal through **SMO**, a transmembrane protein, to regulate gene transcription by repressing or activating **Gli3**, a transcription factor. If SMO is not present, **Sufu** permits the **truncated Gli3 repressor** to block HH-specific gene expression. If SMO is present, activated **full-length Gli2A** translocates to the cell nucleus to regulate HH-specific gene expression (the expression of cyclin D, cyclin E, Myc and Patched).

HH ligands: Sonic (Shh), Indian (Ihh) and Desert (Dhh).

Pathogenesis: Gorlin syndrome, basal cell carcinoma (skin), medulloblastoma.

Wingless (Wnt)/β-catenin signaling

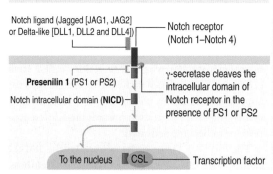

Key functions: Regulation of stem cell differentiation during development through β-catenin–dependent or β-catenin–independent pathways. This pathway integrates signals from other signaling pathways (FGF, TGF-β and BMP).

Pathway: In the β-**catenin-dependent pathway**, **Wnt secretory glycoprotein** binds to FZD receptor and **coreceptors LRP5/LRP6** to stabilize β-catenin in the cytoplasm. Then, β-catenin translocates to the nucleus and stimulates the transcription of Wnt target genes by interacting with the coactivators LEF1 (lymphoid enhancer-binding factor 1) and TCF (T cell factor) 1, TCF3 and TCF4 (not shown). In the β-**catenin independent pathway**, Wnt protein induces G protein-coupled phosphatidylinositol to activate **PKCδ**.

Pathogenesis: Point mutations of β-catenin in human colorectal tumors prevent phosphorylation of the kinase **GSK-3β** (see Chapter 16, Lower Digestive Segment).

Notch signaling

Key functions: The Notch signaling pathway mediated cell-cell communication (juxtacrine cellular signaling) by direct cell-cell contact.

Pathway: Following ligand binding (**JAG1, JAG2, DLL1, DDL3** and **DLL4**), **Notch receptors** (1 to 4) undergo proteolytic cleavage catalyzed by the γ-**secretase** complex that includes **presenilin 1** (PS1) or PS2. The intracellular domain (**NICD**) of Notch receptor is released from the plasma membrane and translocates to the nucleus. In the nucleus, NICD interacts with the transcription factor **CSL** and activates the transcription of target genes (such as *HES* and *HEY* family of transcription factors, not shown) to regulate the expression of other genes.

Pathogenesis: The nuclear accumulation of NICD is obsereved in acute lymphoblastic leukemia and lymphoma. Non-functional Notch receptor and ligands are implicated in the autosomal dominant form of cerebral arteriopathy.

Regenerative medicine by cell reprogramming

Following stress and injury, other tissues, such as the liver, muscle, and the nervous system, can regenerate mature cells. For example, bone marrow stem cells can produce muscle tissue as well as hematopoietic tissue in an appropriate host system (see Chapter 7, Muscle Tissue). Cultured stem cells of the central nervous system are capable of hematopoiesis in transplanted irradiated mouse recipients.

Recall that embryonic stem cells, forming the **inner cell mass (embryoblast)** of the early embryo (the blastocyst), have the potential to differentiate into almost all tissues and organs except the placenta.

Patient-derived pluripotent embryonic stem cells, matching genetically the own cells of a patient, provide an experimental source of medically useful differentiating tissues (such as pancreatic islets for the treatment of diabetes, skin for the treatment of burns

and wounds, regenerating cartilage for the treatment of arthritis, and endothelial cells for the repair of blood vessels affected by arteriosclerosis) and reduce the risk of rejection by the immune system.

Three cell reprogramming methods have been used in culture to produce patient-derived pluripotent embryonic stem cells:

1. To **induce programmed stem cells (iPS)** from mature cells grown in the presence of a transcription factor cocktail.

2. By **somatic cell nuclear transfer (SCNT)**, or **cloning**, consisting in the removal of the nucleus from an egg and replaced with the nucleus of a mature donor somatic cell. As the embryo develops, **nuclear transfer embryonic cells (NT ES)** are removed from the inner cell mass. Note that NT ES are genetically matched to the donor cell.

3. By collecting **blastocysts** from the inner cell

Transforming growth factor-β (TGF-β) signaling
Bone morphogenetic protein (BMP) signaling

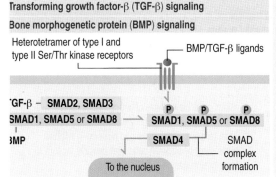

Key functions: BMPs are members of the TGF-β superfamily and regulate cell growth, differentiation, and development in a wide range of biological processes by activating **SMAD proteins**.
Pathway: BMP/TGF-β ligands induce the oligomerization of serine/ threonine receptor kinases and phosphorylation of the cytoplasmic signaling molecules **SMAD2** and **SMAD3** for the **TGF-β pathway**, or **SMAD1/5/8** for the **BMP pathway**. The common **SMAD4** transducer translocates to the nucleus. Activated SMADs regulate several biological processes by cell-specific modulation of transcription.
Pathogenesis: TGF-β is a tumor suppressor of pre-malignant cells but enhances invasion and metastasis of more advanced carcinomas. Mutations of *SMAD4* genes are frequent in gastrointestinal and pancreatic tumors. TGF-β and BMP can be involved in **epithelial-mesenchymal transition (EMT**; see Box 3-F).

Fibroblast growth factor (FGF) signaling

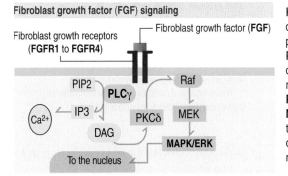

Key functions: The FGF signaling pathway is involved in the regulation of several developmental processes including patterning, morphogenesis, differentiation, cell proliferation or migration.
Pathway: Ligand binding to **tyrosine kinase FGF receptors 1 to 4**, results in the dimerization and subsequent transactivation by phosphorylation of tyrosine residues. The four main activated signaling pathways are: **JAK/STAT** (not shown), **Phosphatidylinositol 3-kinase** (not shown), Phospholipase C-γ (**PLCγ**) and **MAPK/ERK**. MAPK/ERK translocates to the nucleus and phosphorylates specific transcription factors. **PIP2**: phosphatidyl-inositol; **IP3**: inositol-triphosphate; **DAG**: diacylglycerol; **PKCδ**: protein kinase Cδ; **MEK**: MAP kinase or ERK kinase; **MAPK**: mitogen–activated protein kinase; **ERK**: extracellular signal–regulated kinase.

mass of embryos derived from in vitro fertilization (**IVF**) to generate unprogrammed embryonic stem cells (**IVF ES**).

Although human pluripotent stem cells are important for regenerative medicine, there are potential complication derived from the three available approaches. For example, human iPS are not fully reprogrammed and have **epigenetic differences** with NT ES and IVF ES. As we discuss in Chapter 20, Spermatogenesis, **epigenetic** defines the genomic modifications that impact on gene expression without modifying DNA sequence.

At present, IVF ES exhibit properties close to the intact blastocysts but they are **allogenic** (they exhibit properties close to the intact blastocysts but are genetically different and potentially incompatible when transplanted). NT ES are epigenetically stable (like IVF ES) and histocompatible (like iPS).

Cell culture

Cell culture techniques have been a powerful tool for examining the factors that regulate cell growth and for comparing the properties of normal and cancer cells.

Many cells grow in tissue culture, but some are much easier to grow than others. Culture medium contains **salts**, **amino acids**, **vitamins**, and a source of energy such as **glucose**. In addition, most cells require a number of **hormones** or **growth factors** for sustained culture and cell division. These factors are usually provided by addition of **serum** to the culture medium.

For some cell types the components supplied by serum have been identified, and these cells can be grown in **serum-free**, **hormone and growth factor–supplemented medium**. Some of these factors are hormones, such as insulin, and growth factors, including EGF, FGF, and PDGF.

When normal cells are placed in culture in the presence of adequate nutrients and growth factors, they will grow until they cover the bottom of the culture dish, forming a monolayer. Further cell division then ceases. This is called **density-dependent inhibition**

Box 3-F | Epithelial-mesenchymal transition (EMT)

• Epithelial-mesenchymal transition occurs when epithelial cells lose intercellular junctions, adhesion molecules and apical–basolateral polarity and become migratory and even invasive, as in the case of cancer.
• Epithelial cells adopt a mesenchymal phenotype: they establish interactions with the extracellular matrix, lose cell-cell contacts by downregulating the expression of E-cadherin, disrupt their apical-basal polarity and reorganize their cytoskeleton.
• Induction of EMT involves the activation of SNAIL transcription factors to repress E-cadherin and the nuclear translocation of SMAD proteins in response to key transcription factor activation of TGF-β/BMP and Wnt/β-catenin signaling.
• EMT is classified as: (1) **Type 1 EMT**, that takes place during embryonic development. An example are cells of the neural crest that become mobile and migrate and localize into various organs. (2) **Type 2 EMT**, that is observed during fibrosis following tissue injury and inflammation. An example is **fibrogenesis**, that occurs during chronic liver disease and can lead to cirrhosis. (3) **Type 3 EMT**, that occurs in cancer and metastasis when tumor cells disassemble cell-cell contacts.

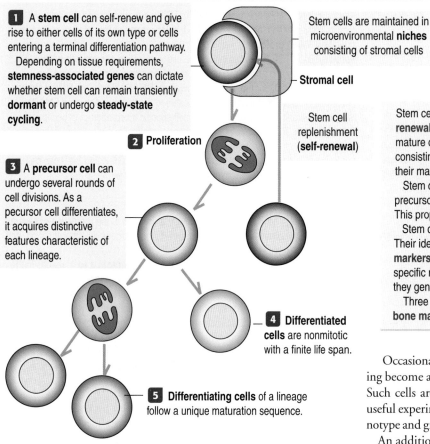

Figure 3-11. Properties of stem cells

1 A **stem cell** can self-renew and give rise to either cells of its own type or cells entering a terminal differentiation pathway.
Depending on tissue requirements, **stemness-associated genes** can dictate whether stem cell can remain transiently **dormant** or undergo **steady-state cycling**.

Stem cells are maintained in microenvironmental **niches** consisting of stromal cells

Stromal cell

Stem cell replenishment (**self-renewal**)

2 Proliferation

3 A **precursor cell** can undergo several rounds of cell divisions. As a precursor cell differentiates, it acquires distinctive features characteristic of each lineage.

4 **Differentiated cells** are nonmitotic with a finite life span.

5 **Differentiating cells** of a lineage follow a unique maturation sequence.

Stem cells have three characteristics: **self-renewal**, **proliferation**, and **differentiation** into mature cells. Stem cells are housed in **niches** consisting of stromal cells that provide factors for their maintenance.

Stem cells of the embryo can give rise to cell precursors that generate all the tissues of the body. This property defines stem cells as **multipotent**.

Stem cells are difficult to identify morphologically. Their identification is based on specific **cell surface markers** (cell surface antigens recognized by specific monoclonal antibodies) and on the lineage they generate following **transplantation**.

Three typical examples are the stem cells of **bone marrow**, **intestine**, and **testes**.

of growth. The cells become quiescent but can be triggered to enter the cell cycle and divide again by an additional dose of growth factor or by replating at a lower cell density.

Cells cultured from a tissue can be kept growing and dividing by regularly replating the cells at lower density once they become confluent. After about 50 cell divisions, however, the cells begin to stop dividing and the cultures become **senescent**.

The number of divisions at which this occurs depends on the age of the individual from which the initial cells were taken. Cells from an embryo, **human embryonic stem cells (HESCs)**, have two unique properties: **self-renewal** (the ability to proliferate indefinitely while maintaining their cellular identity), and **pluripotency** (the ability to differentiate into all the cell types of the embryo). Yet, HESCs share cellular and molecular aspects with tumor cells: rapid proliferation, lack of contact inhibition, genomic instability, high telomerase activity and high expression of oncogenes. When injected into immunodeficient mice, HESCs form **teratomas**, benign tumors consisting of differentiated tissues from all three germinal layers. HESCs can also form **teratocarcinomas**, aggressive tumors representing the malignant equivalents of the teratomas.

Occasionally, cells that would normally stop growing become altered and appear to become **immortal**. Such cells are called a **cell line**. Cell lines are very useful experimentally and still show most of the phenotype and growth characteristics of the original cells.

An additional change known as **transformation** is associated with the potential for **malignant growth**. Transformed cells no longer show normal growth control and have many alterations, such as **anchorage-independent growth**. In contrast, normal cells grow when anchored to a solid substrate.

Cells in culture can be transformed by **chemical carcinogens** or by **infection with certain viruses** (tumor viruses). Tumor viruses will also cause tumors in certain host animals, but in different species they may cause ordinary infections. Cancer cells cultured from tumors also show the characteristics of transformation. We will discuss the role of retroviruses in carcinogenesis at the end of this chapter.

General Pathology: Cellular senescence and cancer
Aging is the gradual decline over time in cell and tissue function that often, not always, decreases the longevity of an individual. Cellular senescence (Latin *senex*, old man or old age) specifies the molecular aspects of loss of function of mitotic cells during aging. Senescence is used interchangeably with aging.

At older age, cellular senescence in humans determines typical pathologies, including atherosclerosis (leading to brain stroke), heart failure, osteoporosis, macular degeneration, cardiopulmonary and renal failure and neurodegenerative diseases such as Alzheimer's and Parkinson's disease.

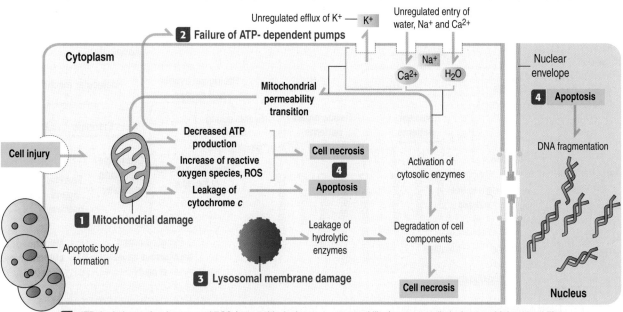

Figure 3-12. Mechanisms of cell injury

1 **ATP depletion** and an **increase of ROS** (superoxide, hydrogen peroxide and hydroxyl radicals) impact on several cellular activities that may lead to necrosis or apoptosis, depending on the type and intensity of an injury and the characteristics of the injured cell.

2 Nonfunctional ATP-dependent pumps fail to regulate the normal influx and efflux of electrolytes and water. An increase in intracellular Ca^{2+} activates cytosolic enzymes (proteases, phospholipases, endonucleases and ATPases) and enhance mitochondrial

permeability (a process called **mitochondrial permeability transition**).

3 **Lysosomal membrane damage** determines the leakage of hydrolytic lysosomal enzymes into the cytosol.

4 Persistence of mitochondrial damage leads to either **necrosis** or **apoptosis** (triggered by the leakage of mitochondrial cytochrome *c*). Activation of caspases, DNA fragmentation and formation of apoptotic bodies take place.

An irreversible arrest in cell proliferation takes place when senescent cells experience DNA damage at telomeres and mitogenic signalling fail to prompt them to resume the cell cycle. In our discussion of mitosis (see Figure 1-51 in Chapter 1, Epithelium), we call attention to the role of **telomerase**, an enzyme that maintains the ends of chromosomes, or **telomeres**.

In normal cells, insufficient telomerase activity limits the number of mitotic divisions and forces the cell into **senescence**. **Telomere shortening and the limited life span of a cell are regarded as potent tumor suppressor mechanisms**. Most human tumors express **human telomerase reverse transcriptase (hTERT)**. The ectopic expression of hTERT in primary human cells confers endless growth in culture. The use of telomerase inhibitors in cancer patients is currently being pursued.

General Pathology: Cell and tissue injury

Cell and tissue injury consists in a number of biochemical and morphologic changes resulting from exogenous or endogenous causes leading to a reversible or irreversible disruption of normal cell function (Figure 3-12).

Exogenous causes of injury include **physical injury** (trauma), **thermal injury** (heat or cold), **radiation injury** (ultraviolet light or ionizing radia-

tion), **chemical injury** (caustic material), **bacterial toxicity** (cholera toxin inducing watery diarrhea), **drug toxicity** (mercury toxicity to the kidneys) and **environmental injury** (air pollutants). **Endogenous** causes of injury include **genetic defects** (inborn errors of metabolism) and **nutritional deficiency** (intestinal malabsorption resulting from celiac disease).

The most relevant causes of cell injury are **hypoxia**, determined by a decrease in the supply of oxygen, and **anoxia**, caused by a complete block in the oxygen supply. Hypoxia and anoxia result from **inadequate oxygen supply** (low concentration of oxygen in air at high altitude, drowning or lung disease), a **failure in oxygen transport in blood** (anemia), a **disruption in blood flow** (ischemia, determined by heart failure), **blood vessel obstruction** (thrombosis or embolism), **disruption in blood supply** (rupture of an aneurysm) or a consequence of **inhibition of cellular respiration** (cyanide poisoning).

Complete ischemia by blockage of an arterial branch of the coronary artery causes **infarction** of the cardiac muscle supplied by that blood vessel. If the occluded blood vessel is reopened soon after ischemic injury (by angioplasty and thrombolysis), injured cardiocytes may recover by **reperfusion**. Irreversibly injured cardiocytes may not recover by reperfusion.

Reperfusion may be detrimental to viable cardio-

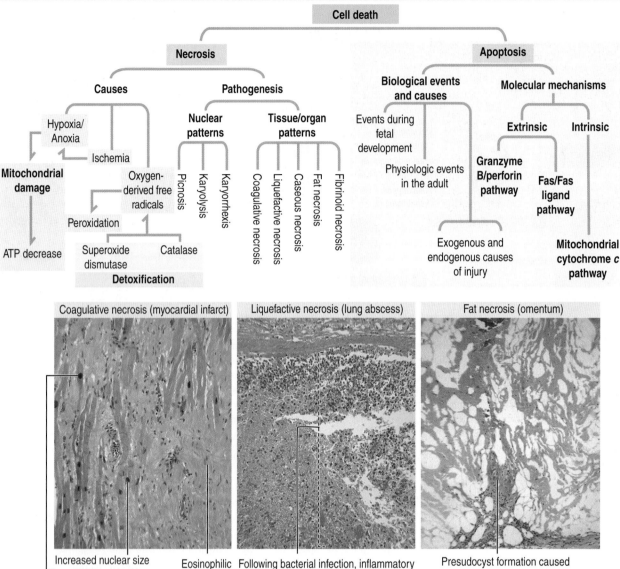

Figure 3-13. Concept Mapping: Cell death, necrosis, and apoptosis

Coagulative necrosis (myocardial infarct)

Increased nuclear size and DNA content in adjacent cardiocytes (hypertrophy)

Eosinophilic anucleated cardiocytes

Liquefactive necrosis (lung abscess)

Following bacterial infection, inflammatory cells accumulate and release enzymes that transform a focal area of lung tissue into a creamy yellow mass called pus

Fat necrosis (omentum)

Presudocyst formation caused by fat necrosis of omental fat. Vascularized connective tissue is observed

cytes at the marginal infarction site by **hemorrhage**, caused by damaged endothelial cells, thus hampering the restoration of blood flow, or by **reactive oxygen species, ROS** (superoxide, hydrogen peroxide and hydroxyl radicals). Free radicals, originated from oxygen metabolism, are active chemical compounds that react with lipids, proteins and DNA. Free radicals damage cell membranes by **lipid peroxidation**, cause DNA breakage and inactivate enzymes by protein crosslinking when protective mechanisms (such as **superoxide dismutase**, **catalase** and **glutathione**) are not functional.

Recall that oxygen is essential for aerobic respiration. Hypoxia disrupts normal oxidative phosphorylation to the point that the capacity of mitochondria to generate ATP is reduced. ATP provides energy for the function of Na^+/K^+ ATPase pumps, necessary for maintaining high concentration of sodium in the extracellular space and high concentration of potassium inside the cell. The unregulated cell influx of sodium, calcium and water from the extracellular space and the leakage of potassium out of the cell result in cell swelling (see Figure 3-12).

Severe cell injury can be monitored by the release of cytoplasmic enzymes into the blood, such as **creatinine kinase** (skeletal or cardiac muscle injury), **aspartate aminotransferase**, AST, and **alanine aminotransferase**, ALT (injured hepatocytes), and **lactate dehydrogenase**, LDH (disrupted cells, including red blood cells).

Figure 3-14. Apoptotic bodies

Scanning electron microscopy

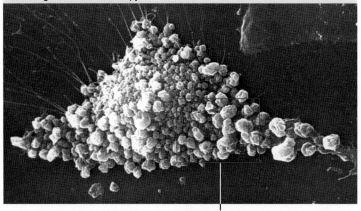

Apoptotic bodies

Transmission electron microscopy

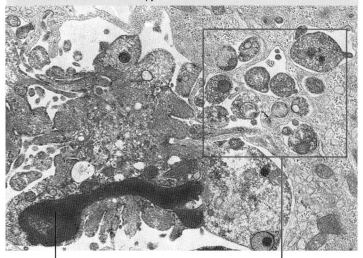

Residual nucleus

Apoptotic bodies containing cell

Depending on the removal or persistence of the cause and the cell type, cell injury can be reversible or irreversible. Irreversible cell injury leads to cell death, or **necrosis** (Greek *nekrós*, dead) or apoptosis.

General Pathology: Necrosis

Necrosis can be recognized by specific microscopic and macroscopic changes (Figure 3-13). Microscopically, in addition to cell membrane breakdown caused by cell swelling, the cell nucleus displays **pyknosis** (Greek *pyknos*, crowded; *osis*, condition; condensation of chromatin), **karyolysis** (Greek *karyon*, nucleus; *lysis*, dissolution; breakdown of chromatin by endonucleases) and **karyorrhexis** (Greek *karyon* + *rhexis*, rupture; presence of fragmented chromatin in the cytoplasm).

Several forms of necrosis can be recognized at the macroscopic level.

1. **Coagulative necrosis**, the most common form of necrosis resulting from vascular occlusion, is characterized by a paler than normal tissue area that retains its overall shape but all cell functions have stopped. The initial inflammatory response (infiltration of neutrophils during the first 24 and 48 hours) is followed days later by the eosinophilic staining of anucleated cell remnants. An example is **myocardial infarct**, caused by ischemia associated to blockage of a branch of the coronary artery (see Figure 3-13).

2. **Liquefactive necrosis** is recognized by the softening of the necrotic tissue caused by hydrolytic lysosomal enzymes released from dead cells and neutrophils. Examples include **brain infarct**, wherein the necrotic tissue is removed by macrophages and the remaining cavity is filled by fluid derived from the surrounding brain interstitial spaces; an **abscess**, a localized purulent infection of the affected organ or tissue, defined by a cavity occupied with **pus** (liquefied tissue previously infiltrated with neutrophils, see Figure 3-13); and **wet gangrene** of extremities, seen in patients with diabetes, resulting from the tissue liquefied action of enzymes released from infecting bacteria (*Clostridium perfringens*).

3. The crumble consistency and opaque aspect of the necrotic tissue in **caseous necrosis**, found tuberculous and histoplasmosis granulomas (nodular inflammatory lesions), mimics cottage cheese.

4. **Fat necrosis** occurs after enzymatic and traumatic injury.

Enzymatic fat necrosis involves adipose tissue within and around the pancreas. The release of lipases from exocrine pancreatic cells during acute pancreatitis destroys the plasma membrane of adipose cells followed by the breakdown of triglycerides into fatty acids. Fatty acids combine with interstitial calcium, giving the necrotic adipose tissue a chalky white appearance by a process called **fat saponification** (Latin *sapon*, soap).

Traumatic fat necrosis is the consequence of traumatic injury (sports and accidents affecting adipose tissue of the breasts, thigh and other locations).

5. **Fibrinoid necrosis** is restricted to the smooth muscle wall of small arteries, arterioles and renal glomeruli affected by autoimmune diseases such as systemic lupus erythematosus. Fibrin-like eosinophilic material impregnates the vascular wall. It can be recognized under the microscope because it does not have distinct macroscopic features.

General Pathology: Apoptosis

Under normal physiologic conditions, cells deprived of survival factors, damaged, or senescent commit suicide through an orderly regulated cell death program called **apoptosis** (Greek *apo*, off; *ptosis*, fall). Viral infection can induce apoptosis to prevent viral replication, viral dissemination or persistent viral infection of the cell. Anticancer drugs as inducers of apoptosis of cancer cells represent a therapeutic strategy.

Figure 3-15. Programmed cell death or apoptosis

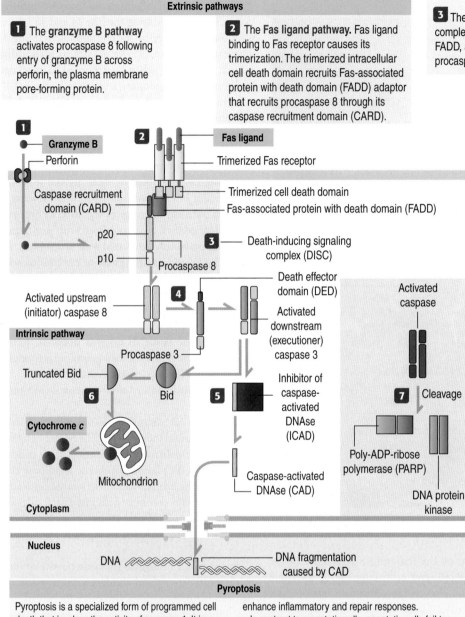

Extrinsic pathways

1 The **granzyme B pathway** activates procaspase 8 following entry of granzyme B across perforin, the plasma membrane pore-forming protein.

2 The **Fas ligand pathway.** Fas ligand binding to Fas receptor causes its trimerization. The trimerized intracellular cell death domain recruits Fas-associated protein with death domain (FADD) adaptor that recruits procaspase 8 through its caspase recruitment domain (CARD).

3 The death-inducing cell signaling complex (DISC) consists of Fas receptor, FADD, and procaspase 8. Within DISC, procaspase 8 becomes active caspase 8.

4 Procaspases consist of two subunits (p10 and p20) and an N-terminal recruitment domain.

Caspases can be upstream initiators with a long N-terminal prodomain called CARD (such as procaspase 8) or downstream executioners with a short N-terminal prodomain called DED (such as procaspase 3). Activated caspases are heterotetramers. Upstream caspases can activate downstream executioner caspases.

5 Activated caspase 8 can cleave ICAD to become CAD, a caspase-activated DNAse. CAD migrates to the nucleus and induces DNA fragmentation.

6 The **cytochrome c pathway.** Activated caspase 8 can cleave Bid, a member of the Bcl-2 family of proteins.

Truncated Bid facilitates the leakage of mitochondrial cytochrome c into the cytoplasm.

7 Activated caspases cleave two DNA repair enzymes (PARP and DNA protein kinase). DNA fragmentation proceeds undisturbed.

Pyroptosis

Pyroptosis is a specialized form of programmed cell death that involves the activity of **caspase 1**. It is characterized by cell swelling, plasma membrane breakdown, and DNA fragmentation. The cytoplasmic content is released into the extracellular space to enhance inflammatory and repair responses.

In contrast to pyroptotic cells, apoptotic cells fail to trigger inflammatory responses because cell components are packaged in apoptotic bodies, and (2) caspase 1 is not involved in the induction of apoptosis.

Apoptosis is different from **necrosis**. As we have seen, necrosis is a nonphysiologic process that occurs after acute injury (for example, in an ischemic stroke). Necrotic cells lyse and release cytoplasmic and nuclear contents into the environment, thus triggering an inflammatory reaction.

Cells undergoing apoptosis lose intercellular adhesion, fragment the chromatin, and break down into small blebs called **apoptotic bodies** (Figure 3-14). Apoptotic bodies are phagocytosed by macrophages and inflammation does not occur.

Apoptotic cell death is observed during normal fetal development. For example, the formation of fingers and toes of the fetus requires the elimination by apoptosis of the tissue between them. During fetal development of the central nervous system, an excess of neurons, eliminated later by apoptosis, is required to establish appropriate connections or synapses between them (see Chapter 8, Nervous Tissue). The regression of the embryonic müllerian duct in the male fetus is triggered by Sertoli cell-derived anti-müllerian hormone, AMH (see Chapter 21, Sperm Transport and Maturation).

In the adult female, the breakdown of the endome-

Figure 3-16. **Role of mitochondria in apoptosis**

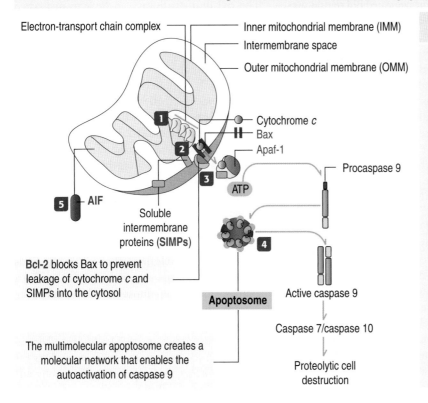

Electron-transport chain complex

Inner mitochondrial membrane (IMM)

Intermembrane space

Outer mitochondrial membrane (OMM)

1

2

3

ATP

5 — AIF

Cytochrome *c*

Bax

Apaf-1

Procaspase 9

Soluble
intermembrane
proteins (**SIMPs**)

4

Bcl-2 blocks Bax to prevent
leakage of cytochrome *c* and
SIMPs into the cytosol

Apoptosome

Active caspase 9

Caspase 7/caspase 10

The multimolecular apoptosome creates a
molecular network that enables the
autoactivation of caspase 9

Proteolytic cell
destruction

Cytochrome *c* in apoptosis

1 Cytochrome *c* shuttles electrons between
electron-chain complexes III and IV. If
cytochrome *c* is not present, electron flow
stops and ATP synthesis does not occur.

2 Cytochrome *c* is located between the IMM
and OMM.

3 Antiapoptotic **Bcl-2** blocks Bax, which
facilitates the release of **cytochrome *c*** and
SIMPs.

4 During apoptosis, **cytochrome *c*** and
**SIMPs are released across the OMM and
interact with apoptosis protease activating
factor-1 (Apaf-1) to form the apoptosome**
(together with **ATP** and **procascapse 9**).

Apaf-1 activates procaspase 9. Caspase 9
activates caspase 7 and caspase 10 leading to
the proteolytic destruction of the cell.

5 **Apoptosis-inducing factor (AIF)** is a
mitochondrial protein that can be released into
the cytoplasm, migrate to the cell nucleus, bind
to DNA and trigger DNA fragmentation in the
absence of caspases.

---

trium during the premenstrual phase and the regression of the corpus luteum in the ovary are determined by a hormonal-regulated ischemia and consequent hypoxia (see Chapter 22, Follicle Development and The Menstrual Cycle).

Mature granulocytes in peripheral blood have a life span of 1 to 2 days before undergoing apoptosis.

The clonal selection of T cells in the thymus (to eliminate self-reactive lymphocytes to prevent autoimmune diseases; see Chapter 10, Immune-Lymphatic System) and cellular immune responses involve apoptosis.

What a nematode worm told us about apoptosis

The genetic and molecular mechanisms of apoptosis emerged from studies of the nematode worm *Caenorhabditis elegans*, in which 131 cells are precisely killed and 959 remain.

In this worm, four genes are required for the orderly cell death program: *ced-3* (for cell death defective-3), *ced-4*, *egl-1* (for egg laying-1), and *ced-9*. The products of the first three genes mediate cell death. The gene *ced-9* is an inhibitor of apoptosis.

The proteins encoded by these four genes in the worm are found in vertebrates. Protein ced-3 is homologous to **caspases**; ced-4 corresponds to **Apaf-1** (for **apoptotic protease activating factor-1**), ced-9 to **Bcl-2** (for B-cell leukemia-2); and egl-1 is homologous to Bcl-2 homology region 3 (BH3)-only proteins.

Extrinsic and intrinsic signals of apoptosis

Extrinsic and intrinsic signals determine cell apoptosis. **Extrinsic signals** bind to cell surface receptors (for example, Fas ligand and granzyme B/perforin) (Figure 3-15). **Intrinsic signals** (for example, the release of cytochrome *c* from mitochondria) can trigger cell death (see Figure 3-15 and Figure 3-16).

Fas receptor (also known as APO-1 or CD95) is a cell membrane protein that belongs to the **TNF receptor family (already discussed in the Cytokine receptor and ligand section)**. Fas receptor has an intracellular cell death domain.

Fas ligand binds to Fas receptor and causes its **trimerization**. Fas ligand initiates programmed cell death by binding to the **Fas receptor** and triggers a cell signaling cascade consisting of the sequential activation of **procaspases** into active **caspases**. The trimerized cell death domain recruits procaspase 8 through the **FADD** (for **Fas-associated protein with death domain**) adaptor and forms a **DISC** (for **death-inducing signaling complex**). DISC consists of Fas receptor, FADD, and procaspase 8.

Procaspase 8 autoactivated at DISC becomes active caspase 8. Active caspase 8 can do two things:

1. It can process procaspase 3 to active caspase 3, which can cleave several cellular proteins, including **ICAD** (for **inhibitor of CAD**) giving rise to CAD. **CAD** (for **caspase-activated DNAse**) is released from ICAD, translocates to the cell nucleus, and breaks down chromosomal DNA.

2. Caspase 8 can cleave **Bid**, a proapoptotic member of the Bcl-2 family. The truncated Bid translocates to mitochondria to release cytochrome *c* into the cytoplasm.

As discussed in Chapter 10, Immune-Lymphatic System, a cytotoxic T cell destroys a target cell (for example, a virus-infected cell) by the activation of procaspase 8 by the combined Fas/Fas ligand and granzyme B/perforin pathways.

Remember that caspase activation, the key event of apoptosis, involves two extrinsic pathways: the Fas/Fas ligand and the granzyme B/perforin pathways and an intrinsic pathway, the mitochondrial cytochrome *c* pathway (see Concept Mapping in Figure 3-13)

Caspases: Initiators and executioners of cell death

Caspases (for **cysteine aspartic acid–specific proteases**) exist as inactive precursors (procaspases), which are activated to produce directly or indirectly cellular morphologic changes during apoptosis.

Procaspases consist of two subunits (**p10** and **p20**) and an N-terminal recruitment domain (see Figure 3-15). Activated caspases are heterotetramers consisting of two p10 subunits and two p20 subunits derived from two procaspases.

Caspases can be **upstream initiators** and **downstream executioners**. Upstream initiators are activated by the cell-death signal (for example, Fas ligand or TNFL). Upstream initiator caspases activate downstream caspases, which directly mediate cell destruction.

Completion of the cell death process occurs when executioner caspases activate the DNA degradation machinery. Caspases cleave two DNA repair enzymes (**poly-ADP–ribose polymerase [PARP]**, and **DNA protein kinase**), and unrestricted fragmentation of chromatin occurs.

As you realize, the key event in caspase-mediated cell death is the regulatory activation of **initiator caspases.**

Upstream (**initiator**) procaspases include procaspases 8, 9, and 10 with a **long** N-terminal prodomain called **CARD** (for **caspase-recruiting domain**). Downstream (**executioner**) procaspases comprise procaspases 3, 6, and 7 with a **short** N-terminal prodomain called **DED** (for **death-effector domain**).

Caspase activation takes place when a caspase-specific regulatory molecule (for example, FADD) binds to the CARD/DED domain. Caspase activation may become out of control and destroy the cell. To prevent this uncontrolled event, inhibitors of apoptosis are available to interact with modulators of cell death, thus preventing unregulated caspase activation.

Intrinsic pathway: Mitochondrial cytochrome *c*

Cytochrome *c* is a component of the mitochondria electron-transporting chain involved in the production of ATP, and also a trigger of the caspase cascade.

The cell death pathway can be activated when cytochrome *c* is released from the mitochondria into the cytoplasm. How does cytochrome *c* leave mitochondria? To answer this question, we need to consider aspects of members of the **Bcl-2 family.**

Bcl-2 family members can have **proapoptotic** or **antiapoptotic** activities. **Bcl-2 and Bcl-xL have antiapoptotic activity. Bax, Bak, Bid, and Bad are proapoptotic proteins**. Bcl-2 is associated with the outer mitochondrial membrane of viable cells and prevents Bax from punching holes in the outer mitochondrial membrane, causing cytochrome *c* to leak out. A balance between proapoptotic Bax and antiapoptotic Bcl-2 proteins controls the release of cytochrome *c*.

In the cytoplasm, leaking cytochrome *c*, in the presence of ATP, **soluble internal membrane proteins (SIMPs)**, and procaspase 9, binds to Apaf-1 to form a complex called an **apoptosome**. The apoptosome determines the activation of **caspase 9**, an upstream initiator of apoptosis (see Figure 3-16). Caspase 9 activates caspase 3 and caspase 7, leading to cell death.

As you can see, exogenous activators, such as Fas ligand and Granzyme B, and the endogenous **mitochondrial permeability transition**, leading to an abrupt release of cytochrome *c,* are three key triggers of apoptosis. However, **AIF** (for **apoptosis-inducing factor**) is a protein of the intermitochondrial membrane space that can be released into the cytoplasm, migrate to the nucleus, bind to DNA, and trigger cell destruction without participation of caspases.

General Pathology: Apoptosis in the immune system

Mutations in the **Fas receptor**, **Fas ligand**, or **caspase 10** genes can cause **autoimmune lymphoproliferative syndrome (ALPS)**. ALPS is characterized by the accumulation of mature lymphocytes in lymph nodes and spleen causing **lymphoadenopathy** (enlargement of lymph nodes) and **splenomegaly** (enlargement of the spleen), and the existence of autoreactive lymphocyte clones producing autoimmune conditions such as **hemolytic anemia** (caused by destruction of red blood cells) and **thrombocytopenia** (reduced number of platelets).

General Pathology: Apoptosis in neurodegenerative diseases

Neurologic diseases are examples of the mechanism of cell death. For example, an **ischemic stroke** can cause an **acute neurologic disease** in which necrosis and activation of caspase 1 are observed. Necrotic cell death occurs in the center of the infarction, where the damage is severe. Apoptosis may be observed at the periphery of the infarction, because the damage is not severe due to collateral blood circulation. Pharmaco-

Figure 3-17. Necroptosis

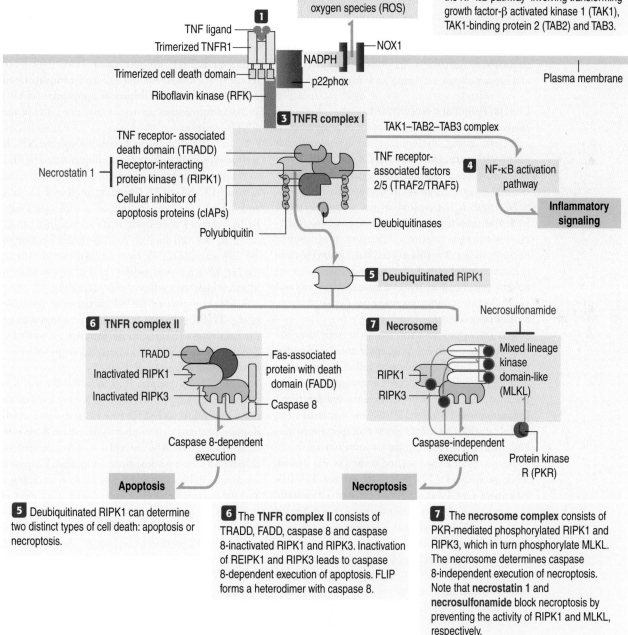

1 Binding of tumor necrosis factor ligand to tumor necrosis factor receptor 1 (TNFR1) causes a conformational change enabling the intracellular assembly of the **TNFR complex I.**

2 RFK links theTNFR1 cell death domain to p22phox, NADPH and NADPH oxidase 1 (NOX1) to induces necroptosis by generating non-mitochondrial **ROS** from the plasma membrane.

3 The **TNFR complex I** consists of the proteins TRADD, RIPK1, cIAPs, TRAF2 and TRAF5. RIPK1 and TRAF2 and TRAF5 are ubiquitinated by cIAPs.

4 In the presence of polyubiquitinated RIPK1, the TNFR complex can activate the NF-κB pathway involving transforming growth factor-β activated kinase 1 (TAK1), TAK1-binding protein 2 (TAB2) and TAB3.

2 Non-mitochondrial reactive oxygen species (ROS)

TNF ligand
Trimerized TNFR1
NOX1
NADPH
Trimerized cell death domain
p22phox
Plasma membrane
Riboflavin kinase (RFK)

3 TNFR complex I

TAK1–TAB2–TAB3 complex

TNF receptor- associated death domain (TRADD)
Receptor-interacting protein kinase 1 (RIPK1)
Necrostatin 1
Cellular inhibitor of apoptosis proteins (cIAPs)
Polyubiquitin
TNF receptor-associated factors 2/5 (TRAF2/TRAF5)
Deubiquitinases

4 NF-κB activation pathway

Inflammatory signaling

5 Deubiquitinated RIPK1

Necrosulfonamide

6 TNFR complex II

TRADD
Inactivated RIPK1
Inactivated RIPK3
Fas-associated protein with death domain (FADD)
Caspase 8

Caspase 8-dependent execution

Apoptosis

7 Necrosome

RIPK1
RIPK3
Mixed lineage kinase domain-like (MLKL)

Caspase-independent execution
Protein kinase R (PKR)

Necroptosis

5 Deubiquitinated RIPK1 can determine two distinct types of cell death: apoptosis or necroptosis.

6 The **TNFR complex II** consists of TRADD, FADD, caspase 8 and caspase 8-inactivated RIPK1 and RIPK3. Inactivation of REIPK1 and RIPK3 leads to caspase 8-dependent execution of apoptosis. FLIP forms a heterodimer with caspase 8.

7 The **necrosome complex** consists of PKR-mediated phosphorylated RIPK1 and RIPK3, which in turn phosphorylate MLKL. The necrosome determines caspase 8-independent execution of necroptosis. Note that **necrostatin 1** and **necrosulfonamide** block necroptosis by preventing the activity of RIPK1 and MLKL, respectively.

logic treatment with caspase inhibitors can reduce tissue damage leading to neurologic improvement.

Caspase activation is associated with the fatal progression of **chronic neurodegenerative diseases. Amyotrophic lateral sclerosis (ALS)** and **Huntington's disease** are two examples.

ALS consists in the progressive loss of motor neurons in the brain, brainstem, and spinal cord. A mutation in the gene encoding **superoxide dismutase 1 (*SID1*)** has been identified in patients with familial ALS. Activated caspase 1 and caspase 3 have been found in spinal cord samples of patients with ALS.

Motor neurons and axons die and reactive microglia and astrocytes are present. We come back to ALS in Chapter 8, Nervous Tissue.

Huntington's disease is an autosomal dominant neurodegenerative disease characterized by a movement disorder (**Huntington's chorea**). The disease is caused by a mutation in the protein **huntingtin**. Huntingtin protein fragments accumulate and aggregate in the neuronal nucleus and transcription of the *caspase 1* gene is upregulated. Caspase 1 activates caspase 3 and both caspases cleave the allelic wild-type form of huntingtin, which becomes depleted. As the disease progresses, Bid is activated and releases mitochondrial cytochrome *c*. Apoptosomes are assembled and further caspase activation leads to neuronal death.

General Pathology: Necroptosis

We learned that apoptosis is a form of **programmed** cell death during development and disease and that necrosis is an **unregulated** process of cell death. However, necrosis can take place in a **regulated** manner by the molecular mechanism of **necroptosis**.

Necroptosis is involved in the pathogenesis of ischemic-reperfusion injury, stroke, neurodegeneration and viral infection. Therefore, programmed necroptosis is a desirable process to be intercepted in the treatment of ischemia-reperfusion, neurodegeneration, inflammatory bowel disease and bacterial and viral infection, conditions that display morphologic aspects of necrosis.

It is important to stress from the start that the death domain-containing **receptor-interacting protein kinase 1** (**RIPK1**) has emerged as an important upstream regulator that exerts a strategic control at the crossroad of two important events: **cell death** and **inflammation**. Therefore, RIPK1 is a significant and useful target for developing new therapies for pathologic processes involving inflammation and cell death.

Necroptosis can be initiated at the **Fas/Fas ligand**, **TNF receptor 1** (TNFR1), cell surface **Toll-like receptors** (see Chapter 10, Immune-Lymphatic System), and the **cytoplasmic viral RNA sensor DAI** (for DNA-dependent activator of interferon regulatory factors).

As we have seen, Fas/Fas ligand activate the apoptotic machinery involving initiator and execution caspases and mitochondrial release of cytochrome *c*. The most characterized pathway leading to necroptosis is initiated by TNF ligand binding to TNFR1 (Figure 17). It can lead to cell survival, apoptosis or necroptosis.

Necroptosis involves:

1. **The activity of ubiquitinated or deubiquitinated RIPK3.**

2. An **execution phase** involving the **necrosome**, a phosphorylated protein multicomplex that includes

RIPK1 and RIPK3 in addition to the **mixed lineage kinase domain-like** (**MLKL**) **protein complex**. The execution phase does not involve caspase 8. In fact the function of caspase 8 is inhibited. The outcome of necroptosis is the disintegration of mitochondria, lysosomes and plasma membrane, including the production of non-mitochondrial ROS.

Figure 3-17 illustrates the different pathways following binding of TNFL to TNFR1. Note the following:

1. Upstream signaling elements of apoptosis and necroptosis are shared and regulated in opposing ways. Note that **TNFR complex I** includes **ubiquitinated RIPK1, ubiquitinated** TRAF (for TNF receptor-associated factors) 2 and **ubiquitinated** TRAF 5. **Cellular inhibitors of apoptosis** (cIAPs) and **deubiquitinases** are regulatory molecules of the TNFR complex I.

2. The TNFR complex I signals through the **NF-kB activation pathway**. It requires **ubiquitinated** RIPK1 to recruit transforming growth factor-β activated kinase 1 (TAK1), TAK1-binding protein 2 (TAB2) and TAB3. As you realize, ubiquitin sequesters RIPK1 thereby preventing it from engaging in cell death so that cell survival can take place because of **NF-kB activation.** We have already seen details of the NF-kB activation pathway and its significance in immunologic and inflammatory signaling.

3. Deubiquitinated RIPK1 dictates the assembly of the **TNFR complex II** (leading to **apoptosis**) or the **necrosome** (leading to **necroptosis**). Essentially, deubiquitinated RIPK1 relinquishes its pro-survival function and triggers cell death.

4. The **TNFR complex II** includes RIPK1, RIPK3. **TRADD** (the adapter protein TNFR-associated death domain), to link to **FADD** (the Fas-associated death domain protein) that binds to **procaspase 8. As** you recall, procaspase 8 is autocatalytically activated to **caspase 8** following homodimer formation. Caspase 8 inactivates RIPK1 and RIPK3 by proteolytic cleavage and the caspase-dependent executioner machinery is ready for apoptosis.

5. The necrosome is assembled when there is no activation or function of caspase 8. The necrosome consists of phosphorylated RIPK1, RIPK3 and MLKL by the action of protein kinase R (PKR).

6. Plasma membrane channels release ROS to provoke swelling of necroptotic cells leading to a breakdown of the plasma membrane. Note that riboflavin kinase (RFK) links the death domain of TNRF1 to p22phox, a subunit of NADPH oxidases, including NADPH oxidase 1 (NOX1), to produce ROS.

7. **Necrostatin 1** prevents the deubiquitination of RIPK1. Consequently, RIPK1 retaining a polyubiquitin chain is not available for organizing the necrosome. Necrostatin 1 has a protective effect in

experimental models of brain ischemia. **Necrosulfonamide** inhibits MLKL and prevents the activity of the necrosome. Necroptosis inhibitors have clinical-therapeutic relevance in transplantation of solid organs by preventing harmful immunologic responses and reducing proinflammatory parenchymal responses that may activate rejection.

8. Apoptosis and necroptosis may occur in the same tissue.

General Pathology: Mitochondrial permeability transition

We have previously referred to mitochondrial permeability transition when we discussed the molecular biology of cell injury (see Figure 3-12).

Mitochondrial permeability transition is a process that induces regulated cell death necrosis mediated by **cyclophilin D**, a mitochondrial matrix protein. **Cyclosporine**, an immunosuppressant drug widely used in organ transplantation to prevent rejection, blocks cyclophilin to prevent mitochondrial permeability transition as a means to reduce inflammatory responses and necroptosis, thus improving graft survival and protection from ischemia-reperfusion injury.

Mitochondrial permeability transition occurs by the opening of the **permeability transition pore.** The permeability transition pore consists of the voltage-dependent anion channel (in the outer mitochondrial membrane), the adenine-nucleotide translocase (in the inner mitochondrial membrane) and cyclophilin D (in the mitochondrial matrix).

A prolonged opening of permeability transition pores determines a sudden increase in the permeability of the inner mitochondrial membrane to ions and small molecular mass solutes. This condition determines osmotic swelling of the mitochondrial matrix and breakdown of the outer mitochondrial membrane.

General Pathology: Intracellular degradation

The intracellular degradation of organelles and residual or misfolded proteins (Figure 3-18) can occur by:

1. The **autophagy pathway.**
2. The **ubiquitin-proteasome pathway.**
3. The **mitophagy signaling pathway.**

The autophagy pathway involves the sequestration of cytoplasmic components within **autophagosomes**. The ubiquitin-proteasome pathway utilizes a catalytic multisubunit structure, the 26S proteasome, that recognizes ubiquitinated proteins for degradation.

The autophagy pathway is a self-degradation and cytoprotective process involved in the turnover of cytoplasmic organelles as an adaptation to declining nutrient resources or as a form of cell death (when the intensity and duration of stress are excessive).

Autophagy and apoptosis often occur in the same cell, with autophagy preceding apoptosis.

The ubiquitin-proteasome pathway pursues the degradation of proteins that have already accomplished a specific function (such as specific cyclins during the cell cycle) or proteins that have folded incorrectly because of faulty translation or encoded by defective genes. As we have seen, the apoptosis pathway is concerned with the turnover of entire cells. While apoptosis and the ubiquitin-proteasome activities take place in the cytosol, autophagy occurs within a sealed compartment, the autophagosomes, with the assistance of lysosomes.

The mitophagy signaling pathway eliminates damaged mitochondria to maintain normal cell function. Defects in mitochondria function are the cause of reactive oxidative stress (ROS) and specific neurodegenerative disorders, such as some familial forms of Parkinson's disease.

Autophagy pathway

The process of autophagy starts with, the **phagophore**, a cytomembrane derived from the endoplasmic reticulum, Golgi or plasma membrane. The phagophore expands, surrounds and encloses a cytoplasmic components (such as mitochondria, see Figure 3-18) that is captured within a double membrane structure, the **autophagosome**. Lysosomes fuse with the autophagosome to form an **autolysosome (also called autophagolysosome)** where autophagic degradation takes place by the activity of lysosomal acid hydrolases. Lysosomal permeases and transporter proteins export the breakdown products back to the cytoplasm. As you can see, autophagy is a cellular cleansing and recycling pathway. Progressive dysfunction of autophagy is likely to lead to aging.

The autophagy pathway includes the following steps:

1. **Cytomembrane selection to become a phagosome**. Autophagy starts with the formation of a membranous phagophore, usually at endoplasmic reticulum-mitochondria contact sites (see Figure 3-18). Multiple protein components participate in the initiation of a phagophore. The **ULK1 complex**, with kinase activity, triggers **mTOR complex** (a negative autophagy regulator), to initiate autophagy by selecting a cytomembrane to become a phagophore, the precursor of an autophagosome. Then a complex of autophagy (Atg) proteins (Atg5-Atg12) conjugate and interact with LC3 (protein light chain 3) at the phagophore (see Figure 3-18).

2. **Formation of an autophagosome.** The phagophore double membrane extends and encloses at random or selectively an organelle or cell component for degradation within the autophagosome. Recycling of the Atg5-Atg12/Atg16L and some LC3 takes place.

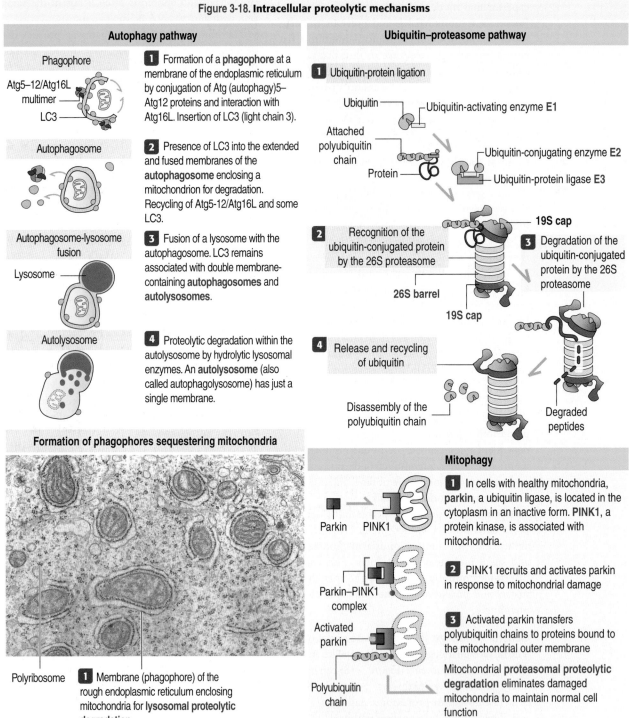

Figure 3-18. Intracellular proteolytic mechanisms

Autophagy pathway

Phagophore

Atg5–12/Atg16L multimer
LC3

1 Formation of a **phagophore** at a membrane of the endoplasmic reticulum by conjugation of Atg (autophagy)5–Atg12 proteins and interaction with Atg16L. Insertion of LC3 (light chain 3).

Autophagosome

2 Presence of LC3 into the extended and fused membranes of the **autophagosome** enclosing a mitochondrion for degradation. Recycling of Atg5-12/Atg16L and some LC3.

Autophagosome-lysosome fusion

Lysosome

3 Fusion of a lysosome with the autophagosome. LC3 remains associated with double membrane-containing **autophagosomes** and **autolysosomes**.

Autolysosome

4 Proteolytic degradation within the autolysosome by hydrolytic lysosomal enzymes. An **autolysosome** (also called autophagolysosome) has just a single membrane.

Formation of phagophores sequestering mitochondria

Polyribosome

1 Membrane (phagophore) of the rough endoplasmic reticulum enclosing mitochondria for **lysosomal proteolytic degradation**.

Ubiquitin–proteasome pathway

1 Ubiquitin-protein ligation

Ubiquitin
Ubiquitin-activating enzyme **E1**
Attached polyubiquitin chain
Ubiquitin-conjugating enzyme **E2**
Protein
Ubiquitin-protein ligase **E3**

2 Recognition of the ubiquitin-conjugated protein by the 26S proteasome

19S cap

26S barrel

19S cap

3 Degradation of the ubiquitin-conjugated protein by the 26S proteasome

4 Release and recycling of ubiquitin

Disassembly of the polyubiquitin chain

Degraded peptides

Mitophagy

Parkin   PINK1

1 In cells with healthy mitochondria, **parkin**, a ubiquitin ligase, is located in the cytoplasm in an inactive form. **PINK1**, a protein kinase, is associated with mitochondria.

Parkin–PINK1 complex

2 PINK1 recruits and activates parkin in response to mitochondrial damage

Activated parkin

3 Activated parkin transfers polyubiquitin chains to proteins bound to the mitochondrial outer membrane

Polyubiquitin chain

Mitochondrial **proteasomal proteolytic degradation** eliminates damaged mitochondria to maintain normal cell function

---

3. **Formation of an autolysosome.** A lysosome fuses with the autophagosome and various lysosomal enzymes initiate the breakdown of proteins, lipids and nucleic acids. LC3 remains associated with the autophagosome double membrane and the autolysosome single membrane.

We indicated that the mTOR is a negative autophagy regulator. Hypoxia and a decrease in ATP intracellular levels release the autophagy inhibition activity of mTOR. In contrast, the abundance of nutrients and growth factors keeps mTOR's cytoprotective autophagy inhibitory activity.

Ubiquitin–proteasome pathway

The ubiquitin–proteasome pathway involves four successive regulated steps (see Figure 3-18):

1. The attachment of a chain of ubiquitin molecules to a protein substrate by an enzymatic cascade.

Figure 3-19. Concept Mapping: Neoplasia

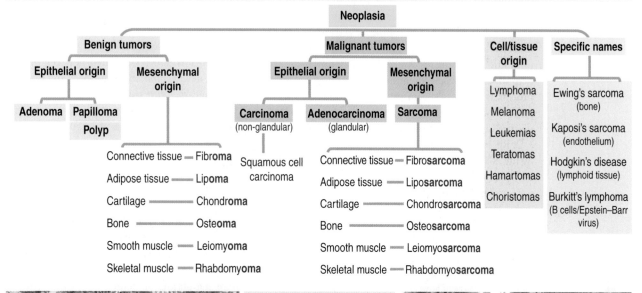

Neoplasia

Benign tumors
- **Epithelial origin**
  - Adenoma
  - Papilloma
  - Polyp
- **Mesenchymal origin**
  - Connective tissue — Fibr**oma**
  - Adipose tissue — Lip**oma**
  - Cartilage — Chondr**oma**
  - Bone — Oste**oma**
  - Smooth muscle — Leiomy**oma**
  - Skeletal muscle — Rhabdomy**oma**

Malignant tumors
- **Epithelial origin**
  - **Carcinoma** (non-glandular)
    - Squamous cell carcinoma
  - **Adenocarcinoma** (glandular)
- **Mesenchymal origin**
  - **Sarcoma**
    - Connective tissue — Fibro**sarcoma**
    - Adipose tissue — Lipo**sarcoma**
    - Cartilage — Chondro**sarcoma**
    - Bone — Osteo**sarcoma**
    - Smooth muscle — Leiomyo**sarcoma**
    - Skeletal muscle — Rhabdomyo**sarcoma**

Cell/tissue origin
- Lymphoma
- Melanoma
- Leukemias
- Teratomas
- Hamartomas
- Choristomas

Specific names
- Ewing's sarcoma (bone)
- Kaposi's sarcoma (endothelium)
- Hodgkin's disease (lymphoid tissue)
- Burkitt's lymphoma (B cells/Epstein–Barr virus)

Adenomatous polyp (colon)

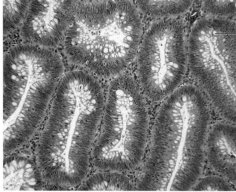

Goblet cells

Glandular benign neoplasm consisting of dysplastic intestinal epithelium with abundant goblet cells and a vascularized stroma. Adenomas are the precursors of nearly all colorectal cancers. Adenomas may be sessile, perduncular or flat with a tubular or villous architecture and a grade of dysplasia.

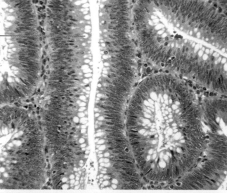

Squamous cell carcinoma (larynx)

Metastasis of squamous cell carcinoma (lymph node)

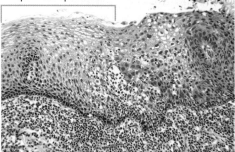

Relatively intact stratified squamous epithelium

Basement membrane

Chronic granulomatous inflammatory reaction in the lamina propria

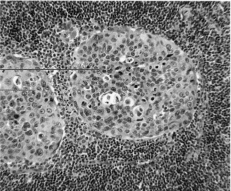

Melanoma (skin)

Epidermis

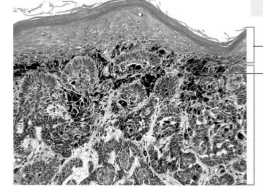

Epidermis

Melanin

Invasive pigmented (melanin) melanoma in the dermis

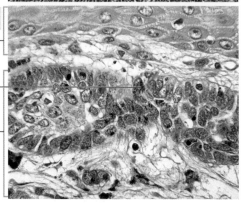

First, **E1**, the ubiquitin-activating enzyme, activates ubiquitin in the presence of ATP to form a thioester bond. Then, **E2**, the ubiquitin-conjugating enzyme, uses the thioester bond to conjugate activated ubiquitin to the target protein. E2 transfers the activated ubiquitin to a lysine residue of the substrate with the help of **E3**, a specific ubiquitin-protein ligase. This process is repeated several times to generate a long polyubiquitin chain attached to the substrate protein destined for degradation in the **26S proteasome**.

2. Recognition of the ubiquitin-conjugated protein by the 26S proteasome. A protein subunit (designated S5a) in the 19S cap of the proteasome acts as a receptor for the polyubiquitin chain.

3. Degradation of the ubiquitin-conjugated protein into oligopeptides in the 26S barrel, the inner proteolytic chamber of the proteasome, in the presence of ATP.

4. The release and recycling of ubiquitin.

The 26S proteasome is a giant (~2000 kd) multimeric protease present in the nucleus and cytoplasm. Structurally, the 26S proteasome consists of a barrel-shaped core capped by two structures that recognize ubiquitinated proteins. Protein degradation occurs within a chamber of the barrel-shaped core. As we have indicated, proteins degraded by the 26S proteasome include proteins involved in the regulation of the cell cycle (cyclins), transcription factors, and the processing of antigens involved in the activation of inflammatory and immune responses.

Mitophagy signaling pathway

The mitophagy signaling pathway pursues the disposal of damaged mitochondria and involves two enzymes (see Figure 3-18):

1. **Parkin**, a **ubiquitin ligase** that is located in the cytoplasm in an inactive form.

2. **PINK1**, a **protein kinase**, associated with the outer mitochondrial membrane.

In response to mitochondrial damage, PINK1 recruits and activates parkin.

Activated parkin exerts its ubiquitin ligase activity by transferring polyubiquitin to proteins attached to the outer mitochondrial membrane. Ubiquitin-tagged proteins are recognized by the proteasomal proteolytic machinery to initiate mitochondrial degradation.

Note that the goal of the parkin-PINK1 complex is to eliminate defective mitochondria. If the parkin-PINK1 complex is defective, dysfunctional mitochondrial are not cleared and cell function is compromised. Parkinson's disease is an example of a neurodegenerative disease caused by mitochondrial dysfunction determined by mutations in the ubiquitin ligase parkin and protein kinase PINK1.

Also note the clear difference of the lysosomal–based autophagy pathway and ubiquitin-proteasome–based mitophagy signaling pathway executed during the removal of aged or damaged mitochondria.

General Pathology: Neoplasia

Neoplasia means poorly regulated new cell growth (Greek *neos*, new; *plasma*, things formed) and the term is interchangeable with **tumor** (Latin *tumor*, swelling). **Cancer** (Latin, a crab) is a malignant neoplasm or malignant tumor. The cells of origin derive from the three embryonic layers (ectoderm, mesoderm and endoderm)

Two types of tumors are considered from a clinical perspective: **benign tumors** and **malignant tumors**. A benign tumor is characterized by localized active growth and results in the development of a cellular mass, or tumor, with similar structural, and sometimes, functional features resembling the cells of origin.

Benign neoplasms or benign tumors are for the most part encapsulated, grow slowly and do not spread at a distance by invading blood or lymphatic vessels. However, benign tumors can compress adjacent tissues (for example, compression of the urethra by a prostatic benign tumor or a benign tumor of the brain stem). A benign tumor can grow in the lumen of an organ (for example, the intestine) and cause an obstruction.

A malignant tumor can be **differentiated**, resembling the tissue of origin, **poorly differentiated**, by retaining some of the characteristics of the tissue of origin, and **undifferentiated or anaplastic**, when the cell or tissue origin cannot be identified.

Tumor staging system (TNM: **tumors/nodes/metastases**) is based on three parameters (Cuthbert Dukes [1890-1977] staging for colorectal cancer):

1. The **size of the tumor** and the **degree of local invasion (T)**.

2. The involvement of **regional lymph nodes (N)**.

3. The presence of **metastasis (M)**.

For example, T1, N0, M0 signifies small tumor, no regional lymph node involved and absence of metastases.

Most **carcinomas** (Greek *karkinoma*, cancer; *oma*, tumor) are malignant neoplasms of epithelial cell origin (ectoderm and endoderm). An **adenocarcinoma** is a malignant tumor resembling glandular pattern. **Sarcomas** (Greek *sarkoma*, fleshly excrescence; *oma*, tumor) are malignant neoplasms of mesenchyme (mesoderm) origin (Figure 3-19).

In general, carcinomas develop from a **dysplasia** (Greek *dys*, difficult; *plasis*, a molding), a process that involves genetic alterations and the participation of diverse cellular signaling pathways (see Box 3-D).

Dysplasia occurs in epithelial tissues. It is defined by an increase in the rate of mitosis, lack of complete cell

Box 3-G | Proto-oncogenes and tumor suppressor proteins in human cancers

• **Chronic myelogenous leukemia:** The **c-abl** proto-oncogene translocated from chromosome 9 to chromosome 22 (called the **Philadelphia chromosome**) encodes a fusion protein with constitutive active tyrosine kinase activity.
• **Burkitt's lymphoma:** The **c-myc** proto-oncogene is translocated from chromosome 8 to chromosome 14. This translocation places c-myc under the control of an active immunoglobulin locus *(immunoglobulin heavy-chain gene, Cm)* and detached from its normal regulatory elements. Burkitt's lymphoma is endemic in some parts of Africa and affects mainly children or young adults. It generally involves the maxilla or mandible. It responds to chemotherapy.
• **p53:** Inactivation of this **tumor suppressor protein**, a transcription factor expressed in response to DNA damage (see Chapter 1, Epithelium), is associated with 50% to 60% of human cancers. Inactive p53 enables the progression through the cell cycle of cells containing damaged DNA.

differentiation and abnormal cell-cell relationships. **Dysplasia can progress into carcinoma in situ and then to invasive tumor.**

Carcinoma in situ is restricted to an epithelial layer without breaking through the basement membrane to reach the subjacent connective tissue. Carcinomas in situ are usually found in the uterine cervix, skin, and breast, localized in the lactiferous ducts (intraductal carcinoma) or in the mammary lobular tissue (intralobular carcinoma).

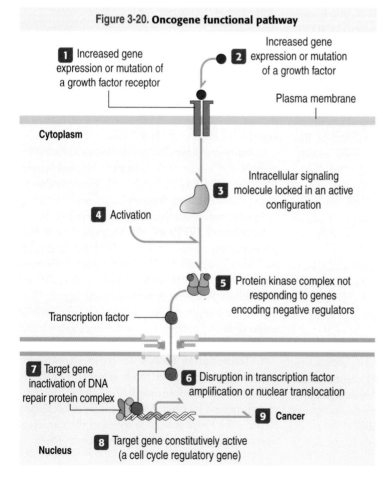

Figure 3-20. Oncogene functional pathway

Neoplastic adenomatous polyps have similar features of carcinoma in situ and are precursors of carcinomas in some organs such as colon (see Chapter 16, Lower Digestive Segment). A polyp grows outwards from an epithelial surface, representing a neoplasm (adenoma) or an inflammatory process.

In addition to **local invasion**, carcinoma cells spread through lymphatic vessels, giving rise to **metastases in lymph nodes**. Some carcinoma cells invade blood vessels to produce **hematogenous metastases**. Metastasis (Greek *meta*, on the midst of; *stasis*, placing), or **secondary tumors**, originate from cells detached from a **primary tumor**.

Sarcomas originate in mesenchyme-derived soft tissues, are locally invasive and spread predominantly through blood vessels. Sarcomas progenitor cells are not restricted by a basement membrane like epithelial cell progenitors. Sarcomas consist of fusiform cells, whereas carcinomas tend to retain an epithelial configuration stabilized by cell junctions and cell adhesion molecules.

Note in Figure 3-19 the designation of benign and malignant tumors of mesenchymal origin.

Figure 3-19 also shows the designation of a number of tumors that do not conform with the carcinoma and sarcoma designation. They are named on the basis of their cell or tissue origin:

1. **Lymphomas**, when they originate in the lymphoid system.
2. **Melanoma**, when the cell of origin is the melanocyte.
3. **Leukemias** (Greek *leukos*, white; *haima*, blood), when the malignancy develops from multipotential stem cells or committed progenitor cells and spreads through the body after crossing endothelial cell barriers. Hematopoietic neoplasms can arise from a preceding **myelodysplasia**, an equivalent to epithelial dysplasia.
4. **Teratoma**, when benign or malignant tumoral cells derive from the three embryological layers (ectoderm, mesoderm and endoderm), the male and female gonads or non-gonadal sites.
5. **Hamartomas**, when developmental abnormalities (such as hemangiomas) produce tumoral masses in a normal site (skin).
6. **Choristomas**, when tissue overgrowth takes place in an aberrant site and mimics a tumor. Choristomas can be localized in the head and neck region (pharynx, oral cavity and middle ear). Several different tissue types can occur in the oral cavity as choristomas (cartilage, bone, glial tissue and thyroid tissue).

In addition, a number of tumors are identified by the name of the discoverer (see Figure 3-19). For example, **Ewing's sarcoma**, a bone tumor highly sensitive to radiation therapy that affects children and young adults, belongs to the group of Ewing's Sar-

Box 3-H | **Proto-oncogenes and oncogenes**

- A **proto-oncogene** is a normal gene encoding a regulatory protein of the cell cycle, cell differentiation, or a cell-signaling pathway. Proto-oncogenic proteins mimic growth factors, hormone receptors, G proteins, intracellular enzymes, and transcription factors.
- An **oncogene** is a **mutated proto-oncogene** that encodes an **oncoprotein** able to disrupt the normal cell cycle and to cause cancer.
- Proto-oncogenes and oncogene are designated by an **italicized three-letter name**. An oncogene present in a virus has the prefix **v**. A proto-oncogene present in a cell has the prefix **c**.
- A protein encoded by a proto-oncogene or oncogene has the same three-letter designation as the proto-oncogene or oncogene; however, the letters are not italicized and the first letter is capitalized.
- **Anti-oncogenes** are also called **tumor suppressor genes**. Uncontrolled activity of a tumor suppressor gene product results in constitutive activation of cell growth (uncontrolled cell division), leading to cancer.

coma Family of Tumor (ESFT). ESFT is characterized by a translocation between chromosomes 11 and 22, t(11;22) of a gene in chromosome 22, that encodes the Ewing sarcoma gene (EWS), and the transcription factor encoding gene FLI1 from chromosome 11. The result is a new fused gene, EWA/FLI, encoding an abnormal protein.

Burkitt's lymphoma is described in Box 3-G. Details on **Hodgkin's disease** or lymphoma are included in Chapter 10, Immune-Lymphatic System. **Kaposi's sarcoma** (a tumor originated in endothelial cells caused by human herpesvirus 8 [HHV8], also known as Kaposi's sarcoma-associated herpesvirus [KSHV]) is discussed in Chapter 12, Cardiovascular System.

General Pathology: Proto-oncogenes, oncogenes, and tumor suppressor genes

Mutations of proto-oncogenes and tumor suppressor genes lead to cancer. The mutated version of a proto-oncogene (Greek *prōtos*, first; *genos*, birth) (see Box 3-H) is called oncogene (Greek *onkos*, bulk, mass).

Mutations of proto-oncogenes are **dominant** because the mutation of a single allele can lead to cellular transformation. In contrast, the mutation of a tumor suppressor gene is **recessive**: both alleles of a tumor suppressor gene must be mutated for cell transformation to take place.

Oncogenes express **constantly** active products leading to unregulated cell growth and differentiation, the two properties of cancer cells. A cell becomes **transformed** when it changes from regulated to unregulated growth.

Mutations can be in the gene sequence (point mutations, deletions, insertions or gene amplification) or by **chromosomal translocation or chromosomal fusion** (by placing a gene in a different regulatory environment). Note that the terms proto-oncogenes and oncogenes are not interchangeable.

Figure 3-20 integrates the six major categories of oncogene products within the oncogene functional pathway.

Oncogene genes are involved in several **regulatory functions** as (Figure 3-21):

1. **Growth factors.**
2. **Growth factor receptors.**
3. **Signal transduction molecules.**
4. **Transcription factors.**
5. **Other factors.**

1. **Growth factors:** Oncogene-derived proteins are capable to induce the abnormal proliferation of nearby cells (paracrine), distant cells (endocrine) or their own (autocrine). Examples are **platelet-derived growth factor** (PDGF) released from platelets during coagulation and the **Wingless family** of secreted glycoproteins (see Box 3-D)

2. **Growth factor receptors** (receptor tyrosine kinases): As we have already seen earlier in this chapter, tyrosine kinases add phosphate groups to tyrosine residues in target proteins to switch them on or off. When a cell surface receptor is constitutively tyrosine phosphorylated (in the absence of a ligand), it transmits signals inside the cell leading to cancer. Examples are the **epidermal growth factor receptor (EGFR)**, **platelet-derived growth factor receptor (PDGFR)**, **vascular endothelial growth factor receptor (VEGFR)**, **human epidermal growth factor receptor 2 (HER2)**, and **c-kit receptor** (involved in the migration of mast cells to the connective tissue and the colonization of the gonadal ridges by primordial germ cells during development).

3. **Signal transducer molecules**, including:
Cytoplasmic tyrosine kinases. Examples of intracellular oncogenes with tyrosine kinase activity include the *c-abl* gene in **chronic myeloid leukemia** and the **Src family** (see Box 3-G).

Cytoplasmic serine/threonine kinases. Examples include **Raf kinase**, that activates a second kinase, MEK (see The Ras, Raf and MAP kinase pathway) and **cyclin-dependent kinases**, discussed in Chapter 1, Epithelium, in our discussion of the cell cycle.

Regulatory GTPases. An example is the **Ras protein,** a membrane associated GTP binding/GTPase. After interacting with Raf cytoplasmic protein serine kinase, Ras breaks down GTP into GDP and a phosphate following activation by the ligands EGF or TGF-β. Ras protein, acting as an on/off switch in major signaling pathways, stimulates cell growth and proliferation.

4. **Transcription factors:** Oncogenes coding for sequence-specific DNA binding proteins include *myb* (for avian myeloblastosis virus) and *ets* (for E26 transformation specific). An example for transcription factor is the *c-myc* gene, that regulates the transcription of genes inducing cell proliferation.

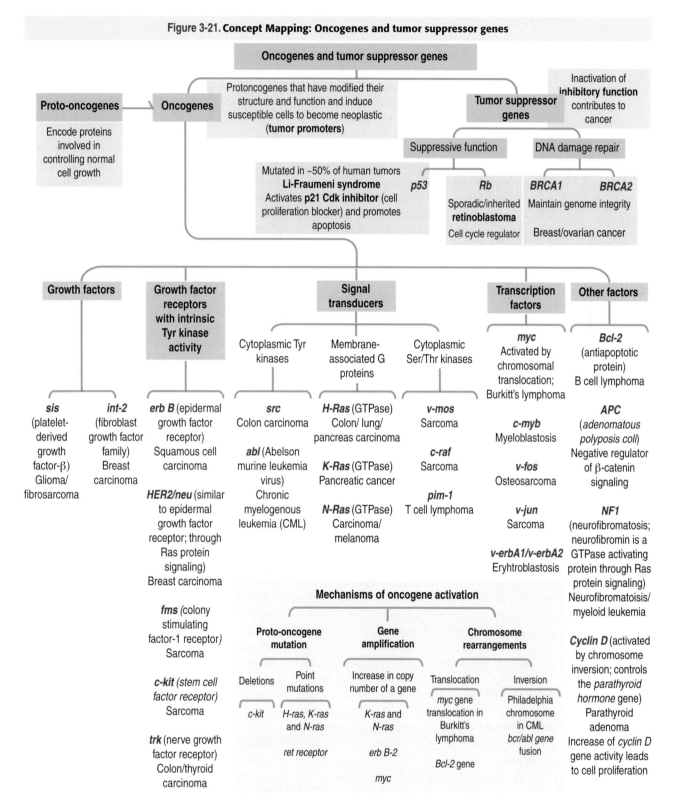

Figure 3-21. Concept Mapping: Oncogenes and tumor suppressor genes

The *c-myc* gene is an example of proto-oncogene activation by chromosomal translocation. The *c-myc* gene is translocated to one of the immunoglobulin loci in Burkitt's lymphomas (see Box 3-G). The *c-myc* gene is a target of the APC/β-catenin/Tcf pathway in colon carcinoma cells (see Chapter 16, Lower Digestive Segment).

5. **Other factors**, inluding the activation of the oncogene *Bcl-2,* associated with mitochondrial membranes, can block apoptosis, as we have already discussed; the *APC* gene, a negative regulator of β-catenin signaling in *Adenomatous polyposis coli*, and others (see Figure 3-21).

Tumor suppressor genes encode proteins that under normal conditions prevent the development of tumors. In general, they inhibit the cell cycle. When this inhibitory function is lost because of a mutation of a tumor suppressor gene, a condition known as **loss-of-function** mutations, cancer development occurs. As indicated above, a mutation in tumor suppressor genes is recessive because inactivation of both alleles is required in an individual cell.

Tumor suppressor genes include the **p53 gene** the **retinoblastoma (Rb)** gene (see Chapter 1, Epithelium). Their function is to regulate the cell cycle.

An additional group includes the **BRCA1** and **BRCA2 genes**, tumor suppressor genes associated with breast and ovarian cancer. Their function is to maintain DNA integrity.

The gene products encoded by the *BRCA1* and *BRCA2* genes are nuclear proteins that co-localize with RAD-51 at sites of DNA damage and participate in homologous recombination repair of double-stranded breaks.

A loss of *BRCA1* or *BRCA2* gene function encodes defective protein products resulting in the accumulation of genetic defects that can lead to cancer. We come back to the role of *BRCA1* and *BRCA2* genes in breast cancer in Chapter 23, Fertilization, Placentation, and Lactation.

Identification of oncogenes in retroviruses

Although most animal viruses destroy the cells they infect, several types of viruses are able to establish a long-term infection, in which the cell is not killed. This stable virus–host cell interaction perpetuates the viral information in the cell, usually by direct insertion into cellular DNA.

The first oncogenes to be identified came from the study of **retroviruses**. All vertebrate animals, including humans, inherit genes related to retroviral genes and transmit them to their progeny. These are called **endogenous proviruses**, whereas those that infect a cell are called **exogenous proviruses**.

Cancer viruses isolated from every type of vertebrate animal induce a wide variety of tumors and belong to several virus types: **RNA-containing tumor viruses**, called **retroviruses**, and **DNA-containing tumor viruses**, including the **polyomaviruses**, the **papillomaviruses**, the **adenoviruses**, and the **herpesviruses**.

RNA-containing retroviruses have a distinct cell cycle. In the initial stages of infection, the **viral RNA is copied into DNA** by the viral enzyme **reverse transcriptase**. Once synthesized, the viral DNA molecule is transported into the nucleus and inserted randomly as a **provirus** at any one of the available sites of host chromosomal DNA. Proviruses contain signals for the regulation of their own viral genes, but such signals can be transmitted to the proto-oncogene, forcing it to produce larger than normal amounts of RNA and a protein.

Retroviruses and polyomaviruses have received the most attention because they carry one or two genes that have specific cancer-inducing properties: so-called **viral oncogenes**. Retroviruses and polyomaviruses like cellular genes, are subject to mutations. A group of such mutants of **Rous sarcoma virus (RSV**; species of origin: chicken) has proved useful for determining the role of the **viral gene v-src**. The *src*-like sequences in normal cells constitute a **cellular gene called c-src**, a **proto-oncogene**.

The **viral *src*** derives directly from the **cellular *src***. A precursor of RSV seems to have acquired a copy of c-src during infection of a chicken cell. **c-src is harmless but its close relative, v-src, causes tumors and transform cells after RSV infection**. A chicken fibroblast produces about 50 times more src RNA and protein than an uninfected fibroblast containing only the c-*src* gene. The c-*src* gene assumed great significance when it was recognized that many other retroviruses carry oncogenes, often different from v-*src*. Each of these genes is also derived from a distinct, normal cellular precursor.

The classification of genes as proto-oncogenes is based on the understanding that mutant forms of these genes participate in the development of cancer (see Box 3-G). However, proto-oncogenes serve different biochemical functions in the control of normal growth and development.

RSV-infected cells produce a 60-kd protein. This protein was identified as the product that the **v-*src* gene** uses to transform cells. It was named **p60$^{v\text{-}src}$**. This protein can function as a **protein kinase** and, within a living cell, many proteins can be phosphorylated by **Src kinase** activity. The target for phosphorylation is **tyrosine** residues.

Cell transformation by the v-*src* oncogene causes a tenfold increase in total cellular phosphotyrosine in cellular target proteins restricted to the inner side of the **cell membrane**. Many other proteins encoded by proto-oncogenes or involved in control of cell growth function like the Src protein, such as protein kinases, are often specific for tyrosine.

• Cell signaling is the mechanism by which cells respond to chemical signals. Signaling molecules are either secreted or expressed on the cell surface of cells. When a signaling molecule binds to its receptor, it initiates intracellular reactions to regulate cell proliferation, differentiation, cell movements, metabolism, and behavior.

• There are several cell signaling mechanisms:
(1) Endocrine signaling involves a hormone secreted by an endocrine cell and transported through blood circulation to act on a distant target.
(2) Paracrine signaling is mediated by molecules acting locally to regulate the function of a neighboring cell.
(3) Autocrine signaling consists in cells responding to signaling molecules that are produced by themselves.
(4) Neurotransmitter signaling is a specific form of paracrine signaling involving neurons and neurotransmitter molecules released at a synapse.
(5) Neuroendocrine signaling consists in a neuroendocrine cell releasing a hormone into the bloodstream in response to a stimulus released from an axon terminal.
Cell signaling requires negative or positive feedback action to regulate the release of the targeting hormone or ligand.

• Hormones or ligands can be:
(1) Steroid hormones (for example, cholesterol-derived testosterone, estrogen, progesterone, and corticosteroids).
(2) Peptide hormones (for example, insulin, neuropeptides secreted by neurons, and

growth factors). Steroid hormones bind to cytosol and nuclear receptors. Nonsteroid signaling molecules, such as thyroid hormone, vitamin D_3, and retinoids (vitamin A), bind to intracellular receptors.
Peptide hormones and growth factors bind to a cell surface receptor.
Several specific signaling molecules exist:
(1) Epinephrine can be a neurotransmitter and also a hormone released into the bloodstream.
(2) Eicosanoids and leukotrienes (derived from arachidonic acid) are lipid-containing signaling molecules, which bind to cell surface receptors.

• Nitric oxide is a signaling molecule of very short half-life (seconds). Nitric oxide is synthesized from arginine by the enzyme nitric oxide synthase. Nitric oxide can diffuse across the plasma membrane but it does not bind to a receptor. Its major function is the regulation of the activity of intracellular enzymes. One of the relevant functions of nitric oxide is the dilation of blood vessels. Nitroglycerin, an agent used in the treatment of heart disease, is converted to nitric oxide, which increases heart blood flow by dilation of the coronary artery.

• After binding to a cell surface receptor, peptide hormones or growth factors activate intracellular targets downstream of the receptor.
(1) G protein–coupled receptors consist of three subunits (α, β and γ) forming a complex. The α subunit binds GDP (guanosine diphosphate) and regulates G protein activity. When a signaling molecule binds to its receptor, the α subunit of the associated G protein dissoci-

ates, releases GDP, and binds GTP (guanosine triphosphate) to activate an adjacent target molecule.
(2) Tyrosine kinases can be a transmembrane protein or present in the cytosol. The first form is called tyrosine kinase receptor; the second form is known as nonreceptor tyrosine kinase. Binding of a ligand to tyrosine kinase receptor produces its dimerization resulting in autophosphorylation of the intracellular domain. Downstream molecules with SH2 (Src homology 2) domains bind to the catalytic kinase domain of tyrosine kinase receptor. The activity of tyrosine kinase receptor can be disrupted by inducing unregulated autophosphorylation in the absence of a ligand. Tyrosine kinase activity can be inhibited by imatinib mesylate, a molecule with binding affinity to the adenosine triphosphate (ATP)-binding domain of the catalytic domain. Imatinib is used in the treatment of chronic myeloid leukemia, chronic myelomonocytic leukemia, systemic mastocytosis, and mast cell leukemias.
(3) Cytokine receptors are a family of receptors that stimulate intracellular protein tyrosine kinases, which are not intrinsic components of the receptor. Ligand binding to cytokine receptors triggers receptor dimerization and cross-phosphorylation of the associated tyrosine kinases. Members of the cytokine receptor–associated tyrosine kinase family are the Src family and the Janus kinase family (JAK).
(4) Receptors can be linked to enzymes such as protein tyrosine phosphatases and protein serine and threonine kinases. Tyrosine phosphatases remove tyrosine phosphate groups from phosphotyrosine and

Concept mapping | **Cell Signaling**

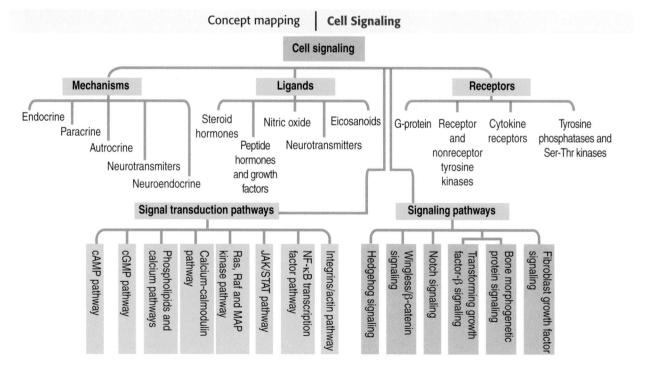

arrest signaling started by tyrosine phosphorylation. Members of the transforming growth factor-β (TGF-β) family are protein kinases that phosphorylate serine and threonine residues. Ligand binding to TGF-β induces receptor dimerization and the serine- or threonine-containing intracellular domain of the receptor cross-phosphorylates the polypeptide chains of the receptor.

• Following ligand binding, most receptors activate intracellular enzymes to transmit and amplify a signal.

(1) The cAMP (cyclic adenosine monophosphate) pathway results from the formation of cAMP (known as a second messenger) from ATP by the enzyme adenylyl cyclase. The intracellular effects of cAMP are mediated by cAMP-dependent protein kinase (also known as protein kinase A). Inactive cAMP-dependent protein kinase is a tetramer composed of two regulatory subunits (the binding site of cAMP) and two catalytic subunits. The enzyme phosphodiesterase degrades cAMP. Upon cAMP binding, the catalytic subunits dissociate and each catalytic subunit phosphorylates serine residues on target proteins or migrates to the cell nucleus.

In the cell nucleus, the catalytic subunit phosphorylates the transcription factor CREB (CRE-binding protein) bound to CRE (the cAMP response element), and specific gene activity is induced.

(2) The cGMP (cyclic guanosine monophosphate) pathway uses guanylate cyclase to produce cGMP, which is degraded by a cGMP-dependent phosphodiesterase. Photoreceptors of the retina use cGMP to convert light signals to nerve impulses.

(3) The phospholipase C–Ca²⁺ pathway consists in the production of second messengers from the phospholipid phosphatidylinositol 4.5-bisphosphate (PIP_2). Hydrolysis of PIP_2 by phospholipase C (PLC) produces two second messengers: diacylglycerol and inositol 1,4,5-triphosphate (IP_3). Diacylglycerol and IP_3 stimulate protein kinase C (protein serine and threonine kinases) and the mobilization of Ca^{2+}. Protein kinase C activates protein kinases of the MAP (mitogen activated protein) kinase pathway to phosphorylate transcription factors.

(4) The Ca^{2+}-calmodulin pathway consists in the activation of calmodulin, a Ca^{2+}-dependent protein, when Ca^{2+} concentration increases and binds to calmodulin. You should note that the phospholipase C–Ca^{2+} and Ca^{2+}-calmodulin pathway regulates Ca^{2+} concentration by Ca^{2+} release from intracellular storage as well as entry into the cell from the extracellular space.

(5) The MAP kinase pathway involves serine and threonine MAP kinases. The extracellular signal–regulated kinase (ERK) family is a MAP kinase acting through either tyrosine kinase or G protein–associated receptors. The activation of ERK is mediated by two protein kinases: Raf and MEK (MAP kinase or ERK kinase). Raf interacts with rat sarcoma virus (Ras) protein, a key element of the group of oncogenic proteins.

Raf phosphorylates MEK which activates ERK, and then phosphorylated ERK activates nuclear (Elk-1) and cytosolic target proteins. Two other MAP kinases are JNK and p38 MAP kinases.

(6) The JAK-STAT pathway regulates transcription factors. Signal transducer and activators of transcription (STAT) proteins are transcription factors with an SH2 domain and present in the cytoplasm in an inactive state. Ligand binding to a cytokine receptor determines the attachment of STAT to the receptor associated Janus kinase (JAK), a tyrosine kinase, through their SH2 domain. Phosphorylated STAT dimerizes and translocates to the cell nucleus to activate gene transcription.

(7) The NF-κB (for nuclear factor involved in the transcription of the κ light chain gene in B lymphocytes) transcription factor pathway is stimulated by protein kinase C and is involved in immune responses. When inactive, the NF-κB heterodimer is bound to the inhibitory subunit I-κB and remains in the cytoplasm. Phosphorylation of I-κB, triggered by I-κB kinase, results in the destruction of I-κB by the 26S proteasome and the nuclear translocation of the NF-κB heterodimer to activate gene transcription.

(8) The integrin-actin pathway transmits outside-in mechanical and chemical signals initiated in the extracellular matrix to the cell interior mediated by intermediary proteins linking actin to integrin heterodimers.

• There are specific signaling pathways with roles in embryonic and fetal development, body axis patterning, cell migration and cell proliferation. They include:

(1) Hedgehog (HH) signaling.
(2) Wingless (Wnt)/β-catenin signaling.
(3) Notch signaling; (4) Transforming growth factor-β (TGF-β) signaling.
(5) Bone morphogenetic protein signaling, a member of the TGF-β superfamily.
(6) Fibroblast growth factor signaling.

All of them utilize diverse regulatory steps and crosstalk mechanisms, including transcription factors that translocate from the cytoplasm to the nucleus.

• Stem cells have three properties:
(1) Self-renewal.
(2) Proliferation.
(3) Differentiation.
Stem cells, housed in a distinct microenvironment called stem cell niche, can give rise to cell precursors that generate tissues of the body.

The functional state of stem cells is governed by stemness. Stemness is the characteristic gene expression profile of different stem cells not observed in ordinary, non-stem cells.

Stem cells are present in the intestinal epithelium, the epidermis of the skin, the hematopoietic tissue, and spermatogenic cells.

• Human pluripotent cells and cell replacement therapies are the pursuit of regenerative medicine.

Three cell reprogramming methods have been used to produce pluripotent embryonic stem cells:

(1) Induced programmed stem cells (iPS) using a transcription factor cocktail.
(2) Somatic cell nuclear transfer (SCNT), or cloning, to produce genetically matched nuclear transfer embryonic cells (NT ES) removed from the inner cell mass of embryos.
(3) Blastocysts from the inner cell mass of embryos derived from in vitro fertilization (unprogrammed embryonic stem cells, IVF ES).

IVF ES exhibit properties close to the intact blastocysts but they are allogenic (they exhibit properties close to the intact blastocysts but are genetically different and potentially incompatible when transplanted). NT ES are epigenetically stable (like IVF ES) and histocompatible (like iPS).

• Cell culture procedures demonstrate that:
(1) Cells stop growing when they cover entirely the surface of a culture dish. This is called density-dependent inhibition of growth.
(2) Cultured cells can continue growing until they stop dividing. The cells have become senescent.
(3) Tumor cells can become immortal and their growth in culture is endless. Such cells can establish a cell line.
(4) Transformed cells have a malignant growth potential and exhibit anchorage-independent growth. In contrast, normal cells grow attached to a substrate.

• Aging is the gradual decline over time in cell and tissue function that often, not always, decreases the longevity of an individual. Cellular senescence specifies the molecular aspects of loss of function of mitotic cells during aging. For example, telomerases maintain the end of the chromosomes, the telomeres. Insufficient telomerase activity forces cells into senescence. Telomere shortening is a potent tumor suppressor mechanism. Most tumor express human telomerase reverse transcriptase (hTERT) and the growth of their cells in culture is endless.

• Cell injury consists in a number of biochemical and morphologic changes resulting from exogenous or endogenous causes leading to a reversible or irreversible disruption of normal cell function. Hypoxia (a decrease in the supply of oxygen) or anoxia (a complete block in oxygen supply) trigger cell injury. Ischemia is a major cause of cell injury. Complete ischemia by blockage of an arterial branch of the coronary artery causes infarction of the cardiac muscle supplied by that blood vessel. If the occluded blood vessel is reopened soon after ischemic injury (by angioplasty and thrombolysis), injured cardiocytes may recover by reperfusion.

• Oxygen is essential for oxidative phophorylation involved in ATP production by mitochondria. Increased mitochondrial permeability is a typical feature of mitochondrial damage. Impaired mitochondrial function results in a decrease in ATP production, increase of reactive oxygen species (ROS; superoxide, hydrogen peroxide and hydroxyl radicals) and leakage of cytochrome *c* (the trigger of the intrinsic apoptosis pathway). ATP deficiency affects the function of ATP-dependent pumps at the plasma membrane, resulting in a significantly unregulated influx of calcium, sodium and water and an efflux of potassium. Excess of intracellular calcium, together with a leakage of lysosomal hydrolytic enzymes (due to lysosomal membrane permeability), activate cytosolic enzymes, which degrade cell components and continue enhancing mitochondrial permeability.

Depending on the type and time of injury and the characteristics of an injured cell, injury can be reversible or irreversible.

Irreversible cell injury determines cell death by necrosis (unregulated process of cell death) or apoptosis (regulated process of cell death).

Necrosis can be recognized by microscopic and macroscopic changes. Microscopic changes include a breakdown of cell membranes, cell swelling and nuclear changes (pyknosis, karyolysis, and karyorrhexis).

Macroscopic changes include:
(1) Coagulative necrosis.
(2) Liquefactive necrosis.
(3) Caseous necrosis.
(4) Fat necrosis.
Fibrinoid necrosis of the wall of blood vessels can be detected microscopically.

• Apoptosis or programmed cell death can be determined by external and internal signals.
Two **extrinsic pathways** are:
(1) The granzyme B/perforin pathway.
(2) The Fas receptor/Fas ligand pathway.
The **intrinsic pathway** consists in the leakage of mitochondrial cytochrome *c* into the cytosol.

The end point of all three pathways is the activation of procaspases to caspases, the initiators and executors of cell death.

A defect in the activity of Fas receptor, Fas ligand, and caspases can cause the autoim-mune lymphoproliferative syndrome (ALPS), characterized by the abnormal and excessive accumulation of lymphocytes in the lymph nodes and spleen.

Aberrant activation of caspases is associated with neurodegenerative disease, such as **amyotrophic lateral sclerosis** (ALS) and **Huntington's disease.**

• Necroptosis is a regulated form of necrosis involving a molecular mechanism distinct from necrosis and apoptosis. Necrotic cell death is dependent on receptor-interacting protein kinase 3 (RIPK3).

Necroptosis has pathophysiologic relevance in myocardial infarction and stroke, atherosclerosis, ischemia–reperfusion injury, pancreatitis, and inflammatory bowel diseases.

Two significant differences are:
(1) Necroptosis has inflammation as an alternative to necrotic cell death through the NF-κB activation pathway.
(2) Necrotic cell death can take place by either a caspase-dependent mechanism (apoptosis) or caspase-independent mechanism (necroptosis).

• The proteolysis of residual and misfolded proteins or the disposal of aged organelles, like mitochondria, can occur by:
(1) The autophagy pathway, starting with a phagophore sourrounding and enclosing the disposable organelle to be degraded by lysosomes.
(2) The ubiquitin–26S proteasome pathway requires the attachment of a polyubiquitin chain to proteins marked for degradation by the ~2000-kd 26S proteasome protease.
(3) The mitophagy signaling pathway, concerned with the disposal of defective or non-functional mitochondria utilizing parkin, a ubiquitin ligase, and PINK1, a protein kinase. The final elimination step of the polyubiquitinated target involves the 26S proteasome.

• Neoplasia (tumor) can be:
(1) Benign or malignant.
(2) Epithelial or non-epithelial (mesenchyma)–derived.
Benign epithelial tumors include papillomas and adenomatous polyps.

Malignant epithelial tumors are called carcinomas (epithelial-type) or adenocarcinomas (glandular-type).

Sarcomas are mesenchyme-derived tumors. Review the terminology using Figure 3-19.

Carcinomas can spreads by local invasion or through lymphatic vessels, giving rise to metastases in lymph nodes.

Sarcomas usually spread by hematogenous metastases (predominantly through blood vessels).

• Proto-oncogenes express growth factors, growth factor receptors, signal transduction molecules, nuclear transcription factors and other factors. An oncogene results from the mutation of a proto-oncogene. Oncogenes determine unregulated cell growth and a cell then becomes transformed.

Tumor suppressor genes encode proteins that under normal conditions prevent the development of tumors by inhibiting the potentially malignant cell cycle. Cancer develops when this inhibitory function is not present (loss-of-function).

The first oncogenes to be identified were the retroviruses (RNA-containing viruses) with cancer-inducing properties (viral oncogenes).

DNA-containing viruses (polyomaviruses, the papillomaviruses, the adenoviruses, and the herpesviruses) can induce tumors.

The chicken cell Rous sarcoma virus (RSV) includes the viral gene *v-src*. The proto-oncogene equivalent in normal cells is *c-src*. The *v-src* gene encodes the protein p60^{v-src}, which functions as a tyrosine protein kinase.

Cell transformation by the *v-src* oncogene results in a significant increase in total cell phosphotyrosine.

4. Connective Tissue

The connective tissue provides the supportive and connecting framework (or stroma) for all the other tissues of the body. The connective tissue is formed by cells, fibers and the extracellular matrix (ECM). The ECM (ground substance) represents a combination of collagens, noncollagenous glycoproteins, and proteoglycans surrounding the cells of connective tissue. The resident cell of the connective tissue is the fibroblast. Immigrant cells to the connective tissue include macrophages, mast cells, and plasma cells. The connective tissue has important roles in immune and inflammatory responses, and tissue repair after injury.

Classification

Unlike epithelial cells, which are almost free of intercellular material, **connective tissue cells are widely separated by components of the ECM.** In addition, epithelial cells lack direct blood and lymphatic supply, whereas connective tissue is directly supplied by blood and lymphatic vessels and nerves.

The classification of the connective tissue into specific types is based on the proportion of three of its components: **cells, fibers,** and **ECM.**

Connective tissue can be classified into three major groups:

1. **Embryonic connective tissue** (or mesenchyme, Figure 4-1).
2. **Adult connective tissue** (Figure 4-1).
3. **Special connective tissue** (Figure 4-2).

Embryonic connective tissue derives from the mesoderm during early embryonic development. This type of connective tissue, found primarily in the **umbilical cord,** consists predominantly of stellate-shaped **mesenchymal cells** producing a **hydrophilic ECM** with a jelly-like consistency. Because of this consistency, it is also called **mucoid connective tissue** or **Wharton's jelly.**

Adult connective tissue has considerable structural diversity because **the proportion of cells to fibers varies from tissue to tissue.** This variable cell-to-fibers ratio is the basis for the subclassification of adult connective tissue into two types of connective tissue proper:

1. **Loose** (or **areolar**) **connective tissue**
2. **Dense connective tissue**

Loose connective tissue contains **more cells than collagen fibers** and is generally found surrounding blood vessels, nerves, and muscles. This type of connective tissue facilitates dissection as performed by anatomists, pathologists, and surgeons.

Dense connective tissue contains **more collagen fibers than cells.** When the collagen fibers are preferentially oriented, as in tendons, ligaments, and the cornea, the tissue is called **dense regular connective tissue.** When the collagen fibers are randomly oriented, as in the dermis of the skin and submucosa of the alimentary tube, the tissue is called **dense irregular connective tissue.**

Adult connective tissue includes **reticular** and **elastic connective tissue** that predominate in specific organs.

Reticular connective tissue (Figure 4-2) contains reticular fibers, which form the **stroma** of organs of the lymphoid-immune system (for example, lymph nodes and spleen), the hematopoietic bone marrow, and the liver. This type of connective tissue provides a delicate meshwork to allow passage of cells and fluid.

Elastic connective tissue (Figure 4-2) contains irregularly arranged **elastic fibers** in ligaments of the vertebral column or concentrically arranged **sheets** or **laminae** in the wall of the aorta. This type of connective tissue provides **elasticity.**

The **special connective tissue** category comprises types of connective tissue with special properties not observed in the embryonic or adult connective tissue proper. There are four types of special connective tissue (Figure 4-2):

1. **Adipose tissue.**
2. **Cartilage.**
3. **Bone.**
4. **Hematopoietic tissue (bone marrow).**

Adipose tissue has more cells (called **adipose cells** or **adipocytes**) than collagen fibers and ECM. This type of connective tissue is the most significant energy storage site of the body.

Cartilage and **bone,** also regarded as **special connective tissue,** are traditionally placed in separate categories. Essentially, cartilage and bone are dense connective tissues with specialized cells and ECM. An important difference is that cartilage has a **noncalcified ECM,** whereas the ECM of bone is **calcified.** These two types of specialized connective tissue fulfill weight-bearing and mechanical functions that are discussed later (see Cartilage and Bone). The **hematopoietic tissue** is found in the marrow of selected bones. This type of connective tissue is discussed in Chapter 6, Blood and Hematopoiesis.

Figure 4-1. Classification of connective tissue

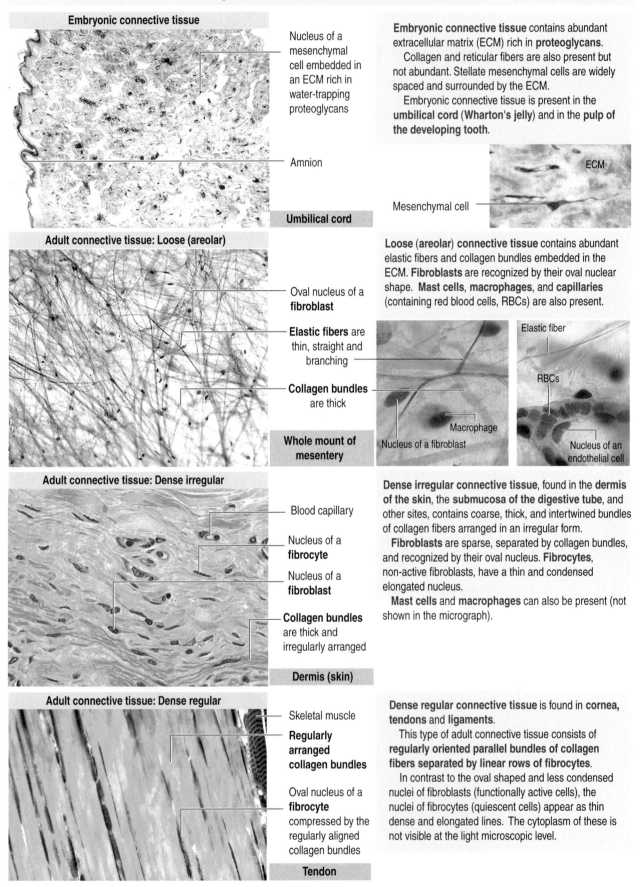

Embryonic connective tissue

Umbilical cord

Nucleus of a mesenchymal cell embedded in an ECM rich in water-trapping proteoglycans

Amnion

Embryonic connective tissue contains abundant extracellular matrix (ECM) rich in **proteoglycans**.

Collagen and reticular fibers are also present but not abundant. Stellate mesenchymal cells are widely spaced and surrounded by the ECM.

Embryonic connective tissue is present in the **umbilical cord** (**Wharton's jelly**) and in the **pulp of the developing tooth**.

ECM

Mesenchymal cell

Adult connective tissue: Loose (areolar)

Whole mount of mesentery

Oval nucleus of a **fibroblast**

Elastic fibers are thin, straight and branching

Collagen bundles are thick

Loose (areolar) connective tissue contains abundant elastic fibers and collagen bundles embedded in the ECM. **Fibroblasts** are recognized by their oval nuclear shape. **Mast cells**, **macrophages**, and **capillaries** (containing red blood cells, RBCs) are also present.

Elastic fiber

RBCs

Macrophage

Nucleus of a fibroblast

Nucleus of an endothelial cell

Adult connective tissue: Dense irregular

Dermis (skin)

Blood capillary

Nucleus of a **fibrocyte**

Nucleus of a **fibroblast**

Collagen bundles are thick and irregularly arranged

Dense irregular connective tissue, found in the **dermis of the skin**, the **submucosa of the digestive tube**, and other sites, contains coarse, thick, and intertwined bundles of collagen fibers arranged in an irregular form.

Fibroblasts are sparse, separated by collagen bundles, and recognized by their oval nucleus. **Fibrocytes**, non-active fibroblasts, have a thin and condensed elongated nucleus.

Mast cells and **macrophages** can also be present (not shown in the micrograph).

Adult connective tissue: Dense regular

Tendon

Skeletal muscle

Regularly arranged collagen bundles

Oval nucleus of a **fibrocyte** compressed by the regularly aligned collagen bundles

Dense regular connective tissue is found in **cornea**, **tendons** and **ligaments**.

This type of adult connective tissue consists of **regularly oriented parallel bundles of collagen fibers separated by linear rows of fibrocytes**.

In contrast to the oval shaped and less condensed nuclei of fibroblasts (functionally active cells), the nuclei of fibrocytes (quiescent cells) appear as thin dense and elongated lines. The cytoplasm of these is not visible at the light microscopic level.

Figure 4-2. Classification of connective tissue

Adult connective tissue: Reticular tissue

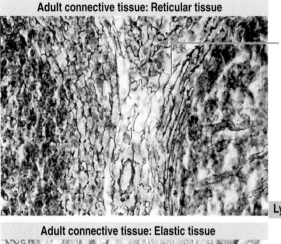

Lymphatic nodule

Reticular fibers (type III collagen) can be identified in the stroma of this lymphatic nodule after impregnation with **silver salts**. Reticular fibers are **argyrophilic**.

Reticular connective tissue is characteristic of **lymphatic tissues (lymph node and spleen)** and **liver**.

Reticular fibers, synthesized by fibroblasts (also called **reticular cells**), are thin and wavy structures.

Adult connective tissue: Elastic tissue

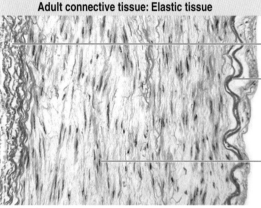

Artery

Elastic fibers are arranged in concentric sheets in the wall of this artery. In this section, elastic lamellae appear as wavy pink bands.

Smooth muscle cells

Elastic connective tissue is characteristic of **the walls of large blood vessels** and **ligaments**.

Elastic fibers in the wall of a blood vessel, are synthesized by **smooth muscle cells** and form **fenestrated lamellae** or **membrane sheet** in a concentric arrangement around the lumen.

Special types of connective tissue

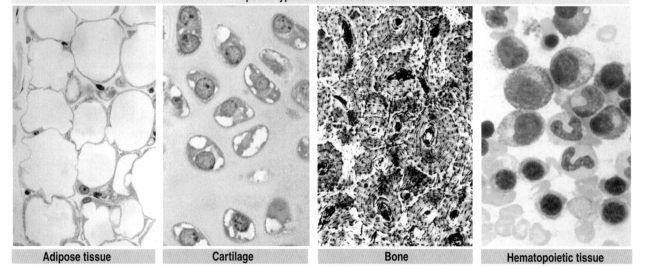

Adipose tissue | **Cartilage** | **Bone** | **Hematopoietic tissue**

Components of connective tissue

The connective tissue consists of:

1. **Cells**, including the **fibroblast**, the resident cell, and immigrant cells, the **macrophage**, the **mast cell** and the **plasma cell**.

2. Fibers (**collagen, elastic** and **reticular fibers**).

3. **ECM components**.

We discuss first how the fibroblast produces distinct types of fibers and ECM.

Fibroblast

Fibroblast, the permanent cell component of the connective tissue, can produce collagens and elastic fibers as well as ECM.

Under light microscopy, the **fibroblast** appears as a spindle-shaped cell with an elliptical nucleus. The cytoplasm is generally not resolved by the light microscope.

Under **electron microscopy**, the fibroblast shows

• **Type I collagen**
Present in **bone**, **tendon**, **dentin**, and **skin** as banded fibers with a transverse periodicity of 64 nm. This type of collagen provides tensile strength.
• **Type II collagen**
Observed in **hyaline** and **elastic cartilage** as fibrils thinner than type I collagen.
• **Type III collagen**
Present in the **reticular lamina of basement membranes**, as a component of reticular fibers (30 nm in diameter). **This is the first collagen type synthesized during wound healing and then is replaced by type I collagen.**

Reticular fibers can be better recognized after impregnation with silver salts because reticular fibers are **argyrophilic** (silver-loving; Greek *argyros*, silver). Silver impregnation is a valuable tool in pathology for the recognition of distortions in the distribution of reticular fibers in alterations of lymphoid organs. Reticular fibers, and collagens in general, are glycoproteins and can be recognized with the **periodic acid–Schiff (PAS) reaction** because of their carbohydrate content.
• **Type IV collagen**
Present in the **basal lamina**. This type of collagen does not form bundles. Single molecules of type IV collagen bind to one of the type IV collagen-binding sites of laminin.
• **Type V collagen**
Observed in **amnion** and **chorion** in the fetus and in muscle and tendon sheaths. **This type of collagen does not form banded fibrils.**

the typical features of a protein-secreting cell: a well-developed rough endoplasmic reticulum and a Golgi apparatus.

The fibroblast synthesizes and continuously secretes proteoglycans, glycoproteins and the precursor molecules of various types of collagens and elastic fibers.

Different types of collagen proteins and proteoglycans can be recognized as components of the **basement membrane**. As you may remember, **type IV collagen is found in the basal lamina** and **type III collagen** appears in the **reticular lamina** as a component of **reticular fibers** (see Boxes 4-A and 4-B). Heparan sulfate proteoglycans and the fibronectin, two additional products of the fibroblast, are present in the basement membrane. The protein collagen is a component of collagen and reticular fibers but elastic fibers lack collagen.

• The so-called **reticular cell** is in fact a fibroblast that synthesizes reticular fibers containing type III collagen. Reticular fibers form the stroma of bone marrow and lymphoid organs.
• The **osteoblast (bone)**, **chondroblast (cartilage)**, and **odontoblast (teeth) also synthesize collagen**. These cell types are fibroblast equivalents in their respective tissues. Therefore, the synthesis of collagen is not limited to the fibroblast in connective tissue. In fact, **epithelial cells synthesize type IV collagen**.
• **A fibroblast may simultaneously synthesize more than one type of collagen**.
• **Smooth muscle cells**, found in the wall of arteries, intestine, the respiratory bronchial tree, and uterus, **can synthesize types I and III collagen**.

Collagen: Synthesis, secretion, and assembly

Collagens are generally divided into two categories: **fibrillar collagens** (forming fibrils with a characteristic banded pattern), and **nonfibrillar collagens** (see Box 4-C).

The synthesis of collagen starts in the rough endoplasmic reticulum (RER) following the typical pathway of synthesis for export from the cell (Figure 4-3).

Preprocollagen is synthesized with a **signal peptide** and released as **procollagen** within the cisterna of the RER. **Procollagen** consists of three polypeptide α chains, lacking the signal peptide, assembled in a **triple helix**.

Hydroxyproline and **hydroxylysine** are typically observed in collagen. Hydroxylation of proline and lysine residues occurs in the RER and requires ascorbic acid (vitamin C) as a cofactor. Inadequate wound healing is characteristic of **scurvy**, caused by a vitamin C deficiency.

Packaging and secretion of **procollagen** take place in the Golgi apparatus. Upon secretion of procollagen, the following three events occur in the extracellular space:

1. Enzymatic (**procollagen peptidase**) removal of most of the nonhelical endings of procollagen to give rise to soluble **tropocollagen** molecules.

2. Self-aggregation of tropocollagen molecules by a stepwise overlapping process to form **collagen fibrils**.

3. Cross-linking of tropocollagen molecules, leading to the formation of **collagen fibers**. **Lysyl oxidase**

• Collagen is a three-chain fibrous protein in which the α chains coil around each other (called a coiled-coil structure) like the strands of a rope. This triple-helix molecular organization generates a protein with considerable tensile strength.
• In **fibrillar collagen** (types I, II, III, and V), the completely processed molecule contains one triple helix, which accounts for almost the entire length of each molecule. Multiple triple helices of collagen fibers are aligned end-to-end and side-by-side in a regular arrangement. As a result, collagen fibers form dark and light periodic bands observed with the electron microscope.
• In **nonfibrillar collagens**, such as **type IV collagen**, several shorter triple-helical segments are separated by non-helical triple domains and the N-terminal and C-terminal globular domains are not cleaved during protein processing.
• **Collagens form aggregates** (fibrils, fibers, or bundles) either alone or with extracellular matrix components. **Collagen fibrils and fibers** can be visualized with the electron microscope but not with the light microscope. **Collagen bundles** can be identified with the light microscope.

Figure 4-3. Synthesis of collagen

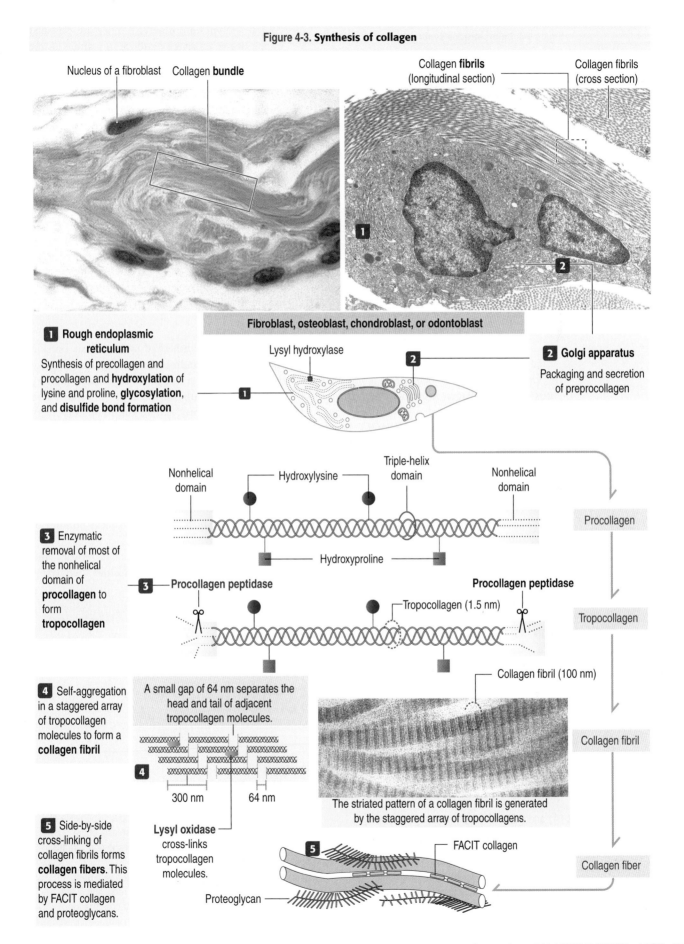

Nucleus of a fibroblast Collagen **bundle**

Collagen **fibrils** (longitudinal section)

Collagen fibrils (cross section)

1 **Rough endoplasmic reticulum**

Synthesis of precollagen and procollagen and **hydroxylation** of lysine and proline, **glycosylation**, and **disulfide bond formation**

Fibroblast, osteoblast, chondroblast, or odontoblast

Lysyl hydroxylase

2 **Golgi apparatus**

Packaging and secretion of preprocollagen

Nonhelical domain   Hydroxylysine   Triple-helix domain   Nonhelical domain

Procollagen

Hydroxyproline

3 Enzymatic removal of most of the nonhelical domain of **procollagen** to form **tropocollagen**

3 **Procollagen peptidase**   **Procollagen peptidase**

Tropocollagen (1.5 nm)

Tropocollagen

4 Self-aggregation in a staggered array of tropocollagen molecules to form a **collagen fibril**

A small gap of 64 nm separates the head and tail of adjacent tropocollagen molecules.

4

300 nm   64 nm

Collagen fibril (100 nm)

The striated pattern of a collagen fibril is generated by the staggered array of tropocollagens.

Collagen fibril

5 Side-by-side cross-linking of collagen fibrils forms **collagen fibers**. This process is mediated by FACIT collagen and proteoglycans.

Lysyl oxidase cross-links tropocollagen molecules.

5

FACIT collagen

Proteoglycan

Collagen fiber

Figure 4-4. Ehlers-Danlos syndromes

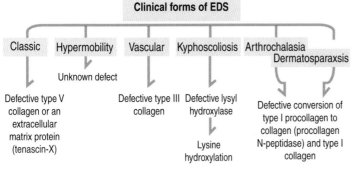

• A group of clinically and genetically diverse group of disorders resulting from defects in the synthesis and/or structure of collagen.
• Abnormal collagen is devoid of tensile strength and skin is hyperextensible and vulnerable to trauma. The joints are hypermobile.
• Collagen defects extend to blood vessels and the internal organs resulting in tissue rupture or detachment (retina).

Clinical forms of EDS

Classic	Hypermobility	Vascular	Kyphoscoliosis	Arthrochalasia Dermatosparaxsis

Defective type V collagen or an extracellular matrix protein (tenascin-X)

Unknown defect

Defective type III collagen

Defective lysyl hydroxylase → Lysine hydroxylation

Defective conversion of type I procollagen to collagen (procollagen N-peptidase) and type I collagen

catalyzes cross-links between tropocollagens.

Groups of collagen fibers orient along the same axis to form **collagen bundles**. The formation of collagen bundles is guided by proteoglycans and other glycoproteins, including **FACIT** (for fibril-associated collagens with interrupted helices) collagens.

Pathology: Ehlers-Danlos syndrome

Ehlers-Danlos syndrome (Figure 4-4) is clinically characterized by **hyperelasticity of the skin** and **hypermobility of the joints**.

The major defect resides in the synthesis, processing, and assembly of collagen. Several clinical subtypes are observed. They are classified by the degree of severity and the mutations in the collagen genes. For example, the vascular type form of Ehlers-Danlos syndrome, caused by a mutation in the *COL3A1* gene, is associated with severe vascular alterations leading to the development of varicose veins and spontaneous rupture of major arteries. A deficiency in the synthesis of type III collagen, prevalent in the walls of blood vessels, is the major defect. Arthrochalasia and dermatosparaxsis types of Ehlers-Danlos syndrome display congenital dislocation of the hips and marked joint hypermobility. Mutations in the *COL1A1* and *COL1A2* genes (Figure 4-5), encoding type I collagen, and *procollagen N-peptidase* gene disrupt the cleavage site at the N-terminal of the molecule and affect the conversion of procollagen to collagen in some individuals.

Elastic fibers

Elastic fibers are synthesized by **fibroblasts** (in skin and tendons), **chondroblasts** (in elastic cartilage of the auricle of the ear, epiglottis, larynx, and auditory tubes), and **smooth muscle cells** (in large blood vessels like the aorta and in the respiratory tree). Like collagen, the synthesis of elastic fibers involves both the RER and the Golgi apparatus (Figure 4-6).

Proelastin, the precursor of elastin, is cleaved and secreted as **tropoelastin**. In the extracellular space, tropoelastin interacts with **fibrillins 1 and 2 and fibulin 1** to organize **elastic fibers** (0.1-0.2 μm in diameter), which aggregate to form **bundles of elastic fibers**.

Tropoelastin contains a characteristic but uncommon amino acid: **desmosine**. Two lysine

Figure 4-5. Molecular defects of collagen

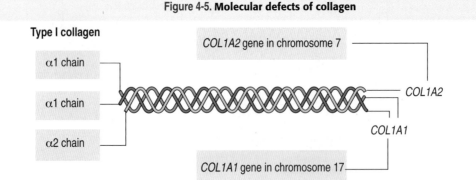

A mutation in *COL1A1* and *COL1A2* genes, encoding the α1 and α2 chains of type I collagen, respectively, involves cleavage sites for the N-terminal region of the molecule and interferes with the conversion of procollagen to collagen. This leads to defective cross-linking and a consequent reduction in the tensile strength of tendons (rich in type I collagen). This mutation is observed in some clinical forms of **Ehlers-Danlos syndrome**.

Strickler syndrome is characterized by myopia, hypoplasia of the lower jaw, and arthritis associated with dysplasia of the epiphyses. Type II collagen is abundant in cartilage and vitreous humor (eye). The *COL2A1* gene is mutated.

Osteogenesis imperfecta type I is associated with bone fragility. *COL1A1* point mutations determine a reduction in the production of type I collagen required for normal ossification.

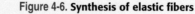

Figure 4-6. Synthesis of elastic fibers

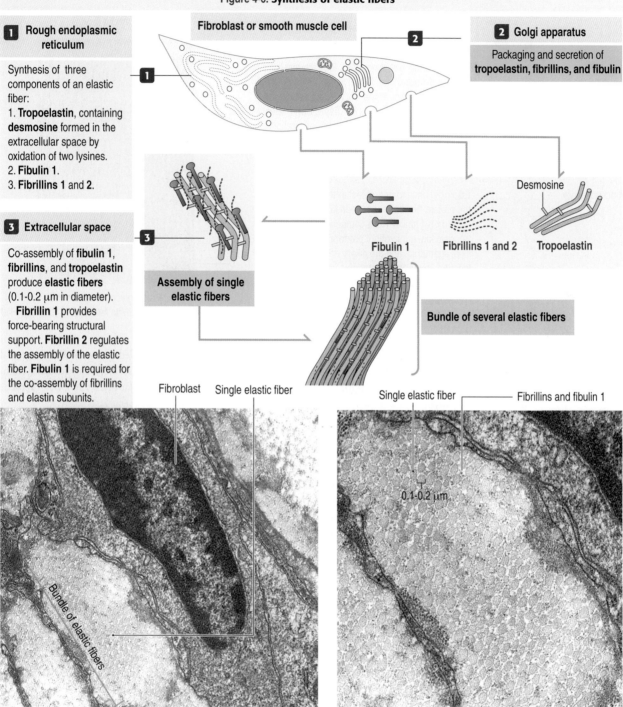

1 Rough endoplasmic reticulum

Synthesis of three components of an elastic fiber:
1. **Tropoelastin**, containing **desmosine** formed in the extracellular space by oxidation of two lysines.
2. **Fibulin 1**.
3. **Fibrillins 1** and **2**.

Fibroblast or smooth muscle cell

2 Golgi apparatus

Packaging and secretion of **tropoelastin, fibrillins, and fibulin**

3 Extracellular space

Co-assembly of **fibulin 1**, **fibrillins**, and **tropoelastin** produce **elastic fibers** (0.1-0.2 μm in diameter).
Fibrillin 1 provides force-bearing structural support. **Fibrillin 2** regulates the assembly of the elastic fiber. **Fibulin 1** is required for the co-assembly of fibrillins and elastin subunits.

Fibulin 1   Fibrillins 1 and 2   Tropoelastin

Desmosine

Assembly of single elastic fibers

Bundle of several elastic fibers

Fibroblast   Single elastic fiber

Single elastic fiber   Fibrillins and fibulin 1

0.1-0.2 μm

Bundle of elastic fibers

residues of tropoelastin are oxidized by lysyl oxidase to form a desmosine ring that cross-links two tropoelastin molecules. Cross-linking enables the stretching and recoil of tropoelastin, like rubber bands.

Elastic fibers are produced during embryonic development and in adolescence but not so much in adults. Although elastic fibers are resilient during human life, many tissues decrease elasticity with age, in particular the skin, which develops wrinkles.

Under the light microscope, elastic fibers stain black or dark blue with **orcein**, a natural dye obtained from lichens.

Under the electron microscope, a cross section of a single elastic fiber shows a dense core surrounded by microfibrils of **fibulin 1** and **fibrillins** (see Figure 4-6).

Pathology: Marfan syndrome

Marfan syndrome is an autosomal dominant disorder

Figure 4-7. Defective fibrillin

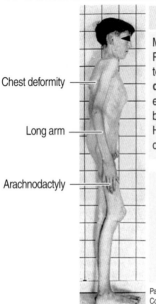

Marfan syndrome

Marfan syndrome is an autosomal dominant disorder. Patients are tall, with long arms, legs, fingers, and toes (**arachnodactyly**). **Mitral valve prolapse**, **dilation of the root of the aorta** (detected by echocardiography), and **aortic dissection** (detected by MRI) are typical cardiovascular manifestations. Heart-related complications may shorten the life span of people with Marfan syndrome.

Etiology: an inherited defect in the gene encoding the protein **fibrillin-1** is responsible for the Marfan syndrome. Fibrillin-1 is a component of tropoelastin, a microfibril predominant in the aorta, skin, ligaments, and the ciliary zonular fibers of the lens. An increase in proteoglycans between the elastic lamellae weakens the wall of the aorta.

Chest deformity

Long arm

Arachnodactyly

Patient with Marfan syndrome from McKusick VA: Heritable Disorders of Connective Tissue, 4th ed. St. Louis, Mosby, 1972.

Tunica media (aorta)

Elastic fibers

Proteoglycans replace the elastic lamellae

Microscopy from Weidner N, Cote RJ, Suster S, Weiss LM: Modern Surgical Pathology, St. Louis, Saunders, 2003.

in which the elastic tissue is weakened. Defects are predominantly observed in three systems: the **ocular**, **skeletal**, and **cardiovascular systems**. The **ocular defects** include **myopia** and **detached lens** (ectopia lentis). The skeletal defects (Figure 4-7) include long and thin arms and legs (**dolichostenomelia**), hollow chest (**pectus excavatum**), scoliosis, and elongated fingers (**arachnodactyly**).

Cardiovascular abnormalities are life-threatening. Patients with Marfan syndrome display **prolapse of the mitral valve** and **dilation of the ascending aorta**. Dilation of the aorta and peripheral arteries may progress to **dissecting aneurysm** (Greek *aneurysma*, widening) and rupture.

Medical treatment, such as administration of β-adrenergic blockers to reduce the force of systolic contraction in order to diminish stress on the aorta, and limited heavy exercise, increase the survival rate of patients with Marfan syndrome.

Defects observed in Marfan syndrome are caused by poor recoiling of the elastic lamellae dissociated by an increase in proteoglycans (see Figure 4-7). In the skeletal system, the periosteum, a relatively rigid layer covering the bone, is abnormally elastic and does not provide an oppositional force during bone development, resulting in skeletal defects.

A mutation of the *fibrillin 1* gene on chromosome 15 is responsible for Marfan syndrome. Fibrillin is present in the aorta, suspensory ligaments of the lens (see Chapter 9, Sensory Organs: Vision and Hearing), and the periosteum (see Bone).

A homologous *fibrillin 2* gene is present on chromosome 5. Mutations in the *fibrillin 2*

gene cause a disease called congenital contractural arachnodactyly. This disease affects the skeletal system, but ocular and cardiovascular defects are not observed.

Macrophages

Macrophages have **phagocytic** properties and derive from **monocytes**, cells formed in the bone marrow (Figure 4-8).

Monocytes circulate in blood and migrate into the connective tissue, where they differentiate into macrophages. Macrophages have specific names in certain organs; for example, they are called **Kupffer cells** in the liver, **osteoclasts** in bone, and **microglial cells** in the central nervous system. Macrophages migrate to the site of inflammation, attracted by certain mediators, particularly C5a (a member of the complement cascade; see Chapter 10, Immune-Lymphatic System).

Macrophages in the connective tissue have the following structural features:

1. They contain abundant **lysosomes** required for the breakdown of phagocytic materials.

2. Active macrophages have numerous **phagocytic vesicles** (or **phagosomes**) for the transient storage of ingested materials.

3. The nucleus has an irregular outline.

Macrophages of the connective tissue have three major functions:

1. **To turn over senescent fibers and ECM material.**

2. To **present antigens to lymphocytes as part of inflammatory and immunologic responses** (see Chapter 10, Immune-Lymphatic System).

3. **To produce cytokines** (for example, **interleukin-1**,

Figure 4-8. Macrophages

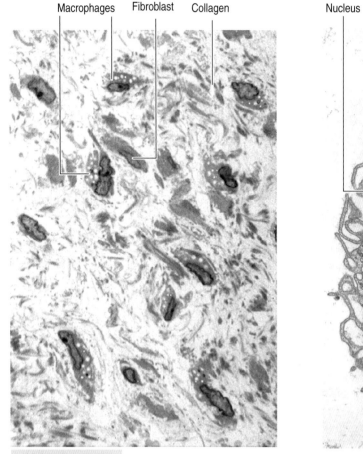

Macrophages   Fibroblast   Collagen

Light microscopy

Nucleus   Mitochondrion

Electron microscopy

Vesicle   Secondary lysosome (active)   Primary lysosome (inactive)   Filopodia

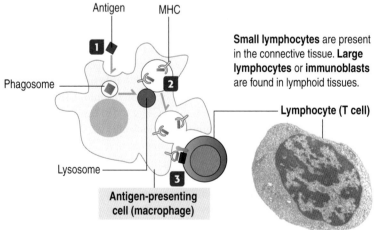

Antigen   MHC

Phagosome

Lysosome

Antigen-presenting cell (macrophage)

Lymphocyte (T cell)

Small lymphocytes are present in the connective tissue. **Large lymphocytes** or **immunoblasts** are found in lymphoid tissues.

Macrophages as antigen-presenting cells

1 A macrophage takes up an antigen that is stored within a phagocytic vesicle (phagosome).

2 A lysosome fuses with the phagosome and the antigen is broken down into small peptide fragments, which bind to a receptor molecule, called the **major histocompatibility complex (MHC)**.

3 The phagocytic vesicle fuses with the plasma membrane, and the antigen is presented to a **lymphocyte** (T cell derived from the thymus).

---

an activator of helper T cells, and **tumor necrosis factor ligand**, an inflammatory mediator (see Chapter 3, Cell Signaling).

Mast cells

Like macrophages, **mast cells** (*Mastzellen*; German, *mast*, fattening) originate in the **bone marrow** from myeloid precursor cells lacking cytoplasmic granules

but expressing the **c-kit receptor** (a tyrosine kinase), its ligand **stem cell factor** and FcεRI, the high affinity receptor for immunoglobulin E.

Mature mast cells can release abundant proteases and proteoglycans stored in granules as well as newly synthesized lipid-derived mediators (leukotrienes) after stimulation by chemokines and cytokines.

Mast cells and basophils circulating in blood derive from the same myeloid progenitor in the bone marrow. Basophils leave the bone marrow with cytoplasmic granules; mast cells acquire them later when they rich their final destination. Mast cells express α4β7 integrin, involved in the relocation or homing process.

There are two populations of mast cells:

1. **Connective tissue mast cells (CTMCs)**, that migrate and locate around blood vessels and nerve endings of the connective tissue.

2. **Mucosa mast cells (MMCs)**, that associate with T cells, predominantly in the lamina propria of the mucosae of the intestine and lungs.

An important distinction is that CTMCs are T cell–independent in contrast to MMCs, whose activities are T cell–dependent.

The **mast cell** is the source of **vasoactive mediators** contained in **cytoplasmic granules** (Figure 4-9). These granules contain **histamine**, **heparin**, and **chemotactic mediators** to attract monocytes, neutrophils, and eosinophils circulating in blood to the site of mast cell activation.

Leukotrienes are vasoactive products of mast cells. **Leukotrienes are not present in granules; instead, they are released from the cell membrane of the mast cells as metabolites of arachidonic acid** (see Chapter 3, Cell Signaling).

CTMCs differ from MMCs in the number and size of **metachromatic** (see Box 4-D) cytoplasmic granules, which tend to be more abundant in CTMCs. In addition, intestinal MMCs contain **mast cell chymase protein MCP-1** (a chymotryptic peptidase), whereas CTMCs lack this protease but express MCP-4 (a chymase), MCP-5 (an elastase), MCP-6 and MCP-7 (tryptases) and CPA3 (mast cell carboxypeptidase A). These mast cell proteases have a **pro-inflammatory** action.

Although CTMCs and MMCs have the same cell precursor, the definitive structural and functional characteristics of mast cells are acquired on the site of differentiation (connective tissue or mucosae).

General Pathology: Mast cells and allergic hypersensitivity reactions

The secretion of specific vasoactive mediators plays an important role in the regulation of vascular permeability and bronchial smooth muscle tone during **allergic hypersensitivity reactions** (for example, in **asthma**, **hay fever**, and **eczema**).

The surface of **mast cells** and **basophils** contains immunoglobulin E (IgE) receptors (**FcεRI**). Antigens bind to two adjacent FcεRI receptors and the mast cell becomes IgE-sensitized (see Figure 4-9). An IgE-sensitized mast cell releases Ca^{2+} from intracellular storage sites as well as the content of the cytoplasmic granules by a process known as **degranulation**.

The release of histamine during asthma (Greek *asthma*, panting) causes dyspnea (Greek *dyspnoia*, difficulty with breathing) triggered by the histamine-induced spasmodic contraction of the smooth muscle surrounding the bronchioles and the hypersecretion of goblet cells and mucosal glands of bronchi.

During **hay fever**, histamine increases vascular permeability leading to **edema** (excessive accumulation of fluid in intercellular spaces).

Mast cells in the connective tissue of skin release leukotrienes that induce increased vascular permeability associated with **urticaria** (Latin *urtica*, stinging nettle), a transient swelling in the dermis of the skin.

Plasma cells

The plasma cell, which derives from the differentiation of **B lymphocytes** (also called **B cells**), synthesizes and secretes a single class of immunoglobulin (Figure 4-10). We discuss in Chapter 10, Immune-Lymphatic System, details of the origin of plasma cells.

Immunoglobulins are glycoproteins, and therefore plasma cells have the three structural characteristics of cells active in protein synthesis and secretion:

1. A well-developed **rough endoplasmic reticulum**

2. An extensive **Golgi apparatus**

3. A prominent **nucleolus**

At the light microscopic level, most of the cytoplasm of a plasma cell is basophilic because of the large amount of ribosomes associated with the endoplasmic reticulum. A clear area near the nucleus is slightly **acidophilic** and represents the Golgi apparatus. The nucleus has a characteristic cartwheel configuration created by the particular distribution of heterochromatin.

Extracellular matrix

The ECM is a combination of **collagens**, **noncollagenous glycoproteins**, and **proteoglycans** surrounding cells and fibers of the connective tissue.

Recall that the **basement membrane** contains several ECM components such as **laminin**,

---

Box 4-D | Metachromasia: Highlights to remember

• The granules of the mast cell have a staining property known as **metachromasia** (Greek *meta*, beyond; *chroma*, color).

• After staining with a metachromatic dye, such as **toluidine blue**, the mast cell granules stain with a color that is different from the color of the dye (purple-red instead of blue).

• This phenomenon is determined by a change in the electronic structure of the dye molecule after binding to the granular material. In addition, mast cell granules are PAS positive because of their glycoprotein nature.

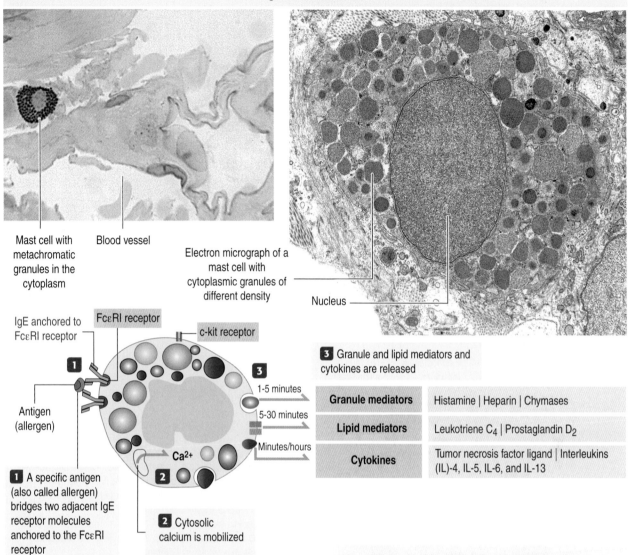

Figure 4-9. Mast cell

Mast cell with metachromatic granules in the cytoplasm

Blood vessel

Electron micrograph of a mast cell with cytoplasmic granules of different density

Nucleus

IgE anchored to FcεRI receptor

FcεRI receptor

c-kit receptor

Antigen (allergen)

Ca²⁺

1 A specific antigen (also called allergen) bridges two adjacent IgE receptor molecules anchored to the FcεRI receptor

2 Cytosolic calcium is mobilized

3 Granule and lipid mediators and cytokines are released

1-5 minutes

5-30 minutes

Minutes/hours

Granule mediators	Histamine | Heparin | Chymases
Lipid mediators	Leukotriene C_4 | Prostaglandin D_2
Cytokines	Tumor necrosis factor ligand | Interleukins (IL)-4, IL-5, IL-6, and IL-13

Nonactivated mast cells contain abundant granules storing **histamine, proteases**, and **proteoglycans**.

Histamine is formed by decarboxylation of histidine.

Proteoglycans contribute to the packaging and storage of histamine and proteases (mainly tryptase and chymase).

Chymases (mast cell specific serine proteases, MCPs) are unique of mast cells. They are not present in basophils.

After activation, binding of a specific antigen to two adjacent FcεRI receptors, mast cells:

1. Release histamine, proteases, and proteoglycans.

2. Synthesize mediators derived from **arachidonic acid** through the **cyclooxygenase**, and **lipoxygenase** pathways.

Cyclooxygenase (**prostaglandin D_2**) and lipoxygenase (**leukotriene C_4**) metabolites are **not present in granules**. These metabolites are important inflammatory mediators.

fibronectin, various types of **collagen**, and **heparan sulfate proteoglycan**. In addition, epithelial and nonepithelial cells have receptors for ECM constituents. An example is the family of **integrins** with binding affinity for laminin and fibronectin. Integrins interact with the cytoskeleton (F-actin), strengthening cell interactions with the ECM by establishing focal contacts or modifying cell shape or adhesion.

Several noncollagenous glycoproteins of the ECM mediate interactions with cells and regulate the assembly of ECM components. Noncollagenous glycoproteins have a widespread distribution in several connective tissues, although cartilage and bone contain specific types of noncollagenous glycoproteins. We study them later when we discuss the processes of **chondrogenesis** (formation of cartilage) and **osteogenesis** (bone formation).

Proteoglycan aggregates (Figure 4-11) are the major components of the ECM. Each proteoglycan consists of **glycosaminoglycans** (**GAGs**), proteins complexed with polysaccharides.

GAGs are linear polymers of disaccharides with sulfate residues. GAGs control the biological

Figure 4-10. **Plasma cell**

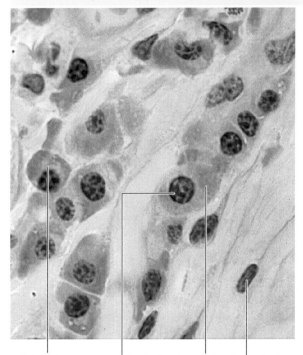

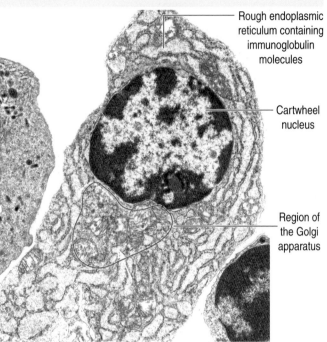

Rough endoplasmic reticulum containing immunoglobulin molecules

Cartwheel nucleus

Region of the Golgi apparatus

Golgi region | Cartwheel nucleus | Rough endoplasmic reticulum | Nucleus of a fibroblast

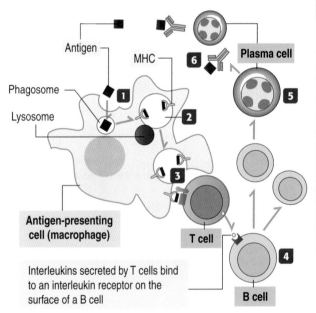

Antigen

MHC

Phagosome

Lysosome

Plasma cell

Antigen-presenting cell (macrophage)

T cell

Interleukins secreted by T cells bind to an interleukin receptor on the surface of a B cell

B cell

Origin of a plasma cell

1 An antigen is taken up by a macrophage (antigen-presenting cell).

2 The antigen is stored in a phagosome, which fuses with a lysosome. Within an acidic pH microenvironment, lysosomal hydrolytic enzymes become active and break down the antigen into small peptides. Small peptides bind to **MHC molecules** inserted in the membrane of the phagosome.

3 The phagcytic vesicle fuses with the plasma membrane and the **peptide-MHC is exposed to T cells**, which bind to the antigenic peptide and secrete cytokines or interleukins.

4 Interleukins bind to adjacent **B cells**, which are induced to divide by mitosis to increase their cell number.

5 B cells differentiate into immunoglobulin-secreting plasma cells.

6 Specific **immunoglobulins bind to free antigen** in the extracellular space to neutralize the damaging effect.

A more detailed analysis of the antigen-presenting cell and T cell–B cell interaction are discussed in Chapter 10, Immune-Lymphatic System.

functions of proteoglycans by establishing links with cell surface components, growth factors, and other ECM constituents.

Different types of GAGs are attached to a **core protein** to form a proteoglycan. The core protein, in turn, is linked to a **hyaluronan molecule** by a **linker protein**. The hyaluronan molecule is the axis of a **proteoglycan aggregate**. Proteoglycans are named according to the prevalent GAG (for example, **proteoglycan chondroitin sulfate, proteoglycan dermatan sulfate, proteoglycan heparan sulfate**).

The **embryonic connective tissue** of the umbilical cord (**Wharton's jelly**) is predominantly ECM material surrounding the two umbilical arteries and the single umbilical vein.

Proteoglycans have extremely high charge density and, therefore, significant osmotic pressure. These attributes enable a connective tissue bed to resist compression because of the very high swelling capacity of these molecules. The umbilical blood vessels, crucial elements for fetal-maternal fluid, gas, and nutritional exchange, are surrounded by a

Figure 4-11. Proteoglycan aggregate

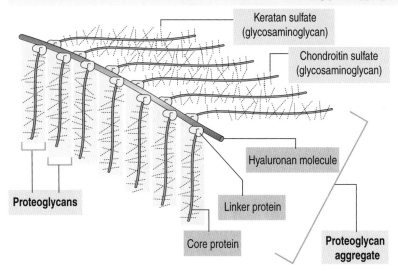

Keratan sulfate (glycosaminoglycan)

Chondroitin sulfate (glycosaminoglycan)

Hyaluronan molecule

Proteoglycans

Linker protein

Core protein

Proteoglycan aggregate

Proteoglycans are extracellular protein complexes of glycosaminoglycans

Proteoglycan aggregates are formed by:
1. An axial **hyaluronan molecule**.
2. **Core proteins** attached to the hyaluronan molecule by a **linker protein**.
3. **Glycosaminoglycans** attached to a core protein.

Several chains of glycosaminoglycans bound to the core protein form a proteoglycan. The molecular mass of a proteoglycan is about 10^8 kd.

proteoglycan-enriched type of connective tissue to provide resistance to compression.

General Pathology: Degradation of the extracellular matrix

The ECM can be degraded by **matrix metalloproteinases (MMPs;** also called **matrixins),** a family of zinc-dependent proteases **secreted as pro-enzymes (zymogens)** proteolytically activated in the ECM. The activity of MMPs in the extracellular space can be specifically balanced by **tissue inhibitors of MMPs (TIMPs) during tissue remodeling.**

The expression of MMP genes can be regulated by inflammatory cytokines, growth factors, hormones, cell–cell and cell–matrix interaction. Humans have 23 MMP genes

The degradation of the ECM occurs normally during the development, growth, tissue repair and wound healing. However, excessive degradation of the ECM is observed in several pathologic conditions such as rheumatoid arthritis, osteoarthritis, chronic tissue ulcers and cancer. Tumor invasion, metastasis, and tumor angiogenesis require the participation of MMPs whose expression increases in association with tumorigenesis.

Members of the family of MMPs include several subgroups based on their substrates (Figure 4-12):

1. **Collagenases (MMP-1, MMP-8,** and **MMP-13)** degrade types I, II, and III collagens and other ECM proteins. MMP-1 is synthesized by fibroblasts, chondrocytes, keratinocytes, monocytes, and macrophages, hepatocytes, and tumor cells. MMP-8 is stored in cytoplasmic granules of polymorphonuclear leukocytes and released in response to a stimulus. MMP-13 can degrade several collagens (types I, II, III, IV, IX, X, and XI), laminin and fibronectin, and other ECM components.

2. **Gelatinases (MMP-2** and **MMP-9)** can degrade a number of ECM molecules including type IV, V and XI collagens, laminin and aggrecan core protein. Similar to collagenases, MMP-2, but not MMP-9, can digest type I, II and III collagens. Gelatinases are produced by alveolar macrophages.

3. **Stromelysins** MMP-3 and MMP-10 digest a number of ECM molecules, but MMP-11 activity is very weak toward ECM molecules. Stromelysins degrade basement membrane components (type IV collagen and fibronectin).

4. **Matrilysins (MMP-7** and **MMP-26).** MMP-7 is synthesized by epithelial cells and cleaves cell surface molecules such as pro–α-defensin, Fas-ligand, pro–tumor necrosis factor ligand, and E-cadherin. MMP-26 is expressed in normal endometrial cells and some carcinoma cells.

5. **Membrane-type MMPs (MT-MMPs)** include two categories:
- Transmembrane proteins (MMP-14, MMP-15, MMP-16, and MMP-24).
- Glycosylphosphatidylinositol (GPI)-anchored proteins (MMP-17 and MMP-25).

MT-MMPs are activated intracellularly and are active enzymes on the cell surface.

A number of MMPs are not grouped within the above categories:

1. **Metalloelastase (MMP-12)** is expressed by macrophages, hypertrophic chondrocytes and osteoclasts.

2. **MMP-19,** also called **rheumatoid arthritis synovial inflammation,** digests components of basement membranes. MMP-19 is found in the activated lymphocytes and plasma cells from patients with rheumatoid arthritis.

3. **Enamelysin (MMP-20)** is expressed in **ameloblasts** (enamel–producing cells of the developing tooth) and digests amelogenin.

Figure 4-12. **Concept Mapping: MMPs and TIMPs**

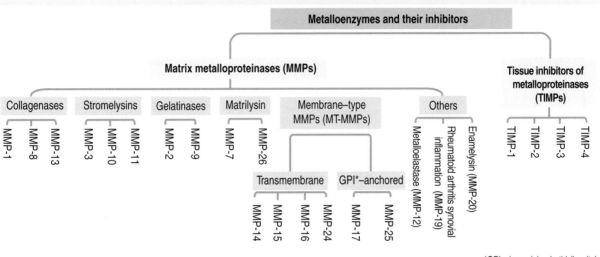

*GPI, glycosylphophatidylinositol

TIMPs (TIMP-1, TIM-2, TIMP-3 and TIMP-4) are inhibitors of MMPs. TIMP-3 is a major regulator of MMP activities.

MMPs are a target of therapeutic intervention to inhibit tumor invasion and metastasis. We come back to this topic in Chapter 23, Fertilization, Placentation, and Lactation, when we discuss the significance of metalloproteinases during the early stages of embryo implantation in the endometrial stroma or decidua.

General Pathology: Molecular biology of tumor invasion

As discussed in the Neoplasia section of Chapter 3, Cell Signaling, invasion and metastasis are two important events of carcinoma (Greek *karkinoma*, from *karkinos*, crab, cancer + *oma*, tumor), a tumor derived from epithelial tissues.

Adenoma is a structurally benign tumor of glandular epithelial cell origin lacking invasive and metastatic properties. Malignant carcinomas may arise from benign adenomas. For example, a small benign adenoma or **polyp** of the colon can become an invasive carcinoma.

Sarcoma (Greek *sarx,* flesh + *oma*) is a tumor derived from the connective tissues (muscle, bone, cartilage) and mesodermal cells. For example, fibrosarcoma derives from fibroblasts and osteosarcoma originates from bone.

Invasion is defined by the **breakdown of the basement membrane** by tumor cells and implies the transition from precancer to cancer. **Metastasis** is the spread of tumor cells throughout the body through blood and lymphatic vessels, generally leading to death. Figure 4-13 illustrates and describes the initial events of tumor cell invasion.

Many carcinomas produce members of the matrix metalloproteinase family to degrade various types of collagen as we have seen in the preceding section. Normal tissues produce tissue inhibitors of metalloproteinases that are neutralized by carcinoma cells. Tumors that behave aggressively are capable of overpowering the protease inhibitors.

One critical event during metastasis is angiogenesis, the development of blood vessels. Blood vessels supply oxygen and nutrients required for tumor growth. Angiogenesis is stimulated by tumor cells, in particular the proliferation of capillary endothelial cells forming new capillaries in the tumoral growth. In Chapter 12, Cardiovascular System, we discuss the mechanism of action and targets of endostatin and angiostatin, two new proteins that inhibit angiogenesis.

Adipose tissue or fat

There are two classes of adipose tissue:

1. **White fat**, the major **reserve of long-term energy and also an endocrine tissue**

2. **Brown fat**, which participates in thermogenesis

Similar to fibroblasts, chondroblasts, osteoblasts and myoblasts, white fat and brown fat adipose cells derive from a mesenchymal stem cells in a process known as **adipogenesis.**

Adipogenesis

Adipogenesis requires the activation of the master adipogenic regulator, the DNA binding **peroxisome proliferator-activated receptor-γ (PPARγ)**, in the presence of insulin and glucocorticoids (Figure 4-14).

Preadipocytes can follow two different cell differentiation pathways:

1. One pathway results in the formation of white fat preadipocytes directly from mesenchymal stem cells.

Figure 4-13. Tumor invasion and metastasis

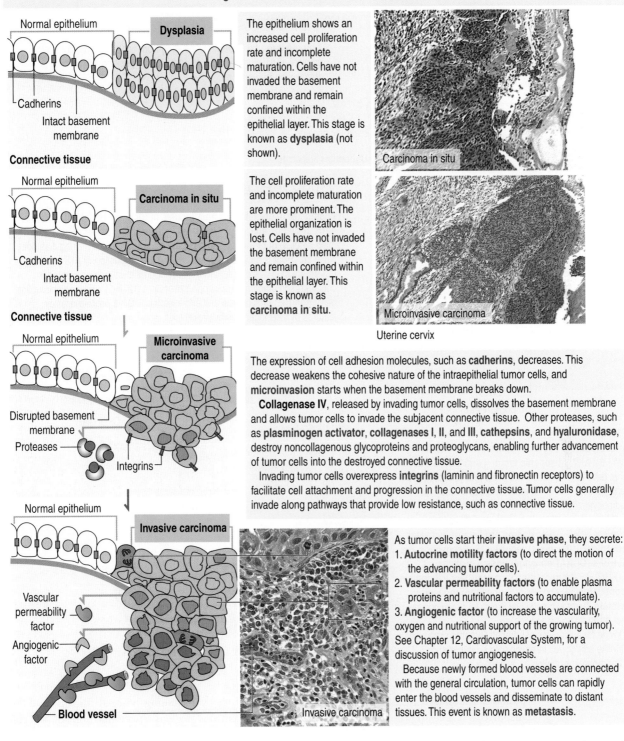

Normal epithelium | **Dysplasia**

Cadherins
Intact basement membrane

Connective tissue

The epithelium shows an increased cell proliferation rate and incomplete maturation. Cells have not invaded the basement membrane and remain confined within the epithelial layer. This stage is known as **dysplasia** (not shown).

Normal epithelium | **Carcinoma in situ**

Cadherins
Intact basement membrane

Connective tissue

The cell proliferation rate and incomplete maturation are more prominent. The epithelial organization is lost. Cells have not invaded the basement membrane and remain confined within the epithelial layer. This stage is known as **carcinoma in situ**.

Carcinoma in situ

Microinvasive carcinoma

Uterine cervix

Normal epithelium | **Microinvasive carcinoma**

Disrupted basement membrane
Proteases
Integrins

The expression of cell adhesion molecules, such as **cadherins**, decreases. This decrease weakens the cohesive nature of the intraepithelial tumor cells, and **microinvasion** starts when the basement membrane breaks down.

Collagenase IV, released by invading tumor cells, dissolves the basement membrane and allows tumor cells to invade the subjacent connective tissue. Other proteases, such as **plasminogen activator**, **collagenases I, II**, and **III**, **cathepsins**, and **hyaluronidase**, destroy noncollagenous glycoproteins and proteoglycans, enabling further advancement of tumor cells into the destroyed connective tissue.

Invading tumor cells overexpress **integrins** (laminin and fibronectin receptors) to facilitate cell attachment and progression in the connective tissue. Tumor cells generally invade along pathways that provide low resistance, such as connective tissue.

Normal epithelium | **Invasive carcinoma**

Vascular permeability factor
Angiogenic factor
Blood vessel

Invasive carcinoma

As tumor cells start their **invasive phase**, they secrete:
1. **Autocrine motility factors** (to direct the motion of the advancing tumor cells).
2. **Vascular permeability factors** (to enable plasma proteins and nutritional factors to accumulate).
3. **Angiogenic factor** (to increase the vascularity, oxygen and nutritional support of the growing tumor). See Chapter 12, Cardiovascular System, for a discussion of tumor angiogenesis.

Because newly formed blood vessels are connected with the general circulation, tumor cells can rapidly enter the blood vessels and disseminate to distant tissues. This event is known as **metastasis**.

2. The other pathway generates myoblasts and brown fat preadipocytes from a common **MYF5⁺PAX7⁺** (**myogenic factor 5⁺ and paired-box 7⁺**) precursor. Therefore, white fat and brown fat precursor cells diverge in early development.

The differentiation of white fat preadipocytes into end-stage adipocytes is driven by **PPARγ** and **C/EBPs** (CCAAT/enhancer-binding proteins). The differentiation of the **MYF5⁺PAX7⁺** myoblast/ brown fat preadipocyte precursor into brown fat preadipocytes requires also PPARγ in addition to **BMP7** (bone morphogenetic protein 7) and **PRDM16** (transcriptional co-regulator PR domain-containing 16). PRDM16 is essential for brown fat adipogenesis.

BMP7 and PRDM16 are not involved in white fat adipogenesis. Preadipocytes committed to adipogenesis activate the expression of genes

Figure 4-14. Adipogenesis

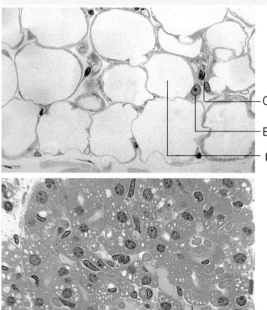

Unilocular adipocyte (white fat)

A **single large fat inclusion**, resulting from coalescing multiple lipid droplets, pushes the nucleus to an eccentric position. Fat in this preparation is unstained.

- Capillary
- Eccentric nucleus
- **Unilocular** adipocyte

Multilocular adipocyte (brown fat)

Aggregates of epithelial-like **multilocular, mitochondria-rich adipocytes surrounded by abundant blood vessels** are characteristic of brown fat. The main function of brown fat is to dissipate energy instead of storing it as does white fat. Heat is generated by uncoupling the production of ATP from the movement of H^+ across the inner mitochondrial membrane down the concentration gradient. **Uncoupling protein-1 (UCP-1)** activates uncoupling. **Mitochondrial biogenesis** and expression of **UCP-1 protein** are key features of thermogenesis by brown fat.

- **Multilocular** adipocyte
- Blood vessels

Adipogenesis

Mesenchymal stem cells give rise to white fat **preadipocytes** and a common precursor expressing MYF5+PAX7+ (**myogenic factor 5 and paired box 7**) that drive differentiation into **brown fat preadipocytes** and **muscle cells**. Therefore, white and brown fat adipocytes derive from different precursors.

White fat preadipocytes and brown fat preadipocytes express PPARγ (**peroxisome proliferator–activated receptor-γ**), the master regulator of adipogenesis and C/EBPs (**CCAAT/enhance-binding proteins**).

PRDM16 (**transcriptional co-regulator PR domain-containing 16**) and BMP7 (**bone morphogenetic protein 7**) are expressed by brown fat preadipocytes but not white fat preadipocytes.

White fat adipocytes can transdifferentiate into brown fat–like adipocytes following cold exposure and β-adrenergic signaling.

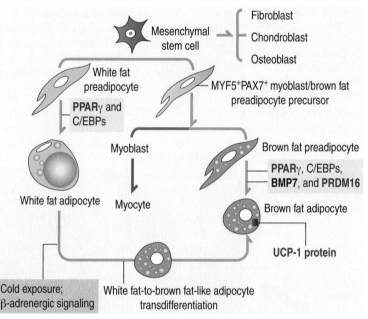

typical of the adipocyte phenotype, such as **glucose transporter** 4 (GLUT4) protein, **fatty acid binding protein-4**, **leptin** and **adiponectin** (Figure 4-15).

In the presence of cold exposure and β-adrenergic signaling, white fat adipocytes can transdifferentiate into brown fat-like adipocytes expressing **UCP-1** (**uncoupling protein 1**), a mitochondrial protein that increases thermogenesis by dissociation of oxidative phosphorylation from energy production.

Adipogenesis occurs during both the prenatal and postnatal states of the individual and is reduced as age increases. White fat is distributed throughout the body surrounding visceral organs and in subcutaneous regions. Accumulation of visceral fat during obesity correlates with insulin resistance (type 2 diabetes) and inflammation. Weight loss is associated with a decrease in adipocyte size without affecting adipocyte cell numbers. Brown fat is found in paravertebral, supraclavicular, and periadrenal sites.

Lipid storage and breakdown

During white fat adipogenesis, adipocytes synthesize **lipoprotein lipase** and begin to

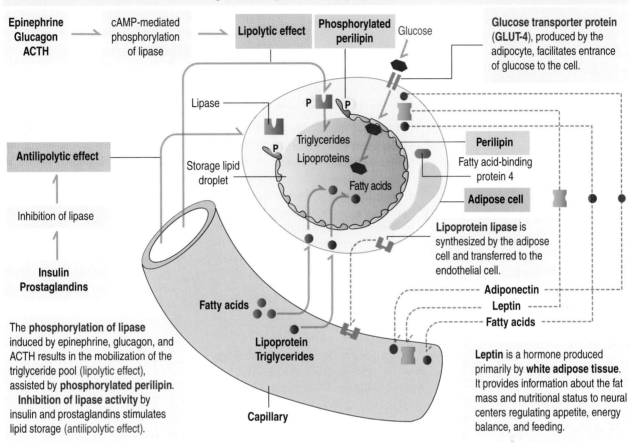

Figure 4-15. Regulation of adipocyte function

Epinephrine Glucagon ACTH → cAMP-mediated phosphorylation of lipase → **Lipolytic effect**

Phosphorylated perilipin

Glucose

Glucose transporter protein (GLUT-4), produced by the adipocyte, facilitates entrance of glucose to the cell.

Lipase

Storage lipid droplet

Triglycerides
Lipoproteins

Fatty acids

Perilipin
Fatty acid-binding protein 4

Adipose cell

Antilipolytic effect

Inhibition of lipase

Insulin Prostaglandins

Lipoprotein lipase is synthesized by the adipose cell and transferred to the endothelial cell.

Fatty acids

Lipoprotein Triglycerides

Capillary

Adiponectin
Leptin
Fatty acids

Leptin is a hormone produced primarily by **white adipose tissue**. It provides information about the fat mass and nutritional status to neural centers regulating appetite, energy balance, and feeding.

The **phosphorylation of lipase** induced by epinephrine, glucagon, and ACTH results in the mobilization of the triglyceride pool (lipolytic effect), assisted by **phosphorylated perilipin**.
  Inhibition of lipase activity by insulin and prostaglandins stimulates lipid storage (antilipolytic effect).

accumulate fat in small cytoplasmic droplets. Small droplets fuse to form a single large lipid-storage droplet, a characteristic of mature **unilocular** (Latin *unus*, single; *loculus*, small place) **adipocytes** (see Figure 4-14).

The single lipid-storage droplet pushes the nucleus to an eccentric position and the adipocyte assumes a "signet-ring" appearance. **In histologic sections, capillaries appear as single structures that may contain blood cell elements, whereas adipocytes form aggregates.**

The surface of lipid droplets is surrounded by the protein **perilipin**. Phosphorylated perilipin changes its conformation, thus enabling lipase-mediated breakdown and release of lipids. **Each perilipin-coated lipid droplet is in contact with the cytosol;**

it is not surrounded by a cytomembrane. Therefore, lipid droplets are classified as cell **inclusions**. Aggregates of fat droplets can be visualized by histochemistry under specific technical conditions (see Box 4-E).

Lipid droplets contain about 95% triglycerides rich in carotene, a lipid-soluble pigment that gives the so-called white fat a yellowish color. Adipocytes synthesize **lipoprotein lipase**. Lipoprotein lipase is transferred to endothelial cells in the adjacent blood vessels to enable the passage of fatty acids and triglycerides into the adipocytes.

The blood supply to white fat, mainly capillaries, is not as extensive as in brown fat.

The **storage of lipids** in mature adipocytes is regulated by the antilipolytic effect of **insulin** and **prostaglandins** resulting in the inhibition of lipase. The **breakdown and release of lipids** is regulated by the lipolytic effect of **epinephrine**, **glucagon**, and **adrenocorticotropic hormone** (ACTH) as a result of the phosphorylation of lipase and perilipin (see Figure 4-15). Adipose tissue is innervated by the sympathetic nervous system.

Adipocytes **of brown fat** contain many lipid-storage droplets (**multilocular**; Latin *multus*, many; *loculus*, small place). Brown fat is mostly decreased during childhood and is supplied by abundant blood

---

Box 4-E | Fat in histologic sections

- Fat is usually dissolved by solvents (xylene) used during paraffin embedding. Only the nucleus and a narrow cytoplasmic rim, surrounding a central empty space, can be visualized.
- Fat that is fixed and stained with osmium tetroxide appears brown. This reagent is also used for the visualization of lipid-rich myelin in nerves (see Chapter 8, Nervous Tissue).
- Alcoholic solutions of fat-soluble dyes (such as Sudan III or Sudan black) can also be used for the detection of aggregates of fat droplets in frozen sections.

vessels and sympathetic adrenergic nerve fibers. Lipochrome pigment and abundant mitochondria, rich in cytochromes, give this type of fat a brownish color.

As stated initially, the main function of brown fat is to dissipate energy in the form of heat (thermogenesis) in cold environments as a protective mechanism in the newborn. Thermogenesis by brown fat cells has two requirements (see Figure 4-14):

1. Mitochondrial biogenesis
2. The expression of **UCP-1**

As we briefly mentioned in Chapter 2, Epithelial Glands, in our discussion on UCP transporters in mitochondria, UCP-1 dissipates the proton gradient established across the inner mitochondrial membrane when electrons pass along the electron-transport chain. Thermogenesis occurs because UCP-1 allows the reentry of protons down their concentration gradient into the mitochondrial matrix and uncouples respiration from ATP production.

Clinical significance: Obesity

Obesity is a disorder of energy balance. It occurs when energy intake exceeds energy expenditure. Protection against obesity without consideration of energy intake results in an increase in circulating levels of triglycerides, and excessive accumulation of fat in liver (**steatosis**). The metabolic activities of adipocytes have very significant clinical consequences. An increase in visceral adiposity is associated with a higher risk of insulin resistance (see Chapter 19, Endocrine System), **dyslipidemia** (alteration in blood fat levels), and cardiovascular disease.

One of the secreted products of adipocytes is

leptin, a 16-kd protein encoded by the *ob* gene. Leptin is released into the circulation and acts peripherally to regulate body weight. Leptin acts on hypothalamic targets involved in appetite and energy balance. Leptin-deficient mice (*ob/ob*) are obese and infertile. Both conditions are reversible with leptin administration.

The leptin receptor in hypothalamic target cells shares sequence homology with cytokine receptors. During inflammation, the release of the cytokines **interleukin-1** and **tumor necrosis factor ligand** increases leptin in serum, an indication that leptin interacts with cytokines to influence responses to infection and inflammatory reactions. Infections, injury, and inflammation up-regulate leptin gene expression and serum protein levels. As we discuss later, leptin has a role in bone formation.

Adiponectin (30-kd) modulates a number of metabolic processes, including glucose regulation and fatty acid breakdown. Obesity is associated with decreased adiponectin. Adiponectin has potential antiatherogenic and anti-inflammatory properties.

Cartilage

Like the fibroblast and the adipocyte, the **chondroblast** derives from a mesenchymal stem cell. Chondroblasts contain lipids and glycogen, a well-developed RER (basophilic cytoplasm), and Golgi apparatus (Figure 4-16). The proliferation of chondroblasts results in growth of the cartilage.

Similar to typical connective tissue, the **cartilage consists of cells embedded in ECM surrounded by the perichondrium.** The perichondrium is formed by a layer of undifferentiated cells that can differentiate into chondroblasts.

In contrast to typical connective tissue, the cartilage is **avascular** and cells receive nutrients by diffusion through the ECM (see Box 4-F). At all ages, chondrocytes have significant nutritional requirements. Although they rarely divide in the adult cartilage, they can do so to enable healing of bone fractures (see Box 4-G).

Growth of cartilage (chondrogenesis)

Cartilage grows by two mechanisms (Figure 4-17 and Figure 4-18):

1. By **interstitial growth**, from chondrocytes **within the cartilage** (see Figure 4-17).

2. By **appositional growth**, from undifferentiated cells **at the surface of the cartilage, or perichondrium** (see Figure 4-18).

During chondrogenesis, chondroblasts produce and deposit **type II collagen** fibers and ECM (**hyaluronic acid** and **GAGs**, mainly chondroitin sulfate and keratan sulfate) until chondroblasts are separated and trapped within spaces in the matrix

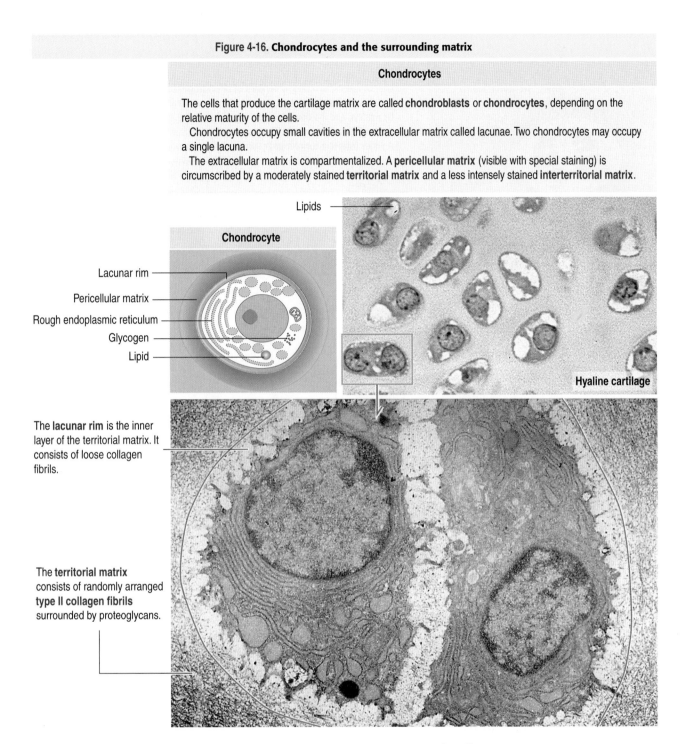

Figure 4-16. Chondrocytes and the surrounding matrix

Chondrocytes

The cells that produce the cartilage matrix are called **chondroblasts** or **chondrocytes**, depending on the relative maturity of the cells.

Chondrocytes occupy small cavities in the extracellular matrix called lacunae. Two chondrocytes may occupy a single lacuna.

The extracellular matrix is compartmentalized. A **pericellular matrix** (visible with special staining) is circumscribed by a moderately stained **territorial matrix** and a less intensely stained **interterritorial matrix**.

Lipids

Chondrocyte

Lacunar rim

Pericellular matrix

Rough endoplasmic reticulum

Glycogen

Lipid

Hyaline cartilage

The **lacunar rim** is the inner layer of the territorial matrix. It consists of loose collagen fibrils.

The **territorial matrix** consists of randomly arranged **type II collagen fibrils** surrounded by proteoglycans.

called **lacunae** (Latin *lacuna*, small lake). The cells are then called **chondrocytes**. The space between the chondrocyte and the wall of the lacuna seen in histologic preparations is an artifact of fixation.

The matrix in close contact with each chondrocyte forms a bluish (with hematoxylin and eosin), metachromatic (see Box 4-D), or PAS-positive basket-like structure called the **territorial matrix**.

Each cluster of chondrocytes, known as an **isogenous group**, is enclosed by the territorial matrix and separated from each other by a wider and pale **interterritorial matrix**.

Types of cartilage

There are three major types of cartilage (Figure 4-19):

1. **Hyaline cartilage.**
2. **Elastic cartilage.**
3. **Fibrocartilage.**

Hyaline cartilage is the most widespread cartilage in humans. Its name derives from the clear appearance of the matrix (Greek *hyalos,* glass).

In the fetus, hyaline cartilage forms most of the skeleton before it is reabsorbed and replaced by bone by a process known as **endochondral ossification**.

Figure 4-17. Chondrogenesis: Interstitial growth

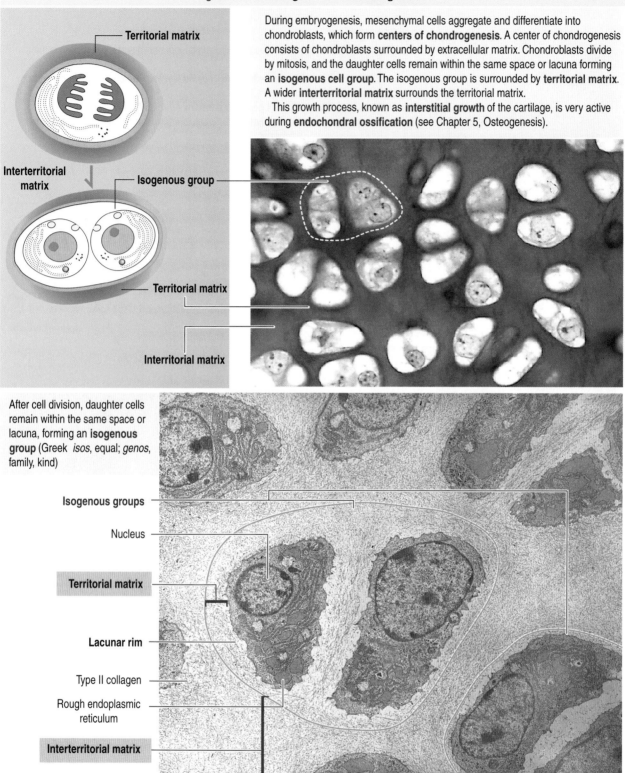

During embryogenesis, mesenchymal cells aggregate and differentiate into chondroblasts, which form **centers of chondrogenesis**. A center of chondrogenesis consists of chondroblasts surrounded by extracellular matrix. Chondroblasts divide by mitosis, and the daughter cells remain within the same space or lacuna forming an **isogenous cell group**. The isogenous group is surrounded by **territorial matrix**. A wider **interterritorial matrix** surrounds the territorial matrix.

This growth process, known as **interstitial growth** of the cartilage, is very active during **endochondral ossification** (see Chapter 5, Osteogenesis).

Territorial matrix

Interterritorial matrix

Isogenous group

Territorial matrix

Interritorial matrix

After cell division, daughter cells remain within the same space or lacuna, forming an **isogenous group** (Greek *isos*, equal; *genos*, family, kind)

Isogenous groups

Nucleus

Territorial matrix

Lacunar rim

Type II collagen

Rough endoplasmic reticulum

Interterritorial matrix

In adults, hyaline cartilage persists as the nasal, laryngeal, tracheobronchial, and costal cartilage. **The articular surface of synovial joints** (knees, shoulders) **is hyaline cartilage and does not participate in endochondral ossification.** Articular surfaces are not lined by an epithelium.

The hyaline cartilage contains:
1. **Cells** (chondrocytes)
2. **Fibers** (type II collagen synthesized by chondrocytes)
3. **ECM** (also synthesized by chondrocytes)
Chondrocytes have the structural characteristics

Figure 4-18. Chondrogenesis: Appositional growth

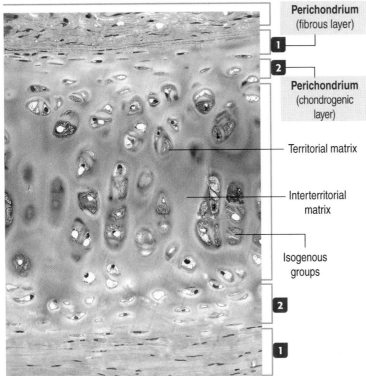

Surrounding connective tissue

Perichondrium (fibrous layer)

1

2

Perichondrium (chondrogenic layer)

Territorial matrix

Interterritorial matrix

Isogenous groups

2

1

1 The **outermost cells** of the developing cartilage are spindle-shaped and clustered in a regular fibrous layer called **perichondrium**, a transitional zone between cartilage and the surrounding general connective tissue.

2 The **inner cells of the perichondrium**, the **chondrogenic layer**, differentiate into **chondroblasts**, which synthesize and secrete **type II collagen** precursors and other extracellular matrix components.

By this mechanism, new layers of cells and extracellular matrix are added to the surface of the cartilage by the process of **appositional growth**, and the overall size of the cartilage increases. This process increases the size of the initial **anlagen** (German *anlagen*, plan, outline) of the future skeleton.

A mutation in the gene expressing the **transcription factor Sox9** causes **campomelic dysplasia** in humans consisting in bowing and angulation of long bones, hypoplasia of the pelvic and scapular bones, abnormalities of the vertebral column, a decrease in the number of ribs, and craniofacial abnormalities. **Sox9 controls the expression of type II collagen and the proteoglycan aggrecan.**

Sox9-null chondrogenic cells remain in the perichondrium and do not differentiate into chondrocytes. Other members of the Sox family participate in chondrogenesis.

Sox9 participates in male sex determination (see Chapter 21, Sperm Transport and Maturation).

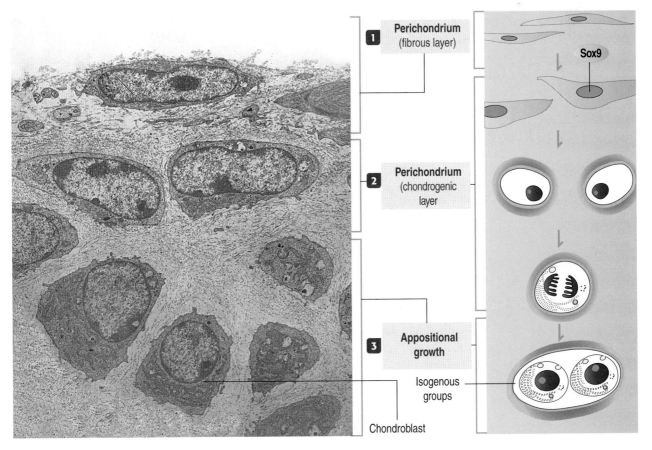

Perichondrium (fibrous layer)

1

Sox9

Perichondrium (chondrogenic layer

2

Appositional growth

3

Isogenous groups

Chondroblast

Figure 4-19. Types of cartilage

Hyaline cartilage

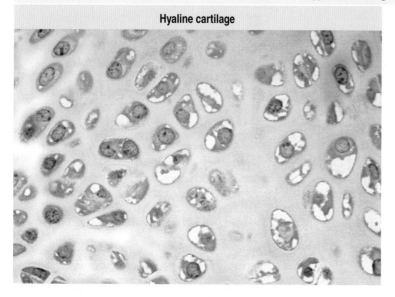

Hyaline cartilage has the following features:
It is **avascular**.

It is surrounded by **perichondrium** (except in articular cartilage). The perichondrium has an **outer fibrous layer**, an **inner chondrogenic layer** and **blood vessels**.

It consists of chondrocytes surrounded by territorial and interterritorial matrices containing **type II collagen** interacting with proteoglycans.

It occurs in the **temporary skeleton of the embryo, articular cartilage** (see Box 4-H) and the **cartilage of the respiratory tract** (nose, larynx, trachea and bronchi) and costal cartilages.

Elastic cartilage

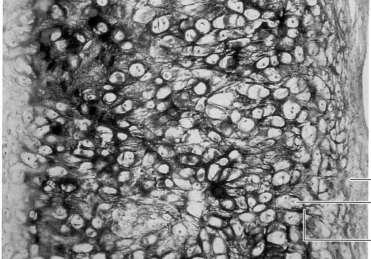

Elastic cartilage has the following features:
It is **avascular**.

It is surrounded by **perichondrium**.

It consists of chondrocytes surrounded by territorial and interterritorial matrices containing **type II collagen** interacting with proteoglycans and **elastic fibers**, which can be stained by **orcein** for light microscopy.

It occurs in the **external ear, epiglottis**, and **auditory tube**.

—— Perichondrium

—— Chondrocytes

—— Elastic fibers

Fibrocartilage

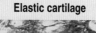

Fibrocartilage has the following features:
It is generally **avascular**.

It **lacks a perichondrium**.

It consists of **chondrocytes** and **fibroblasts** surrounded by **type I collagen** and a less rigid extracellular matrix. Fibrocartilage is considered an intermediate tissue between hyaline cartilage and dense connective tissue.

It predominates in the **intervertebral disks, articular disks of the knee, mandible, sternoclavicular joints**, and **pubic symphysis**.

Chondrocytes aligned
along the lines of stress

Box 4-H | **Cartilage of the joints**

- The specialized extracellular matrix of hyaline cartilage has a dual role:
 1. It acts like a **shock absorber**, because of its stiffness and elasticity.
 2. It provides a **lubricated surface for movable joints**.
  The lubrication fluid (hyaluronic acid, immunoglobulins, lysosomal enzymes, collagenase in particular, and glycoproteins) is produced by the **synovial lining of the capsule of the joint**.
- The analysis of the **synovial fluid** is valuable in the diagnosis of joint disease.

of a protein-secreting cell (well-developed RER and Golgi apparatus, and large nucleolus) and store lipids and glycogen in the cytoplasm. Chondrocytes are coated by a pericellular matrix, surrounded by the territorial and interterritorial matrices, respectively. A lacunar rim separates the cell from the territorial matrix.

The surface of hyaline cartilage is covered by the **perichondrium**, a fibrocellular layer that is continuous with the periosteal cover of the bone and that blends into the surrounding connective tissue. **Articular cartilage lacks a perichondrium.**

The perichondrium consists of two layers (see Figure 4-18):

1. An **outer fibrous layer**, which contains fibroblasts producing bundles of type I collagen and elastin.

2. An **inner layer**, called the **chondrogenic layer**, formed by elongated chondrocytes aligned tangentially to the perichondrium of the cartilage.

The ECM contains hyaluronic acid, proteoglycans (rich in the GAGs chondroitin sulfate and keratan sulfate) and a high water content (70% to 80% of its weight). **Aggrecan** is a large proteoglycan (about 2500 kd) characteristic of cartilage. It provides a hydrated gel-like structure that facilitates the load-bearing properties of cartilage.

Box 4-I | **Sox9 transcription factor**

- Genes encoding proteins that turn on (activate) or turn off (repress) other genes are called **transcription factors**. Many transcription factors have common DNA-binding domains and can also activate or repress a single target gene as well as other genes (a cascade effect). Therefore, mutations affecting genes encoding transcription factor have pleiotropic effects (Greek *pleion*, more; *trope*, a turning toward).
- Examples of transcription factor genes include homeobox-containing genes, high mobility group (HMG)-box–containing genes, and the T-box family.
- The HMG domain of Sox proteins can bend DNA, and facilitate the interaction of enhancers with a distantly located promoter region of a target gene.
- Several *Sox* genes act in different developmental pathways. For example, Sox9 protein is expressed in the gonadal ridges of both genders but is up-regulated in males and down-regulated in females before gonadal differentiation. Sox9 also regulates chondrogenesis and osteogenesis and the expression of type II collagen by chondroblasts. Mutations of the *Sox9* gene cause skeletal defects (**campomelic dysplasia**), and **sex reversal** (XY females).

The **transcription factor Sox9** (for sex determining region Y–box 9) is required for the expression of cartilage-specific ECM components such as type II collagen and the proteoglycan aggrecan. Sox9 activates the expression of the *COL2A1* gene.

A lack of Sox9 expression prevents the chondrogenic layer to differentiate into chondrocytes (see Box 4-I). Mutations in the *Sox9* gene cause the rare and severe dwarfism called **campomelic dysplasia** (see Figure 4-18). We come back to Sox9 to stress its role of enabling mesenchymal stem cells to become preosteoblasts.

The structure of the **elastic cartilage** is similar to that of hyaline cartilage except that the ECM contains abundant **elastic fibers** synthesized by chondrocytes. Elastic cartilage predominates in the auricle of the external ear, a major portion of the epiglottis and some of the laryngeal cartilages. The specialized matrix of the cartilage has remarkable flexibility and the ability to regain its original shape after deformation.

Unlike hyaline cartilage, **fibrocartilage** is opaque, the matrix contains **type I collagen fibers**, the **ECM has a low concentration of proteoglycans and water** and it **lacks a perichondrium**.

Fibrocartilage has great tensile strength and forms part of the intervertebral disk, pubic symphysis, and sites of insertion of tendon and ligament into bone.

The fibrocartilage is sometimes difficult to distinguish from dense regular connective tissue of some regions of tendons and ligaments. Fibrocartilage is distinguished by **characteristic chondrocytes within lacunae, forming short columns** (in contrast to flattened fibroblasts or fibrocytes lacking lacunae, surrounded by the dense connective tissue and ECM). You may like to compare tendon in Figure 4-1 and fibrocartilage in Figure 4-19 to see the structural differences.

Bone

Bone is a rigid inflexible connective tissue in which the ECM has become impregnated with salts of calcium and phosphate by a process called **mineralization**. Bone is highly vascularized and metabolically very active.

The functions of bone are:

1. **Support and protection of the body and its organs.**

2. **A reservoir for calcium and phosphate ions.**

Macroscopic structure of mature bone

Two forms of bone can be distinguished based on the gross appearance (Figure 4-20), :

1. **Compact or dense bone.**

2. **Spongy, trabecular or cancellous bone.**

Compact bone appears as a solid mass. Spongy

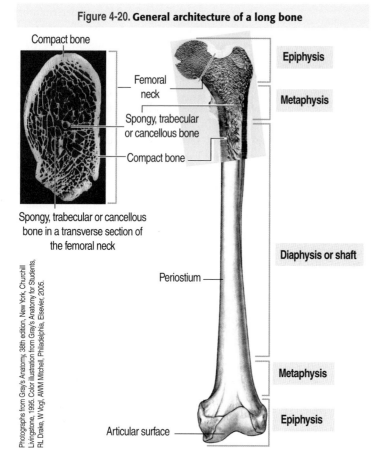

Figure 4-20. General architecture of a long bone

Compact bone

Spongy, trabecular or cancellous bone in a transverse section of the femoral neck

Femoral neck

Spongy, trabecular or cancellous bone

Compact bone

Periostium

Articular surface

Epiphysis

Metaphysis

Diaphysis or shaft

Metaphysis

Epiphysis

Photographs from Gray's Anatomy, 38th edition, New York, Churchill Livingstone, 1995. Color illustration from Gray's Anatomy for Students, RL Drake, W Vogl, AWM Mitchell, Philadelphia, Elsevier, 2005.

bone consists of a network of bony spicules or trabeculae delimiting spaces occupied by the bone marrow.

In long bones, such as the femur, the **shaft** or **diaphysis** consists of compact bone forming a hollow cylinder with a central marrow space, called the **medullary** or **marrow cavity**.

The ends of the long bones, called **epiphyses**, consist of spongy bone covered by a thin layer of compact bone.

In the growing individual, epiphyses are separated from the diaphysis by a cartilaginous **epiphyseal plate**, connected to the diaphysis by spongy bone. A tapering transitional region, called the **metaphysis**, connects the epiphysis and the diaphysis. Both the epiphyseal plate and adjacent spongy bone represent the **growth zone**, responsible for the increase in **length** of the growing bone.

The **articular surfaces**, at the ends of the long bones, are covered by hyaline cartilage, the **articular cartilage**. Except on the articular surfaces and at the insertion sites of tendons and ligaments, most bones are surrounded by the **periosteum**, a layer of specialized connective tissue with osteogenic potential.

The marrow wall of the diaphysis, the **endosteum**, and the spaces within spongy bone are lined by **osteoprogenitor cells**, with osteogenic potential.

Microscopic structure of mature bone

Two types of bone are identified on the basis of the microscopic three-dimensional arrangement of the collagen fibers:

1. **Lamellar or compact bone**, typical of the mature bone, displays a **regular alignment of collagen fibers**. This bone is mechanically strong and forms slowly.

2. **Woven bone**, observed in the developing bone, is characterized by an **irregular alignment of collagen fibers**. This bone is mechanically weak, is formed rapidly and is then replaced by lamellar bone. Woven bone is produced during the repair of a bone fracture.

The **lamellar bone** consists of **lamellae**, largely composed of **bone matrix**, a mineralized substance deposited in layers or lamellae, and osteocytes, each one occupying a cavity or **lacuna** with radiating and branching **canaliculi** that penetrate the lamellae of adjacent lacunae.

The lamellar bone displays four distinct patterns (Figure 4-21):

1. The **osteons** or **haversian systems**, formed by concentrically arranged lamellae around a longitudinal vascular channel. About 4 to 20 lamellae are concentrically arranged around the haversian canal.

2. The **interstitial lamellae**, observed between osteons and separated from them by a thin layer known as the **cement line**.

3. The **outer circumferential lamellae**, visualized at the external surface of the compact bone under the periosteum.

4. The **inner circumferential lamellae**, seen on the internal surface subjacent to the endosteum.

The **vascular channels** in compact bone have two orientations with respect to the lamellar structures:

1. The longitudinal **haversian canal**, housing capillaries and postcapillary venules in the center of the osteon (Figures 4-21 to 4-23).

2. The transverse or oblique **Volkmann's canals**, connecting haversian canals with one another, containing blood vessels derived from the bone marrow and some from the periosteum.

Periosteum and endosteum

During embryonic and postnatal growth, the **periosteum** consists of:

1. An **inner layer of preosteoblasts (or osteoprogenitor cells)**, in direct contact with bone. In the adult, the periosteum contains quiescent connective tissue cells that retain their osteogenic potential in case of bone injury and repair. The inner layer is the **osteogenic layer** (see Figure 4-21).

2. An **outer layer** rich in blood vessels, some of them entering Volkmann's canals, and thick anchoring collagen fibers, called **Sharpey's fibers**,

Figure 4-21. Haversian system or osteon

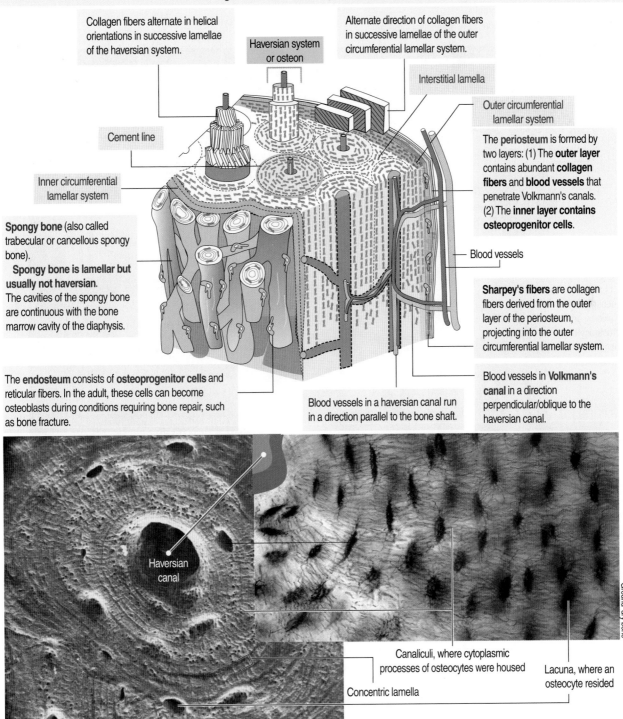

Collagen fibers alternate in helical orientations in successive lamellae of the haversian system.

Haversian system or osteon

Alternate direction of collagen fibers in successive lamellae of the outer circumferential lamellar system.

Interstitial lamella

Cement line

Outer circumferential lamellar system

Inner circumferential lamellar system

The **periosteum** is formed by two layers: (1) The **outer layer** contains abundant **collagen fibers** and **blood vessels** that penetrate Volkmann's canals. (2) The **inner layer contains osteoprogenitor cells**.

Spongy bone (also called trabecular or cancellous spongy bone).
  Spongy bone is lamellar but usually not haversian.
The cavities of the spongy bone are continuous with the bone marrow cavity of the diaphysis.

Blood vessels

Sharpey's fibers are collagen fibers derived from the outer layer of the periosteum, projecting into the outer circumferential lamellar system.

The **endosteum** consists of **osteoprogenitor cells** and reticular fibers. In the adult, these cells can become osteoblasts during conditions requiring bone repair, such as bone fracture.

Blood vessels in a haversian canal run in a direction parallel to the bone shaft.

Blood vessels in **Volkmann's canal** in a direction perpendicular/oblique to the haversian canal.

Haversian canal

Ground dry bone

Canaliculi, where cytoplasmic processes of osteocytes were housed

Concentric lamella

Lacuna, where an osteocyte resided

Scanning electron micrograph courtesy of Richard G. Kessel, Iowa City, Iowa

---

that penetrate the outer circumferential lamellae.

The **endosteum** covers the spongy walls and extends into all the cavities of the bone, including the haversian and Volkmann's canals. It consists of osteoprogenitor cells, reticular stromal cells of the bone marrow and connective tissue fibers.

As discussed in Chapter 6, Blood and Hematopoiesis, preosteoblasts and osteoblasts in

the endosteum contribute hematopoietic cytokines to the bone marrow microenvironment, the **endosteal niche**, essential for hematopoietic stem cell proliferation and maturation.

Bone matrix
The **bone matrix** consists of organic (35%) and inorganic (65%) components.

Figure 4-22. **Organization of compact bone: Osteon**

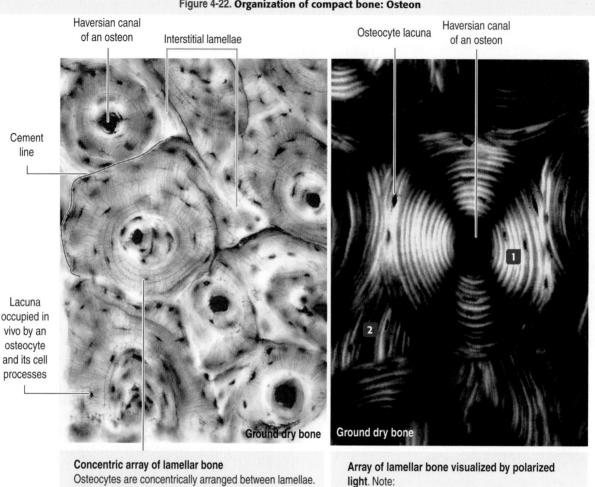

Concentric array of lamellar bone
Osteocytes are concentrically arranged between lamellae.
Osteocytes of adjacent lamellae are interconnected by
cell processes lodged in canaliculi.

Array of lamellar bone visualized by polarized
light. Note:
1 The concentric array of the lamellae.
2 The banding distribution of interstitial lamellae.

The **organic component** contains **type I collagen fibers** (90%); **proteoglycans**, enriched in **chondroitin sulfate**, **keratan sulfate** and **hyaluronic acid**, and **noncollagenous proteins**.

The **inorganic component of the bone** is represented predominantly by deposits of **calcium phosphate** with the crystalline characteristics of **hydroxyapatite**. The crystals are distributed along the length of collagen fibers through an assembly process assisted by noncollagenous proteins.

Type I collagen is the predominant protein of the bone matrix. In mature lamellar bone, collagen fibers have a highly ordered arrangement with changing orientations with respect to the axis of the haversian canal in successive concentric lamellae (see Figure 4-21).

Noncollagenous matrix proteins synthesized by osteoblasts and with unique properties in the mineralization of bone include **osteocalcin**, **osteopontin**, and **osteonectin**. The synthesis of osteocalcin (5.8 kd) and osteopontin (44 kd; also known as bone sialoprotein I) increases following stimulation with the active vitamin D metabolite, 1α,25-dihydroxycholecalciferol. Vitamin K induces amino acid carboxylation of osteocalcin to enable its calcium binding properties. Osteopontin participates in the anchoring of osteoclast to bone by the formation of a sealing zone before bone resorption. Osteonectin (32 kd) binds to type I collagen and hydroxyapatite.

Osteocalcin, osteopontin, and osteonectin are not exclusively bone effectors. For example, undercarboxylated osteocalcin (the hormone form) stimulates the proliferation and insulin secretion by B cells of the pancreatic islets of Langerhans.

We discuss later that osteoblasts regulate osteoclast differentiation by **osteoprotegerin**, **RANKL**, and **macrophage colony-stimulating factor**.

Cellular components of bone

Bone contains cells of two different lineages:

1. The **osteoblast**, of mesenchymal origin.

2. The **osteoclast**, derived from a monocyte precursor.

Figure 4-23. **Osteocytes are connected to each other by cell processes**

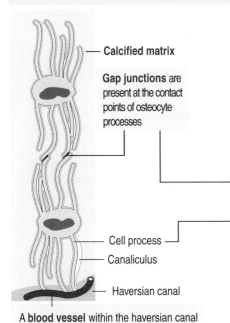

- Calcified matrix

Gap junctions are present at the contact points of osteocyte processes

- Cell process
- Canaliculus

- Haversian canal

A **blood vessel** within the haversian canal provides nutrients to osteocytes.

Nutrients are transported through a chain of cell processes away from the haversian canal, toward osteocytes located far from the canal.

The transport of the canalicular system is limited to a distance of about 100 μm.

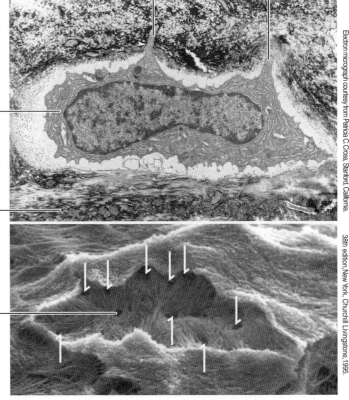

Photograph from: Gray's Anatomy, 38th edition. New York, Churchill Livingstone, 1995.

Cell processes are embedded within canaliculi, spaces surrounded by mineralized bone. Extracellular fluid within the lumen of the canaliculi transports molecules by passive diffusion.

Cell processes entering canaliculi

Electron micrograph courtesy from Patricia C. Cross, Stanford, California.

An **osteocyte**, trapped in the calcified matrix, occupies a space or lacuna. Osteocytes are responsible for maintenance and turnover of the bone matrix.

Calcified bone matrix

The wall of an **osteocyte lacuna** shows several openings of canaliculi (arrows) occupied in vivo by cell processes of an osteocyte housed in the space surrounded by calcified bone matrix.

Scanning electron micrograph from: Gray's Anatomy, 38th edition.New York, Churchill Livingstone, 1995.

The osteoblast

Osteoblasts are epithelial-like cells with cuboidal or columnar shapes, forming a monolayer covering all sites of active bone formation.

Osteoblasts are highly polarized cells: they deposit **osteoid**, the **nonmineralized organic matrix of the bone**, along the osteoblast-bone interface.

Osteoblasts initiate and control the mineralization of the osteoid.

In electron micrographs, osteoblasts display the typical features of cells actively engaged in protein synthesis, glycosylation, and secretion. Their specific products include **type I collagen**, **osteocalcin**, **osteopontin**, and **osteonectin** as well as several

Figure 4-24. **Function of the osteoblast**

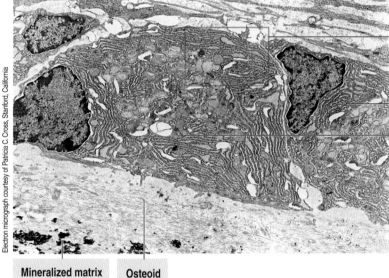

Electron micrograph courtesy of Patricia C. Cross, Stanford, California

Prominent rough endoplasmic reticulum

Osteoblasts

Osteoblasts produce multiple **hematopoietic cytokines**, including granulocyte-colony stimulating factor, macrophage-colony stimulating factor, granulocyte-macrophage-colony stimulating factor and interleukins.

Mineralized matrix | Osteoid

Osteoblasts derive from osteoprogenitor cells. Osteocytes are the most mature or terminally differentiated cells of the osteoblastic lineage.

Osteoblasts synthesize the organic matrix of bone, the **osteoid**, and control the mineralization of the matrix.

Alkaline phosphatase is an **ectoenzyme** (a cell surface protein) that hydrolyzes monophosphate esters at high pH. This enzyme disappears when the osteoblast ceases protein synthesis and becomes embedded in the mineralized bone matrix as an osteocyte.

Vitamin D_3 (1α,25-dihydroxycholecalciferol) regulates the expression of **osteocalcin**, a protein with high binding affinity for hydroxyapatite.

Growth hormone stimulates the production of **IGF-1** in hepatocytes. IGF-1 stimulates the growth of long bones at the level of the epiphyseal plates.

The major protein products of an osteoblast are:

1. **Type 1 collagen**. Osteoid consists of type I collagen and proteoglycans. As a typical protein-producing cell, the osteoblast has a well-developed rough endoplasmic reticulum.

2. Several **noncollagenous proteins**. They include: **RANKL**, the ligand for receptor for activation of nuclear factor kappa (κ) B (RANK), present in osteoclast precursor cells; **osteocalcin**, required for bone mineralization; **osteopontin**, to mediate the formation of the osteoclast sealing zone; and **osteoprotegerin**, a RANKL-binding "decoy" protein.

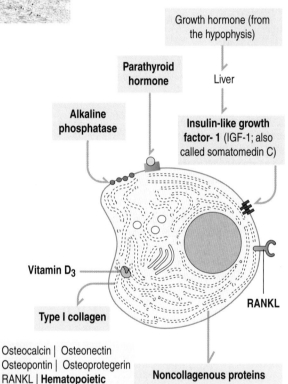

Growth hormone (from the hypophysis)

Parathyroid hormone

Alkaline phosphatase

Liver

Insulin-like growth factor- 1 (IGF-1; also called somatomedin C)

Vitamin D_3

Type I collagen

RANKL

Osteocalcin | Osteonectin
Osteopontin | Osteoprotegerin
RANKL | **Hematopoietic cytokines**

Noncollagenous proteins

hematopoietic cytokines (Figure 4-24).

Osteoblasts give a strong cytochemical reaction for **alkaline phosphatase** that disappears when the cells become embedded in the matrix as osteocytes.

When bone formation is completed, osteoblasts flatten out and transform into osteocytes embedded in the mineralized bone matrix.

Osteocytes are highly branched cells with their body occupying small spaces, or **lacunae**, between lamellae. Small channels, the **canaliculi**, course through the lamellae and interconnect neighboring lacunae. Cell processes of adjacent osteocytes are found within canaliculi. They are connected to each other by **gap junctions** (see Figure 4-23).

Nutrient materials diffuse from a blood vessel within the haversian canal through the canaliculi into the lacunae. As you can see, the delicate network of osteocytes depends not only on intercellular communication across gap junctions but also on the mobilization of nutrients and signaling molecules along the **extracellular** environment of the canaliculi extending from lacuna to lacuna.

The life of an osteocyte depends on this nutrient diffusion process and the life of the bone matrix depends on the osteocyte. Osteocytes can remain alive for years provided that vascularization is steady.

Figure 4-25. Osteoblast differentiation

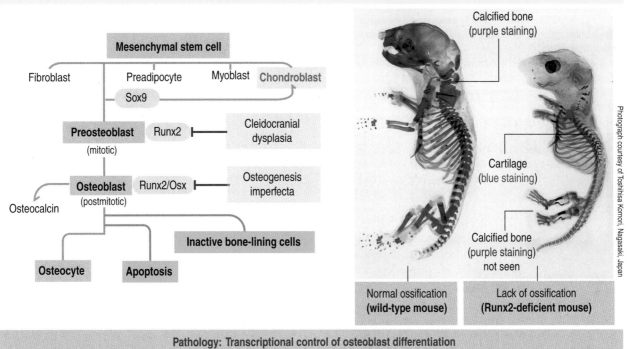

Mesenchymal stem cell

Fibroblast — Preadipocyte — Myoblast — **Chondroblast**

Sox9

Preosteoblast — Runp2 — Cleidocranial dysplasia
(mitotic)

Osteoblast — Runx2/Osx — Osteogenesis imperfecta
(postmitotic)

Osteocalcin

Inactive bone-lining cells

Osteocyte — **Apoptosis**

Calcified bone (purple staining)

Cartilage (blue staining)

Calcified bone (purple staining) not seen

Normal ossification **(wild-type mouse)**

Lack of ossification **(Runx2-deficient mouse)**

Photograph courtesy of Toshihisa Komori, Nagasaki, Japan

Pathology: Transcriptional control of osteoblast differentiation

Osteoblasts derive from a mesenchymal stem cell that gives rise to muscle cells, adipocytes, fibroblasts, and chondroblasts.

Three osteoblast specific genes encoding **transcription factors,** control the differentiation of the osteoblast progeny: (1) *Sox9* (for sex determining region Y–box 9), determines the differentiation of the mesenchymal progenitor into **preosteoblasts** and **chondroblasts**; (2) *Runx2* (for Runt homeodomain protein 2), induces the differentiation of the mitotically-active preosteoblasts into post-mitotic **osteoblasts** and, together with Osx, controls the expression of osteocalcin. Undercarboxylated osteocalcin is a specific secretory protein that enters the blood circulation to possibly stimulate insulin secretion by pancreatic β cells and testosterone production by Leydig cells. (3) *Osterix (Osx)*, encoding a zinc finger transcription factor, is required for the differentiation of osteoblasts into osteocytes and the function of osteocytes and chondroblasts.

Runx2-deficient mice have a skeleton consisting of cartilage without any indication of osteoblast differentiation represented by bone formation and mineralization. In addition, because osteoblasts regulate the formation of osteoclasts, Runx2-deficient mice lack osteoclasts.

Patients with **cleidocranial dysplasia** (hypoplastic clavicles and delayed ossification of sutures of certain skull bones) have a *Runx2* type of gene mutation.

A loss of Osx expression affects osteoblast differentiation, resulting in ectopic cartilage formation under the perichondrium at the diaphysis, where the bone collar develops. Osx-deficient patients have "brittle bone disease" (**osteogenesis imperfecta**).

Regulation of Sox9, Runx2 and Osx transcription factor expression by cell signaling pathways

The expression of the transcription factors Sox9, Runx2 and Osx is regulated by several cell signaling pathways: (1) Hedgehog signaling, mediated by Indian hedgehog protein, is required for the differentiation of Runx2+/Osx+ osteoblasts. (2) Notch signaling inhibits osteoblast differentiation by down regulation of Osx activation. (3) Wnt/β-catenin signaling stimulates osteoblast differentiation by Osx activation. (4) Bone morphogenetic protein signaling promotes the transition of Runx2+ preosteoblasts to Runx2+/Osx+ osteoblast by enhancing the expression of Runx2 and Osx. (4) Fibroblast growth factor signaling regulates Runx2+ preosteoblast proliferation and Runx2+/Osx+ osteoblast differentiation. Review in Chapter 3, Cell Signaling, the details of the indicated cell signaling pathways.

Pathology: Differentiation of the preosteoblast to osteoblast to osteocyte

Mesenchyme stem cells are the precursors of **preosteoblasts** as well as fibroblasts, adipocytes, muscle cells, and chondroblasts. Mitotically-active preosteoblasts give rise to post-mitotic **osteoblasts**. Then, a subset of osteoblasts differentiate into **osteocytes**, trapped within the mineralized osteoid.

Other osteoblasts undergo apoptosis or become just quiescent bone-lining cells (Figure 4-25).

Sox9 triggers the differentiation of mesenchymal stem cells into preosteoblasts (see Box 4-I and Figure 4-25). The differentiation of preosteoblasts into osteoblasts is controlled by the transcription factors **Runx2** (for Runt homeodomain protein 2) and **Osterix (Osx)**.

The *Runx2* gene is the earliest and most specific indicator of osteogenesis. Together with the *Osx* transcription factor gene, the *Runx2* gene modulate the expression of **osteocalcin**, a specific secretory protein expressed by postmitotic osteoblasts. Osteocalcin is a biochemical marker of the osteogenesis process.

The expression of *Runx2* and *Osx* genes is regulated by hedgehog (HH), Notch, Wnτ/b-catenin, bone morphogenetic protein (BMP) and fibroblast growth factor (FGF) signaling pathways (see Figure 4-25).

Runx2-deficient mice develop to term and have a skeleton consisting of cartilage (see Box 4-J). There is no indication of osteoblast differentiation or bone formation in these mice. In addition, Runx2-deficient mice lack osteoclasts. As we will discuss soon, osteoblasts produce proteins that regulate the formation of osteoclasts.

Consistent with the skeletal observations in the Runx2-deficient mice is a condition in humans known as **cleidocranial dysplasia (CCD)**. CCD is characterized by hypoplastic clavicles, delayed ossification of sutures of certain skull bones, and mutations in the *Runx2* gene.

Leptin, a peptide synthesized by **adipocytes** with binding affinity to its receptor in the hypothalamus, **negatively** regulates bone formation by a central mechanism. The leptin-hypothalamic control mechanism inhibits the production and release of **serotonin**. Mice deficient in leptin or its receptor have a considerably higher bone mass than wild-type mice. In fact, patients with generalized **lipodystrophy** (absence of adipocytes and white fat) exhibit **osteosclerosis** (increased bone hardening) and accelerated bone growth.

The osteoclast

Osteoclasts do not belong to the mesenchyme stem cell lineage. Instead, osteoclasts derive from **monocyte precursors** originated in bone marrow.

Monocytes reach the bone through the blood circulation and fuse into multinucleated cells with as many as 30 nuclei to form osteoclasts by a process regulated by osteoblasts (see Osteoclastogenesis).

Osteoclasts have three essential functions:

1. **Bone remodeling by the process of bone turnover**. This process involves removal of bone matrix at several sites, followed by its replacement with new bone by osteoblasts.

2. **Proper shaping of the bones.**

3. **Extension of the medullary spaces to enable hematopoiesis.**

The osteoclast is a large (up to 100 μm in diameter) and highly polarized cell that occupies a shallow concavity called **Howship's lacuna** or the **subosteoclastic acidic compartment** (Figures 4-26 and 4-27). Osteoclasts are found in cortical (compact) bone, within the haversian canals, and on the surfaces of trabeculae of cancellous (spongy) bone.

After attachment to the target bone matrix, osteoclasts generate a secluded acidic compartment required for bone resorption. The acidic compartment consists of two essential components:

1. The **ruffled border**, a plasma membrane specialization with many folds producing a large surface area for several important functional events: the release of H^+ and lysosomal protease **cathepsin K** and **matrix metalloproteinase-9 (MMP-9)** and the internalization of degraded bone matrix products into coated vesicles and vacuoles for material elimination. Remember that osteoclasts are an example of a cell type with **secretory lysosomes** represented by the release of cathepsin K into the subosteoclastic compartment.

2. The **sealing zone** is assembled around the apical circumference of the osteoclast to seal off the bone resorption lacuna. The sealing zone consists of plasma membrane associated with **actin filaments** and $\alpha_v\beta_3$ **integrin** and the protein **osteopontin**.

The cytoplasm of the osteoclast is very **rich in mitochondria, acidified vesicles** and **coated vesicles**. The membrane of the acidified vesicles contains H^+-ATPase; mitochondria are the source of adenosine triphosphate (ATP) to drive the H^+-ATPase pumps required for the **acidification of the subosteoclastic compartment** for the subsequent activation of cathepsin K and MMP-9.

Bone resorption involves first the dissolution of the inorganic components of the bone (**bone demineralization**) mediated by H^+-ATPase (adenosine triphosphatase) within an acidic environment, followed by enzymatic degradation of the organic matrix (consisting of type I collagen and noncollagenous proteins) by cathepsin K and MMP-9,

Figure 4-26 provides functional details of an osteoclast. Note that the mechanism of acidification

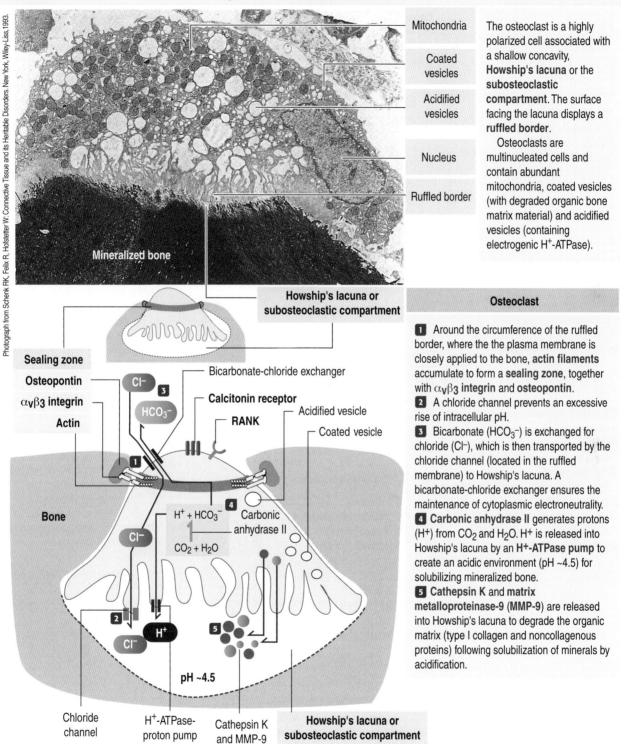

Figure 4-26. Function of the osteoclast

Mitochondria

Coated vesicles

Acidified vesicles

Nucleus

Ruffled border

Mineralized bone

The osteoclast is a highly polarized cell associated with a shallow concavity, **Howship's lacuna** or the **subosteoclastic compartment**. The surface facing the lacuna displays a **ruffled border**.

Osteoclasts are multinucleated cells and contain abundant mitochondria, coated vesicles (with degraded organic bone matrix material) and acidified vesicles (containing electrogenic H⁺-ATPase).

Howship's lacuna or subosteoclastic compartment

Sealing zone

Osteopontin

$\alpha_V\beta_3$ integrin

Actin

Bicarbonate-chloride exchanger

Cl^-

HCO_3^-

Calcitonin receptor

RANK

Acidified vesicle

Coated vesicle

Bone

Cl^-

$H^+ + HCO_3^-$

$CO_2 + H_2O$

Carbonic anhydrase II

Cl^-

H^+

pH ~4.5

Chloride channel

H^+-ATPase-proton pump

Cathepsin K and MMP-9

Howship's lacuna or subosteoclastic compartment

Osteoclast

1 Around the circumference of the ruffled border, where the the plasma membrane is closely applied to the bone, **actin filaments** accumulate to form a **sealing zone**, together with $\alpha_V\beta_3$ **integrin** and **osteopontin**.

2 A chloride channel prevents an excessive rise of intracellular pH.

3 Bicarbonate (HCO_3^-) is exchanged for chloride (Cl^-), which is then transported by the chloride channel (located in the ruffled membrane) to Howship's lacuna. A bicarbonate-chloride exchanger ensures the maintenance of cytoplasmic electroneutrality.

4 **Carbonic anhydrase II** generates protons (H^+) from CO_2 and H_2O. H^+ is released into Howship's lacuna by an **H⁺-ATPase pump** to create an acidic environment (pH ~4.5) for solubilizing mineralized bone.

5 **Cathepsin K** and **matrix metalloproteinase-9 (MMP-9)** are released into Howship's lacuna to degrade the organic matrix (type I collagen and noncollagenous proteins) following solubilization of minerals by acidification.

of Howship's lacuna by osteoclasts is similar to the production of HCl by parietal cells in the stomach (see Chapter 15, Upper Digestive Segment).

When the osteoclast is inactive, the ruffled border disappears and the osteoclast enters into a resting phase. Osteoclasts are transiently active in response to a metabolic demand for the mobilization

of calcium from bone into blood. Osteoclast activity is directly regulated by **calcitonin** (synthesized by **C cells** of the thyroid follicle), **vitamin D₃**, and regulatory molecules produced by osteoblasts.

Osteoclastogenesis (osteoclast differentiation)
Osteoclastogenesis is triggered by two specific

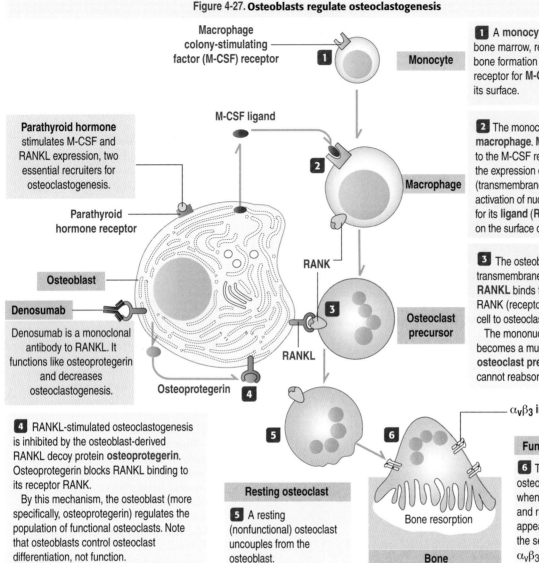

Figure 4-27. Osteoblasts regulate osteoclastogenesis

Macrophage colony-stimulating factor (M-CSF) receptor

1

Monocyte

1 A **monocyte**, derived from bone marrow, reaches an area of bone formation and remodeling. A receptor for **M-CSF** is expressed on its surface.

M-CSF ligand

Parathyroid hormone stimulates M-CSF and RANKL expression, two essential recruiters for osteoclastogenesis.

Parathyroid hormone receptor

2

Macrophage

2 The monocyte becomes a **macrophage**. **M-CSF ligand** binds to the M-CSF receptor and induces the expression of **RANK** (transmembrane receptor for activation of nuclear factor kappa B) for its **ligand** (**RANKL**) expressed on the surface of osteoblasts.

RANK

Osteoblast

Denosumab

Denosumab is a monoclonal antibody to RANKL. It functions like osteoprotegerin and decreases osteoclastogenesis.

RANKL

Osteoprotegerin

3

Osteoclast precursor

3 The osteoblast-expressed transmembrane protein ligand **RANKL** binds to the osteoclast RANK (receptor) and commits the cell to osteoclastogenesis.

The mononucleated monocyte becomes a multinucleated **osteoclast precursor**, which still cannot reabsorb bone.

4

4 RANKL-stimulated osteoclastogenesis is inhibited by the osteoblast-derived RANKL decoy protein **osteoprotegerin**. Osteoprotegerin blocks RANKL binding to its receptor RANK.

By this mechanism, the osteoblast (more specifically, osteoprotegerin) regulates the population of functional osteoclasts. Note that osteoblasts control osteoclast differentiation, not function.

5

Resting osteoclast

5 A resting (nonfunctional) osteoclast uncouples from the osteoblast.

6

Bone resorption

Bone

$\alpha_v\beta_3$ **integrin**

Functional osteoclast

6 The maturation of osteoclasts is completed when the sealing zone and ruffled border appear. The formation of the sealing zone requires $\alpha_v\beta_3$ integrin.

molecules produced by the **osteoblast**:

1. **Macrophage colony-stimulating factor (M-CSF)**.

2. **Nuclear factor kappa B (NF-κB) ligand (RANKL)**.

The osteoclast precursor, derived from the monocyte-macrophage, responds to M-CSF, required for the survival and proliferation of the precursor (Figure 4-27).

RANKL is a member of the **tumor necrosis factor (TNF) superfamily**. RANKL binds to **RANK receptor** on the surface of the osteoclast precursor. RANKL binding determines RANK trimerization and the recruitment of an adaptor molecule called **TRAF6** (for TNF receptor–associated factor 6). TRAF6 stimulates a downstream signaling cascade, including the nuclear relocation of two transcription factors: **NF-κB** and **NFATc1** (**for nuclear factor–activated T cells c1**). In the nucleus, these two

transcription factors activate genes triggering the differentiation of the osteoclast precursor (Figure 4-28).

Osteoblasts synthesize **osteoprotegerin**, a protein with high binding affinity for RANKL. Osteoprotegerin is a soluble "decoy" protein that binds to RANKL and prevents RANK-RANKL interaction. By this mechanism, **osteoprotegerin modulates the osteoclastogenic process**.

Parathyroid hormone stimulates the expression of RANKL so the pool of RANKL increases relative to osteoprotegerin. An excess of parathyroid hormone enhances osteoclastogenesis, resulting in an elevation of calcium levels in blood caused by increased bone resorption (see Chapter 19, Endocrine System). **Denosumab**, a monoclonal antibody to RANKL, functions like osteoprotegerin, thus preventing bone loss caused by excessive osteoclast differentiation and activity stimulated by parathyroid hormone.

Figure 4-28. RANK-RANKL signaling

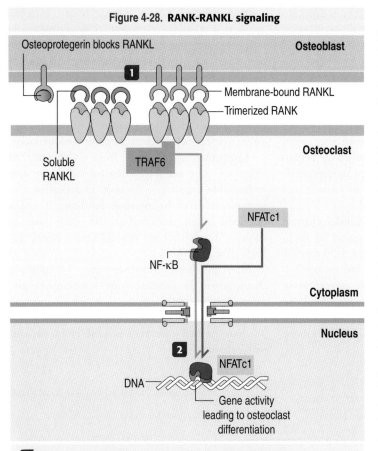

Osteoprotegerin blocks RANKL — Osteoblast

Membrane-bound RANKL
Trimerized RANK

Soluble RANKL

Osteoclast

TRAF6

NFATc1

NF-κB

Cytoplasm

Nucleus

NFATc1

DNA

Gene activity leading to osteoclast differentiation

1 Binding of membrane-bound or soluble RANKL to RANK determines RANK trimerization followed by the recruitment of adaptor molecules, in particular **TRAF6** (for TNF [tumor necrosis factor] receptor–associated factor).

2 The nuclear translocation of the osteoclastogenic transcription factors **NFATc1** (for nuclear factor–activated T cells c1) and **NF-κB** (nuclear factor kappa B), stimulate gene activity to activate osteoclast differentiation.

Pathology: Osteoporosis, osteopetrosis, and osteomalacia

Osteoporosis (Greek *osteon*, bone; *poros*, pore; *osis*, condition) is defined as the loss of bone mass leading to bone fragility and susceptibility to fractures.

The major factor in osteoporosis is the deficiency of the sex steroid **estrogen** that occurs in postmenopausal women. In this condition, the amount of reabsorbed old bone, due to an **increase in the number of osteoclasts**, exceeds the amount of formed new bone. This accelerated turnover state can be reversed by estrogen therapy and calcium and vitamin D supplementation. Osteoporosis and osteoporotic fractures are also observed in men.

Osteoporosis is asymptomatic until it produces skeletal deformity and bone fractures (typically in the spine, hip and wrist). The **vertebral bones** are predominantly **trabecular bone** surrounded by a thin rim of compact bone. Therefore, they may be crushed or may wedge anteriorly, resulting in pain and in a reduction in height. Elderly persons with osteoporosis may have a hip fracture when they fall.

Bisphosphonate drugs decrease fracture by inhibiting bone resorption and increasing bone mass. **Whole body mechanical vibrations (WBD)** treatment stimulates bone formation mediated by direct osteocyte signaling effects and indirect bone stimulation through skeletal muscle activation.

WBD therapy consists in the patient standing on a motorized oscillating platform that produces vertical accelerations, which are transmitted from the feet to muscles and bones to improve the structure of trabecular structure and the thickness of the cortical bone.

The diagnosis of osteoporosis is made radiologically or, preferentially, by measuring bone density by dual-energy x-ray absorptiometry (DEXA). DEXA measures photon absorption from an x-ray source to estimate the amount of bone mineral content.

The realization that RANKL plays a major contribution in osteoclast development and in bone resorptive activity stimulated the development of pharmaceutical agents to arrest skeletal disorders.

A monoclonal antibody to RANKL, called **denosumab** (Amgen), functions like osteoprotegerin. The antibody has been administered subcutaneously every 3 months for 1 year in postmenopausal women with severe osteoporosis determined by low bone mineral density detected by DEXA. Denosumab mimics the function of osteoprotegerin and decreases bone resorption, as determined by measuring in urine and serum of bone-collagen degradation products and increased bone mineral density at 1 year. A concern with denosumab anti-RANKL treatment is the expression of RANKL-osteoprotegerin in cells of the immune system (dendritic cells and B and T cells).

Osteopetrosis (Greek *osteon*, bone; *petra*, stone; *osis*, condition) is a clinical syndrome caused by a failure of osteoclasts to remodel bone. Their role was established by studies of the *op/op* mouse, which does not express M-CSF, lacks osteoclasts, and has an increase in bone mass as in osteopetrosis. For comparison, **osteosclerosis** is an increase in bone mass due to enhanced **osteoblastic activity**.

Autosomal recessive osteopetrosis (ARO), the most severe and life threatening form of the disorder, becomes apparent in early infancy. ARO is caused by a deficiency of the carbonic anhydrase II enzyme, associated with renal tubular acidosis and cerebral calcifications. Severe anemia and infections are related to bone marrow failure due to the **occlusion of marrow spaces**. Compression of cranial nerves determines hearing and vision loss and paralysis of facial muscles.

Intermediate autosomal osteopetrosis (IAO) can have either an autosomal dominant or an autosomal recessive pattern of inheritance. Detected in childhood, this form of osteopetrosis does not display severe bone marrow abnormalities although anemia and bone fracture, in addition to abnormal organ calcifications, are observed.

Autosomal dominant osteopetrosis (ADO), also called Albers-Schönberg disease, is the most prevalent and mildest type of the disorder when compared to ARO and IAO. Multiple bone factures and scoliosis (abnormal curvature of the spine) are characteristic. Because of its relatively benign clinical condition, many patients are asymptomatic and the condition is only detected by coincidental radiographic examination.

Mutations of the *CLCN7* (chloride channel voltage sensitive 7) gene are responsible for about 75% of cases of ADO. Note in Figure 4-26 that the chloride channel contributes to the transport of Cl⁻ to the subosteoclastic reabsorption compartment so an acidic pH can be achieved for effective bone resorption. Also, note that carbonic anhydrase II plays an essential role in osteoclast-mediated bone resorption.

Osteomalacia (Greek *osteon*, bone; *malakia*, softness) is a disease characterized by a progressive softening and bending of the bones. Softening occurs because of a defect in the mineralization of the osteoid due to lack of vitamin D or renal tubular dysfunction (see Chapter 14, Urinary System). In the young, a defect in mineralization of cartilage in the growth plate (see Chapter 5, Osteogenesis), causes a defect called rickets (juvenile osteomalacia).

Osteomalacia can result from a deficiency of vitamin D (for example, intestinal malabsorption) or heritable disorders of vitamin D activation (for example, renal 1α-hydroxylase deficiency in which calciferol is not converted to the active form of vitamin D, calcitriol; see vitamin D in Chapter 19, Endocrine System).

Although bone fractures are a common characteristic in patients with osteomalacia and osteoporosis, note that there is defective osteogenesis in osteomalacia in contrast to bone weakening of a previous normal osteogenesis process in patients with osteoporosis.

Essential concepts | Connective Tissue

• Connective tissue provides support, or stroma, to the functional component, or parenchyma, of tissues. The functions of connective tissue include the storage of metabolites, immune and inflammatory responses and tissue repair after injury.
Connective tissue consists of thee basic components: cells, fibers and extracellular matrix (called ground substance). The proportion of these three components contributes to the classification of connective tissue.
Connective tissue can be classified into three major groups:
(1) Embryonic connective tissue.
(2) Adult connective tissue.
(3) Special connective tissue (including adipose tissue, cartilage, bone, and hematopoietic tissue).
The embryonic connective tissue, or mesenchyme, consists predominantly of extracellular matrix. The umbilical cord contains this type of connective tissue, also called mucoid connective tissue or Wharton's jelly.
The adult connective tissue can be subclassified as:
(1) Loose or areolar connective tissue (more cells than fibers, found in the mesentery or lamina propria of mucosae).
(2) Dense connective tissue (more collagen fibers, arranged in bundles, than cells). The latter is subdivided into two categories:
• Dense irregular connective tissue (with a random orientation of collagen bundles, found in the dermis of the skin).
• Dense regular connective tissue (with an orderly orientation of collagen bundles, found in tendon).

An extension of the adult connective tissue classification is based on which fibers predominate. Reticular connective tissue contains abundant reticular fibers (type III collagen). Elastic connective tissue, found in the form of sheets or laminae in the wall of the aorta, is rich in elastic fibers.

• There are two major classes of cells in the connective tissue:
(1) The resident fibroblasts.
(2) The immigrant macrophages, mast cells and plasma cells.
The fibroblast synthesizes the precursor molecules of various types of collagens and elastin and proteoglycans.
Collagen synthesis proceeds in an orderly sequence. Procollagen, the initial collagen precursor which contains hydroxyproline and hydroxylysine, is secreted by fibroblasts in the form of a triple helix flanked by nonhelical domains. Procollagen peptidase cleaves the nonhelical domains and procollagen becomes tropocollagen. Tropocollagen molecules self-assemble in a staggered array in the presence of lysyl oxidase to form a cross-banded collagen fibril. Side-by-side linking of collagen fibrils, a process mediated by proteoglycans and a form of collagen with interrupted triple helices (called FACIT), results in the assembly of collagen fibers. What you see in the light microscope are bundles of collagen fibers.
Keep In mind that not only fibroblasts can produce collagens. Osteoblasts, chondroblasts, odontoblasts and smooth muscle cells can also synthesize collagens. Even epithelial cells can synthesize type IV collagen. You have

already seen that the basement membrane contains type IV collagen in the basal lamina and type III collagen in the reticular lamina.
Defects in the processing of procollagen and tropocollagen and the assembly of collagen fibrils give rise to variations of the Ehlers-Danlos syndrome, characterized by hyperelasticity of the skin and hypermobility of the joints.
Elastin, the precursor of elastic fibers, is also synthesized and processed sequentially. Fibroblasts or smooth muscle cells secrete desmosine- and isodesmosine-containing pro-elastin, which is partially cleaved to give rise to tropoelastin. These cells also produce fibrillin 1 and 2 and fibulin 1. Tropoelastin, fibrillins and fibulin 1 assemble into elastic fibers that aggregate to form bundles of elastic fibers.
A defect in fibrillin 1 affects the assembly of mature elastic fibers, a characteristic of Marfan syndrome.
Macrophages derive from monocytes produced in the bone marrow. A typical property of macrophages is phagocytosis. Their function in connective tissue is the turnover of fibers and extracellular matrix and, most important, the presentation of antigens to lymphocytes as an essential step of immune and inflammatory reactions.
Mast cells also originate in the bone marrow from precursors expressing c-kit receptor, stem cell factor (a c-kit receptor ligand) and FcεRI, a receptor for immunoglobulin E.
There are two populations of mast cells:
(1) Connective tissue mast cells (CTMCs).
(2) Mucosa mast cells (MMCs).
Mast cells acquire metachromatic granules

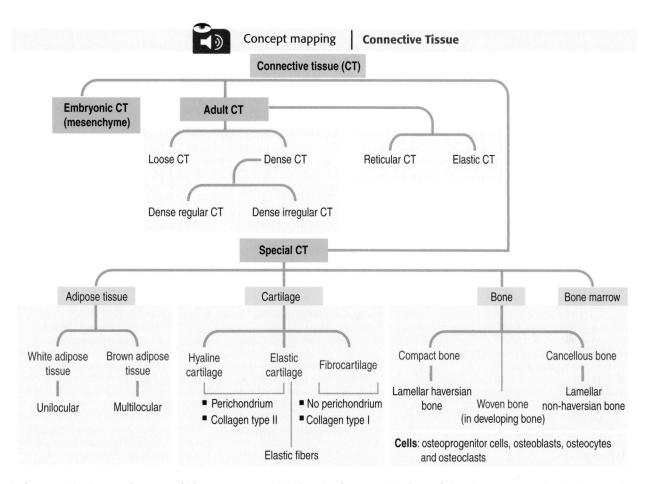

Connective tissue (CT)

Embryonic CT (mesenchyme)

Adult CT

Loose CT — Dense CT — Reticular CT — Elastic CT

Dense regular CT — Dense irregular CT

Special CT

Adipose tissue — Cartilage — Bone — Bone marrow

White adipose tissue — Brown adipose tissue

Unilocular — Multilocular

Hyaline cartilage — Elastic cartilage — Fibrocartilage

- Perichondrium
- Collagen type II

- No perichondrium
- Collagen type I

Elastic fibers

Compact bone — Cancellous bone

Lamellar haversian bone — Woven bone (in developing bone) — Lamellar non-haversian bone

Cells: osteoprogenitor cells, osteoblasts, osteocytes and osteoclasts

in the connective tissue and mucosa, which stain with a color that is different from the color of the dye. The granules contain vasoactive mediators (histamine, heparin, and chemotactic mediators), chymases and other proteases. Granules are released, by a process called degranulation, when a specific antigen (or allergen) dimerizes two adjacent IgE molecules anchored to FcεRI receptors and cytosolic calcium is released from intracellular storage sites. Leukotrienes are vasoactive agents not present in granules; they are metabolites of the plasma membrane–associated arachidonic acid. Like most vasoactive agents, they induce an increase in vascular permeability leading to edema.

Mast cells and basophils circulating in blood derive from the same progenitor in the bone marrow.

Mast cells play a role in allergic hypersensitivity reactions associated with asthma, hay fever, and eczema.

Plasma cells derive from the differentiation of B lymphocytes (B cells). Three characteristics define the structure of a plasma cell: a well-developed rough endoplasmic reticulum, an extensive Golgi apparatus, and a prominent nucleolus. These features define the plasma cell as an actively protein-producing cell, whose main product are immunoglobulins.

The **extracellular matrix** is a combination of collagens, noncollagenous glycoproteins, and proteoglycans.

Proteoglycan aggregates are the major

components. Each proteoglycan consists of a core protein attached to a linear hyaluronan molecule by a linker protein. Attached to the core protein are numerous glycosaminoglycan chains (keratan sulfate, dermatan sulfate and chondroitin sulfate). The extracellular matrix is maintained by a balance of matrix metalloproteinases (MMPs) and tissue inhibitors of metalloproteinases (TIMPs). MMPs are zinc-dependent proteases, which include collagenases, stromelysins, gelatinases, matrilysin and membrane-type MMPs.

• Tumor invasion of the connective tissue. Malignant cells originated in a lining epithelium (carcinoma) or a glandular epithelium (adenocarcinoma) can break down the basement membrane and invade the underlying connective tissue.

The histologic sequence of epithelial tumor invasion starts with dysplasia (increased cell proliferation and incomplete cell maturation), followed by carcinoma in situ (loss of epithelial normal organization within the limits of the basement membrane), microinvasive carcinoma (decreased expression of cadherins and breakdown of the basement membrane) and invasive carcinoma.

Cessation in the expression of cadherins weakens the cohesive nature of the epithelial tumor. The production of proteinases allows the tumor cells to invade and attach to components of the connective tissue. Then, tumor cells produce autocrine motility factors, to enable tumor cell motility; vascular permeability

factors, to ensure a supply of nutrients; and angiogenic factors, to increase the vascular support of the growing tumors. Finally, tumor cells can produce chemokine molecules on their surface that facilitate their transendothelial migration to metastasize.

• **Adipose tissue** or fat is a special type of connective tissue. There are two types of adipose tissue:

(1) White fat, the major reserve of long-term energy.

(2) Brown fat, a thermogenic type of fat.

Mesenchymal stem cells give rise to white fat preadipocytes and common myoblast/brown fat preadipocyte precursors. Note that white fat and brown fat derive from different precursors.

The master regulator of adipogenesis is **PPARγ** (peroxisome proliferator-activated receptor-γ). White fat can transdifferentiate into brown fat-like adipocytes following cold exposure and β-adrenergic signaling.

Adipocytes synthesize lipoprotein lipase. Lipoprotein lipase is transferred to endothelial cells in the adjacent blood vessels to enable the passage of fatty acids and triglycerides into the adipocytes.

Fat can accumulate in a single lipid-storrage droplet (unilocular) or multiple small lipid droplets (multilocular). White fat is unilocular; brown fat is multilocular.

Fat can break down by a lipolytic effect consisting in the activation of the enzyme lipase by epinephrine, glucagon or ACTH. Fat deposits can increase by inhibition of lipase activity (antilipolytic effect) determined by insulin and prostaglandins.

The surface of lipid droplets is surrounded by the protein perilipin. Phosphorylated perilipin changes its conformation and enables lipolysis by lipases.

Leptin, a peptide produced by adipocytes, regulates appetite, energy balance, and feeding. Leptin-deficient mice are obese and infertile, conditions that are reversible when leptin is administered to the mutants.

Adipocytes in brown fat contain abundant mitochondria. An important mitochondrial component is uncoupling protein-1 (UCP-1), a protein that allows the reentry of protons down their concentration gradient in the mitochondrial matrix, a process that results in the dissipation of energy in the form of heat (thermogenesis).

• **Cartilage** is another special type of connective tissue. Like adipocytes, chondroblasts derive from mesenchymal stem cells. Like a typical connective tissue member, cartilage consists of cells, fibers, and extracellular matrix. Chondroblasts and chondrocytes produce type II collagen (except in fibrocartilage, where chondrocytes produce type I collagen) and the proteoglycan aggrecan.

There are three major types of cartilages:
(1) Hyaline cartilage.
(2) Elastic cartilage.
(3) Fibrocartilage.

Cartilage lacks blood vessels and is surrounded by the perichondrium (except in fibrocartilage and articular hyaline cartilage, which lack a perichondrium). The perichondrium consists of two layers: an outermost fibrous layer, consisting of elongated fibroblast-like cells and blood vessels, and the innermost chondrogenic cell layer.

Chondrogenesis (cartilage growth) takes place by two mechanisms:
(1) Interstitial growth (within the cartilage).
(2) Appositional growth (at the perichondrial surface of the cartilage).

During interstitial growth, centers of chondrogenesis, consisting of chondroblasts located in lacunae and surrounded by a territorial matrix, divide by mitosis without leaving the lacunae and form isogenous groups. Isogenous groups are separated from each other by an interterritorial matrix. Interstitial growth is particularly prevalent during endochondral ossification.

During appositional growth, the cells of the perichondrial chondrogenic layer differentiate into chondroblasts following activation of the gene encoding the transcription factor Sox9. New layers are added to the surface of the cartilage by appositional growth.

A lack of Sox9 gene expression causes campomelic dysplasia characterized by bowing and angulation of long bones, hypoplasia of the pelvis and scapula, and abnormalities of the vertebral column.

• **Bone**. Macroscopically, a mature long bone consists of a shaft or diaphysis, and two epiphyses at the endings of the diaphysis. A tapering metaphysis links each epiphysis to the diaphysis. During bone growth, a cartilaginous growth plate is present at the epiphysis-metaphysis interface. After growth, the growth plate is replaced by a residual growth line.

The diaphysis is surrounded by a cylinder of compact bone housing the bone marrow. The epiphyses consist of spongy or cancellous bone covered by a thin layer of compact bone. The periosteum covers the outer surface of the bone (except the articular surfaces and the tendon and ligament insertion sites). The endosteum lines the marrow cavity.

Microscopically, there is:
(1) Lamellar bone, with a regular alignment of collagen fibers, typical of mature bone.
(2) Woven bone, with an irregular alignment of collagen fibers, observed in the developing bone.

A cross section of a compact bone shows the following components:
(1) The periosteum, formed by an outer connective tissue layer pierced by periosteal blood vessels penetrating Volkmann's canals feeding each osteon or haversian system. The inner periosteal layer attaches to bone by Sharpey's fibers derived from the outer periosteal layer.
(2) The outer circumferential lamellae.
(3) Osteons or haversian systems, cylindrical structures parallel to the longitudinal axis of the bone. Blood vessels are present in the central canal, which is surrounded by concentric lamellae. Each lamella contains lacunae and radiating canaliculi occupied by osteocytes and their cell processes. Osteocyte cytoplasmic processes are connected to each other by gap junctions. A fluid containing ions is present in the lumen of the canaliculi.
(4) The inner circumferential lamellae.
(5) Spongy bone (trabecular or cancellous bone), consisting of lamellae lacking a central canal (lamellar bone but no haversian system), extending into the medullary cavity.
(6) The endosteum, a lining of osteoprogenitor cells supported by reticular fibers. You can regard the endosteum as also the "capsule" of the bone marrow.

• The two major cell components of bone are the osteoblast and the osteoclast. Osteoblasts derive from mesenchyme stem cells. Osteoclasts are monocyte-derived cells from the bone marrow.

The **osteoblast** is a typical protein-producing cell whose function is regulated by parathyroid hormone and IGF-1 (produced in liver following stimulation by growth hormone). Osteoblasts synthesize type I collagen, noncollagenous proteins, and proteoglycans. These are the components of the bone matrix or osteoid deposited during bone formation.

In mature bone, the bone matrix consists of about 35% organic components and about 65% inorganic components (calcium phosphate with the crystalline characteristics of hydroxyapatite).

There are several noncollagenous proteins produced by osteoblasts that you should remember: macrophage colony- stimulating factor (M-CSF), RANKL, osteoprotegerin, osteocalcin, osteonectin and osteopontin. The first three play an essential role in osteoclastogenesis. Osteoclacin is a blood biochemical marker of osteogenesis. Osteonectin binds to type I collagen and hydroxyapatite. Osteopontin contributes to the development of the sealing zone during osteoclast bone resorption activity.

Under the influence of the transcription factor Sox9, mesenchymal stem cells give rise to preosteoblasts, the mitotically–active osteoprogenitor cells expressing the transcription factor Runx2. Preosteoblasts differentiate into postmitotic osteoblasts expressing the transcription factors Runx2 and Osterix (Osx).

Osteoblasts can follow three differentiation routes:
(1) To become osteocytes.
(2) To remain as quiescent bone-lining cells.
(3) To undergo apoptosis.

Note that the osteoblast differentiation process requires the participation of three transcription factors: Sox9, Runx2, and Osx.

Runx2-deficient mice have a skeleton consisting of cartilage and lack osteoclasts. In humans, cleidocranial dysplasia, characterized by hypoplastic clavicles and delayed ossification of sutures of certain skull bones, is associated with defective expression of the *Runx2* gene.

The function of **osteoclasts** is regulated by calcitonin, produced by C cells located in the thyroid gland. Active osteoclasts, involved in bone resorption, are highly polarized cells. The free domain has a sealing zone, a tight belt consisting of $\alpha_v\beta_3$ integrin with its intracellular domain linked to F-actin and the extracellular domain attached to osteopontin on the bone surface.

The domain associated to the subosteoclastic compartment (Howship's lacunae) displays a ruffled plasma membrane (ruffled border). The cytoplasm contains mitochondria, coated vesicles and acidified vesicles. The osteoclast is a multinucleated cell resulting from the fusion of several monocytes during osteoclastogenesis.

You should be aware that the bone marrow contains megakaryocytes that may be confused with the osteoclasts. Osteoclasts are intimately associated to bone and are multinucleated; megakaryocytes are surrounded by hematopoietic cells and their nucleus is multilobed.

Howship's lacuna is the site where bone is removed by an osteoclast. Bone removal occurs in two phases: First, the mineral component is mobilized in an acidic environment (~pH 4.5); second, the organic component is degraded by cathepsin K.

Carbonic anhydrase II in the cytoplasm of the osteoclast produces protons and bicarbonate from CO_2 and water. The acidified vesicles, with H^+-ATPase in their membranes, are inserted in the ruffling border. With the help of mitochondrial ATP, H^+ are released through the H^+-ATPase pump into Howship's lacuna and the pH becomes increasingly acidic.

Bicarbonate escapes the cell through a bicarbonate-chloride exchanger; chloride entering the osteoclast is released into the lacuna. Because of the significant H^+ transport, a parallel bicarbonate-chloride ion transport mechanism is required to maintain intracellular electroneutrality.

• Osteoclastogenesis. The osteoclast precursor is a member of the monocyte-macrophage lineage present in the adjacent bone marrow. Osteoblasts recruit monocytes and differentiate them into osteoclasts, the cell in charge of bone remodeling and mobilization of calcium.

Osteoclastogenesis consists of several phases under strict control by the osteoblast. Osteoblasts produce:

(1) M-CSF, that binds to the M-CSF receptor on the monocyte surface and the monocyte becomes a macrophage.

(2) The macrophage expresses RANK, a transmembrane receptor for the ligand RANKL produced by the osteoblast, and becomes an osteoclast precursor.

(3) RANK-RANKL interaction commits the osteoclast precursor to osteoclastogenesis. RANKL binding trimerizes RANK, which recruits TRAF6 to promote the nuclear translocation of NFATc1 and NF-κB to activate osteoclast differentiation.

(4) Osteoprotegerin, also produced by the osteoblasts, binds to RANKL to prevent RANK-mediated association of the osteoclast precursor. This event can stop osteoclastogenesis (it does not stop osteoclast function).

(5) The osteoclast precursor becomes a resting osteoclast waiting to attach to bone and become a functional osteoclast.

(6) An osteoclast becomes functional when $\alpha_v\beta_3$ integrin binds to osteopontin and begins the formation of the sealing zone. Then, the H^+-ATPase-containing acidified vesicles are transported by motor proteins associated to microtubules to the ruffling border. The acidification of Howship's lacuna starts with the activation of carbonic anhydrase II.

• Osteoporosis, osteopetrosis and osteomalacia are bone pathologic conditions.

Osteoporosis is the loss of bone mass leading to bone fragility and susceptibility to fractures. The major factor in osteoporosis is the deficiency of the sex steroid estrogen that occurs in postmenopausal women. Because an increase in the number of osteoclasts exceeds the amount of formed new bone, the monoclonal antibody denosumab, with binding affinity to RANKL, functions like osteoprotegerin (blocking the interaction of RANKL with RANK receptor) to reduce further differentiation of the osteoclast precursor.

Osteopetrosis is a clinical syndrome caused by a failure of osteoclasts to remodel bone. A mutation of the gene encoding M-CSF prevents the differentiation of osteoclasts.

Osteomalacia is characterized by a progressive softening and bending of the bones. Softening occurs because of a defect in the mineralization of the osteoid due to lack of vitamin D or renal tubular dysfunction.

5. Osteogenesis

Bone, including associated ligaments, tendons and articular cartilage, withstand the forces of compression, tension and shear stress. Bone develops by replacement of a preexisting connective tissue. The two processes of bone formation–osteogenesis or ossification–observed in the embryo are: (1) intramembranous ossification, in which bone tissue is laid down directly in embryonic connective tissue or mesenchyme, and (2) endochondral ossification, in which bone tissue replaces a preexisting hyaline cartilage, the template–or anlage–of the future bone. In addition to a description of the two major processes of ossification, this chapter addresses pathologic conditions, such as the sequence of bone fracture healing, metabolic and hereditary disorders and rheumatoid arthritis, within an integrated histologic and clinical context.

Intramembranous ossification

The mechanism of bone formation during intramembranous and endochondral ossification is essentially the same: **A primary trabecular network, called primary spongiosa, is first laid down and then transformed into mature bone.** But there is a difference in the nature of the template that becomes bone: a mesenchymal template is the starting point of intramembranous ossification, in contrast to a cartilage template of endochondral ossification.

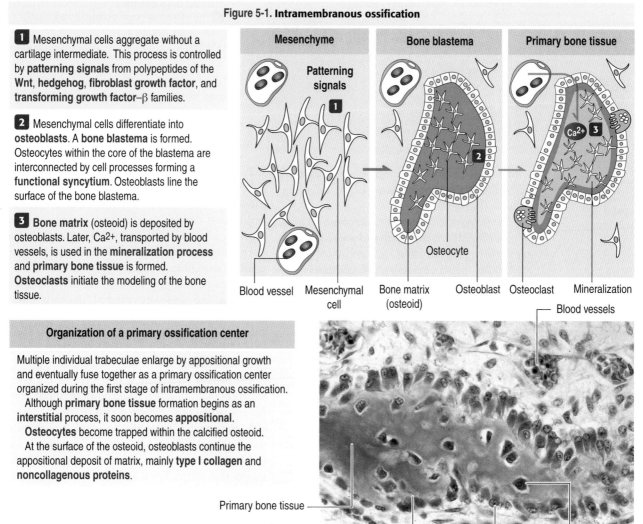

Figure 5-1. Intramembranous ossification

1 Mesenchymal cells aggregate without a cartilage intermediate. This process is controlled by **patterning signals** from polypeptides of the **Wnt, hedgehog, fibroblast growth factor,** and **transforming growth factor**–β families.

2 Mesenchymal cells differentiate into **osteoblasts**. A **bone blastema** is formed. Osteocytes within the core of the blastema are interconnected by cell processes forming a **functional syncytium.** Osteoblasts line the surface of the bone blastema.

3 **Bone matrix** (osteoid) is deposited by osteoblasts. Later, Ca^{2+}, transported by blood vessels, is used in the **mineralization process** and **primary bone tissue** is formed. **Osteoclasts** initiate the modeling of the bone tissue.

Organization of a primary ossification center

Multiple individual trabeculae enlarge by appositional growth and eventually fuse together as a primary ossification center organized during the first stage of intramembranous ossification.

Although **primary bone tissue** formation begins as an **interstitial** process, it soon becomes **appositional.**

Osteocytes become trapped within the calcified osteoid.

At the surface of the osteoid, osteoblasts continue the appositional deposit of matrix, mainly **type I collagen** and **noncollagenous proteins**.

Figure 5-2. Intramembranous ossification

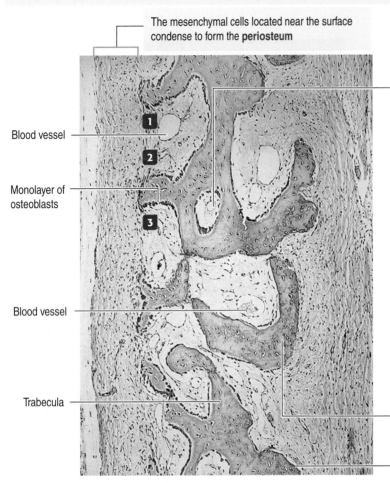

The mesenchymal cells located near the surface condense to form the **periosteum**

Blood vessel

Monolayer of osteoblasts

Blood vessel

Trabecula

The continued deposition of bone on trabecular surfaces determines the occlusion of the intertrabecular spaces, and **compact bone is formed**.

In other areas, the thickening of the trabeculae does not occur and the connective tissue in the intertrabecular space differentiates into **hematopoietic tissue**. The primary spongiosa persists as **cancellous bone**.

Intramembranous ossification

The frontal and parietal bones and parts of the occipital, temporal, mandible, and maxilla bones develop by intramembranous ossification. Intramembranous ossification requires:

1 A **well-vascularized primitive connective tissue**.

2 Bone formation is **not preceded** by the formation of a **cartilage**.

3 An aggregate of mesenchymal stem cells differentiates **directly** into osteoid-producing osteoblasts.

Osteoblasts organize thin trabeculae of **woven bone**, forming an irregular network called **primary spongiosa**.

Acidophilic osteoid

Intramembranous ossification of certain parts of the skull and the clavicle occurs in the following sequence (Figure 5-1):

1. The embryonic connective tissue (mesenchyme) becomes highly vascularized and mesenchymal stem cells aggregate while still embedded in an extracellular matrix containing collagen fibers and proteoglycans.

Box 5-A | From preosteoblasts to osteoblasts to osteocytes

• Mesenchymal stem cells differentiate into preosteoblasts and then into osteoblasts for bone formation when they express the transcription factor Runx2 and later, at a more advanced stage of differentiation, Runx2 and osterix.

• The differentiation of osteoblasts to osteocytes requires the expression of Runx2 and osterix.

• The differentiation of mesenchymal stem cells into chondrocytes occurs when the gene encoding **Sox9** is expressed. During endochondral ossification (as we will see later), chondrocytes undergo hypertrophy. The transition from cell cycling chondrocyte to hypertrophic chondrocyte is stimulated by Runx2 but inhibited by Sox9.

• Putting things together, Runx2 has a role in chondrocytic and osteoblastic differentiation. Runx2 and Osterix specify the differentiation of osteoblasts to osteocytes. A lack of osterix gene expression affects osteoblastic differentiation but not chondrocyte maturation. An example is **cleidocranial dysplasia** with defects in intramembranous and endochondral ossification.

2. Aggregated mesenchymal stem cells **directly** differentiate into **osteoblasts** that begin to secrete **osteoid** or **bone matrix** (see Box 5-A). Numerous ossification centers develop and eventually fuse, forming a network of anastomosing **trabeculae** resembling a sponge, the so-called **spongy bone** or **primary spongiosa**.

3. Because collagen fibers in the newly formed trabeculae are **randomly** oriented, the early intramembranous bone is described as **woven bone**, in contrast with the **regularly** oriented collagen fibers of the **lamellar or compact bone** formed later during bone remodeling.

4. Calcium phosphate is deposited in the bone matrix or osteoid, which is laid down by **apposition**. No interstitial bone growth occurs.

5. Bone matrix mineralization leads to two new developments (Figure 5-2): the entrapment of osteoblasts as **osteocytes** within the mineralized bone matrix that is remodeled by the bone resorptive **osteoclasts**, and the partial closing of the perivascular channels, which assume the new role of **hematopoiesis** by conversion of mesenchymal stem cells into blood-forming cells.

Osteocytes remain connected to each other by

Figure 5-3. Endochondral ossification: Primary ossification center

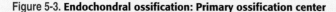

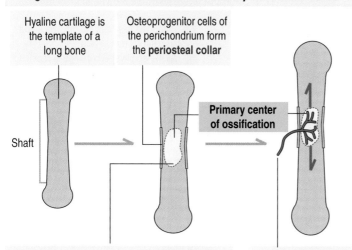

Hyaline cartilage is the template of a long bone

Osteoprogenitor cells of the perichondrium form the **periosteal collar**

Shaft

Primary center of ossification

Proliferation of chondrocytes followed by their hypertrophy at the midpoint of the shaft initiates the formation of the **primary ossification center**. Hypertrophic chondrocytes secrete **vascular endothelial cell growth factor** to induce sprouting of blood vessels from the perichondrium.
Then, **calcification of the matrix** and **apoptosis of hypertrophic chondrocytes** occur.

Blood vessels, forming the **periosteal bud**, branch in opposite directions

cytoplasmic processes enclosed within narrow tunnels called **canaliculi**. New osteoblasts are generated from preosteoblasts, the osteoprogenitor cells, located adjacent to the blood vessels.

The final developmental events include:

1. **The conversion of woven bone to lamellar (compact) bone**. In lamellar bone, the newly synthesized collagen fibers are aligned into bundles with a regular orientation. Lamellae arrange in concentric rings around a central blood vessel occupying the haversian canal form **osteons** or **haversian systems**. Membranous bones remain as spongy bone in the center, the **diploë**, enclosed by an outer and an inner layer of lamellar compact bone.

2. The condensation of the external and internal connective tissue layers to form the **periosteum** and **endosteum**, respectively, containing osteoprogenitor cells.

At birth, bone development is not complete, and the bones of the skull are separated by spaces (**fontanelles**) housing osteogenic tissue. The bones of a young child contain woven and lamellar bony matrix.

Endochondral ossification

Endochondral ossification is the process by which **skeletal cartilage templates** are replaced by bone. Bones of the extremities, vertebral column, and pelvis (the appendicular skeleton) derive from a hyaline cartilage template.

As in intramembranous ossification, a **primary ossification center** is formed during endochondral ossification (Figure 5-3). Unlike intramembranous ossification, this center of ossification starts when proliferated chondrocytes deposit an extracellular matrix containing type II collagen.

Shortly thereafter, chondrocytes in the central region of the cartilage undergo hypertrophy and synthesize **type X collagen**, a marker for hypertrophic chondrocytes. **Angiogenic factors** secreted by hypertrophic chondrocytes (**vascular endothelial cell growth factor** [**VEGF**]) induce the invasion of blood vessels from the perichondrium to form a nascent bone marrow cavity.

These events result in the formation of the **primary ossification center**. Hypertrophic chondrocytes undergo apoptosis as **calcification of the matrix** in the middle of the shaft of the cartilage template takes place.

At the same time, the inner perichondral cells exhibit their initial osteogenic potential, and a thin **periosteal collar** of bone is formed around the midpoint of the shaft, the **diaphysis**. Consequently, the primary ossification center ends up located inside a cylinder of bone. The periosteal collar, formed under the periosteum by apposition, consists of woven bone. The periosteal collar is later converted into compact bone.

The following sequence of events defines the next steps of endochondral ossification (Figure 5-4):

1. **Blood vessels** invade the space formerly occupied by the hypertrophic chondrocytes, and they branch and project toward either end of the center of ossification. Blind capillary ends extend into spaces formed within the calcified cartilage.

2. **Osteoprogenitor cells (preosteoblasts)** and hematopoietic stem cells reach the core of the calcified cartilage through the perivascular connective tissue surrounding the invading blood vessels. Then, preosteoblasts differentiate into osteoblasts that aggregate on the surfaces of the calcified cartilage and begin to deposit **bone matrix (osteoid)**.

3. At this developmental step, a **primary center of ossification**, defined by the **periosteal collar** and the center of ossification in the interior of the cartilage template, is organized at the diaphysis.

Secondary centers of ossification develop later in the **epiphyses**.

The **growth in length of the long bones** depends on the growth of the hyaline cartilage while the center of the cartilage is being replaced by bone at the equidistant zones of ossification.

Secondary centers of ossification

Up to this point, we have analyzed the development of primary centers of ossification in the diaphysis of long bones that occurs by the third month of fetal life.

After birth, **secondary centers of ossification** develop in the **epiphyses** (see Figure 5-4). As in the diaphy-

Figure 5-4. Endochondral ossification: Secondary ossification centers

The **metaphysis** is the portion of the diaphysis nearest to the epiphyses. The **epiphyseal cartilaginous growth plate** between the metaphysis and the epiphysis will eventually be replaced by bone. The bone at this site is particularly dense and is recognized as an **epiphyseal line**. **Indian hedgehog (Ihh)**, a member of the hedgehog protein family, stimulates chondrocyte proliferation in the growth plate and prevents chondrocyte hypertrophy.

4 Blood vessels from the diaphysis and epiphysis intercommunicate.
5 All the epiphyseal cartilage is replaced by bone, except for the **articular surface**.

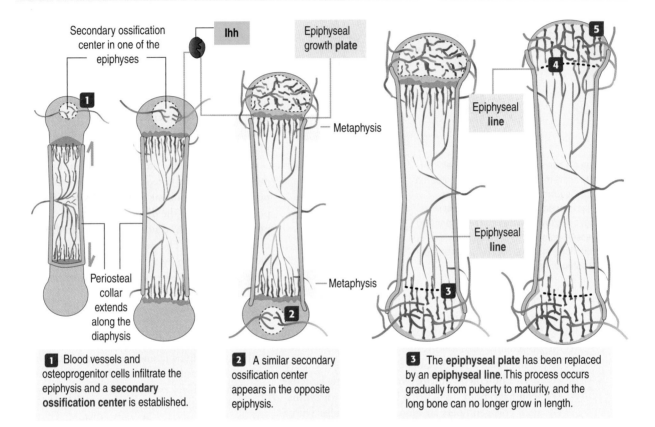

1 Blood vessels and osteoprogenitor cells infiltrate the epiphysis and a **secondary ossification center** is established.

2 A similar secondary ossification center appears in the opposite epiphysis.

3 The **epiphyseal plate** has been replaced by an **epiphyseal line**. This process occurs gradually from puberty to maturity, and the long bone can no longer grow in length.

sis, the space occupied by hypertrophic chondrocytes is invaded by blood vessels and preosteoblasts from the perichondrium. Most of the hyaline cartilage of the epiphyses is replaced by the spongy bone, except for the **articular cartilage** and a thin disk, the **epiphyseal growth plate**, located between the epiphyses and the diaphysis. The epiphyseal growth plate is responsible for subsequent growth in length of the bone by a mechanism that we discuss later.

Zones of endochondral ossification

We have seen that the deposition of bone in the center of the diaphysis is preceded by an erosion process in the hyaline cartilage template (see Figures 5-3 and 5-4). This center of erosion, defined as the **primary ossification center**, extends in opposite directions of the template, coinciding with the formation of a bony collar.

The bony collar provides strength to the midsection of the diaphysis or shaft as the cartilage is weakened by the gradual removal of the cartilage before its replacement by bone.

The continuing process of cartilage erosion and bone deposition can be visualized histologically (Figure 5-5). **Four major zones** can be distinguished, starting at the end of the cartilage and approaching the zone of erosion:

1. The **reserve zone** is a site composed of primitive hyaline cartilage and is responsible for the growth in length of the bone as the erosion and bone deposition process advances.

2. The **proliferative zone** is characterized by the active mitotic activity of chondrocytes aligning as cellular **stacks** parallel to the long axis of the cartilage template (Figures 5-6 and 5-7).

3. The **hypertrophic zone** is defined by **chondrocyte apoptosis** and **calcification** of the territorial matrix surrounding the columns of previously proliferated chondrocytes.

Despite their structurally collapsing appearance (see Figure 5-7), postmitotic hypertrophic chondrocytes play an important role in bone growth. Hypertrophic chondrocytes have the following functional characteristics:

Figure 5-5. Endochondral ossification: Four major zones

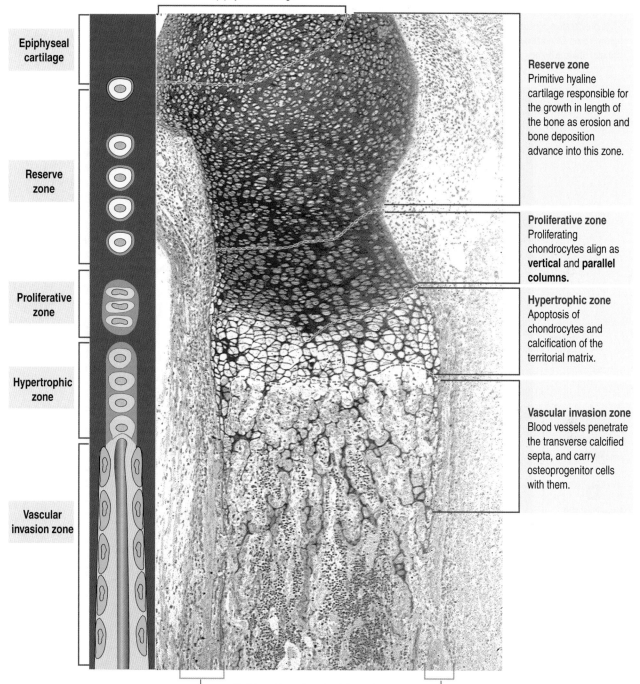

Epiphyseal cartilage

Epiphyseal cartilage

Reserve zone

Proliferative zone

Hypertrophic zone

Vascular invasion zone

Reserve zone
Primitive hyaline cartilage responsible for the growth in length of the bone as erosion and bone deposition advance into this zone.

Proliferative zone
Proliferating chondrocytes align as **vertical** and **parallel columns.**

Hypertrophic zone
Apoptosis of chondrocytes and calcification of the territorial matrix.

Vascular invasion zone
Blood vessels penetrate the transverse calcified septa, and carry osteoprogenitor cells with them.

Perichondrium changing into periosteum

• To direct the **mineralization of the surrounding cartilage matrix.**

• To **attract blood vessels** through the secretion of vascular endothelial growth factor (VEGF).

• To recruit **macrophages** (called **chondroclasts**) to degrade the cartilage matrix.

• To instruct **adjacent chondrocytes of the perichondrium to change into preosteoblasts and continue forming the bone collar.**

• To **produce type X collagen**, a marker of hypertrophic chondrocytes.

• To undergo **apoptosis** when their task is accomplished.

As a result of chondrocyte hypertrophy, the longitudinal and transverse septa separating adjacent proliferating chondrocytes appear thinner due to a compression effect. A calcification process is visualized along the **longitudinal and transverse septa.**

Figure 5-6. Endochondral ossification: Zones of proliferation, hypertrophy, and vascular invasion

1 **Proliferative zone**

The proliferative zone contains **flattened chondrocytes in columns** or clusters parallel to the growth axis. Chondrocytes are separated by the territorial matrix. All the chondrocytes within a cluster share a common territorial matrix.

The names of the zones reflect the predominant activity. The limits between the zones are not precise.

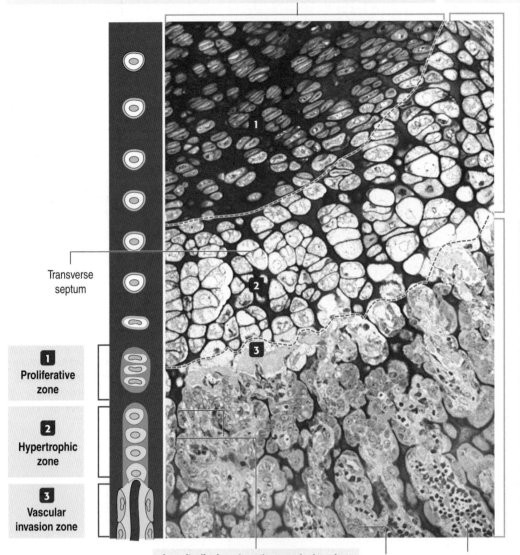

2 **Hypertrophic zone**

Hypertrophic chondrocytes calcify the matrix, synthesize **type X collagen**, attract blood vessels by secreting **vascular endothelial growth factor**, instruct perichondral cells to become osteoblasts to form the **bone collar,** and undergo apoptosis.

3 **Vascular invasion zone**

Blood vessels penetrate the **transverse septa** of the last hypertrophic chondrocyte layer and form vascular spaces with blood (lacunae).

The **longitudinal septa**, corresponding to the interterritorial matrix, are not degraded by the vascular invasion.

Osteoblasts beneath the sites of vascular invasion begin to deposit osteoid along the **longitudinal septa** forming **trabecular bone**.

Transverse septum

1 **Proliferative zone**

2 **Hypertrophic zone**

3 **Vascular invasion zone**

Longitudinal septa at the vascular invasion zone are the first sites where osteoblasts begin to deposit bone matrix (osteoid)

Osteoblasts

Blood cells

The deepest zone, proximal to the vascular invasion zone, consisting of thinner and disrupted transverse calcified septa, faces the blind end of capillary sprouts (Figure 5-8) of the developing bone marrow cavity containing hematopoietic cells.

4. The **vascular invasion zone,** an angiogenic process stimulated by VEGF produced by hypertrophic chondrocytes, is the site where blood vessels penetrate the fragmented transverse septa and carry with them migrating preosteoblasts and osteoclast-like resorptive chondroclasts.

Preosteoblasts give rise to osteoblasts that begin lining the surfaces of the exposed cores of calcified cartilage (stained blue, basophilic, in the light microscopy photograph in Figures 5-6 and 5-8) and initiate the deposition of **osteoid** (stained pink, acidophilic, in Figure 5-8). The cartilage longitudinal struts are gradually replaced by bone spicules

The deposit of osteoid denotes the beginning of osteogenesis and results in the formation of **bone spicules** (with a calcified cartilage matrix core) and, later, their conversion into **trabeculae** (consisting of

Figure 5-7. **Endochondral ossification: Zones of proliferation and hypertrophy**

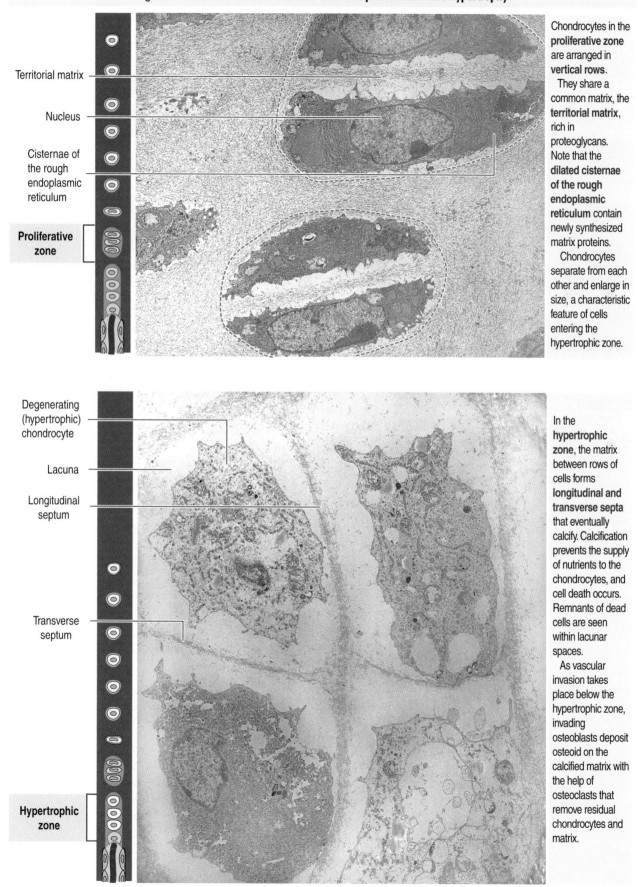

Territorial matrix

Nucleus

Cisternae of the rough endoplasmic reticulum

Proliferative zone

Chondrocytes in the **proliferative zone** are arranged in **vertical rows**.

They share a common matrix, the **territorial matrix**, rich in proteoglycans. Note that the **dilated cisternae of the rough endoplasmic reticulum** contain newly synthesized matrix proteins.

Chondrocytes separate from each other and enlarge in size, a characteristic feature of cells entering the hypertrophic zone.

Degenerating (hypertrophic) chondrocyte

Lacuna

Longitudinal septum

Transverse septum

Hypertrophic zone

In the **hypertrophic zone**, the matrix between rows of cells forms **longitudinal and transverse septa** that eventually calcify. Calcification prevents the supply of nutrients to the chondrocytes, and cell death occurs. Remnants of dead cells are seen within lacunar spaces.

As vascular invasion takes place below the hypertrophic zone, invading osteoblasts deposit osteoid on the calcified matrix with the help of osteoclasts that remove residual chondrocytes and matrix.

Figure 5-8. Endochondral ossification: Zones of hypertrophy and vascular invasion

Unmineralized osteoid contains type I collagen fibers and proteoglycans

Calcified cartilage matrix (**longitudinal septum**)

A capillary sprout, in contact with hypertrophic chondrocytes, has penetrated a transverse septum.

Disrupted **transverse septum** of the territorial matrix undergoing mineralization.

Nucleus

Osteoblast

Hematopoietic tissue in the developing bone marrow

Osteoblasts are lining a longitudinal septum and start to deposit osteoid on the calcified cartilage matrix.

Vascular invasion zone

Osteoid denoted by dotted lines along the **calcified cartilage matrix** (dark purple staining).

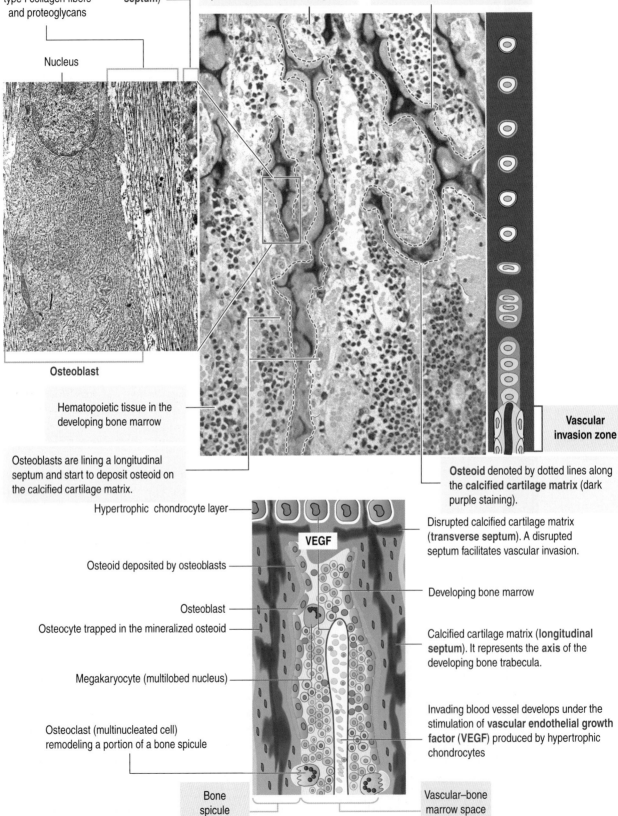

Hypertrophic chondrocyte layer

VEGF

Osteoid deposited by osteoblasts

Osteoblast

Osteocyte trapped in the mineralized osteoid

Megakaryocyte (multilobed nucleus)

Osteoclast (multinucleated cell) remodeling a portion of a bone spicule

Bone spicule

Disrupted calcified cartilage matrix (**transverse septum**). A disrupted septum facilitates vascular invasion.

Developing bone marrow

Calcified cartilage matrix (**longitudinal septum**). It represents the **axis** of the developing bone trabecula.

Invading blood vessel develops under the stimulation of **vascular endothelial growth factor** (**VEGF**) produced by hypertrophic chondrocytes

Vascular–bone marrow space

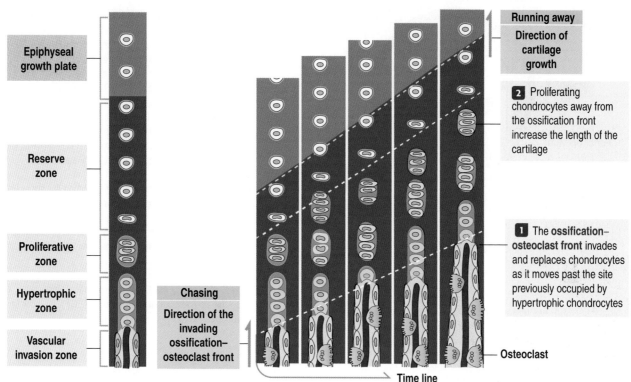

a core of bone lamellae and entrapped osteocytes but lacking calcified cartilage matrix). As a consequence, **woven bone** appears in the midsection of the developing bone.

Growth in length of the diaphysis

The ossification process advances bidirectionally toward the equidistant hypertrophic zones as the bone marrow cavity increases in width by the combined loss of cartilage and remodeling of the newly formed bone spicules by osteoclasts.

Imagine endochondral osteogenesis as an invading process consisting of an ossification front that advances by replacing hypertrophic chondrocytes while osteoclasts are engaged in the remodeling of nascent bone spicules and enlarging the bone marrow cavity (Figure 5-9).

In response to the invasion front, chondrocytes of the proliferating zone, supplied by chondrocytes of the reserve zone adjacent to the epiphyseal growth plate, continue to divide and delay their conversion into hypertrophic chondrocytes, thus keeping a distance from the osteogenic-osteoclast invasion front.

Consequently, the shaft or diaphysis grows in length by keeping intact and active the cartilage of the epiphyseal growth plate, located between the diaphysis and epiphysis of the bone.

How does the growth plate manage to keep running away from the chasing invading ossification-osteoclast front?

Hedgehog signaling: The epiphyseal growth plate and dwarfism

Indian hedgehog (Ihh), a member of the hedgehog family of proteins, is expressed by **early hypertrophic chondrocytes** within the endochondral template.

Ihh has the following signaling functions (Figure 5-10):

1. To stimulate adjacent perichondrial chondrocytes to express RUNX2 and differentiate into osteoblasts to continue forming the bone collar.

2. Also, to stimulate perichondrial chondrocytes to produce and secrete **parathyroid hormone–related peptide (PTHrP)**.

PTHrP has two functions:

1. PTHrP binds to its receptor (**PTHrPr**) on the surface of chondrocytes of the **reserve zone** to **stimulate** their proliferation.

2. PTHrP also binds to chondrocytes of the **proliferative zone** to **inhibit** their differentiation into hypertrophic chondrocytes.

Essentially, Ihh maintains the pool of proliferating chondrocytes in the epiphyseal growth plate by delaying their hypertrophy. A feedback loop between Ihh and PTHrP regulates the balance between proliferating and hypertrophic chondrocytes.

At the end of the growing period, the epiphyseal growth plate is gradually eliminated and a continuum is established between the diaphysis and the epiphyses. No further growth in length of the bone is possible once the epiphyseal growth plate disappears.

Figure 5-10. Growth plates and bone growth in length

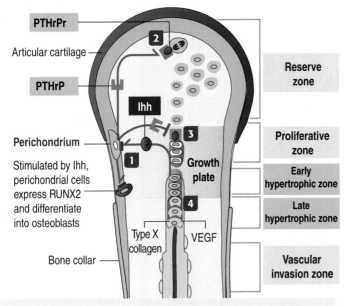

PTHrPr

Articular cartilage

PTHrP

Perichondrium

Stimulated by Ihh, perichondral cells express RUNX2 and differentiate into osteoblasts

Bone collar

Ihh

1

2

3

Growth plate

4

Type X collagen

VEGF

Reserve zone

Proliferative zone

Early hypertrophic zone

Late hypertrophic zone

Vascular invasion zone

Growth of the epiphyseal growth plate cartilage

1 **Indian hedgehog (Ihh)** protein, secreted by chondrocytes of the **early hypertrophic zone**, signals the synthesis and secretion of **parathyroid hormone–related protein (PTHrP)** by cells of the chondrogenic layer of the perichondrium (epiphysis).

Ihh has two functions: (1) regulation of the formation of the bone collar by stimulating the expression of RUNX2, thus promoting the differentiation of perichondrial cells into osteoblasts; (2) stimulation of PTHrP secretion by perichondrial cells.

2 PTHrP binds to its receptor (**PTHrPr**) on the surface of chondrocytes of the **reserve zone** to **stimulate their proliferation**.

3 PTHrP also binds to chondrocytes of the proliferative zone to **inhibit their differentiation into hypertrophic chondrocytes**.

4 Chondrocytes of the **late hypertrophic zone** secrete **type X collagen**, a marker of differentiation, and **vascular endothelial growth factor (VEGF)**, an inducer of vascular invasion.

Note that PTHrP has **opposite effects** to ensure the maintenance of the growth plate and longitudinal growth of long bones. Growth plate inactivation occurs at puberty when the height of the individual is determined. Growth plate inactivation is the direct result of an increase of **estrogen secretion** at puberty in both women and men.

Achondroplasia (ACH) is the most common skeletal dysplasia causing short-limb dwarfism. Skeletal defects are determined by a decrease in the proliferation and differentiation of chondrocytes. Fibroblast growth factor receptor 3 (FGFR3), a receptor tyrosine kinase, normally controls a signal that stops chondrogenesis. Mutations in the gene encoding FGFR3 are identified in patients with ACH. Mutations cause FGFR3 to become overactive, stopping the proliferation and differentiation of chondrocytes.

Clinical significance: Metaphyseal chondrodysplasia

Mutations of the genes encoding PTHrP and PTHrPr give rise to **Jansen's disease** or **metaphyseal chondrodysplasia**.

Circulating **parathyroid hormone cannot compensate for PTHrP deficiencies** because the avascular nature of the cartilage makes parathyroid hormone circulating in blood relatively inaccessible to chondrocytes.

A lack of expression of Ihh protein in mutant mice results in dwarfism and absence of endochondral ossification. In contrast, intramembranous ossification does not appear to require Ihh signaling. Ossification of the skull bones is normal in Ihh-null mice.

Conversion of a bone trabecula into an osteon

As the bone grows in length, new layers of bone are laid down under the periosteum of the diaphysis by **appositional growth**. Simultaneous gradual erosion of the inner wall of the diaphysis results in a width increase of the marrow cavity. As a result, the overall width of the shaft or diaphysis increases but the walls does not increase proportionally in thickness.

How does the trabecular organization of the developing bone by endochondral ossification change into the form of haversian systems or osteons?

The stalactite-like **spicules** formed during endochondral ossification change into **trabeculae**. Remember that a spicule consists of a longitudinal core of calcified cartilage coated by osteoid produced by osteoblasts lining the surface. In contrast, a trabecula lacks the calcified cartilage core; instead it contains an osteocyte lamellar core lined by osteoblast depositing osteoid on the surface.

Trabeculae are then converted into osteons, each consisting of a bone cylinder with a central longitudinal tunnel housing a blood vessel. Blood vessels at the exterior of the shaft derive from periosteal blood vessels and branches of the nutrient artery are provided at the endosteal site.

The following sequence is observed during **the trabecula–to–osteon conversion** (Figure 5-11):

1. The **longitudinal edges** of a trabecula are the boundary of a **groove**. The groove contains a blood vessel (derived from the initial vascular invasion zone). The ridges and grooves are lined by osteoblasts that continue depositing osteoid. The wall of the trabecula contains entrapped osteocytes within mineralized osteoid.

As a result of the ridges growing toward one another, the groove is converted into a tunnel lined by osteoblasts and the blood vessel becomes trapped inside a tunnel. The blood vessel interconnects with a similar vessel of an adjacent tunnel through perforating spaces leading to a **Volkmann's canal**.

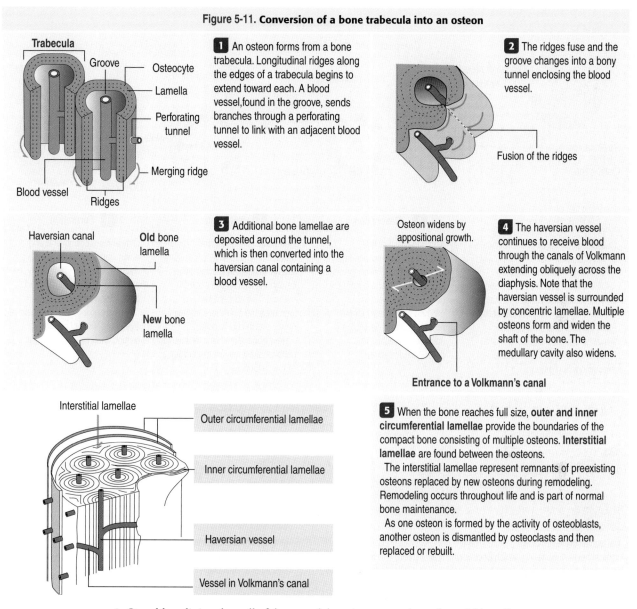

Figure 5-11. Conversion of a bone trabecula into an osteon

1 An osteon forms from a bone trabecula. Longitudinal ridges along the edges of a trabecula begins to extend toward each. A blood vessel, found in the groove, sends branches through a perforating tunnel to link with an adjacent blood vessel.

Trabecula
Groove
Osteocyte
Lamella
Perforating tunnel
Merging ridge
Blood vessel
Ridges

2 The ridges fuse and the groove changes into a bony tunnel enclosing the blood vessel.

Fusion of the ridges

3 Additional bone lamellae are deposited around the tunnel, which is then converted into the haversian canal containing a blood vessel.

Haversian canal
Old bone lamella
New bone lamella

Osteon widens by appositional growth.

4 The haversian vessel continues to receive blood through the canals of Volkmann extending obliquely across the diaphysis. Note that the haversian vessel is surrounded by concentric lamellae. Multiple osteons form and widen the shaft of the bone. The medullary cavity also widens.

Entrance to a Volkmann's canal

Interstitial lamellae
Outer circumferential lamellae
Inner circumferential lamellae
Haversian vessel
Vessel in Volkmann's canal

5 When the bone reaches full size, **outer and inner circumferential lamellae** provide the boundaries of the compact bone consisting of multiple osteons. **Interstitial lamellae** are found between the osteons.

The interstitial lamellae represent remnants of preexisting osteons replaced by new osteons during remodeling. Remodeling occurs throughout life and is part of normal bone maintenance.

As one osteon is formed by the activity of osteoblasts, another osteon is dismantled by osteoclasts and then replaced or rebuilt.

2. Osteoblasts lining the wall of the tunnel deposit by apposition new concentric lamellae and convert the structure into an osteon. **Unlike the osteons, Volkmann's canals are not surrounded by concentric lamellae.**

3. Appositional growth continues adding lamellae under the periosteum, which with time become the **outer circumferential lamellae** surrounding the entire shaft.

A modeling–remodeling process occurs through the balancing activities of the bone-forming osteoblasts and the bone-resorbing osteoclasts. At the end of the process, the outer circumferential lamellae becomes the boundary of the multiple haversian systems and interstitial lamellae fill the spaces between the haversian systems or osteons.

4. Osteoblasts lining the inner surface of the bone, the **endosteum**, develop the **inner circumferential lamellae** by a similar mechanism described for the

outer circumferential lamellae.

The crevices between the cylindrical osteons and osteons and outer and inner circumferential lamellae contain **interstitial lamellae** corresponding to remnants of the older lamellae derived from bone remodeling.

Bone remodeling

Bone remodeling is the continuous replacement of old bone by newly formed bone throughout life and occurs at random locations. The purpose of remodeling is:

1. To establish the optimum of bone strength by repairing microscopic damage (called microcracking).

2. To maintain calcium homeostasis.

Microcracking, caused by minor trauma, can be limited to just a region of an osteon. For example, damage to canaliculi interconnecting osteocytes

Figure 5-12. Bone remodeling

Compact bone remodeling (within an osteon)

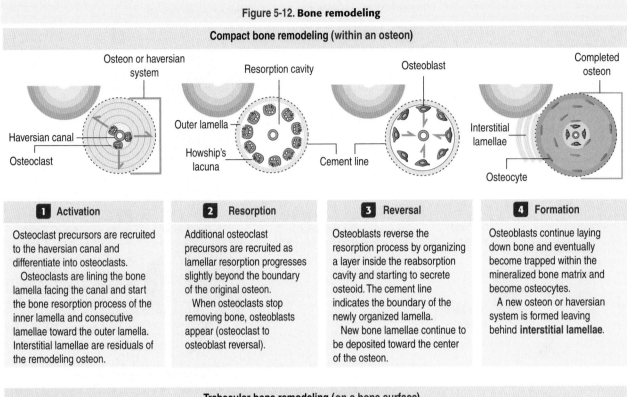

1 Activation	**2** Resorption	**3** Reversal	**4** Formation
Osteoclast precursors are recruited to the haversian canal and differentiate into osteoclasts. Osteoclasts are lining the bone lamella facing the canal and start the bone resorption process of the inner lamella and consecutive lamellae toward the outer lamella. Interstitial lamellae are residuals of the remodeling osteon.	Additional osteoclast precursors are recruited as lamellar resorption progresses slightly beyond the boundary of the original osteon. When osteoclasts stop removing bone, osteoblasts appear (osteoclast to osteoblast reversal).	Osteoblasts reverse the resorption process by organizing a layer inside the reabsorption cavity and starting to secrete osteoid. The cement line indicates the boundary of the newly organized lamella. New bone lamellae continue to be deposited toward the center of the osteon.	Osteoblasts continue laying down bone and eventually become trapped within the mineralized bone matrix and become osteocytes. A new osteon or haversian system is formed leaving behind **interstitial lamellae**.

Trabecular bone remodeling (on a bone surface)

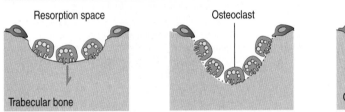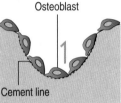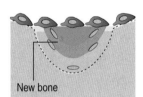

Trabecular bone remodeling occurs on the bone surface, in contrast to cortical bone remodeling, which occurs within an osteon. The trabecular endosteal surface is remodeled by this mechanism similar to cortical bone remodeling: osteoclasts create a resorption space limited by a cement line. Then osteoblast line the cement line surface and start to deposit osteoid until new bone closes the resorption space.

disrupts osteocyte cell-cell communication, leading to cell death. Microcracking can be repaired by the osteoclast-osteoblast remodeling process illustrated at the top of Figure 5-12. If the architecture of the osteon is defective, as in osteoporosis, microcracking becomes widespread and a complete bone fracture may occur.

Under normal conditions, the same amount of resorbed bone is replaced by the same volume of new bone. If the volume of resorbed bone is not completely replaced by new bone, the tissue becomes weakened and a risk of spontaneous fractures arises.

There are two forms of bone remodeling:

1. **Compact bone remodeling.**
2. **Trabecular bone remodeling.**

Compact bone remodeling is the resorption of an old haversian system followed by the organization of a new haversian system (see Figure 5-12).

Trabecular bone remodeling occurs on the endosteal bone surface (see Figure 5-12), in contrast to cortical bone remodeling, that occurs inside an osteon.

Note a significant difference between compact bone remodeling and trabecular bone remodeling: **the remodeled trabecular bone remains lamellar but not haversian.** In other words, lamellae are not enclosing a blood vessel as in the haversian systems that characterize compact bone remodeling.

General Pathology: Bone fracture and healing

Traumatic bone fracture are common during childhood and in the elderly. **Pathologic fractures** are independent of trauma and associated with a bone alteration, such as osteoporosis or a genetic collagen defect such as osteogenesis imperfecta. **Stress fractures** are caused by inapparent minor trauma (microcracking) during the practice of sports.

Fractures can be:

1. **Complete fractures,** when the bone fragments are separated from each other.
2. **Comminuted fractures,** when a complete fracture produces more than two bone fragments.

Figure 5-13. Bone fracture healing

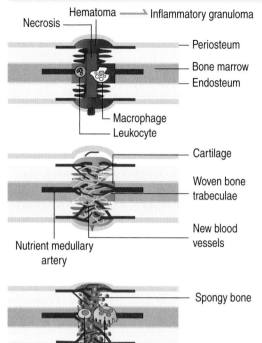

Hematoma/inflammatory phase

Accumulation of blood between the fracture ends, under the periosteum and the bone marrow space. The periosteum opposite to the trauma impact site may be torn. Osteocytes and marrow cells undergo cell death and necrotic material is observed in the immediate fracture zone. An inflammatory response follows. Macrophages and polymorphonuclear leukocytes migrate into a fibrin scaffold and an inflammatory granuloma is formed. The fracture is stabilized.

Reparative phase: Soft callus formation

Cells derived from the periosteum and endosteum initiate the repair of the fracture. Periosteal-derived capillary buds extend into the inflammatory granuloma. The nutrient medullary artery also contributes capillaries. Cartilage is formed and a soft callus contributes to the stability of the bone fractured ends. Woven bone, in the form of trabeculae, gradually replaces the cartilage. Mineralization of the woven bone is observed.

Reparative phase: Hard callus formation

Osteoblasts, derived from osteoprogenitor cells, are active. The ends of the fracture become enveloped by the periosteal (external) and internal hard callus and a clinical union can be visualized. Yet, the reparative process is not complete: the necrotic ends of the fractured bone, and even portions of the hard callus, are being reabsorbed. In addition, woven bone needs to be replaced by compact bone.

Remodeling phase

Osteoclasts reabsorb excessive and missplaced trabeculae and new bone is laid down by osteoblasts to construct compact bone along the stress lines. New haversian systems or osteons and Volkmann's canals are formed to house blood vessels.

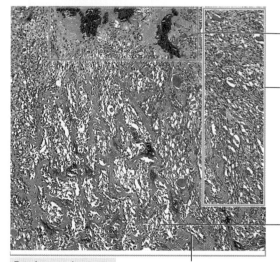

Repair woven bone area. Osteoid with embedded osteocytes. Osteoblasts are aligned along the periphery of the osteoid

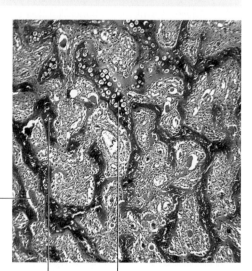

Mineralization of bone deposited on calcified cartilage. Calcified cartilage. Hard callus formation

3. **Open** or **compound**, when the fractured bone ends penetrates the skin and soft tissues.

4. **Simple or closed fractures**, when the skin and soft tissues are intact.

Pott's fracture consists in the fracture of the distal end of the fibula and injury to the distal end of the tibia. **Colles' fracture** is the fracture of the radius close to the wrist.

The healing of a simple fracture involves the following phases (Figure 5-13):

1. **Hematoma/inflammatory phase.** Bleeding and accumulation of blood at the fracture site occurs (**hematoma**) because of massive disruption of blood vessels housed in the haversian and Volkmann's canals.

Swelling, pain and an inflammatory process starts immediately. Macrophages, monocytes, lymphocytes, and polymorphonuclear cells, as well as fibroblasts, are attracted to the fracture site. The result is the formation of **granulation tissue** that bulges over the edges of the fractured bone and connects the fragments.

The development of this temporary granuloma is seen during the first week after fracture. Cytokines released by inflammatory cells and platelets recruit osteprogenitor cells from the periosteum and endosteum to the temporary granuloma, whose appropriate formation and stability require proper immobilization in the form of bracing.

2. **Reparative phase: cartilagenous soft callus** (Latin *callus*, hard skin) **phase**. Phagocytic cells start the removal of dead cells and damaged bone tissue. Capillaries infiltrate the granulation tissue and osteoprogenitor cells give rise to osteoblasts at the periosteal and endosteal sites that, together with fibroblasts, initiate the healing process. A s**oft callus** consisting of **noncalcified cartilage** connects the two ends of the fractured bone.

About 3 to 4 weeks after the injury, periosteal and endosteal-derived osteoblasts penetrate and replace the soft cartilaginous callus with woven bone.

Osteoblast penetration starts from each end of the fractured fragments and a distinct collar, consisting of woven bone typical of cancellous bone, is formed around the fragments.

3. **Reparative phase: hard bone callus phase.** The union of the fragments is achieved by the development of a **hard bone callus.** Osteoblasts deposit osteoid that is calcified and woven bone is formed.

4. **Remodeling phase.** This repair process is still in progress 2 to 3 months after the injury. Excess material of the bone callus is removed by osteoclasts and woven bone is replaced by lamellar compact bone between and around the bone fragments.

General Pathology: Metabolic and hereditary bone disorders

As we have learned, ossification results from the balanced processes of bone formation and resorption mediated by osteoblasts and osteoclasts, respectively, under the control of local regulatory factors and blood-borne signaling molecules, including **parathyroid hormone**, **vitamin D₃**, and **calcium**.

Excessive resorption causes **osteoporosis**, accounting for most non-traumatic bone fractures. Defective bone resorption causes osteopetrosis, characterized by dense but usually fragile bones.

A number of metabolic/dietary and hereditary conditions can alter the skeleton by affecting osteogenesis, bone remodeling or disturbing the mineralization of the bone matrix (Figure 5-14).

Rickets and **osteomalacia** are a group of bone diseases characterized by a **defect in the mineralization of the bone matrix** (osteoid), most often caused by a **lack of vitamin D₃**. Rickets is observed in children and produces skeletal deformities. Osteomalacia is observed in adults and is caused by poor mineralization of the bone matrix.

We have already stressed the medical significance of the RANK-RANKL signaling pathway as a pharmacologic target in the treatment of **osteoporosis** by controlling osteoclastogenesis.

Osteopetrosis includes a group of hereditary diseases characterized by **abnormal osteoclast function**. The bone is abnormally brittle and breaks like a soft stone. The marrow canal is not developed, and most of the bone is woven because of absent remodeling.

We have already discussed a mutation in the *colony-stimulating factor-1* gene whose expression is required for the formation of osteoclasts (see Bone in Chapter 4, Connective Tissue).

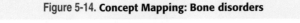

Figure 5-14. Concept Mapping: Bone disorders

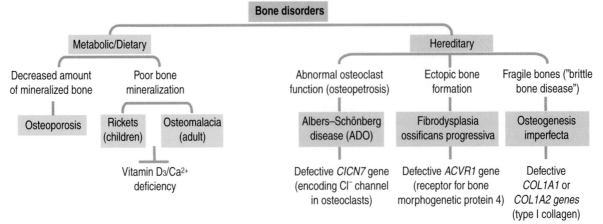

Figure 5-15. **Joints and arthritis**

| Normal joint | | Developing normal joint |

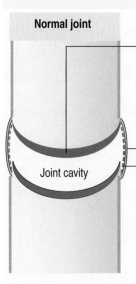

Articular cartilage
Hyaline cartilage. It lacks perichondrium and is not lined by the synovial membrane.

Joint capsule
It consists of dense connective tissue with blood vessels, lined by the **synovial membrane**. The capsule is continuous with the periosteum and is attached to the edges of the articular cartilage.

Synovial membrane
A layer of vascular connective tissue covered by 1–3 layers of **synovial cells**. There is **no basal lamina**. Capillaries are fenestrated. The **synovial fluid** is a capillary ultrafiltrate that contains the glycoprotein **lubricin** produced by synovial cells. Lubricin reduces wear to bone cartilage.

Joint cavity

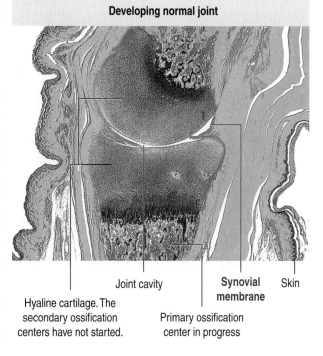

Joint cavity   **Synovial membrane**   Skin

Hyaline cartilage. The secondary ossification centers have not started.

Primary ossification center in progress

A clinical variant of autosomal dominant osteopetrosis (ADO), also known as **Albers-Schönberg disease**, is caused by different mutations in the *CICN7* gene encoding the **chloride channel in osteoclasts**. Recall that Cl⁻ is required to acidify the Howship's resorption lacunae environment for the activation of secretory cathepsin K enzyme. Review in Chapter 4, Connective Tissue, details of osteoclast function and the discussion on osteopetrosis.

Fibrodysplasia ossificans progressiva (FOP) is a very rare autosomal dominant disorder of the connective tissue. The main clinical features are **skeletal malformations** (hands and feet) present at birth and the **ossification of soft tissues** (muscles of the neck and back) precipitated by trauma. Ectopic bone formation also occurs in ligaments, fasciae, aponeuroses, tendons, and joint capsules.

Patients with FOP have a mutation in the gene encoding **activin receptor type 1A (ACVR1)**, a receptor for **bone morphogenetic protein 4 (BMP4)**. An early clinical indication of FOP is a short big toe malformation detected in the newborn. BMPs are members of the transforming growth factor–β superfamily with a role in the development of bone and other tissues.

The ACVR1 mutation consists in the substitution of histidine for arginine at position 206 of the 509-amino-acids-long ACVR1. This single amino acid substitution results in the abnormal constitutive activation of ACVR1 leading to the transformation of connective tissue and muscle tissue into a secondary skeleton. A poor prognosis is determined by the involvement of thoracic muscles, leading to respiratory failure.

Osteogenesis imperfecta is a genetic disorder characterized by fragile bones and fractures ("brittle bone disease"). Additional defects include hearing loss, scoliosis, curved long bones, blue sclera, dentinogenesis imperfecta, and short stature. This condition is caused by a dominant mutation to genes encoding type I collagen (*COL1A1* or *COL1A2*). In patients with osteogenesis imperfecta, **bisphosphonate** drugs reduce bone fracture by inhibiting bone resorption and increasing bone mass and **whole body mechanical vibrations** treatment stimulates bone formation.

Figure 5-16. Synovial membrane

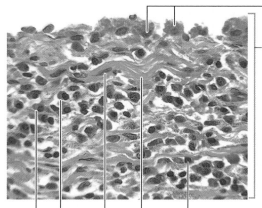

Synovial cells

The **synovial membrane** normally consists of a lining of one or two cell layers of synovial cells and underlying loose connective tissue. The synovial-lining cells are designated **type A (macrophage-like synovial cells)** and **type B (fibroblast-like synovial cells)**.

Plasma cells   Fibroblast   Lymphocyte

Collagen bundle

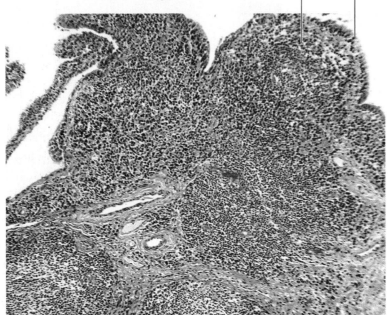

Figure 5-17. Rheumatoid arthritis

Sinovial villi proliferation over the articular cartilage and bone to form the pannus. Inflammatory granuloma within the joint causes degeneration and destruction of the articular cartilage.

Synovial cells

Hyperplasia of the synovial cell lining and subjacent infiltration by lymphocytes and plasma cells surrounding prominent synovial blood vessels

Synovial blood vessel

Rheumatoid arthritis is a chronic inflammatory disease characterized by the presence of activated CD4+ T cells **1**, plasma cells, macrophages **2**, and **synovial cells** **3** changing the synovial membrane lining into villus-type inflammatory tissue called **pannus**. Within the pannus, cellular responses lead to release of collagenase and metalloproteases **4** and other effector molecules.

The initial cause of rheumatoid arthritis is a peptide antigen presented to T cells (CD4+) which, in turn, release **interleukin-15** to activate synovial macrophages normally present in the synovial membrane.

Synovial macrophages secrete **proinflammatory cytokines**, **tumor necrosis factor ligand** and **interleukins-1 and -6**, to induce the proliferation of synovial cells, which then release **collagenase** and **matrix metalloproteases**. Neutrophils contribute **prostaglandins**, **proteases**, and **reactive oxygen species** targeted to the destruction of the **articular cartilage** and subjacent **bone tissue**. The chronic destruction of the articular cartilage, erosion of the periarticular periosteal bone by activated osteoclasts and the hypertrophy of the synovial membrane are characteristic features of rheumatoid arthritis.

Thickening of the synovial membrane (**pannus**) followed by its hypertrophy and hyperplasia (synovial villi) and replacement by connective tissue

Rheumatoid arthritic joint

Antigen-presenting cell (MHC-II)

Interleukin-15

Tumor necrosis factor ligand and interleukins-1 and -6

1 T cell (CD4+)

2 Macrophage

3 Synovial villi

5 Periarticular bone erosion

4 Collagenase and metalloprotease

Chondrocyte apoptosis

Prostaglandins, proteases and reactive oxygen species

Osteoclast

Joints

Bones are interconnected by articulations, or joints, that permit movement.

There are three types of joints:

1. **Synarthroses** permit little or no movement (cranial bones, ribs, and the sternum).

2. **Amphiarthroses** enable slight movement (intervertebral disks and bodies).

3. **Diarthroses** permit free movement.

In a **diarthroidal joint** (Figure 5-15), a **capsule** links the ends of the bones. The **capsule** is lined by a **synovial membrane** that encloses the **articular** or **synovial cavity**. The **synovial cavity** has **lubricin**, a synovial fluid glycoprotein necessary for reducing wear to the hyaline cartilage covering the opposing articular surfaces.

The **articular cartilage** is almost typical hyaline cartilage except that it **lacks a perichondrium** and has a unique collagen fiber organization in the form of overlapping arches. Collagen arcades sustain the mechanical stress on the joint surfaces.

The **joint capsule** consists of **two layers**:

1. An outer layer of dense connective tissue with blood vessels and nerves.

2. An inner layer, called the **synovial membrane**, covered by one to two layers of **synovial cells** overlying the connective tissue (Figure 5-16).

There are two classes of synovial cells:

1. **Type A macrophage-like synovial cells.**
2. **Type B fibroblast-like synovial cells.**

There is no basal lamina separating synovial cells from the connective tissue. The connective tissue contains a rich network of **fenestrated capillaries**.

Synovial fluid is a combined product of the synovial cells and the ultrafiltrate of the capillaries. The fluid is rich in **hyaluronic acid**, **glycoproteins**, and **leukocytes**.

Pathology: Rheumatoid arthritis

Rheumatoid arthritis is a chronic inflammatory and destructive autoimmune disease of the joints of unknown cause. Synovitis, the inflammatory process of the synovial membrane, occurs when leukocytes infiltrate the synovial compartment.

The production of cytokines by synovial cells is a key factor in the pathogenesis of rheumatoid arthritis. The initial event is the recruitment of activated CD4$^+$ T cells across synovial vessels. Activated CD4$^+$ T cells stimulate the production of **tumor necrosis factor ligand (TNFL)**, **interleukin-2 (IL-2)**, and **interleukin-6 (IL-6)**, and the secretion of **collagenase** and **metalloproteinases** (in particular MMP-1, 3, 8, 13, 14, and 16), by monocytes, macrophages, and fibroblast-like synovial cells.

TNFL and IL-1 can be detected in synovial fluid of patients with rheumatoid arthritis. TNFL and IL-1 stimulate fibroblast-like synovial cells, osteoclasts, and chondrocytes to release cartilage and bone-destroying MMPs.

Tissue inhibitors of MMPs (TIMPs) are unable to reverse the joint destructive cascade. Neutrophils synthesize prostaglandins, proteases and reactive oxygen species, contributors to synovitis. TNFL, IL-1, and IL-6 are key cytokines driving the build up of synovial inflammatory tissue in rheumatoid arthritis (Figure 5-17).

A proliferative process (hyperplasia) of the synovial cell lining, together with a loss in the expression of wear protective lubricin, leads to the destruction of the articular cartilage by apoptosis of chondrocytes, followed by destruction of the subjacent bone. Bone erosion, a result from osteoclast invading the periosteum adjacent to the articular surface, is detected in 80% of the affected patients within 1 year after diagnosis. Osteoclasts are activated by synovial cytokines.

Rheumatoid arthritis is characterized by the production of the autoantibodies **rheumatoid factor** and **anti–citrullinated protein antibody (ACPA)**:

1. Rheumatoid factor is a highly affinity autoantibody against the Fc domain of immunoglobulins. Rheumatoid factor has a dual role: it is a diagnostic marker of rheumatoid arthritis and also participates in its pathogenesis.

2. A post-translational conversion of the amino acid arginine into citrulline modifies the folding of citrullinated proteins that become a selective target of the immune system. ACPA-positive patients disease have a less favorable evolution than those that are ACPA-negative.

IL-6 stimulates the activation of local CD4$^+$ T cells that, in turn, stimulate B cells to differentiate into **plasma cells** that produce the autoantibodies rheumatoid factor and ACPA.

From a clinical perspective, rheumatoid arthritis cause **systemic illness**, including cardiovascular, pulmonary, and skeletal disorders caused by inflammatory mediators (cytokines and immune complexes) circulating in blood.

Essential concepts	Osteogenesis

• There are two processes of osteogenesis (bone formation or ossification):
  (1) Intramembranous bone formation.
  (2) Endochondral bone formation.
  Both processes have a common aspect: the transformation of a primary trabecular network (also called primary spongiosa) into mature bone. However, they differ in the starting point: intramembranous bone formation consists in the transformation of a mesenchymal template into bone; endochondral ossification consists in the replacement of preexisting hyaline cartilage template into bone.

• **Intramembranous bone formation** is characteristic of skull flat bones. The following sequence is observed:
  (1) Aggregates or mesenchymal condensations are formed in several sites.

  (2) Mesenchymal cells differentiate into osteoblasts to form the bone blastema originated by interstitial growth.
  (3) bone matrix or osteoid, containing type I collagen and noncollaginous proteins, is deposited by osteoblasts.
  (4) blood-borne calcium is deposited in the osteoid, which becomes calcified (mineralized).
  (5) osteoblasts become enclosed in the mineralized matrix and differentiate into osteocytes, connected to each other by cellular processes forming a network.
  (6) new osteoblasts appear along the surface of the primary bone tissue or primary ossification center, forming a trabecula.
  Several trabeculae enlarge by appositional growth and fuse together to form woven bone. Note that intramembranous bone formation starts as interstitial growth and continues by appositional growth.
  The final steps include the conversion of woven bone in the outer and inner layers into compact or lamellar bone of haversian type (concentric lamellae around a space containing blood vessels). The center of the membranous bone remains as spongy bone, called diploë. The external and internal connective layers become the periosteum and endosteum, respectively.

• **Endochondral bone formation** is characteristic of long bones, vertebral column, and pelvis. The following sequence is observed:
  (1) Chondrocytes in the center of the hyaline cartilage template become hypertrophic and start synthesizing type X collagen, vascular endothelial cell growth factor (VEGF).

(2) Blood vessels from the perichondrium invade the hypertrophic cartilage center, whose matrix becomes calcified; the primary ossification center is established.

(3) The inner perichondrial cells form a thin periosteal collar at the midpoint of the shaft or diaphysis. The periosteal collar forms woven bone—by the intramembranous bone formation process—under the future periosteum.

(4) Blood vessels invade the space formerly occupied by hypertrophic chondrocytes and preosteoblasts and hematopoietic cells arrive through the perivascular tissue.

(5) Preosteoblasts differentiate into osteoblasts, which align along the calcified cartilage matrix and begin to deposit osteoid forming stalactite-like spicules. The primary ossification center now consists of two components: the periosteal collar and the center of ossification in the interior of the cartilage template.

• Two steps will follow:

(1) The growth in length of the future long bone.

(2) The development of secondary centers of ossification in the epiphyses.

The growth in length of the long bones depends on the interstitial growth of the hyaline cartilage while the center of the cartilage is being replaced by bone. The secondary centers of ossification consist in the replacement of hyaline cartilage by spongy bone, except the articular cartilage and a thin disk, the epiphyseal growth plate, in the metaphyses (linking the diaphysis to the epiphyses).

The epiphyseal growth plate retains the capacity of chondrogenesis and, after puberty, is replaced by the epiphyseal line. Chondrogenesis of the growth plate and the formation of the bony collar are regulated by Indian hedgehog (Ihh) secretory protein in a paracrine manner.

Ihh, secreted by chondrocytes of the early hypertrophic zone of the hyaline cartilage template adjacent to the growth plate, signal perichondral cells to express RUNX2 and become osteoblast to continue forming the bony collar. In addition, Ihh stimulates the synthesis of parathyroid hormone-related peptide (PTH rP) by cells of the chondrogenic layer of the perichondrium.

PTHrP does two things: First, it binds to the PRHrP receptor on the surface of chondrocytes of the reserve zone of the growth plate to stimulate their proliferation; second, it binds to chondrocytes of the proliferative zone to prevent their hypertrophy. Essentially, PTHrP keeps the developmental potential of the growth plate active until the individual's programmed bone length has been completed.

• Endochondral bone formation consists of four major histologic zones:

(1) The reserve zone, composed of hyaline cartilage "running away" from the "chasing" ossification front, the vascular invasion zone and the bone resorptive activity of osteoclasts.

(2) The proliferative zone, characterized by the mitotic activity of chondrocytes, forming stacks of isogenous groups, also running away from the chasing vascular invasion zone.

(3) The hypertrophic zone, the "facilitator" of the vascular invasion zone by producing VEGF, recruiting macrophage-like chondroclasts to destroy the calcified cartilage matrix, and producing type X collagen, an imprint of their hypertrophic nature.

(4) The vascular invasion zone, the site where blood vessels sprouts, penetrating the transverse calcified cartilage septa, carry preosteoblasts and hematopoietic cells. A characteristic of this zone are the spicules, which will become trabeculae.

A spicule consists of a longitudinal core of calcified cartilage coated by osteoid produced by osteoblasts lining the surface. A trabecula is an osteocyte lamellar core (instead of a calcified cartilage core), covered by osteoblast depositing osteoid on the surface.

Trabeculae, built by osteoblasts and remodeled by osteoclasts, results in the formation of woven or cancellous bone.

Woven bone will change into a lamellar bone of the haversian system type using the blood vessel as the axial center for the concentric deposit and organization of lamellae.

Recall that osteoblasts have two major tasks: to continue forming bone, until they become sequestered in the lacunae as osteocytes, and to direct osteoclastogenesis by the RANK-RANKL signaling pathway.

• The conversion of bone trabeculae into osteons consists in the following steps:

Longitudinal ridges of a trabecula advance toward one another and enclose the periosteal blood vessel, creating a tunnel that houses a blood vessel. The blood vessels will become the center of a haversian system or osteon. Blood is supplied by transverse blood vessels occupying the Volkmanns's canals. Keep in mind that the haversian system has concentric lamellae; the Volkmann's canal does not.

Appositional bone growth continues under the periosteum to form the outer circumferential lamellae. Osteoblasts lining the endosteum form the inner circumferential lamellae, also by appositional bone growth.

The shaft or diaphysis grows in width by apposition consisting in new compact bone being laid down under the periosteum. At the same time, woven bone is gradually reabsorbed at the inner side, or endosteum, of the shaft and the width of the marrow cavity increases. Consequently, the shaft becomes wider but the walls, formed by compact bone, does not increase significantly in thickness. Keep in mind that woven bone, persisting at the endosteal surface, is lamellar but not haversian.

• Bone remodeling is a continuous and random process consisting in the replacement of newly formed bone and old bone

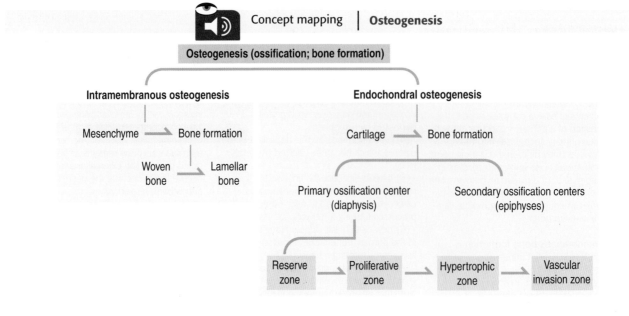

Concept mapping | Osteogenesis

Osteogenesis (ossification; bone formation)

Intramembranous osteogenesis

Mesenchyme → Bone formation

Woven bone

Lamellar bone

Endochondral osteogenesis

Cartilage → Bone formation

Primary ossification center (diaphysis)

Secondary ossification centers (epiphyses)

Reserve zone → Proliferative zone → Hypertrophic zone → Vascular invasion zone by a resorption-production sequence involving the combined participation of osteoblasts and osteoclasts.

There are two forms of bone remodeling:
(1) Cortical bone remodeling.
(2) Trabecular bone remodeling.

Cortical bone remodeling occurs in an old haversian system followed by the reorganization of a new one. Osteoclasts begin eroding the lamella facing the central canal until they reach the outermost lamella. Residual lamellae of the ongoing degradation process are pushed in between the existing intact osteons, forming the interstitial lamellae. The osteoclasts disappear and osteoblasts begin the reconstruction process by constructing new lamellae from the periphery to the central canal where a blood vessel is located. The starting point of the reconstruction of a new osteon is marked by the cement line, a structure that absorbs microcracking created by load forces acting on bone.

Trabecular bone remodeling follows the same osteoclast resorption and osteoclast-osteoblast reversal sequence. A major difference is that this process occurs on the bone surface instead of in an osteon.

• **Bone fractures** take place when pathologic and traumatic fractures occur.

Fractures can be:
(1) Complete fractures (when the bone fragments are separated from each other).
(2) Comminuted fractures (when a complete fracture produces bones broken into more than two fragments).
(3) Open or compound fractures (when the fractured bone ends penetrates the skin and soft tissues).
(4) Simple or closed fractures (when the skin and soft tissues are intact).

A few type of fractures are designated by specific names. For example, Pott's fracture consists in the fracture of the distal end of the fibula and injury to the distal end of the tibia. Colles' fracture is the fracture of the radius close to the wrist.

The healing of a fracture involves the following phases:
(1) Hematoma/inflammatory phase. Bleeding and an inflammatory process lead to the formation of temporary granulation tissue during the first week after fracture. The bone fragments are connected and proper immobilization is required.
(2) Reparative phase (soft callus). A soft noncalcified cartilagenous callus connects the two ends of the fractured bone.

(3) Reparative phase (hard bone callus). Osteoblasts deposit osteoid that is calcified and woven bone is formed.
(4) Remodeling phase (2 to 3 months after the injury). Excess material of the bone callus is removed by osteoclasts and woven bone is replaced by lamellar compact bone.

• **Metabolic and hereditary bone disorders** include:

Rickets (children) and osteomalacia (adults) are a group of bone diseases characterized by a defect in the mineralization of the bone matrix (osteoid), most often caused by a lack of vitamin D_3.

Osteopetrosis includes a group of hereditary diseases characterized by abnormal or nonexisting osteoclast function. A clinical variant, autosomal dominant osteopetrosis (ADO), also known as Albers-Schönberg disease, is caused by mutations in the *CICN7* gene encoding the chloride channel in osteoclasts.

Osteoporosis is a degenerative bone disease in which the osteoclast-driven bone degradation process is not fully compensated by the same bone production volume by osteoblasts.

Fibrodysplasia ossificans progressiva (FOP) is an inherited disorder of the connective tissue consisting in the aberrant ossification of muscle tissue and connective tissue and skeletal malformations. A mutation in the receptor ACVR1 (activin receptor type 1A) of bone morphogenetic protein leads to the unregulated activation of the receptor and the deposit of bone in nonskeletal tissues.

Osteogenesis imperfecta is a genetic disorder defined by fragile bones and fractures ("brittlebone disease"). Additional defects include hearing loss, scoliosis, curved long bones, blue sclera, dentinogenesis imperfecta and short stature. This condition is caused by a dominant mutation to genes encoding type I collagen (*COL1A1* [α-1 chain peptide] or *COL1A2* [α-2 chain peptide]). Missense mutations leading to a defective peptide chain results in abnormalities in most of the collagen triple helix.

• **Joints** can be classified into:
(1) Synarthroses, which permit little or no movement.
(2) Amphiarthroses, which enable slight movement.
(3) Diarthroses, which permit free movement.

A diarthrodial joint consists of a vascularized outer layer of dense connective tissue capsule

continuous with the periosteum. The capsule surrounds the joint and encloses the synovial cavity, containing fluid produced by the lining cells of the synovial membrane.

• **Rheumatoid arthritis** is a chronic inflammatory and destructive autoimmune disease of the joints of unknown cause.

Synovitis, the inflammatory process of the synovial membrane, occurs when leukocytes infiltrate the synovial compartment. The production of cytokines by synovial cells is a key factor in the pathogenesis of rheumatoid arthritis.

A proliferative process (hyperplasia) of the synovial cell lining, together with a loss in the expression of synovial protective lubricin, causes the destruction of the articular cartilage by apoptosis of chondrocytes, followed by destruction of the subjacent bone.

Bone erosion, a result from osteoclast invading the periosteum adjacent to the articular surface, is detected in 80% of the affected patients within 1 year after diagnosis. Osteoclasts are activated by synovial cytokines.

Synovitis occurs when leukocytes infiltrate the synovial compartment. The initial event is triggered by the activation of CD4+ T cells by an undetermined antigen.

CD4+ T cells and antigen-presenting cells induce the villus-like proliferation of synovial cells (called pannus) and the production of tumor necrosis factor ligand, interleukins, collagenases, and metalloproteinases (proinflammatory effectors), which continue triggering an inflammatory response by synovial cells.

Rheumatoid arthritis is characterized by the production of autoantibodies:
(1) Rheumatoid factor.
(2) Anti-citrullinated protein antibody (ACPA).

Rheumatoid factor is a highly affinity autoantibody against the Fc domain of immunoglobulins. Rheumatoid factor has a dual role:
(1) It is a diagnostic marker of rheumatoid arthritis
(2) It also has participates in its pathogenesis.

A post-translational conversion of the amino acid arginine into citrulline modifies the folding of citrullinated proteins that become a selective target of the immune system. ACPA-positive patients disease have a less favorable evolution than those that are ACPA-negative.

6. Blood and Hematopoiesis

Blood, a specialized type of connective tissue, consists of plasma, erythrocytes, leukocytes, and platelets. Blood offers valuable diagnostic information about normal body functions and pathologic alterations because of its biochemical composition and easy access. Hematopoiesis, the self-renewal and differentiation of multipotent stem cells in bone marrow, is responsible for the release of end-stage mature cells into the blood circulation (~1 x 10^9 erythrocytes and ~1 x 10^8 leukocytes every hour). Bone marrow microenvironments, or niches, enable colonies of hematopoietic cells to fullfil their commitment of producing and maintaining a steady number of mature cell populations and platelets in blood. This chapter describes the structural and functional characteristics of blood cells, their development, and the distribution of progenitor cells in specific hematopoietic niches.

Blood

Blood consists of **cells** and **plasma**. These components may be separated by centrifugation when blood is collected in the presence of anticoagulants. The sedimented red blood cells (RBCs) constitute about **42%–47%** of blood volume. This percentage of erythrocyte volume is the **hematocrit** (Greek, *haima*, blood; *krino*, to separate). Sitting on top of the erythrocyte layer is the **buffy coat** layer, which contains **leukocytes** (Greek *leukos*, white; *kytos*, cell) and **platelets**. The translucent supernatant fraction above the packed RBCs is plasma. Normal adult blood volume measures **5 to 6 L**.

Plasma

Plasma is the fluid component of blood (Figure 6-1). Plasma contains salts and organic compounds (including amino acids, lipids, vitamins, proteins, and hormones). In the absence of anticoagulants, the cellular elements of blood, together with plasma

proteins (mostly **fibrinogen**), form a clot in the test tube. The fluid portion is called **serum**, which is essentially fibrinogen-free plasma.

Red blood cells (erythrocytes)

RBCs, also called erythrocytes (Greek *erythros*, red; *kytos*, cell), are non-nucleated, biconcave-shaped cells measuring about **7.8 µm** in diameter (unfixed). RBCs lack organelles and consist only of a plasma membrane, its underlying cytoskeleton (Figure 6-2), hemoglobin, and glycolytic enzymes.

RBCs (average number: **4 to 6 x 10^6 per mm³**) circulate for **120 days**. Senescent RBCs are removed by phagocytosis or destroyed by **hemolysis** in the spleen. RBCs are replaced in the circulation by **reticulocytes**, which complete their hemoglobin synthesis and maturation 1 to 2 days after entering the circulation. Reticulocytes account for **1% to 2%** of circulating RBCs. RBCs transport oxygen and carbon dioxide and are confined to the circulatory system.

Pathology: RBC cytoskeletal and hemoglobin abnormalities

The main determinant of **anemia** in **hemolytic anemias** is **RBC destruction**. Normal RBC destruction takes place in spleen but acute and chronic RBC hemolysis occurs within blood vessels as the result of **membrane cytoskeleton**, **metabolic** or **hemoglobin** abnormalities.

1. Defects of the membrane cytoskeleton: **Elliptocytosis** and **spherocytosis** are alterations in the shape of RBCs caused by defects in the membrane cytoskeleton. **Elliptocytosis**, an autosomal dominant disorder characterized by the presence of oval-shaped RBCs, is caused by defective self-association of spectrin subunits, defective binding of spectrin to ankyrin, protein 4.1 defects, and abnormal glycophorin (see Figure 6-2).

Spherocytosis is also an autosomal dominant condition involving a deficiency in **spectrin**. RBCs are spherical, of different diameter and many of them

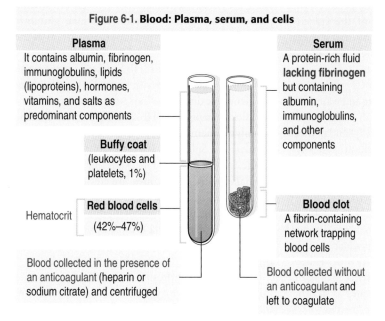

Figure 6-1. Blood: Plasma, serum, and cells

Plasma
It contains albumin, fibrinogen, immunoglobulins, lipids (lipoproteins), hormones, vitamins, and salts as predominant components

Buffy coat
(leukocytes and platelets, 1%)

Hematocrit

Red blood cells
(42%–47%)

Blood collected in the presence of an anticoagulant (heparin or sodium citrate) and centrifuged

Serum
A protein-rich fluid **lacking fibrinogen** but containing albumin, immunoglobulins, and other components

Blood clot
A fibrin-containing network trapping blood cells

Blood collected without an anticoagulant and left to coagulate

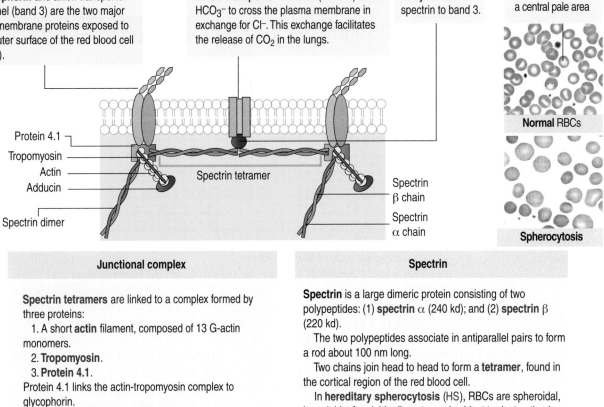

Figure 6-2. Cell membrane of a red blood cell

Glycophorin and anion transporter channel (band 3) are the two major transmembrane proteins exposed to the outer surface of the red blood cell (RBC).

Anion transporter channel (band 3) allows HCO_3^- to cross the plasma membrane in exchange for Cl^-. This exchange facilitates the release of CO_2 in the lungs.

Ankyrin anchors spectrin to band 3.

Normal RBCs show a central pale area

Normal RBCs

Protein 4.1
Tropomyosin
Actin
Adducin

Spectrin tetramer

Spectrin dimer

Spectrin β chain

Spectrin α chain

Spherocytosis

Junctional complex

Spectrin tetramers are linked to a complex formed by three proteins:
  1. A short **actin** filament, composed of 13 G-actin monomers.
  2. **Tropomyosin**.
  3. **Protein 4.1**.
Protein 4.1 links the actin-tropomyosin complex to glycophorin.
  Adducin is a **calmodulin-binding protein** that stimulates the association of actin with spectrin.

Spectrin

Spectrin is a large dimeric protein consisting of two polypeptides: (1) **spectrin** α (240 kd); and (2) **spectrin** β (220 kd).
  The two polypeptides associate in antiparallel pairs to form a rod about 100 nm long.
  Two chains join head to head to form a **tetramer**, found in the cortical region of the red blood cell.
  In **hereditary spherocytosis** (HS), RBCs are spheroidal, less rigid, of variable diameter and subject to destruction in the spleen. This alteration is caused by cytoskeletal abnormalities involving sites of interactions between **spectrin** α and β and **protein 4.1**.

Micrographs from Hoffbrand AV, Pettit JE: Color Atlas of Clinical Hematology, 3rd ed., London, Mosby, 2000.

lack the typical central pale area seen in normal RBCs (see Figure 6-2). The common clinical features of elliptocytosis and spherocytosis are **anemia**, **jaundice** (resulting from increased bilirubin production), and **splenomegaly** (enlargement of the spleen). **Splenectomy** is usually curative, because the spleen is the primary site responsible for the destruction of elliptocytes and spherocytes.

2. Metabolic defects: Normal RBCs produce energy to maintain cell shape, electrolyte and water content by metabolizing glucose through the glycolytic (Embden-Meyerhof glycolytic pathway) and pentose phosphate (hexose monophosphate shunt) pathways.

The most abundant phosphate in RBC is 2,3-diphosphoglycerate (2,3-DPG), involved in the release of oxygen from hemoglobin. The enzyme glucose 6-phosphate dehydrogenase (G6PD) protects the membrane and hemoglobin from oxidant damage, a frequent metabolic cause of intravascular hemolysis caused by severe infection, hepatitis or diabetic ketoacidosis observed in the presence of **G6PD deficiency**. **Pyruvate kinase deficiency** is another metabolic defect found in hemolytic anemia.

3. Hemoglobin defects: Hemoglobin genetic defects ($\alpha_2\beta S_2$) cause **sickle cell anemia** and **thalassemia** (Greek *thalassa*, sea; observed in populations along the Greek and Italian coasts). **Sickle cell anemia** results from a point mutation in which **glutamic acid** is replaced by **valine** at the sixth position in the β-globin chain.

Defective hemoglobin (Hb S) tetramers aggregate and polymerize in deoxygenated RBCs, changing the biconcave disk shape into a rigid and less deformable sickle-shaped cell. Hb S leads to severe **chronic hemolytic anemia** and **obstruction of postcapillary venules** (see Spleen in Chapter 10, Immune-Lymphatic System).

Thalassemia syndromes are heritable anemias characterized by defective synthesis of either the α or β chains of the normal hemoglobin tetramer ($\alpha_2\beta_2$). The specific thalassemia syndromes are designated by the affected globin chain: α-**thalassemia** and β-**thalassemia.**

Thalassemia syndromes are defined by anemia caused by defective synthesis of the hemoglobin molecule and hemolysis.

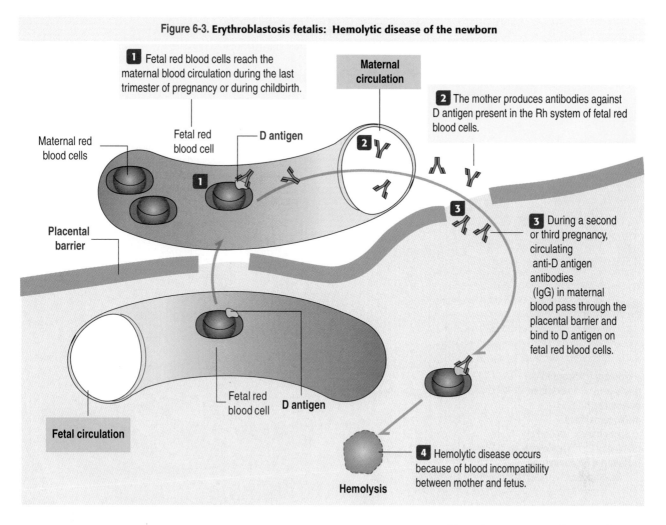

Figure 6-3. Erythroblastosis fetalis: Hemolytic disease of the newborn

1 Fetal red blood cells reach the maternal blood circulation during the last trimester of pregnancy or during childbirth.

Maternal circulation

2 The mother produces antibodies against D antigen present in the Rh system of fetal red blood cells.

Maternal red blood cells

Fetal red blood cell

D antigen

Placental barrier

3 During a second or third pregnancy, circulating anti-D antigen antibodies (IgG) in maternal blood pass through the placental barrier and bind to D antigen on fetal red blood cells.

Fetal red blood cell   D antigen

Fetal circulation

4 Hemolytic disease occurs because of blood incompatibility between mother and fetus.

Hemolysis

Clinical significance: Hemoglobin A1c (glycated hemoglobin) and diabetes mellitus

A valuable clinical indicator of average **plasma glucose concentration** is the measurement of **hemoglobin A1c** (glycohemoglobin or glycated [coated] hemoglobin). Glucose links to hemoglobin A1 in a non-enzymatic irreversible reaction.

The normal range for the hemoglobin A1c is between 4% and 5.6%. Hemoglobin A1c levels between 5.7% and 6.4% indicate increased risk of diabetes mellitus, and levels of 6.5% or higher indicate diabetes mellitus. Determination of glycated hemoglobin is an efficient way to assess pre-diabetes or diabetes mellitus conditions as well as the treat-

ment to achieve long-term regulation of serum glucose levels to prevent cardiovascular, renal, and retinal complications.

Clinical significance: Erythroblastosis fetalis

Erythroblastosis fetalis is an antibody-induced hemolytic disease in the newborn that is caused by blood group incompatibility between mother and fetus (Figure 6-3 and Box 6-A). This incompatibility occurs when the fetus inherits RBC antigenic determinants that are foreign to the mother. ABO and Rh blood group antigens are of particular interest.

Essentially, the mother becomes sensitized to blood group antigens on **red blood cells**, which can reach maternal circulation during the last trimester of pregnancy (when the cytotrophoblast is no longer present as a barrier, as we discuss in Chapter 23, Fertilization, Placentation, and Lactation) or during childbirth. Within the Rh system, **D antigen** is the major cause of Rh incompatibility. The initial exposure to the Rh antigen during the first pregnancy does not cause erythroblastosis fetalis because **immunoglobulin M (IgM)** is produced. IgMs cannot cross the placenta because of their large size.

Box 6-A | Hemolysis in erythroblastosis fetalis

• The hemolytic process in erythroblastosis fetalis causes hemolytic anemia and jaundice.
• Hemolytic anemia causes hypoxic injury to the heart and liver, leading to generalized edema (hydrops fetalis; Greek *hydrops*, edema).
• Jaundice causes damage to the central nervous system (German *kernicterus*, jaundice of brain nuclei).
• Hyperbilirubinemia is significant, and unconjugated bilirubin is taken up by the brain tissue.

Figure 6-4. **Neutrophil**

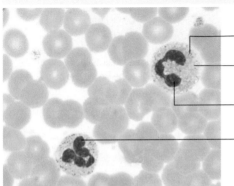

- Specific (secondary) granules
- Primary granules
- Trilobed nucleus
- Tetralobed nucleus

Neutrophils represent 50% to 70% of total leukocytes (the most abundant leukocyte in a normal blood smear). They measure 12 to 15 μm in diameter with a very pale pink cytoplasm (close in color to the erythrocyte).

Neutrophils contain **primary granules** that can barely be resolved, and smaller **specific (secondary) granules**.

The nucleus (stained dark blue) is usually segmented into three to five indented lobes.

Granular contents of a neutrophil

Neutrophils, so called because of the appearance of their cytoplasmic granules following **Wright-Giemsa staining**, migrate to the sites of infection where they recognize and phagocytose bacteria. Migration and ingestion require substances contained in the cytoplasmic granules.

Primary (or **azurophilic**) **granules** contain **elastase**, **defensins**, and **myeloperoxidase**.

Secondary (or **specific**) **granules** contain **lysozyme**, **lactoferrin**, **gelatinase**, and other **proteases**.

The weak staining properties of secondary granules are responsible for the cytoplasmic light-colored appearance.

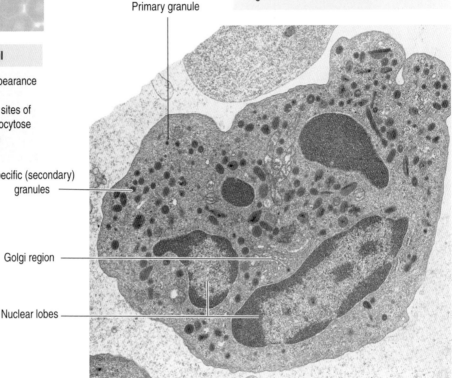

Primary granule

- Specific (secondary) granules
- Golgi region
- Nuclear lobes

Subsequent exposure to D antigen during the second or third pregnancy leads to a strong **immunoglobulin G (IgG)** response (IgGs can cross the placenta).

Rh-negative mothers are given anti-D globulin soon after the delivery of an Rh-positive baby. Anti-D antibodies mask the antigenic sites on the fetal RBCs that may have leaked into the maternal circulation during childbirth. This prevents long-lasting sensitization to Rh antigens.

Leukocytes

Leukocytes (**6 to 10 × 10³ per mm³**; see Box 6-B) are categorized as either **granulocytes (containing primary, and specific or secondary cytoplasmic granules,** Box 6-C) or **agranulocytes (containing only primary granules)**.

In response to an appropriate stimulus, leukocytes may leave the bloodstream (**diapedesis**) and enter the connective tissue by the **homing** mechanism (see Figure 6-9).

Granulocytes

These phagocytic cells have a **multilobed nucleus** and measure **12 to 15 μm** in diameter. Their average lifespan varies with cell type. Three types of granulocytes can be distinguished by their cytoplasmic granules:

1. **Neutrophils** (Figure 6-4). These cells have

Box 6-B | Blood cells/μL or mm³

Erythrocytes	4-6 × 10⁶	
Leukocytes	6000 to 10,000	
Neutrophils	5000	(60% to 70%)
Eosinophils	150	(2% to 4%)
Basophils	30	(0.5%)
Lymphocytes	2400	(28%)
Monocytes	350	(5%)
Platelets	300,000	
Hematocrit	42%–47%	

Figure 6-5. **Eosinophil**

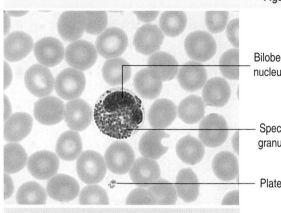

Bilobed nucleus

Specific granules

Platelets

Eosinophils represent 1% to 5% of total leukocytes. They measure 12 to 15 μm in diameter.

Their cytoplasm contains large, refractile specific granules that appear bright red and are clearly discernible.

The nucleus of the eosinophil is typically bilobed.

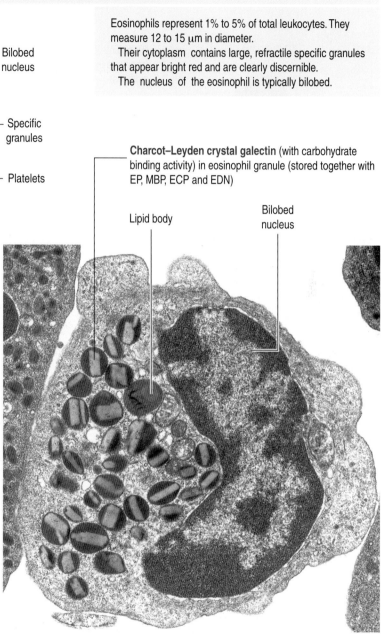

Charcot–Leyden crystal galectin (with carbohydrate binding activity) in eosinophil granule (stored together with EP, MBP, ECP and EDN)

Lipid body

Bilobed nucleus

Granular contents of an eosinophil

Eosinophil peroxidase (EP)
It binds to microorganisms and facilitates their killing by macrophages.
Major basic protein (MBP)
1. It is the predominant component of the crystalline center of the eosinophil granule.
2. It binds to and disrupts the membrane of parasites (binding is mediated by its Fc receptor).
3. It causes basophils to release histamine by a Ca2+-dependent mechanism.
Eosinophil cationic protein (ECP)
1. It neutralizes heparin.
2. Together with MBP, it causes the fragmentation of parasites.
Eosinophil–derived nerurotoxin (EDN)
Secretory protein with ribonuclease and antiviral activity

Other products of eosinophils

Cytokines (Interleukins (IL)-2 to IL-6 and others), **enzymes** (acid phosphatase, collagenase histaminase, catalase and others) and **growth factors** (vascular endothelial growth factor (VEGF), nerve growth factor (NGF), stem cell factor (SCF) and others)
Lipid bodies (leukotrienes, prostaglandins)

Box 6-C | **Primary and specific granules**

• Primary and specific (secondary) granules contain enzymes. Tertiary granules have been described; they produce proteins (cathepsin and gelatinase), which enable neutrophils to attach to other cells and aid the process of phagocytosis.
• Peroxidase is a marker enzyme of primary granules. The presence of alkaline phosphatase and a lack of peroxidase characterize the secondary granules.
• Why are primary granules azurophilic with the Wright blood stain method? Because primary granules contain sulfated glycoproteins that presumably account for this deep-blue (azure) staining.

a multilobed nucleus. Their cytoplasm contains secondary (specific) and primary granules (see Box 6-C). In stained smears, neutrophils appear very pale pink. Neutrophils, which constitute **50% to 70%** of circulating leukocytes, have a lifespan of **6 to 7 hours** and may live for up to **4 days** in the connective tissue.

After leaving the circulation through postcapillary venules, neutrophils act to eliminate opsonized bacteria or limit the extent of an inflammatory reaction in the connective tissue. The mechanism of bacterial opsonization and the relevant role of neutrophils in acute inflammation are discussed in Chapter 10, Immune-Lymphatic System.

Enzymes contained in the primary granules (**elastase, defensins** and **myeloperoxidase**) and secondary

Figure 6-6. **Basophil**

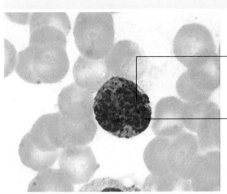

Basophils represent less than 1% of total leukocytes, so they may be difficult to find.

Their specific granules are large and stain dark blue or purple. Basophils also contain a few primary granules.

The nucleus, which is typically bilobed, is often obscured by the specific granules.

Bilobed nucleus (obscured by the granules)

Specific (secondary) granules

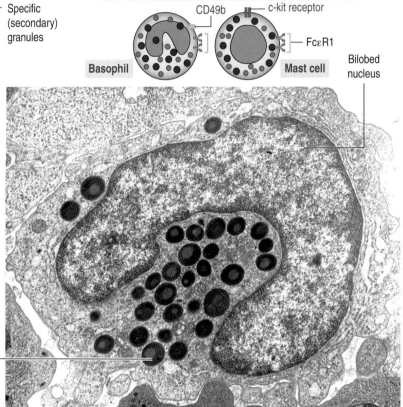

Granular contents of a basophil

Basophils contain large cytoplasmic granules with **sulfated** or **carboxylated acidic proteins** such as heparin. They stain dark blue with the **Wright-Giemsa stain**.

Basophils, similar to **mast cells** in the connective tissue, express on their surface **IgE receptors (FcεR1)** but differ in the expression of **c-kit receptor** and **CD49b**. Both release histamine to mediate allergic reactions when activated by antigen binding.

An increase in the number of basophils (more than 150 basophils/μL) is called basophilia and is observed in acute hypersensitivity reactions, viral infections, and chronic inflammatory conditions, such as rheumatoid arthritis and ulcerative colitis.

Cytoplasmic granules

granules (**lactoferrin, gelatinase, lysozyme** and other **proteases**), specific receptors for **C5a** (produced by the complement system pathway, see Chapter 10, Immune-Lymphatic System), and **L-selectin**, and **integrins** (with binding affinity to endothelial cell ligands such as **intercellular-adhesion molecules 1 and 2 [ICAM-1 and ICAM-2]**) enable the antibacterial and homing function of neutrophils (see Figure 6-9).

2. **Eosinophils** (Figure 6-5). Eosinophils have a characteristic bilobed nucleus. Their cytoplasm is filled with large, refractile granules that stain red in blood smears and tissue sections. The various components of the eosinophil granules and other secretory molecules are listed in Figure 6-5. Eosinophil degranulation occurs in response to cytokines (such as interferon-γ and chemokine ligand 11, CCL11) binding to eosinophil surface receptors. Cytokine **interleukin-5 (IL-5)** is a major regulator of eosinophil function.

Eosinophils constitute **1%** to **5%** of circulating leukocytes and have a half-life of about 18 hours.

Eosinophils leave the circulation, recruited to the connective tissue by IL-5. These cells are the first line of defense against **parasites** and also participate in triggering **bronchial asthma** (see Figure 6-10 and Chapter 13, Respiratory System).

3. **Basophils** (Figure 6-6). These granulocytes contain large, **metachromatic** cytoplasmic granules that often obscure the bilobed nucleus.

Basophils represent only **1%** of circulating leukocytes. Basophils complete their maturation in bone marrow. In contrast, mast cells enter connective tissue or mucosae as immature cells lacking cytoplasmic granules. In addition, basophils and mast cells differ in the presence of c-kit receptor and CD49b but share FcεR1: basophils are c-kit⁻FcεR1⁺ CD49b⁺; mast cells are c-kit⁺FcεR1⁺CD49b⁻.

Basophils have a short lifespan (about 60 hours), whereas mast cells survive for weeks and months. The relationship between basophil and mast cell lineages is further discussed in the Hematopoiesis section of this chapter.

Figure 6-7. **Lymphocyte**

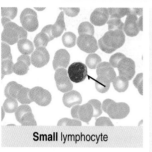

Small lymphocyte

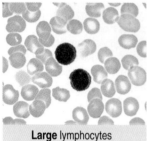

Large lymphocytes

Lymphocytes are relatively abundant, accounting for 20% to 40% of total leukocytes. In circulating blood, lymphocytes may range from approximately 7 to12 μm in diameter. However, the typical lymphocyte in a normal blood smear is small, about the size of a red blood cell.

The nucleus of a **small lymphocyte** is densely stained, with a round or slightly indented shape (*pointer*). The nucleus occupies most of the cell, reducing the cytoplasm to a thin basophilic rim.

Large lymphocytes have a round, slightly indented nucleus surrounded by a pale cytoplasm. Occasionally, a few primary granules (lysosomes) may be present.

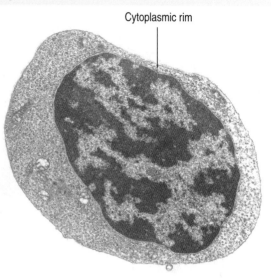

Cytoplasmic rim

Small lymphocytes represent 97% of the population of circulating lymphocytes. Note that the nucleus is surrounded by a thin cytoplasmic rim. **Large lymphocytes** represent 3% of the population of circulating lymphocytes.

Lymphocytes are divided into two categories: **B lymphocytes**, produced in the bone marrow, and **T lymphocytes**, also produced in the bone marrow but that complete their maturation in the thymus.

A less abundant class is the **natural killer cell**.

During fetal development, the **yolk sac**, **liver**, and **spleen** are sites where lymphocytes originate. In postnatal life, the **bone marrow** and **thymus** are the **primary lymphoid organs** where lymphocytes develop before they are exposed to antigens.

Secondary lymphoid organs are the **lymph nodes**, the **spleen**, and lymphoid aggregates of the gastrointestinal and respiratory tracts.

Basophils play a role in immediate (**bronchial asthma**) and type 2 hypersensitivity in response to allergens (**allergic skin reaction**) and parasitic worms (**helminths**).

Figure 6-8. **Monocyte**

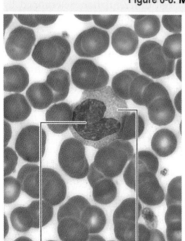

Kidney-shaped nucleus   Small cytoplasmic granules

Monocytes (2% to 8% of total leukocytes) are the largest leukocytes, ranging in size from 15 to 20 μm.

The eccentrically placed nucleus is typically kidney shaped and contains fine strands of chromatin.

The abundant cytoplasm stains pale gray-blue and is filled with small lysosomes that give a fine, granular appearance.

Monocytes travel briefly in the bloodstream and then enter the peripheral tissue where they are transformed into macrophages and survive a longer time.

Macrophage-derived monocytes are more efficient phagocytic cells than neutrophils.

Agranulocytes

Agranulocytes include **lymphocytes** and **monocytes.** Agranulocytes have a round or indented nucleus. They contain only lysosomal-type, **primary granules.**

Lymphocytes are either large (**3%** of lymphocytes; 7 to 12 μm) or small (**97%** of lymphocytes; **6 to 8 μm** (Figure 6-7) cells. In either case, the nucleus is round and may be slightly indented. The cytoplasm is basophilic, often appearing as a thin rim around the nucleus (see Figure 6-7). A few primary granules may be present. Lymphocytes may live for a few days or several years.

Lymphocytes are divided into two categories:

1. **B lymphocytes** (also called **B cells**) are produced and mature in bone marrow. Antigen-stimulated B cells differentiate into antibody-secreting **plasma cells.**

2. **T lymphocytes** (also called **T cells**) are produced in bone marrow but complete their maturation in the **thymus.** Activated T cells participate in **cell-mediated immunity** (for additional details, see Chapter 10, Immune-Lymphatic System).

Monocytes (Figure 6-8) can measure **15 to 20** μm in diameter. Their nucleus is kidney shaped or oval. Cytoplasmic granules are small and may not be resolved on light microscopy.

Figure 6-9. **Homing and inflammation**

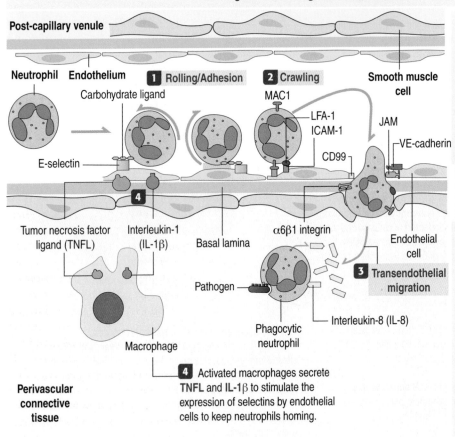

Figure 6-9. Homing and inflammation

1 Rolling and adhesion
Leukocytes (neutrophil in the diagram) establish reversible binding between selectins induced on the endothelial cell surface and carbohydrate ligands on the neutrophil surface. This binding is not strong and the cell keeps rolling.

2 Crawling
A strong interaction occurs between the neutrophil and the endothelial cell. This interaction is mediated in part by intercellular adhesion molecules **ICAM-1** on the endothelium and **LFA-1** (lymphocyte function–associated antigen 1) and **MAC1** (αMβ2 integrin/macrophage antigen 1).

3 Transendothelial migration
Neutrophils migrate across the endothelium along an **IL-8** concentration gradient produced by phagocytic neutrophils. **CD99** contributes to diapedesis by up-regulating laminin-binding α6β1 integrin. Infiltrating neutrophils disrupt the interaction of junctional adhesion molecules (**JAM**) and vascular endothelial cadherins (**VE-cadherin**).

Monocytes circulate in blood for **12 to 100 hours** and then enter the connective tissue. In the connective tissue, monocytes differentiate into macrophages, which are involved in bacterial phagocytosis, antigen presentation, and clean-up of dead cell debris. In bone, monocytes differentiate into **osteoclasts** under the control of osteoblasts (see Chapter 4, Connective Tissue).

Pathology: Leukemias

Leukemias are the most common neoplastic diseases of leukocytes. They are characterized by the neoplastic proliferation of one or more cell lineages in bone marrow, frequent circulation of neoplastic cells in peripheral blood and reduction in the development of normal red blood cells and platelets.

There are acute and chronic leukemias. Acute leukemias consist in the massive proliferation of immature cells with respect to bone marrow cells and rapid progression of the disease.

Acute leukemias are classified as **acute lymphoblastic leukemias** (ALL), when derived from lymphoid cells and **acute myeloblastic leukemias** (AML), when derived from myeloid, erythroid and megakaryocytic cell progenies.

Anemia (caused by a depletion of red blood cell formation), **infections** (determined by a decline in the formation of normal leukocytes) and **bleeding** (a reduction in the number of platelets) are relevant features.

The diagnosis is based on the microscopic examination of bone marrow samples. ALL affects mainly children; AML affects adults.

The **French-American-British (FAB) classification**, includes different types of acute leukemias according to the degree of cell differentiation determined by the cytochemical detection of cell markers: **L1** to **L3** (lymphoid–ALL) and **M1** to **M7** (myeloid–AML).

Chronic leukemias are classified as **lymphocytic**, **myeloid** and **hairy-cell** type leukemias. They are characterized by a lesser proliferation of immature cells and slow progression of the disease.

Chronic lymphocytic leukemia (CLL) is mainly observed in adults (50 years and older). A predominant proliferation of B cells and a large number of abnormal lymphocytes in peripheral blood are predominant features. Lymphoadenopathy and splenomegaly are a common clinical findings.

Chronic myeloid leukemia (CML) is regarded as a myeloproliferative condition (proliferation of abnormal bone marrow stem cells) affecting adults. Patients develop hepatosplenomegaly and leukocytosis (excessive myelocytes, metamyelocytes and neutrophils in peripheral blood). After a chronic phase of about five

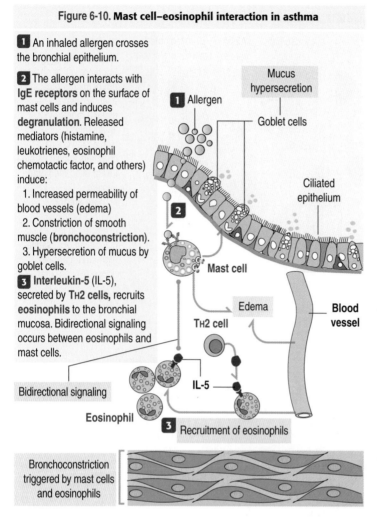

Figure 6-10. Mast cell–eosinophil interaction in asthma

1 An inhaled allergen crosses the bronchial epithelium.

2 The allergen interacts with **IgE receptors** on the surface of mast cells and induces **degranulation**. Released mediators (histamine, leukotrienes, eosinophil chemotactic factor, and others) induce:
  1. Increased permeability of blood vessels (edema)
  2. Constriction of smooth muscle (**bronchoconstriction**).
  3. Hypersecretion of mucus by goblet cells.

3 **Interleukin-5** (IL-5), secreted by TH2 cells, recruits **eosinophils** to the bronchial mucosa. Bidirectional signaling occurs between eosinophils and mast cells.

Bidirectional signaling

Eosinophil

Bronchoconstriction triggered by mast cells and eosinophils

Mucus hypersecretion

1 Allergen

Goblet cells

Ciliated epithelium

2

Mast cell

Edema

TH2 cell

Blood vessel

IL-5

3 Recruitment of eosinophils

---

years, the disease can change into an acute leukemia, requiring stem cell bone marrow transplantation.

Patients with CML usually have the **Philadelphia chromosome**, a reciprocal translocation between the long arms of chromosomes 9 and 22, designated t(9;22)(q34;q11). A fusion gene is created by placing the *abl* gene on chromosome 9 (region q34) to a part of the *bcr* (breakpoint cluster region) gene on chromosome 22 (region q11). The fusion gene (*abl/bcr*) encodes a tyrosine kinase involved in cell transformation leading to a neoplastic phenotype. The drug **imatinib** is a specific tyrosine kinase inhibitor. We come back to imatinib and tyrosine kinases inhibition at the end of this chapter.

Hairy-cell leukemia (HCL) is a rare type of B cell leukemia. The cells look hairy because of multiple thin cytoplasmic projections. Splenomegaly, lymphadenopathy, and recurrent infections are common findings. A relationship between HCL and exposure to the herbicide Agent Orange has been recorded.

General Pathology: Leukocyte recruitment and inflammation

We have studied in Chapter 1, Epithelium, the mo-lecular principles of homing (or leukocyte recruitment). We now expand the concept of leukocyte recruitment by studying the **mechanism of migration of phagocytic neutrophils to the site of infection and inflammation** (Figure 6-9).

Rapid movement of circulating leukocytes across post-capillary venular walls from the bloodstream to the connective tissue in response to injury and infection is essential to the actions of the immune system. Neutrophil recruitment takes place at permissive sites, marked by chemotactic factors released by pathogen-derived endotoxins and guided by host chemokines bound to endothelial cell surfaces.

The **first step** is the binding of carbohydrate ligands on the surface of the neutrophil to endothelial selectins (E selectin). Binding determines rolling and adhesion of the neutrophil to an endothelial cell surface.

The **second step**, crawling and transendothelial migration, demands a stronger interaction of neutrophil with the endothelium. This interaction is mediated by the activation integrins by the neutrophil. **Integrin LFA-1** (also known as αLβ2 integrin or lymphocyte function–associated antigen 1) and **MAC1** (also known as αMβ2 integrin or macrophage antigen 1) interacts with **ICAM-1** on the endothelial cell surface. Note that β2 integrin subunit is common to LFA-1 and MAC1. ICAM-1 is induced by inflammatory cytokines **tumor necrosis factor ligand** and **interleukin-1β** (IL-1β) produced by activated macrophages present at the site of inflammation.

Preparing neutrophils for squeezing between adjacent endothelial cells (paracellular migration) or through endothelial cells (transcellular migration), requires the chemoattractant **interleukin-8**. It is produced by inflammatory cells (for example, neutrophils).

Transendothelial migration, or **diapedesis**, is facilitated by disrupting the interaction of endothelial cell adhesion molecules such as **junctional adhesion molecules (JAMs)**, **vascular endothelial cell cadherin** (**VE-cadherin**) and **CD99**. The up-regulation of α6β1 **integrin** by **CD99**, produced by endothelial cells, facilitates penetration of the vascular basal membrane and the smooth muscle cell layer. After breaching the basement membrane and the smooth muscle cell layer, neutrophil display motility involving membrane protrusions and the rearrangement of the actin cytoskeleton.

In the acute inflammation site, neutrophils migrate in an ameboid fashion that is intrinsic and relatively independent from the inflammation environment. A detailed account of the contribution of neutrophils to acute inflammation is presented in Chapter 10, Immune-Lymphatic System.

Pathology: Leukocyte adhesion deficiency (LAD)

As shown in Figure 6-9, selectin-carbohydrate inter-

Figure 6-11. **Platelets**

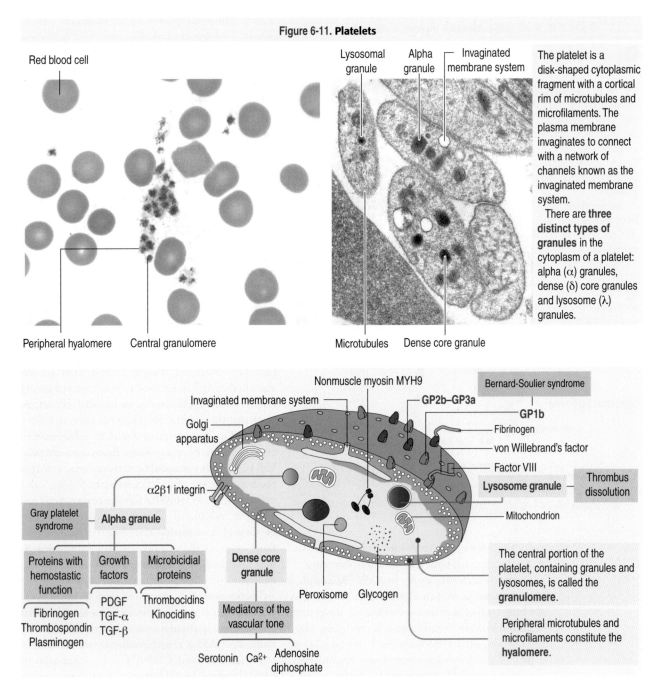

Red blood cell

Lysosomal granule Alpha granule Invaginated membrane system

The platelet is a disk-shaped cytoplasmic fragment with a cortical rim of microtubules and microfilaments. The plasma membrane invaginates to connect with a network of channels known as the invaginated membrane system.

There are **three distinct types of granules** in the cytoplasm of a platelet: alpha (α) granules, dense (δ) core granules and lysosome (λ) granules.

Peripheral hyalomere Central granulomere

Microtubules Dense core granule

Nonmuscle myosin MYH9

Bernard-Soulier syndrome

Invaginated membrane system

GP2b–GP3a

GP1b

Golgi apparatus

Fibrinogen

von Willebrand's factor

Factor VIII

$\alpha2\beta1$ integrin

Lysosome granule — Thrombus dissolution

Gray platelet syndrome **Alpha granule**

Mitochondrion

Proteins with hemostastic function | Growth factors | Microbicidial proteins

Dense core granule

The central portion of the platelet, containing granules and lysosomes, is called the **granulomere.**

Fibrinogen Thrombospondin Plasminogen

PDGF TGF-α TGF-β

Thrombocidins Kinocidins

Mediators of the vascular tone

Peroxisome Glycogen

Peripheral microtubules and microfilaments constitute the **hyalomere.**

Serotonin Ca^{2+} Adenosine diphosphate

actions and integrins (mostly $\beta1$ and $\beta2$ integrins) are required for the transendothelial migration of leukocytes across a venule wall into extravascular areas of inflammation.

Three leukocyte adhesion deficiencies have been described, both characterized by a defect in wound healing, recurrent infections, fever and marked leukocytosis (increase in the number of leukocytes in blood).

Leukocyte adhesion deficiency type I (LAD I) is caused by a defect of the $\beta2$ subunit (also called **CD18**) present in LFA-1 and MAC1 integrins. As a consequence, neutrophils are unable to leave blood vessels because of a defect in the recruitment mecha-

nism. As you recall, LFA-1 and MAC1 are required for binding to endothelial ICAM1, a necessary step for transendothelial migration. In these patients, inflammatory cell infiltrates are devoid of neutrophils. A delay in the separation of the umbilical cord at birth is a classic indication of LAD I.

In leukocyte adhesion deficiency type II (LAD II), the fucosyl-containing ligands for selectins are absent due to a hereditary defect of endogenous fucose metabolism. Individuals with LAD II have reduced intrauterine or postnatal growth and severe mental retardation recognized shortly after birth. LAD III is determined by mutations in **kindlin** (associated with the intracellular domain of β integrin subunit).

Pathology: Mast cell–eosinophil interaction in asthma

We have already seen that mast cells and eosinophils are immigrant cells of the connective tissue. These two cell types have a significant role in the pathogenesis of asthma.

Asthma, a condition in which extrinsic (allergens) or intrinsic (unknown) factors trigger reversible airway obstruction and airway hyperreactivity, provides a good example of mast cell–eosinophil interaction.

Eosinophils are recruited to the bronchial mucosa by cytokine **IL-5** released from activated TH2 cells (a subset of helper T lymphocytes). IL-5 binds to interleukin-5 receptor subunit-α (IL-5Rα) on eosinophils to induce their degranulation.

Two IL-5-specific monoclonal antibodies, mepolizumab and reslizumab, block the binding of IL-5 to IL-5Rα. Initial clinical trials show that these antibodies, administered together with steroids, decrease by 50% the number of eosinophils in the bronchial mucosa and by 0% in sputum. These observations stress the significance of IL-5 in eosinophilic asthma pathogenesis.

There is bidirectional signaling between mast cells and eosinophils in the bronchial mucosa (Figure 6-10).

Mast cells and eosinophils release mediators to enhance mucus hypersecretion (leading to the formation of mucus plugs), edema and bronchoconstriction (determining with time hypertrophy and hyperplasia of the bronchiolar smooth muscle layer). Bronchoconstriction causes airway narrowing and interference of air flow.

Pathology: Eosinophilic esophagitis

Eosinophils are usually found in the gastrointestinal tract, predominantly in the cecum, but seldom in the esophagus. However, esophageal dysfunction, including dysphagia and abdominal pain, correlates with the increase of eosinophils in the esophageal mucosa.

Dysregulated eosinophilia appears to depend on the excessive production of IL-5 and IL-13 by TH2 cells and the presence of the eosinophil chemoattractant chemokine ligand 26 (CCL26) in the inflammatory area of the esophagus.

Fungal and insect allergens appear to trigger eosinophilic esophagitis. The treatment consists in controlling with steroids the inflammatory associated process and blocking IL-5 with the specific monoclonal antibody mepolizumab.

Platelets

Platelets are small (**2 to 4** μm) cytoplasmic discoid fragments derived from the **megakaryocyte** (Figure 6-11) under the control of **thrombopoietin**, a 35- to 70-kd glycoprotein produced in the kidneys and liver.

Megakaryocytes develop cytoplasmic projections that become **proplatelets**, which fragment into platelets. This differentiation process takes 7 to 10 days. **Platelets bind and degrade thrombopoietin, a mechanism that regulates platelet production.**

The plasma membrane is coated by **glycoprotein 1b (GP1b)** and **GP2b-GP3a**, involved in the attachment of platelets to **von Willebrand's factor**. Adhesion of platelets to the vascular endothelium, in turn, is mediated by von Willebrand's factor that also carries **factor VIII** coagulation factor, whereas **fibrinogen** binds to GP2b-GP3a (see Figure 6-11).

The plasma membrane of a platelet invaginates to form a system of **cytoplasmic channels**, called the **invaginated membrane system**, an arrangement that enables the adsorption of clotting factors and also serves as conduits for the release of secretory products stored in granules in thrombin-activated platelets. **Integrin α2β1** is present in the plasma membrane.

The central region of the platelet, the **granulomere**, contains mitochondria, rough endoplasmic reticulum, the Golgi apparatus, and three distinct types of granules:

1. **Alpha (α) granules,** that store proteins involved in hemostatic functions, including **platelet adhesion** (fibrinogen, thrombospondin, vitronectin, laminin and von Willebrand factor), **blood coagulation** (plasminogen and α₂-plasmin inhibitor), **growth factors for endothelial cell repair** (platelet-derived growth factor [PDGF], transforming growth factor-α [TGF-α] and TGF-β) and **microbicidal proteins** (thrombocidins and kinocidins).

2. **Dense (δ) core granules**, containing mediators of vascular tone (serotonin, adenosine diphosphate [ADP] and phosphate).

3. **Lysosomal (λ) granules**, containing hydrolytic enzymes participating in the dissolution of thrombi.

The periphery of the platelet, the **hyalomere**, contains microtubules and microfilaments that regulate platelet shape change, motility toward the sites of injury and infection and release of granule contents.

We indicate that alpha granules contain microbicidal proteins. Platelets can interact with microbial

---

Box 6-D | Hemophilia

- **Hemophilia** is a common hereditary disease associated with serious bleeding due to an inherited deficiency of **factor VIII** or **factor IX**.
- The genes for these blood coagulation factors lie on the X chromosome, and when mutated, they cause the X-linked recessive traits of **hemophilia A** and **B**. Hemophilia affects males, with females as carriers.
- A reduction in the amount or activity of **factor VIII**, a protein synthesized in the liver, causes **hemophilia A**. A deficiency in **factor IX** determines **hemophilia B**.
- Major trauma or surgery can determine severe bleeding in all hemophiliacs and, therefore, a correct diagnosis is critical. Plasma-derived or genetically engineered recombinant factors are available for the treatment of patients with hemophilia.
- **von Willebrand's disease**, the most frequent bleeding disorder, is also hereditary and related to a deficient or abnormal **von Willebrand's factor**.

Figure 6-12. Blood clotting or hemostasis

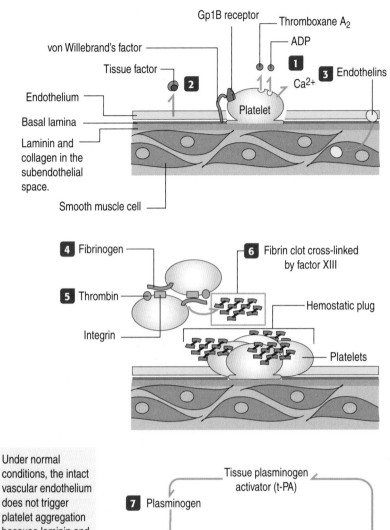

Phase I: Adhesion of platelets to the subendothelium of an injured blood vessel

1 **Activated platelets** release: adenosine diphosphate (**ADP**), to attract other platelets to the site of injury, **thromboxane A₂**, to cause vasoconstriction and platelet aggregation, and **Ca²⁺**, to participate in clotting.

2 **Endothelial cells** release **tissue factor**, which binds to factor VIIa to convert factor X into factor Xa and initiate the common pathway of blood clotting. Von Willebrand's factor binds to **glycoprotein 1B (Gp1B) platelet receptor** to facilitate the attachment of platelets to collagen and laminin in the subendothelial space.

3 **Endothelins**, peptide hormones secreted by endothelial cells, stimulate smooth muscle contraction and proliferation of endothelial cells and fibroblasts to accelerate the repair process.

Phase II: Aggregation of platelets to form a hemostatic plug

4 **Fibrinogen** in plasma binds to activated integrin receptors, and platelets are bridged to each other.

5 **Thrombin**, bound to its receptor on the platelet surface, acts on **fibrinogen** to cleave fibrinopeptides and form a fibrin monomer.

6 **Fibrin monomers** aggregate to form a soft fibrin clot. **Factor XIII** cross-links fibrin monomers. Platelets and fibrin form a hemostatic plug.

Phase III: Platelet procoagulation activity terminates with the removal of the fibrin clot

7 **Plasminogen** (a plasma protein) is converted to **plasmin** (a protease) by **tissue plasminogen activator** (produced by injured endothelial cells and subendothelial connective tissue).

8 **Plasmin** dissolves the fibrin clot.

Under normal conditions, the intact vascular endothelium does not trigger platelet aggregation because laminin and collagen are not exposed.

Endothelial cells secrete prostacyclin, a potent inhibitor of platelet aggregation and secretion of ADP.

---

pathogens and play a significant role in host defense against infection mediated by **thrombocidins**, released from platelets by thrombin stimulation, and chemokine-like **kinocidins**, known to recruit leukocytes to sites of infection.

As you can see, platelets link hemostasis with inflammation and immunity by sensing tissue injury or infection and releasing antimicrobial and wound-healing proteins. Note that the key activators of platelets are signals released from the site of injury or infection.

Platelet host defense functions emphasize the value of platelet transfusion when confronting infection

and sepsis. In fact, morbidity and mortality due to *Staphylococcus aureus* correlate with inherited platelet disorders, including Gray platelet syndrome, and with thrombocytopenia (see below).

Pathology: Platelets and coagulation disorders

About **300,000** platelets per microliter of blood circulate for **8** to **10** days. Platelets promote blood clotting and help to prevent blood loss from damaged vessels.

Purpura (Latin *purpura*, purple) designates a color patch or spot on the skin caused by bleeding. Spots less than 3 mm in diameter are called **petechiae**; spots larger than 1 cm in diameter are called **ecchymoses**.

Figure 6-13. **Phases of blood clotting**

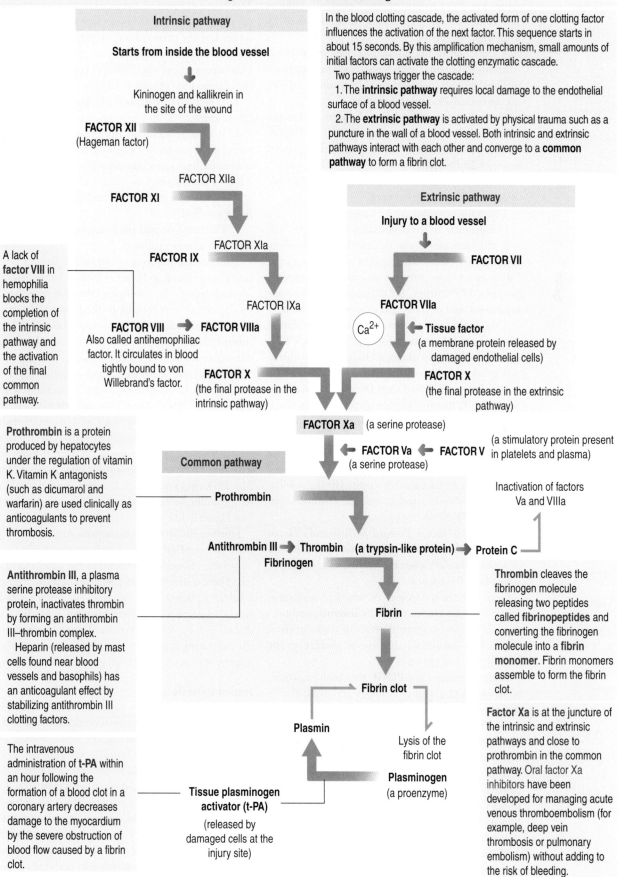

Intrinsic pathway

Starts from inside the blood vessel

Kininogen and kallikrein in the site of the wound

FACTOR XII (Hageman factor)

FACTOR XIIa

FACTOR XI

FACTOR XIa

FACTOR IX

FACTOR IXa

FACTOR VIII → **FACTOR VIIIa**
Also called antihemophiliac factor. It circulates in blood tightly bound to von Willebrand's factor.

FACTOR X (the final protease in the intrinsic pathway)

A lack of **factor VIII** in hemophilia blocks the completion of the intrinsic pathway and the activation of the final common pathway.

In the blood clotting cascade, the activated form of one clotting factor influences the activation of the next factor. This sequence starts in about 15 seconds. By this amplification mechanism, small amounts of initial factors can activate the clotting enzymatic cascade.

Two pathways trigger the cascade:

1. The **intrinsic pathway** requires local damage to the endothelial surface of a blood vessel.

2. The **extrinsic pathway** is activated by physical trauma such as a puncture in the wall of a blood vessel. Both intrinsic and extrinsic pathways interact with each other and converge to a **common pathway** to form a fibrin clot.

Extrinsic pathway

Injury to a blood vessel

FACTOR VII

FACTOR VIIa

Ca^{2+}

Tissue factor (a membrane protein released by damaged endothelial cells)

FACTOR X (the final protease in the extrinsic pathway)

FACTOR Xa (a serine protease)

FACTOR Va ← **FACTOR V** (a stimulatory protein present in platelets and plasma)
(a serine protease)

Common pathway

Prothrombin

Prothrombin is a protein produced by hepatocytes under the regulation of vitamin K. Vitamin K antagonists (such as dicumarol and warfarin) are used clinically as anticoagulants to prevent thrombosis.

Antithrombin III → Thrombin (a trypsin-like protein) → Protein C
Fibrinogen

Inactivation of factors Va and VIIIa

Antithrombin III, a plasma serine protease inhibitory protein, inactivates thrombin by forming an antithrombin III–thrombin complex.

Heparin (released by mast cells found near blood vessels and basophils) has an anticoagulant effect by stabilizing antithrombin III clotting factors.

Fibrin

Thrombin cleaves the fibrinogen molecule releasing two peptides called **fibrinopeptides** and converting the fibrinogen molecule into a **fibrin monomer**. Fibrin monomers assemble to form the fibrin clot.

Fibrin clot

Plasmin

Lysis of the fibrin clot

Plasminogen (a proenzyme)

The intravenous administration of **t-PA** within an hour following the formation of a blood clot in a coronary artery decreases damage to the myocardium by the severe obstruction of blood flow caused by a fibrin clot.

Tissue plasminogen activator (t-PA) (released by damaged cells at the injury site)

Factor Xa is at the juncture of the intrinsic and extrinsic pathways and close to prothrombin in the common pathway. Oral factor Xa inhibitors have been developed for managing acute venous thromboembolism (for example, deep vein thrombosis or pulmonary embolism) without adding to the risk of bleeding.

Widespread and symmetrical petechiae and ecchymoses are characteristic of the **Henoch–Schönlein syndrome**, an allergic purpura reaction caused by drug hypersensitivity.

A reduction in the number of platelets in blood (**thrombocytopenia**) leads to increased susceptibility to bleeding and increased morbidity and mortality due to bacterial or fungal infection.

Thrombocytopenia is defined by a decrease in the number of platelets to less than 150,000/μL of blood. **Spontaneous bleeding** is observed with a platelet count of 20,000/μL.

Thrombocytosis defines an increase in the number of platelets circulating in blood.

Thrombocytopenia can be caused by:

1. A **decrease in the production of platelets**.

2. An **increase in the destruction of platelets**, determined by **antibodies** against platelets or megakaryocyte antigens (**autoimmune thrombocytopenic purpura, ITP**), **drugs**, for example, penicillin, sulfonamides, and digoxin, and **cancer chemotherapy**.

3. **Aggregation of platelets in the microvasculature** (**thrombotic thrombocytopenic purpura, TTP**), probably a result of pathologic changes in endothelial cells producing procoagulant substances.

Deficiency of GP1b–**factor IX** complex, or of **von Willebrand's factor**, a protein associated with factor VIII, leads to two congenital bleeding disorders, **Bernard-Soulier syndrome** and **von Willebrand's disease**, respectively (see Figures 6-11 to 6-13; see Box 6-D).

These two diseases are characterized by the inability of giant platelets to attach to vascular subendothelial surfaces.

The **GP1b–factor IX–von Willebrand's factor complex is relevant for the aggregation and adhesion of normal platelets when they are exposed to injured subendothelial tissues.**

Gray platelet syndrome, an inherited autosomal recessive disease characterized by **macrothrombocytopenia** (thrombocytopenia with increased platelet volume), is due to a reduction or absence in the content of alpha granules.

Alpha granules store **PDGF** that enables platelet adhesiveness and wound healing when secreted during an injury. Platelets have a gray appearance.

MYH9 (myosin heavy chain 9)-related disorders are also associated with macrothrombocytopenia. A defect in the *MYH9* gene, which encodes nonmuscle myosin heavy chain IIA (an isoform expressed in platelets and neutrophils). Defective *MYH9* determines the premature initiation of proplatelet formation within the bone marrow, producing fewer and shorter proplatelets.

We discuss later in this chapter the mechanism of megakaryocyte development and platelet formation.

Pathology: Hemostasis and blood clotting

The blood clotting or coagulation cascade depends on the sequential activation of proenzymes to enzymes and the participation of endothelial cells and platelets to achieve **hemostasis** or arrest of bleeding. Hemostasis occurs when fibrin is formed to reinforce the platelet plug (Figure 6-12).

The blood clotting cascade has the following characteristics:

1. It is dependent on the presence of inactive precursor proteases (for example, factor XII) that are converted into active enzymes (for example, factor XIIa) by proteolysis.

2. It is composed of intrinsic and extrinsic pathways (see Figure 6-13).

3. The extrinsic and intrinsic pathways converge into the common pathway.

The **extrinsic pathway** is triggered by damage outside a blood vessel and is set in motion by the release of tissue factor. The **intrinsic pathway** is stimulated by damage to components of the blood and blood vessel wall. It is induced by contact of factor XII to subendothelial collagen. This contact results from damage to the wall of a blood vessel.

Extrinsic and intrinsic pathways converge to a crucial step in which **fibrinogen is converted to fibrin**, which forms mesh that enables platelets to attach. The convergence starts with the activation of factor X to factor Xa, together with activated factor Va, resulting in the cleavage of **prothrombin** to **thrombin**. The initial hemostatic plug consists of a platelet scaffold for the conversion of prothrombin to thrombin, which changes fibrinogen into fibrin (see Figure 6-12).

Fibrinogen, produced by hepatocytes, consists of three polypeptide chains, which contain numerous negatively charged amino acids in the amino terminal. These characteristics allow fibrinogen to remain soluble in plasma. After cleavage, the newly formed **fibrin** molecules aggregate forming a mesh. We discuss in Chapter 10, Immune-Lymphatic System, the facilitating function of a fibrin meshwork to the migration of neutrophils during acute inflammation.

Hematopoiesis
Hematopoietic niches

In the **fetus**, hematopoiesis (Greek *haima,* blood; *poiein,* to make) starts during the first trimester in islands of hematopoiesis found in the **yolk sac**. The islands develop from **hemangioblasts**, the progenitors of both hematopoietic and endothelial cells.

Fetal hematopoiesis continues after the second trimester in the **liver** and then in the **spleen**. During the seventh month of intrauterine life, the **bone marrow** becomes the primary site of hematopoiesis, where it remains during adulthood. In the adult, an

Figure 6-14. Bone marrow: Structure and vascularization

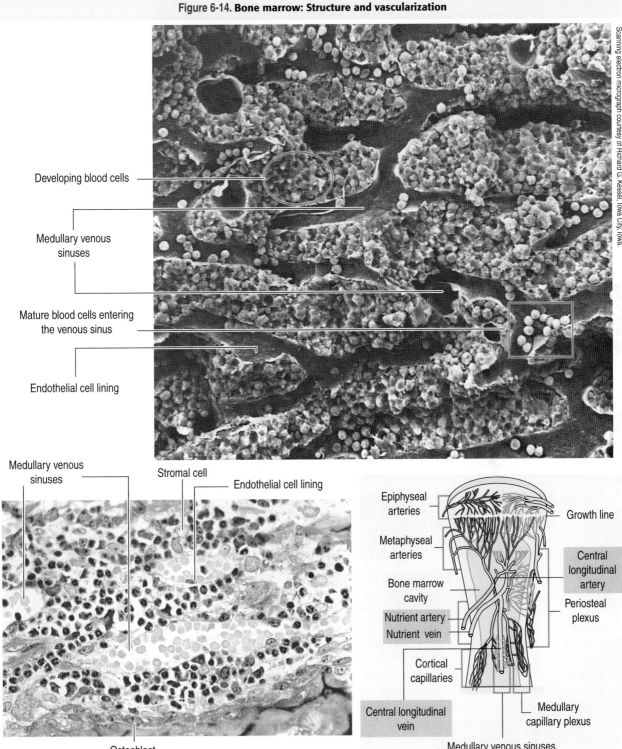

Developing blood cells

Medullary venous sinuses

Mature blood cells entering the venous sinus

Endothelial cell lining

Medullary venous sinuses

Stromal cell

Endothelial cell lining

Osteoblast

Epiphyseal arteries

Growth line

Metaphyseal arteries

Central longitudinal artery

Bone marrow cavity

Periosteal plexus

Nutrient artery

Nutrient vein

Cortical capillaries

Medullary capillary plexus

Central longitudinal vein

Medullary venous sinuses

The bone marrow can be **red** because of the presence of erythroid progenies, or **yellow**, because of adipose cells. Red and yellow marrow may be interchangeable in relation to the demands for hematopoiesis. In the adult, red bone marrow is found in the skull, clavicles, vertebrae, ribs, sternum, pelvis, and ends of the long bones of the limbs.

Blood vessels and nerves reach the bone marrow by piercing the bony shell. The **nutrient artery** enters the midshaft of a long bone and branches into the **central longitudinal artery**, which

gives rise to a **medullary capillary plexus** continuous with the **medullary venous sinuses** and connected to cortical capillaries. Cortical capillaries and medullary capillaries extend into Volkmann's canals and haversian canals.

The venous sinuses empty into the **central longitudinal vein**. Periosteal blood vessels give rise to periosteal plexuses connected to medullary capillaries and medullary venous sinuses.

Figure 6-15. Bone marrow: Structure

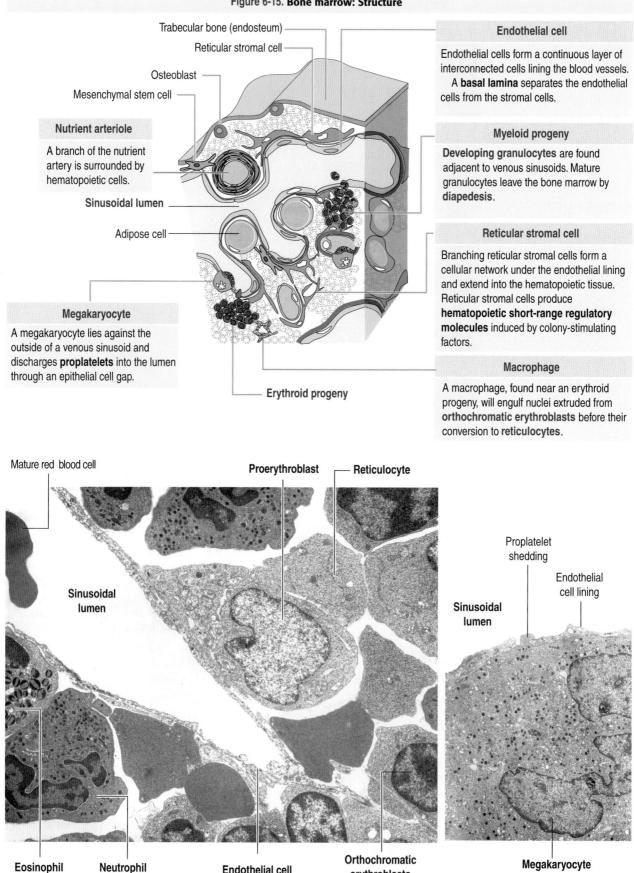

Trabecular bone (endosteum)

Reticular stromal cell

Osteoblast

Mesenchymal stem cell

Nutrient arteriole

A branch of the nutrient artery is surrounded by hematopoietic cells.

Sinusoidal lumen

Adipose cell

Megakaryocyte

A megakaryocyte lies against the outside of a venous sinusoid and discharges **proplatelets** into the lumen through an epithelial cell gap.

Erythroid progeny

Endothelial cell

Endothelial cells form a continuous layer of interconnected cells lining the blood vessels. A **basal lamina** separates the endothelial cells from the stromal cells.

Myeloid progeny

Developing granulocytes are found adjacent to venous sinusoids. Mature granulocytes leave the bone marrow by **diapedesis**.

Reticular stromal cell

Branching reticular stromal cells form a cellular network under the endothelial lining and extend into the hematopoietic tissue. Reticular stromal cells produce **hematopoietic short-range regulatory molecules** induced by colony-stimulating factors.

Macrophage

A macrophage, found near an erythroid progeny, will engulf nuclei extruded from **orthochromatic erythroblasts** before their conversion to **reticulocytes**.

Mature red blood cell

Proerythroblast   **Reticulocyte**

Sinusoidal lumen

Proplatelet shedding

Endothelial cell lining

Sinusoidal lumen

Eosinophil   Neutrophil   Endothelial cell   Orthochromatic erythroblasts   Megakaryocyte

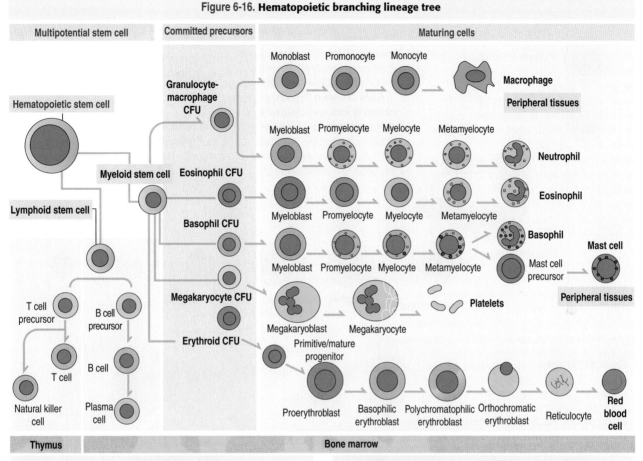

Figure 6-16. Hematopoietic branching lineage tree

The bone marrow consists of: (1) **Hematopoietic stem cells (HSCs)**, multipotential cells capable of self-renewal. (2) **Committed precursor cells** (myeloid stem cell and lymphoid stem cell). (3) **Maturing cells**. Maturing cells develop from cells called **colony-forming units (CFUs)**. The myeloid stem cell gives rise to CFUs responsible for the regeneration of red blood cells (**erythroid CFUs**), platelets (**megakaryocyte CFUs**),

basophils and mast cells (**basophil CFUs**), and eosinophils (**eosinophil CFUs**). Monocytes and neutrophils derive from a common committed progenitor cell (**granulocyte-macrophage CFU**). The **lymphoid stem cell** generates the **B cell** progeny in the **bone marrow** and **T cell** progenies in the **thymus**. They are discussed in detail in Chapter 10, Immune-Lymphatic System.

approximate volume of 1.7 L of marrow contains 10^{12} hematopoietic cells, producing about 1×10^9 RBCs and about 1×10^8 leukocytes every hour.

The bone marrow consists of two microenvironmental domains, called **niches**:

1. The **vascular niche**.

2. The **endosteal niche**.

Niches provide physical support, soluble factors, and cell-mediated interactions to regulate cell self-renewal, differentiation and quiescence of hematopoietic stem cells (HSCs).

Under normal conditions, niches enable the balanced, or homeostatic, cell self-renewal and differentiation of HSCs. Under pathologic conditions, such as **myelodysplasia**, **aging** or **bone marrow malignancies**, niches can alter or restrain normal hematopoiesis.

The vascular niche

The **vascular niche** consists of **blood vessels** sur-

rounded by a distinct population of non-hematopoietic stromal cells, including **mesenchymal stem cells, adipose cells, endothelial cells, reticular stromal cells, and macrophages** (Figures 6-14 to 6-16).

The cytokines secreted by these cells can regulate HSCs. The perivascular space contains extracellular matrix proteins, such as type IV collagen, fibronectin, fibrinogen and von Willebrand factor, that in conjunction with cytokines, regulate the HSC population.

The vascular niche provides a microenvironment for the short-term proliferation and differentiation of HSCs. As discussed in Chapter 10, Immune-Lymphatic System, progenitors of B cells develop in **immune cell niches**, with the participation of osteoblasts, CAR cells (see below), reticular stromal cells and sinusoidal endothelial cells.

The bone marrow is highly vascularized. It is supplied by the **central longitudinal artery**, derived from the **nutrient artery**. **Medullary capillary plexuses**

Figure 6-17. Erythroid lineage

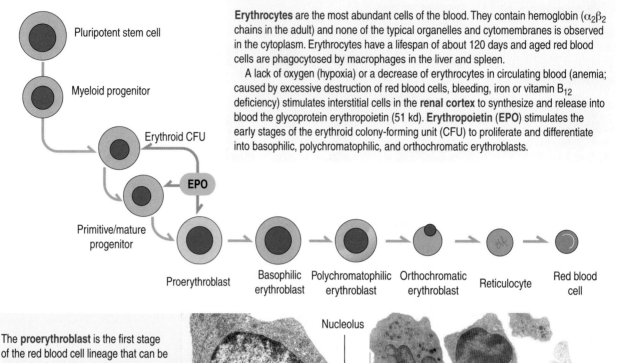

Pluripotent stem cell

Myeloid progenitor

Erythroid CFU

EPO

Primitive/mature progenitor

Proerythroblast

Basophilic erythroblast

Polychromatophilic erythroblast

Orthochromatic erythroblast

Reticulocyte

Red blood cell

Erythrocytes are the most abundant cells of the blood. They contain hemoglobin ($\alpha_2\beta_2$ chains in the adult) and none of the typical organelles and cytomembranes is observed in the cytoplasm. Erythrocytes have a lifespan of about 120 days and aged red blood cells are phagocytosed by macrophages in the liver and spleen.

A lack of oxygen (hypoxia) or a decrease of erythrocytes in circulating blood (anemia; caused by excessive destruction of red blood cells, bleeding, iron or vitamin B_{12} deficiency) stimulates interstitial cells in the **renal cortex** to synthesize and release into blood the glycoprotein erythropoietin (51 kd). **Erythropoietin (EPO)** stimulates the early stages of the erythroid colony-forming unit (CFU) to proliferate and differentiate into basophilic, polychromatophilic, and orthochromatic erythroblasts.

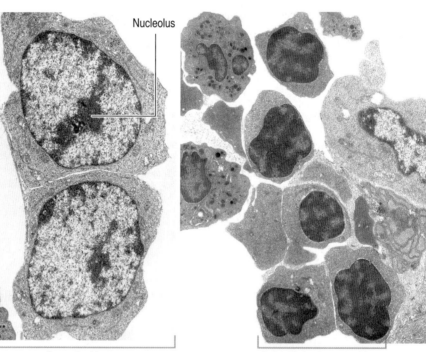

Nucleolus

The **proerythroblast** is the first stage of the red blood cell lineage that can be recognized. It derives from a mature progenitor following stimulation with **erythropoietin**. **Nucleoli are present**. The cytoplasm contains abundant free polyribosomes involved in the synthesis of **hemoglobin**.

The synthesis of hemoglobin proceeds into **basophilic**, **polychromatophilic**, and **orthochromatophilic erythroblasts**.

As hemoglobin accumulates in the cytoplasm, the nucleus of the differentiating erythroblasts is reduced in size, chromatin condenses, and free ribosomes decrease. The orthochromatophilic erythroblast displays maximum chromatin condensation.

Proerythroblasts

Orthochromatic erythroblasts

and **periosteal capillary plexuses** are interconnected. **Medullary sinusoids** drain into the **central longitudinal vein** before leaving through the **nutrient vein** (see Figure 6-14).

Mature hematopoietic cells translocate through the sinusoid wall by active **transendothelial migration,** into the sinuses (see Figure 6-15) before entering the circulation through the central vein. Immature hematopoietic cells lack the capacity of transendothelial migration and are retained in the extravascular space by the endothelial cells.

The sinusoids of the marrow are lined by special-ized **endothelial cells** with significant phagocytic activity and a capacity to produce growth factors that stimulate the proliferation and differentiation of hematopoietic cells.

Marrow **reticular stromal cells** produce hematopoietic growth factors and cytokines that regulate the production and differentiation of blood cells.

Adipose cells provide a local source of energy as well as synthesize growth factors. The population of adipose cells increases with age and obesity and following chemotherapy. Adipose cells exert a **negative** regulatory effect on HSCs function.

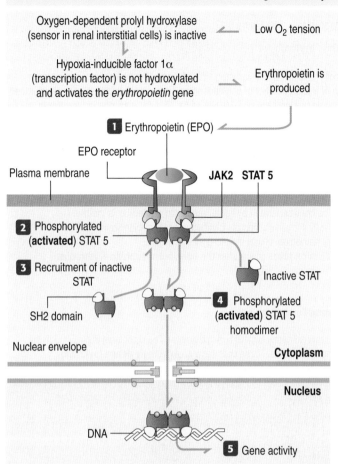

Figure 6-18. Erythropoietin

Oxygen-dependent prolyl hydroxylase (sensor in renal interstitial cells) is inactive ← Low O₂ tension

Hypoxia-inducible factor 1α (transcription factor) is not hydroxylated and activates the *erythropoietin* gene → Erythropoietin is produced

1 Erythropoietin (EPO)

EPO receptor

Plasma membrane

JAK2   STAT 5

2 Phosphorylated (**activated**) STAT 5

3 Recruitment of inactive STAT

SH2 domain

Inactive STAT

4 Phosphorylated (**activated**) STAT 5 homodimer

Nuclear envelope

Cytoplasm

Nucleus

DNA

5 Gene activity

Erythropoietin and the JAK-STAT signaling pathway

1 Erythropoietin (**EPO**), produced by interstitial cells in the renal cortex, is transported to the bone marrow by the blood circulation.

2 In the bone marrow, EPO binds to the **dimerized erythropoietin receptor**, present in early stages of the **erythroid CFU progeny**, and induces binding of cytosolic **STAT 5** (**s**ignal **t**ransducers and **a**ctivators of **t**ranscription 5) protein to **JAK2** (**Ja**nus **k**inase 2), a tyrosine kinase bound to the intracellular domain of the receptor.

3 The inactive (nonphosphorylated) form of STAT 5 contains an **SH2** (**S**rc **h**omology 2) domain. STAT 5 is recruited by JAK2 and binds to it through the SH2 domain. STAT 5 becomes phosphorylated and homodimerizes.

4 The phosphorylated STAT 5 homodimer translocates into the nucleus.

5 After binding to DNA, the phosphorylated STAT 5 homodimer activates the transcription of specific genes required for erythropoiesis.

Marrow **macrophages** remove apoptotic cells, residual nuclei from orthochromatic erythroblasts and megakaryocytes, and exclude particles from entering the marrow.

The endosteal niche

The **endosteal niche**, located at the endosteum–bone marrow interface, consists of preosteoblasts (osteoprogenitor cells), osteoblasts and osteoclasts interacting with HSCs. Type I collagen is the most abundant extracellular component of the endosteal niche.

The endosteal niche is regarded as a site for long-term storage of quiescent HSCs.

Osteoblasts produce multiple hematopoietic cytokines, including **G-CSF** (granulocyte-colony stimulating factor), **M-CSF** (macrophage-colony stimulating factor}, **GM-CSF** (granulocyte-macrophage-colony stimulating factor), **IL-1**, **IL-6**, and **IL-7**. Osteoblasts produce **CXC-chemokine ligand 12** (**CXCL12**) with binding affinity to **CXCR4** (for chemokine receptor type 4). Perivascular reticular stromal cells, called **CAR cells** (for CXCL12-abundant cells) are a major source of CXCL12. The CXCL12-CXCR4 complex is a regulator of the

migration and localization of HSCs in bone marrow. CAR cells, a subpopulation of mesenchymal stem cells, are closely associated with HSCs.

Osteoblasts also express angiopoietin-1, a positive regulator of HSCs, and thrombopoietin (also synthesized in liver and kidney) and osteopontin, that promote HSCs quiescence by stimulating osteoblasts to produce integrins and cadherins to enhance attachment of HSCs to the endosteal surface.

Hematopoietic cell populations

The bone marrow consists of three major populations (see Figure 6-16):

1. **HSCs**, capable of **self-renewal**.
2. **Committed precursor cells**, responsible for the generation of distinct cell lineages.
3. **Maturing cells**, resulting from the differentiation of the committed precursor cell population.

HSCs can self-renew and produce two committed precursor cells that develop into distinct cell progenies:

1. The **myeloid stem cell**.
2. The **lymphoid stem cell**.

Self-renewal is an important property of HSCs. Self-renewal preserves the pool of stem cells and is

Figure 6-19. **Erythroid lineage**

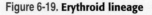

Basophilic cytoplasm

Nucleolus absent

Proerythroblast   See Figure 6-17.

Basophilic erythroblast

A large cell (12 to 16 μm in diameter) with intensely basophilic cytoplasm as an indication of a large number of polyribosomes. The nucleus contains coarsely clumped chromatin and **nucleoli are not usually seen. This cell can divide by mitosis.** Basophilic erythroblasts derive from the proerythroblast.

Hemoglobin

Polyribosomes
Nucleolus absent

Polychromatophilic erythroblasts

These cells may range in diameter from 9 to 15 μm. The nucleus exhibits dense chromatin patches separated by lighter areas. **No nucleolus is visible.** The cytoplasm may contain clumps of polyribosomes (light-blue staining) involved in the synthesis of hemoglobin (light pink-to-gray staining).
No cell division takes place after the polychromatophilic erythroblast.

Hemoglobin (pink staining predominates)

Gradual reduction in cell diameter and increasing nuclear condensation

Eccentric pyknotic nucleus

Orthochromatic erythroblast

This cell is approximately 8 to 10 μm in diameter. The cytoplasm is pink, much the same as the reticulocyte. These cells have an **extremely dense (pyknotic), eccentrically located nucleus. Orthochromatic erythroblasts are postmitotic.**
The transition to reticulocyte is preceded by the extrusion of the condensed nucleus that carries with it a rim of cytoplasm. The extruded nucleus is engulfed by a macrophage.

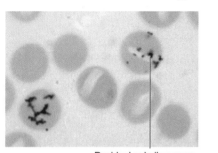

Residual polyribosomes

Reticulocyte

These **anucleated cells** measure approximately 7 to 8 μm in diameter. The cytoplasm is pink like the orthochromatic erythroblast. In regular preparations, these cells appear identical to mature erythrocytes. With **supravital stains**, such as **methylene blue** or **cresyl blue**, a filamentous (reticular) network of polyribosomes becomes visible.
Reticulocytes remain in the bone marrow for 1 or 2 days and then are released into the peripheral blood. Following 1 day of circulation, reticulocytes mature into erythrocytes.

critical for feeding common myeloid progenitor and common lymphoid progenitor into the differentiation or maturation pathway.

HSCs are difficult to identify, mainly because they represent approximately 0.05% of total hematopoietic cells (about 10^6 to 10^7 stem cells). In bone marrow transplantation, only 5% of the normal hematopoietic stem cells are needed to repopulate the entire bone marrow.

HSCs cannot be identified by morphology; they can be recognized by specific cell surface markers (c-kit receptor and Thy-1). Instead, CD34$^+$ committed precursor cell populations, also containing CD34$^-$ HSCs, are generally used for transplantation in the clinical treatment of malignant diseases with chemotherapeutic agents that deplete a certain group of committed precursor cells.

Myeloid and lymphoid stem cells are multipotential cells (see Figure 6-16). They are committed to the formation of cells of the blood and lymphoid organs.

Five **colony-forming units (CFUs)** derive from the myeloid stem cell:

1. The **erythroid CFU**, that produces **red blood cells.**

2. The **megakaryocyte CFU**, that generates **platelets.**

3. The **granulocyte-macrophage CFU**, that produces **monocytes** and **neutrophils.**

4. The **eosinophil CFU.**

5. The **basophil CFU**, that in addition to basophils, produces non-granulated **mast cell precursors** that become granulated mast cells when recruited

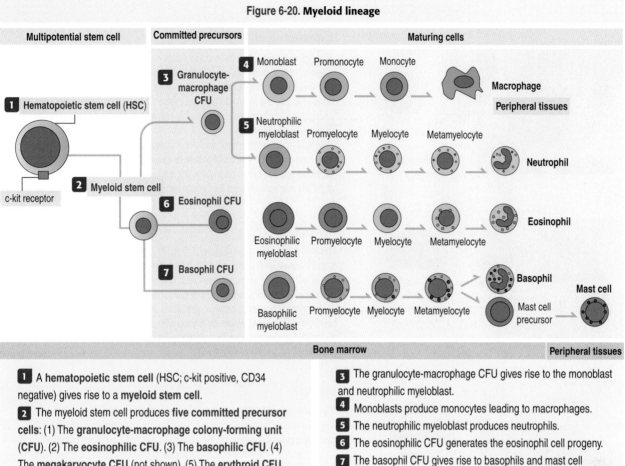

Figure 6-20. Myeloid lineage

Multipotential stem cell	Committed precursors	Maturing cells

1 Hematopoietic stem cell (HSC)

c-kit receptor

2 Myeloid stem cell

3 Granulocyte-macrophage CFU

4 Monoblast — Promonocyte — Monocyte — Macrophage

Peripheral tissues

5 Neutrophilic myeloblast — Promyelocyte — Myelocyte — Metamyelocyte — Neutrophil

6 Eosinophil CFU

Eosinophilic myeloblast — Promyelocyte — Myelocyte — Metamyelocyte — Eosinophil

7 Basophil CFU

Basophilic myeloblast — Promyelocyte — Myelocyte — Metamyelocyte — Basophil / Mast cell precursor — Mast cell

Bone marrow | Peripheral tissues

1 A **hematopoietic stem cell** (HSC; c-kit positive, CD34 negative) gives rise to a **myeloid stem cell**.

2 The myeloid stem cell produces **five committed precursor cells**: (1) The **granulocyte-macrophage colony-forming unit (CFU)**. (2) The **eosinophilic CFU**. (3) The **basophilic CFU**. (4) The **megakaryocyte CFU** (not shown). (5) The **erythroid CFU** (not shown).

3 The granulocyte-macrophage CFU gives rise to the monoblast and neutrophilic myeloblast.

4 Monoblasts produce monocytes leading to macrophages.

5 The neutrophilic myeloblast produces neutrophils.

6 The eosinophilic CFU generates the eosinophil cell progeny.

7 The basophil CFU gives rise to basophils and mast cell precursors. Mast cells mature (granulate) in peripheral tissues.

to connective tissue and mucosae (see Chapter 4, Connective Tissue).

The **lymphoid stem cell** derives from the hematopoietic stem cell and gives rise to T cell and B cell precursors. We study the development and maturation of T cells and B cells in Chapter 10, Immune-Lymphatic System.

Clinical significance: Hematopoietic growth factors
Hematopoietic growth factors control the proliferative and maturational phases of hematopoiesis. In addition, they can extend the life span and function of a number of cells produced in the bone marrow. Several recombinant forms are available for clinical treatment of blood disorders.

Hematopoietic growth factors, also known as **hematopoietic cytokines**, are glycoproteins produced in the bone marrow by endothelial cells, stromal cells, fibroblasts, developing lymphocytes, and macrophages. Hematopoietic growth factors are also produced outside the bone marrow.

There are three major groups of hematopoietic growth factors:

1. **Colony-stimulating factors.**

2. **Erythropoietin** (Figure 6-17) and **thrombopoietin** (Greek *thrombos*, clot; *poietin*, to make).

3. **Cytokines** (primarily **interleukins**).

Colony-stimulating factors are so named because they are able to stimulate committed precursor cells to grow in vitro into cell clusters or colonies. Interleukins are produced by leukocytes (mainly lymphocytes) and affect other leukocytes (paracrine mechanism) or themselves (autocrine mechanism).

Hematopoietic cells express distinct patterns of **growth factor receptors** as they differentiate. Binding of the ligand to the receptor leads to a conformational change, activation of intracellular kinases, and the final induction of cell proliferation (see Chapter 3, Cell Signaling).

We discuss the roles of specific hematopoietic growth factors when we analyze each cell lineage.

Erythroid lineage
Erythropoiesis includes the following sequence (see Figure 6-17): **proerythroblast, basophilic erythroblast, polychromatophilic erythroblast, orthochromatic erythroblast, reticulocyte,** and **erythrocyte.**

The major regulator of erythropoiesis is **erythropoi-**

Figure 6-21. **Myeloid lineage**

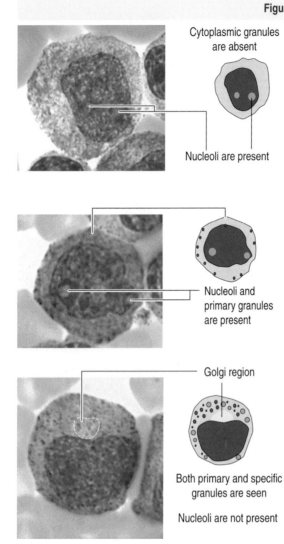

Cytoplasmic granules
are absent

Nucleoli are present

Nucleoli and
primary granules
are present

Golgi region

Both primary and specific
granules are seen

Nucleoli are not present

Golgi region

Myeloblast

Throughout the granulocytic differentiation process (the neutrophilic series is shown), major changes occur in the structure of the nucleus and the content of the cytoplasm. For example, in the myeloblast (10 to 20 μm; a cell usually difficult to identify in Wright-stained preparations), the nucleus is round with uncondensed chromatin and a visible nucleolus. As the cell progresses through the subsequent stages of differentiation, the nucleus becomes indented, then segmented, and the chromatin increases its condensation. **The cytoplasm of the myeloblast is essentially granule-free.** Primary granules appear in the promyelocyte stage, while specific or secondary granules are synthesized by myelocytes.

Promyelocyte

This cell measures approximately 15 to 20 μm in diameter. It has a large, round nucleus with uncondensed chromatin and one or more oval nucleoli. **The synthesis of primary granules, stained red or magenta, occurs exclusively at this stage.** The cytoplasm is basophilic due to the presence of abundant rough endoplasmic reticulum. **Promyelocytes give rise to neutrophilic, eosinophilic, or basophilic myelocytes.** It is not possible in conventional preparations to determine which type of granulocyte will be produced by a given promyelocyte.

Myelocyte

This cell, measuring 12 to 18 μm, has a round or oval nucleus that may be slightly indented; nucleoli are not present. **The basophilic cytoplasm contains primary granules produced in the promyelocyte stage as well as some specific granules, whose synthesis is detected in the myelocyte.** Consequently, the myelocyte cytoplasm begins to resemble that of the mature basophil, eosinophil, or neutrophil. The **myelocyte is the last stage capable of mitosis.** Myelocytes produce a large number of specific granules, but a finite number of primary granules (produced in the promyelocyte) are distributed among daughter myelocytes.

Metamyelocyte

This postmitotic cell measures 10 to 15 μm in diameter. The eccentric, bean-shaped nucleus now contains some condensed chromatin. The cytoplasm closely resembles that of the mature form. The specific granules outnumber the primary granules.

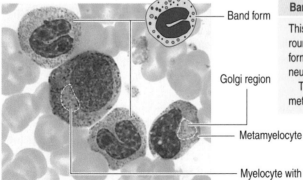

Band form

Golgi region

Metamyelocyte

Myelocyte with Golgi region

Band form

This cell has a diameter of about 9 to 15 μm. The nucleus is U-shaped with rounded ends. Its cytoplasm resembles that of the mature form. Two band form neutrophils are shown together with a myelocyte and a metamyelocyte neutrophil.

The Golgi region can be distinguished in the myelocyte and metamyelocyte.

Figure 6-22. **Myeloid lineage: Cell types**

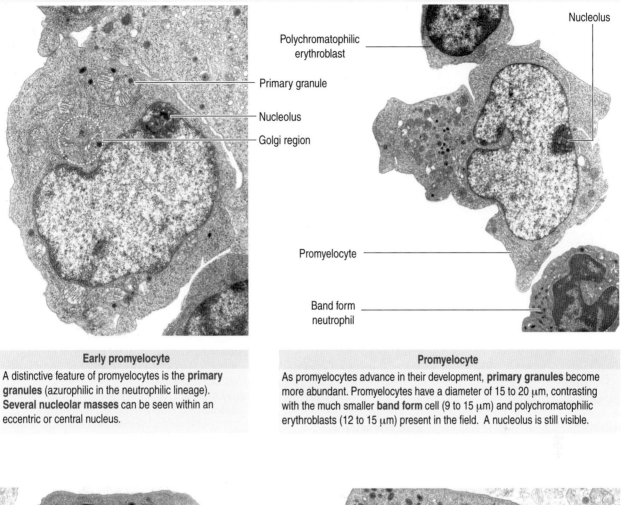

Polychromatophilic erythroblast

Nucleolus

Primary granule

Nucleolus

Golgi region

Promyelocyte

Band form neutrophil

Early promyelocyte

A distinctive feature of promyelocytes is the **primary granules** (azurophilic in the neutrophilic lineage). **Several nucleolar masses** can be seen within an eccentric or central nucleus.

Promyelocyte

As promyelocytes advance in their development, **primary granules** become more abundant. Promyelocytes have a diameter of 15 to 20 μm, contrasting with the much smaller **band form** cell (9 to 15 μm) and polychromatophilic erythroblasts (12 to 15 μm) present in the field. A nucleolus is still visible.

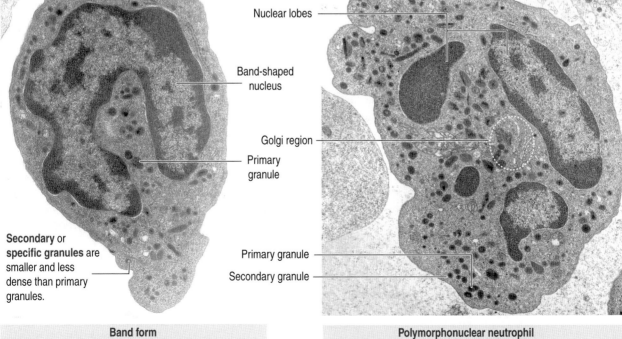

Nuclear lobes

Band-shaped nucleus

Golgi region

Primary granule

Secondary or **specific granules** are smaller and less dense than primary granules.

Primary granule

Secondary granule

Band form

Both **primary** and **secondary** or **specific granules** can be seen in the cytoplasm of this **band form neutrophil**.

Polymorphonuclear neutrophil

Both primary and secondary granules can be seen in the cytoplasm of this cell displaying a **multilobulated nucleus**.

Figure 6-23. Myeloid lineage: Basophil

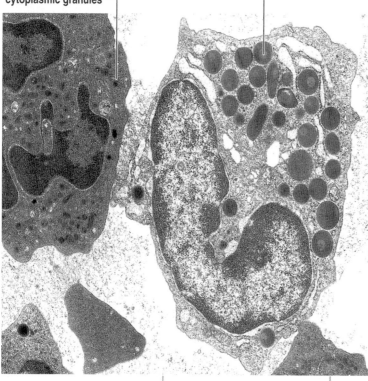

Neutrophil contains **smaller cytoplasmic granules**

Basophil contains **larger granules**

Band form basophil

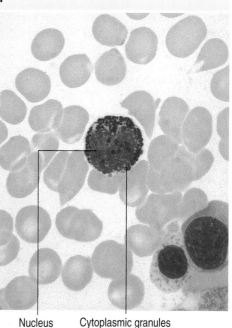

Nucleus   Cytoplasmic granules

Basophils display **large cytoplasmic granules** containing substances that are released to mediate allergic and inflammatory reactions, in particular to affect vascular permeability.

An increase in basophils is seen in **myeloproliferative disorders**. An acute nonlymphocytic leukemia with basophil-like cells is associated with symptoms caused by the release of histamine.

etin (**EPO**) (Figure 6-18), a glycoprotein produced primarily (90%) in the **kidneys** (juxtatubular interstitial cells in the renal cortex) in response to **hypoxia** (a decrease in oxygen level in inspired air or tissues).

Renal juxtatubular interstitial cells sense oxygen levels through **oxygen-dependent prolyl hydroxylase**, a protein that hydroxylates the transcription factor **hypoxia-inducible factor 1α (HIF-1α)** to repress the activity of the *erythropoietin* gene. Under conditions of **low oxygen tension, the hydroxylase is inactive and nonhydroxylated HIF-1α can drive the production of erythropoietin.**

Erythropoietin stimulates the proliferation of erythroid progenitor cells by decreasing the levels of cell cycle inhibitors and increasing cyclins and the antiapoptotic protein $Bclx_L$. Erythropoietin is also produced by neurons and glial cells in the central nervous system and in the retina. The administration of erythropoietin exerts a protective effect on neurons after ischemia (stroke).

Erythropoietin synthesis in **chronic renal diseases** is severely impaired. Recombinant erythropoietin can be administered intravenously or subcutaneously for the treatment of anemia caused by a decrease in the production of erythropoietin by the kidneys.

The effectiveness of erythropoietin treatment can be monitored by an **increase of reticulocytes in circulating blood**. Reticulocytes can be identified by the supravital stain of residual polyribosomes forming a reticular network (Figure 6-19).

Note in Figure 6-17 that polychromatophilic erythroblasts are erythropoietin-independent, mitotically active, and specifically involved in the synthesis of hemoglobin. Derived orthochromatic erythroblasts, reticulocytes, and mature RBCs are postmitotic cells (not involved in mitosis).

Leukopoiesis

Leukopoiesis (Greek *leukos,* white; *poietin,* to make) results in the formation of cells belonging to the **granulocyte** and **agranulocyte** series.

In the current branching lineage tree model of hematopoiesis (see Figure 6-16), the **myeloid stem cell generates the granulocytic neutrophil, eosinophil and basophil progenies**, in addition to megakaryocyte and erythroid progenies.

The **granulocyte lineage** (Figure 6-20) includes the **myeloblast, promyelocyte, myelocyte, metamyelocyte, band cell,** and **mature form.** In the binary lineage tree model, the granulocyte-macrophage precursor gives rise to **neutrophils** and **monocytes.** **Agranulocytes** include **lymphocytes** and **monocytes.**

Figure 6-24. **Origin and fate of monocytes**

Monocytes are recognized by the **indented nucleus**. The cytoplasm displays **lysosomes** that increase in number when **the monocyte becomes a macrophage. Monocytes are the largest cells found in peripheral blood**. They circulate for about 14 hours and then migrate into tissues where they differentiate into a variety of **tissue-specific macrophages.**

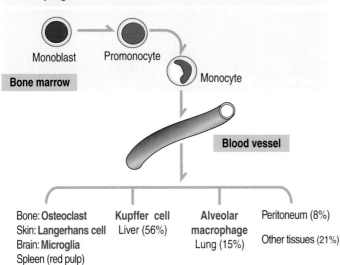

Monoblast → Promonocyte → Monocyte

Bone marrow

Blood vessel

Bone: **Osteoclast**
Skin: **Langerhans cell**
Brain: **Microglia**
Spleen (red pulp)

Kupffer cell
Liver (56%)

Alveolar macrophage
Lung (15%)

Peritoneum (8%)

Other tissues (21%)

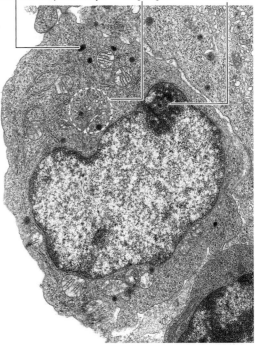

Lysosomes in a promonocyte   Golgi region   Nucleolus

Granulocytes

Neutrophil and macrophage cell lines share a common precursor cell lineage: the granulocyte-macrophage CFU (see Figure 6-20).

Eosinophils and basophils derive from independent eosinophil and basophil CFUs. Neutrophil, eosinophil, and basophil granulocytes follow a similar pattern of proliferation, differentiation, maturation, and storage in the bone marrow. Details of these processes are better recognized for neutrophils, the most abundant granulocyte in the bone marrow and blood. It takes 10 to 14 days for neutrophils to develop from early precursors, but this timing is accelerated in the presence of infections or by treatment with granulocyte colony-stimulating factor (CSF) or granulocyte-macrophage CSF (see below).

Myeloblasts, promyelocytes, and **myelocytes are mitotically dividing cells; metamyelocytes** and **band cells cannot divide** but continue to differentiate (see Figure 6-20).

A typical feature of the maturation of granulocytes are the cytoplasmic **primary** (azurophilic) and **secondary** (specific) **granules** (Figures 6-21 and 6-22).

Myeloblasts are undifferentiated cells lacking cytoplasmic granules. Promyelocytes and myelocytes display primary granules in cells of the neutrophil, eosinophil, and basophil series. Primary granules persist as such throughout the cell differentiation sequence (see Figure 6-22). **Secondary granules appear in myelocytes.**

Eosinophils exhibit the same maturation sequence as neutrophils. Eosinophil-specific granules are larger than neutrophil granules and appear refractile under the light microscope. Eosinophilic granules contain **eosinophil peroxidase** (with antibacterial activity) and several cationic proteins (**major basic protein,** and **eosinophil cationic protein,** with antiparasitic activity). See Figure 6-5 for a listing of proteins associated with eosinophils.

The basophil CFU produces basophils and mast cell precursors, a lineage specification that is regulated by the expression of the transcription factors **GATA-binding protein 2** (GATA2) and **CCAAT/enhancer-binding protein-α** (C/EBPα). Deletion of C/EBPα favors mast cell development, whereas its overexpression induces the development of the basophil lineage. In addition, signalling mediated by **STAT5** (for signal transducer and activator of transcription 5) is essential for the development of basophil precursors in bone marrow.

Basophils are distinguished by their large, coarse, and metachromatic granules that fill the cytoplasm and often obscure the nucleus (Figure 6-23). Like neutrophils and eosinophils, basophils complete their maturation in bone marrow. The granules contain **peroxidase, heparin,** and **histamine** as well as **kallikrein,** a substance that attracts eosinophils. See Figure 6-6 for additional structural and functional features of basophils.

Mast cells leave the bone marrow as immature precursor cells rather than granule-containing mature cells like basophils. Mast cells are found close to blood

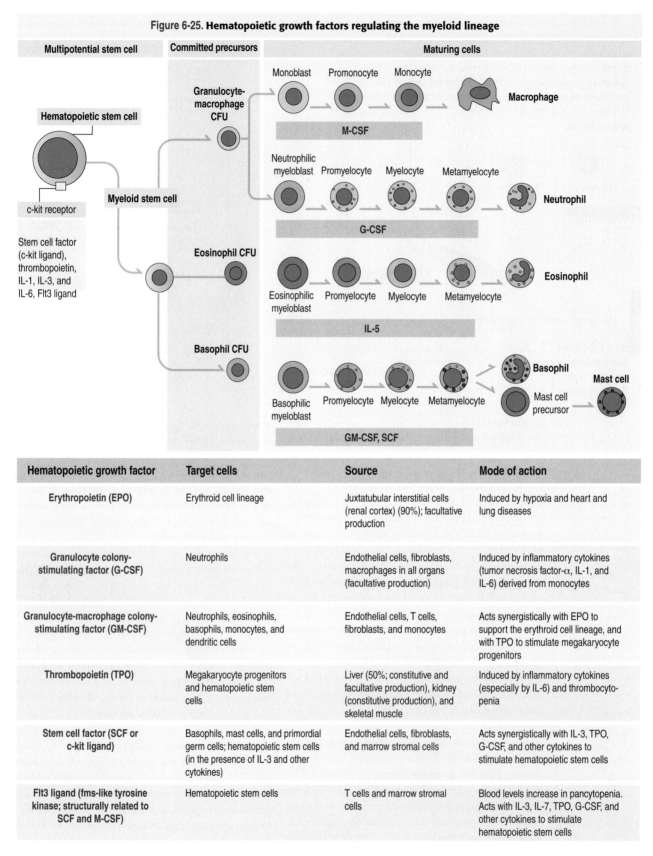

Figure 6-25. Hematopoietic growth factors regulating the myeloid lineage

Hematopoietic growth factor	Target cells	Source	Mode of action
Erythropoietin (EPO)	Erythroid cell lineage	Juxtatubular interstitial cells (renal cortex) (90%); facultative production	Induced by hypoxia and heart and lung diseases
Granulocyte colony-stimulating factor (G-CSF)	Neutrophils	Endothelial cells, fibroblasts, macrophages in all organs (facultative production)	Induced by inflammatory cytokines (tumor necrosis factor-α, IL-1, and IL-6) derived from monocytes
Granulocyte-macrophage colony-stimulating factor (GM-CSF)	Neutrophils, eosinophils, basophils, monocytes, and dendritic cells	Endothelial cells, T cells, fibroblasts, and monocytes	Acts synergistically with EPO to support the erythroid cell lineage, and with TPO to stimulate megakaryocyte progenitors
Thrombopoietin (TPO)	Megakaryocyte progenitors and hematopoietic stem cells	Liver (50%; constitutive and facultative production), kidney (constitutive production), and skeletal muscle	Induced by inflammatory cytokines (especially by IL-6) and thrombocytopenia
Stem cell factor (SCF or c-kit ligand)	Basophils, mast cells, and primordial germ cells; hematopoietic stem cells (in the presence of IL-3 and other cytokines)	Endothelial cells, fibroblasts, and marrow stromal cells	Acts synergistically with IL-3, TPO, G-CSF, and other cytokines to stimulate hematopoietic stem cells
Flt3 ligand (fms-like tyrosine kinase; structurally related to SCF and M-CSF)	Hematopoietic stem cells	T cells and marrow stromal cells	Blood levels increase in pancytopenia. Acts with IL-3, IL-7, TPO, G-CSF, and other cytokines to stimulate hematopoietic stem cells

vessels and have a significant role in vasodilation during hyperemia in acute inflammation.

Immature mast cells in the periphery can be identified by their expression of the **receptor for immunoglobulin E (FcεRI)** and the tyrosine kinase c-**kit recepto**r for **stem cell factor.**

Remember from our discussion in Chapter 4, Connective Tissue, that there are two classes of mature

Figure 6-26. **Megakaryocyte and the origin of platelets**

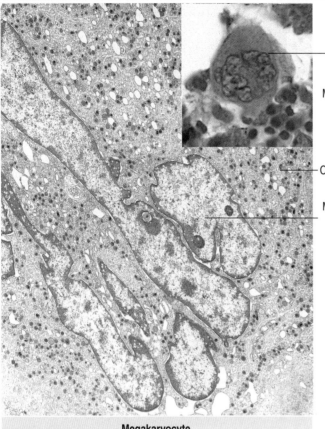

Multilobed nucleus

Cytoplasm

Multilobed nucleus

Alpha granule

Nuclear envelope

Megakaryocyte

Dense core granule   Invaginated membrane system

The development and maturation of a megakaryocyte (in about 5 days) are characterized by the following sequence:
1. **Serial mitotic divisions** (reaching a DNA content up to 128n) **without cell division**, a process known as **endoreduplication**. As a result, a tightly packed, multilobed nucleus is observed.
2. **Cytoplasmic maturation**, characterized by an increase in the number of **dense core granules, alpha granules**, and a network of membrane channels and tubules known as the Invaginated membrane system.
3. **Proplatelet shedding** into sinusoids of the bone marrow.

During the cytoplasmic maturation of a megakaryocyte, the cell membrane invaginates to form channels separating cytoplasmic islands about 3 to 4 μm in diameter.

These platelet demarcation channels eventually coalesce to generate **proplatelets**. Megakaryocytes typically rest next to bone marrow sinusoids (vascular niche) and extend **10 to 20 proplatelet projections at one time** between endothelial cells into the sinusoids where they are shed. **S1P, bound to the S1pr1 receptor**, mediates the extension and shedding of proplatelets.

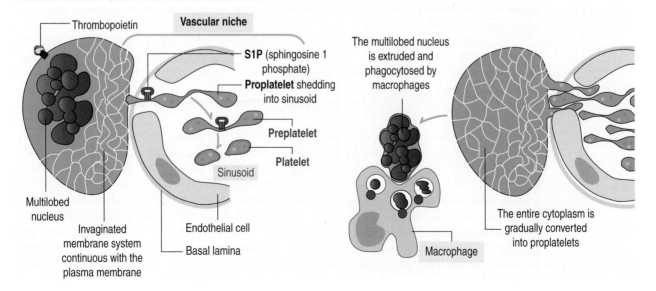

Thrombopoietin

Vascular niche

S1P (sphingosine 1 phosphate)

Proplatelet shedding into sinusoid

Preplatelet

Platelet

Sinusoid

Multilobed nucleus

Invaginated membrane system continuous with the plasma membrane

Endothelial cell

Basal lamina

The multilobed nucleus is extruded and phagocytosed by macrophages

The entire cytoplasm is gradually converted into proplatelets

Macrophage

mast cells: **connective tissue mast cells** (CTMCs; located around blood vessels) and T-cell dependent **mucosal mast cells** (MMCs; in the intestinal villi and respiratory mucosa). CTMCs and MMCs contain subsets of metachromatic granules specifically synthesized during their maturation in local tissues and released upon host response to pathogens.

It is important to stress once more that basophils and mast cells are associated with type 2 immunity, that develops in the presence of TH2 cells, high levels of immunoglobulin E and eosinophilia and in response to allergens and multicellular parasites (helminths).

Agranulocytes: Lymphocytes

Lymphocytes constitute a heterogeneous population of cells that differ from each other in terms of **origin**, **life span**, preferred sites of **localization within lymphoid organs**, **cell surface markers** and **function**.

HSCs gives rise to all hematopoietic cells, including lymphocytes of the B and T cell lineage. **B cells mature in the bone marrow and then migrate to other lymphoid organs. T cells complete their maturation in the thymus and then migrate to specific lymphoid organs.**

A **lymphoblast** gives rise to a **prolymphocyte**, an intermediate stage that precedes the mature **lymphocyte. B and T lymphocytes are nonphagocytic cells. They are morphologically similar but functionally different**, as discussed in Chapter 10, Immune-Lymphatic System.

Lymphoblasts (8 to 12 μm in diameter) are the precursors of the lymphocytes. A lymphoblast has an uncondensed nucleus with a large nucleolus. The cytoplasm contains many polyribosomes and a few cisternae of the endoplasmic reticulum (see Figure 6-7).

Lymphocytes (8 μm in diameter or less) contain a round or slightly indented condensed nucleus. The nucleolus is not visible. The cytoplasm is moderately basophilic and generally devoid of granules.

Monocytes

Monocytes derive from the **granulocyte-macrophage CFU.** We have already discussed that the granulocyte-macrophage CFU gives rise to the neutrophil lineage and the macrophage lineage.

Under the influence of a specific CSF, each precursor cell establishes its own hierarchy: the granulocyte colony-stimulating factor (G-CSF) takes the granulocyte precursor cell into the **myeloblast** pathway; the granulocyte-macrophage colony-stimulating factor (GM-CSF) guides the monocyte precursor cell into the **monoblast** pathway, leading to the production of peripheral blood monocytes and tissue macrophages. Receptors for the macrophage-stimulating factor

(M-CSF) are restricted to the monocyte lineage (see Osteoclastogenesis in Chapter 5, Osteogenesis).

Monoblasts (14 μm in diameter) are morphologically similar to myeloblasts. The monoblast is present in the bone marrow and is difficult to identify with certainty. The cytoplasm is basophilic and the nucleus is large and displays one or more nucleoli. The following cell in the series is the **promonocyte**.

Promonocytes (11 to 13 μm in diameter) contain a large nucleus with a slight indentation and uncondensed chromatin. A nucleolus may be visualized. The basophilic cytoplasm, due to polyribosomes, contains primary granules (lysosomes with **peroxidase**, **arylsulfatase**, and **acid phosphatase**). The primary granules are smaller and fewer than in promyelocytes. **Both monoblasts and promonocytes are mitotically active cells.**

Monocytes (12 to 20 μm in diameter) in the bone marrow and the blood have a large indented nucleus found in the central portion of the cytoplasm (Figure 6-24; see Figure 6-8). Granules (**primary lysosomes**) and small vacuoles are typical features. Lysosomes contain proteases and hydrolases. Monocytes are motile in response to chemotactic signals and attach to microorganisms, a function facilitated by special receptors for the Fc portion of immunoglobulin G and for complement proteins coating the microorganism. Monocytes are active phagocytes.

Macrophages (15 to 80 μm in diameter) constitute a population of blood monocytes. After circulating for 20 to 40 hours, monocytes leave the blood to enter the tissues (lungs, spleen, liver, lymph node, peritoneum, gastrointestinal tract and bone [osteoclasts]), where they become macrophages in response to local conditions.

The structural and functional characteristics of tissue macrophages are discussed in Chapter 4, Connective Tissue. In Chapter 11, Integumentary System, we discuss the antigenic reactivity of monocyte-derived **Langerhans cells** in epidermis. In Chapter 17, Digestive Glands, we explore the important role of **Kupffer cells** in liver function, and in Chapter 10, Immune-Lymphatic System, we examine the phagocytic properties of macrophages in spleen.

Pathology: Colony-stimulating factors and interleukins

G-CSF is a glycoprotein produced by endothelial cells, fibroblasts, and macrophages in different parts of the body. The synthetic form of G-CSF (known as filgrastim or lenograstim) causes a dose-dependent increase of neutrophils in the blood. G-CSF is used for the treatment of **neutropenia** (neutrophil + Greek *penia*, poverty; small numbers of neutrophils in circulating blood) after cancer chemotherapy, after bone marrow transplantation, to facilitate an

Figure 6-27. **c-kit receptor**

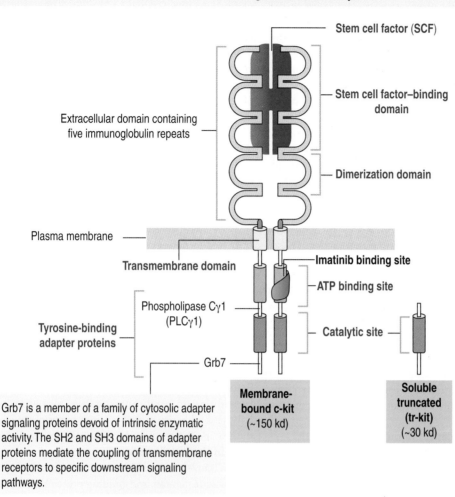

Binding of SCF induces dimerization and autophosphorylation of c-kit, followed by phosphorylation of different substrates.

c-kit exists in two forms: a membrane bound and a soluble truncated form (tr-kit) derived from proteolytic cleavage of the membrane-bound precursor.

Stem cell factor (SCF)

Stem cell factor–binding domain

Extracellular domain containing five immunoglobulin repeats

Dimerization domain

Plasma membrane

Transmembrane domain

Imatinib binding site

ATP binding site

Phospholipase Cγ1 (PLCγ1)

Tyrosine-binding adapter proteins

Catalytic site

Grb7

Membrane-bound c-kit (~150 kd)

Soluble truncated (tr-kit) (~30 kd)

Grb7 is a member of a family of cytosolic adapter signaling proteins devoid of intrinsic enzymatic activity. The SH2 and SH3 domains of adapter proteins mediate the coupling of transmembrane receptors to specific downstream signaling pathways.

Imatinib is an inhibitor of tyrosine kinases with remarkable effects in the treatment of chronic myeloid leukemia.

In the absence of imatinib, a protein substrate will be phosphorylated on tyrosine and initiate a downstream signaling cascade.

In the presence of imatinib (bound to the ATP binding site), a protein substrate is not phosphorylated and the signaling cascade is inhibited.

increase of neutrophils, and in the treatment of chronic neutropenia.

GM-CSF is also a glycoprotein produced by endothelial cells, T cells, fibroblasts, and monocytes that stimulates the formation of neutrophils, eosinophils, basophils, monocytes, and dendritic cells (Figure 6-25). However, GM-CSF is less potent than G-CSF in increasing the levels of neutrophils during neutropenia. As is the case with G-CSF, a synthetic form of GM-CSF (sargramostim or molgramostim) is available for the treatment of neutropenia.

Interleukins have a relevant function in the formation and function of type B and T cells as we discuss in Chapter 10, Immune-Lymphatic System. IL-3 stimulates proliferation of hematopoietic stem cells and acts together with other growth factors, including stem cell factor, thrombopoietin, IL-1, IL-6, and Flt3 (fms-like tyrosine kinase 3) ligand (see Figure 6-25). IL-5 acts specifically on the eosinophil progeny.

Megakaryocytes and platelets

The precursor cell of the platelet (also called **thrombocyte**; Greek *thrombos,* clot) is the **megakaryoblast**, a cell derived from the **megakaryocyte CFU** (see Figure 6-16).

The megakaryoblast (15 to 50 μm in diameter) displays a single kidney-shaped nucleus with several nucleoli. The megakaryoblast enlarges to give rise to the **promegakaryocyte** (20 to 80 μm in diameter) with an irregularly shaped nucleus and a cytoplasm rich in azurophilic granules. The promegakaryocyte forms the mature megakaryocyte located in the vascular niche, adjacent to a sinusoid.

The **megakaryocyte** (50 to 100 μm in diameter; Figure 6-26) contains an irregularly **multilobed nucleus produced by an endomitotic nuclear division process in which DNA replication occurs without cell division (polyploid nucleus).** The DNA content of multilobed nucleus can reach a value of 128n before completing cell maturation in about 5 days and start the formation of platelets. Nucleoli are not detected.

The megakaryocyte can be mistaken for the osteoclast, another large cell in bone that is **multinucleated instead of multilobed.**

The cytoplasm shows a **network of demarcation**

zones formed by the invagination of the plasma membrane of the megakaryocyte. The coalescence of the demarcation membranes results in the formation of **proplatelets released directly into the marrow sinusoidal space** where they fragment into **preplatelets** and then into **platelets**. The formation and release of proplatelet extensions is mediated by **S1P** (for sphingosine 1 phosphate) bound to its receptor **S1pr1**. S1P signaling in the vascular space directly stimulates the release of new platelets.

The entire cytoplasm of the megakaryocyte is gradually converted into proplatelets and its multilobed nucleus is extruded and phagocytosed by macrophages (see Figure 6-26).

Platelets play important roles in maintaining the integrity of blood vessels. Recall the sequential steps of hemostasis following platelet activation (see Figure 6-12).

Finally, megakaryocytes produce and secrete in the bone marrow chemokine C-X-C motif ligand 4 (**CXCL4**) and transforming growth factor-β1 (**TGFβ1**) that regulate the cell cycle activity of HSC. CXCL4 and TGFβ1 increase the number of quiescent HSCs during homeostasis and their decrease stimulates the proliferation of quiescent HSCs. Note that the differentiated megakaryocytes, derived from HSCs, can regulate the pool size of their progenitors.

Clinical significance: Thrombopoietin

Thrombopoietin is produced in the **liver**, has a similar structure to erythropoietin, and stimulates the development of megakaryocytes from the megakaryocyte CFU into platelets. Deficiencies in thrombopoietin cause **thrombocytopenia**. An excess of thrombopoietin causes **thrombocytosis**.

Platelets bind and degrade thrombopoietin, a process that autoregulates platelet production.

Pathology: Stem cell factor (also known as c-kit ligand)

Stem cell factor (SCF) is a ligand protein produced by fetal tissues and reticular stromal cells of the bone marrow. SCF exists in two forms: membrane-associated and soluble forms, the latter generated by proteolytic cleavage of the membrane-associated protein. SCF binds to **c-kit receptor**, a tyrosine kinase.

The **c-kit receptor** has an **extracellular domain** consisting of five immunoglobulin motif repeats responsible for SCF binding and dimerization (Figure 6-27). Binding of SCF induces the dimerization of the c-kit receptor, followed by autophosphorylation. Autophosphorylated c-kit receptor is the docking site of specific signaling molecules.

The **intracellular domain** has an adenosine triphosphate (ATP) binding site and a catalytic site. The tyrosine kinase inhibitor **imatinib** binds to the ATP binding site and prevents the phosphorylation of substrates involved in the activation of downstream signaling. Imatinib shows remarkable results in the treatment of **chronic myeloid leukemia**.

SCF by itself is a weak stimulator of hematopoiesis but makes HSCs responsive to other cytokines (see Figure 6-25). It does not induce the formation of cell colonies by itself. **Flt3** (for fms-like tyrosine kinase 3) ligand is closely related to c-kit receptor and SCF. Similar to SCF, Flt3 ligand acts on the HSC in synergy with thrombopoietin, SCF, and interleukins.

The c-kit receptor is expressed by the c-kit **proto-oncogene**. Mutations in genes expressing c-kit receptor and/or SCF cause:

1. **Anemia.**
2. Defective **development of melanocytes in skin.**
3. Reduced **migration, survival and proliferation of primordial germinal cells in the developing ovaries and testes** (see Chapter 21, Sperm Transport and Maturation).
4. Arrest in the development of **mast cells.**

SCF is potentially useful for the treatment of inherited and acquired disorders of hematopoiesis as well as in bone marrow transplantation.

Pathology: Iron-overload disorders

In addition to erythropoietin, the formation of RBCs is highly dependent on **iron metabolism** and the water-soluble vitamins **folic acid** (folacin) and **vitamin B$_{12}$** (cobalamin).

Iron is involved in the transport of oxygen and carbon dioxide. Several iron-binding proteins store and transport iron, for example, **hemoglobin** in RBCs, **myoglobin** in muscle tissue, **cytochromes** and various **nonheme enzymes.**

Approximately 65–75% of iron is found in the hemoglobin of RBCs in the form of heme. **Heme** is a molecule synthesized in the bone marrow, with one ferrous ion, Fe(II), bound to a tetrapyrrolic ring, and **hematin**, with one ferric ion, Fe(III), bound to a protein. The liver stores about 10–20% of iron in the form of **ferritin.**

Systemic iron levels are controlled by:

1. **Absorption.** Iron is absorbed in the **duodenum.**
2. **Recycling.** Iron recycling of senescent erythrocytes by spleen and liver macrophages is the primary body's iron supply.
3. **Mobilization** of iron stores in the liver.

Mammals do not have a regulated pathway of iron excretion. Instead, this process is controlled by **hepcidin**, an iron regulatory protein.

In blood plasma, iron is bound to **transferrin (Tf)**. Tf delivers iron to cells by binding to their Tf receptors. When there is a defect in Tf or an over-saturation of Tf binding capacity, iron in plasma accumulates in the cytoplasm of parenchymal tissues.

Figure 6-28. Uptake of iron by internalization of transferrin and iron-linked disorders

Iron uptake, storage and intestinal transport

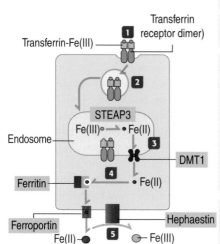

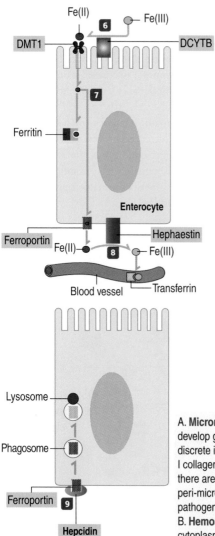

1 The plasma **transferrin (Tf)–Fe(III)** complex binds to a **Tf receptor dimer**

2 The **Tf–Fe(III)–Tf receptor** complex is internalized

3 In the endosomal compartment, the low pH dissociates Fe(III) from Tf bound to the Tf receptor. Fe(III) is converted to Fe(II) by the endosomal reductase **STEAP3**. Fe(II) is released into the cytosol by divalent metal transporter-1 (**DMT1**).

4 Fe(II) is stored to form **ferritin** (non-red blood cells) or incorporated into hemoglobin in red blood cells

5 Fe(II) is exported by **ferroportin** and then converted to Fe(III) by the membrane-associated ferroxidase, **hephaestin**

6 Ferric iron Fe(III) in the diet is converted to ferrous iron Fe(II) by **ferroreductase (DCYTB)** at the brush border of an enterocyte (duodenum–jejunum) and transported into the enterocyte by DMT1

7 Fe(II) attaches to form ferritin or can be transported across the basolateral membrane into blood plasma by ferroportin. Fe(II) is converted to Fe(III) by hephaestin **8**.

9 **Hepcidin** binding to ferroportin prevents iron export. Intracellular store of Fe(II) increases during anemia or hypoxia. Internalized ferroportin is degraded by lysosomes.

A. **Micronodular cirrhosis**. Micronodules develop gradually and they are partitioned into discrete islands by fibrous tissue containing type I collagen. The blue spots indicate iron. Note that there are no inflammation cells in the peri-micronodular space because iron is a toxic pathogen instead of a biological pathogen.
B. **Hemosiderin granules** are seen in the cytoplasm of hepatocytes. They stain blue with **Prussian Blue stain**. Nuclei are stained pink.

Hemochromatosis

Hepcidin, a member of the family of defensins secreted by hepatocytes, regulates the entry of iron into blood plasma.

Hepcidin is encoded by the human gene *HAMP*. **Hepcidin binds to ferroportin and triggers its internalization and lysosomal degradation. Removal of ferroportin from the plasma membrane prevents iron export, leading to increasing levels of iron in the cytoplasm, stored in ferritin.** This negative regulatory mechanism can be modulated during anemia, hypoxia and inflammation.

Iron-overload diseases occur when the amount of iron in plasma exceeds the binding capacity of Tf. Parenchymal tissues, such as liver, take up iron by a Tf-independent mechanism.

Hereditary hemochromatosis (HH) is an iron-overload disease caused by a **genetic defect** in three genes resulting in the abnormal expression of **hepcidin** (HH type 1 [the most common; characterized by liver cirrhosis, fibrosis and diabetes]; HH type 2 [mutation of the Tf receptor gene and decreased expression of hepcidin] and HH type 3 [juvenil hemochromatosis; endocrine and cardiac dysfunction]). HH type 4 is caused by a defective gene encoding ferroportin. **Hemosiderosis** is an **acquired** iron-overload disease.

Micronodular cirrhosis

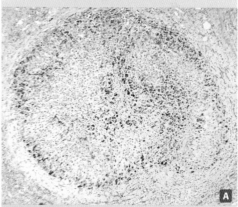

Prussian blue-stained iron deposits in hepatocytes

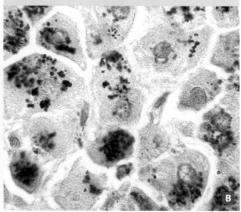

Box 6-E | Anemia

- **Anemia** is a reduction in the mass of circulating red blood cells. It is detected by analysis of peripheral blood (low hemoglobin, low red blood cell count, and low hematocrit). Anemia results in the lack of oxygen-carrying capacity, which is compensated for by a reduction in the affinity of hemoglobin for oxygen, an increase in cardiac output, and an attempt to increase red blood cell production. The most common cause of anemia is **iron deficiency** (low intake, chronic blood loss, or increased demand during pregnancy and lactation).
- Deficiency in **vitamin B$_{12}$** and **folic acid** causes **megaloblastic anemia** (Figure 6-29). This form of anemia is associated with the development of abnormally large red blood cell precursors (**megaloblasts**) that develop into large red blood cells (**macrocytes**). Vitamin B$_{12}$ is normally absorbed in the small intestine after binding to **intrinsic factor**, a glycoprotein secreted by **gastric parietal cells**. The lack of production of intrinsic factor (due to autoimmune atrophic gastritis, or after surgical gastrectomy) results in **pernicious anemia**.

Tf, produced in the liver, and **lactoferrin**, present in maternal milk, are nonheme proteins involved in the **transport of iron** (Figure 6-28). Tf complexed to two Fe(III) ions is called **ferrotransferrin**. Tf devoid of iron is known as **apotransferrin**.

The Tf receptor is a transmembrane dimer with each subunit binding to Fe(III). The internalization of the Tf-Fe(III) complex is dependent on Tf receptor phosphorylation triggered by Ca^{2+}-calmodulin and the protein kinase C complex.

Inside the cell, Fe(III) is released within the acidic endosomal compartment and is converted to Fe(II) by the endosomal ferrireductase **STEAP3**. Fe(II) is then transported out of the endosome into the cytosol by **DMT1** (for divalent metal transporter-1) and either stored in ferritin or incorporated into hemoglobin in RBCs.

The Tf receptor is recycled back to the plasma membrane.

Ferritin is a major protein synthesized in the liver. A single ferritin molecule has the capacity to store up to 4500 iron ions. When the storage capacity of ferritin is exceeded, iron is deposited as **hemosiderin**. Ferritin with little iron is called **apoferritin**.

Fe(II) is exported from the ferritin cell storage by the iron exporter **ferroportin**. The function of ferroportin is tightly controlled by **hepcidin** depending on the body's iron levels. Exported Fe(II) is converted to Fe(III) by the membrane associated ferroxidase, **hephaestin**, and then enters blood circulation (see Figure 8-26).

Hepcidin is a **negative regulator of iron transport** encoded by the human *HAMP* gene. Hepcidin regulates iron homeostasis by down regulating ferroportin, the iron exporter. As a negative regulator, hepcidin major functions are:

1. To sequester iron in tissues.
2. To lower serum iron levels.
3. To reduce iron absorption from the diet.

Upon hepcidin binding to ferroportin, ferroportin is internalized and degraded in lysosomes (see Figure 6-28). Hepcidin-induced internalization of ferroportin determines a **decreased iron efflux** into circulation from duodenal enterocytes, macrophages, and hepatocytes.

Hepcidin expression increases when body iron is abundant and is decreased in iron deficiency.

Under physiologic conditions, the expression of hepatic hepcidin is regulated by several proteins:

1. The **hereditary hemochromatosis protein**, called **HFE** (for **h**igh iron [**Fe**]).

Figure 6-29. Megaloblastic anemia

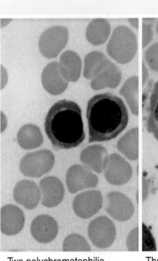

Two polychromatophilic erythroblasts from a healthy adult. Bone marrow smear. May–Grünwald–Giemsa stain.

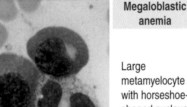

Megaloblastic anemia

Large metamyelocyte with horseshoe-shaped nucleus

Erythroblasts are abundant, larger (megaloblasts) and nuclear chromatin is less condensed

Three polychromatophilic erythroblasts and one large metamyelocyte from a patient with pernicious anemia. Bone marrow smear. May–Grünwald–Giemsa stain.

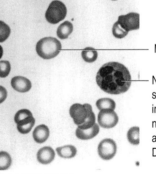

Macrocytic RBC

Neutrophil with seven interconnected nuclear lobes and increased DNA content

The neutrophil has a hypersegmented nucleus. RBCs are macrocytic in a patient with pernicious anemia. Blood smear. May–Grünwald–Giemsa stain.

2. **Tf receptor.**
3. **Hemojuvelin (HJV).**
4. **Bone morphogenic protein 6 (BMP6).**
5. Matriptase-2.
6. Neogenin.
7. **Tf.**

Defective expression of hepcidin will take place when any one of these proteins, in particular HVJ, is missing.

Under hypoxic conditions, the transcription factor **hypoxia-inducible factor 1α (HIF-1α)** binds to the promoter of the *HAMP* gene and blocks the expression of hepcidin. We discussed early on in this chapter the activity of the erythropoietin gene as an inducer of RBC production. We made the point that, under conditions of low oxygen tension, the transcription factor **HIF-1α** becomes active to enhance the production of erythropoietin.

As you can see, the activity of **HIF-1α** is necessary for providing two of the critical elements for erythropoiesis: erythropoietin, and iron.

Iron-overload diseases, such as **hereditary hemochromatosis (HH)**, can occur when misregulation of *HAMP* gene expression takes place. Massive deposits of iron in hepatocytes are very harmful, leading to cirrhosis and liver fibrosis (see Figure 6-28).

HH has been attributed to defects in four genes:

1. **HH type 1**, the most common iron-overload disorder, is characterized by increased absorption and deposition of iron in the liver, heart, pancreas and skin. Cirrhosis, diabetes and heart arrhythmias occur over time. Mutations in the *HFE* gene create a defective hereditary hemochromatosis protein, HFE, that affects the interaction of Tf with the Tf receptor, thereby hampering the regulation of iron absorption.

2. **HH type 2**, also called **juvenile hemochromatosis**, is defined by significant heart and endocrine dysfunction, instead of liver disease. It is prevalent in the first and second decade of life.

HH type 2 is determined by mutations in the *HAMP* gene, encoding hepcidin, or in the *HFE2* gene, encoding HJV, a glycophosphatidylinositol (GPI)-linked membrane protein. Juvenile hemochromatosis patients with HJV mutations have a significant suppression of hepatic hepcidin expression, resulting in a severe iron accumulation in specific organs.

3. **HH type 3**, is caused by a mutation in the *TFR2* gene, encoding Tf receptor 2. The expression of hepcidin is affected by this mutation.

4. **HH type 4**, is also called ferroportin disease and affects macrophages. Mutated ferrroportin fails to be inserted in the plasma membrane or is not effective during iron transport.

Patients with the heritable disorder **hemochromatosis**, characterized by excessive iron absorption and tissue deposits, require periodic withdrawals of blood and the administration of **iron chelators** to facilitate the excretion of complexed iron in the urine.

A **decrease in iron** by excessive menstrual flow or gastrointestinal bleeding determines a reduction in hemoglobin-containing iron. RBCs are smaller (**microcytic anemia**, see below) and underpigmented (**hypochromic anemia**).

Pathology: Vitamin B$_{12}$, megaloblastic anemia, and microcytic anemia

Megaloblastic hematopoiesis is caused by deficiencies in vitamin B$_{12}$ or folic acid. **Folic acid** regulates the **folate metabolism** leading to the increased availability of purines and deoxythymidine monophosphate (dTMP) required for DNA synthesis.

Vitamin B$_{12}$ (known as **extrinsic factor**) binds to **intrinsic factor**, a protein produced by the parietal cells in the gastric glands. The vitamin B$_{12}$–intrinsic factor complex binds to specific receptor sites in the **ileum**, transported across enterocytes, and released in blood, where it binds to the transport protein *trans*-cobalaphilin III.

A decrease in vitamin B$_{12}$, due mainly to insufficient production of intrinsic factor or hydrochloric acid in the stomach, or both, can affect folate metabolism and folate uptake, thereby impairing DNA synthesis in bone marrow.

Vitamin B$_{12}$ deficiency is rare because the liver stores up to a 6-year supply of vitamin B$_{12}$. Under deficiency conditions, the maturation of the erythroid cell progeny slows down, causing abnormally large RBCs (**macrocytes**) with fragile cell membranes, resulting in the destruction of RBCs (**megaloblastic anemia**; see Box 6-E and Figure 6-29).

Microcytic anemias are characterized by RBCs that are smaller than normal. The smaller size is due to a decrease in the production of hemoglobin caused by:

1. **A lack of the** hemoglobin **product**. Thalassemias are diseases of hemoglobin synthesis. Thalassemia subtypes are named after the hemoglobin chain involved.

2. **Limited iron availability and suppression of erythropoietin renal production** by inflammatory cytokines during inflammatory states.

3. **A lack of iron delivery to the heme group of hemoglobin** (iron-deficient anemia), the most common cause. Because of the iron loss through menses, women are at greater risk for iron deficiency than men.

4. **Defects in the synthesis of the heme group** (iron-utilization **sideroblastic anemias**). Sideroblastic anemias are characterized by the presence in bone marrow of **ringed sideroblasts**, erythroid precursors with perinuclear mitochondria loaded with non-heme iron.

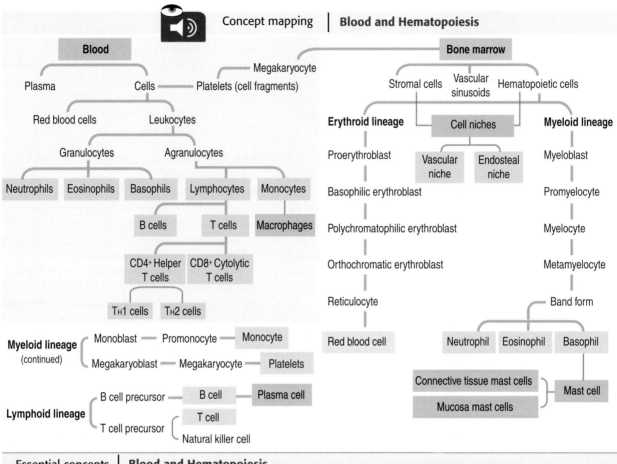

Concept mapping | Blood and Hematopoiesis

Blood
- Plasma
- Cells
  - Red blood cells
  - Leukocytes
    - Granulocytes
      - Neutrophils
      - Eosinophils
      - Basophils
    - Agranulocytes
      - Lymphocytes
        - B cells
        - T cells
          - CD4+ Helper T cells
          - CD8+ Cytolytic T cells
            - TH1 cells
            - TH2 cells
      - Monocytes
        - Macrophages
- Platelets (cell fragments)
- Megakaryocyte

Myeloid lineage (continued)
- Monoblast — Promonocyte — Monocyte
- Megakaryoblast — Megakaryocyte — Platelets

Lymphoid lineage
- B cell precursor — B cell — Plasma cell
- T cell precursor — T cell
  - Natural killer cell

Bone marrow
- Stromal cells
- Vascular sinusoids
- Hematopoietic cells
  - Cell niches
    - Vascular niche
    - Endosteal niche

Erythroid lineage
- Proerythroblast
- Basophilic erythroblast
- Polychromatophilic erythroblast
- Orthochromatic erythroblast
- Reticulocyte
- Red blood cell

Myeloid lineage
- Myeloblast
- Promyelocyte
- Myelocyte
- Metamyelocyte
- Band form
  - Neutrophil
  - Eosinophil
  - Basophil
    - Connective tissue mast cells
    - Mucosa mast cells
      - Mast cell

Essential concepts | Blood and Hematopoiesis

• Blood is a specialized connective tissue consisting of plasma (an equivalent to extra-cellular matrix) and cells. Plasma contains proteins, salts, and organic compounds. Plasma contains fibrinogen; serum, the fluid after blood coagulation, is fibrinogen-free. The cellular elements of the blood are red blood cells (RBCs or erythrocytes) and leukocytes (white blood cells). Platelets are fragments of megakaryocytes.

• RBCs (4 to 6 × 10^6/mm^3; 7.8 μm in diameter) are non-nucleated cells containing hemoglobin, a heme protein involved in the transport of oxygen and carbon dioxide. The plasma membrane contains a cytoskeleton consisting of glycophorin and anion trans-porter channel (band 3), two transmembrane proteins. The protein ankyrin anchors spectrin, a spectin α–spectrin β dimeric protein, to band 3. Spectrin tetramers are linked to a complex of three proteins: F-actin, tropomyo-sin, and protein 4.1. Adducin is a calmodulin-binding protein that favors the association of F-actin to spectrin.
Elliptocytosis (caused by defective self-assembly of spectrin, abnormal binding of spectrin to ankyrin, and abnormal protein 4.1 and glycophorin) and **spherocytosis** (caused by spectrin deficiency) are alterations in the shapes of RBCs. Anemia, jaundice, and splenomegaly are clinical features. **Sickle cell anemia** (glutamic acid replaced by

valine in the β-globin chain) and **thalassemia** (defective globin α or β chains in hemoglobin) are caused by hemoglobin defects. **Chronic hemolytic anemia** is a clinical feature of the two conditions.

A valuable clinical indicator of average plasma glucose concentration in blood is the measure-ment of hemoglobinA1c (glycohemoglobin or glycated). The normal range for the hemoglobin A1c is between 4% and 5.6%.

Erythroblastosis fetalis is an antibody-induced hemolytic disease in the newborn caused by Rh incompatibility between mother and fetus. The Rh-negative mother makes antibodies to D antigen present on the surface of fetal RBCs. During a second or third pregnancy, anti-D antigen antibodies cause hemolysis of fetal RBCs. Anemia and severe jaundice (which causes damage to the brain, a condition known as kernicterus) are clinical manifestations of the fetus.

• Leukocytes (6 to 10 × 10^3/mm^3) are classified as granulocytes (with primary, and specific or secondary cytoplasmic granules) and agranulocytes (containing only primary granules).
There are three types of granulocytes: (1) neutrophils (5 × 10^3/mm^3), (2) eosinophils (1.5 × 10^2/mm^3), and (3) basophils (0.3 × 10^2/mm^3).
Neutrophils (12 to 15 μm in diameter) have

the following characteristics: (1) They contain primary granules (elastase and myeloperoxi-dase), and secondary granules (lysozyme and other proteases). (2) They enter a blood ves-sel by diapedesis and leave blood circulation by the mechanism of homing. (3) The nuclei are segmented (polymorphonucleated cell).

Eosinophils (12 to 15 μm in diameter) have the following features: (1) Cytoplasmic granules contain eosinophil peroxidase (EP; binds to microorganisms to be phagocytosed by macrophages), major basic protein (MBP; a crystalline protein that disrupts the membrane of parasites), eosinophilic cationic protein (ECP; works with MBP to fragment parasites) and eosinophil–derived neurotoxin (EDN; with antiviral activity). (2) They participate in allergic reactions. (3) They have a bilobed nucleus with refractile red cytoplasmic granules con-taining Charcot–Leyden crystal galectin.

Eosinophils and mast cells interact in **asthma**, a condition that causes obstruction of the small-caliber bronchi and bronchioles due to mucus hypersecretion and smooth muscle bronchial constriction.

Eosinophils are usually found in the gastroin-testinal tract, predominantly in the cecum, but seldom in the esophagus. However, esopha-geal dysfunction, including dysphagia and abdominal pain, correlates with the increase of eosinophils in the esophageal mucosa. This condition is known as eosinophilic esophagitis.

Basophils (9 to12 μm in diameter) have the following features: (1) metachromatic coarse cytoplasmic granules and bilobed nucleus. (2) Similar to mast cells, basophils participate in allergic reactions. (3) They may leave blood circulation and enter the connective tissue.

Basophils and mast cells differ in the presence of c-kit receptor and CD49b but share FcεR1receptors.

There are two types of agranulocytes: lymphocytes and monocytes.

Lymphocytes are either large lymphocytes (9 to 12 μm in diameter) or small lymphocytes (6 to 8 μm in diameter).

Lymphocytes are divided into two categories: B lymphocytes (or B cells; originate and differentiate in bone marrow), and T lymphocytes (CD4+ helper T cells and CD8+ cytolytic T cells, that originate in bone marrow but differentiate in thymus). There are two subsets of T cells: TH1 and TH2 cells. We study them in detail in Chapter 10, Immune-Lymphatic System.

Monocytes (12 to 20 μm in diameter) circulate in blood for 12 to 100 hours before entering the connective tissue to become macrophages. Monocytes become osteoclasts in bone under the influence of osteoblasts.

• **Leukemias** are the most common neoplastic diseases of leukocytes. There are acute and chronic leukemias.

Acute leukemias are classified as acute lymphoblastic leukemias (ALL), when derived from lymphoid cells and acute myeloblastic leukemias (AML), when derived from myeloid, erythroid and megakaryocytic cell progenies. The diagnosis is based on the microscopic examination of bone marrow samples. ALL affects mainly children; AML affects adults.

Chronic leukemias are classified as lymphocytic, myeloid and hairy-cell type leukemias. Chronic lymphocytic leukemia (CLL) is mainly observed in adults (50 years and older). Chronic myeloid leukemia (CML) is regarded as a myeloproliferative condition (proliferation of abnormal bone marrow stem cells) affecting adults. Patients with CML usually have the Philadelphia chromosome, a reciprocal translocation between the long arms of chromosomes 9 and 22, designated t(9;22)(q34;q11). The fusion gene (*abl/bcr*) encodes a tyrosine kinase involved in cell transformation leading to a neoplastic phenotype. Hairy-cell leukemia (HCL) is a rare type of B cell leukemia.

• **Homing** or leukocyte recruitment is the mechanism by which neutrophils, lymphocytes, monocytes, and other cells circulating in blood leave a blood vessel to enter the connective tissue or a lymphoid organ or tissue. Homing occurs in two steps:

(1) Selectin-mediated attachment and rolling of a cell on the surface of an endothelial cell.

(2) Integrin-mediated transendothelial migration of the cell. Homing plays a significant role in immune and inflammatory reactions, metastasis, and tissue morphogenesis.

A defect in the integrin β subunit, the cause of **leukocyte adhesion deficiency I (LAD I)**,

prevents migration of leukocytes and defects in wound healing and persistence of inflammation are seen. A defect in carbohydrate ligands for selectins, the cause of **leukocyte adhesion deficiency II (LAD II)**, results in chronic inflammation due to recurrent infections.

• Platelets (3×10^5/mm³; 2 to 4 μm in diameter) are cytoplasmic fragment of mekagaryocytes, cells stimulated by thrombopoietin. Platelets bind and degrade thrombopoietin, a mechanism that regulates platelet production. Cytoplasmic projections, called proplatelets, enter blood circulation and fragment into platelets.

A platelet has a central region, called a granulomere containing mitochondria, rough endoplasmic reticulum, the Golgi apparatus, and three distinct types of granules:

(1) Alpha (α) granules, that store proteins involved in hemostatic functions as well as microbicidal proteins (thrombocidins and kinocidins). Platelets can interact with microbial pathogens and play a significant role in host defense against infection.

(2) Dense (δ) core granules, containing mediators of vascular tone.

(3) Lysosomal (λ) granules, containing hydrolytic enzymes participating in the dissolution of thrombi.

A peripheral region, called a hyalomere, has microtubules and microfilaments and an invaginated membrane system.

The plasma membrane is coated by glycoprotein1b (GP1b) and GP2b-GP3a, involved in the attachment of platelets to von Willebrand's factor. Deficiency of these two proteins, and factors of the blood clotting cascade, causes **bleeding disorders** (GP1b receptor–factor IX: **Bernard-Soulier syndrome**; von Willebrand's factor–factor VIII: **von Willebrand's disease**).

Adhesion of platelets to the vascular endothelium, in turn, is mediated by von Willebrand's factor that also carries factor VIII coagulation factor, whereas fibrinogen binds to GP2b-GP3a.

Platelets promote blood clotting and help to prevent blood loss from damaged vessels. Purpura designates a color patch or spot on the skin caused by bleeding. Spots less than 3 mm in diameter are called petechiae; spots larger than 1 cm in diameter are called ecchymoses. Petechiae and ecchymoses are characteristic of the Henoch–Schönlein syndrome, an allergic purpura reaction caused by drug hypersensitivity.

Thrombocytosis is an increase in circulating platelets. **Thrombocytopenia** is a reduction in the number of platelets (less than 1.5×10^5/mm³) circulating in blood. **Autoimmune thrombocytopenic purpura** (ITP) is caused by antibodies targeting platelets or megakaryocytes, or drugs (penicillin, sulfonamides, and digoxin). **Thrombotic thrombocytopenic purpura** (TTP) is determined by pathologic changes in endothelial cells producing procoagulant substances. This condition leads to the aggregation of platelets in small blood vessels.

• **Blood clotting or hemostasis**. The process involves the conversion of proenzymes (designated factor X) to active enzymes (designated factor Xa) by proteolysis. It is characterized by an extrinsic pathway (initiated by damage outside a blood vessel), and an intrinsic pathway (initiated by damage inside a blood vessel, usually the wall of the vessel). Extrinsic and intrinsic pathways converge to a common pathway in which fibrinogen is converted to fibrin and platelets begin to attach to the fibrin mesh.

Hemophilia is a common hereditary disease associated with serious bleeding due to an inherited deficiency of factor VIII or factor IX.

The genes for these blood coagulation factors lie on the X chromosome, and when mutated, they cause the X-linked recessive traits of hemophilia A and B. Hemophilia affects males, with females as carriers.

A reduction in the amount or activity of factor VIII, a protein synthesized in the liver, causes hemophilia A. A deficiency in factor IX determines hemophilia B.

Major trauma or surgery can determine severe bleeding in all hemophiliacs and, therefore, a correct diagnosis is critical. Plasma-derived or genetically engineered recombinant factors are available for the treatment of patients with hemophilia.

• **Hematopoiesis** is the formation of blood cells in the bone marrow (adult). The bone marrow consists of two microenvironmental domains, called niches:

(1) The vascular niche.

(2) The endosteal niche. Niches provide physical support, soluble factors, and cell-mediated interactions to regulate cell self renewal, differentiation and quiescence of hematopoietic stem cells (HSCs).

The vascular niche is a framework of blood vessels surrounded by a distinct perivascular population of non-hematopoietic cells stromal cells, including mesenchymal stem cells, adipose cells, endothelial cells,abundant reticular stromal cells and macrophages. Marrow reticular stromal cells produce hematopoietic growth factors and cytokines that regulate the production and differentiation of blood cells. Marrow macrophages remove apoptotic cells.

The endosteal niche, located at the endosteum–bone marrow interface, consists of preosteoblasts (osteprogenitor cells), osteoblasts and osteoclasts interacting with HSCs. Osteoblasts produce multiple hematopoietic cytokines, including G-CSF (granulocyte-colony stimulating factor), M-CSF (macrophage-colony stimulating factor}, GM-CSF (granulocyte-macrophage-colony stimulating factor), IL-1, IL-6, and IL-7.

Hematopoietic cell populations. The bone marrow consists of:

(1) HSCs, capable of self-renewal.

(2) Committed precursor cells, responsible for the generation of distinct cell lineages.

(3) Maturing cells, differentiating cells derived from committed precursor cells.

The HSC gives rise to the myeloid stem cell and the lymphoid stem cell.

The myeloid stem cell generates five colony-forming units (CFU):
(1) Erythroid CFU.
(2) Megakaryocyte CFU.
(3) Basophil CFU.
(4) Eosinophil CFU.
(5) Granulocyte-macrophage CFU. The granulocyte-macrophage CFU gives rise to neutrophils and monocytes.

The proliferation and maturation of the CFU is controlled by hematopoietic growth factors (called hematopoietic cytokines) produced by cells of the marrow stromal compartment and outside the bone marrow. There are three major groups of hematopoietic growth factors:
(1) Colony-stimulating factors (CSF).
(2) Erythropoietin (EPO).
(3) Cytokines (mainly interleukins).

• **Erythroid lineage** consists of the following sequence: proerythroblast, basophilic erythroblast, polychromatophilic erythroblast, orthochromatic erythroblast, reticulocyte, and erythrocyte.

EPO is the major regulator; it stimulates the erythroid CFU cell, the derived cell, called mature or primitive progenitor, and the proerythroblast. EPO is produced by juxtaglomerular interstitial cells of the renal cortex. The effectiveness of erythropoietin treatment can be monitored by an increase of reticulocytes in circulating blood.

• **Leukopoiesis** is the development of cells of the granulocyte (neutrophil, basophil, and eosinophil) and agranulocyte (lymphocyte and monocyte) lineage. The granulocyte lineage consists of the following sequence: myeloblast, promyelocyte, myelocyte, metamyelocyte, band cell, and mature form. Neutrophil and macrophage cell lines share a common precursor cell lineage: the granulocyte–macrophage CFU. Eosinophils and basophils derive from independent eosinophil and basophil CFUs. The basophil CFU produces basophils and mast cell precursors, a lineage specification that is regulatedby the expression of the transcription factors GATA-binding protein 2 (GATA2) and CCAAT/enhancer-binding protein-α (C/EBPα).

A characteristic of granulocytes is the appearance in the cytoplasm of primary (azurophilic) granules (promyelocyte and myelocyte), followed by secondary or specific granules (from myelocyte on). Primary granules coexist with secondary or specific granules.

Agranulocytes include lymphocytes and monocytes.

The lymphocyte lineage follows two pathways:
(1) B cells originate and mature in bone marrow.
(2) T cells originate in bone marrow and mature in thymus. A lymphoblast gives rise to a prolymphocyte, which matures as a lymphocyte. B and T cells are morphologically similar but functionally different.

The monocyte lineage derives from the granulocyte-macrophage CFU. A monoblast gives rise to a promonocyte; the final stage is monocyte, which differentiates in connective tissue into macrophage, and in bone differentiates into osteoclast.

Agranulocytes contain primary granules (lysosomes).

• **CSF and interleukins.** G-CSF stimulates the development of neutrophils. GM-CSF stimulates the formation of neutrophils, eosinophils, basophils, monocytes, and dendritic cells (present in lymphoid organs and lymphoid tissues). Interleukins play an important role in the development and function of the lymphoid lineage. Interleukins act synergistically with CSF, SCF, and Flt3 ligand to stimulate the development of the hematopoietic stem cells.

• **Megakaryocyte** (also called thrombocyte, 50 to 100 μm in diameter), the precursor cells of the platelet, derives from the megakaryoblast (15 to 50 μm in diameter), a cell derived from the megakaryocyte CFU. The megakaryocyte has an irregularly multilobed nucleus produced by an endomitotic nuclear division process in which DNA replication occurs without cell division (polyploid nucleus).

The megakaryocyte can be mistaken for the osteoclast, another large cell in bone that is multinucleated instead of multilobed.

The cytoplasm shows a network of demarcation zones formed by the invagination of the plasma membrane. The coalescence of the invaginated membranes results in the formation of proplatelets released directly into the marrow sinusoidal space where they fragment into preplatelets and then into platelets. Platelets play important roles in maintaining the integrity of blood vessels.

• **Stem cell factor** (SCF) is a ligand protein produced by fetal tissues and reticular stromal cells of the bone marrow. SCF binds to c-kit receptor, a tyrosine kinase. SCF makes HSCs responsive to other cytokines.

The c-kit receptor is expressed by the c-kit protooncogene. Mutations in genes expressing c-kit receptor and/or SCF cause: anemia, defective development of melanocytes in skin, reduced migration, survival and proliferation of primordial germinal cells in the developing ovaries and testes and arrest in the development of mast cells.

• **Iron-overload disorders.** In addition to erythropoietin, the formation of RBCs is highly dependent on iron metabolism and the water-soluble vitamins folic acid (folacin) and vitamin B12 (cobalamin).

Several iron-binding proteins store and transport iron, for example, hemoglobin in RBCs, myoglobin in muscle tissue, cytochromes and various nonheme enzymes. Approximately 65–75% of iron is found in the hemoglobin of RBCs in the form of heme. The liver stores about 10–20% of iron in the form of ferritin.

Systemic iron levels are controlled by:
(1) Absorption. Iron is absorbed in the duodenum.
(2) Recycling. Iron recycling of senescent erythrocytes by spleen and liver macrophages is the majority of the body's iron supply.

(3) Mobilization of iron stores in the liver.

In blood plasma, iron is bound to transferrin (Tf). Tf delivers iron to cells that express Tf receptors. Tf, produced in the liver, and lactoferrin, present in maternal milk, are nonheme proteins involved in the transport of iron. Tf bound to two Fe(III) ions is called ferrotransferrin. When Tf is devoid of iron is called apotransferrin.

The internalization of the Tf-Fe(III) complex is dependent on Tf receptor phosphorylation triggered by Ca2+-calmodulin and the protein kinase C complex.

Inside the cell, Fe(III) is released within the acidic endosomal compartment and is converted to Fe(II) by the endosomal ferrireductase STEAP3. Fe(II) is then transported out of the endosome into the cytosol by DMT1 (for divalent metal transporter-1) and either stored in ferritin or incorporated into hemoglobin in RBCs. The Tf receptor complex is recycled back to the plasma membrane.

Ferritin is a major protein synthesized in the liver. When the storage capacity of ferritin is exceeded, iron is deposited as hemosiderin. Ferritin with little iron is called apoferritin.

Fe(II) is exported from the ferritin cell storage by the iron exporter ferroportin. The function of ferroportin is tightly controlled by hepcidin according to the body iron levels. Exported Fe(II) is converted to Fe(III) by the membrane associated ferroxidase, hephaestin, before entering the blood circulation.

Hepcidin is a **negative regulator** of iron transport: hepcidin expression **increases** when body iron is abundant and **decreases** when there is iron deficiency.

Under physiologic conditions, the expression of hepatic hepcidin is regulated by several proteins: the hereditary hemochromatosis protein, called HFE (for high iron [Fe]), Tf receptor, hemojuvelin (HJV), bone morphogenic protein 6 (BMP6), matriptase-2, neogenin and Tf. Defective expression of hepcidin will take place when any one of these proteins, in particular HVJ, is missing.

Under hypoxic conditions, the transcription factor hypoxia-inducible factor 1α (HIF-1α) binds to the promoter of the *HAMP* gene and blocks the expression of hepcidin. Iron-overload diseases, such as **hereditary hemochromatosis (HH)**, can occur when misregulation of *HAMP* gene expression takes place.

Patients with **idiopathic hemochromatosis** absorb and deposit an excess of iron in tissues. A decrease in iron by excessive menstrual flow or gastrointestinal bleeding results in small RBCs (**microcytic anemia**).

• **Megaloblastic hematopoiesis** is caused by deficiencies in vitamin B$_{12}$ or folic acid.

Vitamin B$_{12}$ binds to intrinsic factor produced by parietal cells in the stomach. The vitamin B$_{12}$–intrinsic factor complex binds to a specific receptor site in the ileum (small intestine), absorbed by enterocytes, and released into the bloodstream, where it binds to *trans*-cobalaphilin III, a transport protein. **Megaloblastic anemia** occurs when there are deficiencies of folate and vitamin B$_{12}$.

7. Muscle Tissue

Muscle is one of the four basic tissues. There are three types of muscle: skeletal, cardiac, and smooth. All three types are composed of elongated cells, called muscle cells, myofibers, or muscle fibers, specialized for contraction. In all three types of muscle, energy from the hydrolysis of adenosine triphosphate (ATP) is transformed into mechanical energy. Skeletal muscle disorders (myopathies) can be congenital and also caused by disruption of normal nerve supply, mitochondria dysfunction, inflammation (myositis), autoimmunity (myasthenia gravis), tumors (rhabdomyosarcoma) and injury. Cardiomyopathies affect the blood pumping ability and normal electrical rhythm of the heart muscle. This chapter describes structural aspects of the three types of muscle within a functional and molecular framework conducive to the understanding of the pathophysiology of myopathies.

Skeletal muscle

Muscle cells or fibers form a long multinucleated syncytium grouped in bundles surrounded by connective tissue sheaths and extending from the site of origin to their insertion (Figure 7-1).

The **epimysium** is a dense connective tissue layer ensheathing the **entire muscle**. The **perimysium** derives from the epimysium and surrounds bundles or **fascicles** of muscle cells. The **endomysium** is a delicate layer of reticular fibers and extracellular matrix surrounding **each muscle cell**. Blood vessels and nerves use these connective tissue sheaths to reach the interior of the muscle. An extensive capillary network, flexible to adjust to contraction-relaxation changes, invests individual skeletal muscle cell.

The connective tissue sheaths blend and radiating muscle fascicles interdigitate at each end of a muscle with regular dense connective tissue of the tendon to form a **myotendinous junction**. The tendon anchors into a bone through the periosteal Sharpey's fibers.

Characteristics of the skeletal muscle cell or fiber

Skeletal muscle cells are formed in the embryo by the fusion of myoblasts that produce a postmitotic, multinucleated **myotube**. The myotube matures into the long muscle cell with a diameter of 10 to 100 μm and a length of up to several centimeters.

The plasma membrane of the muscle cell (called the **sarcolemma**) is surrounded by a **basal lamina** and **satellite cells** (Figure 7-2). We discuss the significance of satellite cells in muscle regeneration.

The sarcolemma projects long, finger-like pro-

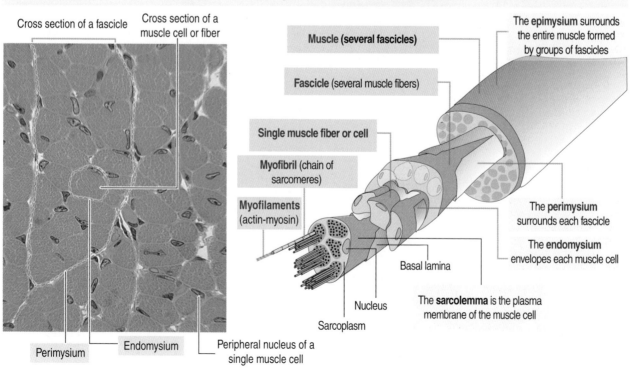

Figure 7-1. General organization of the skeletal muscle

Cross section of a fascicle

Cross section of a muscle cell or fiber

Perimysium

Endomysium

Peripheral nucleus of a single muscle cell

Muscle (several fascicles)

Fascicle (several muscle fibers)

Single muscle fiber or cell

Myofibril (chain of sarcomeres)

Myofilaments (actin-myosin)

The **epimysium** surrounds the entire muscle formed by groups of fascicles

The **perimysium** surrounds each fascicle

The **endomysium** envelopes each muscle cell

Basal lamina

Nucleus

Sarcoplasm

The **sarcolemma** is the plasma membrane of the muscle cell

Figure 7-2. **Skeletal muscle (striated)**

The cytoplasm of the muscle cell or fiber contains an elaborate and regular arrangement of **myofibrils**, each organizing alternating short segments of differing refractive index: **dark A bands and light I bands**.

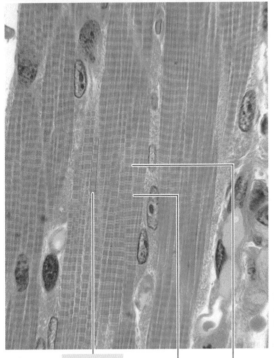

Cross section of a skeletal muscle cell with peripheral nucleus

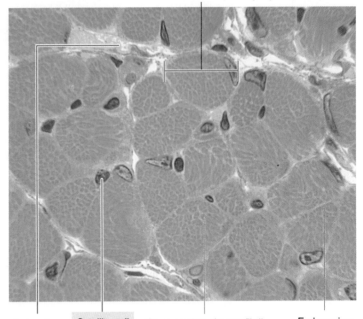

Perimysium   Satellite cell   Cross section of a myofibril   Endomysium

Myofibril   Dark band   Light band

Myofilaments are components of a myofibril. There are two major classes of myofilaments: (1) the thin **actin** filaments; (2) the thicker **myosin** filaments. The cross-banded pattern of striated (skeletal or cardiac) muscle is due to the orderly arrangement of actin and myosin filaments. Actin is the predominant component of the I band. Myosin is the main component of the A band. I and A bands form a **sarcomere**, which extends between two adjacent Z disks.

Peripherally located nucleus   Sarcomere   Z disk (band or line)   Sarcoplasm   **Myofibril**   Sarcolemma coated by basal lamina

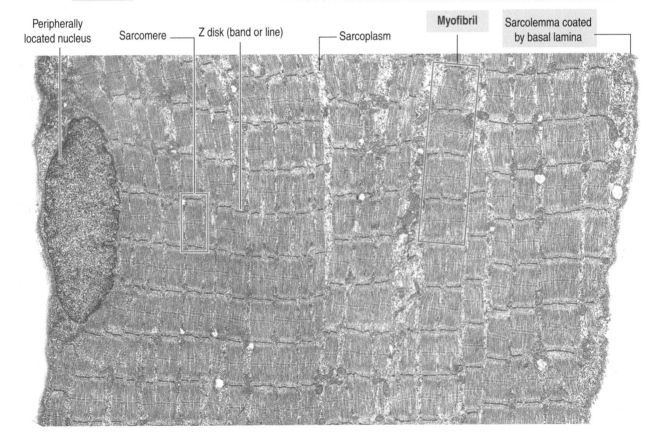

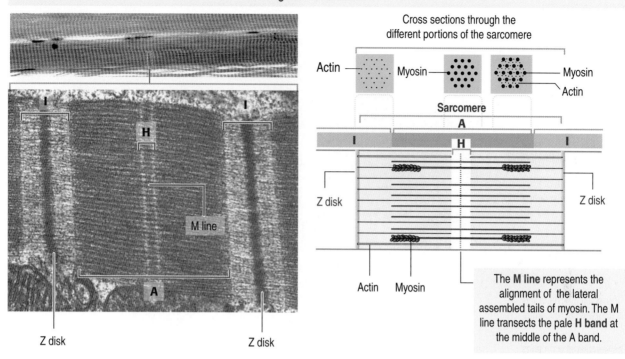

Figure 7-3. Sarcomere

Cross sections through the different portions of the sarcomere

Actin — Myosin Myosin — Actin

Sarcomere

A

I   H   I

Z disk   Z disk

Actin   Myosin

The **M line** represents the alignment of the lateral assembled tails of myosin. The M line transects the pale **H band** at the middle of the A band.

Z disk   Z disk

---

cesses, called **transverse tubules** or **T tubules**, into the cytoplasm of the cell, the **sarcoplasm**. T tubules make contact with membranous sacs or channels, the **sarcoplasmic reticulum**.

The sarcoplasmic reticulum contains high concentrations of Ca^{2+}. The site of contact of the T tubule with the sarcoplasmic reticulum cisternae is called a **triad** because it consists of **two lateral sacs of the sarcoplasmic reticulum and a central T tubule**.

The many nuclei of the muscle fiber are located at the **periphery** of the cell, just under the sarcolemma.

About 80% of the sarcoplasm is occupied by myofibrils surrounded by **mitochondria** (called **sarcosomes**). Myofibrils are composed of two major filaments formed by contractile proteins: **thin filaments** contain **actin**, and **thick filaments** are composed of **myosin** (see Figure 7-2).

Depending on the type of muscle, mitochondria may be found parallel to the long axis of the myofibrils, or they may wrap around the zone of thick filaments. Thin filaments insert into each side of the Z disk (also called **band**, or **line**) and extend from the **Z disk** into the **A band**, where they alternate with thick filaments.

The myofibril: A repeat of sarcomere units

The **sarcomere** is the basic contractile unit of striated muscle (Figure 7-3). Sarcomere repeats are represented by **myofibrils** in the sarcoplasm of skeletal and cardiac muscle cells.

The arrangement of thick (myosin) and thin (actin) myofilaments of the sarcomere is largely responsible for the banding pattern observed under light and electron microscopy (see Figures 7-2 and 7-3). Actin and myosin interact and generate the contraction force. The Z disk forms a **transverse sarcomeric scaffold** to ensure the efficient transmission of the generated force.

Thin myofilaments measure 7 nm in width and 1 μm in length and form the **I band**. Thick filaments measure 15 nm in width and 1.5 μm in length and are found in the **A band**.

The A band is bisected by a light region called the **H band** (see Figures 7-3 and 7-4). The major component of the H band is the enzyme **creatine kinase**, which catalyzes the formation of ATP from creatine phosphate and adenosine diphosphate (ADP). We discuss later how creatine phosphate maintains steady levels of ATP during prolonged muscle contraction.

Running through the midline of the H band is the **M line**. M-line striations correspond to a series of bridges and filaments linking the bare zone of thick filaments. Thin filaments insert into each side of the **Z disk**, whose components include α-**actinin**.

Components of the thin and thick filaments of the sarcomere

F-actin, the thin filament of the sarcomere, is doublestranded and twisted. F-actin is composed of globular monomers (**G-actin**; see Cytoskeleton in Chapter 1, Epithelium).

As you recall, G-actin monomers bind to each other in a head-to-tail fashion, giving the filament polarity, with barbed (plus) and pointed (minus) ends. The

Figure 7-4. Skeletal muscle cell

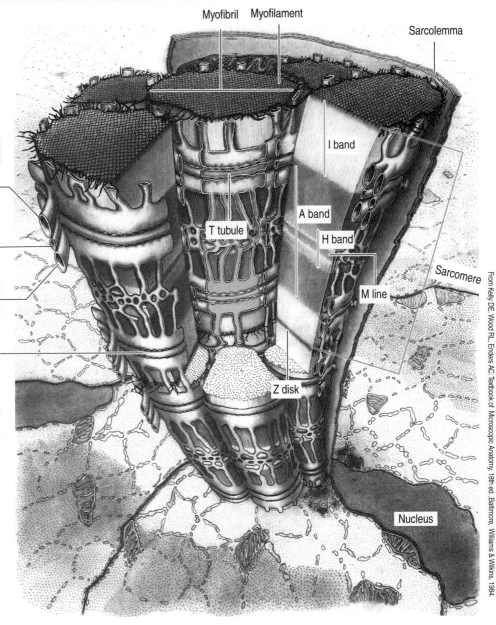

Myofibril   Myofilament

Sarcolemma

Triad (at the A-I junction)

Terminal cisterna of the sarcoplasmic reticulum

Invagination of the sarcolemma (**T tubule**)

Terminal cisterna of the sarcoplasmic reticulum

The sarcolemma projects long, finger-like processes called **transverse tubules**, or **T tubules**, into the fiber. T tubules make contact with membranous sacs or channels, the **sarcoplasmic reticulum**.

I band

A band

H band

T tubule

M line

Sarcomere

Z disk

Nucleus

From Kelly DE, Wood RL, Enders AC: Textbook of Microscopic Anatomy, 18th ed., Baltimore, Williams & Wilkins, 1984.

barbed end of actin filaments inserts into the Z disk.

F-actin forms a complex with tropomyosin and troponins. **Tropomyosin** runs in the groove formed by F-actin strands. Tropomyosin consists of two nearly identical α-helical polypeptides twisted around each other. Each molecule of tropomyosin extends for the length of **seven actin monomers** and binds the **troponin complex** (Figure 7-5).

Troponin is a complex of three proteins: **troponin I, C,** and **T.**

1. **Troponin T** binds the complex to tropomyosin.

2. **Troponin I** inhibits the binding of myosin to actin.

3. **Troponin C** binds Ca^{2+} and is found only in striated muscle.

Myosin II, the major component of the thick filament, has adenosine triphosphatase (ATPase) activity (it hydrolyzes ATP) and binds to F-actin, the major component of the thin filament, in a reversible fashion.

Myosin II consists of two identical **heavy chains** and two pairs of **light chains** (Figure 7-6; see Cytoskeleton in Chapter 1, Epithelium). At one end, each heavy chain forms a globular head. Two different light chains are bound to each head: the **essential light chain** and the **regulatory light chain**.

The globular head has three distinct regions:

1. An actin-binding region.

2. An ATP-binding region.

3. A light chain–binding region.

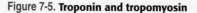

Figure 7-5. Troponin and tropomyosin

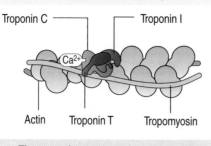

Troponin C — Troponin I

Actin — Troponin T — Tropomyosin

The troponin-tropomyosin-actin complex

Tropomyosin consists of two nearly identical α-helical polypeptides twisted around each other. Tropomyosin runs in the groove formed by F-actin strands. Each molecule of tropomyosin extends for the length of seven actin monomers and binds the troponin complex.

Troponin is a complex of three proteins: **troponin I, C**, and **T**. Troponin T binds the complex to tropomyosin. Troponin I inhibits the binding of myosin to actin. Troponin C binds Ca^{2+} and is found only in striated muscle.

Myosin II, like the other molecular motors kinesins and dyneins, use the chemical energy of ATP to drive conformational changes that generate motile force. As you recall, kinesins and dyneins move along microtubules. Myosins move along actin filaments to drive muscle contraction.

Nebulin (Figure 7-7) is a giant protein (600–900-kd) associated with thin (F-actin) filaments; it inserts into the Z disk and acts as a **stabilizer** required for maintaining the length of F-actin.

Titin (see Figure 7-7) is a very large protein with a molecular mass in the range of millions determined by about 34,000 amino acids. Each molecule associates with thick (myosin) myofilaments and inserts into the Z disk, extending to the bare zone of the myosin filaments, close to the M line.

Titin has the following functions:

1. It controls the assembly of the thick myofilament by acting as a template.

2. It regulates sarcomere elasticity by establishing a spring-like connection between the end of the thick myofilament and the Z disk.

3. It limits the displacement range of the sarcomere in tension.

Z disks are the insertion site of actin filaments of the sarcomere. A component of the Z disk, α-**actinin**, anchors the barbed end of actin filaments to the Z disk.

Desmin is a 55-kd intermediate (10-nm) filaments protein with three major roles essential for the maintenance of the mechanical integrity of the contractile apparatus in skeletal, cardiac, and smooth muscle:

1. Desmin stabilizes myofibrils and nuclei. Desmin filaments encircle the Z disks of myofibrils and are linked to the Z disk and to each other by **plectin** filaments (Figure 7-8). Desmin filaments extend from the Z disk of one myofibril to the adjacent myofibril, forming a supportive latticework. Desmin filaments also extend from the sarcolemma to the nuclear envelope.

2. Desmin links myofibrils to the sarcolema. Desmin inserts into specialized sarcolemma-associated plaques, called **costameres**. Costameres, acting in concert with the dystrophin-associated protein complex, transduce contractile force from the Z disk to the basal lamina, maintain the structural integrity of the sarcolemma, and stabilize the position of myofibrils in the sarcoplasm.

3. Desmin determines the distribution and function of mitochondria in skeletal and cardiac muscle. In the absence of desmin, proper mitochondrial positioning is lost and mitochondrial function is compromised, leading to cell death by either energy deprivation or release of proapoptotic cytochrome *c*.

The heat shock protein α**B-crystallin** protects desmin filaments from stress-induced damage. Desmin, plectin, and αB-crystallin form a mechanical stress protective network at the Z-disk level.

Mutations in these three proteins determines the destruction of myofibrils after repetitive mechanical stress, conducive to the development of dilated cardiomyopathy, skeletal myopathy and smooth muscle defects.

Mechanism of muscle contraction

During muscle contraction, the muscle shortens about one third of its original length. The relevant aspects of muscle shortening are summarized in Figure 7-9 as follows:

1. The **length** of the thick and thin filaments **does not change** during muscle contraction (the length of the A band and the distance between the Z disk and the adjacent H band are constant).

Figure 7-6. Myosin II

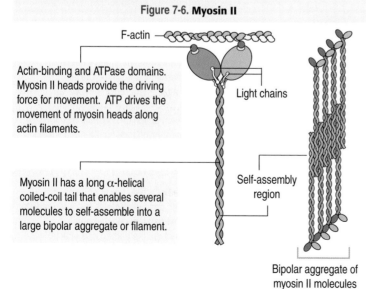

F-actin

Actin-binding and ATPase domains. Myosin II heads provide the driving force for movement. ATP drives the movement of myosin heads along actin filaments.

Light chains

Myosin II has a long α-helical coiled-coil tail that enables several molecules to self-assemble into a large bipolar aggregate or filament.

Self-assembly region

Bipolar aggregate of myosin II molecules

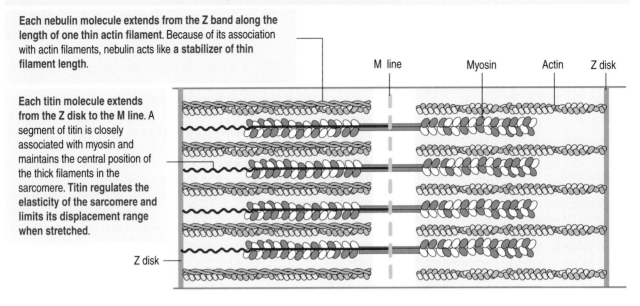

Figure 7-7. Sarcomere: Nebulin and titin

Each nebulin molecule extends from the Z band along the length of one thin actin filament. Because of its association with actin filaments, nebulin acts like **a stabilizer of thin filament length.**

Each titin molecule extends from the Z disk to the M line. A segment of titin is closely associated with myosin and maintains the central position of the thick filaments in the sarcomere. **Titin regulates the elasticity of the sarcomere and limits its displacement range when stretched.**

M line   Myosin   Actin   Z disk

Z disk

2. The **length of the sarcomere decreases** because thick and thin filaments slide past each other (the size of the H band and I band decrease).

3. The force of contraction is generated by the process that moves one type of filament past adjacent filaments of the other type.

Creatine phosphate: A back up energy source
Creatine phosphate is a back up mechanism to maintain steady levels of ATP during muscle contraction. Consequently, the concentration in muscle of free

ATP during prolonged contraction does not change too much.

Figure 7-10 provides a summary of the mechanism of regeneration of creatine phosphate, which takes place in mitochondria and diffuses to the myofibrils, where it replenishes ATP during muscle contraction.

A depolarization signal travels along T tubules
We discussed that the **triad** consists of a transverse T tubule flanked by sacs of the sarcoplasmic reticulum, and that the sarcoplasm of a skeletal muscle cell is

Figure 7-8. Cytoskeletal protective network of a skeletal muscle cell

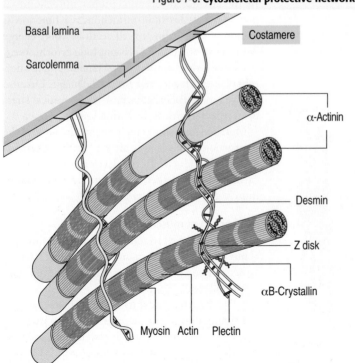

Basal lamina
Sarcolemma
Costamere
α-Actinin
Desmin
Z disk
αB-Crystallin
Myosin   Actin   Plectin

A mechanical stress protective network surrounds each myofibril at the Z disk.

Desmin, an intermediate filament extending from one myofibril to the other and anchored to the sarcolemma, encircles the Z disk of each sarcomere. Desmin inserts into specialized sarcolemma attachment regions known as **costameres**. Desmin filaments facilitate the coordinated contraction of individual myofibrils by holding adjacent myofibrils together and linking them to the sarcolemma.

Plectin links adjacent desmin filaments to each other.

αB-Crystallin, a heat shock protein associated with desmin, protects this intermediate filament from stress-induced damage.

α-Actinin anchors the barbed end of actin filaments to the Z disk.

Figure 7-9. Sarcomere: Muscle contraction and relaxation

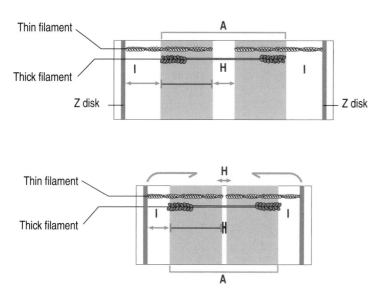

Thin filament
Thick filament
Z disk
A
I H I
Z disk

Resting striated muscle

The A band represents the distribution of the myosin thick filaments. The H band represents the myosin tail regions of the thick filaments not overlapping with thin actin filaments.

Actin thin filaments are attached to the Z disk. Two half–I bands, containing actin thin filaments, are seen at the right and left sides of the Z disk.

Thin filament
Thick filament
H
I I
A

During muscle contraction

The length of the myosin thick and thin actin filaments does not change.

The length of the sarcomere decreases because thick and thin filaments slide past each other. This is demonstrated by **a reduction in the length of the H band and the I band**.

packed with myofibrils (each consisting of a linear repeat of sarcomeres) with abundant mitochondria between them. How does a nerve impulse reach and deliver contractile signals to myofibrils located in the interior of the muscle cell?

An excitation-contraction signal is generated by **acetylcholine**, a chemical transmitter released from a nerve terminal in response to an **action potential**. Acetylcholine diffuses into a narrow gap, called the **neuromuscular junction**, between the muscle and a nerve terminal (Figure 7-11). The action potential spreads from the sarcolemma to the T tubules, which transport the excitation signal to the interior of the

muscle cell. Remember that **T tubules** form rings around every sarcomere of every myofibril **at the A-I junction**.

We discuss later that the companions of the T tubule, the channels of the sarcoplasmic reticulum, contain calcium ions. Calcium ions are released inside the cytosol to activate muscle contraction when the action potential reaches the T tubule. This excitation-contraction sequence occurs in about 15 milliseconds.

Neuromuscular junction: Motor end plate

The neuromuscular junction is a specialized structure formed by motor nerves associated with the target muscle and visible with the light microscope.

Once inside the skeletal muscle, the motor nerve gives rise to several branches. Each branch forms swellings called **presynaptic buttons** covered by **Schwann cells**. Each nerve branch **innervates a single muscle fiber**. The "parent" axon and all of the muscle fibers it innervates form a **motor unit**. Muscles that require fine control have few muscle fibers per motor unit. Very large muscles contain several hundred fibers per motor unit.

When myelinated axons reach the perimysium, they lose their myelin sheath but the presynaptic buttons remain covered with Schwann cell processes. A presynaptic button contains mitochondria and membrane-bound vesicles filled with the neurotransmitter **acetylcholine**. The neurotransmitter is released at dense areas on the cytoplasmic side of the axon membrane, called **active zones**.

Synaptic buttons occupy a depression of the muscle fiber, called the **primary synaptic cleft**. In this region, the sarcolemma is thrown into deep **junctional folds** (**secondary synaptic clefts**). Acetylcholine receptors

Figure 7-10. Creatine cycle during muscle contraction

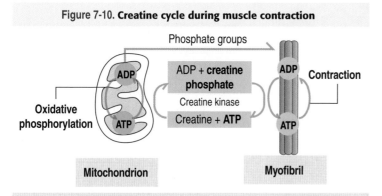

Phosphate groups
Oxidative phosphorylation
ADP
ATP
ADP + creatine phosphate
Creatine kinase
Creatine + **ATP**
ADP
ATP
Contraction
Mitochondrion
Myofibril

Creatine phosphate replenishes ATP levels during muscle contraction

ATP is a source of chemical energy during the interaction of myosin and actin resulting in muscle contraction. When the concentration of ATP decreases, a back up source of energy is the **hydrolysis of creatine phosphate**.

Creatine kinase catalyzes a reversible reaction generating **creatine** and **ATP** from the hydrolysis of creatine phosphate. Newly synthesized creatine phosphate derives from mitochondria and shuttles phosphate groups between mitochondria and the myofibril.

Figure 7-11. **Neuromuscular junction**

Neuromuscular junction: The motor end plate

Motor axons branch at the muscle cell surface. Each branch forms **presynaptic buttons** covered by Schwann cells. Buttons lie over the **motor end plate** region, separated from the sarcolemma by the **synaptic cleft**. Each presynaptic button in the end plate is associated to a **primary synaptic cleft**, a depression of the muscle

fiber formed by deep infoldings of the sarcolemma. **Junctional folds** (or secondary synaptic cleft) derive from the primary cleft. **Acetylcholine** receptors are found at the crest of the **junctional folds**. **Voltage-gated Na^{2+} channels** are found at the bottom of the junctional folds. The **basal lamina** contains **acetylcholinesterase**.

Box 7-A summarizes the functional types of skeletal muscle.

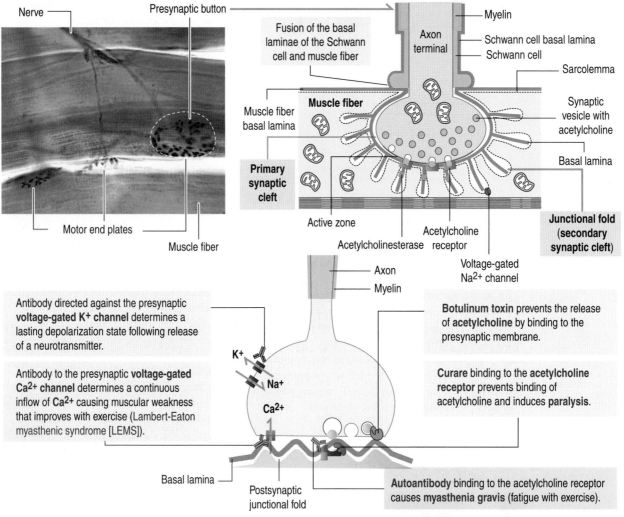

Nerve — Presynaptic button —

Fusion of the basal laminae of the Schwann cell and muscle fiber

Axon terminal

Myelin
Schwann cell basal lamina
Schwann cell
Sarcolemma

Muscle fiber

Muscle fiber basal lamina

Primary synaptic cleft

Synaptic vesicle with acetylcholine

Basal lamina

Active zone

Acetylcholinesterase — Acetylcholine receptor

Junctional fold (secondary synaptic cleft)

Motor end plates

Muscle fiber

Voltage-gated Na^{2+} channel

Axon
Myelin

Antibody directed against the presynaptic **voltage-gated K$^+$ channel** determines a lasting depolarization state following release of a neurotransmitter.

Antibody to the presynaptic **voltage-gated Ca^{2+} channel** determines a continuous inflow of Ca^{2+} causing muscular weakness that improves with exercise (Lambert-Eaton myasthenic syndrome [LEMS]).

K$^+$

Na$^+$

Ca^{2+}

Botulinum toxin prevents the release of **acetylcholine** by binding to the presynaptic membrane.

Curare binding to the **acetylcholine receptor** prevents binding of acetylcholine and induces **paralysis**.

Basal lamina —

Postsynaptic junctional fold

Autoantibody binding to the acetylcholine receptor causes **myasthenia gravis** (fatigue with exercise).

Box 7-A | Functional types of muscle fibers

• A single action potential through a motor unit determines a twitch contraction. Most skeletal muscles consist of muscle fibers of the twitch type capable of postural maintenance or brief bursts of intense activity.

• Most skeletal muscles in humans consist of a combination of different types of muscle fibers difficult to identify in routine histological preparations.

• Three main categories are distinguished. **Type I muscle fibers** are slow-contracting and fatigue-resistant (red fibers; rich in myoglobin and blood supply). **Type IIA muscle fibers** are fast-contracting and moderately fatigue-resistant (white fibers). **Type IIB muscle fibers** are fast-contracting and not fatigue-resistant.

• Type I, type IIA, and type IIB muscle fibers contain myosin heavy-chain isoforms differing in the rate of ATPase activity. ATPase histochemistry enables identification of the different types of muscle fibers.

are located at the crests of the folds and **voltage-gated Na$^+$ channels** are down into the folds (see Figure 7-11).

The basal lamina surrounding the muscle fiber extends into the synaptic cleft. The basal lamina contains **acetylcholinesterase**, which inactivates acetylcholine released from the presynaptic buttons into acetate and choline. The basal lamina covering the Schwann cell becomes continuous with the basal lamina of the muscle fiber.

Clinical significance: Disorders of neuromuscular transmission

Synaptic transmission at the neuromuscular junction can be affected by **curare** and **botulinum toxin** (see Figure 7-11).

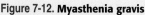

Figure 7-12. **Myasthenia gravis**

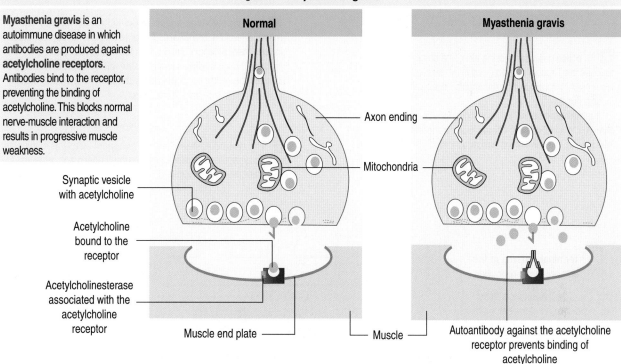

Myasthenia gravis is an autoimmune disease in which antibodies are produced against **acetylcholine receptors**. Antibodies bind to the receptor, preventing the binding of acetylcholine. This blocks normal nerve-muscle interaction and results in progressive muscle weakness.

Normal

Myasthenia gravis

Axon ending

Mitochondria

Synaptic vesicle with acetylcholine

Acetylcholine bound to the receptor

Acetylcholinesterase associated with the acetylcholine receptor

Muscle end plate

Muscle

Autoantibody against the acetylcholine receptor prevents binding of acetylcholine

---

Curare binds to the acetylcholine receptor and prevents binding of acetylcholine. Curare derivatives are used in surgical procedures in which muscle paralysis is necessary.

Botulinum toxin, an exotoxin from the bacterium *Clostridium botulinum*, prevents the release of acetylcholine at the presynaptic end. Muscle paralysis and dysfunction of the autonomous nervous system occur in cases of food poisoning mediated by botulinum toxin.

Myasthenia gravis is an autoimmune disease in which antibodies are produced against acetylcholine receptors (Figure 7-12). Autoantibodies bind to the receptor, preventing the binding of acetylcholine. This blocks normal nerve-muscle interaction and results in progressive muscle weakness.

Calcium controls muscle contraction

In the absence of Ca^{2+}, muscle is relaxed and the troponin-tropomyosin complex blocks the myosin binding site on the actin filament.

When a depolarization signal arrives, Ca^{2+} exits the terminal cisternae of the sarcoplasmic reticulum with the help of the **ryanodine-sensitive Ca^{2+} channel** (Figure 7-13). In the sarcomere, Ca^{2+} binds to troponin C and causes a change in configuration of the troponin-tropomyosin complex. As a result, the myosin-binding site on the actin filament is exposed. Myosin heads bind to the actin filament, and hydrolysis of ATP occurs.

As we have seen, steady levels of ATP rely on the

mitochondrial supply of creatine phosphate and the availability of creatine kinase (see Figure 7-10). **Creatine kinase** is an enzyme found in soluble form in the **sarcoplasm** and also is a component of the **M-line region** of the H band. Creatine kinase catalyzes the transfer of phosphate from creatine phosphate to ADP.

The energy of hydrolysis of ATP produces a change in the position of the myosin head, and the thin filaments are pulled past the thick filaments. Contraction results in the complete overlap of the A and I bands (see Figure 7-9). The contraction continues until Ca^{2+} is removed.

In summary, the sarcoplasmic reticulum, a network of smooth endoplasmic reticulum surrounding each myofibril (see Figure 7-4), stores Ca^{2+}. In response to depolarization signals, the sarcoplasmic reticulum releases Ca^{2+}. When membrane depolarization ends, Ca^{2+} is pumped back into the sarcoplasmic reticulum with the help of **Ca^{2+}-dependent ATPase**, and binds to the protein **calsequestrin** (see Figure 7-13). Contraction can no longer take place.

Pathology: Muscular dystrophies

Muscular dystrophies are a group of congenital muscular diseases characterized by muscle weakness, atrophy, elevation of serum levels of muscle enzymes, and destructive changes of muscle tissue (Figure 7-14).

Muscular dystrophies are caused by a deficiency in the **dystrophin-associated protein (DAP) complex.** The DAP complex consists of **dystrophin** and two

Figure 7-13. **Muscle contraction**

Membrane depolarization

1 An action potential passing along the sarcolemma reaches the T tubule system (triad in the skeletal muscle) responsible for transmitting the impulse deep within the muscle fiber.

Internally, the net negative charge of the membrane changes to a net positive charge. Such **depolarization** initiates the cell contraction cascade.

2 An **L-type voltage-sensitive Ca²⁺ channel** located in the membrane of the **transverse T tubule** changes its conformation in response to depolarization. This conformational change induces the **ryanodine-sensitive Ca²⁺ channel present in the membrane of the sarcoplasmic reticulum** to open and release Ca²⁺ stored in the terminal cisterna.

3 The **ryanodine-sensitive Ca²⁺ channel** (sensitive to the plant alkaloid ryanodine that blocks the channel) opens and releases Ca²⁺ from the sarcoplasmic reticulum store into the **sarcomere**.

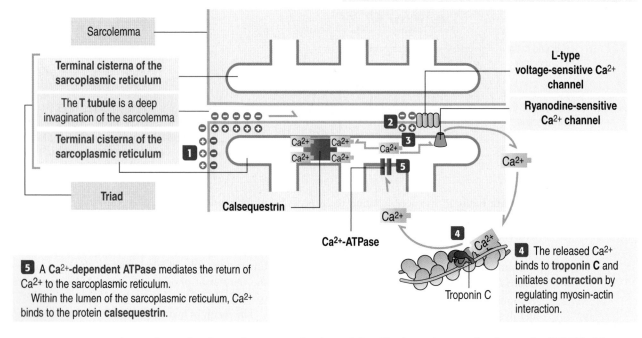

5 A **Ca²⁺-dependent ATPase** mediates the return of Ca²⁺ to the sarcoplasmic reticulum.

Within the lumen of the sarcoplasmic reticulum, Ca²⁺ binds to the protein **calsequestrin**.

4 The released Ca²⁺ binds to **troponin C** and initiates **contraction** by regulating myosin-actin interaction.

subcomplexes: the **dystroglycan complex** (α and β subunits), and the **sarcoglycan complex** (α, β, γ, δ, ε, and ζ subunits; for simplicity, only four subunits are shown in Figure 7-14).

Additional proteins include **syntrophins** (α, β1, β2, γ1, and γ2 subunits), **dystrobrevin**, and **sarcospan**. Dystrophin, syntrophins, and dystrobrevin are located in the sarcoplasm; dystroglycans, sarcoglycans, and sarcospan are transmembrane glycoproteins. Patients with a primary defect in dystroglycans and syntrophins have not been identified.

The most important muscle protein involved in muscular dystrophies is **dystrophin**, a 427-kd cytoskeletal protein associated to F-actin, dystroglycans, and syntrophins (see Figure 7-14). The absence of dystrophin determines the loss of components of the DAP complex. **The function of dystrophin is to reinforce and stabilize the sarcolemma during the stress of muscle contraction** by maintaining a mechanical link between the cytoskeleton and the extracellular matrix.

Deficiencies of dystrophin are characteristic of

Duchenne's muscular dystrophy (DMD). Most patients die young (in their late teens or early twenties) due to an involvement of the diaphragm and other respiratory muscles.

DMD is an X chromosome–linked recessive disorder caused by a mutation in the dystrophin gene. The disorder is detected in affected boys after they begin to walk. Progressive muscle weakness and wasting, sudden episodes of vomiting (caused by delayed gastric emptying), and abdominal pain are observed. A typical laboratory finding is **increased serum creatine kinase levels.**

Muscle biopsies reveal muscle destruction, **absence of dystrophin,** and a **substantial reduction of sarcoglycans,** and other components of the DAP complex, detected by immunohistochemistry.

Heterozygote female carriers may be asymptomatic or have mild muscle weakness, muscle cramps, and elevated serum **creatine kinase** levels. Women with these mutations may give birth to affected males or carrier females.

Sarcoglycanopathies in limb-girdle muscular

Figure 7-14. Muscular dystrophies

A mutation in **laminin-2** (which consists of α, β, and γ chains), causes congenital muscle dystrophy.

The **dystroglycan complex** links dystrophin to laminin-2. Dystroglycan-α binds to the α chain of laminin-2 (called merosin) and dystroglycan-β binds to dystrophin. Patients with a primary defect in dystroglycans have not been identified.

Structural muscle proteins associated with mutations causing myopathies

The **Z disk** is the insertion site of actin filaments of the sarcomere and plays a role in the transmission of tension through the myofibril.

Desmin filaments (intermediate filament protein) encircle the Z disks and are linked to them and to one another by **plectin** filaments. By this association, desmin: (1) **integrates mechanically the contractile action of adjacent myofibrils** and (2) **links the Z disk to the sarcolemma at costamere sites.**

The heat shock protein αB-crystallin protects desmin filaments from stress-dependent damage.

Note that **desmin, plectin, and αB-crystallin form a network around the Z disks**, thus protecting the integrity of the myofibrils during mechanical stress.

Mutations of desmin, plectin, and αB-crystallin cause fragility of the myofibrils and their destruction after continuous stress.

The components of the **sarcoglycan complex** are specific for cardiac and skeletal muscle.

Defects in the components of the complex cause autosomal recessive **limb-girdle muscular dystrophies** (known as **sarcoglycanopathies**).

Dystrophin reinforces and stabilizes the sarcolemma during the stress of muscle contraction by maintaining a link between the cytoskeleton and the extracellular matrix. When dystrophin is absent, the DAP complex is lost and the sarcolemma is disrupted, allowing unregulated calcium entry, which causes necrosis of the muscle fiber.

A deficiency in dystrophin is typical of **Duchenne's muscular dystrophy**, an X-linked recessive condition.

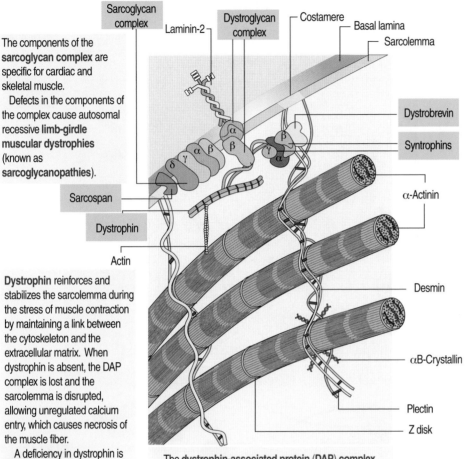

The **dystrophin-associated protein (DAP) complex** includes dystrophin and components of the dystroglycan complex and sarcoglycan complex.

Labels: Sarcoglycan complex, Laminin-2, Dystroglycan complex, Costamere, Basal lamina, Sarcolemma, Dystrobrevin, Syntrophins, α-Actinin, Desmin, αB-Crystallin, Plectin, Z disk, Sarcospan, Dystrophin, Actin

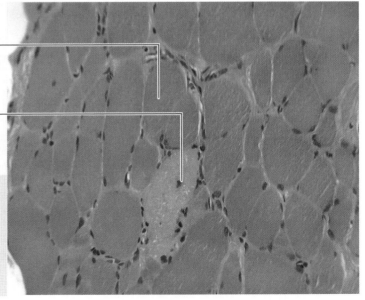

Cross section of a normal skeletal muscle fiber with the characteristic peripheral nucleus.

Degenerating skeletal muscle fiber in the early stages of Duchenne's muscular dystrophy.

Muscular dystrophies are a heterogeneous group of congenital muscle diseases characterized by severe muscle weakness and atrophy and destruction of muscle fibers.

The most important muscle protein involved in muscular dystrophies is **dystrophin**. The absence of dystrophin leads to a loss of the DAP complex (consisting of the subcomplexes **dystroglycan complex** and **sarcoglycan complex**).

Figure 7-15. **Satellite cells and muscle regeneration**

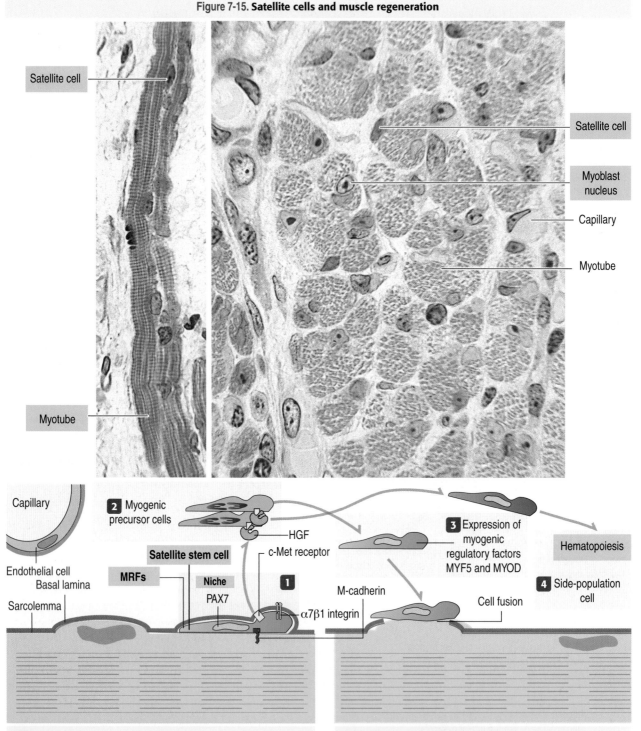

Satellite cell

Satellite cell

Myoblast nucleus

Capillary

Myotube

Myotube

Capillary

Myogenic precursor cells

2

HGF

c-Met receptor

Satellite stem cell

MRFs

Niche

PAX7

Endothelial cell
Basal lamina

Sarcolemma

1

α7β1 integrin

M-cadherin

3 Expression of myogenic regulatory factors MYF5 and MYOD

Hematopoiesis

4 Side-population cell

Cell fusion

1 A basal lamina surrounds both the skeletal muscle cell and associated **satellite stem cells (SCs)**. Mitotically quiescent SCs in the adult are located in a specific **niche** where they can reassume proliferation in response to stress or trauma.

SCs are attached to the basal lamina by α7β1 integrin and to the sarcolemma of the adjacent muscle fiber by M-cadherin. The activation of SCs involves the upregulation of the **myogenic regulatory factors (MRFs)**: (1) the bHLH (basic helix–loop–helix) transcription factor **MYF5**; (2) **MYOD** (myoblast determining protein); (3) **MYG6** (muscle-specific regulatory factor) and (4) **myogenin**. The transcription factor PAX7 regulates the expression of MRFs to induce

the proliferation and self-renewal of SCs. The **c-Met receptor** on the surface of SC has strong binding affinity for the chemotactic agent **HGF (hepatocyte growth factor)**.

2 Daughter cells of the activated SCs, **myogenic precursor cells**, undergo several rounds of cell division. HGF–c-Met binding induces the proliferation of the SCs.

3 Myogenic precursor cells, expressing the MRFs **MYF5** and **MYOD**, fuse with existing skeletal muscle cells or myotubes.

4 A population of stem cells in adult skeletal muscle, called **side-population cells**, has the capacity to differentiate into all major blood cell lineages.

dystrophies have mutations in the genes for α-, β-, γ-, and δ-sarcoglycan that cause defective assembly of the sarcoglycans, thus disrupting their interaction with the other dystroglycan complex proteins and the association of the sarcolemma with the extracellular matrix.

Pathology: Satellite cells and muscle regeneration
Muscle development involves the chain-like alignment and fusion of **committed muscle cell precursors**, the **myoblasts**, to form multinucleated **myotubes**.

Two important events occur during the commitment of the muscle cell precursor to myogenesis:

1. **The muscle cell precursor stops dividing**, determined by the up regulated expression of **myogenic regulatory factors (MRFs), MYF5 and MYOD,** and the **downregulation of PAX7**, a transcription factor.

2. **The muscle cell precursor initiates its terminal differentiation**, triggered by **myogenin** and **MRF4**.

Satellite cells are a resident stem cell population distinct from the myoblasts. They are involved in postnatal skeletal muscle maintenance, repair and regeneration They **are** attached to the surface of the myotubes. A **basal lamina** surrounds the satellite cell and the myotube (Figure 7-15).

Satellite cells occupy a **niche, a specific site where they reside for an indefinite period of time, produce a cell progeny and self-renew.** Satellite cells express α7β1 **integrin**, linking F-actin to the basal lamina, and **M-cadherin**, a calcium-dependent adhesion molecule attaching the satellite cell to the sarcolemma of the subjacent muscle fiber. Capillaries are located close to the satellite cells.

Satellite cells are mitotically **quiescent** in the adult, but can reassume self-renewal and proliferation in response to stress or trauma. **MRF** expression induces the proliferation of satellite cells. The descendants of the activated satellite cells, called **myogenic precursor cells**, undergo multiple rounds of cell division before they can fuse with existing or new myofibers.

Quiescent satellite cells express a receptor on their surface encoded by the proto-oncogene **c-Met**. The c-Met receptor has strong binding affinity for the chemotactic agent **HGF** (hepatocyte growth factor) bound to proteoglycans of the basal lamina. The HGF–c-Met complex up regulates a signaling cascade leading to proliferation of the satellite cells and the expression of MRFs, MYF5 and MYOD.

In addition to satellite cells as progenitors of the myogenic cells in adult skeletal muscle, a population of stem cells in adult skeletal muscle, called **side-population cells**, has the capacity to differentiate into all major blood cell lineages as well as myogenic satellite cells.

Side-population cells are present in bone marrow and may give rise to myogenic cells that can participate in muscle regeneration.

The pluripotent nature of satellite cells and side-population cells raises the possibility of stem cell therapy of a number of muscle injuries and degenerative diseases, including muscular dystrophy.

Neuromuscular spindle and Golgi tendon organ
The central nervous system continuously monitors the position of the limbs and the state of contraction of the various muscles. Muscles have a specialized encapsulated sensor called the **neuromuscular spindle** that contains sensory and motor components (Figure 7-16).

A neuromuscular spindle consists of 2 to 14 specialized striated muscle fibers enclosed in a fusiform sheath or capsule of connective tissue continuous with the endomysium that surrounds each of the muscle fibers. The fibers are 5 to 10 mm long and therefore much shorter than the surrounding contractile muscle fibers.

The specialized muscle fibers in the interior of the neuromuscular spindle are called **intrafusal fibers** to distinguish them from the nonspecialized **extrafusal fibers** (Latin *extra*, outside; *fusus*, spindle), the regular skeletal muscle fibers.

There are two kinds of intrafusal fibers designated by their histologic appearance:

1. **Nuclear bag fiber**, consisting of a nonstriated sensory bag-like region that contains many nuclei.

2. The **nuclear chain fiber**, so-called because its central portion contains a chain-like array of nuclei.

The distal portion of the nuclear bag fiber and nuclear chain fiber is made up of striated muscle components with contractile properties.

The neuromuscular spindle is innervated by two sensory axons. One of these axons is an **Ia fiber**. After crossing the capsule, the Ia fiber loses its myelin sheath and winds around the central portion of the nuclear bag and nuclear chain fibers forming an **annulospiral ending** or **primary sensory ending** (see Figure 7-16) to record the degree of tension of the intrafusal fibers.

The other sensory fiber, **type II sensory fiber**, terminates at the ends of the intrafusal fibers, distant from the midregion, in the form of **flower spay endings** or **secondary sensory ending**.

Motor nerve fibers derive from two types of motor neurons of the spinal cord:

1. The large-diameter **alpha (α) motor neurons**, that innervate the **extrafusal fibers** of muscles, outside the spindle (not shown in Figure 7-16).

2. The small-diameter **gamma (γ) motor neurons**, that innervate the **intrafusal fibers** within the spindle (A γ **motor fiber** shown in Figure 7-16).

The neuromuscular spindle is a receptor for the stretch reflex to adjust the muscle tone. It contributes

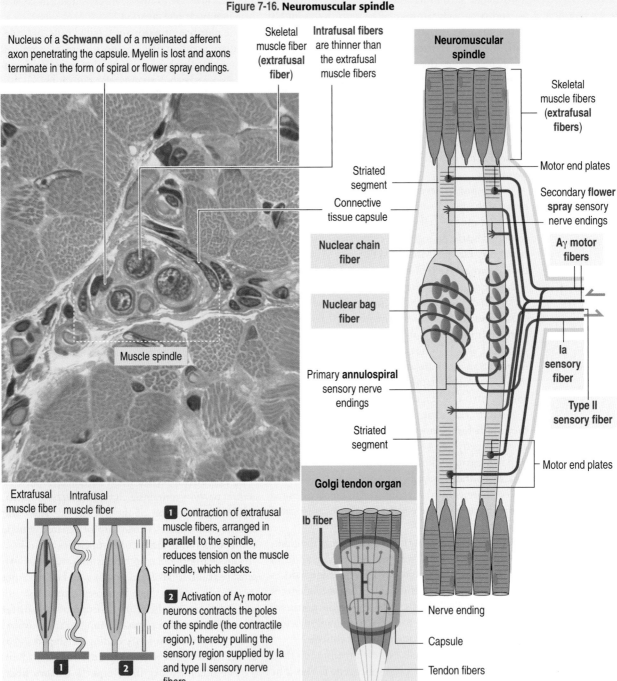

Figure 7-16. Neuromuscular spindle

Nucleus of a **Schwann cell** of a myelinated afferent axon penetrating the capsule. Myelin is lost and axons terminate in the form of spiral or flower spray endings.

Skeletal muscle fiber (**extrafusal fiber**)

Intrafusal fibers are thinner than the extrafusal muscle fibers

Neuromuscular spindle

Skeletal muscle fibers (**extrafusal fibers**)

Motor end plates

Secondary **flower spray** sensory nerve endings

Aγ motor fibers

Striated segment

Connective tissue capsule

Nuclear chain fiber

Nuclear bag fiber

Primary **annulospiral** sensory nerve endings

Striated segment

Ia sensory fiber

Type II sensory fiber

Motor end plates

Muscle spindle

Golgi tendon organ

Extrafusal muscle fiber

Intrafusal muscle fiber

1 Contraction of extrafusal muscle fibers, arranged in **parallel** to the spindle, reduces tension on the muscle spindle, which slacks.

2 Activation of Aγ motor neurons contracts the poles of the spindle (the contractile region), thereby pulling the sensory region supplied by Ia and type II sensory nerve fibers.

Ib fiber

Nerve ending

Capsule

Tendon fibers

---

to the clinical test of **tendon reflexes**, such as the **knee jerk** (rapid extension of the knee following tapping of the patellar tendon).

How does the neuromuscular spindle work? (see Figure 7-16). Intrafusal muscle fibers are in **parallel** with the extrafusal muscle fibers. When the extrafusal muscle fibers contract (shorten), the neuromuscular spindle becomes slack. If the spindle remains slack, no further information about changes in **muscle length** can be transmitted to the spinal cord.

This situation is corrected by a feedback control mechanism by which the sensory region of the spindle

activates gamma motor neurons, which contract the poles of the spindle (the contractile region). Consequently, the spindle stretches.

In addition to the neuromuscular spindle, **Golgi tendon organs** or **neurotendinous spindles** (see Figure 7-16), located at muscle-tendon junctions, provide information about the **tension** or force of contraction of the skeletal muscle.

Each Golgi tendon organ is surrounded by a connective tissue capsule that encloses a few collagen fibers of the tendon. About 12 or more muscle fibers, in series with the adjacent muscle fibers, insert into

Figure 7-17. **Interaction of cardiac muscle cells or cardiocytes**

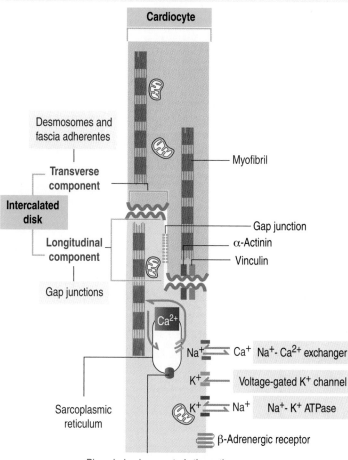

Phospholamban controls the active transport of Ca²⁺ into the lumen of the sarcoplasmic reticulum

the intracapsular tendon fibers. The axon of a **Ib fiber** pierces the caspsule, enters the receptor and branches in contact with the tendon fibers. The sensory endings are stimulated by **tension** in the tendon.

Afferent signals from the Golgi tendon organ reach the spinal cord and an inhibitory signal, from alpha motor neurons, relaxes the corresponding muscle under tension.

This regulatory response protects against the possibility of muscular damage that may result from excessive and strong muscle contraction. Note that, in contrast, the neuromuscular spindle responds to changes in the **length** of the intrafusal fibers.

One last point: the neuromuscular spindle, the Golgi tendon organ and paccinian corpuscles associated with the capsules of the synovial joins are examples of **proprioceptors** (Latin, *proprius*, one's own; *capio*, to take), structures that inform how the body is positioned and moves in space.

Cardiac muscle

Cardiac cells (or **cardiocytes**) are branched cylinders, 85 to 100 μm long, approximately 15 μm in diam-

eter (Figures 7-17 and 7-18), with a **single centrally located nucleus** (Figure 7-19).

The organization of contractile proteins is the same as that found in skeletal muscle. However, the cytomembranes exhibit some differences:

1. T tubules **are found at the level of the Z disk**, and are substantially larger than those of skeletal muscle found at the A-I junction.

2. The sarcoplasmic reticulum is not as extensive as that of skeletal muscle.

3. **Diads**, rather than the triads seen in skeletal muscle, are typical in cardiocytes (see Figure 7-18). A diad consists of a T tubule interacting with just one sarcoplasmic reticulum cisterna (instead of two opposite cisternae, as in skeletal muscle).

4. **Mitochondria are more abundant in cardiac muscle** than in skeletal muscle and contain numerous cristae.

The cardiocytes are joined end-to-end by specialized junctional complexes called **intercalated disks** (see Figure 7-17). Intercalated disks have a steplike arrangement, with **transverse components** that run **perpendicular** to the long axis of the cell and **longitudinal components** running in **parallel** to the cardiocyte for a distance that corresponds to one or two sarcomeres before it turns again to form another transverse component (see Figure 7-18).

The transverse component consists of:

1. **Desmosomes**, which mechanically link cardiac cells.

2. **Fasciae adherentes**, which contain α-**actinin** and **vinculin** and provide an insertion site for the actin-containing thin filaments of the last sarcomere of each cardiocyte (see Figure 7-19).

Gap junctions, restricted to the **longitudinal component** of the intercalated disk, enable ionic communication between cells leading to synchronous muscle contraction.

The terminal fibers of the conducting system of the heart are specialized, glycogen-rich **Purkinje fibers**. Compared with the contractile fibers, Purkinje fibers are larger, paler-stained, and contain fewer myofibrils (see Chapter 12, Cardiovascular System, for additional details).

Clinical significance: Transport proteins on the sarcolemma of cardiocytes

The sarcolemma of the cardiocyte contains specific **transport proteins** (see Figure 7-17) controlling the release and reuptake of ions critical for systolic contractile function and diastolic relaxation.

Active transport of Ca²⁺ into the lumen of the sarcoplasmic reticulum by Ca²⁺-dependent ATPase is controlled by **phospholamban**. The activity of phospholamban is regulated by phosphorylation. Changes in the amount and activity of phospholamban, regulated by **thyroid hormone**, may alter

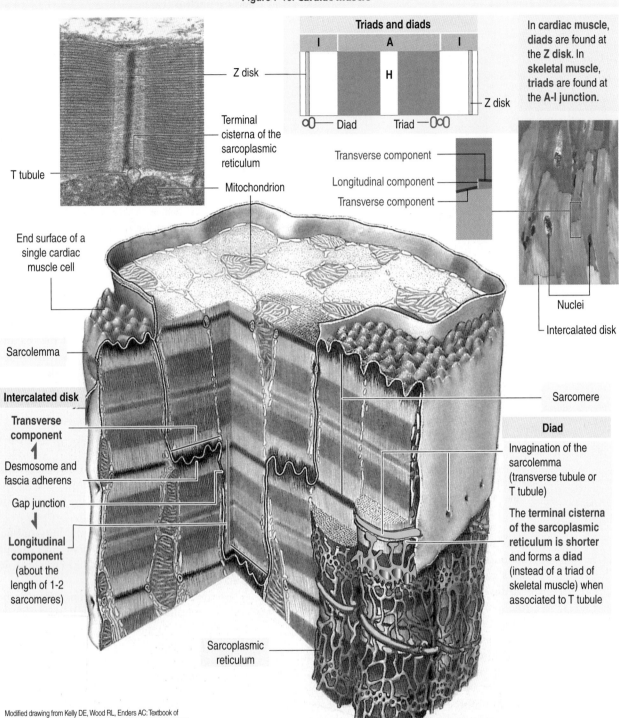

Figure 7-18. **Cardiac muscle**

Triads and diads

In cardiac muscle, **diads** are found at the **Z disk**. In skeletal muscle, **triads** are found at the **A-I junction**.

Z disk

Terminal cisterna of the sarcoplasmic reticulum

T tubule

Mitochondrion

Transverse component

Longitudinal component

Transverse component

Nuclei

Intercalated disk

End surface of a single cardiac muscle cell

Sarcolemma

Intercalated disk

Transverse component

Desmosome and fascia adherens

Gap junction

Longitudinal component (about the length of 1-2 sarcomeres)

Sarcomere

Diad

Invagination of the sarcolemma (transverse tubule or T tubule)

The terminal cisterna of the sarcoplasmic reticulum is shorter and forms a diad (instead of a triad of skeletal muscle) when associated to T tubule

Sarcoplasmic reticulum

Modified drawing from Kelly DE, Wood RL, Enders AC: Textbook of Microscopic Anatomy, 18th Edition, Baltimore: Williams & Wilkins, 1984.

diastolic function during heart failure and thyroid disease. An increase in heart rate and cardiac output is observed in hyperthyroidism. We discuss the role of phospholamban in Graves' disease (hyperthyroidism) in Chapter 19, Endocrine System.

Additional transporters, including the **Na⁺- Ca²⁺ exchanger** and **voltage-gated K⁺ channels**, regulate the intracellular levels of K⁺ and Na⁺. β-**Adrenergic receptor** is also present in the sarcolemma.

General Pathology: Myocardial infarction

Myocardial infarction is the consequence of a loss of blood supply to the myocardium caused by an obstruction of an atherosclerotic coronary artery. The clinical outcome depends on the anatomic region affected and the extent and duration of disrupted blood flow.

Irreversible damage of cardiocytes occurs when the loss of blood supply lasts more than 20 minutes.

Figure 7-19. **Cardiac muscle cell or cardiocyte**

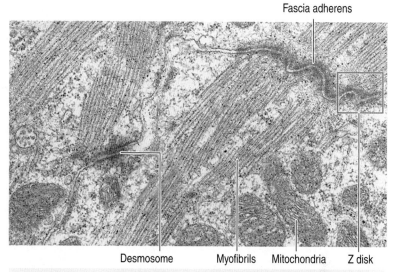

Intercalated disk

Central nucleus

Fascia adherens

Desmosome   Myofibrils   Mitochondria   Z disk

Intercalated disks are unique to cardiac muscle cells. The **transverse component** of the intercalated disk connects adjacent cardiac muscle cells. It is formed by the **fascia adherens** (plural, fasciae adherentes) and **desmosomes**. **Actin** and α-**actinin** attach to the fascia adherens. **Desmin** is linked to the desmosome. The **longitudinal component** of the intercalated disk runs parallel to the myofilaments and the long axis of the cell before it turns again to form another transverse component. **Gap junctions** are the major structures of the longitudinal component (not shown).

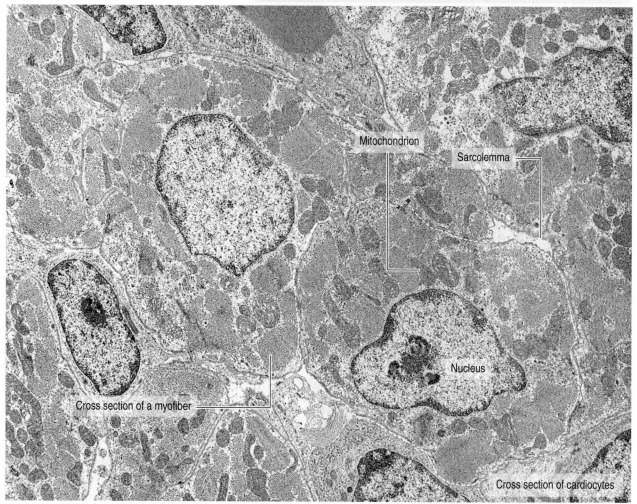

Mitochondrion

Sarcolemma

Nucleus

Cross section of a myofiber

Cross section of cardiocytes

Figure 7-20. **Myocardial infarction**

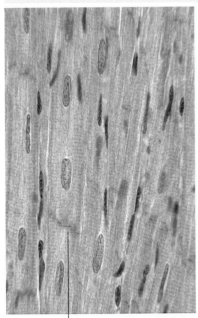

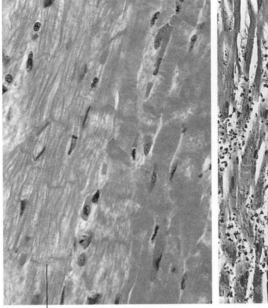

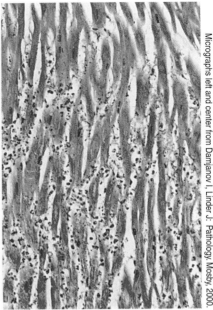

Micrographs left and center from Damjanov I, Linder J: Pathology. Mosby, 2000.

Intercalated disk

Normal cardiac tissue consists of branching and anastomosing striated cardiocytes with a central nucleus and intracellular contractile myofilaments. Intercalated disks join individual cardiocytes.

Myocardial ischemia caused by occlusion of the coronary artery results within the first **24 hours** in the necrosis of cardiocytes.

Cardiocytes display an eosinophilic cytoplasm lacking the characteristic intracellular striations detected in the adjacent unaffected cardiocytes. The nuclei are pyknotic (Greek, *pyknos*, dense, thick; *osis,* condition) and irregularly shaped. Lactic dehydrogenase-1 and creatine kinase MB*, released from dead cardiocytes, are detected in serum.

Serum levels of these enzymes remain elevated days after the myocardial infarction.

Three days later, the necrotic cardiocytes are surrounded by neutrophils.

After 3 weeks (not shown), capillaries, fibroblasts, macrophages, and lymphocytes are observed in the necrotic area. After 3 months, the infarcted region is replaced by scar tissue.

*Creatine kinase (CK) is composed of two dimers, M and B. CK-MM isoenzyme predominates in skeletal muscle and heart. CK-BB is present in brain, lung, and other tissues. CK-MB is characteristic of myocardium.

If blood flow is restored in less than 20 minutes, an event known as **reperfusion**, cardiocyte cell viability is maintained. Timing is critical for implementing early therapy to reestablish blood flow by using thrombolytic agents. The histologic changes of myocardial infarction are summarized in Figure 7-20.

Creatine kinase and its **MB isoenzyme (CK-MB)** are conventional markers of myocardial necrosis. A more sensitive marker is **cardiocyte-specific troponin I** not expressed in skeletal muscle. An increase of troponin I in the serum of patients with acute coronary syndromes provides prognostic information on increased risk of death and enables treatment to decrease further myocardial necrosis.

Smooth muscle

Smooth muscle may be found as sheets or bundles in the walls of the gut, bile duct, ureters, urinary bladder, respiratory tract, uterus, and blood vessels.

Smooth muscle differs from skeletal and cardiac muscle: smooth muscle cells are **spindle-shaped,** **tapering cells** with a **central nucleus** (Figure 7-21).

The perinuclear cytoplasm contains mitochondria, ribosomes, rough endoplasmic reticulum, a Golgi apparatus, a latticework of thick **myosin** filaments, thin actin filaments, and intermediate filaments composed of desmin and vimentin.

Actin and **intermediate filaments** insert into cytoplasmic and plasma membrane–associated structures rich in α-actinin, called **dense bodies.** Polyribosomes, instead of rough endoplasmic reticulum, participate in the synthesis of cytoskeletal proteins (Figures 7-21 and 7-22).

Invaginations of the plasma membrane, called **caveolae,** act as a primitive T tubule system, transmitting depolarization signals to the underdeveloped sarcoplasmic reticulum. The development of caveolae from **lipid rafts** and their diverse roles in several tissues are shown in Figure 7-22.

Smooth muscle cells are linked to each other by **gap junctions**. Gap junctions permit synchronous contraction of the smooth muscle.

Figure 7-21. **Smooth muscle cell**

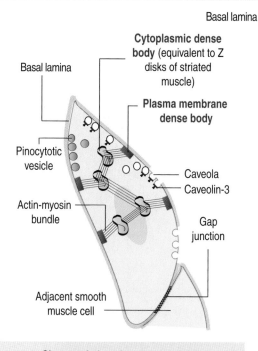

Basal lamina

Cytoplasmic dense body (equivalent to Z disks of striated muscle)

Plasma membrane dense body

Basal lamina

Pinocytotic vesicle

Caveola
Caveolin-3

Actin-myosin bundle

Gap junction

Adjacent smooth muscle cell

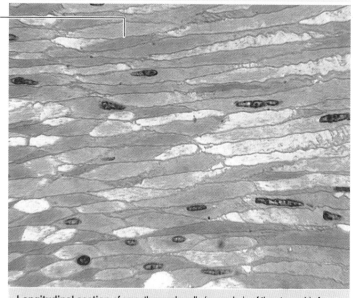

Longitudinal section of smooth muscle cells (muscularis of the stomach). A single oval nucleus is observed in the center of the cells. A **basal lamina** surrounds each smooth muscle cell.

Characteristics of smooth muscle

Smooth muscle is found in the walls of tubular organs, the walls of most **blood vessels**, the iris and **ciliary body** (eye), and **arrector pili muscle** (hair follicles), among other sites. It consists of fusiform individual cells or fibers with a **central nucleus**. Smooth cells in the walls of large blood vessels produce **elastin**.

Caveolae, depressions of the plasma membrane, are permanent structures involved in fluid and electrolyte transport (**pinocytosis**).

Caveolin-3, a protein encoded by a member of the caveolin gene family, is associated with **lipid rafts**. Complexes formed by caveolin-3 bound to **cholesterol** in a lipid raft invaginate and form caveolae. Caveolae detach from the plasma membrane to form **pinocytotic vesicles**.

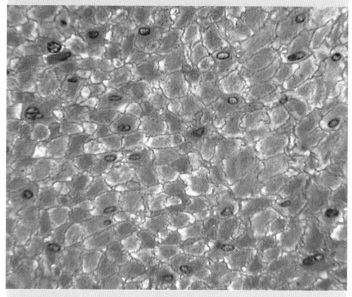

Cross section of smooth muscle cells. Depending on the section level, a central nucleus is observed in some of the muscle cells.

A **basal lamina** surrounds each muscle cell and serves to transmit forces produced by each cell.

Mechanism of smooth muscle contraction

The arrangement of the contractile proteins and the mechanism of contraction of smooth muscle differ from those of skeletal and cardiac muscle:

1. Actin and myosin filaments are not organized in sarcomeres as seen in cardiac and skeletal muscle.

2. **Smooth muscle cells do not contain troponin** but do contain tropomyosin, which binds to and stabilizes actin filaments.

3. Ca^{2+} ions that initiate contraction derive from outside the cell rather than from the sarcoplasmic reticulum.

4. **Myosin light-chain kinase** (instead of troponin, which is not present in smooth muscle cells) is responsible for the Ca^{2+} sensitivity of the contractile fibers in smooth muscle.

We have seen that the sliding of the myosin-actin complex in striated muscle is the basis for contraction (see Figure 7-9).

In smooth muscle, actin filaments and associated myosin attach to cytoplasmic and plasma membrane

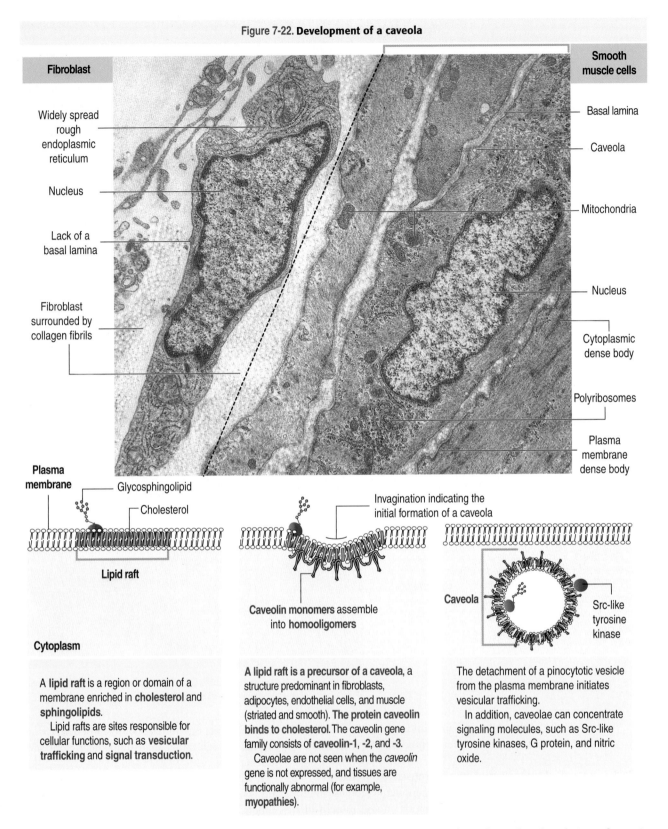

Figure 7-22. Development of a caveola

Fibroblast

Smooth muscle cells

Widely spread rough endoplasmic reticulum

Nucleus

Lack of a basal lamina

Fibroblast surrounded by collagen fibrils

Basal lamina

Caveola

Mitochondria

Nucleus

Cytoplasmic dense body

Polyribosomes

Plasma membrane dense body

Plasma membrane

Glycosphingolipid

Cholesterol

Lipid raft

Cytoplasm

A **lipid raft** is a region or domain of a membrane enriched in **cholesterol** and **sphingolipids**.
Lipid rafts are sites responsible for cellular functions, such as **vesicular trafficking** and **signal transduction**.

Invagination indicating the initial formation of a caveola

Caveolin monomers assemble into **homooligomers**

A lipid raft is a precursor of a caveola, a structure predominant in fibroblasts, adipocytes, endothelial cells, and muscle (striated and smooth). The protein caveolin binds to cholesterol. The caveolin gene family consists of **caveolin-1, -2, and -3**.
Caveolae are not seen when the *caveolin* gene is not expressed, and tissues are functionally abnormal (for example, **myopathies**).

Caveola

Src-like tyrosine kinase

The detachment of a pinocytotic vesicle from the plasma membrane initiates vesicular trafficking.
In addition, caveolae can concentrate signaling molecules, such as Src-like tyrosine kinases, G protein, and nitric oxide.

dense bodies, representing the equivalent of the Z disk of striated muscle. Dense bodies are attached to the plasma membrane through desmin and vimentin intermediate filaments.

When the actin-myosin complex contracts, their attachment to the dense bodies causes cell shortening.

Calcium-dependent phosphorylation of myosin regulatory light chains is responsible for the contraction of smooth muscle. We discuss this mechanism in Chapter 1, Epithelium, when we analyze the role of different myosins in the cell (review Figure 1-32).

Smooth muscle myosin is a **type II myosin**,

consisting of two heavy chains and two pairs of light chains. The myosin molecule is folded when dephosphorylated.

When type II myosin phosphorylates, it unfolds and assembles into filaments. The actin binding site on the myosin head is exposed and myosin can then bind to actin filaments to cause cell contraction.

Smooth muscle can be stimulated to contract by **nervous stimulation**, **hormonal stimulation**, or **stretch**. For example, intravenous **oxytocin** stimulates uterine muscle contractions during labor.

In response to an appropriate stimulus, there is an increase in cytoplasmic Ca^{2+}. Ca^{2+} binds to **calmodulin**. The Ca^{2+}-calmodulin complex activates **myosin light-chain kinase**, which catalyzes phosphorylation of the myosin light chain. When Ca^{2+} levels decrease, the myosin light chain is enzymatically dephosphorylated, and the muscle relaxes.

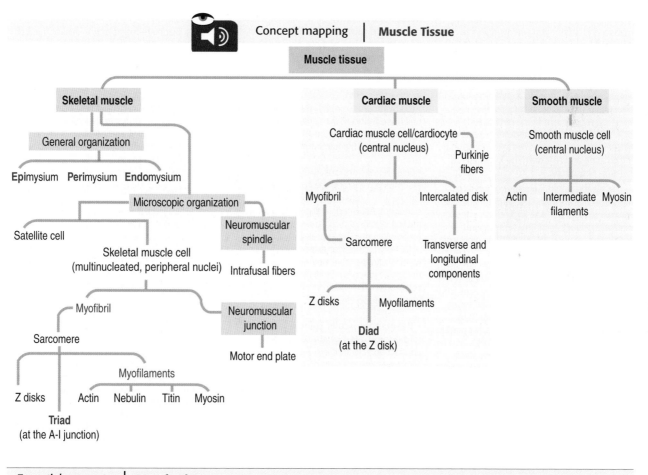

Concept mapping | Muscle Tissue

Essential concepts | Muscle Tissue

- There are three types of muscle:
  (1) Skeletal muscle.
  (2) Cardiac muscle.
  (3) Smooth muscle.
  Skeletal muscle is surrounded by the epimysium, a layer of dense connective tissue. The perimysium, derived from the epimysium, surrounds bundles or fascicles of muscle cells, also called muscle fibers. Each muscle fiber within a fascicle is surrounded by the endomysium, a thin layer of reticular fibers and extracellular matrix closely associated to a basal lamina enveloping each muscle cell.
  Skeletal muscle cells are multinucleated cells, resulting from the fusion of myoblasts.

Each skeletal muscle cell is surrounded by a plasma membrane (called sarcolemma). The sarcolemma is surrounded by a basal lamina and satellite cells.

The sarcolemma projects long processes, called transverse tubules or T tubules, deep into the cytoplasm (called sarcoplasm). The sarcoplasm contains mitochondria (called sarcosomes). Each T tubule is flanked by sacs of the endoplasmic reticulum (called sarcoplasmic reticulum) forming a tripartite structure called a triad, found at the junction of the A band and I band. The nuclei are located at the periphery of the cell. An important component of the sarcoplasm is the myofibril.

A **myofibril** is a linear repeat of **sarcomeres**.

Each sarcomere consists of two major cytoskeletal **myofilaments**: actin and myosin.

Note the difference between myofibril and myofilament. The arrangement of these two myofilaments generates a banding pattern (or striation), characteristic of skeletal and cardiac muscle tissue. There is an A band (dark) and I band (light). The A band is at the center of the sarcomere; the Z disk bisects the I band. The A band is bisected by the H band, which contains creatine kinase. The M line runs through the midline of the H band.

A sarcomere is limited by two adjacent Z disks. Actin inserts into each side of the Z disk. Myosin myofilaments do not attach to the Z disk. Actin is associated with the tropomyosin-troponin complex (formed by troponins I, C, and T) and nebulin. Myosin (called myosin II) consists of two identical heavy chains (with a globular head) and two pairs of light chains. The globular heads have an actin-binding region, and ATP-binding region, and a light chain–binding region. Titin is associated with myosin.

Each Z disk is encircled by the intermediate filament desmin. Desmin filaments are linked to each other by plectin. The desmin-plectin complex forms a lattice with the opposite ends attached to costameres in the sarcolemma. This arrangement stabilizes the myofibrils in the sarcoplasm during muscle contraction.

• During muscle contraction, the length of myosin and actin myofilaments does not change. The length of the sarcomere decreases because actin and myosin slide past each other, represented by a reduction in the width of the I band and H band. ATP is an energy source for muscle contraction. Creatine phosphate (produced in sarcosomes) is a back up mechanism to maintain steady levels of ATP during muscle contraction. Creatine kinase catalyzes a reversible reaction generating creatine and ATP from the hydrolysis of creatine phosphate.

Inside the muscle, a motor nerve gives rise to numerous branches, each innervating a single muscle cell. The motor nerve and its innervating branches form a **motor unit**.

An excitation-contraction signal is produced by the release of acetylcholine from a presynaptic button into a primary synaptic cleft, an invagination on the surface of a muscle cell coated with basal lamina containing acetylcholinesterase. The primary synaptic cleft forms secondary synaptic clefts, also covered by basal lamina. Crests of the secondary synaptic clefts contain acetylcholine receptors.

An action potential depolarizes the sarcolemma, and the action potential travels inside the muscle cell along T tubules, which are in contact with channels of the sarcoplasmic reticulum containing calcium. Calcium ions are released, bind to troponin C, and initiate contraction by regulating myosin-actin interaction. When depolarization ends, calcium ions are pumped back into the sarcoplasmic reticulum channels and bind to calsequestrin.

Botulinum toxin binds to the presynaptic membrane of the nerve terminal and blocks the release of acetylcholine. Curare binds to the acetylcholine receptor, prevents binding of acetylcholine, and induces muscle paralysis. In **myasthenia gravis**, an autoimmune disease that produces fatigue with exercise, autoantibodies bind to the acetylcholine receptor and prevent binding of acetylcholine.

• **Muscular dystrophies** are a group of congenital muscular diseases characterized by muscle weakness, atrophy, serum levels increases of muscle enzymes, and destructive changes in muscle tissue.

The following protein complexes, some of them part of the dystrophin-associated protein (DAP) complex, are present in the sarcoplasm or in the sarcolemma adjacent to the sarcoplasm. They provide mechanical stabilization during muscle contraction:

(1) Dystroglycan complex consists of dystroglycan-α and dystroglycan-β. Dystroglycan-α binds to the α chain of laminin-2, and dystroglycan-β binds to dystrophin. No primary defects in the dystroglycan complex have been identified.

(2) Sarcoglycan complex consists of six transmembrane subunits (α, β, γ, δ, ε, and ζ). **Sarcoglycanopathies** (for example, **limb-girdle muscular dystrophies**) are caused by defects in components of the sarcoglycan complex.

(3) Dystrophin binds the dystroglycan complex to actin in the sarcoplasm. **Duchenne's muscular dystrophy**, an X-linked recessive condition, is caused by a deficiency in dystrophin. The absence of dystrophin results in the loss of syntrophins and other components of the DAP complex.

(4) Dystrobrevin (α and β subunits), present in the sarcoplasm.

(5) Syntrophins (α, β1, β2, γ1, and γ2 subunits) are found in the sarcoplasm and bind to dystrophin and dystrobrevin.

(6) Sarcospan, a transmembrane protein.

• Satellite cells are closely associated to skeletal muscle cells and are covered by a basal lamina. In mature muscle, satellite cells are quiescent. Activated satellite cells activated by trauma or mechanical stress can self-renew and proliferate. The expression of myogenic regulatory factors (for example, Myf5 and MyoD) activates satellite cells, which become myogenic precursor cells (to form muscle cells) or side-population cells (to differentiate into hematopoietic cells).

• The **neuromuscular spindle** is a specialized encapsulated length sensor of muscle contraction. It is supplied by sensory and motor nerves and consists of specialized muscle fibers. Muscle fibers on the interior of the neuromuscular spindle are called intrafusal fibers to distinguish them from the nonspecialized extrafusal fibers, regular skeletal muscle fibers aligned in parallel with the intrafusal fibers.

There are two kinds of intrafusal fibers designated by their histologic appearance:

(1) Nuclear bag fiber, consisting of a non striated sensory bag-like central region that contains many nuclei and striated contractile elements at the ends of the fiber.

(2) Nuclear chain fiber, so-called because its central portion contains a chain-like array of nuclei, also has striated contractile ends.

When extrafusal fibers contract, the neuromuscular spindle becomes slack. This information is transmitted by sensory nerves to the spinal cord, which activates motor neurons that stretch the spindle.

This is the base of the clinical test of tendon reflexes (knee jerk).

In contrast to the neuromuscular spindle, the Golgi tendon organs are located in series with the extrafusal muscle fibers. They provide information about the force of contraction (tension) of the skeletal muscle.

• There are three major types of skeletal muscle fibers: red fibers (involved in maintenance of posture), white fibers (responsible for rapid contraction), and intermediate fibers (a combination of the characteristics of red and white fibers). Muscles contain a mixture of the three types of fibers.

• Cardiac muscle consists of branched cylindrical cells called cardiocytes. They contain a central nucleus and myofibrils in the cytoplasm. The organization of the sarcomere is similar to skeletal muscle. The following differences are observed:

(1) T tubules and short portions of the sarcoplasmic reticulum form diads (instead of triads).

(2) Diads are found at the level of the Z disk (instead of the A-I band junction).

(3) Mitochondria contain abundant cristae.

(4) Cardiocytes are joined end-to-end by intercalated disks.

(5) Intercalated disks display a steplike arrangement with a transverse portion (containing desmosomes and fasciae adherentes), and a longitudinal portion (where gap junctions are located).

A specialized type of cardiac fiber is the Purkinje fiber, a glycogen-rich cell with fewer myofibrils, involved in conductivity.

• Smooth muscle cells are found in the wall of the alimentary tube, urinary excretory passages, respiratory tract, uterus, and blood vessels.

Smooth muscle cells are spindle-shaped, tapering cells, with a central nucleus and surrounded by a basal lamina. We discussed the ability of smooth muscle cells to synthesize and secrete components of collagen and elastic fibers. The cytoplasm contains actin, myosin, and intermediate filaments.

A typical feature of muscle cells are caveolae, regarded as a primitive T tubule system.

Caveolae develop from lipid rafts, a domain in the plasma membrane enriched in cholesterol and sphingolipids. The protein caveolin binds to cholesterol. Caveolae are not seen when the *caveolin* gene is not expressed. The detachment of caveolae forms pinocytotic vesicles, involved in vesicular trafficking and signaling.

• The contraction of smooth muscle cells differs from skeletal and cardiac muscle cells.

Smooth muscle cells lack sarcomeres and troponin, and calcium ions initiate contraction from outside the cell, rather than from the sarcoplasmic reticulum.

Myosin light-chain kinase is responsible for the calcium sensitivity of the contractile actin-myosin component of smooth muscle. An equivalent to the Z disk of striated muscle are the dense bodies.

In response to a stimulus, an increase in cytoplasmic calcium binds to calmodulin. The calcium-calmodulin complex activates myosin light-chain kinase, which catalyzes phosphorylation of the myosin light chain and enables binding of activated myosin to actin.

8. Nervous Tissue

Anatomically, the nervous system can be divided into (1) the central nervous system (CNS) (the brain, spinal cord, and neural parts of the eye) and (2) the peripheral nervous system (PNS) (peripheral ganglia, nerves, and nerve endings connecting ganglia with the CNS and receptors and effectors of the body). The CNS and PNS are morphologically and physiologically different, and these differences are significant in areas such as neuropharmacology. The basic cell components of the CNS are neurons and glia. The PNS contains supporting cells called satellite cells and Schwann cells, analogous to the glial cells of the CNS. This chapter serves as an introduction to the Neuroscience course. In addition, the structure and function of the CNS and PNS are integrated with basic clinical and pathologic concepts of malformations and neurodegenerative diseases. The relevant molecular aspects involved in neurodegenerative diseases are integrated with structure and function.

Development of the nervous system

The CNS develops from the primitive ectoderm (Figure 8-1 and Box 8-A and Box 8-B). A simple epithelial disk, the **neural plate**, rapidly rolls into a hollow cylinder, the **neural tube**. This process is known as **neurulation**.

During this process, a specialized portion of the neural plate, the **neural crest**, separates from the neural tube and the overlying ectoderm. In later development, **the neural crest forms the neurons of the peripheral ganglia and other components of the PNS**. A defect in the closing of the neural tube causes different congenital malformations (see Box 8-C).

Neural crest cells remain separated from the neural tube and differentiate into:

1. The sensory neurons of the dorsal root and cranial nerve ganglia.

2. The sympathetic and parasympathetic motor neurons of the autonomic ganglia.

Some of these cells invade developing visceral organs and form the **parasympathetic** and **enteric ganglia** and the **chromaffin cells of the adrenal medulla**.

The Schwann cells and satellite cells of the dorsal root ganglia also develop from neural crest cells. Schwann cells ensheathe and myelinate the peripheral nerve fibers, and the satellite cells encapsulate the neuronal cell bodies in the dorsal root ganglia.

Figure 8-1. **Early stages of neural tube formation**

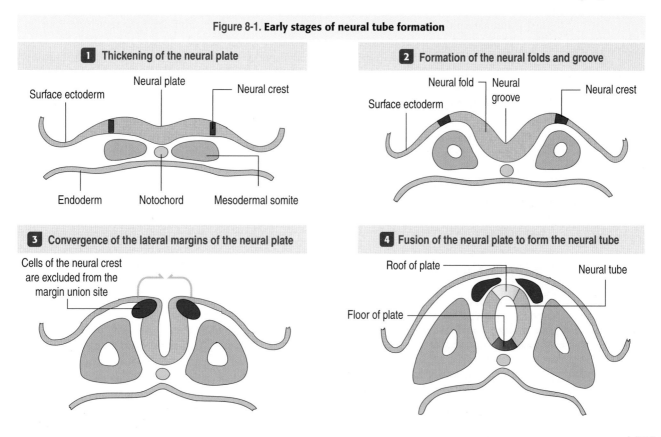

1 Thickening of the neural plate

Surface ectoderm · Neural plate · Neural crest · Endoderm · Notochord · Mesodermal somite

2 Formation of the neural folds and groove

Neural fold · Neural groove · Surface ectoderm · Neural crest

3 Convergence of the lateral margins of the neural plate

Cells of the neural crest are excluded from the margin union site

4 Fusion of the neural plate to form the neural tube

Roof of plate · Neural tube · Floor of plate

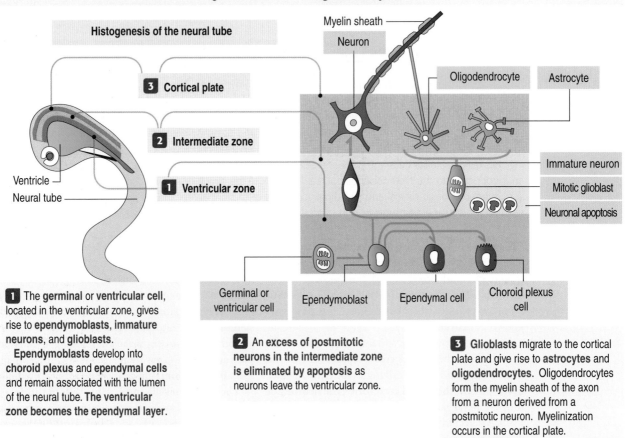

Figure 8-2. Neuronal and glial development

Histogenesis of the neural tube

Myelin sheath
Neuron
Oligodendrocyte
Astrocyte

3 Cortical plate

2 Intermediate zone

Immature neuron
Mitotic glioblast
Neuronal apoptosis

Ventricle
Neural tube
1 Ventricular zone

Germinal or ventricular cell
Ependymoblast
Ependymal cell
Choroid plexus cell

1 The **germinal** or **ventricular cell,** located in the ventricular zone, gives rise to **ependymoblasts, immature neurons,** and **glioblasts.**

Ependymoblasts develop into **choroid plexus** and **ependymal cells** and remain associated with the lumen of the neural tube. **The ventricular zone becomes the ependymal layer.**

2 An **excess of postmitotic neurons in the intermediate zone is eliminated by apoptosis** as neurons leave the ventricular zone.

3 **Glioblasts** migrate to the cortical plate and give rise to **astrocytes** and **oligodendrocytes.** Oligodendrocytes form the myelin sheath of the axon from a neuron derived from a postmitotic neuron. Myelinization occurs in the cortical plate.

The early neural tube consists of a pseudostratified columnar epithelium formed by three zones (Figure 8-2):

1. The **ventricular zone,** where progenitor cells give rise to most cells of the nervous tissue (except microglial cells).

2. The **intermediate zone,** where neurons migrate toward the cortical plate and where excess neurons are destroyed by apoptosis.

3. The **cortical plate,** the future gray matter of the cerebral cortex.

In the ventricular zone, **germinal** or **ventricular cells** proliferate rapidly during early development to give rise to **ependymoblasts** (remaining in the ventricular zone) **and glioblasts** and **postmitotic neurons** (migrating to the intermediate zone).

Immature neurons leave the ventricular zone, migrate to the intermediate zone, lose their capacity to undergo cell division, and differentiate into functional neurons. The neuronal migration mechanism and the consequences of abnormal migration are highlighted in Box 8-D.

During this differentiation process, a selection process, similar to that in the thymus for T cells (see Chapter 10, Immune-Lymphatic System), results in either neuronal heterogeneity or death. Neurons that become postmitotic in the intermediate zone reach the outer layers of the cortical plate and continue their differentiation.

Once the production of immature neurons is complete, the germinal or ventricular cells produce **glioblasts,** which differentiate into **astrocytes, oligodendrocytes,** and **ependymoblasts.** Ependymoblasts give rise to **ependymal cells,** lining the ventricular cavities of the CNS, and **choroid epithelial cells,** which are components of the choroid plexus.

Later, astrocytes develop vascular end-feet attached to blood vessels of the CNS. Coincident with vascularization is the differentiation of **microglia** from monocytes. Microglia respond to injury and become active phagocytic cells.

Box 8-A | Three cell sources of the CNS

• The ectoderm germ cell layer gives rise to three major structures: (1) the **surface ectoderm,** primarily the epidermis of the skin (including hair, nails, and sebaceous glands), lens and the cornea of the eye, anterior pituitary, and tooth enamel; (2) the **neural tube** (brain and spinal cord); and (3) the **neural crest.**
• Cells of the neural crest migrate away from the neural tube and generate components of the peripheral nervous system (Schwann cells and the sympathetic and parasympathetic nervous system), the adrenal medulla, melanocytes of the skin, odontoblasts of the teeth, and neuroglial cells.

Box 8-B | **Brain development**

• By the end of the 4th week, a flexion of the neural tube at the site of the future midbrain marks three regions: the **prosencephalon** (forebrain), **mesencephalon** (midbrain) and **rhombencephalon** (hindbrain). The prosencephalon expands on each side to form the **telencephalon** (cerebral hemispheres). By the 6th week, the **diencephalon**, the remaining part of the prosencephalon, gives rise to the **optic outgrowth** (retina and optic nerve of the eye). See diagram below.

• The **embryonic brainstem** consists at this point of the following components: (1) the **prosencephalon**, that gives rise, as indicated above, to the telencephalon (developing the **cerebral cortex** and **corpus striatum**) and the diencephalon (developing the **thalamus** and **hypothalamus**); (2) the **mesencephalon**, that originates the **midbrain**; and (3) the **rhombencephalon**, that gives rise to the **pons, cerebellum**, and **medulla oblongata**.

• Dilations of the neural canal within the cerebral hemispheres form the **lateral ventricles**, that communicate with the **third ventricle** located within the diencephalon. The **choroid plexus** (formed by a double layer of pia mater called **tela choroidea**) hangs from the roof of the third ventricle. The floor of the third ventricle consists of the **infundibulum**, the **tuber cinereum**, the **mammillary bodies** and the upper end of the midbrain. We come back to this portion of the third ventricle in Chapter 18, Neuroendocrine System, when we discuss the hypophysis. The **aqueduct** of the midbrain communicates the **third** and **fourth ventricles**.

• As shown in Figure 8-2, mitotic activity occurs in the **ventricular zone**, outside the lateral ventricle. Cells migrate to the **cortical plate** of each hemisphere and form the cerebral cortex.

• At the 14th week, **frontal, parietal, occipital** and **temporal lobes** can be identified. The **hippocampus**, a cerebral cortex extension from the medial portion of the hemisphere link, advances into the temporal lobe leaving behind the **fornix**, a trail of fibers. The concavity of the fornix embraces the **choroid fissure** (the insertion line of the **choroid plexus** extending into the lateral ventricle) and the **tail of the caudate nucleus** (whose head is attached to the **thalamus**).

• Major and minor commissures link the cerebral hemispheres: (1) The **corpus callosum**, a much larger commissure extending backward above the fornix, connects the corresponding areas of the cerebral cortex of the hemispheres. (2) The minor **anterior commissure** links the olfactory, or smell, left and right regions as well as the temporal lobes. (3) The **posterior commissure** and the **habenular commissure** are located in front of the pineal gland. (4) The **commissure of the fornix** connect one hippocampus to the other.

• The expanding portions of the cerebral hemispheres contact and fuse with the diencephalon. Consequently, the brainstem consists of three parts: midbrain, pons and medullas oblongata and fibers from the cerebral cortex extend directly to the brainstem. Fibers extending from the thalamus to the cerebral cortex and fibers from the cortex extending into the brainstem, split the **corpus striatum** into the **caudate nucleus** and the **lentiform nucleus**.

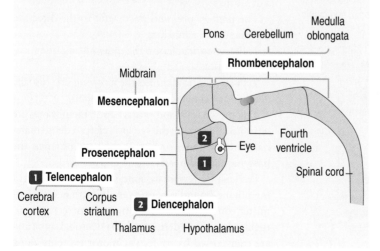

In later development, glioblasts give rise to **oligodendrocytes**, marking the beginning of **myelination** in the CNS. In contrast to neurons, glioblasts and derived glial cells retain the ability to undergo cell division.

The number of neurons in the human brain is in the range of 10^9 to 100^9. Up to 60% to 70% of these are present in the cerebral cortex. Most neurons are present at birth or shortly thereafter. As the brain continues to grow during the postnatal period, the number and complexity of interneuronal connections increase.

Cell types: Neurons

The functional unit of the nervous system is a highly specialized, excitable cell, the nerve cell or **neuron**. Neurons usually consist of three principal components (Figures 8-3 and 8-4):

1. **Soma** or **cell body**.
2. **Dendrites**.
3. **Axon**.

The soma contains the nucleus and its surrounding cytoplasm (also called **perikaryon**; Greek *peri*, around; *karyon*, nucleus).

The dendrites are processes that arise as multiple treelike branches of the soma, forming a **dendritic tree** collectively. The entire surface of the dendritic branches is covered by small protrusions called **dendritic spines**. Dendritic spines establish numerous axonal synaptic connections, as we will see later (see Figure 8-7).

Neurons have a **single axon** originating from the soma at the **axon hillock** and ending in a terminal arborization, the **telodendron**. Each terminal branch of the telodendron has an enlarged ending, the **synaptic terminal** or **synaptic bouton**.

Note that although dendrites and axons branch extensively, axons branch at their distal end (the telodendron), whereas dendrites are multiple extensions of the soma or cell body.

The surface membrane of the soma and the dendritic tree are specialized for the **reception** and **integration** of information, whereas the axon is specialized for the **transmission** of information in the form of an action potential or a nerve impulse.

Types of neurons

Different types of neurons can be identified on the basis of the **number** and **length** of **processes emerging from the soma** (Figure 8-5):

According to the **number of processes**, neurons can be classified as:

1. **Multipolar neurons**, which display **many processes** attached to a polygonal-shaped soma. The processes include a single axon and more than one dendrite. Multipolar neurons are the most abundant

neurons in the nervous system. Pyramidal cells of the cerebral cortex and Purkinje cells and neurons of the cerebellar cortex are two typical examples.

2. **Bipolar neurons** have **two processes**. Bipolar neurons are typical of the visual, auditory, and vestibular systems.

3. **Pseudounipolar neurons** have **only one short process** leaving the cell body. They are localized in sensory ganglia of cranial and spinal nerves. Embry-

onically, pseudounipolar neurons derive from bipolar neuroblasts, and the two neuronal processes fuse during later development (hence the prefix **pseudo**).

Based on the **length of the axon relative to the dendritic tree**, **multipolar neurons** can be subclassified into:

1. **Golgi type I** neurons, when the axon extends beyond the limits of the dendritic tree.

2. **Golgi type II** neurons, when an axon terminates in the immediate area of the cell body and does not extend beyond the limits of the dendritic tree. Small **stellate cells** of the cerebral cortex are Golgi type II cells.

Designation of groups of neurons and axons

In the CNS, functionally and structurally related neurons form aggregates called **nuclei**. An area called the **neuropil** can be found within a **nucleus** and between the neuronal cell bodies. The term neuropil designates an area with packed dendrites, axonal branches with abundant synapses, and glial cells.

Clusters of neurons arranged in a layer form a **stratum**, **lamina** or **layer** (cerebral cortex). When neurons form longitudinal groups, these groups are designated **columns** (see Box 8-E).

Bundles of axons in the CNS are called **tracts**, **fasciculi (bundles)**, or **lemnisci** (for example, the optic tract).

In the PNS, a cluster of neurons forms a **ganglion** (plural **ganglia**). A ganglion can be **sensory** (dorsal root ganglia and trigeminal ganglion) or **motor** (visceromotor or autonomic ganglia). **Axons derived from a ganglion** are organized as **nerves**, **rami** (singular **ramus**), or **roots**.

Synaptic terminals and synapses

The **synaptic terminal** (Figure 8-6) is specialized for the transmission of a chemical message in response to an action potential. The **synapse** is the junction between the **presynaptic terminal** of an axon and a **postsynaptic membrane** receptor surface, generally a dendrite.

The prefixes **pre-** and **post-** refer to the direction of synaptic transmission:

1. **Presynaptic** refers to the transmitting side (usually axonal).

2. **Postsynaptic** identifies the receiving side (usually dendritic or somatic, sometimes axonal).

The presynaptic and postsynaptic membranes are separated by a space: the **synaptic cleft**. A dense material coats the inner surface of these membranes: the **presynaptic and postsynaptic densities**.

Presynaptic terminals contain a large number of membrane-bound **synaptic vesicles** with neurotransmitter contents (40 to 100 nm in diameter) and **mitochondria**. They derive from the neuronal soma and are transported by molecular motor proteins along

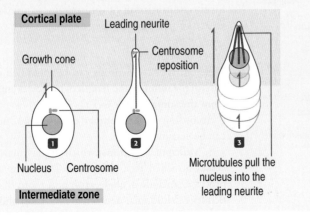

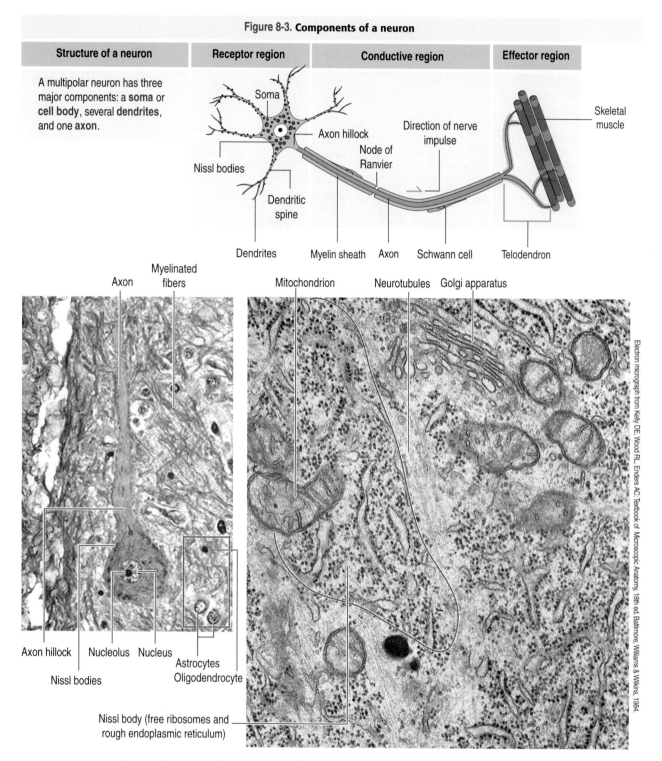

Figure 8-3. **Components of a neuron**

Structure of a neuron	Receptor region	Conductive region	Effector region

A multipolar neuron has three major components: a **soma** or **cell body**, several **dendrites**, and one **axon**.

Soma

Axon hillock

Node of Ranvier

Direction of nerve impulse

Skeletal muscle

Nissl bodies

Dendritic spine

Dendrites   Myelin sheath   Axon   Schwann cell   Telodendron

Axon   Myelinated fibers   Mitochondrion   Neurotubules   Golgi apparatus

Axon hillock   Nucleolus   Nucleus

Nissl bodies

Astrocytes
Oligodendrocyte

Nissl body (free ribosomes and rough endoplasmic reticulum)

Electron micrograph from Kelly DE, Wood RL, Enders AC: Textbook of Microscopic Anatomy, 18th ed. Baltimore, Williams & Wilkins, 1984.

the axon by an **axonal transport** mechanism (Figure 8-7). Presynaptic terminals contain mitochondria, components of the smooth endoplasmic reticulum, microtubules, and a few neurofilaments.

Synapses are classified by their **location on the postsynaptic neuron** (Figure 8-8) as follows:

1. **Axospinous** synapses are axon terminals facing a dendritic spine.

2. **Axodendritic** synapses are axon terminals on the shaft of a dendrite.

3. **Axosomatic** synapses are axon terminals on the soma of a neuron.

4. **Axoaxonic** synapses are axon terminals ending on axon terminals.

Clinical significance: Axonal transport of rabies virus
The role of the axonal cytoskeleton and motor proteins (kinesin and cytoplasmic dynein; see Figure 8-7) was discussed in the Cytoskeleton section of Chapter 1, Epithelium.

Figure 8-4. Components of a neuron

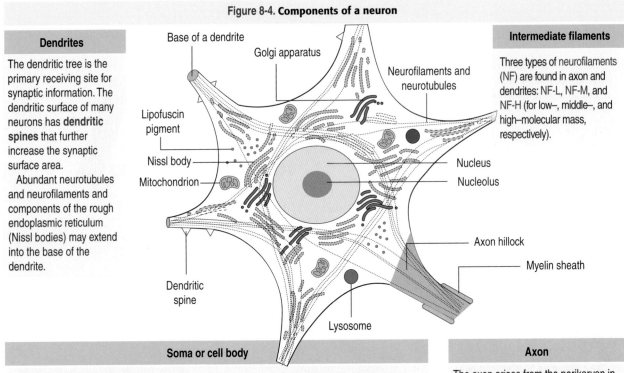

Dendrites

The dendritic tree is the primary receiving site for synaptic information. The dendritic surface of many neurons has **dendritic spines** that further increase the synaptic surface area.

Abundant neurotubules and neurofilaments and components of the rough endoplasmic reticulum (Nissl bodies) may extend into the base of the dendrite.

Intermediate filaments

Three types of neurofilaments (NF) are found in axon and dendrites: NF-L, NF-M, and NF-H (for low–, middle–, and high–molecular mass, respectively).

Base of a dendrite
Golgi apparatus
Neurofilaments and neurotubules
Lipofuscin pigment
Nissl body
Nucleus
Mitochondrion
Nucleolus
Axon hillock
Myelin sheath
Dendritic spine
Lysosome

Soma or cell body

The cell body or soma contains the nucleus and the surrounding cytoplasm or perikaryon. The soma, the trophic center of the neuron, contains organelles for the synthesis of proteins, phospholipids, and other macromolecules. A characteristic feature of the perikaryon is the **abundance of ribosomes**, free or associated with the endoplasmic reticulum. In light microscopic preparations with nucleic acid stains (basophilia), these structures appear as large clumps or **Nissl bodies**. A prominent **Golgi apparatus** and numerous mitochondria also reside in the perikaryon. **Neurotubules** and **neurofilaments** are distinctive features of the perikaryon. These cytoskeletal components extend through the perikaryon into the dendritic and axonal processes. Lysosomes and yellowish-pigmented lipofuscin granules are also present. The nucleus is usually large, with dispersed chromatin (euchromatin) and one or more prominent nucleoli.

Axon

The axon arises from the perikaryon in an area devoid of Nissl substance, the axon hillock. The initial segment of the axon is the site of action potential generation, the trigger zone. Contrary to the gradually tapering dendrite, the diameter of the axon remains constant throughout its length. In myelinated axons, a myelin sheath extends from the initial segment to the telodendron. Many axons have collateral branches.

We emphasize once more the **bidirectional transport of cargos** (including **synaptic vesicles** and **mitochondria**) along the axon:

1. **Kinesin-mediated anterograde axonal transport** of neurotransmitters, from the cell body toward the axon terminal and the plus end of microtubules.

2. **Cytoplasmic dynein-mediated retrograde axonal transport** of growth factors and recycling of axon terminal components from the axon terminal to the cell body and the minus end of microtubules (see Box 8-F).

As you recall, kinesin and dynein motor proteins have a globular motor domain in their heavy subunits that bind to microtubules and hydrolyses adenosine triphosphate (ATP) to propel cargos along the microtubule tracks. Cargos are attached to kinesin by the light subunit of the motor protein. Dynactin is a protein complex involved in the attachment of the cargo to dynein.

There are two types of axonal transport:

1. **Fast axonal transport**, responsible for the movement of vesicles and mitochondria.

2. **Slow axonal transport**, which is responsible for driving cytoplasmic proteins and cytoskeletal proteins for the assembly of microtubules and neurofilaments.

Axonal transport is important in the pathogenesis of neurologic infectious diseases. For example, the **rabies virus** introduced by the bite of a rabid animal

---

Box 8-E | Cerebral cortex

• The cerebral cortex, or pallium (Greek, *pallium*, shell), has a **laminar** (layered) and **columnar** organization that varies from one region to another. Cortex mapping permits to determine the histologic variations of different areas. The map of **Broadmann** divides the cortex into 47 areas.

• The **laminar organization** of neurons varies throughout the cortex. Three cellular laminae are observed in the **paleocortex** of the uncus (olfaction) and **archicortex** of the hyppocampus in the temporal lobe (memory). Six laminae are seen in the **neocortex** (*neopallium*) extending 90% of the brain. They are listed in **Figure 8-5**.

• In the **columnar organization**, neurons extend radially through all laminae. Cell columns, consisting of hundreds of neurons, represent the **functional units** or **modules** of the cortex.

• The main cell types are **pyramidal cells**, **spiny stellate cells**, and **smooth stellate cells**. **Bipolar cells** are found in the external laminae or layers.

Figure 8-5. Types of neurons: Bipolar, pseudounipolar, and multipolar neurons

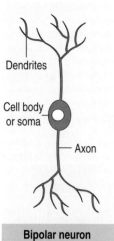

Dendrites

Cell body or soma

Axon

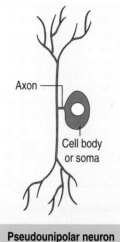

Axon

Cell body or soma

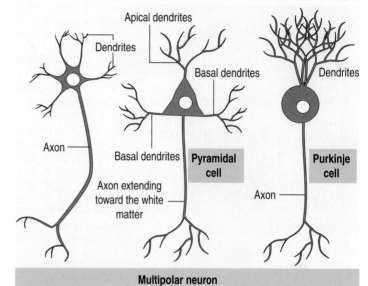

Apical dendrites

Dendrites

Basal dendrites

Dendrites

Axon

Basal dendrites

Pyramidal cell

Purkinje cell

Axon extending toward the white matter

Axon

Bipolar neuron

A single axon emerges from either side of the cell body.

Bipolar neurons are found in sensory structures such as the **retina**, the **olfactory epithelium**, and the **vestibular** and **auditory systems**.

Pseudounipolar neuron

A single axon divides a short distance from the cell body.

The short axon of pseudounipolar neurons (or unipolar) divides into two branches: The peripheral branch carries information from the periphery. The central branch ends in the spinal cord.

These cells are found in **sensory ganglia** of **cranial** and **spinal nerves**.

Multipolar neuron

Many dendrites and a single long axon emerge from the cell body.

Examples of multipolar neurons are the **pyramidal cell** of the cerebral cortex and the **Purkinje cell** of the cerebellar cortex.

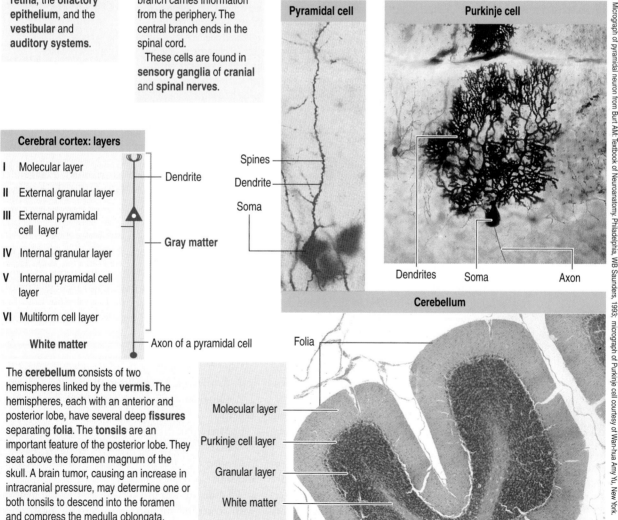

Pyramidal cell

Purkinje cell

Spines

Dendrite

Soma

Dendrites   Soma   Axon

Cerebellum

Cerebral cortex: layers

I   Molecular layer

II   External granular layer

III   External pyramidal cell layer

IV   Internal granular layer

V   Internal pyramidal cell layer

VI   Multiform cell layer

White matter

Dendrite

Gray matter

Axon of a pyramidal cell

Folia

Molecular layer

Purkinje cell layer

Granular layer

White matter

The **cerebellum** consists of two hemispheres linked by the **vermis**. The hemispheres, each with an anterior and posterior lobe, have several deep **fissures** separating **folia**. The **tonsils** are an important feature of the posterior lobe. They seat above the foramen magnum of the skull. A brain tumor, causing an increase in intracranial pressure, may determine one or both tonsils to descend into the foramen and compress the medulla oblongata.

Micrograph of pyramidal neuron from Burt AM: Textbook of Neuroanatomy. Philadelphia, WB Saunders, 1993; micrograph of Purkinje cell courtesy of Wan-hua Amy Yu, New York.

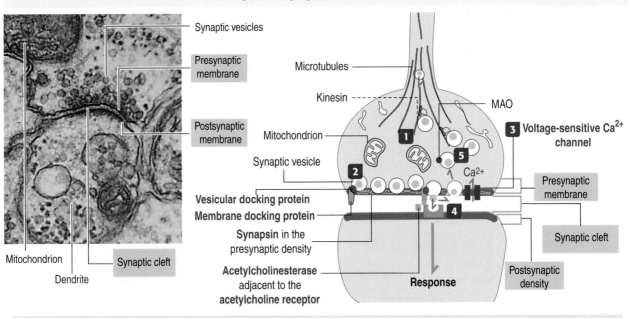

Figure 8-6. Synaptic transmission

Synaptic vesicles

Presynaptic membrane

Postsynaptic membrane

Synaptic cleft

Mitochondrion

Dendrite

Microtubules

Kinesin

MAO

Mitochondrion

Synaptic vesicle

3 Voltage-sensitive Ca²⁺ channel

Ca²⁺

Presynaptic membrane

Vesicular docking protein

Membrane docking protein

Synapsin in the presynaptic density

Synaptic cleft

Acetylcholinesterase adjacent to the **acetylcholine receptor**

Response

Postsynaptic density

Chemical synaptic transmission

1 Neuronal chemical messengers (acetylcholine, glutamate, γ-aminobutyric acid [GABA], and others) are stored in synaptic vesicles and transported to the synaptic terminal by anterograde transport (kinesin-mediated).

2 The membrane of a synaptic vesicle contains **vesicular docking proteins** that attach to **membrane docking proteins** of the presynaptic membrane (rich in **synapsin** filaments).

3 The depolarization of the axon terminal results in a high concentration of Ca²⁺ transported inside the terminal by a

voltage-sensitive Ca²⁺ channel. A surge of Ca²⁺ induces exocytosis of the synaptic vesicle.

4 The released chemical messenger in the synaptic cleft binds to a receptor (cholinergic or adrenergic) on the postsynaptic membrane to transmit information.

The chemical messenger is enzymatically degraded in the cleft (acetylcholine by acetylcholinesterase) or **5** taken up by receptor-mediated endocytosis (norepinephrine) and degraded by the mitochondrial enzyme monoamine oxidase (MAO).

Electron micrograph courtesy of Ilya I. Glezer, New York.

replicates in the muscle tissue from as little as 2 to 16 weeks or longer.

After binding to the **acetylcholine receptor**, the viral particles are mobilized by **retrograde axonal transport** to the cell body of neurons supplying the affected muscle.

The rabies virus continues to replicate within infected neurons and after the shedding of the virions by budding, they are internalized by the terminals of adjacent neurons.

Further dissemination of the rabies virus occurs in the CNS. From the CNS, the rabies virus is transported by **anterograde axonal transport** by the peripheral nerves to the salivary glands. The virus enters the saliva to be transmitted by the bite.

Painful **spasm of the throat muscles on swallowing** accounts for **hydrophobia** (aversion to swallowing water).

The retrograde axonal transport to the CNS of **tetanus toxin**, a protease produced by the vegetative spore form of *Clostridium tetani* bacteria after entering at a wound site, blocks the release of inhibitory mediators at spinal synapses. Spasm contraction of

the jaw muscles (known as **trismus**), exaggerated reflexes, and respiratory failure are characteristic clinical findings.

Glia: The "connective tissue" of the CNS

Glial cells (Greek *glia*, glue) are more numerous than neurons and retain the capacity to proliferate. Most brain tumors, benign or malignant, are of glial origin.

When the CNS is injured, glial cells mobilize, clean up the debris, and seal off the local area, leaving behind a "glial scar" (**gliosis**), which interferes with neuronal regeneration.

Glial cells include:

1. **Astrocytes**, derived from the **neuroectoderm**.

2. **Oligodendrocytes**, derived from the **neuroectoderm**.

3. **Microglia**, derived from the **mesoderm**.

Unlike neurons, glial cells do not propagate action potentials and their processes do not receive or transmit electrical signals.

The **function of glial cells** is **to provide neurons with structural support and maintain local conditions for neuronal function.**

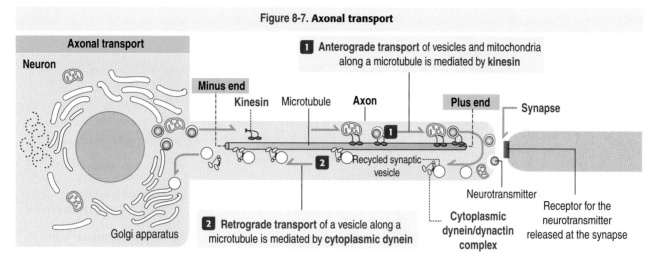

Figure 8-7. Axonal transport

Axonal transport

Neuron

Minus end

Kinesin | Microtubule | **Axon**

Plus end

Synapse

1 Anterograde transport of vesicles and mitochondria along a microtubule is mediated by **kinesin**

Recycled synaptic vesicle

Neurotransmitter

Receptor for the neurotransmitter released at the synapse

Cytoplasmic dynein/dynactin complex

2 Retrograde transport of a vesicle along a microtubule is mediated by **cytoplasmic dynein**

Golgi apparatus

Astrocytes

Astrocytes are observed in the CNS and are divided into two categories:

1. **Fibrous astrocytes**.
2. **Protoplasmic astrocytes**.

Fibrous astrocytes are found predominantly in **white matter** and have long thin processes with few branches. **Protoplasmic astrocytes** reside predominantly in **gray matter** and have shorter processes with many short branches. Astrocytic processes end in expansions called **end-feet** (Figure 8-9).

One of the distinctive features of astrocytes is the presence of a large number of **glial filaments** (**glial fibrillary acidic protein**, a class of intermediate filament studied in Chapter 1, Epithelium). Glial fibrillary acidic protein is a valuable marker for the identification of astrocytes by immunohistochemistry. Nuclei of astrocytes are large, ovoid, and lightly stained.

Most brain capillaries and the inner surface of the pia mater are completely surrounded by **astrocytic end-feet** (see Figure 8-9) forming the **glia limitans** (also called the glial limiting membrane). The close association of astrocytes and brain capillaries suggests a role in the regulation of brain metabolism.

Astrocytes surround neurons and neuronal processes in areas devoid of myelin sheaths (the internodal segments) and form the structural matrix for the nervous system.

Oligodendrocytes and Schwann cells: Myelinization

Oligodendrocytes are smaller than astrocytes and their nuclei are irregular and densely stained. The cytoplasm contains an extensive Golgi apparatus, many mitochondria, and a large number of microtubules. One function of oligodendrocytes is **axonal myelination**.

Several processes of a single oligodendrocytes envelop single axons and form a sheathlike covering (Figure 8-10). **The formation of this sheath is similar to that of Schwann cells in peripheral nerves.**

Myelin sheaths extend from the initial segments of axons to their terminal branches. The segments of myelin formed by individual oligodendrocyte processes are **internodes**. The periodic gaps between the internodes are the **nodes of Ranvier**.

A single oligodendrocyte has many processes and may form 40 to 50 internodes. The nodes of Ranvier are naked segments of axon between the internodal segments of myelin. This region contains a high concentration of voltage-gated sodium channels, essential for the **saltatory conduction** of the action potential. During saltatory conduction in the myelinated axons, the **action potential** "jumps" from one node to the next.

During the formation of the myelin sheath, a cytoplasmic process of the oligodendrocyte wraps around the axon and, after one full turn, the external surface of the glial membrane makes contact with itself,

---

Box 8-F | Neurotransmitters

- Incoming nerve impulses produce focal changes in the **resting membrane potential** of the neuron that spread along the membrane of dendrites and soma.

  Information is conducted along the processes as an electrical excitation (**depolarization**) generated across the cell membrane.
- As the resting membrane potential diminishes, a **threshold level** is reached, **voltage-gated Ca^{2+} channels** open, Ca^{2+} enters the cell, and at that point, the resting potential is reversed: the inside becomes positive with respect to the outside.
- In response to this reversal, the **Na^+ channel** closes and remains closed for the next 1 to 2 msec (the **refractory period**). Depolarization also causes the opening of **K^+ channels** through which K^+ leaves the cell, thus repolarizing the membrane.
- Neuron-to-neuron contacts or **synapses** are specialized for one-way transfer of excitation. Interneuronal communication occurs at a **synaptic junction**, the specialized communication site between the terminal of an axon of one neuron and the dendrite of another.
- When an action potential reaches the axon terminal, a chemical messenger or **neurotransmitter** is released to elicit an appropriate response.

Figure 8-8. Types of synapses

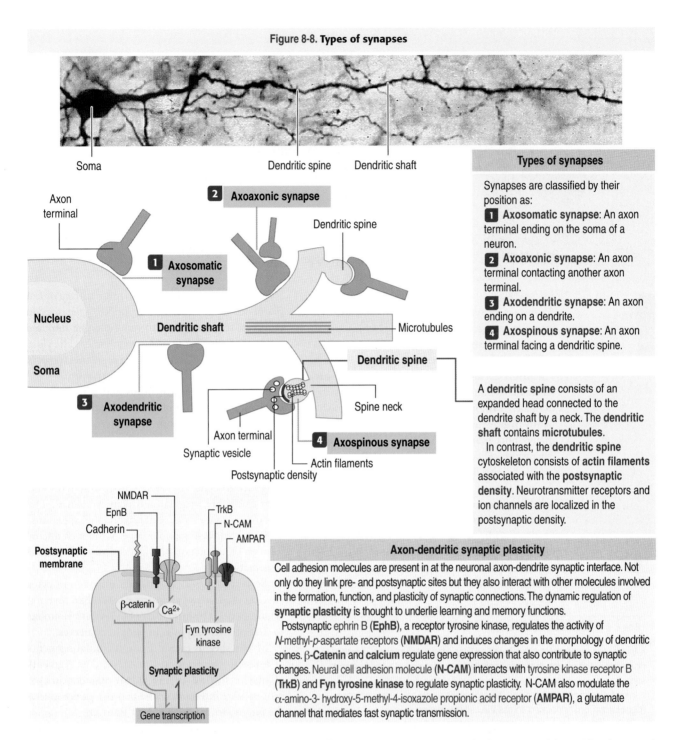

Soma | Dendritic spine | Dendritic shaft

Axon terminal

2 Axoaxonic synapse

Dendritic spine

1 Axosomatic synapse

Nucleus

Dendritic shaft ——— Microtubules

Soma

3 Axodendritic synapse

Dendritic spine

Spine neck

Axon terminal

Synaptic vesicle

4 Axospinous synapse

Actin filaments

Postsynaptic density

NMDAR
EpnB
Cadherin
TrkB
N-CAM
AMPAR

Postsynaptic membrane

β-catenin   Ca²⁺

Fyn tyrosine kinase

Synaptic plasticity

Gene transcription

Types of synapses

Synapses are classified by their position as:
1 **Axosomatic synapse**: An axon terminal ending on the soma of a neuron.
2 **Axoaxonic synapse**: An axon terminal contacting another axon terminal.
3 **Axodendritic synapse**: An axon ending on a dendrite.
4 **Axospinous synapse**: An axon terminal facing a dendritic spine.

A **dendritic spine** consists of an expanded head connected to the dendrite shaft by a neck. The **dendritic shaft** contains **microtubules**.
   In contrast, the **dendritic spine** cytoskeleton consists of **actin filaments** associated with the **postsynaptic density**. Neurotransmitter receptors and ion channels are localized in the postsynaptic density.

Axon-dendritic synaptic plasticity

Cell adhesion molecules are present in at the neuronal axon-dendrite synaptic interface. Not only do they link pre- and postsynaptic sites but they also interact with other molecules involved in the formation, function, and plasticity of synaptic connections. The dynamic regulation of **synaptic plasticity** is thought to underlie learning and memory functions.
   Postsynaptic ephrin B (**EphB**), a receptor tyrosine kinase, regulates the activity of *N*-methyl-*p*-aspartate receptors (**NMDAR**) and induces changes in the morphology of dendritic spines. β-**Catenin** and **calcium** regulate gene expression that also contribute to synaptic changes. Neural cell adhesion molecule (**N-CAM**) interacts with tyrosine kinase receptor B (**TrkB**) and **Fyn tyrosine kinase** to regulate synaptic plasticity. N-CAM also modulate the α-amino-3- hydroxy-5-methyl-4-isoxazole propionic acid receptor (**AMPAR**), a glutamate channel that mediates fast synaptic transmission.

---

forming the **inner mesaxon** (Figure 8-11).

As the oligodendrocyte process continues to spiral around the axon, the external surfaces fuse to form the first **intraperiod line**. At the same time, the cytoplasm is squeezed off from the intracellular space (like toothpaste from a tube), and the cytoplasmic surfaces fuse to form the first **dense line**.

Spiraling continues until the axon is invested with a number of wrappings. The alternate fusion of both the cytoplasmic and external surfaces of the membrane results in an interdigitated double spiral (see Figure 8-11):

1. One spiral of **intraperiod lines** (fused external surfaces with remnant extracellular space).

2. One spiral of **major dense lines** (fused cytoplasmic surfaces).

The dense line terminates when the membrane surfaces separate to enclose the cytoplasm at the surface of the sheath (the **tongue**), and the intraperiod line terminates as the tongue turns away from the sheath.

The **incisures of Schmidt-Lanterman** are seen in longitudinal sections of myelinated nerve fibers in the CNS and PNS. They correspond to areas of residual cytoplasm preserving the viability of myelin.

Figure 8-9. Astrocytes

Pia mater

Glial fibrillary acidic protein (GFAP)

Myelin

3 Glia limitans

2

Axon

Neuron

2 Perivascular feet of astrocytes

1 Protoplasmic astrocyte

Astrocytes

1 Astrocytes are present in the CNS. They are branching cells with cytoplasmic processes ending in expansions called **end-feet**.

2 End-feet cover neurons (dendrites and cell bodies), the inner surface of the pia mater, and every blood vessel of the CNS.

3 Joined end-feet processes coating the pia mater form collectively the **glia limitans (glial limiting membrane)**.

Perivascular end-feet area — Blood capillary — Astrocyte

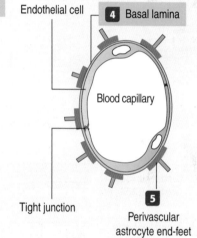

The blood-brain barrier

In the CNS, **capillaries** are lined by continuous endothelial cells linked by **tight junctions**.

Substances can reach the nervous tissue only by crossing through the endothelial cells. However, water, gases, and lipid-soluble molecules can diffuse across endothelial cells.

Tight junctions between endothelial cells are the main components of the blood-brain barrier.
Additional components are:
4 The basal lamina of the endothelial capillaries.
5 The perivascular astrocyte end-feet.

Endothelial cell

4 Basal lamina

Blood capillary

Tight junction

5 Perivascular astrocyte end-feet

As the myelin sheath approaches the node of Ranvier region, an additional ring of cytoplasm separates the cytoplasmic surfaces of the cell membrane. These tongues make contact with the **axolemma**, or surface membrane of the axon, in the paranodal region. Axons branch to form collaterals at a node of Ranvier.

The apposed interdigitating processes of myelinating **Schwann cells** and the incisures of Schmidt-Lanterman are linked by **tight junctions**.

They are called **autotypic tight junctions** because they link plasma membranes of the **same** cell. **Heterotypic tight junctions** are seen between the axolemma (surrounding the axon) and the Schwann cell paranodal cytoplasmic loops adjacent to the node of Ranvier.

Tight junctions contain **claudins** (claudin-1, claudin-2, and claudin-5) and **zonula occludens** (ZO) **proteins** (ZO-1 and ZO-2) (see Figure 8-10).

Tight junctions:

1. Stabilize newly formed wraps of myelin during nerve development.

2. Act as a selective permeability barrier.

3. Restrict the movement of lipids and proteins from specific membrane domains.

Connexin 32 (Cx32) is found in Schwann cells. Cx32 does not form gap junctions with other Schwann cells. Instead, Cx32 predominates in the paranodal membranes and incisures of Schmidt-Lanterman and forms intercellular channels linking portions of the same cell. Mutations in the *Cx32* gene causes **X-linked Charcot-Marie-Tooth disease**, a demyelinating disorder of the PNS characterized by the progressive loss of both motor and sensory functions of the distal legs (see Box 8-G).

Myelin: Protein and lipid components

Myelin in the CNS and PNS is similar in overall protein and lipid composition, except that myelin in the PNS contains more sphingomyelin and glycoproteins. Three proteins are particularly relevant (Figure 8-12):

1. **Myelin basic protein** (MBP).
2. **Proteolipid protein** (PLP).

Figure 8-10. Oligodendrocytes and nodes of Ranvier in the CNS and PNS

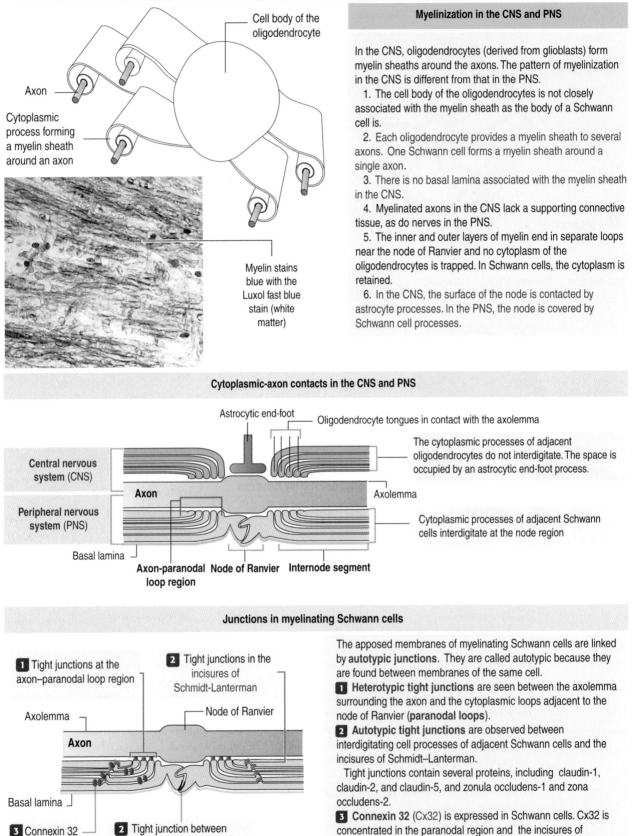

Cell body of the oligodendrocyte

Axon

Cytoplasmic process forming a myelin sheath around an axon

Myelin stains blue with the Luxol fast blue stain (white matter)

Myelinization in the CNS and PNS

In the CNS, oligodendrocytes (derived from glioblasts) form myelin sheaths around the axons. The pattern of myelinization in the CNS is different from that in the PNS.

1. The cell body of the oligodendrocytes is not closely associated with the myelin sheath as the body of a Schwann cell is.

2. Each oligodendrocyte provides a myelin sheath to several axons. One Schwann cell forms a myelin sheath around a single axon.

3. There is no basal lamina associated with the myelin sheath in the CNS.

4. Myelinated axons in the CNS lack a supporting connective tissue, as do nerves in the PNS.

5. The inner and outer layers of myelin end in separate loops near the node of Ranvier and no cytoplasm of the oligodendrocytes is trapped. In Schwann cells, the cytoplasm is retained.

6. In the CNS, the surface of the node is contacted by astrocyte processes. In the PNS, the node is covered by Schwann cell processes.

Cytoplasmic-axon contacts in the CNS and PNS

Astrocytic end-foot

Oligodendrocyte tongues in contact with the axolemma

Central nervous system (CNS)

The cytoplasmic processes of adjacent oligodendrocytes do not interdigitate. The space is occupied by an astrocytic end-foot process.

Axon

Axolemma

Peripheral nervous system (PNS)

Cytoplasmic processes of adjacent Schwann cells interdigitate at the node region

Basal lamina

Axon-paranodal loop region **Node of Ranvier** **Internode segment**

Junctions in myelinating Schwann cells

1 Tight junctions at the axon–paranodal loop region

2 Tight junctions in the incisures of Schmidt-Lanterman

Axolemma

Node of Ranvier

Axon

Basal lamina

3 Connexin 32

2 Tight junction between interdigitating cell processes of adjacent Schwann cells

The apposed membranes of myelinating Schwann cells are linked by **autotypic junctions**. They are called autotypic because they are found between membranes of the same cell.

1 **Heterotypic tight junctions** are seen between the axolemma surrounding the axon and the cytoplasmic loops adjacent to the node of Ranvier (**paranodal loops**).

2 **Autotypic tight junctions** are observed between interdigitating cell processes of adjacent Schwann cells and the incisures of Schmidt–Lanterman.

Tight junctions contain several proteins, including claudin-1, claudin-2, and claudin-5, and zonula occludens-1 and zona occludens-2.

3 **Connexin 32** (Cx32) is expressed in Schwann cells. Cx32 is concentrated in the paranodal region and the incisures of Schmidt-Lanterman. Mutations in the *Cx32* gene determine the demyelinating X-linked Charcot-Marie-Tooth disease.

Figure 8-11. Myelinization

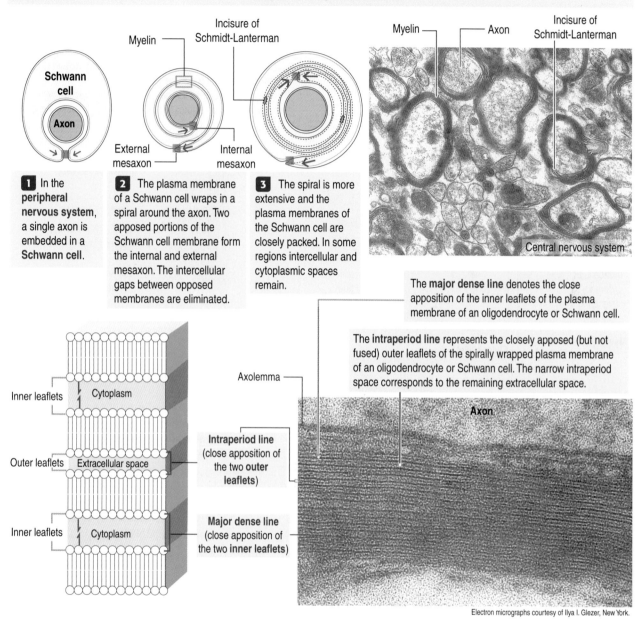

Myelin — Incisure of Schmidt-Lanterman

Schwann cell

Axon

External mesaxon — Internal mesaxon

1 In the **peripheral nervous system**, a single axon is embedded in a **Schwann cell**.

2 The plasma membrane of a Schwann cell wraps in a spiral around the axon. Two apposed portions of the Schwann cell membrane form the internal and external mesaxon. The intercellular gaps between opposed membranes are eliminated.

3 The spiral is more extensive and the plasma membranes of the Schwann cell are closely packed. In some regions intercellular and cytoplasmic spaces remain.

Myelin — Axon — Incisure of Schmidt-Lanterman

Central nervous system

The **major dense line** denotes the close apposition of the inner leaflets of the plasma membrane of an oligodendrocyte or Schwann cell.

The **intraperiod line** represents the closely apposed (but not fused) outer leaflets of the spirally wrapped plasma membrane of an oligodendrocyte or Schwann cell. The narrow intraperiod space corresponds to the remaining extracellular space.

Inner leaflets — Cytoplasm

Outer leaflets — Extracellular space

Inner leaflets — Cytoplasm

Axolemma

Intraperiod line (close apposition of the two **outer** leaflets)

Major dense line (close apposition of the two **inner** leaflets)

Axon

Electron micrographs courtesy of Ilya I. Glezer, New York.

3. Myelin protein zero (MPZ).

MBP is a cytosolic plasma membrane–bound protein present in both the myelin of the PNS and CNS. PLP is a tetraspanin protein found only in the myelin of the CNS. PLP plays a significant role in neural development and is a structural component of myelin. A mutation of the *PLP* gene and its alternatively transcribed DM20 protein causes **Pelizaeus-Merzbacher disease**, an X-linked neuropathy of the group of **leukodystrophies** in which affected males have a reduction of white matter and a reduction in the number of oligodendrocytes. The most common characteristics of Pelizaeus-Merzbacher disease are flickering eyes, and physical and mental retardation.

The predominant protein in myelin of the PNS is **MPZ**, a functional equivalent to PLP in the CNS.

The extracellular domain of two MPZ proteins extends into the extracellular space to establish homophilic interaction with a similar pair of MPZ molecules on an opposite membrane. The **homotetrameric** structure provides intermembrane adhesion essential for the compaction of myelin (see Figure 8-13). The intracellular domain of MPZ participates in a signaling cascade that regulates myelinogenesis. In the CNS, plasma membrane–associated PLPs interact with each other and have a similar stabilizing function.

Proteins of myelin are strong antigens with a role in autoimmune diseases such as **multiple sclerosis** in the CNS and **Guillain-Barré syndrome** in the PNS.

Some axons of the PNS are unmyelinated (see Figure 8-13). A Schwann cell can accommodate several

Figure 8-12. **Structure of myelin**

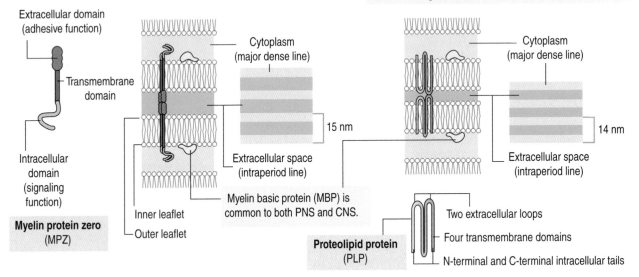

Peripheral nervous system (PNS)

Myelin protein zero (MPZ), synthesized by Schwann cells, interact with each other (homodimers) to stabilize apposed plasma membranes as homotetramers. The intracellular **tail of MPZ** has a signaling function.

Central nervous system (CNS)

In the central nervous system, the homophilic interaction of plasma membrane–associated **proteolipid protein (PLP)** stabilizes adjacent stacks of membranes of oligodendrocytes. PLP has a tetraspanin structure with short and long extracellular loops and two intracellular tails.

axons in individual cytoplasmic invaginations and no myelin is produced.

Pathology: Demyelinating diseases

The integrity of myelin, but not the axon, is disturbed in **demyelinating diseases** affecting the **survival of oligodendrocytes** or the **integrity of the myelin sheath.**

Demyelinating diseases can be:

1. **Immune-mediated.**
2. **Inherited.**

Box 8-G | Charcot-Marie-Tooth disease

• **Charcot-Marie-Tooth disease** is a common and heterogeneous inherited disorder affecting the PNS. The disease is most often an autosomal-dominant syndrome but is genetically heterogeneous.
• The most frequent form is **Charcot-Marie-Tooth disease type 1**, a demyelinating polyneuropathy (with reduced nerve conduction velocity) caused by mutations affecting myelin components. **Charcot-Marie-Tooth disease type 2** is an axonal polyneuropathy (with normal nerve conduction velocity) determined by defects in axonal transport (mutation of a kinesin), membrane trafficking, and protein synthesis.
• **Myelin protein zero (MPZ)** is a member of the immunoglobulin superfamily with a dual role: the compaction of myelin and cell signaling. Myelin in patients with mutations in the *MZP* gene is less compact because of a predominant defect in the extracellular domain of MZP, which is responsible for holding two membranes together. Mutations in the *MZP* gene cause the genetic and clinical variants of **Charcot-Marie-Tooth disease type 1B** and **type 2**.
• A duplication of the *peripheral myelin protein 22* (*PMP22*) gene causes **Charcot-Marie-Tooth disease type 1A**, the most common type of Charcot-Marie-Tooth disease.

---

3. **Metabolic.**
4. **Virus-induced.**

Immune-mediated demyelinating diseases include **multiple sclerosis** and **monophasic demyelinating diseases** (for example, **optic neuritis**).

Multiple sclerosis (Figure 8-14) is characterized by clinically recurrent or chronically progressive neurologic dysfunction caused by multiple areas of demyelination in the CNS, in particular the **brain, optic nerves**, and **spinal cord.**

An immune and inflammatory mediated origin of multiple sclerosis is supported by an increase of immunoglobulin G (IgG) in the cerebrospinal fluid (CSF), and abnormalities of T cell function. Two characteristic pathologic findings are the **multiple sclerosis plaque**, a demyelination lesion of the white matter, and **Creutzfeldt cells**, reactive astrocytes with several nuclear fragments.

An **inherited demyelination** disorder is **adrenoleukodystrophy**, in which **progressive demyelination** is associated with **dysfunction of the adrenal cortex**. The X-linked form of this disease is caused by a mutation of a gene encoding a membrane protein of **peroxisomes**. A defect in this gene leads to the accumulation of **very-long-chain fatty acids (VLCFAs)** in serum (discussed under Peroxisomes in Chapter 2, Epithelial Glands).

Metabolic demyelination disorders include **central pontine myelinolysis**, a syndrome in which neurologic dysfunction is observed following rapid cor-

Figure 8-13. Development of unmyelinated nerves

Unmyelinated nerve fibers

Some axons are unmyelinated. Each Schwann cell is able to house a number of axons occupying individual invaginations of its cytoplasm.

With such an arrangement, the Schwann cell cannot wrap around individual axons and no myelin is produced.

The entire axolemma of such axons is freely exposed to the interstitial tissue, and axons are partially protected by a basal lamina surrounding the supportive Schwann cell.

Nerve impulses along these axons travel continuously and, therefore, less rapidly than saltatory conduction.

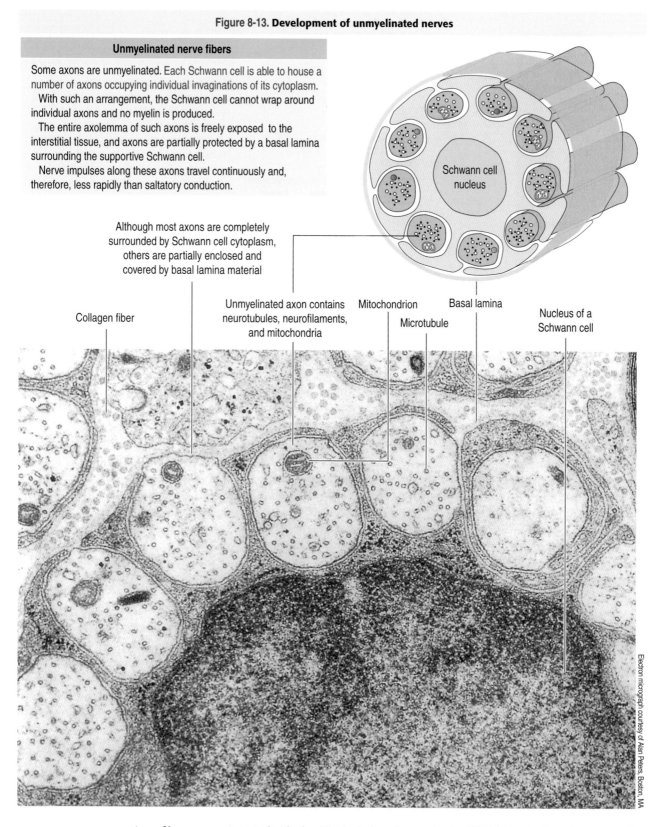

Schwann cell nucleus

Although most axons are completely surrounded by Schwann cell cytoplasm, others are partially enclosed and covered by basal lamina material

Collagen fiber

Unmyelinated axon contains neurotubules, neurofilaments, and mitochondria

Mitochondrion

Microtubule

Basal lamina

Nucleus of a Schwann cell

Electron micrograph courtesy of Alan Peters, Boston, MA

rection of hyponatremia in individuals with alcohol abuse or malnutrition. A typical pathologic finding is the presence of **symmetrical demyelinated lesions in the central pons.**

Vitamin B$_{12}$ deficiency results in demyelination of axons in the CNS (the spinal cord, in particular) and the PNS. **Virus-induced demyelination** can be observed in **progressive multifocal encephalopathy** caused by an opportunistic viral infection of oligodendrocytes in patients with immunodeficiency.

Figure 8-14. Pathogenesis of multiple sclerosis

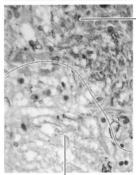

Myelinated axons stained blue with Luxol fast blue

Multiple sclerosis plaque. No myelin staining is detected

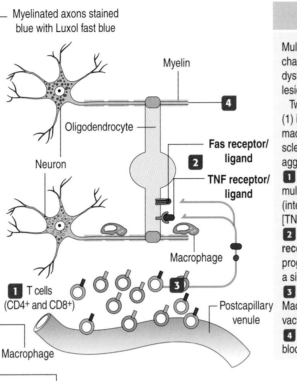

Myelin

Oligodendrocyte

Neuron

4

Fas receptor/ligand

2

TNF receptor/ligand

Macrophage

1 T cells (CD4+ and CD8+)

3

Postcapillary venule

Macrophage

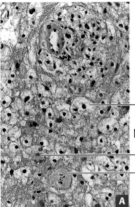

Creutzfeldt cells — T cell

Astrocyte (GFAP–brown stained)

A. Demyelinating axons by macrophages (large cells with foamy cytoplasm). Two reactive astrocytes (**Creutzfeldt cells**) with several nuclear fragments are seen (hematoxylin–eosin, H&E).
B. High magnification view of two Creutzfeldt cells (H&E).
C. Abundant active astrocytes, immunostained for glial fibrillary acidic protein (**GAFP**), present in the demyelinating lesion.

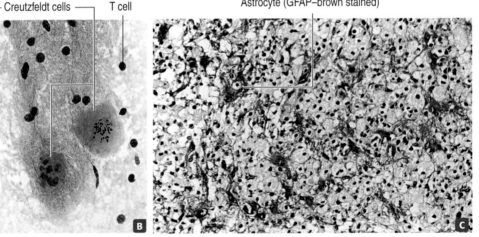

Multiple sclerosis

Multiple sclerosis is a demyelinating disorder characterized by episodes of neurologic dysfunction, separated in **time**, caused by lesions of the white matter, separated in **space**.

Two characteristic microscopic features are: (1) infiltration of inflammatory cells (T cells and macrophages) inside and around multiple sclerosis plaques; and (2) plaques of astrocytic aggregates.

1 **CD8+** and **CD4+ T cells**, recruited to multiple sclerosis lesions, **secrete cytokines** (interleukin-2, tumor necrosis factor ligand [TNFL], and interferon-γ).

2 T cells secrete **Fas ligand** that binds to **Fas receptor** on **oligodendrocytes** to induce their programmed cell death (apoptosis). TNFL exerts a similar apoptotic effect.

3 Macrophages strip myelin off the axons. Macrophages contain myelin in phagocytic vacuoles.

4 Conduction in the demyelinated axon is blocked.

Photographs A-C from Burger PC, Scheithauer BW, Vogel FS: Surgical Pathology of the Nervous System and its Coverings, 4th ed. Philadelphia, Churchill Livingstone, 2002.

Pathology: Neurodegenerative diseases

Degenerative processes of specific groups of neurons of the brain cause movement disorders, dementia syndromes, and autonomic perturbations. Neurodegenerative diseases include:

1. **Amyotrophic lateral sclerosis (ALS)** (Figure 8-15), the most common adult-initiated motor neuron disease, is characterized by progressive degeneration of motor neurons, starting with moderate weakness in one limb and progressing to severe paralysis (swallowing and respiratory disorders), leading to death in about 3 years.

The term **amyotrophic** refers to muscle atrophy. **Lateral sclerosis** refers to the hardness to palpation of the lateral columns of the spinal cord.

Axonal transport defects caused by microtubule disorganization and increased phosphorylation of neurofilaments prevent binding of motor proteins for cargo transport. Consequently, accumulation of vesicles, mitochondria and neurofilaments in the perikaryon determines neuronal dysfunction and axonal atrophy.

In a few familial cases, a mutation in the copper-zinc **superoxide dismutase (*SOD1*)** gene has been reported. Defective SOD1 fails to activate several kinases involved in kinesin-based mitochondrial axonal transport.

2. **Alzheimer's disease**, the most common neurode-

Figure 8-15. Amyotrophic lateral sclerosis

Normal spinal cord (hematoxylin-eosin stain)

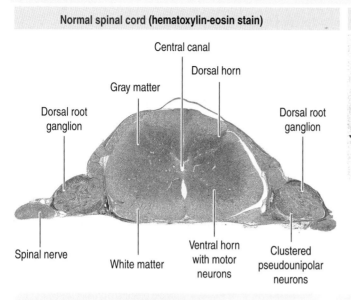

- Central canal
- Dorsal horn
- Gray matter
- Dorsal root ganglion
- Dorsal root ganglion
- Spinal nerve
- White matter
- Ventral horn with motor neurons
- Clustered pseudounipolar neurons

Amyotrophic lateral sclerosis (Luxol fast blue stain)

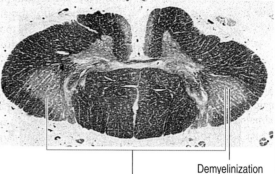

Demyelinization

From Damjanov I, Linder J: Pathology: A Color Atlas, St. Louis, Mosby, 2000.

Symmetrical loss of myelinated fibers in a section of spinal cord (crossed cerebrospinal tracts) from a patient with amyotrophic lateral sclerosis. The preparation was stained for myelin.

Amyotrophic lateral sclerosis (ALS; also known as **Lou Gherig's disease**) is a severe condition characterized by **progressive degeneration of motor neurons of the brainstem and spinal cord**.

Amyotrophic refers to **muscle atrophy**. **Lateral sclerosis** refers to the **hardness to palpation of the lateral columns of the spinal cord** in autopsy specimens. Lateral sclerosis is caused by an increased number of astrocytes (**astrocytic gliosis**) following the degeneration and loss of motor neurons.

ALS is a familial motor neuron disease in 5% to 10% of cases. The others are assumed to be sporadic. Mutations in the gene encoding **superoxide dismutase 1** (**SOD1**) account for 20% of the cases of familial ALS. The remaining 80% are caused by mutations of other genes.

SOD1 is an enzyme that requires copper to catalyze the conversion of toxic superoxide radicals to hydrogen peroxide and oxygen.

The effects of mutant SOD1 result in the disorganization of neurofilaments filaments (NF-L, NF-M, and NF-H; see Figure 8-4). In addition, defective SOD1 fails to activate several kinases involved in the kinesin-based mitochondrial axonal transport. In addition, **axonal transport defects**, caused by microtubule disorganization and increased phosphorylation of neurofilaments, prevent binding of motor proteins for cargo transport. Consequently, vesicles, mitochondria and neurofilaments accumulate in the perikaryon determining neuronal dysfunction and axonal atrophy.

The clinically signs are overactive tendon reflexes, Hoffmann sign (digital reflex: flexion of the terminal phalanx of the thumb following nipping of the nail), Babinski sign (extension of the great toe and abduction of the other toes after plantar stimulation), and clonus (Greek *klonos*, a tumult; muscle contraction and relaxation of a muscle in rapid succession).

Box 8-H | Amyloid deposits

- The conversion of soluble peptide and proteins into **amyloid deposits** is associated with several disorders, including Alzheimer's disease and type II diabetes.
- Amyloid-β protein is produced by endoproteolysis of the amyloid precursor protein (**APP**), a single-transmembrane, receptor-like protein. This is achieved by the sequential cleavage of APP by enzyme complexes designated α-, β- and γ-secretases (see Figure 8-16).
- Three enzymes with α-secretase activity are ADAM9, ADAM10, and ADAM17 (also known as tumor necrosis factor converting enzyme). In Chapter I, Epithelium, we discuss the structure and function of the ADAM family (a disintegrin and metalloproteinase family enzyme).
- The γ-secretase consists of a complex of enzymes composed of presenilin 1 or 2, nicastrin, anterior pharynx defective and presenilin enhancer 2.
- Secretases and ADAMs are **sheddases**. They are involved in regulated intramembrane proteolysis: membrane proteins first shed their ectodomains by membrane-anchored proteases (sheddases), releasing the extracellular domains. Then, the membrane-retained fragment can be cleaved within the transmembrane domains to release hydrophobic peptides (such as amyloid-β) into the extracellular space. α-Secretase (consisting of members of the ADAM family) or β-secretase (also called β-site APP-cleaving enzyme, BACE, see Figure 8-16) are involved in ectodomain shedding of APP.

generative disease, is a progressive cortical dementia affecting language, memory, and vision, as well as emotion or personality.

The predominant lesions are:

1. The accumulation of plaques in the extracellular space consisting of **amyloid** (Greek *amylon*, starch; *eidos*, resemblance) **fibrils** containing β-**amyloid** (Aβ) **peptide**. Amyloid fibrils have a predominant β-sheet structure forming unfolded or partially unfolded conformations of proteins and peptides (Figure 8-16).

Historically, amyloidosis was observed in the mid-19th century as iodide or Congo red–stained deposits in organs of patients who died from this condition.

Amyloid fibrils represent the loss of function of normally soluble, functional peptide and proteins as well as the self-assembly of toxic intermediates.

Keep in mind that the protective mechanisms against amyloid formation include the housekeeping ubiquitin–proteasome and autophagy systems, which prevent the formation and accumulation of misfolded and aggregated polypeptide chains.

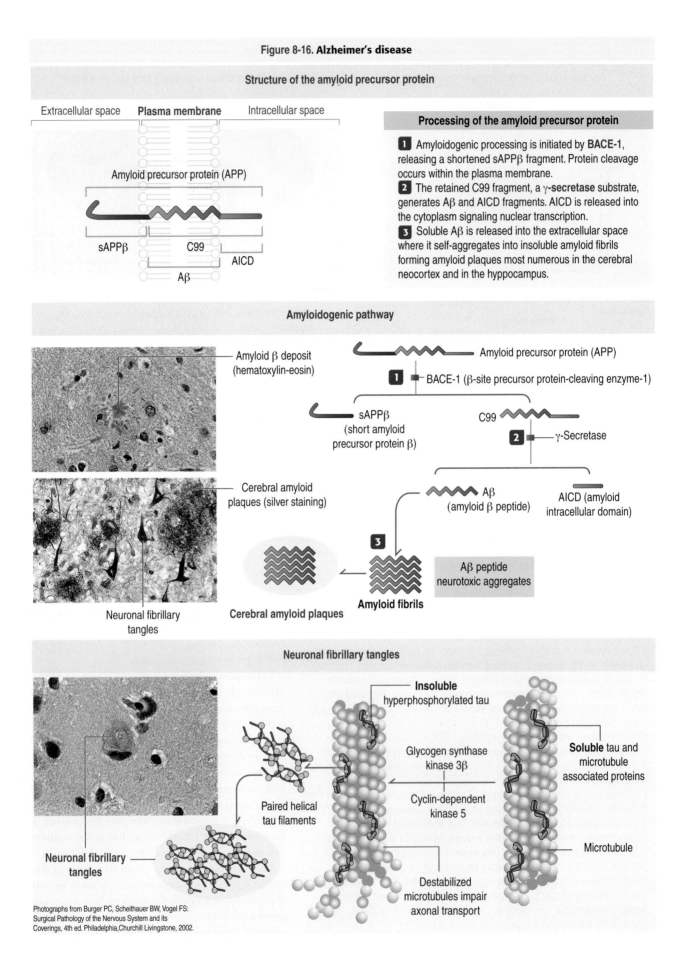

Figure 8-16. Alzheimer's disease

Structure of the amyloid precursor protein

Extracellular space   **Plasma membrane**   Intracellular space

Amyloid precursor protein (APP)

sAPPβ   C99   AICD

Aβ

Processing of the amyloid precursor protein

1 Amyloidogenic processing is initiated by **BACE-1**, releasing a shortened sAPPβ fragment. Protein cleavage occurs within the plasma membrane.

2 The retained C99 fragment, a γ-**secretase** substrate, generates Aβ and AICD fragments. AICD is released into the cytoplasm signaling nuclear transcription.

3 Soluble Aβ is released into the extracellular space where it self-aggregates into insoluble amyloid fibrils forming amyloid plaques most numerous in the cerebral neocortex and in the hyppocampus.

Amyloidogenic pathway

Amyloid β deposit (hematoxylin-eosin)

Cerebral amyloid plaques (silver staining)

Neuronal fibrillary tangles

Amyloid precursor protein (APP)

1 ■— BACE-1 (β-site precursor protein-cleaving enzyme-1)

sAPPβ (short amyloid precursor protein β)

C99

2 ■— γ-Secretase

Aβ (amyloid β peptide)

AICD (amyloid intracellular domain)

3

Amyloid fibrils

Aβ peptide neurotoxic aggregates

Cerebral amyloid plaques

Neuronal fibrillary tangles

Insoluble hyperphosphorylated tau

Glycogen synthase kinase 3β

Cyclin-dependent kinase 5

Soluble tau and microtubule associated proteins

Paired helical tau filaments

Neuronal fibrillary tangles

Microtubule

Destabilized microtubules impair axonal transport

Photographs from Burger PC, Scheithauer BW, Vogel FS: Surgical Pathology of the Nervous System and its Coverings, 4th ed. Philadelphia,Churchill Livingstone, 2002.

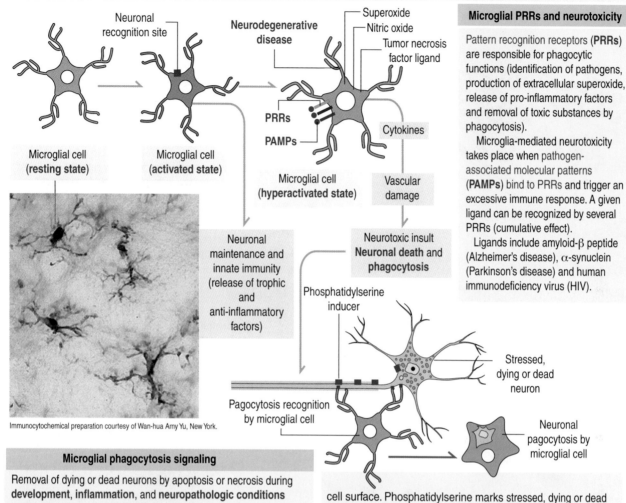

Figure 8-17. Microglial cells

Neuronal recognition site

Neurodegenerative disease

Superoxide
Nitric oxide
Tumor necrosis factor ligand

PRRs
PAMPs

Cytokines

Microglial cell (**resting state**)

Microglial cell (**activated state**)

Microglial cell (**hyperactivated state**)

Vascular damage

Neuronal maintenance and innate immunity (release of trophic and anti-inflammatory factors)

Neurotoxic insult **Neuronal death and phagocytosis**

Phosphatidylserine inducer

Pagocytosis recognition by microglial cell

Stressed, dying or dead neuron

Neuronal pagocytosis by microglial cell

Immunocytochemical preparation courtesy of Wan-hua Amy Yu, New York.

Microglial PRRs and neurotoxicity

Pattern recognition receptors (**PRRs**) are responsible for phagocytic functions (identification of pathogens, production of extracellular superoxide, release of pro-inflammatory factors and removal of toxic substances by phagocytosis).

Microglia-mediated neurotoxicity takes place when pathogen-associated molecular patterns (**PAMPs**) bind to PRRs and trigger an excessive immune response. A given ligand can be recognized by several PRRs (cumulative effect).

Ligands include amyloid-β peptide (Alzheimer's disease), α-synuclein (Parkinson's disease) and human immunodeficiency virus (HIV).

Microglial phagocytosis signaling

Removal of dying or dead neurons by apoptosis or necrosis during **development**, **inflammation**, and **neuropathologic conditions** involve the phagocytic activity of microglial cells, the resident macrophages of the brain and spinal cord.

Microglial cells sense phagocytosis recognition signals, such as phospholipid phosphatidylserine translocated by phosphatidylserine translocases from the inner leaflet of the plasma membrane to the cell surface. Phosphatidylserine marks stressed, dying or dead neurons for removal, thus enabling microglial receptors and opsonins to engulf whole dead neurons or parts of stressed neurons within hours.

Microgliosis is the massive microglial response to tissue damage that can be reparative or destructive (called **reactive microgliosis**).

2. **Neurofibrillary tangles** in the cytoplasm of aging neurons (see Figure 8-16).

3. Progressive **hyppocampal synaptic failure** in correlation with cognitive decline in Alzheimer's disease. In addition, **vascular injury (ischemia)** and **parenchymal inflammation** (activated microglia and reactive astrocytes) enhance the effects of Aβ peptide-containing plaques in the brain.

Plaques and tangles lead to neuronal and white matter loss. Figure 8-16 and Box 8-H summarize and highlight the major molecular events observed in the brains of patients with Alzheimer's disease, in particular the formation of **amyloid plaques**. A disproportion between production and clearance, and accumulation of Aβ peptides may be the initiation factor in Alzheimer's disease.

Neurofibrillary tangles in pyramidal neurons are typical of Alzheimer's disease and other neurodegen-

erative disorders called **tauopathies**.

Alterations in the stabilizing function of **tau**, a microtubule-associated protein, result in the accumulation of twisted pairs of tau in neurons. In normal neurons, **soluble tau** promotes the assembly and stability of microtubules and axonal vesicle transport. **Hyperphosphorylated tau is insoluble**, lacks affinity for microtubules, and self-associates into paired helical filaments (see Figure 8-16).

3. **Parkinson's disease,** the second most common neurodegenerative disease, after Alzheimer's disease. It is characterized clinically by **parkinsonism**, defined by resting tremor, slow voluntary movements (**hypokinetic disorders**), and movements with rigidity. This disease is pathologically defined by **a loss of dopaminergic neurons from the substantia nigra** and elsewhere.

A characteristic pathologic aspect is the presence of

Figure 8-18. Ependyma and choroid plexus

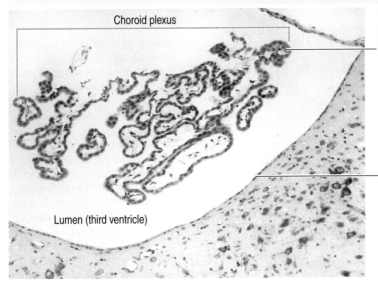

Choroid plexus

Lumen (third ventricle)

Choroid epithelium, formed by cuboidal cells linked by **tight junctions** with apical **microvilli**, infolding of the basal plasma membrane, and abundant mitochondria.
   Choroidal epithelial cells produce cerebrospinal fluid (CSF).

Ependymal epithelium, formed by cuboidal cells linked by **desmosomes**, with apical microvilli and cilia and abundant mitochondria.
   Tanycytes, specialized ependymal cells found in the third ventricle, have basal processes forming end-feet on blood vessels. **Tanycytes are linked to each other and to ependymal cells by tight junctions.**

Glial cell

Central canal (brainstem)

The **central canal** is lined primarily by ependymal cells (**no tanycytes**).

Preparations courtesy of Wan-hua Amy Yu, New York.

Ependyma

The brain ventricles and the central canal of the spinal cord are lined by a simple cuboidal epithelium, the **ependyma**.
   The ependyma consists of two cell types:
   1 **Ependymal cells**, with cilia and microvilli on the apical domain and abundant mitochondria. The basal domain is in contact with astrocytic processes. Ependymal cells are attached to each other by belt desmosomes.
   2 **Tanycytes** (in the third ventricle) are specialized ependymal cells. Two different features are observed:
   1. **Basal processes extend through the astrocytic processes layer to form end-feet on a blood vessel.**
   2. **Tanycytes are attached to each other and to ependymal cells by tight junctions.**

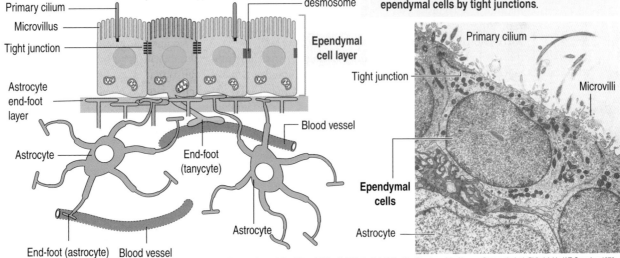

2 Tanycyte   **1** Ependymal cells   Belt desmosome

Primary cilium
Microvillus
Tight junction

Ependymal cell layer

Astrocyte end-foot layer

Blood vessel

Astrocyte   End-foot (tanycyte)   Blood vessel

End-foot (astrocyte)   Blood vessel   Astrocyte

Primary cilium
Tight junction
Microvilli
Ependymal cells
Astrocyte

Electron micrograph from Peters A, Palay SL, Webster H de F: The Fine Structure of the Nervous System, 2nd ed. Philadelphia, WB Saunders, 1976.

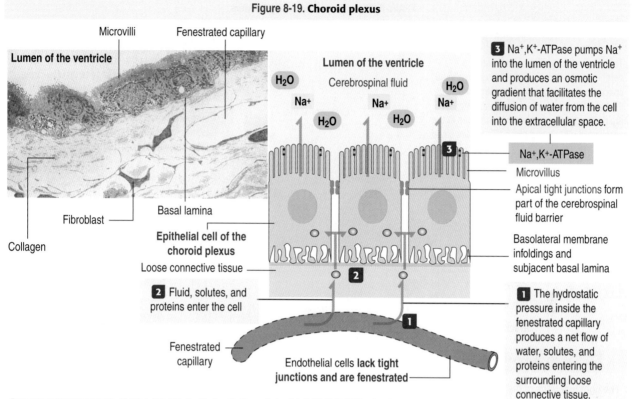

Figure 8-19. Choroid plexus

Microvilli

Fenestrated capillary

Lumen of the ventricle

Fibroblast

Collagen

Basal lamina

Epithelial cell of the choroid plexus

Loose connective tissue

2 Fluid, solutes, and proteins enter the cell

Fenestrated capillary

Endothelial cells **lack tight junctions and are fenestrated**

Lumen of the ventricle

Cerebrospinal fluid

H_2O Na^+ H_2O Na^+ H_2O Na^+ H_2O

3 Na^+,K^+-ATPase pumps Na^+ into the lumen of the ventricle and produces an osmotic gradient that facilitates the diffusion of water from the cell into the extracellular space.

Na^+,K^+-ATPase

Microvillus

Apical tight junctions form part of the cerebrospinal fluid barrier

Basolateral membrane infoldings and subjacent basal lamina

1 The hydrostatic pressure inside the fenestrated capillary produces a net flow of water, solutes, and proteins entering the surrounding loose connective tissue.

Electron micrograph from Peters A, Palay SL, Webster H de F: The Fine Structure of the Nervous System, 2nd ed. Philadelphia, WB Saunders, 1976.

deposits of hyperphosphorylated α-**synuclein** in the cytoplasm of neurons (**Lewy bodies**) and threadlike inclusions in axons (**Lewy neurites**).

Mutations in the *SNCA* gene, encoding α-synuclein, causes **familial autosomal dominant Parkinson's disease**. Permanent phosphorylation of α-synuclein slows down axonal transport.

Another gene associated with a **familial form of Parkinson's disease** is *PARK2* (Parkinson's disease protein 2). *PARK2* encodes the E3 ubiquitin-protein ligase **parkin**. Parkin is involved in the maintenance of mitochondria. Defective mitochondria can trigger the production of reactive oxygen species (ROS) and disrupt cell functions.

How does parkin work? **Mitophagy** is a specific mechanism to eliminate damaged mitochondria by a signaling pathway involving two enzymes: **PINK1** (PTEN [phosphatase and tensin homolog] induced putative kinase 1) and parkin.

Cytoplasmic parkin is inactive when mitochondria are functioning normally, whereas PINK1 is associated with mitochondria. When mitochondria are damaged, parkin links to the outer mitochondrial membrane and its ubiquitin ligase activity is unleashed by PINK1. Activated parkin transfers ubiquitin proteins to proteins bound to the outer mitochondrial membrane to initiate mitophagy, a control process preventing mitochondrial dysfunction.

As we discuss in Chapter 3, Cell Signaling, ubiqui-

tin ligases attach ubiquitin protein chains to proteins, a process called **ubiquitination**, thereby targeting them for degradation by the 26S proteasome.

An impairment in axonal transport, determined by hyperphosphorylated α-synuclein, and the accumulation of damaged mitochondria, caused by mutations in parkin and PINK1, determine high mitochondrial oxidative stress in dopamine neurons, the initial step of the familial forms of Parkinson's disease.

4. **Huntington's disease** is an inherited adult-onset neurodegenerative disorder characterized by muscle incoordination, cognitive decline, and dementia. Huntington's disease and spinal and bulbar muscular atrophy (SBMA; also known as Kennedy disease) belong to the group of **polyglutamine (polyQ) diseases**.

Selected genes are enriched in CAG repeats in the coding region of neuronal genes. SBMA, a male neurodegenerative disease characterized by progressive motor neuron degeneration and bulbar defects (dysarthria [speech disorder] and dysphagia), is caused by a polyQ expansion in the **androgen receptor** protein.

Huntington's disease is caused by a the gene *hun-tingtin (HTT)* containing a number of CAG repeats in the coding region and expressing polyQ HTT protein. Huntington's disease was briefly discussed in Chapter 3, Cell Signaling, within the context of apoptosis involving caspases and cytochrome *c*.

Aggregates of polyQ HTT disrupt axonal transport by inducing microtubule deacetylation. Microtubule

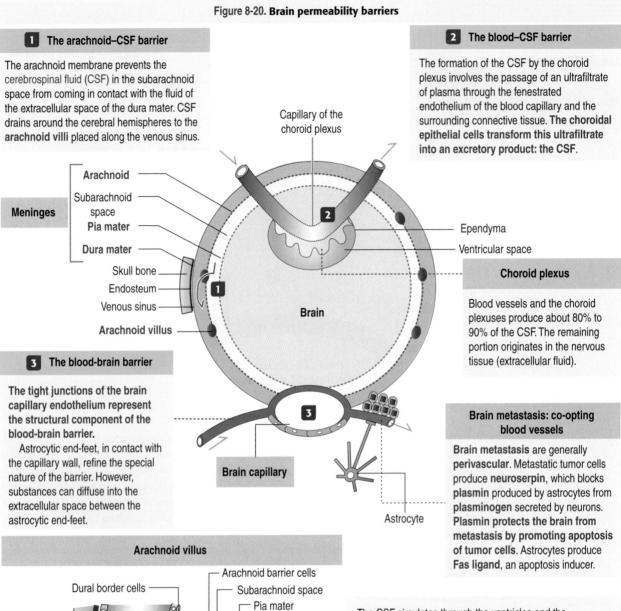

Figure 8-20. Brain permeability barriers

1 The arachnoid–CSF barrier

The arachnoid membrane prevents the cerebrospinal fluid (CSF) in the subarachnoid space from coming in contact with the fluid of the extracellular space of the dura mater. CSF drains around the cerebral hemispheres to the **arachnoid villi** placed along the venous sinus.

2 The blood–CSF barrier

The formation of the CSF by the choroid plexus involves the passage of an ultrafiltrate of plasma through the fenestrated endothelium of the blood capillary and the surrounding connective tissue. **The choroidal epithelial cells transform this ultrafiltrate into an excretory product: the CSF.**

Capillary of the choroid plexus

Arachnoid

Subarachnoid space

Meninges

Pia mater

Dura mater

Skull bone

Endosteum

Venous sinus

Arachnoid villus

Ependyma

Ventricular space

Brain

Choroid plexus

Blood vessels and the choroid plexuses produce about 80% to 90% of the CSF. The remaining portion originates in the nervous tissue (extracellular fluid).

3 The blood-brain barrier

The tight junctions of the brain capillary endothelium represent the structural component of the blood-brain barrier.

Astrocytic end-feet, in contact with the capillary wall, refine the special nature of the barrier. However, substances can diffuse into the extracellular space between the astrocytic end-feet.

Brain capillary

Astrocyte

Brain metastasis: co-opting blood vessels

Brain metastasis are generally **perivascular**. Metastatic tumor cells produce **neuroserpin**, which blocks **plasmin** produced by astrocytes from **plasminogen** secreted by neurons. **Plasmin protects the brain from metastasis by promoting apoptosis of tumor cells.** Astrocytes produce **Fas ligand**, an apoptosis inducer.

Arachnoid villus

Dural border cells

Arachnoid barrier cells

Subarachnoid space

Pia mater

Endosteum

Skull

Endothelium

Brain

Venous sinus   Meninges

The CSF circulates through the ventricles and the subarachnoid space around the central nervous sytsem (CNS). CSF enters the arachnoid space containing **arachnoid villi, protrusions of the arachnoid into the lumen of the venous sinus**, and permeates between or through the endothelial cells lining the venous sinus.

CSF is separated from the blood by the endothelial cell lining of the venous sinus. Blood does not flow from the venous sinus to the subarachnoid space. A blockage of the movement of CSF results in its accumulation in the ventricles and around the brain, a condition known as **hydrocephalus**.

acetylation, a reversible post-translational modification of α-tubulin, is required for the binding of motor protein-cargo complexes to axonal microtubules.

Microglial cells

Microglia comprise about 12% of cells in the brain. They predominate in the gray matter, with higher concentrations in the hippocampus, olfactory telencephalon, basal ganglia, and substantia nigra. Microglial cells exist in a **resting state** characterized by a **branching cytoplasmic morphology**. In response to brain injury or immunologic activity, microglial cells change into an **activated state** characterized by an **ameboidal morphology** accompanied by the up-

Figure 8-21. Peripheral nerve

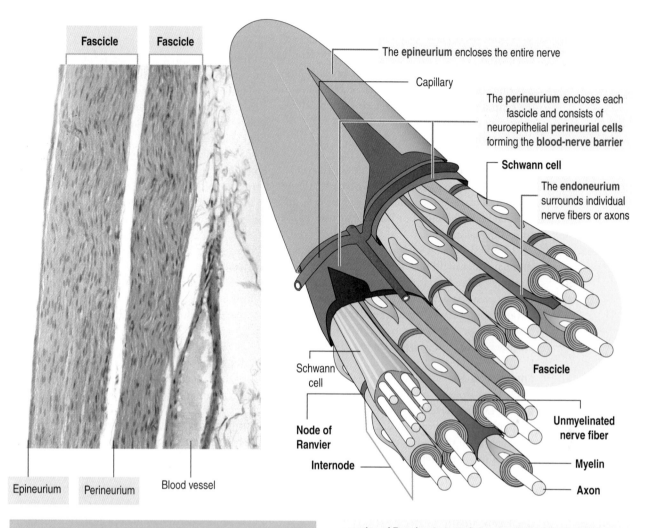

Fascicle **Fascicle**

The **epineurium** encloses the entire nerve

Capillary

The **perineurium** encloses each fascicle and consists of neuroepithelial **perineurial cells** forming the **blood-nerve barrier**

Schwann cell

The **endoneurium** surrounds individual nerve fibers or axons

Schwann cell

Fascicle

Node of Ranvier

Unmyelinated nerve fiber

Internode

Myelin

Axon

Epineurium   Perineurium   Blood vessel

Organization of a peripheral nerve

The **nerve fiber** is the main structural component of a peripheral nerve and consists of an **axon**, **myelin sheath**, and **Schwann cells**.

Nerve fibers are grouped into **fascicles** by connective tissue sheaths. A fascicle contains myelinated and unmyelinated nerve fibers.

Axons contain segments of myelin (**internodes**) separated by nodes of Ranvier. A single Schwann cell provides the myelin sheath for each internode.

The thickness of the myelin sheath is proportional to the diameter of the axon. The wider the axon, the longer the internode distance.

Neuroepithelial cells of the perineurium are joined by tight junctions forming the **blood-nerve barrier**. **Endoneurial capillaries** are lined by continuous endothelial cells linked by tight junctions to contribute to the blood-nerve barrier.

regulation of cell surface molecules, such as **CD14**, major histocompatibility complex (**MHC**) recptors and **chemokine receptors**.

Activated microglial cells participate in brain development by supporting the clearance of neural cells undergoing apoptosis, eliminating toxic debris and enhancing neuronal survival through the release of trophic and anti-inflammatory factors. In the mature brain, microglia facilitate repair by steering the migration of stem cells to the site of inflammation and injury.

Microglial cells may become overactivated and exert neurotoxic effects by the excessive production of cytotoxic substances such as **ROS**, **nitric oxide**, and **tumor necrosis factor ligand**. Activated microglial cells are present in large numbers in neurodegenerative diseases (Alzheimer's disease, Parkinson's disease, multiple sclerosis, amyotrophic lateral sclerosis, Huntington's disease), causing a generalized microglial hyperactivity, a condition called **reactive microgliosis**.

Figure 8-17 provides a summary of the structural and functional aspects of resting, activated and hyperactivated microglial cells.

The distinction between microglia, astrocytes,

and oligodendrocytes is difficult in routine histologic techniques. Immunocytochemical and silver impregnation procedures are commonly used for the identification of glial cells.

Ependyma

Ependyma designates the **simple cuboidal epithelium** covering the surface of the ventricles of the brain and the central canal of the spinal cord. The ependyma consists of two cell types (Figure 8-18):

1. **Ependymal cells.**
2. **Tanycytes.**

Ependymal cells form a simple cuboidal epithelium, lining the ventricular cavities of the brain and the central canal of the spinal cord. These cells differentiate from **germinal** or **ventricular cells** of the embryonic neural tube.

The apical domain of ependymal cells contains abundant **microvilli** and one or more cilia. **Desmosomes** link adjacent ependymal cells. The basal domain is in contact with **astrocytic processes**.

Tanycytes are specialized ependymal cells with basal processes extending between the astrocytic processes to form an end-foot on blood vessels.

Choroid plexus

The choroid plexus produces **cerebrospinal fluid** (**CSF**). During development, the ependymal cell layer comes in contact with the highly vascularized pia mater, forming the **tela choroidea** in the roof of the third and fourth ventricles and along the choroid fissure of the lateral ventricles. These cells differentiate into secretory cells, which in combination with the meningeal blood vessels form the **choroid plexus** (see Figure 8-18).

The cells of the choroid plexus are highly polarized (Figure 8-19). The **apical domain** contains microvilli, and **tight junctions** connect adjacent cells. The **basolateral domain** forms interdigitating folds, and the cell rests on a basal lamina.

Capillaries with fenestrated endothelial cells are located beneath the basal lamina. Macromolecules of the blood plasma can pass freely into the subepithelial space; however, they cannot pass directly into the CSF because of the elaborate interdigitations along the basolateral domain and the apical tight junctions.

Cerebrospinal fluid

The choroid plexuses of the lateral, third, and fourth ventricles produce about 300 mL of CSF every 24 hs.

CSF flows from the lateral ventricles of the brain into the third ventricle through the interventricular foramen. CSF descends to the fourth ventricle through the aqueduct and reaches the brain and spinal subarachnoid space through median and lateral apertures. Some of the CSF descends through the foramen magnum, reaching the lumbar cistern in about 12 hs.

After entering the subarachnoid space, CSF flows outside the CNS into the blood, at the superior sagittal sinus (see Figure 8-20). CSF is transported across the arachnoid epithelium in large vacuoles.

The epithelium of the choroid plexus represents a barrier between the blood and the CSF. Several substances can leave the capillaries of the choroid plexus but cannot enter the CSF.

CSF protects and supports the brain and spinal cord from external forces applied to the skull or vertebral column (cushioning effect).

In addition, the CSF allows the removal of metabolic wastes by continual drainage of the ventricular cavities and subarachnoid space. The volume of CSF varies with the intracranial blood volume. The free communication of CSF among compartments protects against pressure differences.

Lumbar puncture is a procedure to collect a sample of CSF for biochemical analysis and pressure measurement. CSF is collected with a needle inserted obliquely through the interspinous ligament between the third and fourth (L3 and L4) and fourth and fifth (L4 and L5) lumbar vertebrae. The total volume of CSF in an adult is about 120 mL.

Clinical significance: Brain permeability barriers

The brain is supplied with blood from major arteries forming an anastomotic network around the base of the brain. From this region, arteries project into the subarachnoid space before entering the brain tissue.

In the brain, the perivascular space is surrounded by a basal lamina derived from both glial and endothelial cells: the **glia limitans**. Nonfenestrated endothelial cells, linked by tight junctions, prevent the diffusion of substances from the blood to the brain.

Tight junctions represent the structural basis of the blood-brain barrier. This barrier offers free passage to glucose and other selected molecules but excludes most substances, in particular potent drugs required for the treatment of an infection or tumor. If the blood-brain barrier breaks down, tissue fluid accumulates in the nervous tissue, a condition known as **cerebral edema**.

External to the capillary endothelial cell lining is a basal lamina and external to this lamina are the endfeet of the astrocytes.

Although the pericapillary end-feet of astrocytes are not part of the blood-brain barrier, they contribute to its maintenance by transporting fluid and ions from the perineuronal extracellular space to the blood vessels.

Figure 8-20 illustrates details of the three brain permeability barriers:

Figure 8-22. **Peripheral nerve**

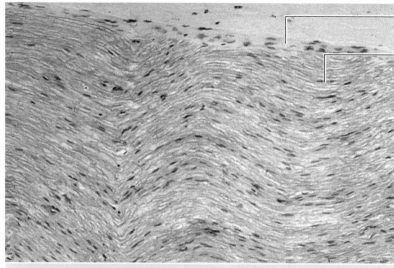

Longitudinal section (hematoxylin-eosin stain)

Perineurium

Nucleus of a Schwann cell

In the PNS, **one Schwann cell forms one segment**, or **internode, of myelin** wrapped around an axon.

A gap, or **node of Ranvier, is visualized at each end of the internode segment.** At the node, interdigitating Schwann cell processes fill the unmyelinated gap.

The surface of the Schwann cell is surrounded by a basal lamina bridging the node of Ranvier.

Nerves elongate during growth, the axon increases in diameter and the layer of myelin becomes thicker.

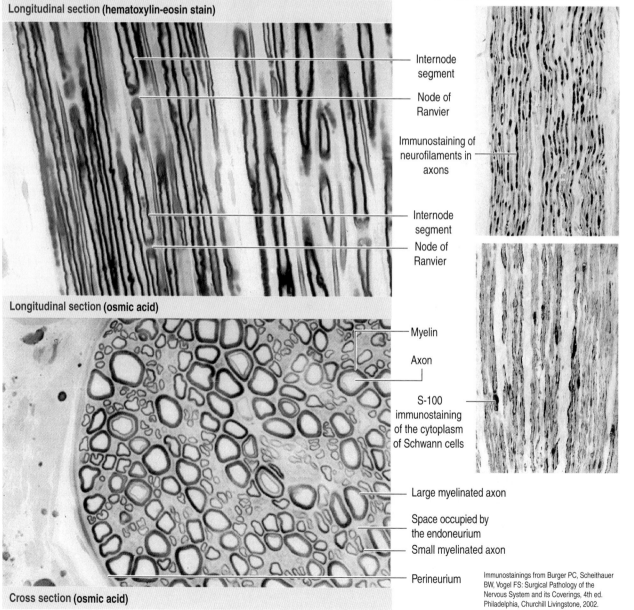

Longitudinal section (osmic acid)

Cross section (osmic acid)

Internode segment

Node of Ranvier

Immunostaining of neurofilaments in axons

Internode segment

Node of Ranvier

Myelin

Axon

S-100 immunostaining of the cytoplasm of Schwann cells

Large myelinated axon

Space occupied by the endoneurium

Small myelinated axon

Perineurium

Immunostainings from Burger PC, Scheithauer BW, Vogel FS: Surgical Pathology of the Nervous System and its Coverings, 4th ed. Philadelphia, Churchill Livingstone, 2002.

Figure 8-23. **Degeneration and regeneration of a peripheral nerve**

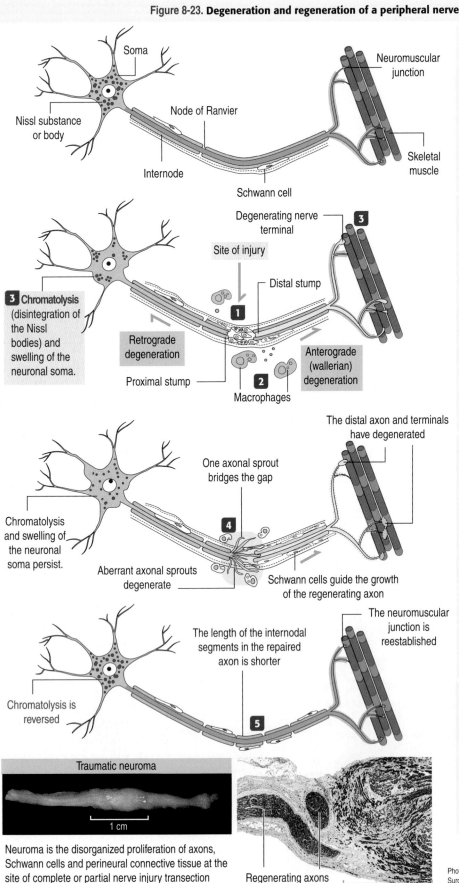

Soma

Neuromuscular junction

Nissl substance or body

Node of Ranvier

Skeletal muscle

Internode

Schwann cell

Degenerating nerve terminal

Site of injury

3

Distal stump

3 **Chromatolysis** (disintegration of the Nissl bodies) and swelling of the neuronal soma.

Retrograde degeneration

1

Anterograde (wallerian) degeneration

Proximal stump

2

Macrophages

The distal axon and terminals have degenerated

One axonal sprout bridges the gap

4

Chromatolysis and swelling of the neuronal soma persist.

Aberrant axonal sprouts degenerate

Schwann cells guide the growth of the regenerating axon

The neuromuscular junction is reestablished

The length of the internodal segments in the repaired axon is shorter

5

Chromatolysis is reversed

Traumatic neuroma

1 cm

Neuroma is the disorganized proliferation of axons, Schwann cells and perineural connective tissue at the site of complete or partial nerve injury transection

Regenerating axons (neurofilament staining)

Neuroma

An intact motor neuron is shown with an axon ending in a neuromuscular junction. The axon is surrounded by a **myelin sheath** and a basal lamina, produced by Schwann cells, and the endoneurium.

The soma of the neuron contains abundant **Nissl bodies** (aggregates of ribosomes attached to the endoplasmic reticulum and free polyribosomes).

1 An injury damages the nerve fiber. Schwann cells undergo mitotic division and bridge the gap between the **proximal** and **distal** axonal stumps.

2 Schwann cells phagocytose myelin. Myelin droplets are extruded from Schwann cells and subsequently are phagocytosed by tissue macrophages.

3 **Chromatolysis** and degeneration of the axon terminals are seen. The distal and proximal segments of the axon degenerate (**anterograde** and **retrograde degeneration**, respectively).

4 The proximal axonal stump generates multiple **sprouts** advancing between Schwann cells. One sprout persists and grows distally (~1.5 mm per day) to reinnervate the muscle. The remaining sprouts degenerate.

In the CNS, degeneration of the axon and myelin is similar and microglial cells remove debris by phagocytosis.

The regeneration process starts but is aborted by the absence of endoneurium and lack of proliferation of oligodendrocytes.

5 Once the regenerated axon reaches the end organ (several months), Schwann cells start the production of myelin. **The internodal segments are shorter.**

The regenerated axon has a reduced diameter (80% of the original diameter) and, therefore, the conduction velocity of the nerve impulse is slower.

Photographs from Burger PC, Scheithauer BW, Vogel FS: Surgical Pathology of the Nervous System and its Coverings, 4th ed. Philadelphia, Churchill Livingstone, 2002.

1. The **arachnoid-CSF barrier**, represented by **arachnoid villi or granulations** distributed along the venous sinus, in particular the **arachnoid barrier cells** linked by tight junctions. Arachnoid villi transfer CSF to the venous system (superior sagittal sinus).

Fluid in the subarachnoid space operates like a shock absorber, which prevents the mass of the brain from compressing nerve roots and blood vessels.

2. The **blood-CSF barrier**, involving tight junctions of the **choroidal epithelium**, is responsible for the production of the CSF. Remember that the tight junctions prevent the paracellular transport of several substances leaving the capillaries of the choroid plexus but unable to enter the CSF.

3. The **blood-brain barrier**, represented by tight junctions sealing the **endothelial** intercellular space.

Obstruction of CSF movement or defective absorption causes an accumulation of fluid in the ventricular spaces and around the brain.

Hydrocephalus is a pathologic condition characterized by an increase in CSF volume and pressure and enlargement of the ventricular space resulting from obstruction of normal CSF circulation. Obstruction of the foramina opening the fourth ventricle to the subarachnoid space is, in most cases, the determinant of hydrocephalus.

The blood-brain barrier is an obstacle for the metastasis of cancerous cells. However, **metastases to the brain** are generally in a **perivascular** location, a condition known as **vascular co-option** of pre-existing vasculature. Metastasis develops and progresses in the absence of angiogenesis.

Metastatic tumor cells produce the protein **neuroserpin**. Neuroserpin blocks **plasmin**, a protein derived from the cleavage of **plasminogen** produced by neurons. Plasmin inhibits spreading of malignant cells along the perivascular space of the brain by triggering the apoptosis of cancer cells.

Astrocytes produce **Fas ligand** (**FasL**), as you remember is an apoptosis inducer, and **plasminogen**

activator, that cleaves neuronal plasminogen into soluble plasmin. In fact, plasmin cleaves FasL, bound to the plasma membrane of astrocytes, into soluble FasL to initiate apoptosis.

The high levels of neuroserpin produced by tumor cells prevent the formation of plasmin and soluble FasL. Consequently, metastatic tumor cells retain the expression of the cell adhesion molecule **L1CAM**, essential for vascular co-option.

Peripheral nervous system

The PNS includes all neuronal elements outside the brain and spinal cord. The peripheral nerves are the **cranial** and **spinal nerves**.

The PNS contains two **supporting cell types**:

1. **Schwann cells**, analogous to the oligodendrocytes of the CNS.

2. **Satellite cells**, Schwann cell–like surrounding the cell bodies of neurons in sensory and autonomic ganglia. We discuss them later.

Individual nerve fibers of the PNS are ensheathed by **Schwann cells** (Figure 8-21). In **myelinated fibers**, individual Schwann cells wrap around the axon, forming a myelin sheath analogous to that of the oligodendrocytes of the CNS (see Figure 8-11). In **unmyelinated fibers**, a single Schwann cell envelops several axons (see Figure 8-13).

There are **two important differences between Schwann cells and oligodendrocytes**:

1. A single Schwann cell forms only one internodal segment of myelin, whereas a single oligodendrocyte may form 40 or 50 internodes.

2. Unmyelinated fibers in the PNS are embedded in Schwann cells, whereas those in the CNS are not ensheathed by oligodendrocytes but may have an investment of astrocytes.

Structure of a peripheral nerve

Connective tissue coverings divide the peripheral nerve into three segments, each with unique structural characteristics (see Figures 8-21 and 8-22):

1. The **epineurium**.
2. The **perineurium**.
3. The **endoneurium**.

The **epineurium** is formed by type I collagen and fibroblasts and covers the entire nerve. It contains arteries, veins and lymphatic vessels.

Within the nerve, the **perineurium** segregates axons into **fascicles**. The perineurium consists of several concentric layers of **neuroepithelial perineurial cells** with two distinct characteristics:

1. A **basal lamina**, consisting of type IV collagen and laminin, surrounds the layers of perineurial cells.

2. Perineurial cells are joined to each other by tight junctions to form a protective diffusion barrier: the **blood-nerve barrier**, responsible for maintaining the

---

Box 8-I | Neurotrophins

• Neurons depend on peripheral structures for their survival. Specific factors, called neurotrophins, are produced by target organs, internalized by nerve endings and transported back to the neuronal soma. Neurotrophins are necessary for the survival of neurons produced in excess during early development, for the growth of their axons and dendrites and for the synthesis of neurotransmitters. Neurotrophins prevent the programmed cell death or apoptosis of neurons.

• Neurotrophins include: nerve growth factor (**NGF**), brain-derived neurotrophic factor (**BDNF**), neurotrophin 3 (**NT-3**), and **NT-4/5**.

• Neurotrophins bind to two specific cell surface receptors: neurotrophin receptor p75 (~75 kd) and tropomyosin receptor kinase (~140 kd; TrkA, B and C). NGF binds preferentially to TrkA. BDNF and NT-4/5 bind to TrkB. NT3 is a ligand for TrkC.

• Neurotrophin signaling activates or represses gene expression.

Figure 8-24. **Sensory and sympathetic ganglia**

Dorsal root ganglia

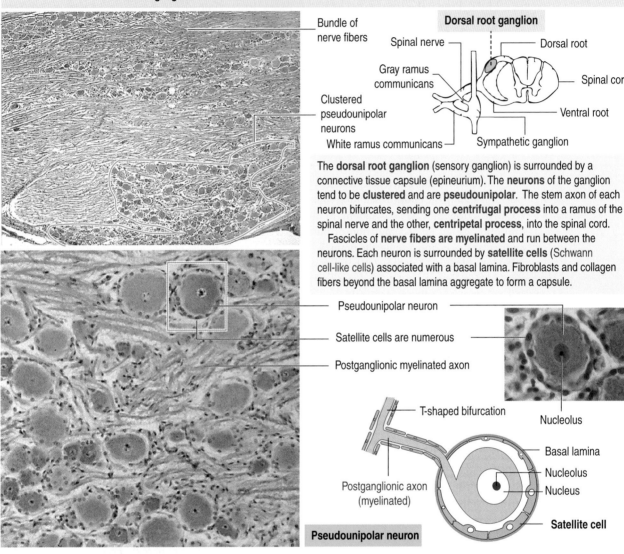

Bundle of nerve fibers

Clustered pseudounipolar neurons

White ramus communicans

Dorsal root ganglion

Spinal nerve — Dorsal root

Gray ramus communicans

Spinal cord

Ventral root

Sympathetic ganglion

The **dorsal root ganglion** (sensory ganglion) is surrounded by a connective tissue capsule (epineurium). The **neurons** of the ganglion tend to be **clustered** and are **pseudounipolar**. The stem axon of each neuron bifurcates, sending one **centrifugal process** into a ramus of the spinal nerve and the other, **centripetal process**, into the spinal cord.

Fascicles of **nerve fibers are myelinated** and run between the neurons. Each neuron is surrounded by **satellite cells** (Schwann cell-like cells) associated with a basal lamina. Fibroblasts and collagen fibers beyond the basal lamina aggregate to form a capsule.

Pseudounipolar neuron

Satellite cells are numerous

Postganglionic myelinated axon

Nucleolus

T-shaped bifurcation

Postganglionic axon (myelinated)

Basal lamina
Nucleolus
Nucleus
Satellite cell

Pseudounipolar neuron

Sympathetic ganglion

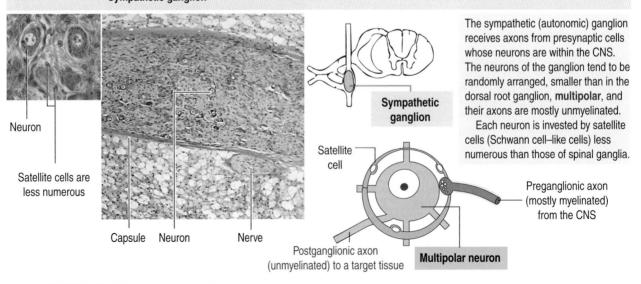

Neuron

Satellite cells are less numerous

Capsule   Neuron   Nerve

Sympathetic ganglion

Satellite cell

Postganglionic axon (unmyelinated) to a target tissue

Multipolar neuron

Preganglionic axon (mostly myelinated) from the CNS

The sympathetic (autonomic) ganglion receives axons from presynaptic cells whose neurons are within the CNS. The neurons of the ganglion tend to be randomly arranged, smaller than in the dorsal root ganglion, **multipolar**, and their axons are mostly unmyelinated.

Each neuron is invested by satellite cells (Schwann cell–like cells) less numerous than those of spinal ganglia.

physiologic microenvironment of the endoneurium.

The **endoneurium** surrounds individual axons and their associated Schwann cells and myelin sheaths. It consists of type III collagen fibrils, a few fibroblasts, macrophages, mast cells and **endoneurial capillaries** between individual the axons lor nerve fibers.

Multiple **unmyelinated axons** are individually encased within recesses of the cytoplasm of Schwann cells. As you remember, unmyelinated axons do not undergo the spiral concentric lamination and myelin formation. For future reference in neuropathology, keep in mind the Luxol fast blue staining method widely used for myelin staining.

Additional components of the blood-nerve barrier are the endothelial cells of the endoneurial capillaries. Endoneurial capillaries derive from the vasa nervorum and are lined by continuous endothelial cells joined by tight junctions.

Pathology: Schwannomas

Schwannomas are benign encapsulated tumors consisting of Schwann cells. Keep in mind that Schwann cells are present in all peripheral nerves. Therefore, schwannomas can be found in many sites (intracranial, intraspinal and extraspinal locations).

Schwannomas can develop at the surface or inside of a nerve fascicle and display spindle cells (called Antoni A pattern) or multipolar cells (called Antoni B pattern), the latter representing the result of a degenerative process. All schwannomas are immunoreactive for S-100 protein (a calmodulin-like cytosolic protein present in cells derived from the neural crest), type IV collagen and laminin. Schwannomas need to be distinguished from **neurofibromas**, that may contain Schwann cells.

Pathology: Segmental demyelination and axonal degeneration

Diseases affecting Schwann cells lead to a loss of myelin, or **segmental demyelination**. Damage to the neuron and its axon leads to **axonal degeneration** (**wallerian degeneration**, first described by the English physiologist Augustus Volney Waller, 1816-1870).

Axonal degeneration (Figure 8-23) may be followed by **axonal regeneration**. Recall from our discussion in Chapter 7, Muscle Tissue, that the **motor unit** is the functional unit of the neuromuscular system. Therefore, segmental demyelination and axonal degeneration affect the motor unit and cause **muscle paralysis** and **atrophy**. Physiotherapy for the paralyzed muscles is necessary to prevent muscle degeneration before regenerating motor axons can reach the motor unit.

Neurotrophins play a significant role in the survival of neurons uncoupled from a peripheral target (see Box 8-I).

Segmental demyelination occurs when the function of the Schwann cell is abnormal or there is damage to the myelin sheath, for example, a traumatic nerve injury. If the nerve fiber is completely severed, the chances of recovery decrease unless a nerve segment is grafted.

The presence of the endoneurium is essential for the proliferation of Schwann cells. Schwann cells guide an axonal sprout, derived from the proximal axonal stump, to reach the end organ (for example, a muscle).

Several sprouts can grow into the connective tissue and, together with proliferative Schwann cells, form a mass called an **traumatic neuroma** (see Figure 8-23). Traumatic neuromas prevent regrowth of the axon after trauma and must be surgically removed to allow reinnervation of the peripheral end organ.

Axonal regeneration is a very slow process. It starts 2 weeks after injury and is completed, if successful, after several months. Schwann cells remyelinate the denuded portion of the axon, but the length of internodal myelin is shorter.

Axonal degeneration results from the primary destruction of the axon by metabolic or toxic damage and is followed by demyelination and degeneration of the neuronal cell body. This process is known as a "**dying back**" neuropathy.

Regeneration of nerve fibers in the CNS is not possible at present because of the following factors:

1. An endoneurium is not present.

2. Oligodendrocytes do not proliferate in contrast to Schwann cells, and a single oligodendrocyte serves a large number of axons.

3. Astrocytes deposit scar tissue (the astrocytic plaque).

Sensory (spinal) ganglia

A cluster of neurons forms a **ganglion** (plural **ganglia**). A ganglion can be **sensory** (dorsal root ganglia and trigeminal ganglion) or **motor** (visceromotor or autonomic ganglia). **Axons derived from a ganglion** are organized as **nerves**, **rami** (singular **ramus**), or **roots**.

Sensory ganglia of the **posterior spinal nerve roots** and the **trunks of the trigeminal, facial, glossopharyngeal, and vagal cranial nerves** have a similar organization (Figure 8-24; see Figure 8-15).

A connective tissue capsule, representing the continuation of the epineurium and perineurium, surrounds each ganglion.

Neurons are **pseudounipolar**, with a single stem **myelinated** process leaving each cell body. The short process bifurcates into a **peripheral centrifugal branch** into one ramus of the spinal nerve and a **centripetal** branch into the spinal cord.

The neuronal cell body is surrounded by a layer of flattened **satellite cells**, similar to Schwann cells and continuous with them as they enclose the peripheral

Figure 8-25. Neurohistochemistry

Methods	Reagents
Basic dyes	
Nissl	Basic dyes (methylene blue, cresyl violet, thionine, hematoxylin)
Metal impregnation methods	
Bielschowsky, Bodian, Cajal, Glees, Nauta	Reduced silver nitrate
Fink-Heimer, Nauta	Reduced silver nitrate
Golgi	Silver nitrate
Myelin stains	
Osmium tetroxide	Osmium tetroxide
Klüver-Barrera	Luxol fast blue, periodic acid–Schiff (PAS), and hematoxylin
Weigert-Pal	Iron-hematoxylin
Glial stains	
Cajal	Gold sublimate
Del Rio Hortega	Silver carbonate
Neurotransmitters	
Induced fluorescence Formaldehyde Glyoxylic acid	
Immunocytochemistry	**Specific antibodies** to neurotransmitters, synthesizing enzymes and neuropeptides
Pathway tracing methods	
Anterograde transport	[³H] **leucine** injected into the soma or perikaryon combined with autoradiography
Retrograde transport	**Horseradish peroxidase** injected near synaptic terminals; the marker is internalized and transported to the perikaryon

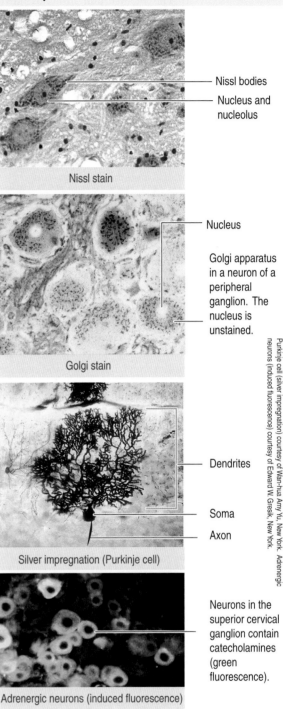

Nissl bodies

Nucleus and nucleolus

Nissl stain

Nucleus

Golgi apparatus in a neuron of a peripheral ganglion. The nucleus is unstained.

Golgi stain

Dendrites

Soma

Axon

Silver impregnation (Purkinje cell)

Neurons in the superior cervical ganglion contain catecholamines (green fluorescence).

Adrenergic neurons (induced fluorescence)

Purkinje cell (silver impregnation) courtesy of Wan-hua Amy Yu, New York. Adrenergic neurons (induced fluorescence) courtesy of Edward W. Gresik, New York.

and central process of each neuron.

Following stimulation of the peripheral sensory receptor, nerve impulse reach the T-bifurcation junction bypassing the neuronal cell body, traveling from the peripheral axon to the centripetal axon.

Autonomic nervous system: Ganglia and plexuses

The main divisions of the autonomic (self-regulating) nervous system (ANS) are:

1. The sympathetic nervous system.
2. The parasympathetic nervous system.
3. The regional autonomic innervation of the heart, enteric nervous system, lower-level bladder controls and the functional innervation of the genital tract.

The controlling neuronal centers, residing in the hypothalamus and brainstem, send fibers to synapse on preganglionic neurons located in the gray matter of the brainstem and spinal cord.

Neurons of the ANS derive from the neural crest and are situated in **ganglia** (a clustering of neurons acting as a transfer site for neuron stimulation), outside the CNS. The ANS consists of elements of the CNS and PNS; the sympathetic and parasympathetic divisions contain ganglia.

Preganglionic neurons, located in the lateral gray horn of the spinal cord at **thoracic and upper lumbar segments levels**, extend **preganglionic fibers, mostly myelinated**, into the corresponding anterior nerve roots and enter the autonomic ganglia of the paravertebral sympathetic chain, outside the CNS.

Some of the preganglionic fibers:

1. Synapse within the nearest ganglion and unmyelinated postganglionic fibers enter spinal nerves of the thoracolumbar region to supply blood vessels and sweat glands in the supply area.

2. Some preganglionic fibers ascend the sympathetic chain and synapse in the superior or middle cervical ganglion or in the **stellate ganglion** (consisting in the fusion of the inferior cervical ganglion and the first thoracic ganglion). Unmyelinated postganglionic fibers extend to the head, neck, and upper limbs as well as the heart and the dilator myoepithelial cells of the iris.

Horner syndrome (Bernard-Horner syndrome) consists in a constricted pupil (**miosis**), **partial ptosis** of the eyelid, and loss of hemifacial sweating (**hemifacial anhidrosis**). It is caused by a disruption in the structure and function of postganglionic neurons in the stellate ganglion.

3. Some preganglionic fibers descend to synapse the lumbar or sacral ganglia. Unmyelinated postganglionic fibers become part of the lumbosacral plexus to reach blood vessels of the skin of the lower limbs.

4. Some preganglionic fibers cross the chain and exit as preganglionic fibers of the thoracic and lumbar splanchnic nerves. The thoracic splanchnic nerves traverse the diaphragm and synapse in the abdominal cavity in the celiac and mesenteric prevertebral ganglia and renal ganglia. Unmyelinated postganglionic fibers reach the gastrointestinal tract, liver, pancreas and the kidneys through the aorta and its branches.

Sensory fibers, detecting pain from viscera, reach the CNS by either or both of the sympathetic and parasympathetic pathways. Their neurons are located in either the spinal ganglion (**dorsal root ganglion**) or the sensory ganglion of several cranial nerves.

In the presence of fear, the sympathetic system stimulates an increase in the heart rate, dilation of the pupils and skin sweating. Blood flow is redirected from the skin and intestinal tract to the skeletal muscle. The sphincters of the urinary and alimentary tracts contract.

The parasympathetic system has a counterbalancing effect of the sympathetic system. It slows down the heart, stimulates intestinal and digestive gland secretory function and accelerates intestinal peristalsis.

Preganglionic fibers exit the CNS from the **craniosacral segment levels**. Fibers exit from the brainstem in four cranial nerves: the oculomotor, facial, glossopharyngeal and vagus and from the sacral segments of the spinal cord.

The **enteric nervous system** consists of two interconnected plexuses within the walls of the alimentary tube:

1. The **myenteric plexus of Auerbach**.
2. The **submucosal plexus of Meissner**.

Each plexus consists of neurons and associated cells, and bundles of nerve fibers passing between plexuses. We discuss the enteric nervous system in Chapter 15, Upper Digestive Segment, and Chapter 16, Lower Digestive Segment.

In summary:

1. Similar to the spinal (sensory) ganglion, sympathetic ganglia are surrounded by a layer of connective tissue continuous with the epineurium and perineurium of the peripheral nerve fiber (see Figures 8-24 and 8-15).

2. The neurons of the sympathetic ganglia are multipolar neurons.

3. The dendrites are contacted by myelinated axons of preganglionic neurons (**white rami**).

4. The axons have a small diameter and are unmyelinated (**gray rami**).

5. Each neuronal cell body is surrounded by Schwann cell–like **satellite cells**, less abundant in sympathetic ganglia when compared to the more abundant satellite cells in dorsal root spinal ganglia.

Neurohistochemistry

The nervous tissue has specialized features not observed in other basic tissues stained with routine staining methods such as hematoxylin-eosin. For example, **basic dyes** can demonstrate the cytoplasmic Nissl substance (ribonucleoproteins) in the cytoplasm of neurons (Figure 8-25).

Reduced silver methods produce dark deposits in various structures of neurons and glial cells. The **Golgi method** is particularly valuable for the study of dendrites. A variant of the Golgi method enables the identification of the cytomembranes and vesicles of the Golgi apparatus.

Myelin stains are based on the use of dyes with binding affinity for proteins bound to phospholipids. An example is Luxol fast blue. They are useful for the identification of tracts of fibers. Combined Nissl and myelin stains are used in neuropathology.

A tracer, such as horseradish peroxidase, injected into a neuron using a micro-pipet, has been used for anterograde transport studies.

Similarly, tracers injected into nerve terminals

can identify the putative neuron by its retrograde transport.

Histochemical techniques are available for the localization of substances (for example, catecholamines, enzymes, and others) present in specific populations of neurons.

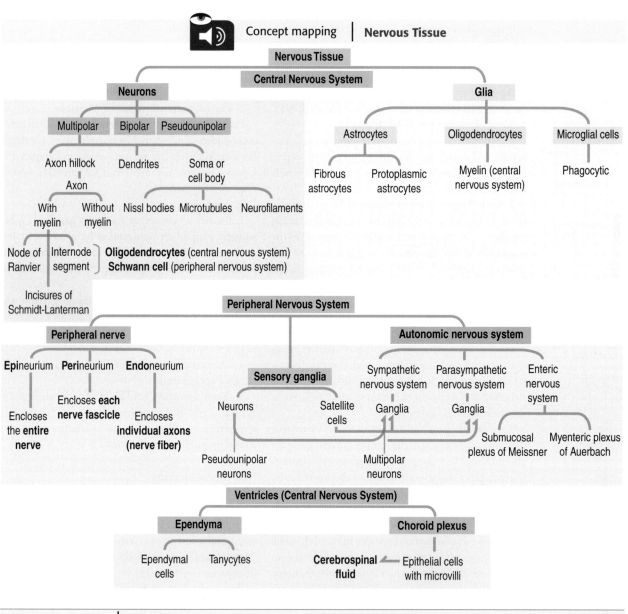

Concept mapping | **Nervous Tissue**

Essential concepts | **Nervous Tissue**

- The nervous system consists of:
  (1) The central nervous system (CNS) (brain, spinal cord, and the neural parts of the eye).
  (2) The peripheral nervous system (PNS) (peripheral ganglia, nerves, nerve endings linking ganglia with the CNS, and receptors and effectors of the body).
  The basic components of the CNS are neurons and glia (astrocytes, oligodendrocytes and microglial cells).
  The PNS includes Schwann cells (peripheral nerves) and satellite cells (ganglia).

- The CNS develops from the primitive ecto-derm. A neural plate folds to form a hollow cylinder, the neural tube (a process known as neurulation).
  A region of the neural tube becomes the neural crest, which forms the neurons of peripheral ganglia and other components of the PNS. In addition, neural crest cells migrate along specific routes and differentiate into melanocytes, smooth muscle, and cartilaginous and skeletal components of the head. Some cells form the medulla of the adrenal gland; others organize the enteric nervous system of the alimentary tube.
  Defects in the closing of the neural tube cause congenital malformation (for example, **spina bifida**, **anencephaly**, and **craniorachischisis**).

- The functional unit of the nervous system is the neuron. A neuron consists of a body (soma or perikaryon), multiple dendrites, and a single axon. Dendrites are covered by dendritic spines. The site of origin of the axon is called the axon hillock. The terminal portion of an axon has branches (called collectively telodendron); each branch has an enlarged synaptic ending or synaptic bouton. The neuronal body contains two important structures:

Nissl body or substance (aggregates of polyribosomes and rough endoplasmic reticulum), and cytoskeletal components (neurofilaments and neurotubules), which extend into the dendritic and axonal processes. Nissl bodies stop at the axon hillock but extend into the base of the dendrites. Neurotubules play a significant role in anterograde and retrograde axonal transport of synaptic vesicles and other molecules, mediated by molecular motor proteins kinesin (anterograde transport) and cytoplasmic dynein (retrograde transport).

• Neurons can be classified according to the **number of processes** as:
(1) Multipolar neurons (a single axon and multiple dendrites; for example, pyramidal cells of the cerebral cortex and Purkinje cells of the cerebellar cortex).
(2) Bipolar neurons (with two processes; found in the sensory system).
(3) Pseudounipolar neurons (a single short process; localized in sensory ganglia of cranial and spinal nerves).
Multipolar neurons can be subclassified according to the **length of processes** as:
(1) Golgi type I neurons (the axon extends beyond the limits of the dendritic tree; for example, pyramidal neurons and Purkinje neurons).
(2) Golgi type II neurons (the axon terminates close to the body and does not extend beyond the limits of the dendritic tree; for example, stellate cells of the cerebral cortex).

• There is a specific nomenclature for groups of neurons and axons:
(1) A nucleus (plural nuclei) is an aggregate of neurons in the CNS.
(2) Neuropil designates the clustering of dendrites, axons, and glial cells within a nucleus and between neuronal bodies.
(3) A stratum or lamina is the aggregate of neurons in a layer.
(4) Bundles of axons in the CNS are called tracts, fasciculi (bundles), or lemnisci.
(5) A ganglion (plural ganglia) is a cluster of neurons in the PNS. A ganglion can be sensory (dorsal root ganglia and trigeminal ganglion) or motor (visceromotor or autonomic ganglia).
(6) Axons derived from a ganglion are organized as nerves, ramus (plural rami), or roots.

• A synapse is the junction between the presynaptic terminal of an axon (transmitting site) and the postsynaptic membrane (receiving site), usually of a dendrite, separated by a synaptic cleft. A presynaptic density (corresponding to specific protein—some of them associated to synaptic vesicles—and channels; the active site of a synaptic ending) and a postsynaptic density (receptors for neurotransmitters) are seen on the corresponding membranes.
Synapses can be:
(1) Axospinous (axon terminal facing a dendritic spine).
(2) Axodendritic (axon terminal on the shaft of a dendrite).

(3) Axosomatic (axon terminal on the soma of a neuron).
(4) Axoaxonic (axon terminal ending on an axon terminal).

• Glial cells include:
(1) Astrocytes (derived from the neuroectoderm).
(2) Oligodendrocytes (derived from the neuroectoderm).
(3) Microglia (derived from the mesoderm).
Astrocytes can be subdivided into fibrous astrocytes (predominant in white matter), and protoplasmic astrocytes (found mainly in gray matter). Astrocytes contain in their cytoplasm the intermediate filament protein glial fibrillary acidic protein.
Brain capillaries and the inner surface of the pia are surrounded by the glia limitans, corresponding to astrocytic end-feet.
Oligodendrocytes are involved in axonal myelination within the CNS. Each oligodendrocyte provides myelin to several axons. The node of Ranvier (flanked by internode segments) is devoid of oligodendrocyte cytoplasm; the space is occupied by an astrocytic end-foot process.
Microglial cells are phagocytic cells and immunoprotect the brain and spinal cord. In response to brain injury or immunologic activity, microglial cells change into an activated state characterized by an ameboidal morphology accompanied by the up-regulation of cell surface molecules.
Microglial cells may become overactivated and exert neurotoxic effects by the excessive production of cytotoxic substances such as ROS, nitric oxide, and tumor necrosis factor ligand. Activated microglial cells are present in large numbers in neurodegenerative diseases (Alzheimer's disease, Parkinson's disease, multiple sclerosis, amyotrophic lateral sclerosis, Huntington's disease), causing a generalized microglial hyperactivity, a condition called reactive microgliosis.
Microglia-mediated neurotoxicity takes place when pathogen- associated molecular patterns (PAMPs) bind to pattern recognition receptors (PRRs) and trigger an excessive immune response. A given ligand can be recognized by several PRRs (cumulative effect).
PRRs are responsible for phagocytic functions (identification of pathogens, production of extracellular superoxide, release of pro-inflammatory factors and removal of toxic substances by phagocytosis).

• **Myelin** is a highly organized multilamellar structure formed by the plasma membrane of oligodendrocytes and Schwann cells.
Myelin surrounds axons and facilitates conduction of a nerve impulse by providing insulation to axons and clustering Na^+ channels in the nodes of Ranvier. This arrangement enables the action potential to jump along nodes by a mechanism called saltatory conduction. Saltatory conduction decreases energy requirements for the transmission of a nerve impulse.

During myelinization, cytoplasmic processes of oligodendrocytes and Schwann cells wrap around the axon. Note a difference: several cytoplasmic processes of an oligodendrocytes wrap around different axons, whereas a Schwann cell supplies only one axon.
Visualization of myelin by electron microscopy reveals two types of densities:
(1) The intraperiod line, representing the close apposition of the external surfaces of the plasma membrane with remnant extracellular space.
(2) The major dense line, corresponding to the apposition of the inner (cytoplasmic) surfaces of the plasma membrane.
The incisures of Schmidt-Lanterman represent residual cytoplasm. The major dense line is slightly thinner in myelin of the CNS.
Proteins of myelin include:
(1) Myelin basic protein (MBP) present in myelin of the CNS and PNS.
(2) Proteolipid protein (PLP) found in myelin of the CNS.
(3) Myelin protein zero (MPZ) the equivalent of PLP in the PNS.
MPZ is responsible for maintaining myelin in a compact state. A mutation of the *PLP* gene and its alternatively transcribed protein DM20 causes Pelizaeus-Merzbacher disease, an X-linked neuropathy affecting males and characterized by a reduction in the white matter.
Proteins of myelin are strong antigens and have a role in the development of **multiple sclerosis** in the CNS and **Guillain-Barré syndrome** in the PNS.
Myelin is separated from the axon by the axolemma, the surface membrane of the axon. Tight junctions (represented by claudins and zonula occludens proteins) are found linking the plasma membranes of the same Schwann cell and adjacent Schwann cell at the level of the node of Ranvier. Gap junctions, containing connexin 32 (Cx32), are present in the region of the incisures of Schmidt-Lanterman. Mutations in the *Cx32* gene determine the **X-linked Charcot-Marie-Tooth disease**, a demyelinating disorder of the PNS.
Multiple sclerosis is a clinically recurrent or chronically progressive neurologic dysfunction caused by multiple areas of demyelination in the CNS, in particular the brain, optic nerves, and spinal cord.
Two characteristic microscopic features are:
(1) Infiltration of inflammatory cells (T cells and macrophages) inside and around multiple sclerosis plaques.
(2) Plaques of astrocytic aggregates.
CD8+ and CD4+ T cells, recruited to multiple sclerosis lesions, secrete cytokines (interleukin-2, tumor necrosis factor ligand [TNFL], and interferon-γ).
T cells secrete Fas ligand that binds to Fas receptor on oligodendrocytes to induce their apoptosis. TNFL exerts a similar apoptotic effect. Demyelinating axons by macrophages with foamy cytoplasm, and reactive astrocytes (Creutzfeldt cells) with several cytoplasmic nuclear fragments are observed.

- The **ependyma** lines the surface of the ventricles (brain) and central canal (spinal cord). It consists of two cell types:

(1) Ependymal cells, a simple cuboidal epithelium with apical microvilli, one or more cilia, linked by desmosomes, and a basal domain in contact with an astrocyte end-foot layer.

(2) Tanycytes, a specialized ependymal cell with a basal cell process making contact with a blood vessel.

The **choroid plexus** produces cerebrospinal fluid (CSF). The plexus consists of epithelial cells linked by tight junctions and with apical microvilli containing Na^+,K^+-ATPase, which pumps Na^+ into the lumen of the ventricle. High Na^+ concentration in the ventricular lumen facilitates the diffusion of water by an osmotic gradient. The basal domain has numerous infoldings.

Hydrostatic pressure inside the subjacent fenestrated capillaries produces a net flow of water, solutes, and proteins. The lining epithelium of the choroid plexus screens and excludes several substances from entering the CSF.

The CSF flows from the fourth ventricle into the brain and spinal subarachnoid space and exits the CNS at the superior sagittal sinus.

- Three **brain permeability barriers** exist:

(1) The arachnoid-CSF barrier, consisting of the arachnoid membrane, which prevents the CSF from coming in contact with the extracellular space of the dura mater, and the arachnoid villi, which enable the CSF to permeate across arachnoid barrier cells and endothelial cells.

(2) The blood-CSF barrier, with a role of the choroid epithelium in selecting protein and solutes that may reach the ventricular space.

(3) The blood-brain barrier, represented by tight junctions sealing the interendothelial space. Astrocyte end-feet in contact with the capillary wall contribute to the barrier.

Brain metastatic tumors can develop and grow in the absence of angiogenesis by co-opting the pre-existing brain vasculature. Metastases to the brain are perivascular.

Metastatic cells avoid apoptosis and co-opt brain vessels by expressing the protein neuroserpin.

Neuroserpin inhibit the production of plasminogen activator by astrocytes, blocking the release of plasmin from plasminogen and the secretion of the apoptosis inducer FAS ligand. Suppression of plasmin and FAS ligand enable metastatic cancer cells to retain adhesion to the brain vasculature, a landmark of vascular co-option.

- The PNS consists of supporting cell types associated to axons extending from neuronal elements of the spinal cord and autonomic and sensory ganglia.

(1) Schwann cells are the equivalent of the oligodendrocytes of the CNS.

(2) Satellite cells surround the cell bodies of neurons in autonomic and sensory ganglia.

Schwann cells can provide a myelin sheath to a myelinated nerve fiber by forming only one internode segment of myelin (a single oligodendrocyte can form several internode segments). In contrast, several unmyelinated nerve fibers can be embedded in the cytoplasm of a single Schwann cell (in the CNS, unmyelinated nerves are ensheathed by astrocytes).

A **peripheral nerve** is covered by layers of connective tissue:

(1) The epineurium covers the entire nerve.

(2) The perineurium separates the nerve into fascicles and consists of neuroepithelial perineurial cells. Perineurial cells are joined to each other by tight junctions to form the protective diffusion barrier: the blood-nerve barrier, responsible for maintaining the physiologic microenvironment of the endoneurium.

(3) The endoneurium surrounds individual axons and their associated Schwann cells.

- **Schwannomas** are benign encapsulated tumors consisting of Schwann cells. Schwannomas can develop at the surface or inside of a nerve fascicle and display spindle cells (called Antoni A pattern) or multipolar cells (called Antoni B pattern), the latter representing the result of a degenerative process. All schwannomas are immunoreactive for S-100 protein.

- Peripheral nerves can be injured (traumatic crush nerve injury) or diseases may affect the function of Schwann cells, leading to a loss of myelin (segmental demyelinization).

A damage to a neuron and its axon causes axonal degeneration, also called wallerian degeneration.

A characteristic of axonal degeneration, caused by toxic or metabolic damage, is chromatolysis, the dispersion of Nissl substance (polyribosomes and rough endoplasmic reticulum) in the neuronal soma, followed by demyelinization.

Segmental demyelinization and axonal degeneration affect the motor unit and cause muscle paralysis. Axonal degeneration may be followed by axonal regeneration in the PNS. Axonal regeneration in the CNS is not feasible because the endoneurium is not present, oligodendrocytes—in contrast to Schwann cells—do not proliferate, and astrocytes deposit scar tissue (astrocytic plaque).

Neuroma is the disorganized proliferation of axons, Schwann cells and perineural connective tissue at the site of complete or partial nerve injury transection

- **Neurodegenerative diseases**.

(1) **Amyotrophic lateral sclerosis** is a motor neuron progressive disease starting with moderate weakness in one limb and progressing to severe paralysis. A mutation in the copper-zinc *superoxide dismutase* gene is frequently seen.

(2) **Alzheimer's disease**, the most common neurodegenerative disorder, is characterized by progressive cortical dementia affecting language and memory. A typical feature is the formation of amyloid plaques containing β-amyloid peptide.

(3) **Parkinson's disease**, the second most frequent after Alzheimer's disease, is caused by a loss of dopaminergic neurons from the substantia nigra. Resting tremor and movements with rigidity are the typical clinical features. A characteristic pathologic aspect is the presence of deposits of hyperphosphorylated α–synuclein in the cytoplasm of neurons (Lewy bodies) and threadlike inclusions in axons (Lewy neurites).

A familial form of Parkinson's disease is PARK2 (Parkinson's disease protein 2).

PARK2 encodes the E3 ubiquitin-protein ligase parkin. Parkin is involved in the maintenance of mitochondria. Defective mitochondria can trigger the production of reactive oxygen species (ROS) and disrupt cell functions.

Mitophagy is a specific mechanism to eliminate damaged mitochondria by a signaling pathway involving two enzymes:

(1) PINK1 (PTEN [phosphatase and tensin homolog] induced putative kinase 1).

(2) Parkin.

The accumulation of damaged mitochondria, caused by mutations in parkin and PINK1, determine high mitochondrial oxidative stress in dopamine neurons, the initial step of the familial forms of Parkinson's disease.

(4) **Huntington's disease**, is a neurodegenerative disease caused by a gene *huntingtin* (*HTT*) containing a number of CAG repeats in the coding region and expressing a so called polyQ HTT protein.

Huntington's disease is characterized by the progressive activation of caspases and cytochrome *c* following accumulation of mutated protein hungtingtin in the neuronal cell nucleus.

- **Sensory ganglia** (dorsal root ganglia) are surrounded by a connective tissue capsule (epineurium). Neurons are clustered and are pseudounipolar. Nerve fascicles contain myelinated nerve fibers. Each neuron is surrounded by satellite cells supported by a basal lamina.

Autonomic ganglia receive preganglionic axons from the CNS and give rise to postganglionic unmyelinated axons. Multipolar neurons are scattered and surrounded by satellite cells (less numerous than those of sensory ganglia).

9. Sensory Organs: Vision and Hearing

The eye can self-focus, adjust for light intensity, and convert light into electrical impulses interpreted by the visual cortex of the brain as detailed images. In humans, the eye is recessed in a bony orbit and is connected to the brain by the optic nerve. The eyeball protects and facilitates the function of the photoreceptive retina, the inner layer of the eyeball harboring photosensitive cells, rods and cones. The ear consists of two anatomic systems designed to amplify sound waves and transmit them to the brain for hearing and for maintaining the sense of body equilibrium by detecting rotation, gravity and acceleration. This chapter provides a comprehensive description of the main histologic components of the eye and ear and addresses pathologic, degenerative, and genetic–based clinical conditions.

Eye

The eyeball consists of **three tunics** or **layers** (Figure 9-1) which, from outside to inside, are:

1. The **sclera** and the **cornea**.
2. The **uvea**.
3. The **retina**.

Three distinct and interconnected chambers are found inside the eyeball: the **anterior chamber**, the **posterior chamber**, and the **vitreous cavity** (see Box 9-A). **Aqueous humor** circulates from the posterior to the anterior chamber. The **lens** is placed in front of the vitreous cavity, which contains **vitreous humor**. The **bony orbit**, the **eyelids**, the **conjunctiva**, and the **lacrimal apparatus** protect the eyeball.

The **ophthalmic artery**, a branch of the internal carotid artery, provides nutrients to the eye and the contents of the orbit. The **superior** and **inferior orbital veins** are the principal venous drainage of the eye. The veins empty into the **intracranial cavernous sinus**.

Development of the eye

A brief summary of the development of the eye is essential to the understanding of the relationship of the various layers in the eyeball. The components of the eye derive from:

1. The surface **ectoderm** of the head.
2. The lateral **neuroectodermal** walls of the embryonic brain in the diencephalon region.
3. The **mesenchyme**.

Figure 9-1. Anatomy of the eye

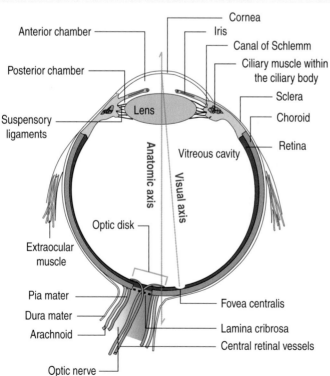

- Anterior chamber
- Posterior chamber
- Suspensory ligaments
- Lens
- Cornea
- Iris
- Canal of Schlemm
- Ciliary muscle within the ciliary body
- Sclera
- Choroid
- Retina
- Anatomic axis
- Visual axis
- Vitreous cavity
- Extraocular muscle
- Optic disk
- Pia mater
- Dura mater
- Arachnoid
- Fovea centralis
- Lamina cribrosa
- Central retinal vessels
- Optic nerve

Box 9-A | The eye: Highlights to remember

- The eye consists of three chambers: (1) The **anterior chamber** is the space between the cornea and the anterior surface of the iris. (2) The **posterior chamber** extends from the posterior surface of the iris to the lens. (3) The **vitreous cavity** or **body** is posterior to the lens and is the largest compartment.
- The human eyeball is roughly spherical with a diameter of about 24 mm. The anterior pole of the eyeball is the center of the **cornea**.
- The posterior pole is located between the **optic disk** and the **fovea**, a shallow depression in the retina. The **anatomic axis** (also called the **optical axis**) is the line connecting the two poles. The **visual axis** joins the apparent center of the pupil and the center of the fovea and divides the eyeball into **nasal** and **temporal halves**.
- The eyeball is surrounded by a soft tissue cushion occupying the bony orbit of the skull. The soft tissue includes loose connective tissue, fat, muscles, blood and lymphatic vessels, nerves, and the lacrimal gland.
- The anterior surface of the eyeball is connected to the integument by the **conjunctiva**, which lines the inner surface of the lids and reflects over the eyeball to the edge of the cornea.

Figure 9-2. Development of the eye

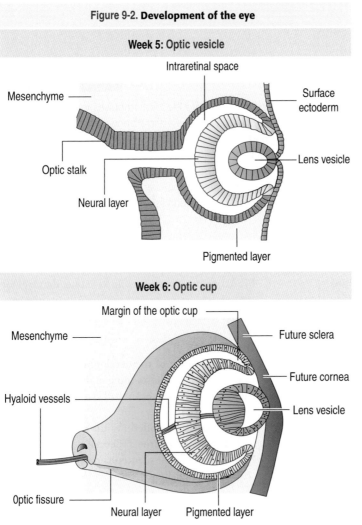

Week 5: Optic vesicle

Mesenchyme
Optic stalk
Neural layer
Intraretinal space
Surface ectoderm
Lens vesicle
Pigmented layer

Week 6: Optic cup

Margin of the optic cup
Mesenchyme
Hyaloid vessels
Optic fissure
Future sclera
Future cornea
Lens vesicle
Neural layer
Pigmented layer

Lateral outpocketings of the right and left sides of the diencephalon give rise to two neuroepithelial **optic vesicles**, each remaining attached to the brain wall by a hollow **optic stalk** (Figure 9-2). The surface ectoderm of the head invaginates into the optical vesicle forming a **lens vesicle** that pinches off. Mesenchyme surrounds both the lens vesicle and the adjacent optic vesicle.

The optic vesicle invaginates and becomes a double-walled **optic cup** (see Figure 9-2). The **optic fissure** forms when the outer layer of the optic cup becomes the **pigmented epithelium**. Cells in the inner layer proliferate and stratify to form the **neural**

Box 9-B | Development of the cornea

- The lens induces the differentiation of the overlying ectoderm. Cells of the mesenchyme secrete types I and II collagen, components of the primary stroma of the cornea.
- **Capillary endothelial cells** migrate into the primary stroma and produce hyaluronic acid, causing the stroma to swell.
- **Mesenchymal cells** in the surrounding space migrate into the stroma and secrete hyaluronidase. The stroma shrinks, and the cornea acquires the correct shape and transparency.

retina. The mesenchyme extending into the invagination of the optic cup acquires a gelatinous consistency and becomes the **vitreous component** of the eye. The **lens vesicle** is kept in place by the free margins of the optic cup and the surrounding mesenchyme.

At the outer surface of the optic cup, the mesenchymal shell differentiates into the vascular **choroid coat** of the eye and the fibrous components of the **sclera** and **cornea** (Figure 9-3; see Box 9-B). Posterior to the lens, the vascular choroid coat forms the **ciliary body**, **ciliary muscle**, and **ciliary processes**. Anterior to the lens, the choroid coat forms the stroma of the **iris**.

The ciliary processes secrete the **aqueous humor** that accumulates first in the **posterior chamber** (between the iris and lens) and then passes into the anterior chamber (between the lens and cornea) across the pupil. The aqueous humor leaves the anterior chamber by entering into the **canal of Schlemm**, linked to the **sinus venosus of the sclera**, a small vein encircling the eye at the anterior edge of the choroid coat or tunica.

Around the rim of the optic cup, the inner and outer layers form the **posterior epithelium** of the **ciliary body** and **iris**. The sphincter and **dilator pupillae muscles** develop from the posterior epithelium.

The inner layer of the optic cup becomes the neural layer of the retina, which differentiates into **photosensory cells**, **bipolar neurons**, and **ganglionic neurons** (including interconnecting **horizontal** and **amacrine cells** and **glial Müller cells**). Axons from the ganglionic neurons form the nerve fiber layer of the retina, which converges on the optic stalk occupying the optic fissure as the **optic nerve**. The optic fissure becomes the escape route from the optic cup (except at its rim).

Outer tunic: Sclera and cornea

The sclera (Figure 9-4) is a 1.0- to 0.4-mm-thick layer of collagen and elastic fibers produced by fibroblasts. The inner side of the sclera faces the choroid, from which it is separated by a layer of loose connective tissue and an elastic tissue network known as the **suprachoroid lamina**. Tendons of the six extrinsic muscles of the eye are attached to the outer surface of the sclera.

Cornea

The cornea is 0.8-1.1 mm thick and has a smaller radius of curvature than the sclera. It is transparent, lacks blood vessels, and is extremely rich in nerve endings. The anterior surface of the cornea is always kept wet with a film of tears retained by microvilli of the apical epithelial cells. The cornea is one of the few organs that can be transplanted without a risk of being rejected by the host's immune system. This success can be attributed to the lack of corneal blood and lymphatic vessels.

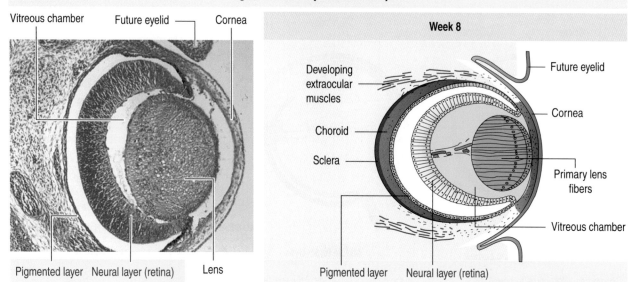

Figure 9-3. Development of the eye

Vitreous chamber | Future eyelid | Cornea

Pigmented layer | Neural layer (retina) | Lens

Week 8

Developing extraocular muscles

Choroid

Sclera

Future eyelid

Cornea

Primary lens fibers

Vitreous chamber

Pigmented layer | Neural layer (retina)

The cornea is composed of five layers (Figure 9-5):

1. The **corneal epithelium**.
2. The **layer** or **membrane of Bowman**.
3. The **stroma** or **substantia propria**.
4. The **membrane of Descemet**.
5. The **corneal endothelium**.

The **corneal epithelium** is a non-keratinized stratified squamous and consists of five to seven layers of cells. Cells of the outer surface have **microvilli** and all cells are connected to one another by desmosomes. The epithelium of the cornea is very sensitive, contains a large number of free nerve endings and has a remarkable wound healing capacity. At the **limbus**, the corneoscleral junction, the corneal epithelium is continuous with that of the conjunctiva.

The cytoplasm of the basal layer cells express keratin 5 and keratin 14 (K5 and K14) that are replaced in the upper layers by corneal-specific K3 and K12. Corneal epithelial cells undergo continuous renewal from **limbus stem cells (LSC)**. LSC migrate transversely from the limbus toward the central cornea. A deficiency in LSC changes the cornea into a nontransparent, keratinized skin-like epithelium leading to partial or complete blindness.

Bowman's layer is 6 to 9 μm thick, consists of type I collagen fibrils, and lacks elastic fibers. This layer is transparent and does not have regenerative capacity. Bowman's layer is the anteriormost part of the corneal stroma, although differently organized. For this reason, it is designated "layer" instead of "membrane." Bowman's layer represents a protective barrier to trauma and bacterial invasion.

The highly transparent **stroma** or **substantia propria** represents about 90% of the thickness of the cornea. Bundles of **types I** and **V collagen** form thin layers regularly arranged in successive planes crossing at various angles and forming a **lattice** that

is highly resistant to deformations and trauma. Fibers and layers are separated by an extracellular matrix rich in **proteoglycans** containing **chondroitin** and **keratan sulfate**.

Nerves in transit to the corneal epithelium are found in the corneal stroma.

Descemet's membrane, one of the thickest basement membranes in the body (5 to 10 μm thick), is produced by the corneal endothelium and contains **type VII collagen**, which forms a hexagonal array of fibers.

The **corneal endothelium** lines the posterior surface of Descemet's membrane and faces the anterior chamber of the eye. It consists of a single layer of squamous epithelial cells, with impermeable intercellular spaces preventing influx of aqueous humor into the corneal stroma. The structural and functional integrity of the corneal endothelium is vital to the maintenance of corneal transparency (see Box 9-C).

Middle tunic: Uvea

The uvea forms the pigmented vascularized tunic of the eye and is divided into three regions (see Figure 9-4; see Box 9-D):

1. The **choroid**.
2. The **ciliary body**.
3. The **iris**.

The **choroid** consists of three layers (Figure 9-6):

1. **Bruch's membrane**, the innermost component of the choroid, consists of a network of collagen and elastic fibers and basal lamina material. Basal laminae derive from the pigmented epithelium of the retina and the endothelia of the underlying fenestrated capillaries.

2. The **choriocapillaris** contains fenestrated capillaries that supply oxygen and nutrients to the outer layers of the retina and the fovea.

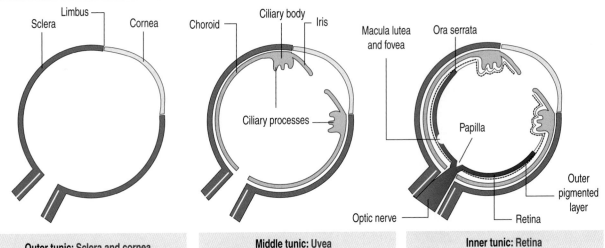

Figure 9-4. **Three tunics of the eye**

Labels: Sclera, Limbus, Cornea, Choroid, Ciliary body, Iris, Ciliary processes, Macula lutea and fovea, Ora serrata, Papilla, Outer pigmented layer, Optic nerve, Retina

Outer tunic: Sclera and cornea

The cornea (Latin *corneus*, horny) is transparent. The rest of the wall of the eye, the **sclera** (Greek *scleros*, hard), is opaque and lined inside by the middle or vascular pigmented layer that absorbs light.

The **limbus** is the zone of transition of the epithelium of the conjunctiva with that of the cornea. The limbus is also the boundary of the transparent cornea with the opaque sclera. The corneoscleral coat:

1. Protects the inner structures of the eye.

2. Together with the intraocular fluid pressure, it maintains the shape and consistency of the eyeball.

Middle tunic: Uvea

In the posterior two thirds of the eye, the vascular layer is called the choroid. In the anterior part of the eye the vascular layer thickens to form the **ciliary body**.

Ciliary processes extend inward from the ciliary body. The vascular layer continues as the iris, whose free edge outlines the **pupil**.

1. The vascular layer is **pigmented**, a property that light-proofs the inner surface of the eye and reduces reflection of the light.

2. Blood vessels travel through the middle layer.

3. Its anterior portion contains smooth muscle: the **muscle of the ciliary body** and the **dilator** and **constrictor of the iris**. The smooth muscle of the ciliary body regulates the tension of the **zonule** or **suspensory ligament** of the lens and, therefore, is an important element in the mechanism of **accommodation**.

Inner tunic: Retina

It consists of two layers: (1) an **outer pigmented layer** (pars pigmentosa) and (2) an **inner retinal layer** (pars nervosa or optica). The retina has a posterior two-thirds light-sensitive zone (pars optica) and an anterior one-third **light-nonsensitive zone** (pars ciliaris and iridica). The scalloped border between these two zones is called the **ora serrata** (Latin *ora*, edge; *serrata*, sawlike).

The retina contains **photoreceptor neurons** (cones and rods), **conducting neurons** (bipolar and ganglion cells), **association neurons** (horizontal and amacrine cells), and a **supporting neuroglial cell**, the Müller cell.

Each eye contains about 125 million rods and cones but only 1 million ganglion cells. The number of cones and rods varies over the surface of the retina. **Only cones are present in the fovea** (0.5 mm in diameter), where fine detail vision is best. Axons from the retinal ganglion cells pass across the surface of the retina, converge on the **papilla** or **optic disk**, and leave the eye through many openings of the sclera (the **lamina cribrosa**) to form the **optic nerve**.

3. The **choroidal stroma** consists of large arteries and veins surrounded by collagen and elastic fibers, fibroblasts, a few smooth muscle cells, neurons of the autonomic nervous system, and melanocytes.

The **ciliary body** (Figure 9-7) is anterior to the ora serrata and represents the ventral projection of both the choroid and the retina. It is made up of two components:

1. The **uveal portion**.

2. The **neuroepithelial portion**.

The **uveal portion** of the ciliary body includes:

1. The continuation of the outer layer of the choroid, known as the **supraciliaris**.

2. The **ciliary muscle**, a ring of smooth muscle tissue that, **when contracted, reduces the length of the circular suspensory ligaments of the lens**; this is known as the **ciliary zonule**.

3. A layer of **fenestrated capillaries** supplying blood to the ciliary muscle.

The **neuroepithelial portion** contributes the two layers of the **ciliary epithelium**:

1. An outer **pigmented epithelial layer**, continuous with the retinal pigmented epithelium. The pigmented epithelial layer is supported by a basal lamina continuous with Bruch's membrane.

2. An inner **nonpigmented epithelial layer**, which is continuous with the sensory retina.

Particular features of these two pigmented and nonpigmented epithelial cell layers are:

1. **The apical surfaces of the pigmented and nonpigmented cells face each other.**

2. The dual epithelium is smooth at its posterior end (pars plana) and folded at the anterior end (pars plicata) to form the **ciliary processes**.

Figure 9-6. **Structure of the choroid**

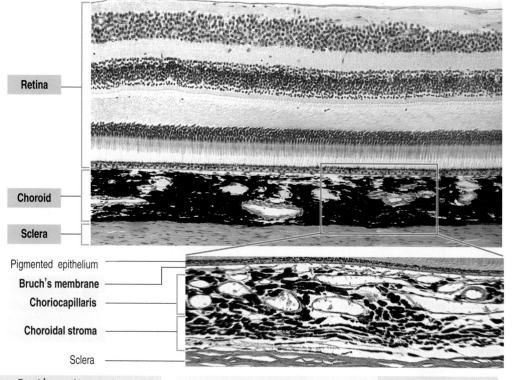

Retina

Choroid

Sclera

Pigmented epithelium

Bruch's membrane

Choriocapillaris

Choroidal stroma

Sclera

Bruch's membrane

Bruch's membrane is formed by:
1. The **basal lamina of the pigmented epithelium** of the retina.
2. Subjacent layers of **collagenous and elastic fibers**.
3. The **basal lamina of endothelial cells** of the underlying capillary network (choriocapillaris).

Choroidal stroma

The stroma contains collagen fibers, some smooth muscle cells, neurons of the autonomic nervous system, blood vessels (arteries and veins), and melanocytes.

Melanocytes are more numerous in heavily pigmented individuals than in persons with light pigment.

Choriocapillaris

Capillaries of the choriocapillaris connect with arteries (branches of the posterior ciliary arteries) and veins (vortex veins) in the choroidal stroma.

The choriocapillaris provides nutrients to the outer layers of the retina.

The accumulation of **proteins** (apolipoprotein E, amyloid protein, complement proteins C5 and C5b-9 complex, and others) in the inner side of Bruch's membrane is called **drusen** (German *Drusen*, stony nodule). A large drusen pushes away the photoreceptors from their blood supply. If the separation is too large, the pigmented epithelium and photoreceptors degenerate.

The earliest indication of **age-related macular degeneration** is the presence of drusen.

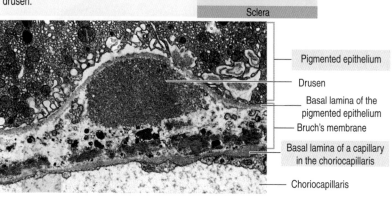

Pigmented epithelium

Drusen

Basal lamina of the pigmented epithelium

Bruch's membrane

Basal lamina of a capillary in the choriocapillaris

Choriocapillaris

Drusen

Photoreceptor cell layer

Pigmented epithelium

Bruch's membrane

Choriocapillaris

Choroidal stroma

Sclera

cells and is the source of new cells of the lens. The posterior epithelium disappears early in the formation of the lens. The anterior epithelium and lens substance are enclosed by the **lens capsule**. There is no epithelial cell layer under the posterior surface of the capsule.

The **lens capsule** is a thick flexible acellular and transparent basement membrane–like structure containing **type IV collagen fibrils** and a **glycosaminoglycan matrix**. Beneath the anterior portion of the capsule is a single layer of **cuboidal epithelial cells** that extend posteriorly up to the equatorial region. In the

Figure 9-7. Ciliary body

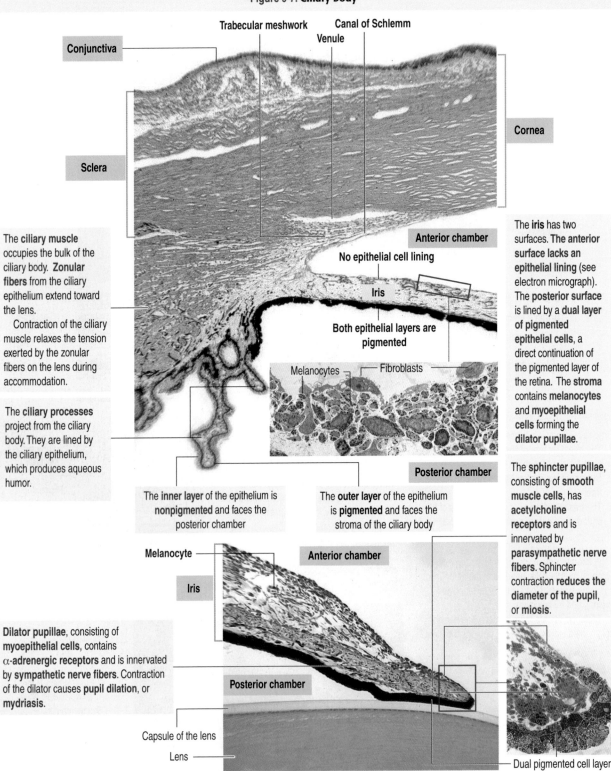

Trabecular meshwork

Canal of Schlemm

Venule

Conjunctiva

Cornea

Sclera

The **ciliary muscle** occupies the bulk of the ciliary body. **Zonular fibers** from the ciliary epithelium extend toward the lens.

Contraction of the ciliary muscle relaxes the tension exerted by the zonular fibers on the lens during accommodation.

The **ciliary processes** project from the ciliary body. They are lined by the ciliary epithelium, which produces aqueous humor.

Anterior chamber

No epithelial cell lining

Iris

Both epithelial layers are pigmented

Melanocytes

Fibroblasts

The **iris** has two surfaces. **The anterior surface lacks an epithelial lining** (see electron micrograph). The **posterior surface** is lined by a **dual layer of pigmented epithelial cells**, a direct continuation of the pigmented layer of the retina. The **stroma** contains **melanocytes** and **myoepithelial cells** forming the **dilator pupillae**.

Posterior chamber

The **inner layer** of the epithelium is **nonpigmented** and faces the posterior chamber

The **outer layer** of the epithelium is **pigmented** and faces the stroma of the ciliary body

The **sphincter pupillae**, consisting of **smooth muscle cells**, has **acetylcholine receptors** and is innervated by **parasympathetic nerve fibers**. Sphincter contraction **reduces the diameter of the pupil**, or **miosis**.

Melanocyte

Anterior chamber

Iris

Dilator pupillae, consisting of **myoepithelial cells**, contains α-**adrenergic receptors** and is innervated by **sympathetic nerve fibers**. Contraction of the dilator causes **pupil dilation**, or **mydriasis**.

Posterior chamber

Capsule of the lens

Lens

Dual pigmented cell layer

The **ciliary epithelium is an extension of the retina beyond the ora serrata and covers the inner surface of the ciliary body**. It consists of two layers: an **inner layer of nonpigmented cells**, a direct continuation of the sensory retina, facing the posterior chamber, and an **outer layer of pigmented cells**, continuous with the retinal pigmented epithelium, in contact with the stroma of the ciliary body.

As the ciliary epithelium approaches the base of the iris, the cells of the inner layer accumulate pigment granules and both layers are pigmented. **Aqueous humor is secreted by the epithelial cells of the ciliary processes** supplied by **fenestrated capillaries**. Zonular fibers, normally associated with the ciliary processes, are not seen in Figure 9-7 but are depicted in Figure 9-11.

Electron micrographs from Hogan MJ, Alvarado JA, Weddell JA: Histology of the Human Eye. Philadelphia, WB Saunders, 1971.

Figure 9-8. Structure of the ciliary epithelium and secretion of aqueous humor

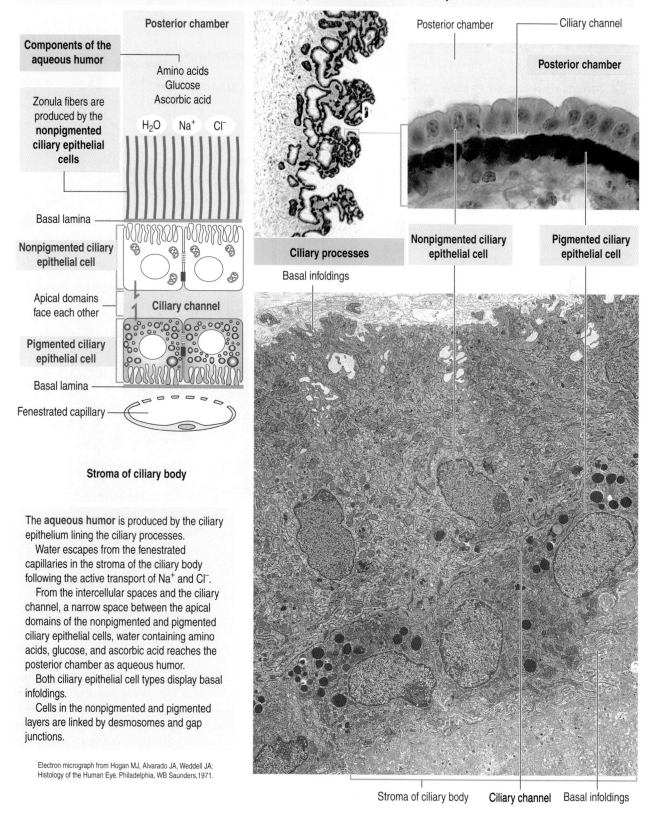

Components of the aqueous humor

Posterior chamber

Amino acids
Glucose
Ascorbic acid

H_2O Na^+ Cl^-

Zonula fibers are produced by the **nonpigmented ciliary epithelial cells**

Basal lamina

Nonpigmented ciliary epithelial cell

Apical domains face each other

Ciliary channel

Pigmented ciliary epithelial cell

Basal lamina

Fenestrated capillary

Stroma of ciliary body

Posterior chamber — Ciliary channel

Posterior chamber

Ciliary processes

Basal infoldings

Nonpigmented ciliary epithelial cell

Pigmented ciliary epithelial cell

Stroma of ciliary body   **Ciliary channel**   Basal infoldings

The **aqueous humor** is produced by the ciliary epithelium lining the ciliary processes.

Water escapes from the fenestrated capillaries in the stroma of the ciliary body following the active transport of Na^+ and Cl^-.

From the intercellular spaces and the ciliary channel, a narrow space between the apical domains of the nonpigmented and pigmented ciliary epithelial cells, water containing amino acids, glucose, and ascorbic acid reaches the posterior chamber as aqueous humor.

Both ciliary epithelial cell types display basal infoldings.

Cells in the nonpigmented and pigmented layers are linked by desmosomes and gap junctions.

Electron micrograph from Hogan MJ, Alvarado JA, Weddell JA: Histology of the Human Eye. Philadelphia, WB Saunders, 1971.

cortical region of the lens, elongated and concentrically arranged cells (called **cortical lens fibers**) **arise from the anterior epithelium at the equator region.** Cortical lens fibers contain a nucleus and organelles.

The nucleus and organelles eventually disappear when the cortical lens fibers approach the center of the lens, **the nuclear lens fiber region.**

Lens cell differentiation consists of the appearance

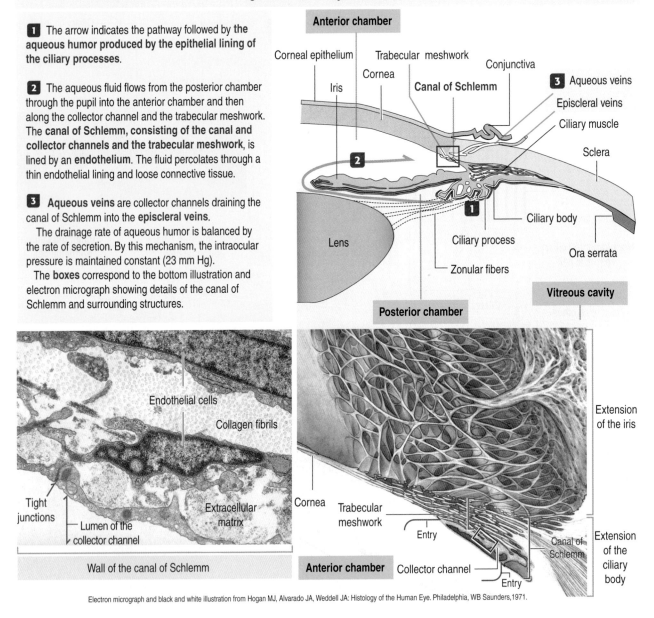

Figure 9-9. **Path of aqueous humor**

1 The arrow indicates the pathway followed by **the aqueous humor produced by the epithelial lining of the ciliary processes.**

2 The aqueous fluid flows from the posterior chamber through the pupil into the anterior chamber and then along the collector channel and the trabecular meshwork. The **canal of Schlemm, consisting of the canal and collector channels and the trabecular meshwork**, is lined by an **endothelium**. The fluid percolates through a thin endothelial lining and loose connective tissue.

3 **Aqueous veins** are collector channels draining the canal of Schlemm into the **episcleral veins**.

The drainage rate of aqueous humor is balanced by the rate of secretion. By this mechanism, the intraocular pressure is maintained constant (23 mm Hg).

The **boxes** correspond to the bottom illustration and electron micrograph showing details of the canal of Schlemm and surrounding structures.

Anterior chamber

Corneal epithelium

Cornea

Iris

Trabecular meshwork

Conjunctiva

Canal of Schlemm

3 Aqueous veins

Episcleral veins

Ciliary muscle

Sclera

Ciliary body

Ciliary process

Ora serrata

Zonular fibers

Lens

Posterior chamber

Vitreous cavity

Endothelial cells

Collagen fibrils

Tight junctions

Lumen of the collector channel

Extracellular matrix

Wall of the canal of Schlemm

Cornea

Trabecular meshwork

Entry

Collector channel

Entry

Canal of Schlemm

Extension of the iris

Extension of the ciliary body

Anterior chamber

Electron micrograph and black and white illustration from Hogan MJ, Alvarado JA, Weddell JA: Histology of the Human Eye. Philadelphia, WB Saunders,1971.

of unique cytoskeletal proteins:

1. **Filensin**, an intermediate filament that contains attachment sites for crystallins.

2. Lens-specific proteins called **crystallins** (α, β, and γ). Filensin and crystallins maintain the conformation and transparency of the lens fiber cell.

Lens cell fibers interdigitate at the medial **suture region**. At these contact sites, gap junctions and some spot desmosomes interlock the opposing cytoplasmic processes. The inner cortical region and the core of the lens consist of older lens fibers lacking nuclei. About 80% of its available glucose is metabolized by the lens.

Clinical significance: Cataracts

Cataracts are an opacity of the lens caused by a change in the solubility of lens proteins as they age. This condition causes high light scattering by the aggregated filensin and crystallins and impairs accurate vision. Cataracts can be cortical, nuclear or posterior subcapsular. Most age-related cataracts are **cortical cataracts**. Cataracts absorb and scatter more light than the normal regions of the lens, producing more light spread and a decrease in contrast of the retinal image. The result is reduced visual acuity.

Cataract surgery consists in a small incision made through the peripheral cornea behind the canal of Schlemm. After opening the anterior lens capsule with a cutting tool, the anterior cortex and nucleus are removed through a suction line. The posterior capsule is left intact. A flexible silicone lens, rolled up as a small tube, is inserted and opens up inside

Figure 9-10. Canal of Schlemm

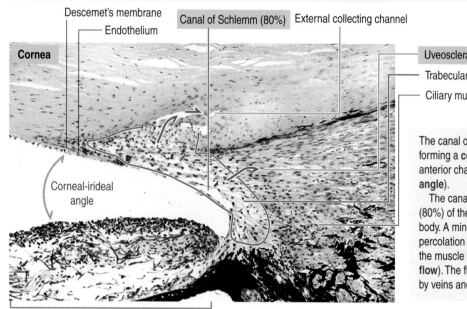

Descemet's membrane
Endothelium
Canal of Schlemm (80%)
External collecting channel

Cornea

Uveoscleral flow (20%)
Trabecular meshwork
Ciliary muscle

Corneal-irideal
angle

Iris

The canal of Schlemm is a modified **annular space** forming a **complete circle** at the apex of the anterior chamber angle (at the **corneal-irideal angle**).

The canal of Schlemm is the major escape route (80%) of the aqueous fluid produced by the ciliary body. A minor draining route (20%) is by fluid percolation into the connective tissue surrounding the muscle fibers of the ciliary body (**uveoscleral flow**). The fluid reaches the sclera and is drained by veins and lymphatics.

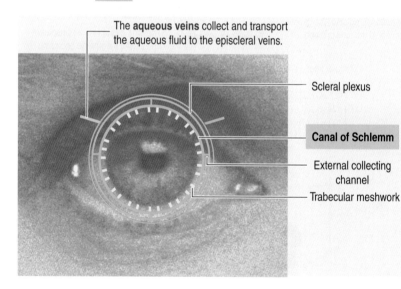

The **aqueous veins** collect and transport the aqueous fluid to the episcleral veins.

Scleral plexus

Canal of Schlemm

External collecting channel

Trabecular meshwork

Clinical significance: Glaucoma

An obstruction in the drainage of aqueous humor leads to an increase in intraocular pressure that gradually damages the retina and causes blindness if untreated. This condition is called **glaucoma** and produces pain and nausea as typical symptoms.

Two forms of glaucoma are recognized: (1) **Open-angle glaucoma**, the most common form, occurs when the trabecular meshwork drains the aqueous humor but the canal of Schlemm is obstructed. (2) **Closed-angle glaucoma** results when the aqueous humor is unable to reach the trabecular meshwork because an inflammatory process of the uvea (uveitis) blocks fluid access to the meshwork drain.

Surgery aimed at restoring aqueous fluid outflow consists of the use of a laser to burn small holes in the trabecular meshwork (**trabeculoplasty**) around the limbus.

the eye to its original shape. The small incision does not require suture on completion of the procedure.

Accommodation

The sharpness of distant and close images focused on the retina depends on the **shape** of the lens (Figure 9-12). **Accommodation** defines the process by which the lens becomes **rounder** to focus the image of a **nearby object** on the retina and **flattens** when the image of a **distant object** is focused on the retina.

Accommodation determines that the distance between the center of the lens and the retina is equivalent to the focal distance needed for the formation of a sharp image on the retina.

Three components contribute to the accommodation process:

1. The **ciliary muscle**.
2. The **ciliary body**.
3. The **suspensory ligaments**, inserted at the equatorial region of the lens capsule.

When the ciliary muscle **contracts**, the ciliary body moves toward the lens. Consequently, the tension of the suspensory ligaments is reduced, and the elastic capsule of the lens enables the lens to acquire a spherical shape. A rounded lens facilitates **close vision**.

When the ciliary muscle **relaxes**, the ciliary body keeps the tension of the suspensory ligaments that pull at the circumference of the lens. Thus, the lens remains flat to enable **distant vision**. This condition is known as **emmetropia** (Greek *emmetros*, in proper measure; *opia,* pertaining to the eye), or normal vision.

Figure 9-11. Lens

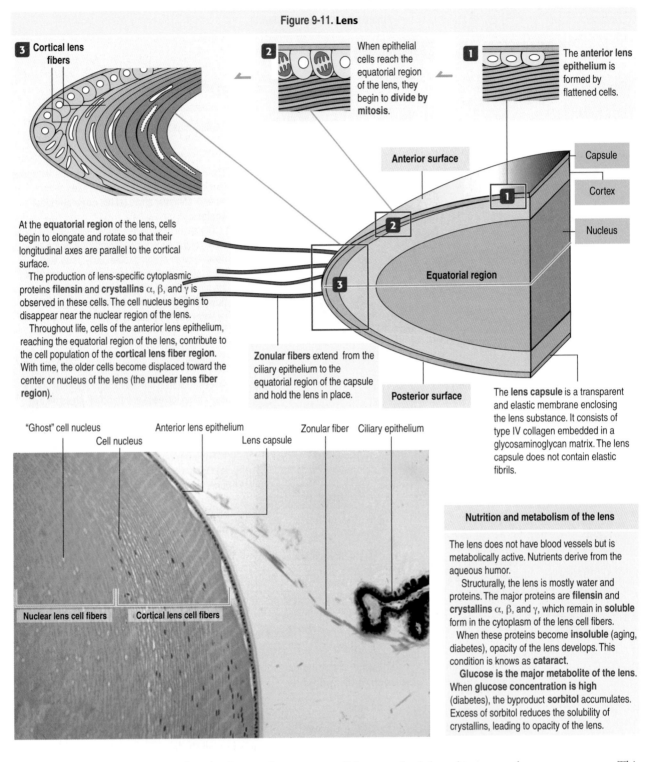

3 Cortical lens fibers

2 When epithelial cells reach the equatorial region of the lens, they begin to **divide by mitosis.**

1 The **anterior lens epithelium** is formed by flattened cells.

Anterior surface

Capsule

Cortex

Nucleus

Equatorial region

At the **equatorial region** of the lens, cells begin to elongate and rotate so that their longitudinal axes are parallel to the cortical surface.

The production of lens-specific cytoplasmic proteins **filensin** and **crystallins** α, β, and γ is observed in these cells. The cell nucleus begins to disappear near the nuclear region of the lens.

Throughout life, cells of the anterior lens epithelium, reaching the equatorial region of the lens, contribute to the cell population of the **cortical lens fiber region**. With time, the older cells become displaced toward the center or nucleus of the lens (the **nuclear lens fiber region**).

Zonular fibers extend from the ciliary epithelium to the equatorial region of the capsule and hold the lens in place.

Posterior surface

The **lens capsule** is a transparent and elastic membrane enclosing the lens substance. It consists of type IV collagen embedded in a glycosaminoglycan matrix. The lens capsule does not contain elastic fibrils.

"Ghost" cell nucleus

Cell nucleus

Anterior lens epithelium

Lens capsule

Zonular fiber   Ciliary epithelium

Nuclear lens cell fibers   Cortical lens cell fibers

Nutrition and metabolism of the lens

The lens does not have blood vessels but is metabolically active. Nutrients derive from the aqueous humor.

Structurally, the lens is mostly water and proteins. The major proteins are **filensin** and **crystallins** α, β, and γ, which remain in **soluble** form in the cytoplasm of the lens cell fibers.

When these proteins become **insoluble** (aging, diabetes), opacity of the lens develops. This condition is knows as **cataract.**

Glucose is the major metabolite of the lens. When **glucose concentration is high** (diabetes), the byproduct **sorbitol** accumulates. Excess of sorbitol reduces the solubility of crystallins, leading to opacity of the lens.

If the eyeball is too deep or the curvature of the lens is not flat enough, the image of a distant object forms in a plane **in front of the retina.** Distant objects are blurry because they are out of focus, but vision at close range is normal. This condition is called **myopia** (Greek *myein,* to shut), or **nearsightedness.**

If the eyeball is too shallow and the curvature of the lens is too flat, the distant image is formed at a plane **behind the retina.** Distant objects are well resolved but objects at a closer range are not. This condition is called **hyperopia** (Greek *hyper,* above), or **farsightedness.**

Older people become farsighted as the lens loses elasticity. This form of hyperopia is known as **presbyopia** (Greek *presbys,* old man).

Accommodation difficulties can be improved by the use of lenses. A diverging lens corrects myopia; a converging lens corrects hyperopia.

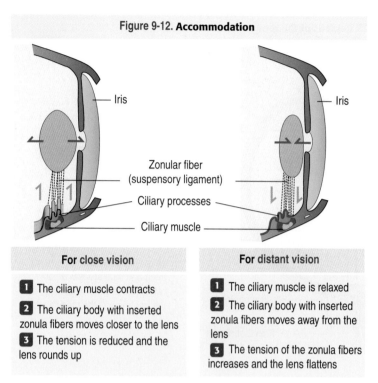

Figure 9-12. Accommodation

Iris

Iris

Zonular fiber
(suspensory ligament)

Ciliary processes

Ciliary muscle

For close vision	**For distant vision**
1 The ciliary muscle contracts	**1** The ciliary muscle is relaxed
2 The ciliary body with inserted zonula fibers moves closer to the lens	**2** The ciliary body with inserted zonula fibers moves away from the lens
3 The tension is reduced and the lens rounds up	**3** The tension of the zonula fibers increases and the lens flattens

Inner layer: Retina

The retina consists of two regions (Figure 9-13):

1. The outer **nonsensory retinal pigmented epithelium**.

2. The inner **sensory retina** (see Box 9-E).

The **nonsensory retinal pigmented epithelium** is a single layer of cuboidal cells extending from the edge of the **optic disk** to the **ora serrata**, where it continues as the pigmented layer of the ciliary epithelium.

The apical domain of the cuboidal nonsensory pigmented epithelium is sealed by **tight junctions** to form the **external retinal barrier** (Figure 9-14).

Granules of **melanin** are present in the apical cytoplasm and apical cell processes. Melanin granules absorb excess light reaching the photoreceptors.

The apical surface contains **microvilli** that surround the outer segments of the photoreceptors (cones and rods).

At this location, the sensory retina and the pigmented epithelium are attached to each other through an amorphous extracellular material, the **interphotoreceptor matrix** (Figure 9-15).

The inner **sensory retina** layer extends from the edge of the **optic disk** to the **ciliary epithelium**.

The sensory retina has two clinically and anatomically important landmarks to remember:

1. The **fovea centralis**, a shallow depression of about 2.5 mm in diameter.

2. The **macula lutea**, a yellow rim surrounding the fovea centralis.

The fovea is the area of the retina where vision is the sharpest and is crossed by the visual axis. We discuss these structures later.

Clinical significance: Detachment of the retina

A separation of the two layers by trauma, vascular disease, metabolic disorders, and aging results in the **detachment of the retina**. Retinal detachment affects the viability of the sensory retina and can be corrected by laser surgery.

The clinical significance of the detachment of the nonsensory retinal pigmented epithelium from the sensory retina is highlighted by the following functions of the pigmented epithelium:

1. The **transport of nutrients from the choroidal blood vessels to the outer layers of the sensory retina**.

2. The **removal of metabolic waste products from the sensory retina**.

3. **Active phagocytosis and recycling of photoreceptor disks shed from the outer segment of the cones and rods**.

4. The **synthesis of basal lamina components of Bruch's membrane** to which the retinal pigmented epithelium is firmly attached.

5. It is essential for **the formation of the photopigment rhodopsin** because it regenerates the bleached photopigment by converting **all-*trans* retinol** into **retinal**, which is returned to the photoreceptor by **interstitial retinoid-binding protein (IRBP)**, a major protein in the interphotoreceptor matrix (see Figure 9-15).

Cell layers of the retina

Four cell groups are found in the **sensory retina** (see Figure 9-14):

1. The **photoreceptor neurons, rods** and **cones**.

2. The **conducting neurons, bipolar** and **ganglion cells**.

3. The **association neurons, horizontal** and **amacrine cells**.

4. The **supporting neuroglial cells, Müller cells**.

Photoreceptor neurons: Rods and cones

Rods (see Figure 9-15) and cones (Figure 9-16) occupy specific regions in the sensory retina. **Cones** are predominant in the **fovea centralis** and perceive color and detail. **Rods** are concentrated at the periphery of the fovea and function in peripheral and dim light vision.

Both rods and cones are elongated cells with specific structural and functional polarity. They consist of two major segments:

1. An **outer segment**.

2. An **inner segment**.

The **outer segment** contains stacks of flat **membranous disks** harboring a photopigment. The disks are infoldings of the plasma membrane that pinch off as they move away from the modified **cilium**, the outer-inner segment connecting region.

The various components of the disks are synthe-

Figure 9-13. **Regions of the retina**

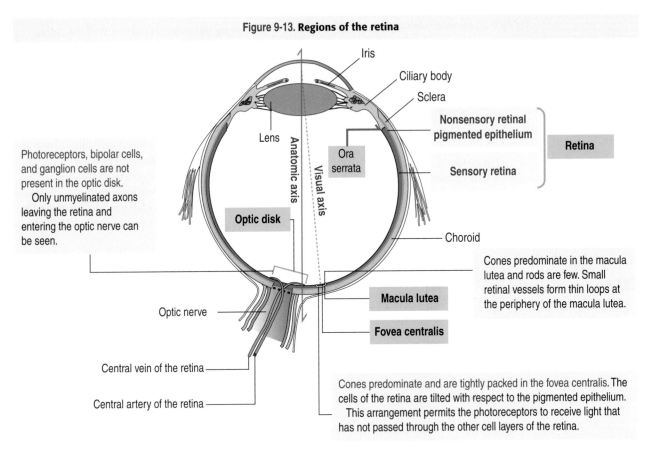

Photoreceptors, bipolar cells, and ganglion cells are not present in the optic disk.

Only unmyelinated axons leaving the retina and entering the optic nerve can be seen.

Iris
Ciliary body
Sclera
Lens
Anatomic axis
Visual axis
Ora serrata
Nonsensory retinal pigmented epithelium
Retina
Sensory retina
Optic disk
Choroid
Cones predominate in the macula lutea and rods are few. Small retinal vessels form thin loops at the periphery of the macula lutea.
Macula lutea
Optic nerve
Fovea centralis
Central vein of the retina
Central artery of the retina
Cones predominate and are tightly packed in the fovea centralis. The cells of the retina are tilted with respect to the pigmented epithelium. This arrangement permits the photoreceptors to receive light that has not passed through the other cell layers of the retina.

sized in the inner segment and are transported by molecular motors (kinesins and cytoplasmic dyneins) along microtubules toward the outer segment across the narrow cytoplasmic bridge containing the modified cilium. We discuss in Chapter 1, Epithelium, details of the mechanism of **intraciliary transport**.

The production and turnover of the disks is continuous. New disks are added near the cilium. Older disks move toward the pigmented epithelium of the retina and once they reach the tip of the outer segment, they are phagocytosed by the cells of the pigmented epithelium. The duration of the disk recycling process is about 10 days.

The **inner segment** displays abundant mitochondria, involved in the synthesis of adenosine triphos-

phate (ATP), the Golgi apparatus, and rough and smooth endoplasmic reticulum. The modified cilium consists of **nine peripheral microtubule doublets** but **lacks the central pair** of microtubules. The terminal portion of the photoreceptors is equivalent to an axon forming synaptic contacts with cytoplasmic processes, **neurites**, of bipolar cells and horizontal cells.

There are three significant **differences between rods and cones**:

1. The **outer segment is cylindrical in the rods and conically shaped in the cones**.

2. The **rods** terminate in a small knob or **rod spherule**, which contacts dendrites of bipolar cells and neurites of horizontal cells. The **cones** end in a thicker **cone pedicle**. The cone pedicle also synapses with bipolar and horizontal cells. The synaptic ending of cones and rods, spherules and pedicles, contains a **synaptic ribbon** surrounded by **synaptic vesicles** (see Box 9-F). In addition, **gap junctions** are present between the terminals of rods and cones. This cone–rod coupling transmits dim light conditions under which only rod photoreceptors are active.

3. Rods contain the photopigment **rhodopsin** (Figure 9-17). Cones contain a similar pigment called **iodopsin**. Rhodopsin operates during night vision. Iodopsin perceives detail and discriminates color (blue, green, and red). Rhodopsin and iodopsin are transmembrane proteins bound to the prosthetic group **11-*cis*-retinal**. The protein lacking the pros-

---

Box 9-E | Retina: Highlights to remember

- The retina derives from the neuroectoderm and represents an extension of the brain. The retina is a stratified layer of nervous cells formed by two layers: (1) the outer **retinal pigmented epithelium** and (2) the inner **sensory retina**.
- The **nonsensory retinal pigmented epithelium** is a **simple cuboidal epithelium** with **melanin** granules.
- The **sensory retina** spans from the margin of the **optic disk** posteriorly to the **ciliary epithelium** anteriorly.
- The optic disk includes the **optic papilla**, formed by protruding nerve fibers passing from the retina into the optic nerve. The optic papilla lacks photoreceptors and represents the **blind spot** of the retina.
- The **fovea centralis** is the area of sharpest vision.

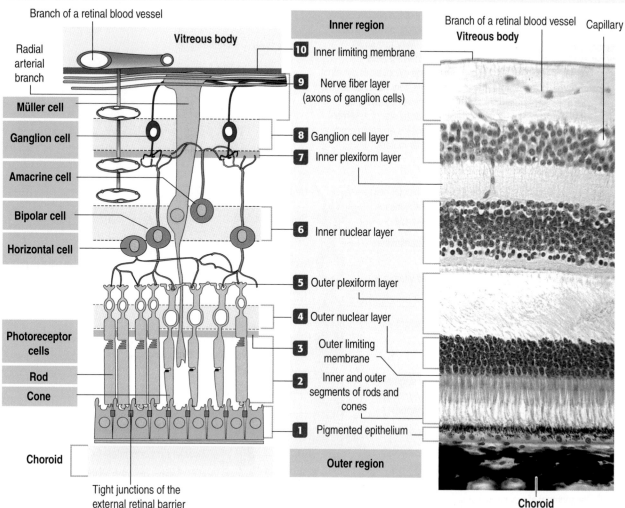

Figure 9-14. Layers of the retina

Branch of a retinal blood vessel

Radial arterial branch

Vitreous body

Müller cell

Ganglion cell

Amacrine cell

Bipolar cell

Horizontal cell

Photoreceptor cells

Rod

Cone

Choroid

Tight junctions of the external retinal barrier

Inner region

Branch of a retinal blood vessel   Capillary
Vitreous body

10 Inner limiting membrane

9 Nerve fiber layer (axons of ganglion cells)

8 Ganglion cell layer

7 Inner plexiform layer

6 Inner nuclear layer

5 Outer plexiform layer

4 Outer nuclear layer

3 Outer limiting membrane

2 Inner and outer segments of rods and cones

1 Pigmented epithelium

Outer region

Choroid

Light passes through several layers of the retina before activating the rod and cone photoreceptor cells. The layers of the retina observed in the photomicrograph are represented in the adjacent diagram. The synapses between the cells of each layer of the retina are also illustrated.

Radial branches from blood vessels (arteries and veins), located on the retinal surface, are interconnected by **capillary beds** present in the inner layers of the retina. **Retinal capillary beds** are lined by **endothelial cells** linked by **tight junctions** creating an internal **blood-retinal barrier**. An **external retinal barrier** is formed by **tight junctions linking the cells of the pigmented epithelium**.

Note that the nuclei of rods and cones are present in the **outer nuclear layer**.

The axons of the cones and rods project into the **outer plexiform layer** and synapse with dendrites of the bipolar cells.

Nuclei of the bipolar cells contribute to the **inner nuclear layer**.

Axons of the bipolar cells synapse with dendrites of the ganglion cells in the **inner plexiform layer**.

Axons of the **ganglion cells** become part of the optic nerve.

Müller cells span most of the retina. The **inner limiting membrane** represents their basal lamina. Their nuclei form part of the inner nuclear layer.

The **outer limiting membrane** corresponds to junctional complexes (**zonula adherens**) between rods, cones, and Müller cells.

Horizontal cells synapse with several rods and cones.

Amacrine cells synapse with axons of bipolar cells and dendrites of ganglion cells.

thetic group is called **opsin** (see Box 9-G).

There are three different photopigments in cones with different light absorbance and sensitive to blue light (420 nm), green light (535 nm), and red light 565 nm), respectively. The isomerization of 11-*cis*-retinal to activated all-*trans*-retinal is identical in rods and cones.

Conducting neurons: Bipolar and ganglion cells
Bipolar cells receive information derived from the interaction of horizontal cells with cone or rod photoreceptors. **Ganglion cells** are the output neurons of the retina; their axons form the optic nerve.

Rod and cone photoreceptors establish chemical synapses with different bipolar cells to separate sig-

Figure 9-15. **Photoreceptors: Rod**

The **modified cilium** connects the inner segment of the photoreceptor cell (the site of synthesis of proteins and other molecules) to the outer segment (containing a stack of disks). The **intraciliary transport** mechanism (see Cytoskeleton in Chapter 1, Epithelium) uses microtubule-based molecular motors (kinesins and cytoplasmic dyneins) to transport proteins, vesicles, and other materials from the inner segment to the outer segment. The modified cilium facilitates the delivery of molecules from a proximal site of synthesis to a distal site of assembly.

The plus/minus polarity of the microtubules enables an anterograde and retrograde transport mechanism through molecular motors.

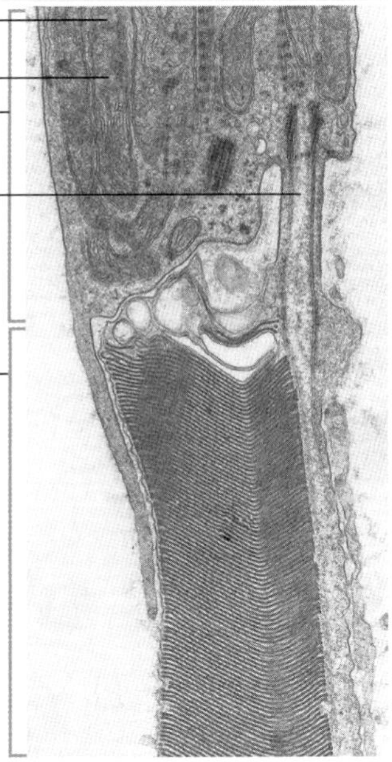

Mitochondria

Inner segment

Modified cilium

Outer segment

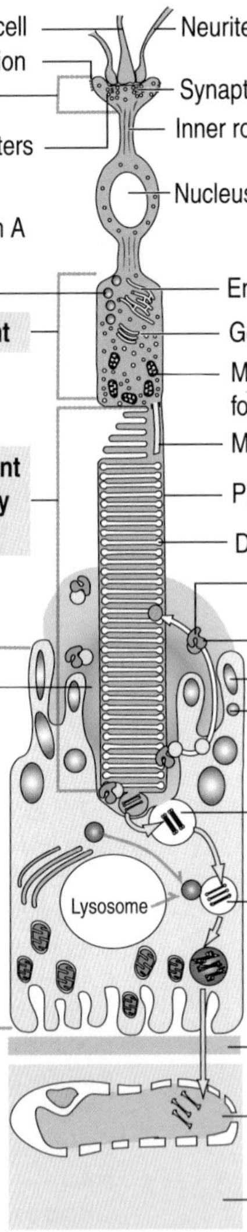

1 **Interphotoreceptor matrix**

A mixture of extracellular proteins, glycoproteins and glycosaminoglycans, link the outer segment of the photoreceptor cell to the pigmented epithelium by means of its viscosity.

A major protein of the matrix is **interstitial retinoid-binding protein (IRBP)**. IRBP transports **retinol** to the pigmented epithelium and returns **retinal** to the photoreceptor.

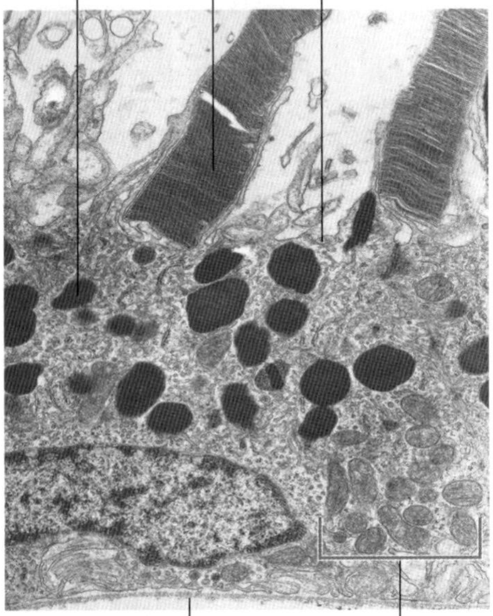

Dendrite of a rod bipolar cell — — Neurite of a horizontal cell
Gap junction — — Synaptic ribbon and vesicles
Spherule —
Neurotransmitters — — Inner rod fiber (axon)
— Nucleus
Stored vitamin A —
— Endoplasmic reticulum
Inner segment — Golgi apparatus
— Mitochondria synthesize adenosine triphosphate required for the assembly of the visual pigment rhodopsin
Outer segment (cylindrically shaped) — Modified cilium
— Plasma membrane
— Disk
— **Interstitial retinoid-binding protein (IRBP)**

2 **Photopigment regeneration**

Apically located melanin granules absorb the light passing through the sensory retina, keeping it from being reflected back inside the eye.

Interphotoreceptor matrix **1**

Outer segment of a photoreceptor

Melanin granule

Pigmented epithelium of the retina

Lysosome

Older disks of the rods are shed and phagocytosed by the pigmented epithelial cells of the retina. Disks are stored in lamellar phagosomes.

Lysosomes fuse with the lamellar phagosome and lysosomal degradation of the disk starts.

Basal lamina (the innermost component of Bruch's membrane

Disk remnants are released into the fenestrated capillaries of the choroid

Choroid

Basal lamina   Mitochondria

2 **Photopigment regeneration**

The bleached photopigment consists of **opsin** and **all-*trans* retinol** (see Figure 9-17). Regeneration of the photopigment consists of the enzymatic conversion **within the pigmented epithelium** of retinol back to 11-*cis* retinal.

Photoreceptors lack the required enzymes. **IRBP** carries all-*trans* retinol produced by bleaching to the pigmented epithelial cells, where it is converted to 11-*cis* retinal, and returns 11-*cis* retinal back to the photoreceptor.

Electron micrographs from Hogan MJ, Alvarado JA, Weddell JA: Histology of the Human Eye. Philadelphia, WB Saunders, 1971.

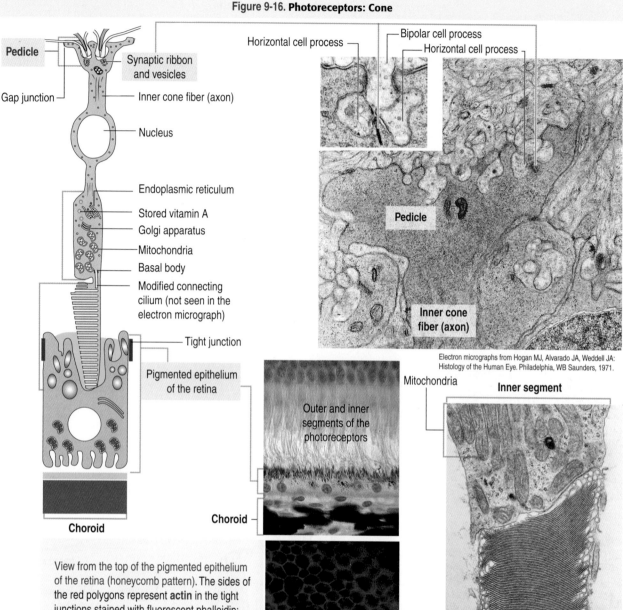

Figure 9-16. Photoreceptors: Cone

Pedicle

Synaptic ribbon and vesicles

Horizontal cell process

Bipolar cell process

Horizontal cell process

Gap junction

Inner cone fiber (axon)

Nucleus

Endoplasmic reticulum

Stored vitamin A

Golgi apparatus

Mitochondria

Basal body

Modified connecting cilium (not seen in the electron micrograph)

Tight junction

Pigmented epithelium of the retina

Choroid

Pedicle

Inner cone fiber (axon)

Electron micrographs from Hogan MJ, Alvarado JA, Weddell JA: Histology of the Human Eye. Philadelphia, WB Saunders, 1971.

Outer and inner segments of the photoreceptors

Choroid

Mitochondria

Inner segment

View from the top of the pigmented epithelium of the retina (honeycomb pattern). The sides of the red polygons represent **actin** in the tight junctions stained with fluorescent phalloidin; the spaces are partially occupied in vivo by the inserted outer segments of the photoreceptors.

Outer segment (conically shaped)

naling into parallel retinal streams. Two major classes of bipolar cells can be distinguished (Figure 9-18):

1. **Rod bipolar cells**, linked to **rod spherules**.
2. **Cone bipolar cells**, linked to **cone pedicles**.

Cone bipolar cells consist of two major classes:

1. The **midget cone bipolar cell**.
2. The **diffuse cone bipolar cell**.

Dendrites of the **diffuse cone bipolar cells** branch within the **outer plexiform layer** and contact several cone pedicles. On the opposite pole, the axon of a diffuse bipolar cell projects into the **inner plexiform**

layer and contacts the dendrites of ganglion cells.

Midget cone bipolar cells synapse with a **single cone pedicle** and a single axon that contacts a **single ganglion cell**.

Essentially, **midget bipolar cells link a single cone to an optic nerve fiber**. In contrast, **diffuse bipolar cells have wider input and output pathways**. The nuclei of the bipolar cells form part of the **inner nuclear layer** of the retina.

Ganglion cells extend their dendrites into the **inner plexiform layer**; the axons form part of the optic

Figure 9-17. **Visual pigment: Rhodopsin**

Photoreceptors respond to light through a process called **bleaching**. During bleaching, the photopigment rhodopsin absorbs a photon and changes chemically into another component less sensitive to light.

Most sensory receptors are depolarized in response to a stimulus and release neurotransmitters. However, when a photoreceptor is activated by light, the plasma membrane becomes **hyperpolarized** and the release of neurotransmitters stops. Hyperpolarization is caused by shutting off the inflow of ions to the photoreceptor.

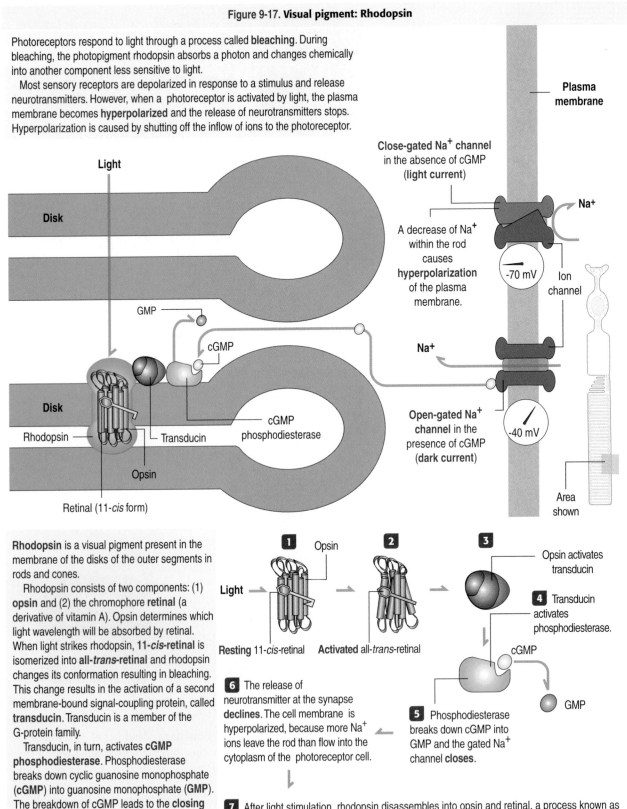

Rhodopsin is a visual pigment present in the membrane of the disks of the outer segments in rods and cones.

Rhodopsin consists of two components: (1) **opsin** and (2) the chromophore **retinal** (a derivative of vitamin A). Opsin determines which light wavelength will be absorbed by retinal. When light strikes rhodopsin, **11-*cis*-retinal** is isomerized into **all-*trans*-retinal** and rhodopsin changes its conformation resulting in bleaching. This change results in the activation of a second membrane-bound signal-coupling protein, called **transducin**. Transducin is a member of the G-protein family.

Transducin, in turn, activates **cGMP phosphodiesterase**. Phosphodiesterase breaks down cyclic guanosine monophosphate (**cGMP**) into guanosine monophosphate (**GMP**). The breakdown of cGMP leads to the **closing of gated Na⁺ channels**, and entry of Na⁺ into the photoreceptor cell is prevented.

Consequently, electronegativity increases inside the plasma membrane and causes hyperpolarization of the entire rod plasma membrane and cease neurotransmitter release.

6 The release of neurotransmitter at the synapse **declines**. The cell membrane is hyperpolarized, because more Na⁺ ions leave the rod than flow into the cytoplasm of the photoreceptor cell.

1 Opsin
Light Resting 11-*cis*-retinal
2 **Activated** all-*trans*-retinal
3 Opsin activates transducin
4 Transducin activates phosphodiesterase.
cGMP
5 Phosphodiesterase breaks down cGMP into GMP and the gated Na⁺ channel **closes**.
GMP

7 After light stimulation, rhodopsin disassembles into opsin and retinal, a process known as **bleaching**. 11-*trans*-retinal is enzymatically converted by cells of the **pigmented epithelium** into all-*cis*-retinal. Then, 11-*cis*-retinal is transported back by **interstitial retinoid-binding protein** to the photoreceptor where it recombines with opsin and rhodopsin molecules are regenerated.

While rhodopsin regeneration is in progress, membrane permeability to Na⁺ returns to normal as cGMP is also synthesized and opens the gated Na⁺ channel.

Figure 9-18. Rod spherules and cone pedicles

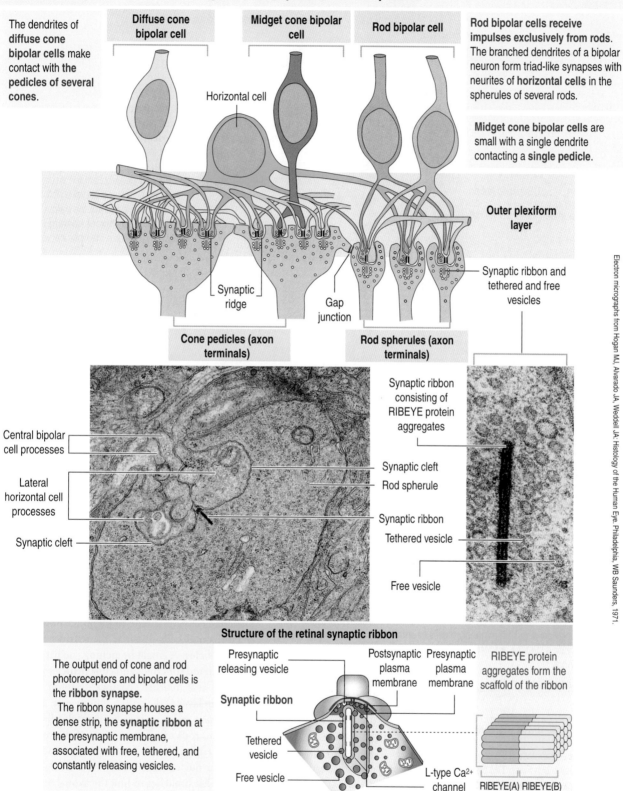

The dendrites of **diffuse cone bipolar cells** make contact with **the pedicles of several cones.**

Diffuse cone bipolar cell

Midget cone bipolar cell

Rod bipolar cell

Horizontal cell

Rod bipolar cells receive impulses exclusively from rods. The branched dendrites of a bipolar neuron form triad-like synapses with neurites of **horizontal cells** in the spherules of several rods.

Midget cone bipolar cells are small with a single dendrite contacting a **single pedicle.**

Outer plexiform layer

Synaptic ridge

Gap junction

Synaptic ribbon and tethered and free vesicles

Cone pedicles (axon terminals)

Rod spherules (axon terminals)

Central bipolar cell processes

Lateral horizontal cell processes

Synaptic cleft

Synaptic ribbon consisting of RIBEYE protein aggregates

Synaptic cleft
Rod spherule

Synaptic ribbon

Tethered vesicle

Free vesicle

Structure of the retinal synaptic ribbon

The output end of cone and rod photoreceptors and bipolar cells is the **ribbon synapse.**

The ribbon synapse houses a dense strip, the **synaptic ribbon** at the presynaptic membrane, associated with free, tethered, and constantly releasing vesicles.

Presynaptic releasing vesicle

Postsynaptic plasma membrane

Presynaptic plasma membrane

RIBEYE protein aggregates form the scaffold of the ribbon

Synaptic ribbon

Tethered vesicle

Free vesicle

L-type Ca^{2+} channel

RIBEYE(A) RIBEYE(B)

Electron micrographs from Hogan MJ, Alvarado JA, Weddell JA: Histology of the Human Eye, Philadelphia, WB Saunders, 1971.

nerve. Two classes of ganglion cells exist:

1. **Diffuse ganglion cells**, contacting several bipolar cells.

2. **Midget ganglion cells**, with their dendrites contacting a single midget bipolar cell. Note that midget ganglion cells receive impulses from cones only.

In Chapter 18, Neuroendocrine System, we discuss in the pineal gland section the presence of a subset of ganglion cells with a function independent of image formation. This subset, called **intrinsically**

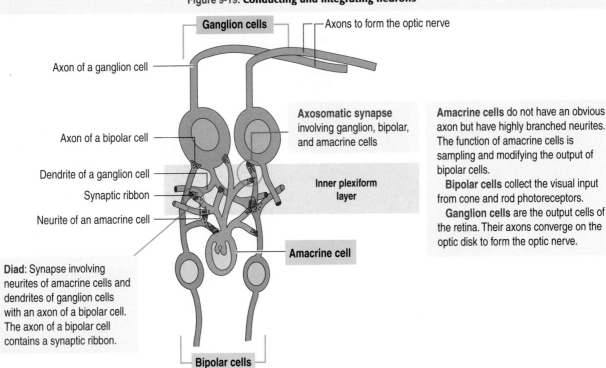

Figure 9-19. Conducting and integrating neurons

Ganglion cells

Axons to form the optic nerve

Axon of a ganglion cell

Axon of a bipolar cell

Dendrite of a ganglion cell

Synaptic ribbon

Neurite of an amacrine cell

Axosomatic synapse involving ganglion, bipolar, and amacrine cells

Inner plexiform layer

Amacrine cell

Diad: Synapse involving neurites of amacrine cells and dendrites of ganglion cells with an axon of a bipolar cell. The axon of a bipolar cell contains a synaptic ribbon.

Bipolar cells

Amacrine cells do not have an obvious axon but have highly branched neurites. The function of amacrine cells is sampling and modifying the output of bipolar cells.
  Bipolar cells collect the visual input from cone and rod photoreceptors.
  Ganglion cells are the output cells of the retina. Their axons converge on the optic disk to form the optic nerve.

---

photosensitive retinal ganglion cells (**ipRGCs**), are **melanopsin-producing ganglion cells**. They are involved in adjusting the internal circadian clock to light and sleep.

Association neurons: Horizontal and amacrine cells
Horizontal cells are retinal neurons forming a network beneath the photoreceptors. They are involved in contrast signaling by averaging visual activity over space and time. **Amacrine cells** are interneurons located in the inner plexiform layer of the retina, at a site where bipolar cells and ganglion cells synapse.

Horizontal and amacrine cells do not have axons or dendrites, only **neuritic processes conducting in both directions**. The nuclei of the horizontal and amacrine cells contribute to the **inner nuclear layer**.

Horizontal cells give rise to **neurites** ending on **cone pedicles**. A single branching neurite synapses with **both rod spherules and cone pedicles** (see Figure 9-18). These neuritic synapses occur in the **outer plexiform layer** of the retina. This neurite and axonal distribution indicates that **horizontal cells integrate cones and rods of adjacent areas of the retina**.

Amacrine cells are found at the inner edge of the **inner nuclear layer**. They have a single neuritic process that branches to link the axonal terminals of the bipolar cells and the dendritic branches of the ganglion cells (Figure 9-19).

Supporting glial cells: Müller cells
The nuclei of Müller cells are located in the **inner nuclear layer**. The cytoplasmic processes extend to

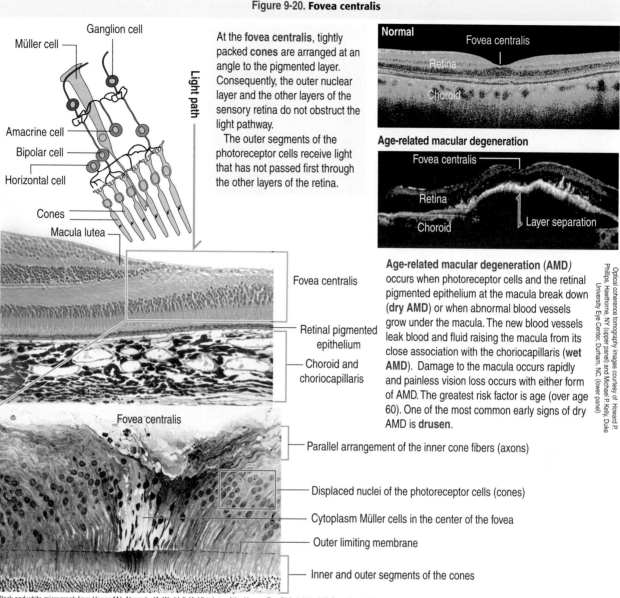

Figure 9-20. **Fovea centralis**

Müller cell

Ganglion cell

Light path

At the **fovea centralis**, tightly packed **cones** are arranged at an angle to the pigmented layer. Consequently, the outer nuclear layer and the other layers of the sensory retina do not obstruct the light pathway.

The outer segments of the photoreceptor cells receive light that has not passed first through the other layers of the retina.

Amacrine cell

Bipolar cell

Horizontal cell

Cones

Macula lutea

Fovea centralis

Retinal pigmented epithelium

Choroid and choriocapillaris

Fovea centralis

Parallel arrangement of the inner cone fibers (axons)

Displaced nuclei of the photoreceptor cells (cones)

Cytoplasm Müller cells in the center of the fovea

Outer limiting membrane

Inner and outer segments of the cones

Normal

Fovea centralis

Retina

Choroid

Age-related macular degeneration

Fovea centralis

Retina

Choroid

Layer separation

Age-related macular degeneration (AMD) occurs when photoreceptor cells and the retinal pigmented epithelium at the macula break down (**dry AMD**) or when abnormal blood vessels grow under the macula. The new blood vessels leak blood and fluid raising the macula from its close association with the choriocapillaris (**wet AMD**). Damage to the macula occurs rapidly and painless vision loss occurs with either form of AMD. The greatest risk factor is age (over age 60). One of the most common early signs of dry AMD is **drusen**.

Optical coherence tomography images courtesy of Howard P. Phillips, Hawthorne, NY (upper panel) and Michael P Kelly, Duke University Eye Center, Durham, NC (lower panel)

Black and white micrograph from Hogan MJ, Alvarado JA, Weddell JA: Histology of the Human Eye. Philadelphia, WB Saunders, 1971.

the **outer** and **inner limiting membrane**. The inner limiting membrane represents the basal lamina of the Müller cells and serves to separate the retina from the vitreous body.

The cytoplasmic processes of Müller cells fill the spaces between photoreceptors and bipolar and ganglion cells. At the outer segment photoreceptor contact sites, a **zonula adherens** and **microvilli** extending from Müller cells stabilize the association between neuronal photoreceptors and glial Müller cells. In addition to glial Müller cells, microglial cells are present in all layers.

Fovea centralis and optic disk

The **fovea centralis**, surrounded by the **macula lutea** (Figures 9-20 and 9-21), is a specialized area of the retina for accurate vision under normal and dim il-

lumination. The **optic disk**, which includes the **optic papilla**, is not suitable for vision.

The **fovea centralis** is located on the **temporal side** of the optic disk. **This area contains abundant cones but lacks rods and capillaries.** The cones synapse with the bipolar cells, both oriented **at an angle** around the margins of the fovea. This histologic feature enables free access of light to the photoreceptors. The **macula lutea** is characterized by a yellow pigment (**lutein** and **zeaxanthin**) in the inner layers surrounding the shallow fovea.

The exit site from the retina of axons derived from ganglion cells is represented by the **optic disk**. The optic disk includes:

1. The **optic papilla**, a protrusion formed by the axons entering the optic nerve.

2. The **lamina cribrosa** of the sclera, pierced by the

Figure 9-21. Optic disk and fovea centralis

Optic disk

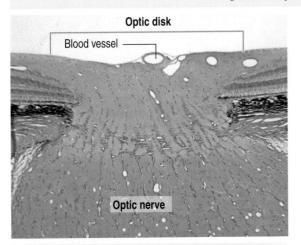

Blood vessel

Optic nerve

Retinal blood vessels can be visualized with an ophthalmoscope or by a **fluorescein angiography**. When **intraocular pressure increases**, the disk of the optic nerve appears **concave**. The disk becomes swollen (**papilledema**) and the veins are dilated when intracranial pressure increases.

Fluorescein angiography (FA) is a valuable test that provides information about the conditions of the retina. FA is performed by injecting a sodium-based fluorescent dye into an arm vein. The dye appears in the blood vessels of the retina in about 10 to 15 seconds. As the dye travels through the retinal blood vessels, a special retinal camera records images. The dye may reveal abnormally leaking blood vessels or the inability of the dye to get through blocked blood vessels. Note that veins are typically larger in diameter than arteries.

The axons of the ganglion cells turn into the **optic nerve** at the **optic disk**, which lacks photoreceptors and corresponds to the **blind spot** of the retina.

The optic disk has a central depression, the **optic cup**, that is pale in comparison with the surrounding nerve fibers. A loss of nerve fibers in glaucoma results in an increase in the optic cup area.

Arterioles and venules radiate in from all directions toward the periphery of fovea

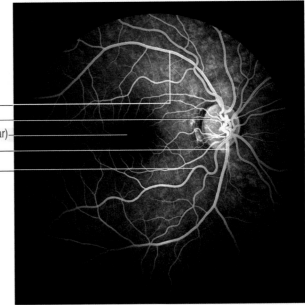

Superior temporal vein
Optic disk
Fovea centralis (avascular)
Inferior temporal vein
Inferior temporal artery

Fluorescein angiogram courtesy of Michael P. Kelly, Duke University Eye Center, Durham, NC.

axons of the optic nerve. Photoreceptors terminate at the edges of the optic disk, which represents the "blind spot" of the retina. **The central artery and vein of the retina pass through the optic disk.**

The eyelids, conjunctiva, and the lacrimal glands
The anterior portion of the eyeball is protected by the eyelids, the conjunctiva, and the fluid produced by the lacrimal gland.

Each **eyelid** consists of two portions (Figure 9-22):

1. An outer **cutaneous portion** lined by a stratified squamous epidermis overlying a loose connective tissue dermis and skeletal muscle (**orbicularis oculi muscle**).

2. An inner **conjunctival portion**, lined by a thin mucous membrane, the **conjunctiva**.

The cutaneous portion contains several skin appendages:

1. **Sweat** and **sebaceous glands**.
2. Three to four rows of stiff hairs, the **eyelashes**, at the eyelid margins. Eyelashes are associated with modified sweat glands known as the **glands of Moll**.

Facing the conjunctival lining is the **tarsal plate**, a fibroelastic dense connective tissue containing large sebaceous **tarsal glands**, also known as **meibomian glands**. Each tarsal gland opens at the margin of the eyelid. The tarsal plate is responsible for the rigidity of the eyelids.

The junction between the cutaneous and conjunctival portions is demarcated clinically by the **sulcus**, a gray line located between the ducts of the meibomian glands and the eyelashes.

The **conjunctiva** is continuous with the skin lining and extends up to the periphery of the cornea. It consists of polygonal to columnar stratified epithelial cells with mucus-secreting goblet cells.

Figure 9-22. Eyelid and its pathology

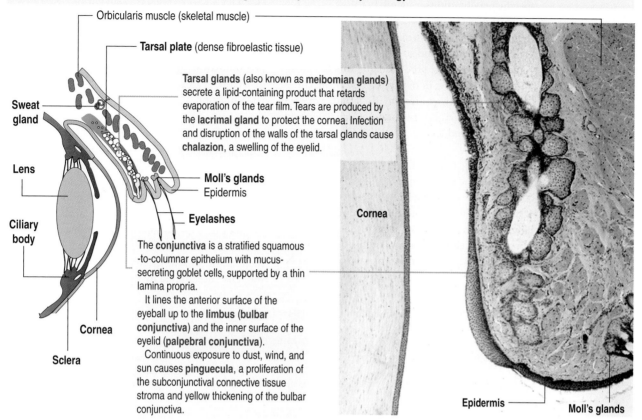

Orbicularis muscle (skeletal muscle)

Tarsal plate (dense fibroelastic tissue)

Tarsal glands (also known as **meibomian glands**) secrete a lipid-containing product that retards evaporation of the tear film. Tears are produced by the **lacrimal gland** to protect the cornea. Infection and disruption of the walls of the tarsal glands cause **chalazion**, a swelling of the eyelid.

Sweat gland

Lens

Moll's glands

Epidermis

Ciliary body

Eyelashes

The **conjunctiva** is a stratified squamous -to-columnar epithelium with mucus-secreting goblet cells, supported by a thin lamina propria.

Cornea

It lines the anterior surface of the eyeball up to the **limbus** (**bulbar conjunctiva**) and the inner surface of the eyelid (**palpebral conjunctiva**).

Sclera

Continuous exposure to dust, wind, and sun causes **pinguecula**, a proliferation of the subconjunctival connective tissue stroma and yellow thickening of the bulbar conjunctiva.

Cornea

Epidermis

Moll's glands

At the corneal rim, the conjunctival epithelium becomes stratified squamous and is continuous with the corneal epithelium. A lamina propria with capillaries supports the lining epithelium.

The **lacrimal gland** produces a fluid, **tears**, that first accumulate in the conjunctival sac and then exit into the nasal cavity through a drainage duct (**nasolacrimal duct**). Tears evaporate in the nasal cavity but can produce a sniffy nose when excessive fluid is produced.

The lacrimal gland (Figure 9-23) is a **tubuloacinar serous gland** with **myoepithelial cells**. It is organized into separate lobes with 12 to 15 independent excretory ducts. Tears enter the excretory canaliculi through the **puncta** and reach the nasolacrimal sac and duct to eventually drain in the inferior meatus within the nasal cavity.

Lacrimal glands receive neural input from:

1. **Parasympathetic nerve fibers**, originating in the pterygopalatine ganglion; **acetycholine receptors** on glandular cells respond to acetylcholine released at the nerve terminals.

2. **Sympathetic nerve fibers**, arising from the superior cervical ganglion.

Blinking produces gentle compression of the lacrimal glands and the release of fluid. Tears keep the surface of the conjunctiva and cornea moist and rinse off dust particles. **Spreading of the mucus secreted by the conjunctival epithelial cells, the oily secretion derived from the tarsal glands, and the continuous blinking of the eyelids prevent rapid evaporation of the tear film.**

Tears contain **lysozyme**, an antibacterial enzyme;

Figure 9-23. Lacrimal gland

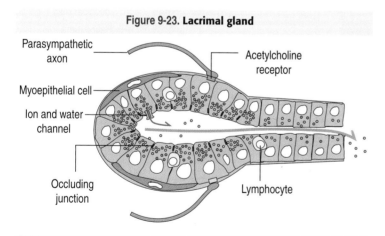

Parasympathetic axon

Acetylcholine receptor

Myoepithelial cell

Ion and water channel

Occluding junction

Lymphocyte

Secretory proteins in tears

Lactoferrin: Bacteriostatic agent. It sequesters iron necessary for bacteria metabolism.
Lysozyme: Bacteriolytic agent. It destroys bacteria.
Secretory immunoglobulin A: Defensive agent. It neutralizes infectious agents.
Tear-specific prealbumin: Unknown function.

lactoferrin; **secretory immunoglobulin A**; and **tear-specific prealbumin** (see Figure 9-23).

Excess production of tears occurs in response to chemical and physical irritants of the conjunctiva, high light intensity, and strong emotions.

A disruption in the production of tears or damage to the eyelids results in the drying out of the cornea (**dry eye** or **keratoconjunctivitis sicca**), which is followed by ulceration, perforation, loss of aqueous humor, and blindness.

Clinical significance: Red eye

A red eye is the most frequent and relatively benign ocular alteration. In some cases, a red eye represents a vision-threatening condition. A **subconjunctival hemorrhage** is the cause of acute ocular redness and can be produced by trauma, bleeding disorders, hypertension, and treatment with anticoagulants. No vision impairment is associated with this disorder.

Conjunctivitis is the most common cause of red eye. The superficial blood vessels of the conjunctiva are dilated and cause edema of the conjunctiva with discharge.

A purulent discharge indicates bacterial infection, predominantly gram-positive organisms. A watery discharge is observed in conjunctivitis caused by viral infection.

Ear

The ear consists of three components (Figure 9-24):

1. The **external ear**, which collects sound and directs it down the ear canal to the tympanic membrane.

2. The **middle ear**, which converts sound pressure waves into mechanical motion of the tympanic membrane. The motion is in turn transmitted to the middle ear ossicles, which reduce the amplitude but increase the force of mechanical motion to overcome the resistance offered by the fluid-filled inner ear.

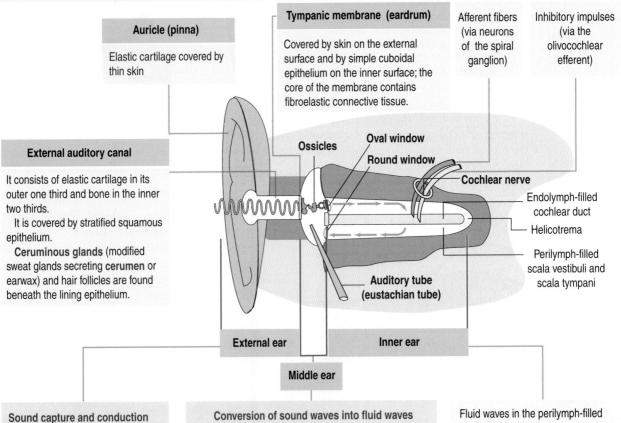

Figure 9-24. **General outline of the external, middle, and inner ear**

Auricle (pinna)

Elastic cartilage covered by thin skin

Tympanic membrane (eardrum)

Covered by skin on the external surface and by simple cuboidal epithelium on the inner surface; the core of the membrane contains fibroelastic connective tissue.

Afferent fibers (via neurons of the spiral ganglion)

Inhibitory impulses (via the olivocochlear efferent)

External auditory canal

It consists of elastic cartilage in its outer one third and bone in the inner two thirds.

It is covered by stratified squamous epithelium.

Ceruminous glands (modified sweat glands secreting **cerumen** or earwax) and hair follicles are found beneath the lining epithelium.

Ossicles

Oval window

Round window

Cochlear nerve

Endolymph-filled cochlear duct

Helicotrema

Perilymph-filled scala vestibuli and scala tympani

Auditory tube (eustachian tube)

External ear

Inner ear

Middle ear

Sound capture and conduction

The sound strikes the tympanic membrane, causing it to vibrate.

Conversion of sound waves into fluid waves

The tympanic membrane vibrates and moves the footplate of the stapes (via the ossicle bone chain) against the oval window.

The in-out movement of the oval window produces waves of pressure in the fluid-containing inner ear.

The tensor tympani and stapedius muscles regulate the amount of energy transmitted from the air to the fluid.

Fluid waves in the perilymph-filled scala vestibuli and scala tympani, caused by oscillatory movements of the stapes against the oval window, result in equal but opposite movements of the round window.

Fluid waves are transmitted to the endolymph-filled cochlear duct, which displaces the basilar membrane and stimulates the hair cells.

Figure 9-25. Development of the inner ear

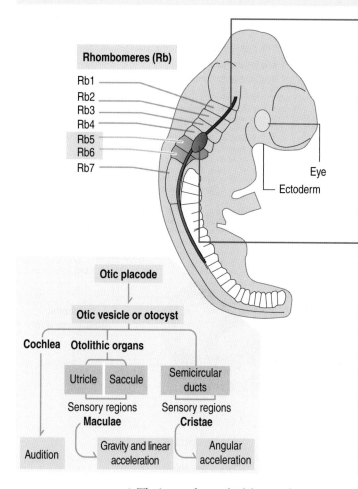

Rhombomeres (Rb)

Rb1
Rb2
Rb3
Rb4
Rb5
Rb6
Rb7

Eye
Ectoderm

Otic placode

Otic vesicle or otocyst

Cochlea | **Otolithic organs**

Utricle | Saccule | Semicircular ducts

Sensory regions **Maculae** | Sensory regions **Cristae**

Audition | Gravity and linear acceleration | Angular acceleration

Tissue and cell sources of the inner ear

The **neural crest cells** give rise to the melanocytes of the stria vascularis in the cochlea and the Schwann cells of the statoacoustic ganglion.

The **somatic ectoderm** gives rise to the otic vesicle responsible for the development of the **membranous labyrinth** (the three semicircular ducts, the utricle and saccule, and the cochlear duct).

Neuroepithelial cells are concentrated in three ampullary crests, two maculae, and one spiral organ.

The **mesenchyme** gives rise to the **otic capsule** (not shown) responsible for the formation of the **osseous labyrinth** (three semicircular canals, vestibule, and cochlea).

Development of the inner ear: otic vesicle

Genes that control hindbrain segmentation or rhombomere (Rb) identity, in particular Rb5 and Rb6, as well as genes expressed in the neural crest cells of the branchial arches control the development of the inner ear.

Under the influence of **fibroblast growth factor-3 (FGF-3)** secreted by Rb5 and Rb6, the otic placode invaginates to form the **otic vesicle** or **otocyst**. FGF receptor-3 is detected in hair cells and their underlying supporting cells in the organ of Corti.

Under the influence of the *Pax-2* (for paired box-2) gene, the otic vesicle elongates to form the dorsal vestibular region and ventral cochlear region. The formation of the **endolymphatic duct** is controlled by FGF-3 secreted by Rb5 and Rb6.

The **semicircular ducts** arise from the vestibular region under the control of the *Prx1* (for periaxin 1) and *Prx2* genes.

3. The **internal ear**, which houses the sensory organs for both hearing and balance, transmits mechanical vibrations to the fluid (the **endolymph**) contained in the **membranous labyrinth** and thereby converts these mechanical vibrations to electrical impulses on the same type of cell for sensory transduction: the **hair cell**.

The inner ear has two systems:

1. The **auditory system** for the perception of sound (hearing).

2. The **vestibular system** for the perception of head and body motion (balance).

External ear

The **auricle** (external ear or pinna) collects sound waves that are conducted across the **external acoustic meatus** to the **tympanic membrane**.

The **auricle** consists of a core of **elastic cartilage** surrounded by skin with hair follicles and sebaceous glands.

The **external acoustic meatus** is a passage extending from the auricle to the eardrum or **tympanic membrane**. The outer one third of this passage is cartilage; the inner two thirds is part of the temporal bone.

Skin lines the cartilage and the bone surfaces. A characteristic feature of this skin lining is the tubular coiled apocrine glands secreting a brown product called **cerumen**. Cerumen waterproofs the skin and protects the external acoustic meatus from exogenous agents such as insects.

Middle ear

The middle ear, or **tympanic cavity**, is an air-filled space in the temporal bone interposed between the tympanic membrane and the structures contained in the inner ear. The main function of the middle ear is the transmission of sound from the tympanic membrane to the fluid-filled structures of the inner ear.

Sound transmission is carried out by the **auditory** or **bony ossicles** (**malleus**, **incus**, and **stapes**) organized in a chainlike fashion by interconnecting small ligaments. In this chain, the arm of the malleus is attached to the **tympanic membrane** at one end; at the other end, the footplate of the stapes is applied to the **oval window** (fenestra vestibuli), an opening of the **bony labyrinth**. The **tensor tympani** (innervated by the trigeminal nerve [cranial nerve V]) and **stapedius muscles** (innervated by the facial nerve [cranial nerve VII]) keep the three auditory ossicles functionally linked.

Figure 9-26. **Membranous labyrinth**

Components of the membranous labyrinth

1 Two small sacs: the **utricle** and the **saccule**.
2 Three **semicircular ducts** open into the utricle. **Ampullae** are dilations connecting the ends of the semicircular ducts to the utricle.
3 Each ampulla contains the **crista ampullaris**. Sensory receptors in the crista ampullaris respond to the position of the head, generating nerve impulses necessary for correcting the position of the body.
4 The **cochlea**.

The sensory receptors of the membranous labyrinth are the **cristae ampullares** in the ampulla of each semicircular duct, the **macula utriculi** in the utricle, the **macula sacculi** in the saccule, and the **organ of Corti** in the cochlea.

The **ductulus reuniens** connects the saccule to the blind end of the cochlea proximal to the **cecum vestibulare**. The opposite blind end of the cochlea is the **cecum cupulare**.

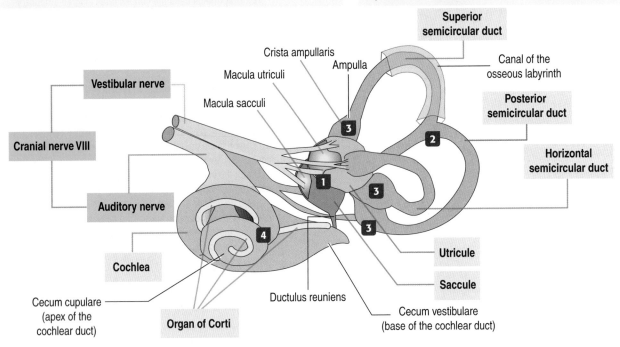

The bony ossicles have two roles:

1. **They modulate the movement of the tympanic membrane.**

2. **They apply force to the oval window, thus amplifying the incoming sound waves.**

Otosclerosis and **otitis media** affect the movements of the ossicles, conditions leading to hearing loss.

The **tympanic cavity** (also called the **tubotympanic recess** or **sulcus**) is lined by a squamous-to-cuboidal epithelium and lacks glands in the supporting connective tissue.

The **tympanic membrane** has an oval shape with a conical depression near the center caused by the attachment of the arm of the malleus. Two differently oriented layers of collagen fibers form the core of the membrane, and the two sides of the membrane are lined by a simple squamous-to-cuboidal epithelium.

The **auditory** or **eustachian tube** links the middle ear with the nasopharynx. Adjacent to the tympanic cavity, the tube is formed by the temporal bone. **Elastic cartilage** continues the bony portion of the tube, which then changes into **hyaline cartilage** near the nasopharynx opening.

A ciliated epithelium with regional variations (low columnar-to-pseudostratified near the nasopharynx) and with mucus-secreting glands lines the bony and cartilaginous segments of the tube.

The **role of the auditory tube** is **to maintain a pressure balance between the tympanic cavity and the external environment.**

Defects in middle ear development include the absence of structural elements, such as the **tympanic ring**, which supports the tympanic membrane and the ossicles. The tympanic ring is derived from mesenchyme of the first pharyngeal arch (malleus and incus) and second pharyngeal arch (stapes), the middle ear muscles, and the tubotympanic recess.

Inner ear: Development of the inner ear

The inner ear and associated cranial ganglion neurons derive from an **otic placode** on the surface of the head.

The placode invaginates and forms a hollow mass of cells called the **otic vesicle**, or **otocyst** (Figure 9-25). Neural crest cells migrate out of the hindbrain and distribute around the otic vesicle. The otic vesicle elongates, forming the dorsal vestibular region and

Figure 9-27. Endolymphatic and perilymphatic spaces

Endolymphatic and perilymphatic ducts

1 Ductules emerging from the utricle and saccule join to form the **endolymphatic duct**.

2 The endolymphatic duct ends in a dilated **endolymphatic sac** located in the subdural space of the brain.

3 The **ductus reuniens** connects the saccule to the base of the membranous coiled **cochlear duct** or **scala media**.

4 The **perilymphatic duct** extends from the vestibular area (which contains the saccule and the utricle) to the subarachnoid space around the brain. The perilymph fluid, with a composition similar to the cerebrospinal fluid, surrounds the membranous labyrinth.

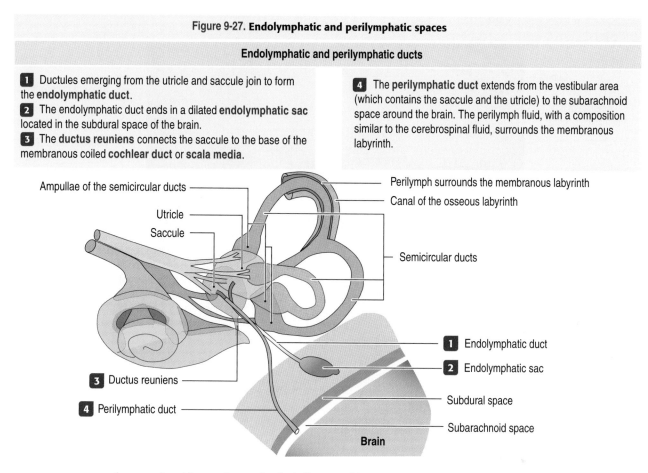

Ampullae of the semicircular ducts

Utricle

Saccule

Perilymph surrounds the membranous labyrinth

Canal of the osseous labyrinth

Semicircular ducts

1 Endolymphatic duct

2 Endolymphatic sac

3 Ductus reuniens

4 Perilymphatic duct

Subdural space

Subarachnoid space

Brain

the ventral cochlear region under the influence of the *Pax-2* (for paired box-2) **gene**. Neither the cochlea nor the spiral ganglion form in the absence of *Pax-2*.

The endolymphatic duct derives from an invagination of the otocyst, regulated by **fibroblast growth factor-3**, secreted by cells in **rhombomeres 5** and **6**. A total of seven rhombomeres, called **neuromeres**, also provide signals for the development of the hindbrain.

Two of the **semicircular ducts** derive from the vestibular region and develop under the control of the *Prx1* (for periaxin 1) and *Prx2* genes. Note that the auditory (cochlea) and vestibular portions (semicircular canals) are under separate genetic control (*Pax-2* and *Prx* genes, respectively).

Figure 9-25 provides the road mapping of the different portions of the inner ear derived from the otic vesicle.

General structure of the inner ear

The inner ear occupies the **osseous labyrinth** within the petrous portion of the temporal bone. The osseous labyrinth contains the **membranous labyrinth** (Figure 9-26), a structure that houses both the **vestibular** and **auditory systems**.

The **vestibular system** consists of two components:

1. Two **sacs** (the **utricle** and **saccule**, also called **otolith organs**).

2. **Three semicircular canals** (superior, horizontal,

and posterior) arising from the **utricle**.

The **auditory system** consists of the **cochlear duct**, lodged in a spiral bony canal anterior to the vestibular system.

The membranous labyrinth contains **endolymph**, a fluid with a high concentration of K^+ and a low concentration of Na^+. **Perilymph** (with a high Na^+ and low K^+ content) is present between the membranous labyrinth and the walls of the osseous labyrinth (Figure 9-27).

Vestibular system

The **semicircular canals** respond to **rotational movements** of the head and body (**angular accelerations**).

The **otolith organs** (saccule and utricle) respond to **translational movements** (**gravity and linear acceleration**).

Sensory cells in the vestibular organ are innervated by afferent fibers of the vestibular branch of the **vestibulocochlear nerve** (cranial nerve VIII). The **labyrinthine artery**, a branch of the anterior inferior cerebellar artery, supplies blood to the labyrinth. The **stylomastoid artery** supplies blood to the semicircular canals.

Semicircular canals

The semicircular ducts are contained within the osseous labyrinth. The three ducts are connected

Figure 9-28. Structure of the crista ampullaris

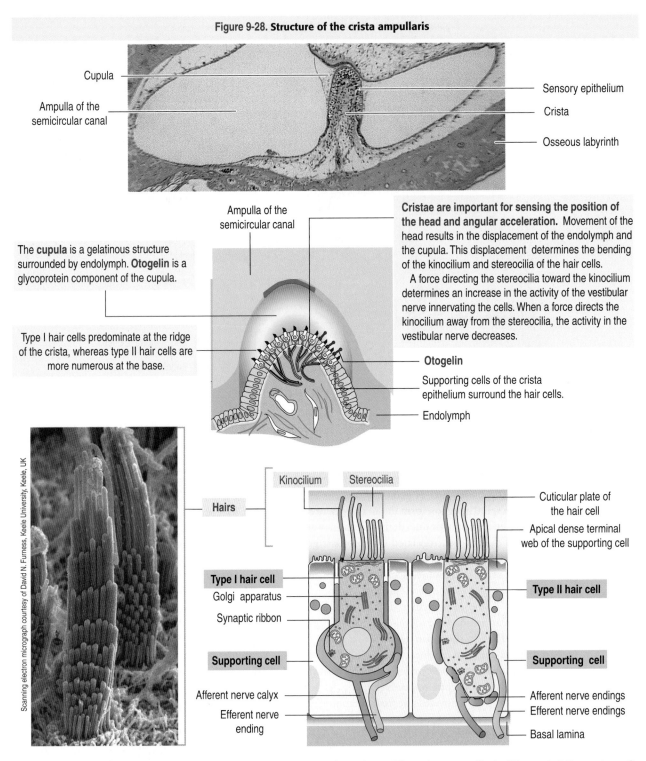

Cupula

Ampulla of the semicircular canal

Sensory epithelium

Crista

Osseous labyrinth

Ampulla of the semicircular canal

The **cupula** is a gelatinous structure surrounded by endolymph. **Otogelin** is a glycoprotein component of the cupula.

Cristae are important for sensing the position of the head and angular acceleration. Movement of the head results in the displacement of the endolymph and the cupula. This displacement determines the bending of the kinocilium and stereocilia of the hair cells.

A force directing the stereocilia toward the kinocilium determines an increase in the activity of the vestibular nerve innervating the cells. When a force directs the kinocilium away from the stereocilia, the activity in the vestibular nerve decreases.

Type I hair cells predominate at the ridge of the crista, whereas type II hair cells are more numerous at the base.

Otogelin

Supporting cells of the crista epithelium surround the hair cells.

Endolymph

Scanning electron micrograph courtesy of David N. Furness, Keele University, Keele, UK

Kinocilium   Stereocilia

Hairs

Cuticular plate of the hair cell

Apical dense terminal web of the supporting cell

Type I hair cell
Golgi apparatus
Synaptic ribbon

Type II hair cell

Supporting cell

Supporting cell

Afferent nerve calyx
Efferent nerve ending

Afferent nerve endings
Efferent nerve endings
Basal lamina

to the utricle. Ducts derived from the utricle and saccule join to form the **endolymphatic duct**. The endolymphatic duct ends in a small dilation called the **endolymphatic sac**, located between the layers of the meninges.

Small dilations, **ampullae**, are present at the semicircular duct–utricle connection sites. Each ampulla has a prominent ridge called the **crista ampullaris**. Cristae are important for sensing the position of the head and angular acceleration.

The crista ampullaris (Figure 9-28) consists of a **sensory epithelium** covered by a gelatinous mass called the **cupula**. The cupula contains **otogelin**, a glycoprotein anchoring the cupula to the sensory epithelium.

The sensory epithelium consists of two cell types (see Figure 9-28):

1. The **hair cells**.
2. The **supporting cells**.

Like all other sensory receptors, hair cells respond

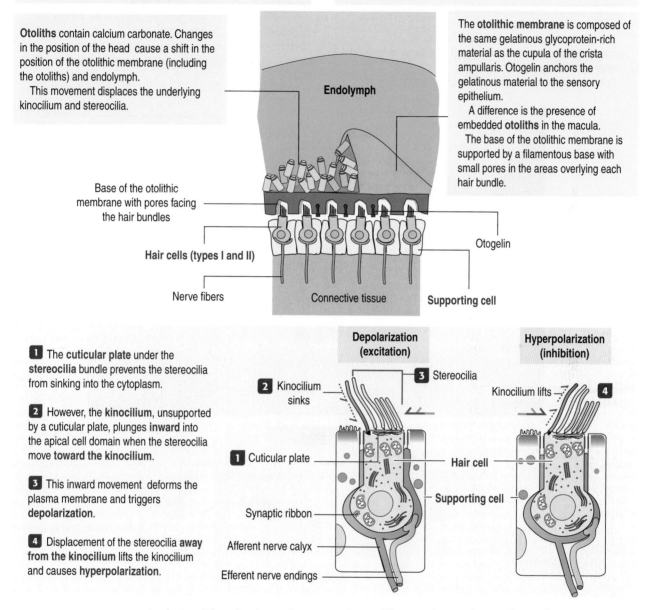

Figure 9-29. Structure of the macula of the saccule and utricle

The **maculae** are sensory receptor areas located in the wall of the **saccule** and **utricle**.

They are concerned with the detection of directional movement of the head. The position of the macula in the utricle is **horizontal** and it is **vertical** in the saccule.

A single layer of supportive cells associated with the basal lamina houses two types of sensory cells: **types I** and **II hair cells**. A long single kinocilium and 50 to 60 stereocilia project from the apical surface of the hair cells.

Otoliths contain calcium carbonate. Changes in the position of the head cause a shift in the position of the otolithic membrane (including the otoliths) and endolymph.

This movement displaces the underlying kinocilium and stereocilia.

The **otolithic membrane** is composed of the same gelatinous glycoprotein-rich material as the cupula of the crista ampullaris. Otogelin anchors the gelatinous material to the sensory epithelium.

A difference is the presence of embedded **otoliths** in the macula.

The base of the otolithic membrane is supported by a filamentous base with small pores in the areas overlying each hair bundle.

Endolymph

Base of the otolithic membrane with pores facing the hair bundles

Hair cells (types I and II)

Otogelin

Nerve fibers

Connective tissue

Supporting cell

Depolarization (excitation)

Hyperpolarization (inhibition)

1 The **cuticular plate** under the **stereocilia** bundle prevents the stereocilia from sinking into the cytoplasm.

2 However, the **kinocilium**, unsupported by a cuticular plate, plunges **inward** into the apical cell domain when the stereocilia move **toward the kinocilium**.

3 This inward movement deforms the plasma membrane and triggers **depolarization**.

4 Displacement of the stereocilia **away from the kinocilium** lifts the kinocilium and causes **hyperpolarization**.

2 Kinocilium sinks

3 Stereocilia

Kinocilium lifts

4

1 Cuticular plate

Hair cell

Supporting cell

Synaptic ribbon

Afferent nerve calyx

Efferent nerve endings

to sustained stimuli by adapting and restoring their sensitivity to threshold **deflections** on a millisecond to sub-millisecond timescale.

The basal surface of the supporting cells is attached to a basal lamina. In contrast, the hair cells occupy a recess in the apical region of the supporting cells and do not reach the basal lamina.

The apical domain of the hair cells contains 60 to 100 hairlike specialized **stereocilia** and a **single kinocilium**. Stereocilia are supported by an actin-containing **cuticular plate**. The free ends of both stereocilia and kinocilia are embedded in the **cupula**.

The cupula attaches to the roof and walls of the ampulla and acts like a partition of the lumen of the ampulla (see Figure 9-28).

The crista ampullaris has two types of hair cells:
1. **Type I hair cells.**
2. **Type II hair cells.**

Both cell types are essentially similar in their internal structure, but differences exist in their shape and innervation:

1. **Afferent nerves**, with terminals containing the neurotransmitters **aspartate** and **glutamate**, enter the spaces separating the supporting cells and **form**

Figure 9-30. **Organization of the macula**

Sensory epithelium of the macula

This epithelium consists of **types I** and **II hair cells** embedded in **supporting cells** touching the basal lamina.

In vivo, kinocilia and stereocilia, extending from the surface of the hair cells, are coated by the **otolithic** (or statoconial) **membrane** containing **otoconia** (Greek "ear dust").

Otoconia are displaced by the endolymph during forward-backward and upward-downward movements of the head (**linear acceleration**).

The sensory epithelium of the macula in the otolithic organs (saccule and utricle) does not respond to head rotation.

The hair cells of the macula are **polarized**: The **kinocilium** is oriented with respect to an imaginary line called the **striola**, which divides the hair cells into two opposite fields.

In the utricule, the kinocilium faces the striola. In the saccule, the kinocilium faces away from the striola.

This orientation determines which population of hair cells will displace their hair bundles in response to a specific movement of the head.

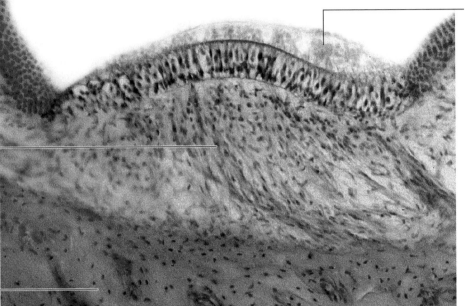

Remnant of the otolithic membrane

The subjacent connective tissue of the macula contains fibers of the vestibular nerve

Bone tissue of the osseous labyrinth

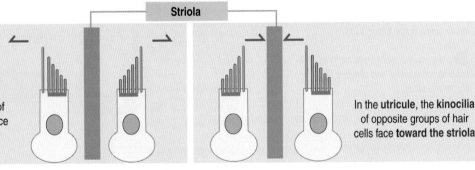

Striola

In the **saccule**, the **kinocilia** of opposite groups of hair cells face **away from the striola**

In the **utricule**, the **kinocilia** of opposite groups of hair cells face **toward the striola**

a **calyx-like network** embracing the rounded basal domain of the type I hair cell. The cytoplasm displays **synaptic ribbons** and associated vesicles (similar to those found in the sensory retina).

2. The nerve endings in contact with the cylindrical type II hair cell do not form a basal calyx. Instead, **simple terminal boutons** can be visualized.

In addition to afferent nerves, both type I and type II hair cells receive **efferent nerve terminals** and have synaptic vesicles containing the neurotransmitter **acetylcholine**. Efferent nerve fibers control the sensitivity of the sensory receptor cells.

Supporting cells and hair cells are associated with each other by apical junctional complexes. Characteristic features of the supporting cells are an **apical dense terminal web** and the presence of **short microvilli**. Supporting cells lack stereocilia and kinocilia, two features typical of hair cells.

Otolithic organs: Utricle and saccule

The utricle and saccule display a sensory epithelium called a **macula** (Figures 9-29 and 9-30). Small ductules derived from the utricle and saccule join to form the **endolymphatic duct** ending in the **endolymphatic**

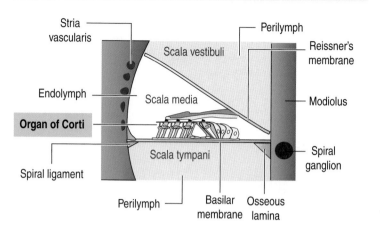

Figure 9-31. Topography of the cochlea

Stria vascularis

Scala vestibuli

Perilymph

Reissner's membrane

Endolymph

Scala media

Modiolus

Organ of Corti

Scala tympani

Spiral ganglion

Spiral ligament

Perilymph

Basilar membrane

Osseous lamina

sac. The **ductus reuniens** links the saccule to the base of the membranous cochlear duct.

Like the sensory epithelium of the crista ampullaris in the semicircular canals, the macula contains hair cells and supporting cells. The characteristics of the hair cells of the macula are described in Figure 9-29.

Note that the macula is covered by a gelatinous substance, the **otolithic membrane**, containing calcium carbonate–protein complexes forming small crystals called **otoliths**. Otoliths are not present in the cupula overlying the hairs of the crista ampullaris.

How do hair cells of the crista ampullaris of the semicircular ducts and the maculae of the utricle and saccule work?

When the position of the cupula and otolithic membrane change in response to movements of the endolymph, it causes displacement of the stereocilia and kinocilium of the hair cells (see bottom of Figure 9-29).

When stereocilia move **toward the kinocilium**, the plasma membrane of the hair cells **depolarizes** and the afferent nerve fibers are **stimulated (excitation)**.

When stereocilia are **deflected away from the kinocilium**, the hair cell **hyperpolarizes** and afferent nerve fibers are **not stimulated (inhibition)**.

One last important point: The hair cells of the macula are **polarized** (see Figure 9-30). The kinocilium is oriented with respect to an imaginary line called the **striola**, which divides the population of hair cells into two opposite fields:

1. In the utricle, the kinocilium faces **toward** the striola.

2. In the saccule, the kinocilium faces **away** from the striola.

These opposite orientations determine which population of hair cells will displace their hair bundles in response to a specific movement of the head.

Again, remember that the cristae ampullares of the semicircular ducts respond to rotational movements of the head and body (**angular acceleration**), whereas

the maculae of the utricle and saccule respond to translational movements (**gravity and linear acceleration**).

Clinical significance: Ménière's disease
Secretory cells in the membranous labyrinth and the endolymphatic sac maintain the ionic balance between endolymph and perilymph (see Figure 9-36).

An **increase in the volume of endolymph** is the cause of **Ménière's disease**, which is characterized by vertigo (illusion of rotational movement in space), nausea, positional **nystagmus** (involuntary rhythmic oscillation of the eyes), vomiting, and ringing in the ears (**tinnitus**).

Cochlea
The cochlear duct is a membranous coiled duct inserted in the bony cochlea. It consists of an **apex** and a **base**. The coiled duct makes about two and two-thirds turns with a total length of 34 mm.

The cochlea has **three spiraling chambers** (Figures 9-31 and 9-32):

1. The **cochlear duct** (also called the **scala media**) represents the central chamber and contains endolymph.

2. Above the cochlear duct is the **scala vestibuli**, starting at the oval window.

3. Below the cochlear duct is the **scala tympani**, ending at the **round window**.

The scalae vestibuli and tympani are filled with perilymph and communicate at the **helicotrema** at the apex of the cochlea (Figure 9-33).

In cross section, the boundaries of the scala media are:

1. The **basilar membrane** at the bottom.

2. The **vestibular** or **Reissner's membrane** above,

3. The **stria vascularis** externally.

The cells and capillaries of the stria vascularis produce endolymph. The **stria vascularis** is lined by a **pseudostratified epithelium** consisting of **basal cells** (of neural crest or mesoderm origin), **intermediate cells** (melanocyte-like cells of neural crest origin) and **marginal cells** (of epithelial cell origin).

Marginal cells contain an ATPase K$^+$ pump involved in K$^+$ release into the endolymph. Basal cells are linked to intermediate cells by gap junctions. Intermediate cells harbor **Kcnj10**, a potassium inwardly rectifying channel, subfamily J, member 10, that generates an endocochlear potential and membrane voltage and produces endolymph. The recycling of K$^+$ions from the hair cells back into the endolymph maintains the appropriate high K$^+$ concentration in the endolymph fluid, critical for normal hair cell function.

The spiraling bony core of the cochlea is the **modiolus**. On the inner side, the spiral osseous lamina projects outward from the modiolus to join the basilar membrane. On the external side, the basilar membrane is continuous with the **spiral ligament**.

Figure 9-32. **Cochlea**

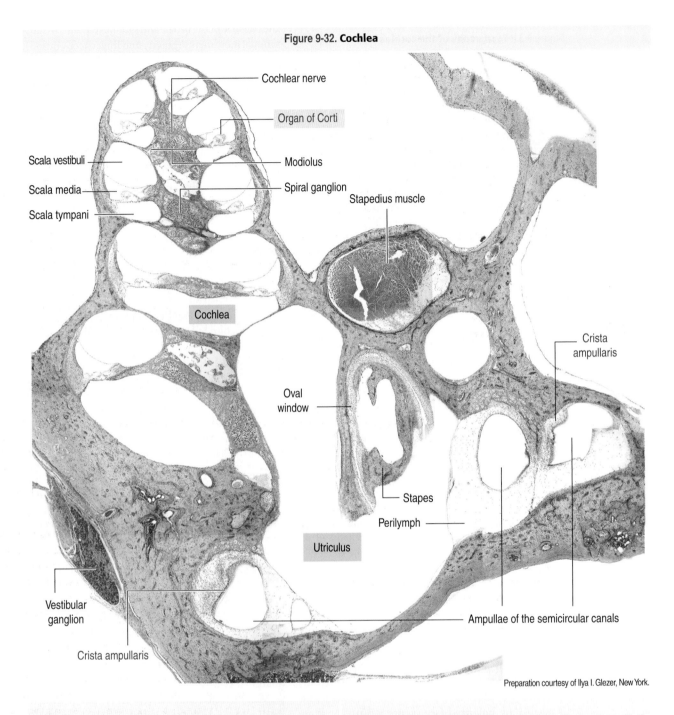

Cochlear nerve

Organ of Corti

Scala vestibuli

Modiolus

Scala media

Spiral ganglion

Scala tympani

Stapedius muscle

Cochlea

Crista ampullaris

Oval window

Stapes

Perilymph

Utriculus

Vestibular ganglion

Ampullae of the semicircular canals

Crista ampullaris

Preparation courtesy of Ilya I. Glezer, New York.

The cochlea (Greek *kochlias*, spiral-shelled snail) is a spiral canal that winds more than two and a half times around a central bony axis, the **modiolus**. Within the bony modiolus is the **cochlear (spiral) ganglion**, spiraling around the inner side of the cochlea. The ganglion contains bipolar neurons: (1) The peripheral processes innervate the hair cells. (2) The central processes enter the core of the modiolus, where they form the cochlear nerve (the cochlear division of cranial nerve VIII).

The membranous portion of the cochlea contains the cochlear duct, or **scala media**. The cochlear duct spans the bony labyrinth dividing it into two separate canals: (1) the **scala vestibuli** and (2) the **scala tympani**.

The **vestibular membrane (Reissner's membrane)** and the **basilar membrane**, two membranes limiting the cochlear duct, separate the

endolymph-filled cochlear duct from the perilymph-filled scala vestibuli and scala tympani.

The lateral wall of the cochlear partition is the **stria vascularis**, a highly vascular tissue that covers a portion of the bony labyrinth and is responsible for the production and maintenance of the unique composition of the **endolymph**.

The cochlear duct does not extend to the apex or cupula of the cochlea but leaves a small opening of communication between the scala vestibuli and scala tympani at the apex, the **helicotrema** (see Figure 9-33). At the base of the cochlea, the stapes on the **oval window** and the membrane of the **round window** (not shown) separate the scala vestibuli and the scala tympani, respectively, from the middle ear cavity.

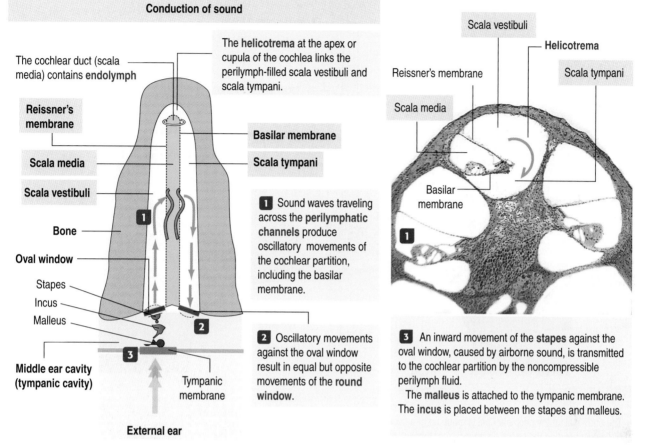

Figure 9-33. Organ of Corti: The sound-transducing component of the inner ear

Conduction of sound

The cochlear duct (scala media) contains **endolymph**

The **helicotrema** at the apex or cupula of the cochlea links the perilymph-filled scala vestibuli and scala tympani.

Reissner's membrane

Basilar membrane

Scala media

Scala tympani

Scala vestibuli

Bone

1 Sound waves traveling across the **perilymphatic channels** produce oscillatory movements of the cochlear partition, including the basilar membrane.

Oval window

Stapes

Incus

Malleus

Middle ear cavity (tympanic cavity)

Tympanic membrane

2 Oscillatory movements against the oval window result in equal but opposite movements of the **round window.**

External ear

Scala vestibuli

Helicotrema

Reissner's membrane

Scala tympani

Scala media

Basilar membrane

3 An inward movement of the **stapes** against the oval window, caused by airborne sound, is transmitted to the cochlear partition by the noncompressible perilymph fluid.

The **malleus** is attached to the tympanic membrane. The **incus** is placed between the stapes and malleus.

Organ of Corti

The **organ of Corti** is the sensory component of the cochlea.

In simple terms, imagine the organ of Corti consisting of a small tunnel (Figure 9-34). The tiny tunnel is flanked by a **single row of inner hair cells (IHCs)** on the side pointing to the modiolus, and **three rows of outer hair cells (OHCs)** on the other side, pointing to the stria vascularis. **Outer and inner pillar cells** form the walls of the tunnels.

OHCs and IHCs, supported by **outer and inner phalangeal cells** respectively, extend from the base to the apex of the cochlea. The **tectorial membrane** extends outward from the **spiral limbus** and covers in part the organ of Corti.

IHCs are the sensory receptors sending most of the neural signals to the central nervous system. OHCs have the mechanical role of amplifying the displacement of the basilar membrane in response to sound waves. The basilar membrane moves the hair cells toward and away from the tectorial membrane.

A relevant component of the hair cells is the **hair bundle** located at their apical domain. A hair bundle is formed by 50 to 150 **stereocilia** in a long-to-short gradient arrangement. **No kinocilium is present in the hair bundle of the cochlea.**

Molecular and mechanical aspects of the hearing process

Each member of the hair bundle, the stereocilium, consists of a core of actin filaments (Figure 9-35). The tip of the actin bundle is the site where actin monomers are added under control of **myosin XVa** in association with the protein **whirlin**. Defects in myosin Va and whirlin cause abnormally short stereocilia.

At the base, the actin bundle is stabilized by the protein **radixin**. Stereocilia within a hair bundle are interconnected by extracellular filaments (**interciliary links**). **Side links** (**myosin VIIa** and associated proteins) connect stereocilia along their shafts. **Tip links** (**cadherin 23**) extend from the tip of a stereocilium to the side of the taller adjacent stereocilium. The tension of the tip link is controlled by **myosin 1c**.

Defects in interciliary links result in **Usher's syndrome**, characterized by disorganization of hair bundles leading to sensorineural deafness of cochlear origin combined with retinitis pigmentosa (loss of vision).

Interciliary links regulate the opening and closing of **mechanoelectrical transduction** (MET) **ion channels**, permeable to Ca^{2+}. Deflection of the hair bundle toward the taller stereocilia side opens the MET channels; displacements in the opposite direction close

Figure 9-34. **Organ of Corti**

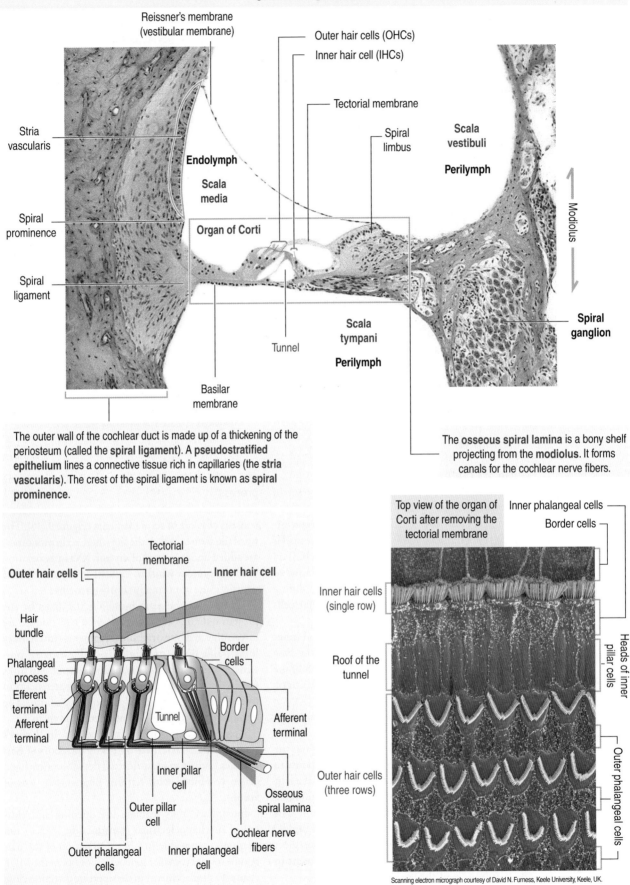

Reissner's membrane
(vestibular membrane)

Outer hair cells (OHCs)

Inner hair cell (IHCs)

Tectorial membrane

Spiral
limbus

Scala
vestibuli

Perilymph

Stria
vascularis

Endolymph

Scala
media

Organ of Corti

Modiolus

Spiral
prominence

**Spiral
ganglion**

Spiral
ligament

Scala
tympani

Perilymph

Tunnel

Basilar
membrane

The outer wall of the cochlear duct is made up of a thickening of the periosteum (called the **spiral ligament**). A **pseudostratified epithelium** lines a connective tissue rich in capillaries (the **stria vascularis**). The crest of the spiral ligament is known as **spiral prominence**.

The **osseous spiral lamina** is a bony shelf projecting from the **modiolus**. It forms canals for the cochlear nerve fibers.

Tectorial
membrane

Inner hair cell

Outer hair cells

Hair
bundle

Border
cells

Phalangeal
process

Efferent
terminal

Tunnel

Afferent
terminal

Afferent
terminal

Inner pillar
cell

Outer pillar
cell

Osseous
spiral lamina

Outer phalangeal
cells

Inner phalangeal
cell

Cochlear nerve
fibers

Top view of the organ of Corti after removing the tectorial membrane

Inner phalangeal cells

Border cells

Inner hair cells
(single row)

Heads of inner
pillar cells

Roof of the
tunnel

Outer hair cells
(three rows)

Outer phalangeal cells

Scanning electron micrograph courtesy of David N. Furness, Keele University, Keele, UK.

Figure 9-35. **Molecular organization of the hair bundle**

Hair bundle, an array of stereocilia arranged in a staircase

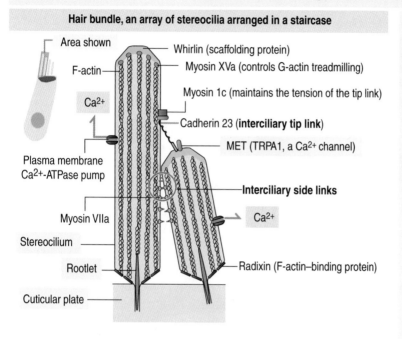

Area shown

Whirlin (scaffolding protein)

F-actin

Myosin XVa (controls G-actin treadmilling)

Ca^{2+}

Myosin 1c (maintains the tension of the tip link)

Cadherin 23 (**interciliary tip link**)

MET (TRPA1, a Ca^{2+} channel)

Plasma membrane Ca^{2+}-ATPase pump

Interciliary side links

Myosin VIIa

Ca^{2+}

Stereocilium

Myosin VIIa

Rootlet

Radixin (F-actin–binding protein)

Cuticular plate

Deflections of the hair bundle are caused by sound vibrations initiated in each eardrum, conducted through the three ossicles in the middle ear, and transmitted within the cochlea as pressure waves. The end result is the displacement of the basilar membrane to elicit an electrical response in hair cells.

Sound-induced motion of the basilar membrane deflects the hair bundles of the hair cells to activate mechanoelectrical transduction (MET) ion channels represented by transient receptor potential channel A1 (TRPA1) linked by an interciliary tip link (for example, Ca^{2+}-dependent cadherin 23). The tension of the tip link is maintained by myosin 1c. Force applied to the interciliary tip link appears to activate TRPA1, which becomes permeable to Ca^{2+}. Plasma membrane Ca^{2+}-ATPase pumps are present. Side links (for example, myosin VIIa) stabilize the cohesion of adjacent hair bundles.

Each hair bundle consists of an F-actin core capped by the scaffolding protein whirlin and associated myosin XVa. G-actin is added at the tip of the stereocilia.

these channels. Interciliary links ensure a uniform response of MET channels. MET Ca^{2+} channels are essential for the conversion of a sound stimulus to an equivalent electrical signal and frequency tuning.

The **tectorial membrane** is an extracellular gel-like matrix contacting the stereocilia bundles of the outer hair cells. It contains types II, V and IX collagens, α- and β-**tectorin** proteins and **otogelin**, also seen in the cupula (crista ampullaris) and otolithic membrane

(maculae). As previously indicated, otogelin is essential for the anchoring of the cupula and otolithic membrane to the sensory epithelium. Conversely, otogelin appears to be dispensable for the anchoring of the tectorial membrane to the spiral limbus.

When the basilar membrane and organ of Corti are displaced by shear forces (Figure 9-36), the hair bundle of OHCs hit the tectorial membrane and the rigid stereocilia are **deflected**; stereocilia do not bend.

Figure 9-36. **Functions of the organ of Corti**

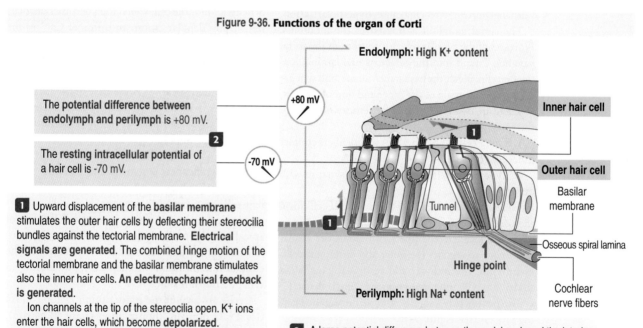

Endolymph: High K^+ content

The **potential difference between endolymph and perilymph is +80 mV.**

2

+80 mV

The **resting intracellular potential** of a hair cell is -70 mV.

-70 mV

Inner hair cell

1

Outer hair cell

Basilar membrane

Tunnel

Osseous spiral lamina

Hinge point

Perilymph: High Na^+ content

Cochlear nerve fibers

1 Upward displacement of the **basilar membrane** stimulates the outer hair cells by deflecting their stereocilia bundles against the tectorial membrane. **Electrical signals are generated.** The combined hinge motion of the tectorial membrane and the basilar membrane stimulates also the inner hair cells. **An electromechanical feedback is generated.**

Ion channels at the tip of the stereocilia open. K^+ ions enter the hair cells, which become **depolarized.** Neurotransmitters released at the basal domain of each hair cell depolarize the afferent cochlear nerve fiber. Signals are relayed to the brain by the VIII cranial nerve.

2 A large potential difference between the endolymph and the interior of the hair cell (150 mV) enhances the response of the cell to the mechanical displacement of the stereocilia.

Figure 9-37. Deafness and balance

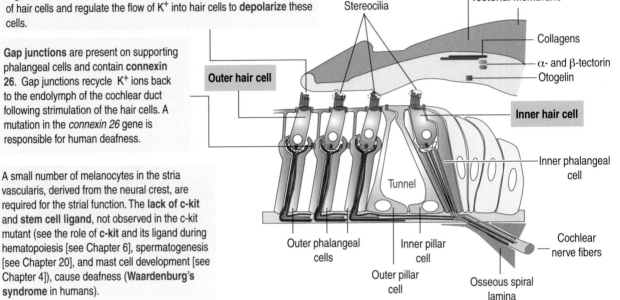

K$^+$ is secreted by cells of the **stria vascularis** into the endolymph. A mutation in the gene encoding a protein of the K$^+$ channel in the intermediate cells of the stria vascularis (*Kcnj10* gene) determines a disruption in the production of endolymph and the degeneration of the organ of Corti. K$^+$ channel proteins are present at the tip of the stereocilia of hair cells and regulate the flow of K$^+$ into hair cells to **depolarize** these cells.

Gap junctions are present on supporting phalangeal cells and contain **connexin 26**. Gap junctions recycle K$^+$ ions back to the endolymph of the cochlear duct following strimulation of the hair cells. A mutation in the *connexin 26* gene is responsible for human deafness.

A small number of melanocytes in the stria vascularis, derived from the neural crest, are required for the strial function. The **lack of c-kit** and **stem cell ligand**, not observed in the c-kit mutant (see the role of **c-kit** and its ligand during hematopoiesis [see Chapter 6], spermatogenesis [see Chapter 20], and mast cell development [see Chapter 4]), cause deafness (**Waardenburg's syndrome** in humans).

Three major proteins of the gel-like tectorial membrane are **collagens types II, V and IX, otogelin**, α-**tectorin**, and β-**tectorin**. A mutation in the genes encoding otogelin and α-tectorin causes deafness.

Stereocilia

Tectorial membrane

Collagens

α- and β-tectorin

Otogelin

Outer hair cell

Inner hair cell

Inner phalangeal cell

Tunnel

Outer phalangeal cells

Inner pillar cell

Outer pillar cell

Osseous spiral lamina

Cochlear nerve fibers

Keep in mind that rigidity is determined at the tip of the stereocilia by a complex group of proteins (see Figure 9-35). Most importantly, stereocilia tension created by deflection opens transduction ion channels.

Deflection of stereocilia toward the **tallest** stereocilia causes **depolarization**. Deflection of stereocilia toward the **shortest** stereocilia causes **hyperpolarization**.

The **spiral ganglion** is housed in the modiolus. Processes of the bipolar sensory neurons of the spiral ganglion extend into the osseous spiral lamina, lose their myelin, pierce the basilar membrane, and synapse on the basal domain of the inner and outer hair cells.

There are two types of bipolar sensory neurons in the spiral ganglion:

1. **Type I cells** (90% to 95%) whose fibers contact inner hair cells.

2. **Type II cells** (5% to 10%) that synapse with outer hair cells.

The neuronal processes of types I and II cells form the cochlear branch of the vestibulocochlear nerve. Olivocochlear efferent fibers run along the basilar membrane to contact the inner and outer hair cells. Neurons of the auditory and vestibular ganglia fail to develop when the *neurogenin 1* gene is deleted.

Two factors play a significant role during the hearing process (see Figure 9-36):

1. The high concentration of K$^+$ in the endolymph and the high concentration of Na$^+$ in the perilymph determine an electrical potential difference. The ion concentration is regulated by the absorptive and secretory activity of the stria vascularis.

2. Fluid movement in the scala tympani induces the movement of the basilar membrane causing the taller stereocilia to be displaced by the tectorial membrane.

As a result, ion channels at the stereocilia tip open driving K$^+$ into the cell, which then becomes depolarized. Upon depolarization, an **influx of Ca^{2+}** to the basal region of the hair cells determines the release of neurotransmitters at the hair cell–cochlear nerve fiber synapse and generation of a stimulus. Note the presence of **ribbon synapses** at the base of the hair cells.

Changes in electrical potential between the perilymph and the hair cells occur in response to the magnitude of sound.

Clinical significance: Deafness and balance
Cytoskeletal components in the apical domain of hair cells are relatively abundant. Hair cells convert mechanical input, determined by the deflection of apical bundles of stereocilia embedded in the tectorial membrane and the otolithic membrane of the cupula, into an electromechanical input leading to synaptic transmission.

In the absence of the transcription factor **Pou4f3** (for POU domain, transcription factor 4, class 3), hair cells express specific markers (including unconventional **myosin VI** and **VIIa**), and both hair cells and spiral ganglion neurons degenerate.

As previously indicated, the tectorial membrane, cupula and otolithic membrane contain α-**tectorin**, β-**tectorin** and otogelin. When the α-tectorin- and otogelin-encoding genes are mutated, deafness and imbalance occur (Figure 9-37).

A mutation in the gene for **connexin 26**, a component of gap junctions on the surface of supporting cells, is responsible for deafness because the recycling of endolymph K⁺ from the intercellular spaces to the stria vascularis is disrupted. Connexin 26 is not present in hair cells.

There are several mouse mutants with a decrease in neural crest–derived melanocytes in the stria vas-cularis. Although the particular role of melanocytes in the stria vascularis is not known, a mutation in the **c-_kit_ gene** (encoding the stem cell factor receptor and its ligand; see Chapter 6, Blood and Hematopoiesis, for a discussion of the c-_kit_ gene) affects the function of the stria vascularis and the mice are deaf.

Waardenburg's syndrome in humans is an autosomal dominant type of congenital deafness associated with pigment abnormalities, such as partial albinism, and abnormal development of the vestibulocochlear ganglion.

Recall that melanocytes have a common origin in the neural crest and are migratory cells.

Essential concepts | **Sensory Organs: Vision and Hearing**

• EYE
The eyeball consists of three tunics (from outside to inside):
(1) Sclera and cornea.
(2) Uvea.
(3) Retina.
Three interconnected chambers are inside the eye:

(1) The anterior chamber (between the corneal endothelium and the anterior surface of the iris).
(2) The posterior chamber (between the posterior surface of the iris and the lens and associated suspensory ligaments of the lens).
(3) The vitreous cavity (from the lens to the retina).

Aqueous humor (produced by the ciliary body) circulates from the posterior to the anterior chambers. Aqueous humor is drained from the trabecular meshwork into the canal of Schlemm located at the corneal-irideal angle.

The eyeball is protected by the bony orbit, the eyelids, conjunctiva, and the lacrimal

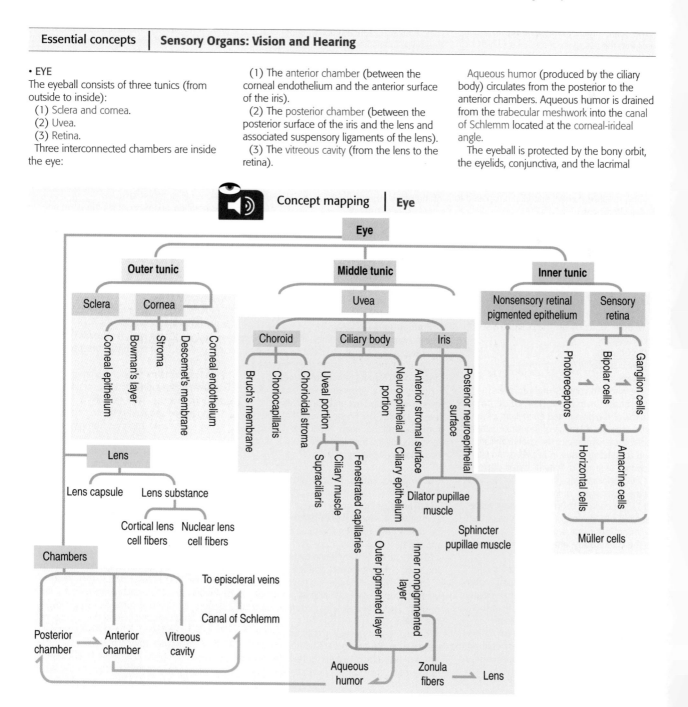

Concept mapping | Eye

apparatus. The ophthalmic artery (a branch of the internal carotid artery) provides nutrients to the eye and the orbit contents.

• The components of the eye derive from three different sites:
(1) The surface ectoderm of the head.
(2) The lateral neuroectodermal walls of the embryonic brain (diencephalon region).
(3) The mesenchyme.
Each optic vesicle, an outpocketing on the right and left sides of the diencephalon, becomes a two-layered optic cup.
The outer layer becomes the pigmented epithelium; the inner neural layer becomes the retina.
The surface of the ectoderm invaginates into the optical vesicle forming the future lens.
The outer surface of the optic cup differentiates into the vascular choroid coat (which gives rise to the ciliary body, ciliary muscle, and ciliary processes), the sclera, and the cornea.
The mesenchyme, extending into the invagination of the optic cup, forms the vitreous component of the eye.

• Outer tunic: Sclera and cornea. The sclera is a thick layer of collagen and elastic fibers produced by fibroblasts. The cornea is a transparent, avascular, and innervated tissue. It consists of five layers:
(1) A stratified corneal epithelium exposed to the environment,
(2) A supporting membrane or layer of Bowman.
(3) A regularly oriented corneal stroma.
(4) The membrane of Descemet.
(5)The corneal endothelium (a simple squamous epithelium in contact with aqueous humor).

• Middle tunic: Uvea. The uvea consists of three regions:
(1) Choroid.
(2) Ciliary body.
(3) Iris.
The choroid consists of three layers:
(1) Bruch's membrane (formed by the basal lamina of the pigmented epithelium of the retina, the basal lamina of fenestrated capillaries corresponding to the choriocapillaris, and connective tissue in between, the site of deposits of amyloid material called drusen).
(2) Choriocapillaris (the source of nutrients to the outer layers of the retina).
(3) The choroid stroma (containing melanocytes, blood vessels, and neurons of the autonomic nervous system).
The ciliary body, anterior to the ora serrata, consists of two portions:
(1) The uveal portion (that includes the supraciliaris portion of the choroid; the ciliary muscle, which controls the curvature of the lens by modifying the length of the suspensory ligaments; and fenestrated capillaries).
(2) The neuroepithelial portion (which contributes two cell layers to the ciliary epithelium: a pigmented cell layer and a nonpigmented cell layer, continuous with the sensory retina.

The apical surfaces of these two layers face each other and secrete aqueous humor).
The iris is a continuation of the ciliary body. It has an anterior surface without epithelial lining (melanocytes and fibroblasts), and a posterior surface lined by a dual layer of pigmented cells. The stroma contains myoepithelial cells (dilator pupillae muscle) and smooth muscle cells (sphincter pupillae).

• The lens is a biconvex, transparent, elastic, and avascular structure kept in place by zonular fibers (extending from the ciliary epithelium and inserting at the equatorial region of the lens capsule).
The lens consists of:
(1) A capsule.
(2) An epithelium.
(3) A lens substance (consisting of cortical and nuclear lens fibers).
Filensin and crystallins (α, β, and γ) are intermediate filament proteins found in the lens. Cataracts, an opacity of the lens, is caused by a change in the solubility of these proteins.

• Accommodation is the process by which the lens becomes rounder (to focus the image of a nearby object on the retina) and flattens (when the image of a distant object is focused on the retina).
Accommodation involves the participation of the ciliary muscle, the ciliary body, and the suspensory ligaments.
When the ciliary muscle contracts, the tension of the ligaments is reduced (because the ciliary body moves closer to the lens), and the lens acquires a spherical shape (close vision).
When the ciliary muscle relaxes, the tension of the ligaments increases (the ciliary body moves away from the lens), and the lens becomes flat (distant vision).
Emmetropia is normal vision. Myopia (or nearsightedness) occurs when the eyeball is too deep or the curvature of the lens is not flat enough for distant vision; the image of a distant object forms in front of the retina.
Hyperopia (or farsightedness) is when the eyeball is too shallow and the curvature of the lens is too flat; the image of a distant object forms behind the retina. Older people become farsighted as the lens loses elasticity, a condition known as presbyopia.

• Inner tunic: Retina. The retina consists of two regions:
(1) The outer nonsensory retinal pigmented epithelium (a single layer of pigmented cuboidal cells extending from the optic disk to the ora serrata).
(2) The inner sensory retina (extending from the optic disk to the ciliary epithelium).
The separation of these two layers, resulting from trauma, vascular disease, metabolic disorders, and aging, results in detachment of the retina.
The pigmented epithelium of the retina is essential for the transport of nutrients from the choroidal blood vessels to the outer layers of the retina, the removal of waste metabolic products from the sensory retina, the phagocytosis and recycling of photoreceptor disks, and the recycling of the photobleached pigment rhodopsin. The basal lamina of the pigmented epithelium is a component of Bruch's membrane.
The sensory retina consists of four cell groups:
(1) Photorecepor neurons (rods and cones).
(2) Conducting neurons (bipolar and ganglion cells).
(3) Association neurons (horizontal and amacrine cells).
(4) Supporting neuroglia Müller cells.
Cells are distributed in 10 layers summarized in Figure 9-14.
There are three distinct nuclear regions:
(1) The outer nuclear layer corresponds to the nuclei of the photoreceptors.
(2) The inner nuclear layer corresponds to the nuclei of bipolar cells, horizontal, and amacrine cells as well as of Müller cells.
(3) The ganglion layer contains the nuclei of the ganglion cells. The plexiform and limiting membranes represent sites of contacts among the retinal cells.
Photoreceptor cells (rods and cones) are elongated and consist of two segments:
(1) An outer segment, which contains flat membranous disks.
(2) An inner segment, the site of synthesis of various cell components.
A modified cilium connects the outer and inner segments. It also provides microtubules for molecular motor proteins (kinesins and cytoplasmic dyneins) to deliver materials to the disk assembly site by the mechanism of intraciliary transport.
The differences between rods and cones are the following:
(1) the outer segment of the rod is cylindrical; in cones it is conical.
(2) Rods terminate in a spherule; cones end in a pedicle. Both endings interact with bipolar and horizontal cells.
(3) Rods contain the photopigment rhodopsin (night vision); cones contain a similar pigment, iodopsin (color vision).
Bipolar and ganglion cells are connecting neurons receiving impulses from photoreceptor cells.
Horizontal and amacrine cells do not have axons or dendrites, only neuritic processes conducting in both directions.
Müller cells are columnar cells that occupy the spaces between photoreceptor and bipolar and ganglion cells. Müller cells contact the outer segment of the photoreceptors, establishing zonulae adherentes and microvilli, corresponding to the outer limiting membrane. The inner limiting membrane represents the basal lamina of Müller cells.
Ribbon synapses, each containing a synaptic ribbon, are found in spherules and pedicles of the photoreceptor cells and in bipolar cells. They are also found in hair cells (inner ear) and pinealocytes (pineal gland).
A synaptic ribbon is a dense strip located at the presynaptic membrane associated with

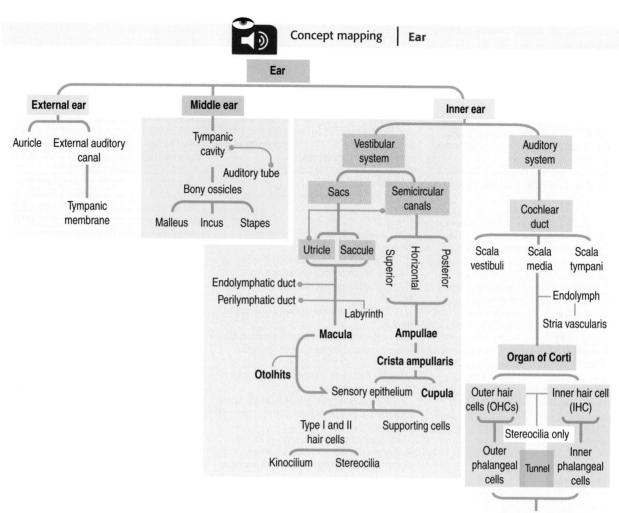

Concept mapping | Ear

Ear

- **External ear**
  - Auricle
  - External auditory canal
    - Tympanic membrane
- **Middle ear**
  - Tympanic cavity
    - Auditory tube
  - Bony ossicles
    - Malleus
    - Incus
    - Stapes
- **Inner ear**
  - Vestibular system
    - Sacs
      - Utricle
      - Saccule
      - Endolymphatic duct
      - Perilymphatic duct
      - Labyrinth
      - **Macula**
        - **Otolhits**
        - Sensory epithelium
    - Semicircular canals
      - Superior
      - Horizontal
      - Posterior
      - **Ampullae**
        - **Crista ampullaris**
        - **Cupula**
        - Type I and II hair cells
          - Kinocilium
          - Stereocilia
        - Supporting cells
  - Auditory system
    - Cochlear duct
      - Scala vestibuli
      - Scala media
        - Endolymph
        - Stria vascularis
      - Scala tympani
      - **Organ of Corti**
        - Outer hair cells (OHCs)
        - Inner hair cell (IHC)
        - Stereocilia only
        - Outer phalangeal cells
        - Tunnel
        - Inner phalangeal cells
        - Tectorial membrane

---

free, tethered and constantly releasing vesicles. RIBEYE protein aggregates form the scaffold of the ribbon.

• The **fovea centralis**, surrounded by the macula lutea, is a specialized area for accurate vision.

The **optic disk** (the exit site of axons derived from ganglion cells and the passage site of blood vessels), including the optic papilla, is not suitable for vision (the blind spot of the retina).

• The **eyelids** consist of two portions:
(1) The outer cutaneous portion.
(2) The inner conjunctival portion.

The cutaneous portion contains sweat and sebaceous glands, and eyelashes associated with glands of Moll. The tarsal plate (fibroelastic connective tissue) faces the conjunctival lining. Large sebaceous glands, called tarsal glands or meibomian glands, open at the margin of the eyelids.

The conjunctiva (polygonal to columnar stratified epithelial lining with mucus-secreting cells) is continuous with the skin and ends at the margin of the cornea, where it becomes stratified squamous epithelium and is continuous with the corneal epithelium.

• The **lacrimal glands** are tubuloacinar serous glands with myoepithelial cells. Blinking produces compression of the lacrimal glands and the release of fluid (tears).

• **EAR**
The ear consists of three portions:
(1) External ear.
(2) Middle ear.
(3) Inner ear.

• The **external ear** consists of the auricle (external ear), which collects sound waves that are conducted across the external acoustic meatus to the tympanic membrane.

• The **middle ear** (or tympanic cavity) is an air-filled space in the temporal bone that contains the auditory or bony ossicles (malleus, incus, and stapes). The arm of the malleus is attached to the tympanic membrane at one end; the footplate of the stapes is applied to the oval window, an opening of the bony labyrinth.

Bony ossicles modulate the movement of the tympanic membrane and apply force to the oval window (to amplify the incoming sound waves).

Otitis media and **otosclerosis** affect the movement of the ossicles and can lead to hearing loss.

The auditory or eustachian tube (elastic cartilage changing to hyaline cartilage) links the middle ear to the nasopharynx. It maintains a pressure balance between the tympanic cavity and the external environment.

• The **inner ear** occupies the osseous labyrinth, which contains the membranous labyrinth.

The membranous labyrinth houses the vestibular and auditory systems. The membranous labyrinth contains endolymph (high concentration of K$^+$ and low concentration of Na$^+$). Perilymph (high concentration of Na$^+$ and low concentration of K$^+$) is present between the osseous labyrinth and the membranous labyrinth.

• The **vestibular system** consists of:
(1) Two sacs (utricle and saccule).
(2) Three semicircular canals: superior, horizontal, and posterior, arising from the utricle.

Ampullae are present at the semicircular canal–utricle connection site.

The endolymphatic duct derives from the utricle and saccule and fuses into a single duct, which terminates in a small dilation, the endolymphatic sac, located between the layers of the meninges.

An increase in the volume of endolymph causes **Ménière's disease**, characterized by vertigo, nausea, positional nystagmus, vomiting, and tinnitus (ringing in the ears).

Each ampulla has a crista, an elevation covered by sensory epithelium consisting of type I and II hair cells and supporting cells, topped by the cupula, a gelatinous substance surrounded by endolymph.

Semicircular canals respond to rotational movements of the head and body (angular acceleration).

Hair cells have an apical domain containing 60 to 100 stereocilia (supported by an actin-containing cuticular plate) and a single kinocilium. The free ends of the stereocilia and kinocilium are embedded in the cupula.

The maculae of the utricle and saccule respond to translational movements (gravity and linear acceleration). Maculae consist of a sensory epithelium (type I and II hair cells and supporting cells) topped by the otolithic membrane, a gelatinous substance similar to cristae, except for the presence of otoliths containing calcium carbonate.

Remember that when the position of the cupula and otolithic membrane change in response to movements of the endolymph, it causes displacement of the stereocilia and kinocilium of the hair cells.

When stereocilia move toward the kinocilium, the plasma membrane of the hair cells depolarizes and the afferent nerve fibers are stimulated (excitation).

When stereocilia are deflected away from the kinocilium, the hair cell hyperpolarizes and afferent nerve fibers are not stimulated (inhibition).

Remember also that the hair cells of the macula are polarized. The kinocilium is oriented with respect to an imaginary line called the striola, which divides the population of hair cells into two opposite fields:

(1) In the utricle, the kinocilium faces toward the striola.

(2) In the saccule, the kinocilium faces away from the striola.

• The **auditory system** consists of the cochlea, a coiled duct.

The cochlea has three spiraling chambers:

(1) The cochlear duct (called scala media).

(2) The scala vesibuli, starting at the oval window.

(3) The scala tympani, ending at the round window.

The scala vestibuli and scala tympani contain perilymph and communicate at the helicotrema.

The stria vascularis, located externally of the cochlear duct, produces endolymph.

The modiolus, located internally in the spiraling bony axis of the cochlea, houses the spiral ganglion.

The organ of Corti is the sensory epithelium of the cochlea. It contains hair cells and supporting cells. Instead of a cupula found in the crista and macula, the sensory epithelium of the cochlea is in contact with the tectorial membrane (consisting of collagens, α- and β-tectorin, and otogelin).

The organ of Corti consists of two groups of hair cells:

(1) Inner hair cell (IHC). Single row.

(2) Outer hair cells (OHCs). Three rows.

IHC and OHCs are separated from each other by the tunnel. The tunnel is limited by outer and inner pillar cells. Hair cells are supported by phalangeal cells.

The apical hair bundle of hair cells of the cochlea lack kinocilia but have stereocilia.

Each stereocilium of the hair bundle consists of a core of actin filaments. The tip of the actin bundle is the site where actin monomers are added. Stereocilia within a hair bundle are interconnected by extracellular filaments (interciliary links). Interciliary links regulate the opening and closing of mechano-electrical transduction (MET) ion channels, permeable to Ca^{2+}.

• **Deafness** occurs when α-tectorin and otogelin are defective in the tectorial membrane, connexin 26 is not present in gap junctions linking cochlear supporting cells, and the vestibulocochlear ganglion is not developed (**Waardenburg's syndrome**). Defects in interciliary links result in **Usher's syndrome**, characterized by disorganization of hair bundles leading to sensorineural deafness of cochlear origin combined with retinitis pigmentosa (loss of vision).

10. Immune-Lymphatic System

The natural physical barriers of epithelia prevent infection by blocking entry of pathogens into the body. When pathogens compromise the defensive nature of an epithelial barrier, cellular components of the immune system are recruited to combat the invading pathogen or antigens. The immune system consists of innate (natural) and adaptive or acquired responses interacting to confront and neutralize infectious diseases. Leukocytes, in particular neutrophils, provide the first line of defense during acute inflammation. Lymphocytes and macrophages confront pathogens during chronic inflammation. In this chapter, we analyze the structure and function of primary and secondary lymphoid organs and their involvement in general and specific defensive actions.

Components of the lymphatic system
The lymphatic system includes **primary** and **secondary lymphoid organs**.

The primary lymphoid organs produce the cell components of the immune system (Figure 10-1).
They are:
1. The **bone marrow**.

2. The **thymus**.

The secondary lymphoid organs are the sites where immune responses occur.
They include:
1. The **lymph nodes**.
2. The **spleen**.
3. The **tonsils**.

Figure 10-1. Lineage origin of the lymphoid progeny within the context of hematopoiesis

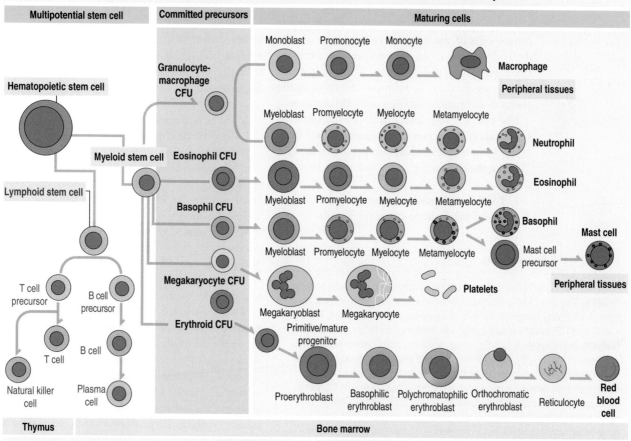

The cells of the immune system arise from the hematopoietic stem cell in the bone marrow. We discussed in Chapter 6, Blood and Hematopoiesis, that hematopoietic stem cells divide to produce two specialized stem cells: **lymphoid stem cell**, which generates B and T lymphocytes, and a **myeloid stem cell**, which gives rise to leukocytes, erythrocytes, megakaryocytes, and macrophages.

B lymphocytes (B cells) differentiate in the bone marrow, When activated outside the bone marrow, B cells differentiate into antibody-secreting **plasma cells**. **T lymphocytes** (T cells) differentiate in the **thymus** into cells that can activate other cells of the immune system (helper cells) or kill bacteria- or virus-infected cells (cytolytic or cytotoxic cells). **CFU**: colony-forming unit.

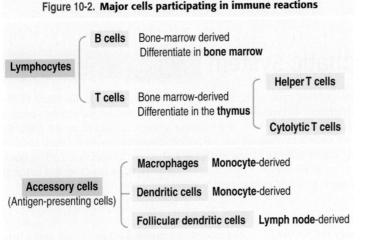

Figure 10-2. Major cells participating in immune reactions

Lymphocytes
- **B cells** — Bone-marrow derived. Differentiate in **bone marrow**
- **T cells** — Bone marrow-derived. Differentiate in the **thymus**
  - **Helper T cells**
  - **Cytolytic T cells**

Accessory cells (Antigen-presenting cells)
- **Macrophages** — Monocyte-derived
- **Dendritic cells** — Monocyte-derived
- **Follicular dendritic cells** — Lymph node-derived

4. Aggregates of lymphocytes and antigen-presenting cells in the **lung** (bronchial-associated lymphoid tissue, BALT) and the mucosa of the **digestive tract** (gut-associated lymphoid tissue, GALT), including **Peyer's patches**.

The lymphatic system is widely distributed because pathogens can enter the body at any point.

The main function of the **lymphoid organs**, as components of the immune system, is to protect the body against invading **pathogens** or **antigens** (bacteria, viruses, and parasites). The basis for this defense mechanism, or **immune response**, is the ability to distinguish **self** from **nonself substances**.

The **two key cell components of the immune system** are **lymphocytes** and **accessory cells** (Figure 10-2). Lymphocytes include two major cell groups:

1. **B cells**, responding to cell-free and cell-bound antigens.

2. **T cells**, subdivided into two categories: **helper T cells** and **cytolytic** or **cytotoxic T cells**. T cells

respond to cell-bound antigens presented by specific molecules.

After leaving the two **primary** organs (bone marrow and thymus), mature B and T cells circulate in the blood until they reach one of the various **secondary lymphoid organs** (lymph nodes, spleen, and tonsils).

B and T cells can leave the bloodstream through specialized venules called **high endothelial venules**, so called because they are lined by tall endothelial cells instead of the typical squamous endothelial cell type.

The **accessory cells** include two monocyte-derived cell types: **macrophages** and **dendritic cells**. An example of a dendritic cell is the **Langerhans cell** found in the epidermis of the skin. A third type, the **follicular dendritic cell**, is present in lymphatic nodules of the lymph nodes. Follicular dendritic cells differ from ordinary dendritic cells in that they do not derive from a bone marrow precursor.

Before we start our discussion of the origin, differentiation, and interaction of lymphocytes and accessory cells, we need to define the characteristics of the immune system. Then, we will be able to integrate the structural aspects of each major lymphatic organ with the specific characteristics of the immune responses.

Types of immunity

Immunity in general is the reaction of cells and tissues to foreign (nonself) substances or **pathogens** including bacterial, viral, and parasite antigens. Two types of immunity are distinguished:

1. Innate or natural immunity.

2. Adaptive or acquired immunity (Figure 10-3).

Innate or **natural immunity of the newborn** is the simplest mechanism of protection. It does not require previous exposure to a pathogen and elicits rapid responses by macrophages and dendritic cells.

Toll-like receptors (TLRs; see Box 10-A) initiate innate immunity against components of invading pathogens (such as nucleic acids, proteins, lipids and polysaccharides). Different TLRs recognize distinct types of conserved microbial structures, a condition that provides specificity to the innate response.

We discuss later in this chapter that the **complement system**, consisting of serum proteins, membrane-bound regulators and receptors, is also a key mechanism of innate defense triggered rapidly upon infection. Stimulation of macrophages and dendritic cells by activated TLRs and the complement system leads to the production and secretion of proinflammatory cytokines, thereby initiating an inflammatory response.

Adaptive or acquired immunity develops when an individual is exposed to a pathogen with the aims of eliminating the pathogen as well as the generation of immunologic memory.

To achieve adaptive or acquired immunity, it is

Box 10-A | Toll-like receptors

- Toll-like receptors (**TLRs**) recognize pathogen-associated molecular patterns (**PAMPs**). The term PAMPs designates proteins associated with a wide spectrum of pathogens recognized by cells of the innate or natural immune system.
- Activated TLR activate in turn the **NF-κB transcription factor pathway** (see Necroptosis in Chapter 3, Cell Signaling), which regulates cytokine expression. Activation of the NF-κB pathway links innate and adaptive immune responses by stimulating the production of proinflammatory cytokines, such as interleukines and tumor necrosis factor ligand, and chemokines, as well as triggering the expression of costimulatory molecules (CD40, CD80, and CD86).
- The intracellular domain of the TLR has structural homology with the cytoplasmic region of interleukin-1 receptors. It is known as **Toll-interleukin-1 receptor domain**, or **TIR domain**, and participates in signaling by recruiting downstream proteins.
- The extracellular region of the TLR contains leucine-rich repeat (LLR) motifs, whereas the extracellular domain of interleukin receptors contains three immunoglobulin-like domains. LLR is involved in the recognition of PAMPs facilitated by accessory proteins (for example, lipopolysaccharides).

Figure 10-3. Types of immunity

Immunity
- **Innate or natural immunity** (Toll-like receptors and complement system)
- **Adaptive or acquired immunity**
  - **Humoral immunity** (antibody-mediated: plasma cells)
  - **Cell-mediated immunity** (T cells, B cells and antigen-presenting cells)

Acquisition of immunity
- **Passive immunity**
  - Maternal antibodies transferred across the placenta to fetus
  - Antibodies of immunized animals (rabies, tetanus)
  - Antitoxins (diphtheria)
- **Active immunity** (post disease)
  - T cells

necessary to select lymphocytes (**clonal selection**) from a vast repertoire of cells bearing antigen-specific receptors generated by a mechanism known as **gene rearrangement**. You can regard adaptive immunity as the perfection of innate or natural immunity because it recognizes vital components of the microorganism utilizing a limited number of **pattern-recognition receptors** expressed on all cells of a given type (**nonclonal**) and independent of immunologic memory.

Adaptive or acquired immunity involves two types of responses to an antigen (or pathogen):

1. The **first response** is mediated by **antibodies** produced by plasma cells, the final differentiation product of B cells as we have seen in Chapter 4, Connective Tissue. This response is known as **humoral immunity** and operates against antigens located outside a cell or bound to its surface. When antibodies bind to an antigen or toxins produced by a pathogen, they can facilitate the phagocytic action of macrophages or recruit leukocytes and mast cells to take advantage of their cytokines and mediators, respectively, and strengthen a response. Humoral immunity results in persistent antibody production and production of memory cells.

2. The **second response requires the uptake of a pathogen by a phagocyte**. An intracellular pathogen is not accessible to antibodies and requires a cell-mediated response, or **cell-mediated immunity**. T cells, B cells, and antigen-presenting cells are the key players in cell-mediated immunity.

A consequence of adaptive or acquired immunity is the protection of the individual when a second encounter with the pathogen occurs. This protection is specific against the same pathogen and, therefore, adaptive or acquired immunity is also called **specific immunity**.

Passive immunity is a temporary form of immunity conferred by serum or lymphocytes transferred from an immunized individual to another individual who has not been exposed or cannot respond to a pathogen. The transfer of maternal antibodies to the fetus is a form of passive immunity that protects newborns from infections until they can develop active immunity. **Active immunity** is the form of immunity resulting from exposure to a pathogen.

Properties of adaptive or acquired immunity

Both humoral and cell-mediated immunity developed against foreign pathogens have the following characteristics:

1. **Specificity**: Specific domains of an antigen are recognized by individual lymphocytes. We will see later how cell membrane receptors on lymphocytes can distinguish and respond to subtle variations in the structure of antigens offered by an antigen-presenting cell. This molecular interaction between cells is known as **immunologic synapse**.

2. **Diversity**: Lymphocytes utilize a gene rearrangement mechanism to modify their antigen receptors in such a way that they can recognize and respond to a large number and types of antigenic domains.

3. **Memory**: The exposure of lymphocytes to an antigen results in two events: their antigen-specific clonal expansion by mitosis, as well as the generation of reserve **memory cells**. Memory cells can react more rapidly and efficiently when exposed again to the same antigen.

4. **Self-limitation**: An immune response is stimulated by a specific antigen. When the antigen is neutralized or disappears, the response ceases.

5. **Tolerance**: An immune response pursues the removal of a non-self antigen while being "tolerant" to self-antigens. Tolerance is achieved by a selection mechanism that eliminates lymphocytes expressing receptors specific for self-antigens. A failure of self-tolerance (and specificity) leads to a group of disorders called **autoimmune diseases**.

Development and maturation of B cells in bone marrow

The bone marrow is the site of origin of B and T cells from a lymphoid stem cell. In Chapter 6, Blood and Hematopoiesis, we discuss developmental aspects of the myeloid and erythroid lineages from a hematopoietic stem cell. The same hematopoietic stem cell gives rise to a **lymphoid stem cell** that generates precursors for B cells and T cells (see Figure 10-1). **B cells mature in the bone marrow,** whereas **the thymus is the site of maturation of T cells.**

Stem B cells in the bone marrow proliferate and mature in a microenvironmental **niche** provided by bone marrow **stromal cells** producing **interleukin-7 (IL-7)** (Figure 10-4).

During maturation, B cells express on their surface

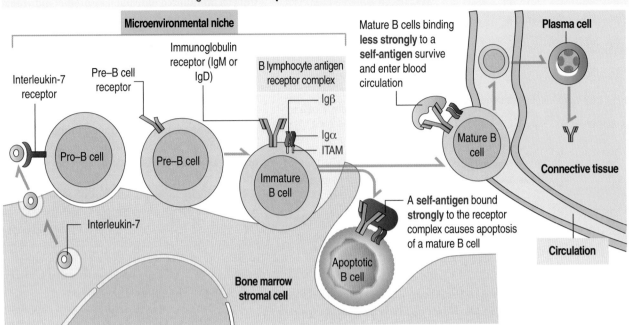

Figure 10-4. Development of B cells in bone marrow

immunoglobulins **M** (IgM) or **D** (IgD) interacting with two additional proteins linked to each other, **immunoglobulins α (Igα)** and **β (Igβ)**. The cell surface IgM or IgD, together with the conjoined **Igα** and **Igβ**, form the **B cell antigen receptor complex**. The intracellular domains of Igα and Igβ contain a tyrosine-rich domain called **immunoreceptor tyrosine-based activation motif (ITAM)**.

Binding of an antigen to the B lymphocyte antigen receptor complex induces the phosphorylation of tyrosine in the ITAM, which, in turn, activates transcription factors that drive the expression of genes required for further development of B cells.

Self-antigens present in the bone marrow test the antigen-binding specificity of IgM or IgD on B cell surfaces. This is a required testing step before B cells can continue their maturation, enter peripheral lymphoid tissues, and interact with foreign (non-self) antigens. **Self-antigens** binding **strongly** to two or more IgM or IgD receptor molecules on B cells induce **apoptosis**. **Self-antigens** with a **weaker binding affinity** for the B cell antigen receptor complex enable the survival and maturation of these B cells when ITAMs of IgM- or IgD-associated Igα and Igβ transduce signaling events, resulting in further differentiation of B cells and the entrance of mature B cells into the circulation.

Major histocompatibility complex (MHC) and human leukocyte antigens (HLA)

The presentation of antigens to T cells is carried out by specialized proteins encoded by genes in the major histocompatibility locus and present on the surface of antigen-presenting cells, the macrophages.

Antigen-presenting cells survey the body, find and internalize antigens by phagocytosis, break them down into antigenic peptide fragments, and bind them to **major histocompatibility complex (MHC)** molecules (Figure 10-5) so that the **antigen peptide fragment–MHC complex** can be exposed later on the surface of the cells.

The *MHC* gene locus expresses gene products responsible for the rejection of grafted tissue between two genetically incompatible hosts.

There are two types of **mouse** MHC gene products: **class I MHC** and **class II MHC**.

1. Class I MHC consists of two polypeptide chains: an α **chain**, consisting of three domains (α_1, α_2, and α_3) encoded by the *MHC* gene locus, and β_2-**microglobulin**, not encoded by the *MHC* gene locus.

Antigens are housed in a cleft formed by the α_1 and α_2 domains. **CD8**, a coreceptor on the surface of **cytolytic T cells**, binds to the α_3 domain of class I MHC.

2. Class II MHC consists of two polypeptide chains, an α chain and a β chain. Both chains are encoded by the *MHC* gene locus. The α_1 and β_1 domains form an antigen-binding cleft. **CD4**, a coreceptor on the surface of **helper T cells**, binds to the β_2 domain of class II MHC.

CD4 and CD8 are cell surface identifiers, members of the **cluster of differentiation** or **designation** (abbreviated as **CD**). See Box 10-B.

All nucleated cells express class I MHC molecules. Class II MHC molecules are restricted mainly to antigen-presenting cells (macrophages, dendritic cells, and B cells), thymic epithelial cells of the thymus, and endothelial cells.

The MHC-equivalent molecules in the **human** are designated **human leukocyte antigens** (**HLAs**). HLA molecules are structurally and functionally homologous to mouse MHC molecules and the gene locus is present on human chromosome 5 (β_2-microglobulin is encoded by a gene on chromosome 15).

The **class I MHC locus encodes** three major proteins in the human: **HLA-A**, **HLA-B**, and **HLA-C**. The **class II MHC locus encodes HLA-DR** (R for antigenically related), **HLA-DQ**, and **HLA-DP** (Q and P preceding R in the alphabet).

T cell receptor

In addition to MHC molecules, subsets of T cells have cell surface receptors that enable each of them to recognize a different antigen–MHC combination. Antigen recognition involves an **immunologic synapse** mechanism consisting in the formation of stable antigen-presenting cell–T cell adhesiveness followed by an activating signaling cascade by T cells (see Box 10-C).

The receptor that recognizes specific antigenic peptides presented by class I and class II MHC molecules is the **T cell receptor** (**TCR**). TCR acts together with accessory cell surface molecules, the **coreceptors**, to stabilize the binding of antigen-presenting cells to T cells. Developing T cells express unique TCRs generated by random rearrangement of a variety of gene segments. These randomly produced TCRs

provide the diversity required to identify numerous foreign peptides.

The TCR consists of two disulfide-linked transmembrane polypeptide chains: the α **chain** and the β **chain** (see Figure 10-5). A limited number of T cells have a TCR composed of γ and δ chains. Each α and β chain consists of a **variable** (**Vα** and **Vβ**) domain and a **constant** (**Cα** and **Cβ**) domain. When compared with the immunoglobulin molecule, the Vα and Vβ domains are structurally and functionally similar to the antigen-binding fragment (Fab) of immunoglobulins.

The TCR molecule is associated with two proteins, CD3 and ζ (not shown in Figure 10-5), forming the **TCR complex**. CD3 and ζ have a signaling role and are present in all T cells. CD3 contains the ITAM cytoplasmic domain previously mentioned as part of the B cell antigen receptor complex and involved in signaling functions.

CD4 and CD8 coreceptors

CD4 and CD8 are T cell surface proteins interacting selectively with class II MHC and class I MHC molecules, respectively. When the TCR recognizes an antigen bound to the cleft of MHC, CD4 or CD8 coreceptors cooperate in the activation of T cell function (see Figure 10-5).

CD4 and CD8 are members of the immunoglobulin (Ig) superfamily. In Chapter 1, Epithelium, we discuss the function and structure of cell adhesion molecules belonging to the Ig superfamily.

Members of the Ig superfamily have a variable number of extracellular Ig-like domains. The two terminal Ig-like domains of CD4 bind to the β_2 domain of the class II MHC (see Figure 10-5). The single Ig-like domain of CD8 binds to the α_3 domain of the class I MHC.

Thus, **CD4$^+$ helper T cells recognize antigens associated with class II MHC, and CD8$^+$ cytolytic T cells (cytolytic thymus-derived lymphocytes [CTL]) respond to antigens presented by class I MHC** (Figure 10-6).

T cell maturation in the thymus: Positive and negative selection

Two initial events take place in the thymus during T cell maturation:

1. A sequence rearrangement of the gene encoding protein components of the **TCR**.

2. The transient coexistence of TCR-associated **coreceptors CD4 and CD8**.

When precursor cells, derived from the bone marrow, enter the **cortex** of the thymus, they lack surface molecules typical of mature T cells. Because **they still do not express CD4 and CD8, they are called "double-negative" T cells** (Figure 10-7).

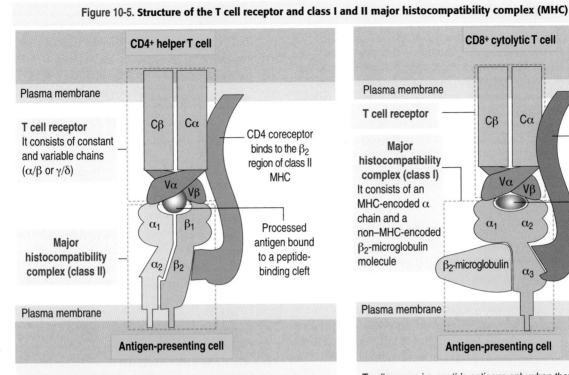

Figure 10-5. Structure of the T cell receptor and class I and II major histocompatibility complex (MHC)

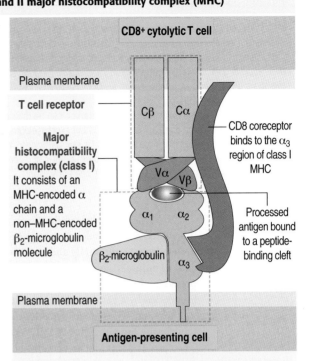

CD4+ helper T cell recognize an antigen presented by class II MHC molecules.

Each class II MHC molecule consists of a single extracellular peptide-binding cleft formed by a pair of MHC-encoded immunoglobulin-like chains. The α_1 and β_1 regions of each chain, anchored to the membrane of the antigen-presenting cell, interact to form the peptide-binding cleft.

Coreceptor CD4 binds to the β_2 region of class II MHC.

T cells recognize peptide antigens only when they are presented bound to MHC. **CD8+ cytolytic T cells recognize an antigen presented by class I MHC molecules. Helper T cells recognize an antigen in association with class II MHC molecules.** This property is called **MHC restriction.**

Class I MHC is a heterodimer consisting of a plasma membrane, anchored α chain, an attached β_2-microglobulin and a bound antigen peptide.

Coreceptor CD8 binds to the α_3 region of class I MHC.

After interacting with **thymic epithelial cells,** the stroma components of the thymus, double-negative T cells proliferate, differentiate, and express the first T cell–specific molecules: TCR and coreceptors CD4 and CD8.

As we have already seen, TCR consists of two pairs

of subunits: **αβ chains** or **γδ chains** (see Figure 10-5). Each chain can vary in sequence from one T cell to another. This variation is determined by the random combination of gene segments and has a bearing on which foreign antigen T cells can recognize.

Maturation of T cells proceeds through a stage where **both CD4 and CD8 coreceptors and low levels of TCR are expressed by the same cell.** These cells are known as **"double-positive" T cells.**

Double-positive T cells **can** or **cannot** recognize self-MHC expressed by thymic epithelial cells in the cortex of the thymus. Selected T cells must be **self-MHC–restricted** and **self-tolerant.** Those cells that can recognize self-MHC eventually mature and express one of the two coreceptor molecules (CD4 or CD8) and become **"single-positive" T cells (clonal selection).** Double-positive cells that cannot recognize self-MHC fail the positive selection and are discarded (**clonal deletion**).

There is an additional test for the selected self-MCH–restricted T cells: only those **T cells that can recognize foreign peptides and self-MHC survive.** If T cells bind to **body's tissue-specific antigens**

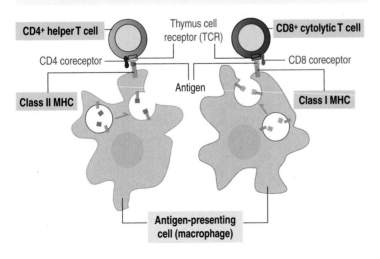

Figure 10-6. General features of helper and cytolytic T cells

Figure 10-7. Maturation of T cells in the thymus

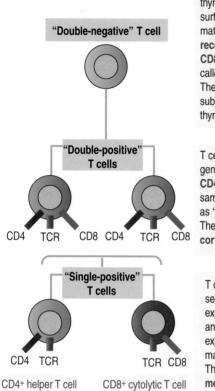

"Double-negative" T cell

Precursor cells entering the thymus from the bone marrow lack surface molecules typical of mature T cells: **thymus cell receptor** (TCR), and **CD4** and **CD8 coreceptors**. These cells are called **"double-negative" T cells**. These cells are seen in the subcapsular **cortex region** of the thymus.

"Double-positive" T cells

CD4   TCR   CD8   CD4   TCR   CD8

T cells begin to rearrange the gene encoding TCR and express **CD4 and CD8 coreceptors** by the same cell. These cells are known as **"double-positive" T cells**. These cells are seen deeper in the **cortex** of the thymus.

"Single-positive" T cells

CD4   TCR   TCR   CD8

CD4+ helper T cell   CD8+ cytolytic T cell

T cells whose receptors bind self-MHC molecules lose expression of **either CD4 or CD8** and increase the level of expression of TCR. These are mature **"single-positive" T cells**. These cells are seen in the **medulla** of the thymus.

(**self-molecules**), they are eliminated by apoptosis and cleared by macrophages.

So, where are the testing foreign and self-peptides coming from?

Branching and interconnected thymic cortical epithelial cells in the **cortex** of the thymus synthesize and present **self** and **non-self peptides** to the previously selected T cells shown to be self-MHC-restricted and self-tolerant. Only those **T cells that can recognize foreign (non-self) peptides and self-MHC survive**.

After completing the positive selection tests in the cortex of the thymus, T cells need to fullfil an additional requirement in the medulla of the thymus.

The **medulla** of the thymus houses **thymic medullary epithelial cells** that produce **cytokines** involved in optimizing the **negative selection of potentially autoreactive T cells**.

When T cells complete their development in the thymus, they enter the bloodstream and migrate to the peripheral lymphoid organs in search of an antigen on the surface of an **antigen-presenting cell**. We come back to additional details of the T cell maturation saga in our discussion of the thymus.

How do CD4+ helper T cells help?

CD4+ helper T cells are activated when they rec-

ognize the antigen peptide–class II MHC complex (Figure 10-8).

In the presence of cells with antigen peptide bound to class II MHC, CD4+ helper T cells proliferate by mitosis and secrete **cytokines**, also called **interleukins**. These chemical signals, in turn, attract B cells, which also have receptor molecules of single specificity on their surface (**immunoglobulin receptor**). Unlike helper T cells, B cells can recognize free antigen peptides without MHC molecules.

When activated by interleukins produced by the proliferating helper T cells, B cells also divide and differentiate into **plasma cells secreting immunoglobulins**. Secreted immunoglobulins diffuse freely, bind to antigen peptides to neutralize them, or trigger their destruction by enzymes or macrophages.

Plasma cells synthesize **only one class of immunoglobulin** (several thousand immunoglobulin molecules per second; lifetime of a plasma cell is from 10 to 20 days). Five classes of immunoglobulins are recognized in humans: **IgG, IgA, IgM, IgE,** and **IgD** (see Box 10-D). Abnormal plasma cells may accumulate in bones and bone marrow, causing bone destruction and affecting the production of normal blood cells. This pathologic condition is called **multiple myeloma** (see Box 10-E).

Some T and B cells become **memory cells**, ready to eliminate the same antigen if it recurs in the future. The **secondary immune response** (re-encounter with the same antigen that triggered their production) is more rapid and of greater magnitude. Memory cells recirculate for many years and provide a surveillance system directed against foreign antigens.

T cell subsets: T$_H$1 and T$_H$2 cells and cytolytic or cytotoxic T cells

We have seen that B cells can differentiate into immunoglobulin-secreting plasma cells under the influence of cytokines produced by CD4+ helper T cells.

B cells can present antigens, thus allowing direct interaction with T cells, which produce and secrete cytokines for plasma cell development. Plasma cells are **effector cells**; they use antibodies to neutralize extracellular pathogens. In contrast, T cells are primary effector cells for controlling or killing intracellular pathogens.

There are T cell subsets: T$_H$1 and T$_H$2 **cells**, derived from CD4+ T cells in the presence of specific cytokines, and **CD8+ cytolytic T cells**.

1. T$_H$1 cells participate in delayed-type hypersensitivity reactions (discussed later in this chapter) and the regulation of immune responses caused by **intracellular pathogens** (viruses, certain bacteria, or single-cell parasites) with the significant participation of macrophages. Interferon-γ, produced by T$_H$1 cells, stimulates the differentiation of T$_H$1 cells but suppresses the proliferation of T$_H$2 cells.

Figure 10-8. Helper T cells

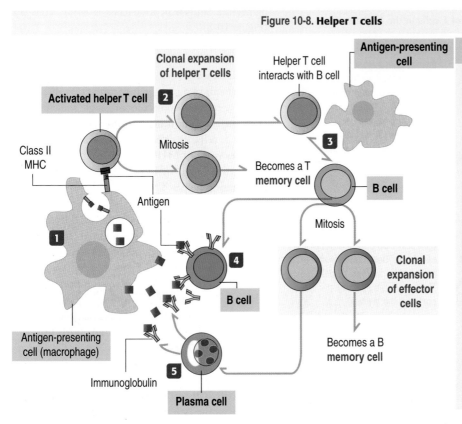

Activated helper T cell

Class II MHC

Antigen

Antigen-presenting cell (macrophage)

Immunoglobulin

Plasma cell

Clonal expansion of helper T cells

Mitosis

2

1

5

4

B cell

Helper T cell interacts with B cell

Becomes a T memory cell

Mitosis

3

Antigen-presenting cell

B cell

Clonal expansion of effector cells

Becomes a B memory cell

How CD4+ helper T cells help

1 A macrophage, acting as an antigen-presenting cell, processes a phagocytosed antigen that is then bound to class II MHC and presented to a helper T cell (cell-mediated immunity).

2 An activated helper T cell divides by mitosis to increase the population of helper T cells at the site of antigen presentation.

3 Helper T cells interact with B cells in the presence of an antigen-presenting cell to induce (1) immediate access of B cells to free antigen in the extracellular space and (2) proliferation of B cells.

4 B cells with cell surface-specific immunoglobulin arrive at the site to rapidly neutralize free antigen.

5 B cells differentiate into plasma cells that secrete immunoglobulin to block free antigen (humoral immunity).

---

2. TH2 cells are involved in immune responses observed in patients with **helminthic** (Greek *helmins*, worm) **intestinal parasites**. TH2 cells produce interleukin-4 (IL-4) and interleukin-13 (IL-13), among other cytokines, and determine the production of immunoglobulin E by plasma cells to activate the responses of mast cells, basophils, and eosinophils.

TH2-derived IL-4 and IL-10 suppress the activation of TH1 cells. As you can see, each subset produces cytokines that inhibit development of the other subset.

The activation of macrophage responses is minimal in TH2-driven immune responses.

3. **Cytolytic or cytotoxic T cells** display **TCR** and **CD8 coreceptor**. CD8+ cytolytic T cells recognize **class I MHC** on antigen-presenting cells.

They are involved in antigen-specific, MHC-restricted cytotoxicity and in the killing of intracellular pathogens that are not accessible to secreted antibodies. Cell killing is caused by the release of **perforin** or **Fas ligand** as already discussed

We return to the clinical significance of helper and cytolytic T cells when we discuss their involvement in the pathology of human immunodeficiency virus-type 1 (HIV-1) infection, allergy, and cancer immunotherapy.

How do CD8+ cytolytic T cells kill?

Another function of CD4+ helper T cells is **to secrete cytokines to stimulate the proliferation of** CD8+ **cytolytic T cells** that recognize the antigen peptide–class I MHC complex on the surface of antigen-presenting cells.

CD8+ cytolytic T cells initiates a **target cell destruction** process (Figure 10-9) by:

Box 10-D | Immunoglobulins

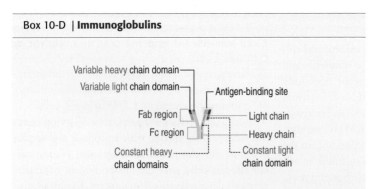

Variable heavy chain domain

Variable light chain domain

Antigen-binding site

Fab region

Light chain

Fc region

Heavy chain

Constant heavy chain domains

Constant light chain domain

• An immunoglobulin (**Ig**) molecule or antibody is composed of four polypeptide chains: two identical light chains and two identical heavy chains. One light chain is attached to one heavy chain by a disulfide bond. The two heavy chains are attached to each other by disulfide bonds.

• Heavy and light chains consists of amino terminal variable regions that participate in antigen recognition (Fab region) and carboxyl terminal constant regions. The constant region (Fc region) of the heavy chains mediate effector functions.

• Immunoglobulins can be membrane-bound or secreted.

• Types of immunogloblins: IgA forms dimers linked by a J chain and participate in mucosal immunity. IgD is a receptor for antigens of inmature B cells. IgE participates in mast cell and basophil activation (degranulation). IgG is the most abundant immunogloblin and the only one to cross the placental barrier. It participates in opsonization, a mechanism that enhances phagocytosis of pathogens. IgM molecules normally exist as pentamers.

Figure 10-9. Cytolytic T cells

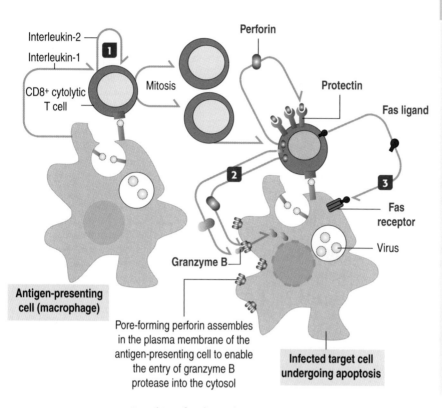

Interleukin-2

Interleukin-1

CD8+ cytolytic T cell

Mitosis

Perforin

Protectin

Fas ligand

Fas receptor

Virus

Granzyme B

Antigen-presenting cell (macrophage)

Pore-forming perforin assembles in the plasma membrane of the antigen-presenting cell to enable the entry of granzyme B protease into the cytosol

Infected target cell undergoing apoptosis

How CD8+ cytolytic T cells kill

1 A CD8+ cytolytic T cell binds to an antigen-presenting cell and is activated by interleukin-1 produced by the antigen-presenting cell (paracrine mechanism), and by interleukin-2, produced by the cytolytic T cell (autocrine mechanism). The cytolytic T cell divides by mitosis to increase the cell population.

2 In the presence of an antigen-presenting cell containing a pathogen antigen (a virus), cytolytic T cells release **protein pore-forming perforin** to kill the infected target cell. The CD8+ cytolytic T cell protects itself with **protectin**, a cell surface molecule that binds perforin. However, the infected antigen-presenting cell lacks protectin and is vulnerable to the action of perforin. Perforin facilitates the delivery of **pro-apoptotic granzyme B proteases** to the target cell.

3 **Fas ligand**, released by the cytolytic T cell and bound to the Fas receptor, together with granzyme destroy by **apoptosis** the target cell.

1. Attaching firmly to the antigen-presenting cell with the help of integrins and cell adhesion molecules (CAMs) on the cell surface of the target cell.

2. Inducing cell membrane damage by the release of pore-forming proteins (called **perforins**).

These pores facilitate the unregulated entry of the pro-apoptotic protease **granzyme**, water, and salts. The cytolytic T cell protects itself by a membrane protein, **protectin**, that inactivates perforin, blocking its insertion into the cytolytic T cell membrane.

CD8+ cytolytic T cells can also destroy target cells by the **Fas-Fas ligand mechanism** seen during **apoptosis** (see Chapter 3, Cell Signaling). When the cytolytic T cell receptor recognizes an antigen on the surface of a target cell, Fas ligand is produced in the cytolytic T cell. The interaction of Fas ligand with the trimerized Fas receptor on the target cell surface (see Figure 10-9) triggers the apoptotic cascade by activation of procaspases into caspases that determine cell death.

Natural killer cells

Natural killer cells destroy virus-infected cells and tumor cells, but this activity **does not depend on antigen activation**. Natural killer cells do not belong to the T or B cell types (they do not express TCR).

Human natural killer cells have **CD56 receptors** as well as **inhibitory** and **activating receptors** interacting respectively with class I MHC and activating ligand of normal cells. Target cells lacking class I MHC activate the destructive function of natural killer cells. The mechanism by which natural killer cells destroy target cells is described in Figure 10-10.

Clinical significance: Acquired immunodeficiency syndrome

The **acquired immunodeficiency syndrome (AIDS)** is caused by HIV-1 and is characterized by significant immunosuppression associated with opportunistic

---

Box 10-E | Multiple myeloma

• Multiple myeloma is caused by the abnormal growth of plasma cells in **bone marrow** and **bone**. An excessive grow of malignant plasma cells in bone and marrow causes bone fractures and prevents the production of normal blood cells in the marrow. Anemia, abnormal bleeding and high risk of infections may develop. Compression of the spinal cord by myeloma cells growing in vertebra can cause back pain, numbness, or paralysis.

• Myeloma cells produce an excessive amount of an abnormal immunoglobulin, called **Bence Jones protein**, present in serum and urine. Renal failure may occur because of the accumulation of immunoglobulins in the kidneys.

• Bone marrow transplantation (**autologous**, from the same patient, or **allogenic**, from a healthy and compatible donor) is a form of treatment in patients resistant or nonresponsive to chemotherapy. First, the bone marrow of the recipient is depleted with very high doses of chemotherapy and low doses of radiation therapy, and then followed by the administration of donor's marrow cells into the blood of the patient. Hematopoietic stem cells will then localize in bone marrow and repopulate it.

Figure 10-10. Natural killer cells

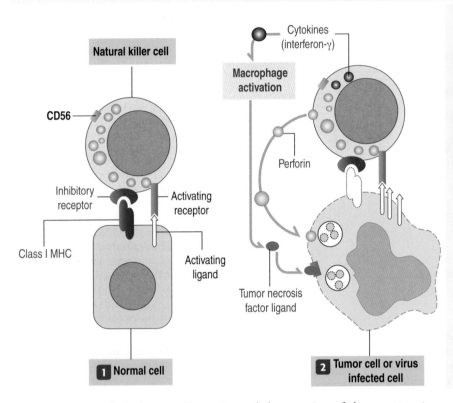

Natural killer (NK) cells comprise about 10% of lymphocytes in the blood and peripheral lymphoid organs. NK cells express CD56, inhibitory and activating surface receptors and abundant cytoplasmic granules containing perforin.

1 When NK cells interact with normal cells expressing class I MHC and activating ligand, the inhibitory receptors of NK cells bind to class I MHC molecules and the activating receptors bind to the activating ligands. No cell killing occurs.

2 NK cells are activated when the inhibitory receptor fails to be neutralized by class I MHC not expressed by tumor cells or virus infected cells. In addition, an excess of activating ligand in the target cell enhances the function of the activating receptor in NK cells. Activated NK cells respond by releasing perforin toward the target cell and secreting cytokines to activate macrophages to become more effective in killing target cells through tumor necrosis factor ligand.

infections, malignancies, and degeneration of the central nervous system.

HIV infects macrophages, dendritic cells, and predominantly CD4-bearing helper T cells. HIV is a member of the lentivirus family of animal retroviruses and causes long-term latent cellular infection.

HIV includes two types, designated HIV-1 and HIV-2. HIV-1 is the cause of AIDS. The genome of the infectious HIV consists of two strands of RNA enclosed within a core of viral proteins and surrounded by a lipid envelope derived from the infected cell. HIV particles are present in blood, semen, and other body fluids. Transmission is by sexual contact or needle injection.

The viral lipid envelope contains glycoproteins designated **gp41** and **gp120**, encoded by the *env* viral sequence.

After binding to the CD4 protein of the host cell,

gp120 changes its conformation and binds to the **chemokine host-cell receptor** (CCR5 or CXCR4). The glycoprotein gp41 mediates HIV-cell fusion to permit viral entry.

Figure 10-11 presents a summary of the cellular events associated with HIV infection. Box 10-F summarizes the steps of the HIV reproductive cycle.

Antiretroviral therapy (**ART**) based on the reproductive cycle of the virus, reduces and almost completely blocks HIV-1 transmission to uninfected individuals. For example, the fusion inhibitor, enfuvirtive, blocks fusion between gp41 and CD4. The CCR5 coreceptor antagonist, maraviroc, prevents gp120-mediated viral binding to CCR5.

A relevant event of HIV infection is the destruction of CD4$^+$ helper T cells responsible for the initiation of immune responses, leading to the elimination of HIV infection. **CD8$^+$ cytolytic T cells** (that attach to virus-infected cells) and **B cells** (that give rise to antibody-producing plasma cells) represent an acquired or adaptive response to HIV infection. Antibodies to HIV antigens are detected within 6 to 9 weeks after infection.

General Pathology: Hypersensitivity reactions

Hypersensitivity is a distinct immune response resulting in harmful host reactions rather protection against a pathogen. There are four types of hypersensitivity reactions:

1. **Type 1 hypersensitivity**, involving IgE and

Box 10-F | **HIV reproductive cycle**

• The life cycle of a retrovirus begins when the virus binds and enters a cell and introduces its genetic material (RNA) and proteins into the cytoplasm.
• The genome of a typical retrovirus includes three coding regions: **gag, pol,** and **env**, specifying, respectively, proteins of the viral core, the enzyme **reverse transcriptase**, and constituents of the viral coat.
• In the cytoplasm, reverse transcriptase converts viral RNA into DNA which is then inserted into cellular DNA. This process is called **integration.**
• The provirus DNA directs the synthesis of viral proteins and RNA.
• Viral proteins and RNA assemble and new viral particles bud off from the cell.

Figure 10-11. **Immune system and HIV infection**

HIV reproductive cycle

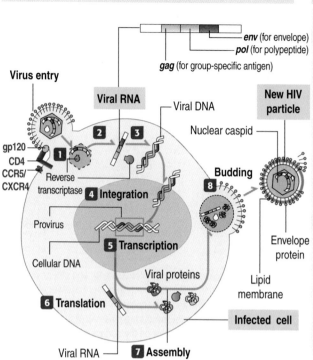

- **env** (for envelope)
- **pol** (for polypeptide)
- **gag** (for group-specific antigen)

Virus entry

Viral RNA

Viral DNA

New HIV particle

Nuclear caspid

gp120
CD4
CCR5/
CXCR4

Reverse transcriptase

Budding

4 Integration

Provirus

5 Transcription

Cellular DNA

Viral proteins

Envelope protein

Lipid membrane

6 Translation

Infected cell

Viral RNA

7 Assembly

Acquired immunodeficiency syndrome (AIDS)

The human immunodeficiency virus type 1 (HIV-1) can infect and destroy immune cells.

CD4, the coreceptor of helper T cells, is a receptor for the HIV-1 envelope protein **glycoprotein 120 (gp120)** that, after a conformation change, binds to chemokine host-cell coreceptor **CCR5** or **CXCR4**. CD4 is also expressed on the surface of macrophages, they can also be infected by this virus.

The virus can replicate within host cells for many years before symptoms are detected (clinical latency) (see Box 10-F for an explanation of steps of the HIV reproductive cycle). The early indication of HIV-1 infection is the presence of antibodies to **gp120**, a viral envelope protein, and against **p24**, a core protein.

During the early phase of HIV-1 infection, infected helper T cells are destroyed and replenished. When the rate of destruction exceeds the replenishing capacity of CD4 cells, cell-mediated immunity is compromised and the patient is susceptible to fatal opportunistic infections. The CD4 helper T cell count is the best indicator of the time-course progression of AIDS.

CD4 helper T cells are destroyed either by a cytotoxic effect determined by HIV-1 infection or by the direct action of cytolytic T cells.

Blood banks screen blood donation for antibodies to gp120. However, the level of antibody may be low, particularly during the early phase of infection. **Antiretroviral therapy (ART)**, based on the biological features of the virus, almost reduces or completely blocks HIV-1 transmission.

Responses of the immune system to HIV infection

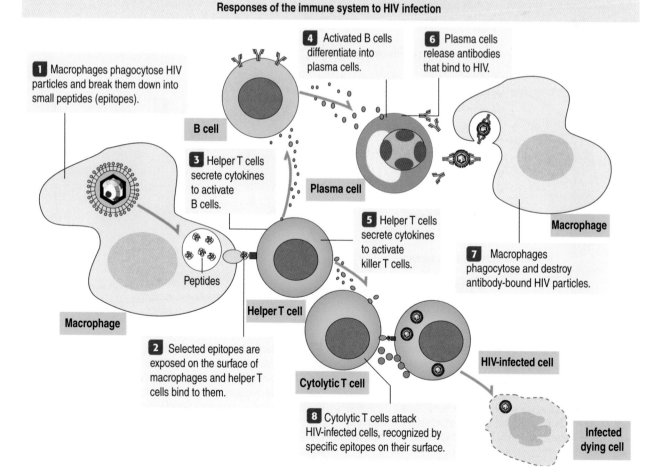

1 Macrophages phagocytose HIV particles and break them down into small peptides (epitopes).

4 Activated B cells differentiate into plasma cells.

6 Plasma cells release antibodies that bind to HIV.

B cell

3 Helper T cells secrete cytokines to activate B cells.

Plasma cell

Macrophage

5 Helper T cells secrete cytokines to activate killer T cells.

7 Macrophages phagocytose and destroy antibody-bound HIV particles.

Peptides

Macrophage

Helper T cell

2 Selected epitopes are exposed on the surface of macrophages and helper T cells bind to them.

Cytolytic T cell

HIV-infected cell

Infected dying cell

8 Cytolytic T cells attack HIV-infected cells, recognized by specific epitopes on their surface.

Figure 10-12. **Type 1 hypersensitivity reactions. Allergy**

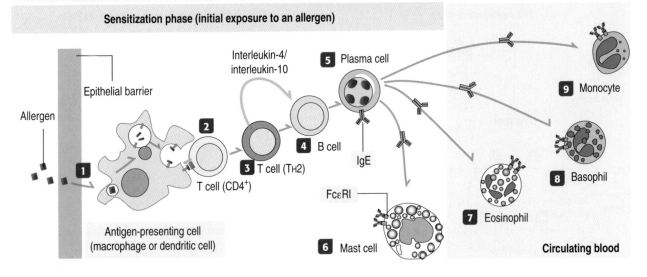

Sensitization phase (initial exposure to an allergen)

Allergens trigger allergy, an immune response in which immunoglobulin E (IgE) antibodies play a significant role.

1 This response develops when an allergen breaks a protective barrier (such as an epithelial layer).

2 The antigen is presented by an antigen-presenting cell to a helper T cell.

3 Depending on the nature of the allergen, one helper T cell subtype (either TH1 or TH2) is recruited to drive the production of IgE. Intestinal helminthic parasites involve the actions of TH2 cells.

4 TH2 cells produce interleukin-4, interleukin-10, and other cytokines to induce the proliferation of B cells and development of other effector cells (mast cells, basophils, and eosinophils).

5 B cells differentiate into IgE-producing plasma cells.

6 IgE binds to the FcεRI receptor on the surface of mast cells (an immigrant cell to the connective tissue).

7 8 9 Eosinophils, basophils, and monocytes (circulating in blood) also express FcεRI receptors and bind IgE.

TH1 cells (not shown) produce interferon-γ in response to viral infection.

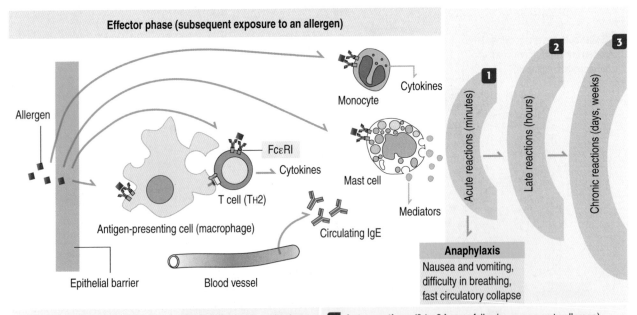

Effector phase (subsequent exposure to an allergen)

Anaphylaxis
Nausea and vomiting, difficulty in breathing, fast circulatory collapse

A subsequent exposure to the same allergen following sensitization finds antigen-presenting cells, TH2 cells, and monocytes with FcεRI receptors on their surfaces. IgE can bind without delay to FcεRI receptors that aggregate and trigger cell signaling responses. Receptor aggregation induces three types of reactions:

1 **Acute reaction** (anaphylaxis, acute asthmatic response) within **seconds to minutes**, triggered by mediators released by mast cells and basophils.

2 **Late reactions** (**2 to 6 hours** following exposure to allergen) attract circulating eosinophils, basophils, and TH2 cells to the site.

3 **Chronic reactions** can develop over **days and weeks** and determine alterations in the structure and function of the affected tissue (for example, respiratory pathology in asthma) caused by a number of cytokines, mediators, and inflammatory agents. Corticosteroids are required to suppress inflammation determined by chronic reactions.

allergens leading to the degranulation of mast cells or basophils (see Chapter 4, Connective Tissue). **Allergy** refers to immune responses characterized by the participation of **IgE** bound to a special receptor, designated **FcεRI**. When an antigen or **allergen** binds to two adjacent IgE molecules, it induces aggregation of the IgE molecules and associated FcεRI receptors. This event results in a signaling cascade that leads to the release of mediators and cytokines (Figure 10-12).

Note that there are two phases:

1. **Sensitization phase**, following an initial exposure to an allergen.

2. **Effector phase**, after a suibsequent exposure to an allergen. Also note that two subsets of helper T cell, T_H1 and T_H2, can trigger distinct responses when activated by specific antigens.

2. **Type 2 hypersensitivity** reactions are caused by antibodies directed against plasma membrane-bound antigens resulting in cytolysis. Type 2 hypersensitivity may involve the complement system (see below). Examples are **autoimmune hemolytic anemia** and Rh incompatibility leading to **erythroblastosis fetalis** (see Chapter 6, Blood and Hematopoiesis).

3. **Type 3 hypersensitivity** is determined by the formation of soluble antigen-antibody complexes that activate the complement system. An example is the **Arthus reaction** in response to intradermal injection of antigen (significant neutrophil infiltrate, erythema [redness of the skin] and edema). Type 3 hypersensitivity, and the resulting inflammatory injury caused by antigen-antibody complex deposition on synovial membranes, are seen in rheumatoid arthritis (see Chapter 5, Osteogenesis), infectious arthritis and systemic lupus erythematosus.

4. **Type 4 hypersensitivity**, also called **delayed hypersensitivity**, involves antigen–T cell–macrophage interactions determining the formation of a **granuloma**. **Tuberculosis, leprosy, sarcoidosis** and **contact dermatitis** are clinical examples.

The **Mantoux reaction** in the tuberculin skin test is a classic delayed hypersensitivity reaction. The injection of purified protein derivative from *Mycobacteria tuberculosis* into the skin of an individual sensitized to tuberculosis (by exposure or infection) result in the activation of sensitized CD4⁺ helper cells that secrete cytokines recruiting and activating macrophages. This local reaction is manifested by erythema and edema in the injected skin site within 48 hours.

A chronic granuloma represents an amplified tissue reaction that develops in response to a sustained immune response to released antigens rather than to the triggering pathogen itself. Helper T cells or cytotoxic T cells, macrophages and multinucleated giant cells are the hallmark of chronic granulomas.

We come back to Type 4 hypersensitivity and chronic granuloma when we address the process of chronic inflammation.

General Pathology: Complement system

The main function of the complement system is to enable the **direct destruction of pathogens or target cells by phagocytes** (macrophages and neutrophils) by a mechanism known as **opsonization** (Greek *opsonein*, to buy provisions) **by producing proteolytic enzyme complexes** (Figure 10-13).

Complement provides a rapid and efficient mechanism for eliminating pathogens to prevent tissue injury or chronic infection. Host tissues have cell surface–anchored regulatory proteins, which can inhibit complement activation and prevent unintended damage.

The complement system consists of about 20 plasma proteins, synthesized mainly in the liver, that complement, or enhance, a tissue response to pathogens. Several components of this system are **proenzymes** converted to active enzymes.

Activation of the complement cascade can be triggered by:

1. Antibodies bound to a pathogen (**classic pathway**).

2. Binding of mannose-binding lectin to a bacterial carbohydrate moiety (**lectin pathway**).

3. By spontaneous activation of C3, a proenzyme (inactive precursor) of the complement sequence (**alternative pathway**).

The critical molecule of the complement cascade is **C1**, a hexamer, called **C1q**, with binding affinity to the **Fc region** of an immunoglobulin. C1q is also associated with two molecules, **C1r** and **C1s**.

When the globular domains of C1q bind to the Fc regions of immunoglobulins already bound to the surface of a pathogen, C1r is activated and converts C1s into a serine protease. **Activation of C1s marks the first step of the complement activation cascade.**

The **second step** is the cleavage of complement protein C4 by C1s. Two fragments are produced:

1. The small fragment C4a is discarded.

2. The large fragment C4b binds to the pathogen surface.

The **third step** occurs when complement protein C2 is cleaved by C1s into C2a (discarded) and C2b. C2b binds to the already bound C4b, forming the **complex C4b-2b**, also called **C3 convertase**, on the surface of a pathogen.

The **fourth step** takes place when complement protein **C3** is cleaved by C3 convertase into C3a (discarded) and C3b. C3b binds to C3 convertase. The **C4b-2b-3b complex**, now designated **C5 convertase**, cleaves complement protein C5 into C5a (discarded) and C5b. C5b binds to C5 convertase.

The **last steps** consist in the binding of the opsonized pathogen to complement receptors on the surface of the phagocyte. Additional complement proteins are C6, C7, C8, and C9. C9 binds to the protein complex and forms the **membrane attack**

Figure 10-13. **Complement system**

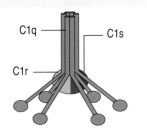

C1q — C1s
C1r

C1 is the first component of the complement activation pathway.
C1 consists of three components:
1. **C1q**, a molecule with six rod domains, each ending as a globular head.
2. **C1r**, a proenzyme.
3. **C1s**, a substrate for C1r, converted into a protease upon activation of C1r.

C3a and **C5a** are **proinflammatory fragments**, which recruit leukocytes to sites of infection and activate them.

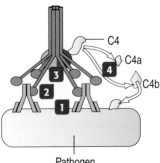

C4
C4a
C4b
3
2
1
4

Pathogen
Classic pathway

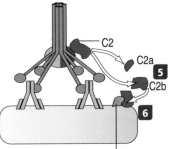

C2
C2a
C2b
5
6

C4b-2b complex
or C3 convertase

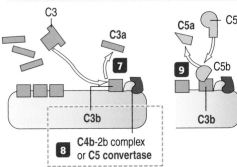

C3
C3a
7
C3b

8 C4b-2b complex or **C5 convertase**

C5a — C5
9
C5b
C3b

1 Immunoglobulins (Igs) bind to the surface of a pathogen (for example, a bacterium).

2 The globular domain of C1q binds to the Fc region of the Ig (one globular domain per Ig).

3 C1q binding activates C1r, which in turn activates C1s. This conversion generates a serine protease that initiates the complement cascade.

4 Protease C1s cleaves complement protein C4 into two fragments: C4a and C4b. C4b binds to the surface of the pathogen.

The complement system is activated immediately in the presence of a pathogen. It provides a rapid and efficient way for eliminating pathogens and triggering inflammation.
  Membrane **complement regulatory proteins (CRegs)** are important modulators of tissue injury in many autoimmune and inflammatory diseases. CRegs protect bystander cells from unintended harm.

5 C1s cleaves complement protein C2 into two fragments: C2a and C2b.

6 C2b binds to the already bound **C4b** forming the C4b-2b complex, or **C3 convertase**.

Opsonic fragments **C3b** and **C4b** label the target pathogen for elimination by phagocytes.

10 The complement cascade, resulting in the **opsonization of the pathogen**, enables phagocytic cells (macrophages and neutrophils) to take up and destroy pathogens.

11 Complement components bind to **complement receptors** on the surface of phagocytes and are taken up.
  Complement proteins C6, C7, C8, and C9 (not shown) participate in the lysis of certain pathogens by forming a lytic pore called the **membrane attack complex (MAC)**.

7 C3 convertase cleaves complement protein C3 into two fragments: **C3a** and **C3b**. One C3 convertase can cleave about 1,000 C3 molecules into C3b.

8 Several C3b molecules bind to C3 convertase (forming the **C4b-2b-3b** complex or **C5 convertase**) or to the surface of the pathogen. C3b is the major **opsonin** of the complement system.

9 Protein C5 binds to the C3b component of C5 convertase and is cleaved into **C5a** and **C5b**. Opsonization of the pathogen is complete.

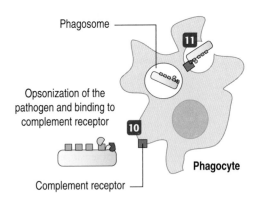

Phagosome
11

Opsonization of the pathogen and binding to complement receptor
10

Complement receptor

Phagocyte

CRegs are membrane proteins. CRegs include **CD55**, **CD46**, and **CD59**. They act by preventing the activity of convertases and enabling inactivating proteases to block completion of the assembly of the cell lytic MAC.

complex (**MAC**), a cytolytic pore that directly initiates the cell destruction process.
  The complement system has the following specific characteristics important to remember:

1. Complement fragments C3a and C5a, produced by the enzymatic cascade, have **proinflammatory** activity.
2. Complement fragments C3a and C5a recruit

leukocytes to the infection site, which become activated and activate other cells.

3. Other fragments (C3b and C4b), mark targets for destruction by phagocytes.

4. Destruction of a pathogen is mediated by the final assembly of the **MAC**, a **transmembrane cytolytic pore**.

5. **Complement regulators (CRegs**; for example, **CD55, CD46, and CD59**) regulate the production of complement fragments, accelerate the decay of the already produced fragments, and block the final cytolytic action of the MAC by preventing its assembly. **CRegs are cell surface–anchored proteins that protect host cells from unintended damage by the activated complement cascade. CD59 blocks the destructive action of the MAC by preventing the binding of C9 to C8. CD59** also modulates the activity of T cells.

6. **Paroxysmal nocturnal hemoglobinuria (PNH)** determines episodes of hemolysis represented by dark urine and anemia, stomach and back pain, and formation of blood clots. **Red blood cells lack CD59** and are susceptible to destruction by the complement system. Therapeutic means to prevent or arrest the complement cascade are being developed to treat patients with PNH.

General Pathology: Inflammation

Invading pathogens (bacteria, virus, parasites and foreign objects) can cause localized tissue damage leading to an inflammatory response.

Acute inflammation is the initial non-specific reaction to tissue damage. If the damage persists and the destruction of the tissue (necrosis) continues, an **immune response** develops with the characteristics of **chronic inflammation.**

When a pathogen is neutralized and removed, the damaged area can be cleared and replaced by tissue with similar structure and function, a process called **restoration** or **regeneration,** If the damaged area is severe and extensive or the damaged tissue cannot regenerate, the affected area is replaced by **scar tissue** by a process called **fibrous repair.** When a pathogen persists and an infection process occurs, tissue destruction continues and concurrent immune responses and fibrous repair take place by the process of chronic inflammation.

Acute inflammation

Two events define the pathogenesis of acute inflammation:

1. **Responses of the microvasculature to injury.** Vasodilation allows increased blood flow into the damaged tissue (a condition called **hyperemia**). Mast cells, basophils and platelets release **histamine.** Endothelial cells release **nitric oxide** to relax the smooth muscle cells of the blood vessel wall to increase blood flow.

Enhanced vascular permeability of capillaries and venules results in the accumulation of fluid, or **exudate**, in the interstitial space, leading to tissue swelling. An exudate is interstitial fluid with high protein content, in particular fibrin. A **transudate** is interstitial fluid with low protein content. An **effusion** is excess of fluid in body cavities (peritoneum, pleura and pericardium).

Fibrin derives from **fibrinogen**. Fibrinogen is cleaved by **thrombin** into **fibrinopeptides** and **fibrin monomers** that are then assembled to form a **fibrin meshwork**. Fibrin provides a framework for the migration of neutrophils and also induces the expression of **chemokines**, members of the family of cytokines that induces **chemotaxis** in adjacent cells (see Chapter 3, Cell Signaling). Chemotaxis is the mechanism that directs the displacement of cells when specific signaling molecules are present in their surrounding environment.

These microvasculature events are represented by the four classical clinical signs of inflammation formulated by Celsus in First Century AD: *rubor* (redness), *tumor* (swelling), *calor* (heat) and *dolor* (pain). Hyperemia is responsible for the first three signs. Pain is determined by released specific local mediators and fluid compression of nerve endings.

2. **Recruitment of neutrophils to the injury site** (Figure 10-14)). Chemotactic factors produced by resident macrophages recruit **neutrophils** from circulating blood into the injured tissue.

As described in Chapter 1, Epithelium and Chapter 6, Blood and Hematopoiesis, neutrophils migrate to the injury site by the process of **homing.** Homing consists in the recruitment of leukocytes (in particular neutrophils, lymphocytes and monocytes) from peripheral blood to specific sites.

Homing is initiated by changes on the endothelial surface triggered by inflammatory mediators, including cytokines (**tumor necrosis factor ligand** and **IL-1**) produced by **resident macrophages** and **leukotrienes**, released by **mast cells.**

Recall that homing is essentially a recruitment cascade involving tethering, rolling, adhesion, crawling and transmigration of leukocytes. Tethering, rolling and adhesion to endothelial cell surfaces involve **selectins** bound to selectin ligand glycoconjugates on the surface of leukocytes. As leukocytes are rolling, they are activated by their contact with chemokines bound to the endothelial surface.

The selectin phase is followed by the crawling and transendothelial migration of leukocytes toward the extravascular space. **Integrins** (LFA1 [lymphocyte function–associated antigen 1] and **MAC1** [macrophage antigen 1]), expressed by neutrophils, bind

Figure 10-14. Function of neutrophils in acute inflammation

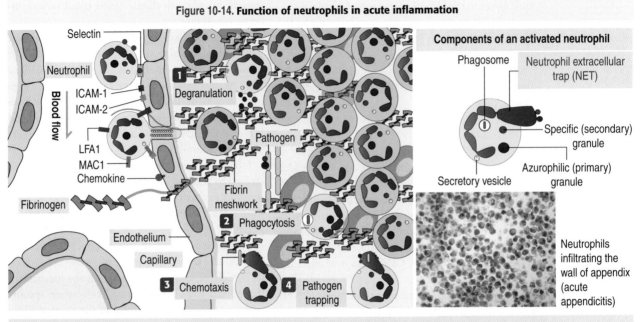

Components of an activated neutrophil

Phagosome — Neutrophil extracellular trap (NET)

Specific (secondary) granule

Azurophilic (primary) granule

Secretory vesicle

Neutrophils infiltrating the wall of appendix (acute appendicitis)

Neutrophil recruitment and function in acute inflammation

Hyperemia: Recruitment of neutrophils to an injured site starts with an increase in blood flow (hyperemia) and vascular leakage initiated by the release of **histamine** from **mast cells**, **basophils**, and **platelets**. A vasodilation effect is triggered by **nitric oxide** produced by endothelial cells causing smooth muscle cells of the blood vessel wall to relax. **Fibrinogen** is cleaved by **thrombin** into **fibrin monomers** that are assembled into a **fibrin meshwork** at the acute inflammation site.

Neutrophil extravasation: This process involves **tethering**, **rolling**, **adhesion**, **crawling**, and **transmigration** on an endothelial surface conditioned by pro-inflammatory mediators. Changes on the surface of the endothelium are stimulated by histamine, leukotrienes and pro-inflammatory cytokines (tumor necrosis factor ligand and interleukin-1) released by **resident macrophages** and **mast cells** when pathogens emerge. **Chemokines** on the endothelium stabilize the attachment of pro-inflammatory cytokines.

Selectins are rapidly synthesized by endothelial cells and bind to glycosylated ligands on the recruiting neutrophil to initiate tethering (capture) and rolling. Adhesion starts with the expression of the **integrin LAF1** (lymphocyte function-associated antigen 1) and **MAC1** (macrophage antigen 1) by neutrophils and intercellular cell

adhesion molecules **ICAM1** and **ICAM2** by endothelial cells. At the endothelial arrest site, neutrophils extend pseudopods containing a reorganized actin cytoskeleton. Finally, neutrophils cross the endothelium (predominantly between endothelial cells but also through an endothelial cell) and the basement membrane within 7 to 20 minutes, guided by a chemokine gradient.

The following neutrophil events occur in the acute inflammation site:

1 Degranulation: release of protease-like proteins and enzymes present in azurophilic (primary) granules and specific (secondary) granules.

2 Phagocytosis: pathogens are taken up into phagosomes.

3 Chemotaxis: in the presence of chemokines, neutrophils approach pathogens for phagocytosis.

4 Pathogen trapping: neutrophils expose to the extracellular space intracellular structures known as **neutrophil extracellular traps (NETs)**. A NET consists of a DNA-histone complex and associated antimicrobial proteins (including myeloperoxidase, lactoferrin, cathepsin, defensins and bacterial permeability proteins) involved in trapping and immobilization of pathogens, possibly killing.

---

to endothelial cell surface molecules ICAM 1 and ICAM2 (intercellular cell adhesion molecule 1 and 2).

As you recall from Chapter 6, Blood and Hematopoiesis, neutrophils have cytoplasmic **azurophilic (primary) granules** containing myeloperoxidase and defensins, and **specific (secondary) granules** harboring lactoferrin and gelatinase.

Gelatinase degrades extracellular matrix components to allow the migration of neutrophil. Neutrophils also contain **secretory vesicles**, that upon activation, release their contents to the cell surface for cell adhesion to integrins.

Neutrophils can eliminate pathogens by several mechanisms:

1. **Phagocytosis**, involving antibacterial proteins released from cytoplasmic granules into phagosomes.

2. Release of **neutrophil extracellular traps (NETs)**, to trap pathogens to prevent spreading and facilitate subsequent phagocytosis.

A NET consists of a core of DNA-histones and attached enzymes released from azurophilic and specific granules (see Figure 10-14).

3. **Degranulation**, to kill pathogens directly. Protease-like proteins and enzymes responsible for the production of reactive oxygen species, contained in cytoplasmic granules, have the capacity of direct killing or incapacitate microorganisms.

Resolution of acute inflammation: fibrous repair

The resolution of acute inflammation pursues two objectives:

1. The protection of the host from excessive tissue damage.

2. To prevent amplification of acute inflammatory responses towards chronic inflammation.

Resolution of acute inflammation encompasses an anti-inflammatory phase and a pro-resolving phase.

During the **anti-inflammatory phase**, anti-inflammatory mediators (such as IL-10), are released. In addition, the pro-inflammatory activity of the **nuclear factor (NF)-κB pathway** is down regulated. You may like to review details of the NF-κB pathway in Chapter 3, Cell Signaling, with particular reference to inflammatory signaling as an alternate pathway to necroptosis.

The recruitment of neutrophils to the inflammation site is slowed down by IL-1 and chemokine receptor antagonists as well as by the clearance of tumor necrosis factor ligand from the endothelial cell surface.

The **pro-resolving phase** involves a switch of the pro-inflammatory activities of neutrophils and macrophages to anti-inflammatory activities. Neutrophils produce **pro-resolving mediators**, including **protectins**; macrophages secrete **maresins** (from **ma**crophage mediator in **res**olving **in**flammation).

Pro-resolving inflammation mediators arrest neutrophil migration and recruit **monocytes**, the macrophage precursors, to assist in the phagocytosis of dead neutrophils and the removal of fibrin and necrotic cells of the inflammation site.

Healing and tissue repair are stimulated by combining the effects of the anti-inflammatory and pro-resolving phases.

Healing involves the formation of **granulation tissue**. The damaged tissue is replaced new capillaries (angiogenesis), macrophages and fibroblasts. Continued proliferation of fibroblasts, depositing type III collagen, and the acquisition of smooth muscle cells by blood vessels (venules and arterioles), result in the organization of **fibrovascular granulation tissue**. Type III collagen is replaced by bundles of type I collagen forming a **collagenous scar. Basically, the fibrin-containing exudate is being replaced first by granulation tissue and subsequently by a fibrous scar by a process called fibrous repair** (Figure 10-15).

In Chapter 5, Osteogenesis, you studied how a bone fracture is repaired. The fibrous repair process as described above will not provide strong bone repair.

Additional steps, including chondrogenesis and osteogenesis, are required to form mineralized bone, the **callus**, to connect the two ends of a broken bone. The callus is later reorganized to restore bone structure before the fracture.

Types of acute inflammation

Three types of acute inflammation, based on the type of exudate or effusion, are considered:

1. **Suppurative acute inflammation**, when neutrophils and debris of dead cells predominate and the affected tissue is liquefied by neutrophil-derived proteolytic enzymes to produce **pus**. Acute appendicitis and recurring otitis media in children are examples of suppurative acute inflammation.

Specific bacteria produce suppurative acute inflammation that can evolve into a **pustule** (at the

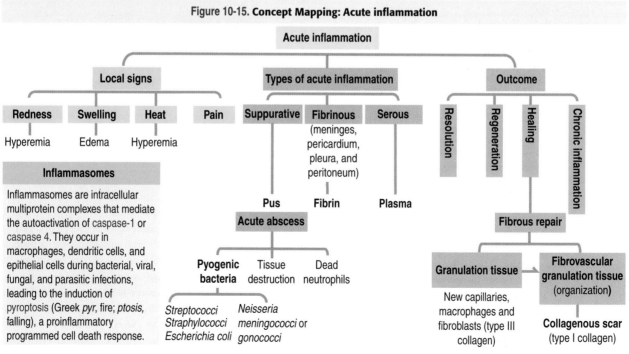

Figure 10-15. Concept Mapping: Acute inflammation

Figure 10-16. Concept Mapping: Acute and chronic inflammation compared

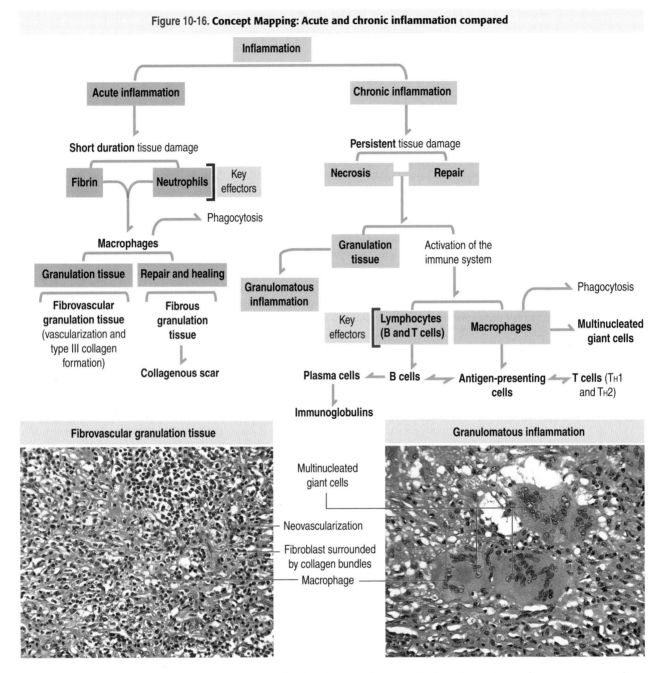

Fibrovascular granulation tissue

Granulomatous inflammation

Multinucleated
giant cells

Neovascularization

Fibroblast surrounded
by collagen bundles
Macrophage

skin surface) or an **abscess**, an enclosed collection of purulent tissue. Bacteria producing localized suppuration are called **pyogenic** (pus-producing).Some of them are listed in Figure 10-15.

2. **Fibrinous acute inflammation**, when **fibrin** is the predominate component of the fluid or **effusion** deposited on the surface of the meninges, peritoneum, pleura and pericardium. A fibrous repair process, converting the fibrinous effusion into scar tissue, causes the thickening of the affected surface and even the possible occlusion of a space (such the pericardial space).

3. **Serous acute inflammation**, when plasma-derived fluid has a **low protein content**. The **transudate** of a blister of the skin, caused by a burn, viral or toxic

agent (poison ivy, poison oak, or poison sumac), or **effusion** of fluid in pleural, peritoneal and pericardial cavities (caused by congestive heart failure or blocked blood or lymphatic vessels) are examples of serous acute inflammation.

Chronic inflammation

The persistence of tissue damage caused by a pathogen can determine chronic inflammation, a process in which tissue necrosis and repair are simultaneous and persistent for many years.

A **chronic peptic ulcer** is an example of chronic inflammation determined by the persistence of a pathogen (*Helicobacter pylori*), excessive production of gastric acid or the effect of nonsteroidal anti-

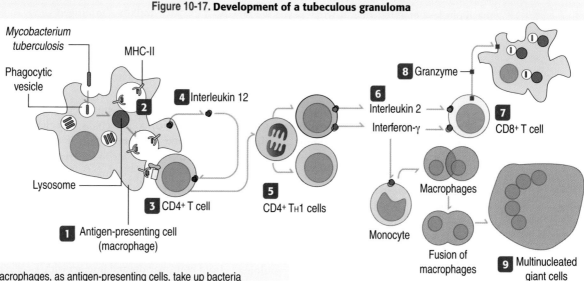

Figure 10-17. Development of a tuberculous granuloma

Mycobacterium tuberculosis

MHC-II

Phagocytic vesicle

4 Interleukin 12

2

Lysosome

3 CD4+ T cell

1 Antigen-presenting cell (macrophage)

5 CD4+ TH1 cells

8 Granzyme

6 Interleukin 2

Interferon-γ

7 CD8+ T cell

Macrophages

Monocyte

Fusion of macrophages

9 Multinucleated giant cells

1 Macrophages, as antigen-presenting cells, take up bacteria (*Micobacterium tuberculosis*) into a phagocytic vesicle.
2 After a self-preserving bacteria-induced delay of 2 to 3 days (that enables bacteria to replicate within the macrophage), lysosome fuses with the vesicle forming a phagosome. Fragments of the bacterium are attached to **MHC-II** (major histocompatibility complex type II) and exposed to the extracellular environment.
3 A **CD4+ T cell** binds to the exposed antigen.
4 The macrophage secretes **interleukin 12** that stimulates the proliferation of the CD4+ T cell **5**.
6 **CD4+ TH1 cells** are produced and secrete **interleukin 2** and **interferon-γ** to activate **CD8+ T cells** **7** to target granzyme protease to macrophages harboring bacteria **8**.
9 After several weeks, recruited **monocytes** are stimulated by **interferon-γ** and become **macrophages**. Macrophages fuse to form **multinucleated giant cells** (known as **Langhans' cells** in tuberculosis infection). These events define **type 4 hypersensitivity** or **delayed type hypersensitivity**.

Granuloma

Langhan's cell

Fibroblast zone

Lymphocyte zone

Macrophage zone with multinucleated giant cells (indicators of type 4 [delayed] hypersensitivity)

Caseous necrosis

Sarcoidosis granuloma in a lymph node. Caseous necrosis is not present. The predominant cells are macrophages and multinucleated giant cells. Few lymphocytes are observed inside the granuloma. A connective tissue boundary is seen in contact with lymphocytes of the lymph node (*).

Multinucleated giant cells

inflammatory drugs (see Chapter 15, Upper Digestive Segment).

Added to the characteristic cellular and tissue aspects of acute inflammation is the involvement in chronic inflammation of the **immune system** represented by **lymphocytes** and **macrophages**.

Macrophages have a dual function: they are phagocytic cells, clearing necrotic tissue and dead cells, and also antigen-presenting cells as part of their immunologic function. From a histopathologic perspective, chronic inflammation displays fibrous repair, represented by fibrous granulation tissue, overlapping with lymphocytes and macrophages (Figure 10-16). **Lymphocytes**, **macrophages** and

plasma cells are regarded the typical combination of **chronic inflammatory cells**.

We have seen that neutrophils are the main effector cells in acute inflammation. Macrophages, derived from monocytes in the presence of interferon-γ, have a prevalent function in chronic inflammation.

In certain diseases, the granuloma is the hallmark of chronic inflammation, a structural pattern that defines **granulomatous inflammation**. As part of **granulomas**, macrophages acquire an epithelial-like pattern and fuse to form **multinucleated giant cells**.

A granuloma (Figure 10-17) consists of a typical central necrotic zone surrounded by a la zone of activated epithelial-like macrophages coexisting with multinucleated giant cells. Surrounding the macrophage-containing zone are lymphocytes (CD4⁺ T cells) and then a limiting fibroblast-collagen zone establishing a capsule-like boundary with the surrounding tissue. The development of a tubeculous granuloma is shown in Figure 10-17.

What causes a granulomatous inflammation?

1. The pathogen can elicit a significant immune response (lymphocytes interacting with macrophages/antigen-presenting cell) but without significant pathogenic potential. Human diseases that fullfil this condition are **tuberculosis** (produced by *Mycobacterium tuberculosis*); leprosy (caused by *Mycobacterium leprae*); and syphilis (produced by *Treponema pallidum*).

The physical and biochemical characteristics of the central zone of a granuloma depends on the pathogen. For example, the **tuberculous granuloma** has a central **caseation** soft cheese-like mass zone surrounded by scattered multinucleated giant cells called **Langhans' cells**. The **sarcoidosis granuloma**, displays a fibrosis center and the multinucleated giant cells may contain calcified spherical deposits, called **Schaumann bodies**.

2. The nature of the pathogen, a non-biological foreign body, such as silicone in lungs, that is resistant to the action of enzymes released by neutrophils, or an unknown pathogen in the disease **sarcoidosis** (affecting lungs, lymph nodes [see Figure 10-17], spleen and liver).

Lymphoid organs

Lymphoid organs are the sites where immune responses occur. The major lymphoid organs are:

1. The **lymph nodes**.
2. The **thymus**.
2. The **spleen**.

Lymph nodes

The function of lymph nodes is to filter the lymph, maintain and differentiate B cells, and house T cells. Lymph nodes detect and react to lymph-borne antigens.

A lymph node is surrounded by a capsule, and the parenchyma is divided into a **cortex** and a **medulla** (Figure 10-18). The **capsule** consists of dense irregular connective tissue surrounded by adipose tissue. The capsule at the convex surface of the lymph node is pierced by numerous **afferent lymphatic vessels**. Afferent lymphatic vessels have **valves** to prevent the reflux of lymph entering a lymph node.

The **cortex** has two zones:

1. The **outer cortex**, containing **lymphoid follicles**.
2. The **deep or inner cortex**, housing **CD4⁺ helper T cells** and **venules** lined by **high endothelial cells**. The deep or inner cortex is a zone in which mainly CD4⁺ helper T cells interact with B cells to induce

their proliferation and differentiation when exposed to a specific lymph-borne antigen.

A **lymphoid follicle** (Figure 10-19) consists of:

1. A **mantle** (facing the cortex),

2. A **germinal center** containing mainly proliferating B cells or **lymphoblasts**, resident **follicular dendritic cells (FDCs)**, migrating **dendritic cells**, **macrophages**, and supporting **reticular cells**, which produce reticular fibers (type III collagen).

A **primary lymphoid follicle** lacks a mantle and germinal center. A **secondary lymphoid follicle** has a mantle and a germinal center. The mantle and germinal center **develop in response to antigen stimulation**.

FDCs are branched (hence the name **dendritic**) cells forming a network within the lymphoid follicle. In contrast to migrating dendritic cells, which derive from bone marrow and interact with T cells, resident FDCs do not derive from a bone marrow cell precursor. FDCs are observed at the edge of the germinal centers and interact with mature B cells. FDCs trap antigens on their surface for recognition by B cells.

Activated B cells, with high-affinity surface Igs migrate to the medullary cords and differentiate into plasma cells secreting IgM or IgG into the medullary sinuses and efferent lymphatic vessels (see Figure 10-19).

The interaction of mature B cells with FDCs rescues the B cell from apoptosis. Only B cells with low-affinity surface immunoglobulin are induced to apoptosis. Macrophages in the lymphoid follicle remove by phagocytosis apoptotic B cells.

Lymphatic sinuses are spaces lined by endothelial cells. They are located under the capsule (**subcapsular sinus**) and along trabeculae of connective tissue derived from the capsule and entering the cortex (**paratrabecular sinus**). Highly phagocytic macrophages are distributed along the subcapsular and paratrabecular sinuses to remove particulate matter present in the percolating lymph. Lymph entering the paratrabecular sinus through the subcapsular sinus percolates to the medullary sinuses and exits through a single efferent lymphatic vessel. Lymph in the subcapsular sinus can bypass the paratrabecular and medullary sinuses and exit through the efferent lymphatic vessel.

High endothelial venules (HEVs) (see Figure 10-18), located in the inner or deep cortex, are the sites of entry of most B and T cells into the lymph node.

The **medulla** is surrounded by the cortex, except at the region of the **hilum** (see Figure 10-18). The hilum is a concave surface of the lymph node where **efferent lymphatic vessels** and a single **vein** leave and an **artery** enters the lymph node.

The medulla consists of two major components:

1. **Medullary sinusoids**, spaces lined by endothelial cells surrounded by reticular cells and macrophages.

Figure 10-18. **Lymph node**

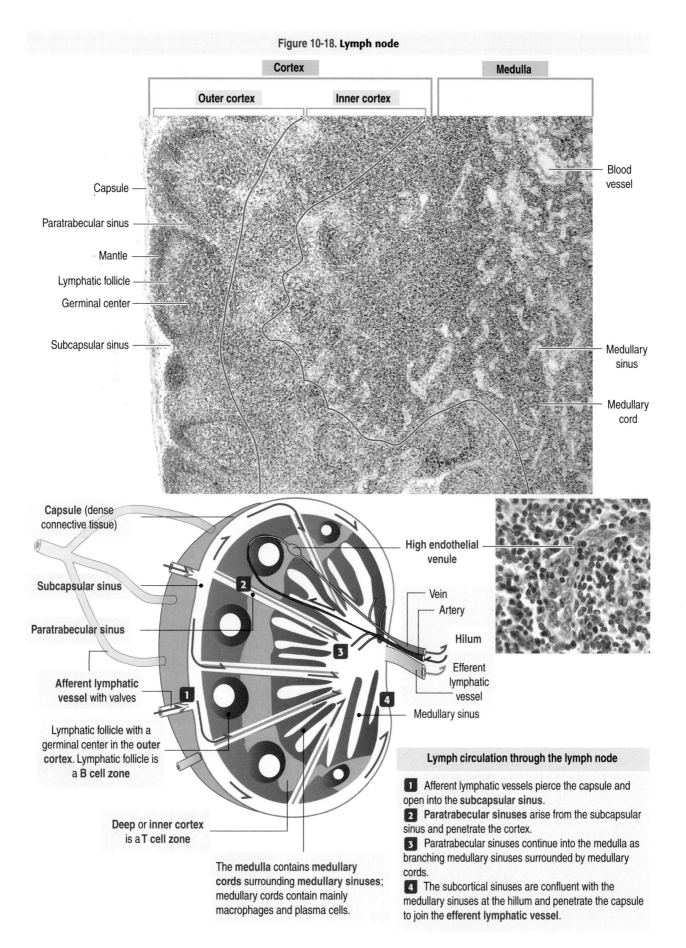

Cortex | **Medulla**

Outer cortex | **Inner cortex**

Capsule

Paratrabecular sinus

Mantle

Lymphatic follicle

Germinal center

Subcapsular sinus

Blood vessel

Medullary sinus

Medullary cord

Capsule (dense connective tissue)

Subcapsular sinus

Paratrabecular sinus

Afferent lymphatic vessel with valves

Lymphatic follicle with a germinal center in the **outer cortex**. Lymphatic follicle is a **B cell zone**

Deep or **inner cortex** is a **T cell zone**

The **medulla** contains **medullary cords** surrounding **medullary sinuses**; medullary cords contain mainly macrophages and plasma cells.

High endothelial venule

Vein
Artery

Hilum

Efferent lymphatic vessel

Medullary sinus

Lymph circulation through the lymph node

1 Afferent lymphatic vessels pierce the capsule and open into the **subcapsular sinus**.

2 **Paratrabecular sinuses** arise from the subcapsular sinus and penetrate the cortex.

3 Paratrabecular sinuses continue into the medulla as branching medullary sinuses surrounded by medullary cords.

4 The subcortical sinuses are confluent with the medullary sinuses at the hillum and penetrate the capsule to join the **efferent lymphatic vessel**.

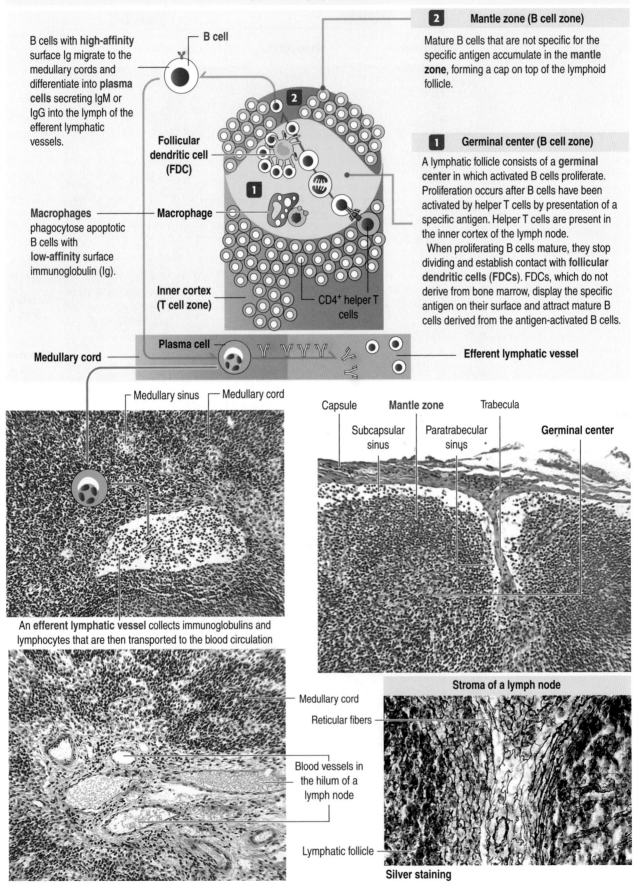

Figure 10-19. Lymphatic follicle

B cell

B cells with **high-affinity** surface Ig migrate to the medullary cords and differentiate into **plasma cells** secreting IgM or IgG into the lymph of the efferent lymphatic vessels.

Follicular dendritic cell (FDC)

Macrophages phagocytose apoptotic B cells with **low-affinity** surface immunoglobulin (Ig).

Macrophage

Inner cortex (T cell zone)

CD4⁺ helper T cells

2 **Mantle zone (B cell zone)**

Mature B cells that are not specific for the specific antigen accumulate in the **mantle zone**, forming a cap on top of the lymphoid follicle.

1 **Germinal center (B cell zone)**

A lymphatic follicle consists of a **germinal center** in which activated B cells proliferate. Proliferation occurs after B cells have been activated by helper T cells by presentation of a specific antigen. Helper T cells are present in the inner cortex of the lymph node.

When proliferating B cells mature, they stop dividing and establish contact with **follicular dendritic cells (FDCs)**. FDCs, which do not derive from bone marrow, display the specific antigen on their surface and attract mature B cells derived from the antigen-activated B cells.

Medullary cord

Plasma cell

Efferent lymphatic vessel

Medullary sinus — Medullary cord

An **efferent lymphatic vessel** collects immunoglobulins and lymphocytes that are then transported to the blood circulation

Capsule | **Mantle zone** | Trabecula
Subcapsular sinus | Paratrabecular sinus | **Germinal center**

Medullary cord

Blood vessels in the hilum of a lymph node

Stroma of a lymph node

Reticular fibers

Lymphatic follicle

Silver staining

Box 10-G | **Lymph flow and dendritic cell migration**

- Terminal afferent lymphatic vessels, transporting lymph to the lymph nodes, derive from collecting lymphatic vessels.
- Terminal afferent lymphatic vessels penetrate the connective tissue cortex of a lymph node and empty their content in the subcapsular sinus.
- The flow of lymph into lymph nodes is regulated by smooth muscle cells present in the wall of collecting lymphatic vessels (intrinsic pumping activity) and by movements in the surrounding tissue (passive extrinsic activity).
- Collecting lymphatic vessels have valves that allow unidirectional flow of lymph and cells (for example, dendritic cells and leukocytes) from lymph node to lymph node. Valves prevent the backflow of lymph processed in the preceding lymph node.
- Dendritic cells are highly mobile. They are distributed as sentinels in the periphery to monitor the presence of foreign antigens. They relocate to secondary lymphoid organs, lymph nodes in particular, to interact with memory T cells present in the deep cortex. An example is the Langerhans cell present in epidermis.

2. **Medullary cords**, with B cells, macrophages, and **plasma cells**. Activated B cells migrate from the cortex, enter the medullary cords and become plasma cells (see Figure 10-19). This is a strategic location, because plasma cells can secrete immunoglobulins directly into the lumen of the medullary sinuses without leaving the lymph node.

Pathology: Lymphadenitis and lymphomas

Lymph nodes constitute a defense site against lymph-borne microorganisms (bacteria, viruses, parasites) entering the node through afferent lymphatic vessels. This defense mechanism depends on the close interaction of B cells in the follicle nodules with CD4$^+$ T cells in the inner cortex.

In Chapter 12, Cardiovascular System, we indicate

that the interstitial fluid, representing plasma filtrate, is transported into blind sacs corresponding to lymphatic capillaries.

This interstitial fluid, entering the lymphatic capillaries as **lymph**, flows into collecting lymphatic vessels becoming afferents to regional lymph nodes (see Box 10-G). Lymph nodes are linked in series by the lymphatic vessels in such a way that **the efferent lymphatic vessel of a lymph node becomes the afferent lymphatic vessel of a downstream lymph node in the chain.**

Soluble and particulate antigens drained with the interstitial fluid, as well as antigen-bearing dendritic cells in the skin (Langerhans cells; see Chapter 11, Integumentary System), enter the lymphatic vessels and are transported to lymph nodes.

Antigen-bearing dendritic cells enter the CD4$^+$ helper T cell–rich inner cortex. Soluble and particulate antigens are detected in the percolating lymph by resident macrophages and dendritic cells strategically located along the subcapsular and paratrabecular sinuses.

When the immune reaction is acute in response to locally drained bacteria (for example, infections of the teeth or tonsils), local lymph nodes enlarge and become painful because of the distention of the capsule by cellular proliferation and edema. This condition is known as **acute lymphadenitis**.

Lymphomas are tumors of the lymphoid tissue in the form of tissue masses. **Lymphocytic leukemia** designates lymphoid tumors involving the bone marrow.

Most of the lymphomas are of B cell origin (80%); the remainder are of T cell origin. Lymphomas include **Hodgkin's lymphoma** (Figure 10-20) and

Figure 10-20. **Hodgkin's lymphoma**

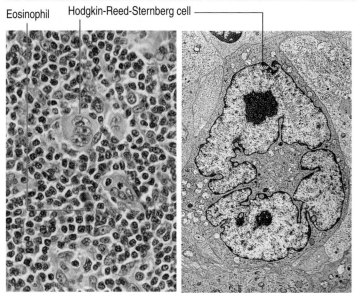

Eosinophil — Hodgkin-Reed-Sternberg cell

Hodgkin's lymphoma: a B cell lymphoma

Hodgkin's lymphoma (HL) is one of the most frequent lymphomas and often affects young adults. A characteristic histologic feature of the classic form of HL is the Hodgkin-Reed-Sternberg (HRS) cell, a tumor cell of germinal center B cell origin. The HRS cell does not express most B cell antigens, such as CD20, CD79A, CD19 and CD22 and immunoglobulins. Instead, HRS cells express molecules not normally seen by B cells, such as CD30, CD15, CD70, and others.

In about 40% of cases, HRS cells are infected by **Epstein-Barr virus**, indicating an important role of this virus in HL pathogenesis. HRS cells are multinucleated or multilobulated with nuclear eosinophilic inclusions.

HRS cells secrete cytokines that attract eosinophils and CD4$^+$ T cells. The latter stimulate the growth of HRS cells in the lymphatic tissue.

Histology image from Hoffbrand AV, Pttit JE: Color Atlas of Clinical Hematology. 3rd Edition. Philadelphia, Mosby, 2000
Electron microscopy image from Damjanov I, Linder J: Pathology: A Color Atlas. Philadelphia, Mosby, 2000

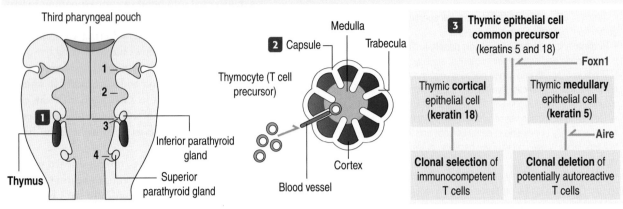

Figure 10-21. Development of the thymus

Third pharyngeal pouch

1
2
3
4

1

Thymus

Inferior parathyroid gland

Superior parathyroid gland

Medulla

2 Capsule — Trabecula

Thymocyte (T cell precursor)

Cortex

Blood vessel

3 Thymic epithelial cell common precursor (keratins 5 and 18)

Foxn1

Thymic **cortical** epithelial cell (keratin 18)

Thymic **medullary** epithelial cell (keratin 5)

Aire

Clonal selection of immunocompetent T cells

Clonal deletion of potentially autoreactive T cells

1 The thymus rudiments originate from the caudal region of the endodermic **third pharyngeal pouch** on each side, proliferate, migrate to the thorax, and become connected by connective tissue.

Parathyroid gland tissue, developing from the same pouch, migrates with the thymus and becomes the inferior parathyroid glands. The superior parathyroid glands originate from the fourth pharyngeal pouch. The numbers 1 to 4 indicate the pharyngeal pouches.

2 A **capsule** forms from the neural crest mesenchyme. Capsule-derived trabeculae extending into the future corticomedullary region of the thymus divide the thymus into **incomplete lobules**.

By 14 weeks, thymocyte precursors arrive from bone marrow through blood vessels, after interconnected **thymic epithelial cells** form a three-dimensional network and **macrophages** are present. By 17 weeks, the thymus is beginning to produce T cells.

3 Thymic epithelial cells play important functions in clonal selection and clonal deletion of differentiating T cells:

1. A common precursor (keratins 5 and 18) gives rise to thymic cortical (keratin 18) and medullary (keratin 5) epithelial cells.

2. Thymic epithelial cells express two essential transcription factors: **Foxn1** (for forkedhead box N1), and **aire** (for autoimmune regulator). **Foxn1** is essential for the differentiation of thymic epithelial cells. **Aire** promotes the expression of a portfolio of tissue-specific cell proteins by thymic **medullary** epithelial cells, which normally do not express these proteins. These proteins permit the identification and disposal of autoreactive T cells. A mutation of the aire gene in humans causes autoimmune polyendocrinopathy–candidiasis–ectodermal dystrophy (APECED).

non-Hodgkin's lymphomas. They are clinically characterized by nontender enlargement of localized or generalized lymph nodes (nodal disease).

The **Hodgkin-Reed-Sternberg cell,** found in classic Hodgkin's lymphoma, is a large multinucleated or multilobulated tumor cell of B cell origin surrounded by T cells, eosinophils, plasma cells, and macrophages (mixed celullarity).

Another group in the lymphoma category includes the **plasma cell tumors,** consisting of plasma cells, the terminally differentiated B cells. Plasma cell tumors (**multiple myeloma**) originate in bone marrow and cause bone destruction with pain due to fractures (see Box 10-E).

Thymus
Development of the thymus

A brief review of the development of the thymus facilitates an understanding of the structure and function of this lymphoid organ.

The **mesenchyme** from the pharyngeal arch gives rise to the capsule, trabeculae, and vessels of the thymus (Figure 10-21). The **thymic epithelial rudiment** attracts **bone marrow–derived thymocyte precursors, dendritic cells,** and **macrophages** required for normal thymic function.

During **fetal life,** the thymus contains lymphocytes derived from the liver. T cell progenitors formed in the bone marrow during hematopoiesis enter the thymus as **immature thymocytes** and mature to become immunocompetent T cells (predominantly $CD4^+$ or $CD8^+$), that are then carried by the blood into lymph nodes, spleen, and other lymphatic tissues (Figure 10-18).

The thymus in humans is fully developed before birth. The production of T cells is significant before puberty. After puberty, the thymus begins to involute and the production of T cells in the adult decreases. The progenies of T cells become established, and immunity is maintained without the need to produce new T cells.

A significant difference from the lymph node and the spleen is that **the stroma of the thymus consists of thymic epithelial cells** organized in a dispersed network to allow for intimate contact with developing **thymocytes,** the T cell precursors arriving from bone marrow. In contrast to the thymus, the stroma of the lymph node and the spleen contains reticular cells and reticular fibers but not epithelial cells.

There are two important aspects during the development of the thymus with relevance to tolerance for self-antigens and autoimmune diseases:

1. **A single precursor cell gives rise to thymic cortical and medullary epithelial cells** (see Figure 10-21).

The transcription factor **Foxn1** (for forkhead box N1) **regulates the differentiation of cortical and medullary thymic cells**, which starts before the arrival of thymocyte precursors from bone marrow.

Differentiation includes the expression of cytokeratins and establishment of desmosome intercellular linkages. In contrast to the stratified squamous epithelium of the epidermis, thymic epithelial cells form an open network that enables a close contact with thymocytes.

A mutation of the *Foxn1* gene produces **nude** and **athymic mice**. In an analogous fashion to thymic epithelial cells, *Foxn1* regulates the differentiation of epidermal keratinocytes (see Chapter 11, Integumentary System).

2. The transcription factor **aire** (for autoimmune regulator) enables the expression of tissue-specific self-proteins by thymic **medullary** epithelial cells. The expression of these proteins permits the **elimination of T cells that recognize specific tissue antigens** (autoreactive T cells).

The human autosomal disorder called **autoimmune polyendocrinopathy–candidiasis–ectodermal dystrophy (APECED)** is associated with a mutation in the *aire* gene (see Figure 10-21 and Box 10-H).

Thymic cortical epithelial cells are involved in the **clonal selection** of T cells. **Medullary epithelial cells** are involved in the **clonal deletion** of potentially autoreactive T cells.

Box 10-H | *Aire* gene and autoimmunity

• The human autosomal disorder autoimmune polyendocrinopathy–candidiasis–ectodermal dystrophy (APECED), also known as autoimmune polyendocrine syndrome type 1 (APS-1), is characterized by the autoimmune destruction of endocrine organs, the inability to eliminate *Candida* yeast infection, and the development of ectodermal dystrophic tissue.
• The production of tissue-specific antibodies and an inflammatory reaction confined to specific structures in several organs (for example, retina, ovary, testis, stomach, and pancreas) are associated with one of the several mutations of the *aire* gene.
• The transcription factor aire enables the expression of several tissue-specific antigens (e.g., thyroglobulin, insulin, retinal S–antigen, zona pellucida glycoprotein in the ovary, proteolipid protein in the central nervous system) by thymic medullary epithelial cells. These self-proteins permit the disposal of autoreactive T cells in the medulla of the thymus.
• In aire-deficient individuals, self-proteins are not expressed, and autoreactive T cells are exported to the periphery. The mechanism of self-tolerance is not operational, because self-reactive T cells are not eliminated by clonal deletion.

Clinical significance: DiGeorge syndrome

DiGeorge syndrome is an **inherited immunodeficiency disease** in which thymic epithelial cells fail to develop. The thymus and parathyroid glands are rudimentary or absent. The cause is a deletion of genes from chromosome 22 (22q11.2 deletion syndrome).

Patients have congenital heart defects, hypoparathyroidism (with low calcium levels in blood), cleft palate, behavioral and psychiatric problems, and increased susceptibility to infections.

When thymic epithelial cells fail to organize the thymus, bone marrow–derived T cell precursors cannot differentiate. Thymic epithelial cells express MHC class I and class II molecules on their surface, and these molecules are required for the clonal selection of T cells. Their absence in DiGeorge syndrome affects the production of functional T cells. The development of B cells is not affected in DiGeorge syndrome.

The **nude (athymic) mouse** is a strain of mice lacking the expression of the **transcription factor Foxn1** necessary for the differentiation of thymic epithelial cells and epidermal cells involved in the normal development of the thymus and **hair follicles**. The nude mouse is the equivalent of DiGeorge syndrome.

Structure of the thymus

The thymus consists of **two lobes** subdivided into **incomplete lobules**, each separated into an **outer cortex** and a **central medulla** (Figure 10-22).

A connective tissue **capsule** with small arterioles surrounds the lobules. The capsule projects **septa** or **trabeculae** into the organ. Blood vessels (**trabecular arterioles** and **venules**) within the trabeculae gain access to the thymic epithelial stroma (Figure 10-23).

The **cortex** contains **thymic epithelial cells** forming an interconnected three-dimensional network supported by collagen fibers. Thymic epithelial cells, linked to each other by **desmosomes**, surround capillaries.

A **dual basal lamina** is present in the space between epithelial cells and capillaries. One basal lamina is produced by the cortical thymic epithelial cells. The other basal lamina is of endothelial cell origin. Macrophages may also be present in proximity (Figure 10-24).

Thymic cortical epithelial cells, basal laminae, and endothelial cells form the **functional blood-thymus barrier** (see Figure 10-24). Macrophages adjacent to the capillaries ensure that antigens escaping from blood vessels into the thymus do not react with developing T cells in the cortex, thus preventing the risk of an autoimmune reaction.

Most T cell development takes place in the cortex. In the outer area of the cortex adjacent to the capsule, double-negative thymocytes proliferate and begin the process of gene rearrangement leading to the expres-

Figure 10-22. Thymus

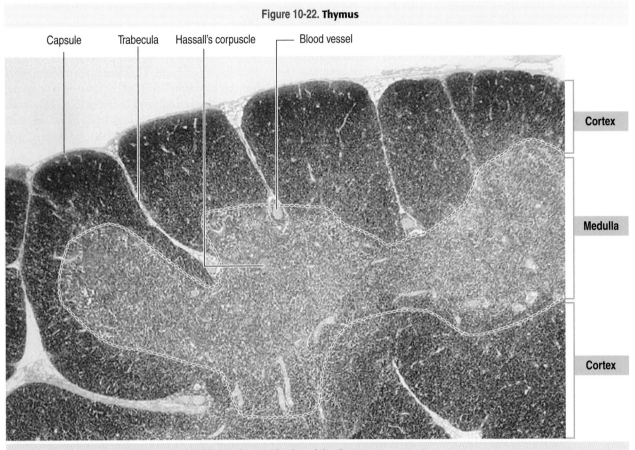

Capsule Trabecula Hassall's corpuscle Blood vessel

Cortex

Medulla

Cortex

Histologic organization of the thymus

The thymus consists of several incomplete lobules. Each lobule contains an independent **outer cortical region**, but the **central medullary region is shared by adjacent lobules**. **Trabeculae**, extensions of the capsule down the **corticomedullary region**, form the boundary of each lobule.

The **cortex** consists of stromal cells and developing T cells (thymocytes), macrophages, and thymic cortical epithelial cells.

MHC classes I and **II** molecules are present on the surface of the cortical epithelial cells.

The characteristic deep-blue nuclear staining of the cortex in histologic preparations reflects the predominant population of T cells as compared with the less basophilic medulla containing a lower number of thymocytes.

Hassall's corpuscles are a characteristic component of the **medulla**. Hassall's corpuscles are not seen in the cortex.

sion of the pre-TCR along with coreceptors CD4 and CD8 (see Figure 10-7 and Figure 10-23).

Deep in the cortex, maturing T cells are double-positive (CD4$^+$ and CD8$^+$) and become receptive to peptide-MHC complexes. The process of **positive selection** of T cells now starts in the presence of thymic cortical epithelial cells expressing both MHC class I and class II molecules on their surface. MHC class II molecules are required for the development of CD4$^+$ T cells; MHC class I molecules are necessary for the development of CD8$^+$ T cells.

T cells that recognize self-MHC molecules but not self-antigens are allowed to mature by positive selection. T cells unable to recognize MHC molecules are not selected and are eliminated by **programmed cell death**, or **apoptosis**.

T cells that recognize both self-MHC and self-antigens (produced by thymic medullary epithelial cells under the regulation of the *aire* gene) are eliminated

by **negative selection** (**clonal deletion**), a task carried out by dendritic cells and macrophages.

About 95% of the developing T cells die within the cortex of the thymus without ever maturing. Double-positive T cells undergo apoptosis within three days in the absence of a surviving signal; trophic signaling enables the progression to single-positive. Within 1 week, single-positive cells will be eliminated by apoptosis unless they receive a positive signal for survival and export to the periphery.

The **medulla** of one lobule is continuous with the medulla of an adjacent lobule. The medulla displays **mature T cells** migrating from the cortex. Maturation of T cells is completed in the medulla and functional T cells enter postcapillary venules in the corticomedullary junction to exit the thymus (see Figure 10-23).

Thymic epithelial cells populate the medulla, many of them forming **Hassall's corpuscles**. Hassall's corpuscles are thymic epithelial cells forming onion-

Figure 10-23. Thymus

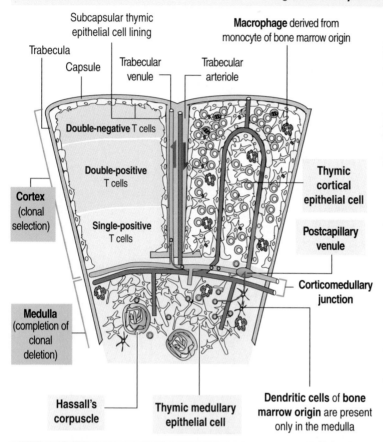

Subcapsular thymic epithelial cell lining
Trabecula
Capsule
Trabecular venule
Trabecular arteriole
Macrophage derived from monocyte of bone marrow origin
Double-negative T cells
Double-positive T cells
Thymic cortical epithelial cell
Cortex (clonal selection)
Single-positive T cells
Postcapillary venule
Medulla (completion of clonal deletion)
Corticomedullary junction
Hassall's corpuscle
Thymic medullary epithelial cell
Dendritic cells of **bone marrow origin** are present only in the medulla

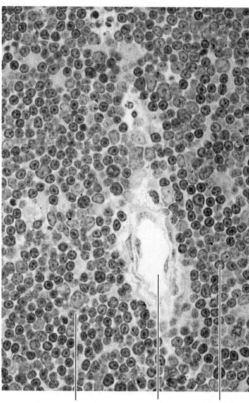

Cortical epithelial cell | Capillary | Developing thymocyte

Hassall's corpuscles

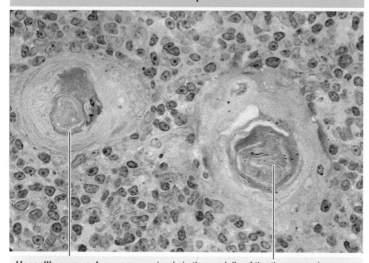

Hassall's corpuscles are present only in the medulla of the thymus and are composed of closely packed whorls of epithelial cells representing **highly keratinized** medullary epithelial cells.

Hassall's corpuscles produce **cytokine thymic stromal lymphopoietin**, which stimulates thymic dendritic cells that in turn complete the maturation of single-positive T cells to optimize negative selection.

Histology of the thymus

The functional thymus consists of two cell populations: **stromal cells** and **developing T cells**.

Stromal cells include (1) the **subcapsular thymic epithelial cells** also lining the trabeculae and perivascular spaces; (2) the **thymic cortical epithelial cells**; (3) the **thymic medullary epithelial cells** that give rise to **Hassall's corpuscles**; (4) **macrophages** present in both cortex and medulla, involved in the removal of apoptotic T cells eliminated during clonal selection and deletion; and (5) **dendritic cells** of bone marrow origin, confined to the medulla.

Developing T cells include T cells at different stages of maturation:

Immature T cells, **double-negative T cells**, enter the cortex of the thymus through blood vessels and proliferate in the subcapsular area.

Double-positive T cells move to the outer cortex where they are confronted with epithelial cells with cell surface MHC classes I and II molecules for **clonal selection**.

Single-positive T cells migrate to the inner cortex.

The majority of T cells (80% to 85%) are in the cortex. The medulla contains the remaining 15% to 20% of T cells undergoing **clonal deletion** (elimination of autoreactive T cells).

like layers (see Figure 10-23). Hassall's corpuscles produce **cytokine thymic stromal lymphopoietin**, which stimulates thymic dendritic cells to complete the maturation of single-positive T cells to optimize

negative selection and ensure tolerance.

Note that **the blood-thymus barrier is not present in the medulla** and that **Hassall's corpuscles can be seen only in the medulla.**

Figure 10-24. The blood-thymus barrier

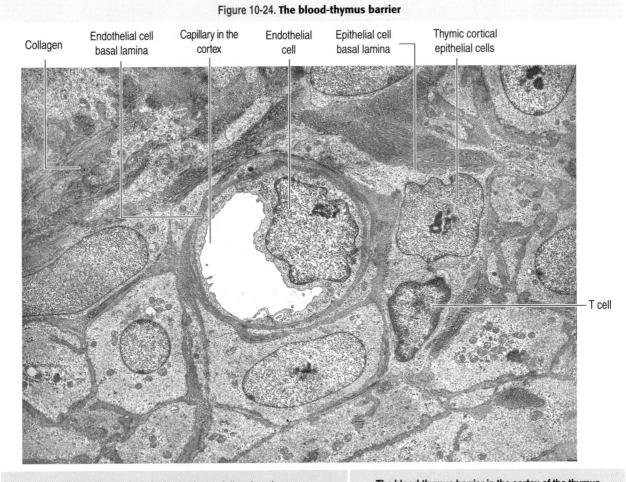

Collagen

Endothelial cell basal lamina

Capillary in the cortex

Endothelial cell

Epithelial cell basal lamina

Thymic cortical epithelial cells

T cell

Postcapillary venule in the corticomedullary junction

Lumen of the **postcapillary venule**

Endothelial cell

Epithelial cell

Maturing T cells

Mature T cells, completing their differentiation under the guidance of thymic medullary epithelial cells, migrate across the endothelium into the lumen of a corticomedullary postcapillary venule.

The blood-thymus barrier in the cortex of the thymus

Endothelial cell basal lamina

Desmosome

Tonofilaments

Thymic cortical epithelial cell surrounded by a basal lamina

Capillary in the **cortex** of the thymus lined by continuous endothelial cells

T cell

Macrophage

The **blood-thymus barrier** consists of thymic cortical epithelial cells joined by desmosomes, dual basal laminae produced by thymic cortical epithelial cells and endothelial cells, and capillary endothelial cells linked by tight junctions.

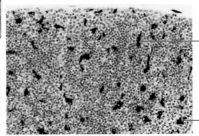

Abundant macrophages in the cortex of the thymus

Immunohistochemistry panel from Martín-Lacave I, García-Caballero T: Atlas of Immunohistochemistry. Madrid, Spain. Ed. Díaz de Santos, 2012.

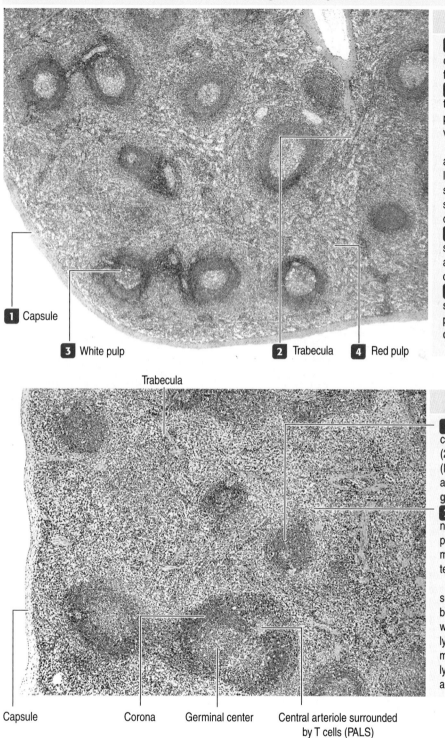

Figure 10-25. Spleen

General organization of the spleen

1 The spleen is surrounded by a **capsule** containing collagen, elastic fibers, and smooth muscle fibers.

2 Branching trabeculae derived from the capsule enter the spleen parenchyma. Trabecular arteries and veins are found in the trabecula.

The spleen does not have a cortex and a medulla and it has no afferent lymphatic vessels. The **stroma** of the spleen is composed of **reticular fibers** supporting the two major components of the spleen:

3 The **white pulp**, consisting of splenic nodules with B and T cells, antigen-presenting cells, and plasma cells.

4 The **red pulp**, consisting of **splenic sinusoids** filled with blood and plates of lymphoid tissue, the **splenic cords**.

1 Capsule

3 White pulp

2 Trabecula

4 Red pulp

Trabecula

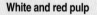

White and red pulp

1 The **white pulp** consists of four components: (1) the **central arteriole**; (2) the periarteriolar lymphoid sheath (**PALS**); (3) a **corona** formed by B cells and antigen-presenting cells; and (4) a **germinal center**.

2 The **red pulp** surrounds the splenic nodules (white pulp). The white and red pulp interact at the **marginal zone** where most branches of the central arteriole terminate in a **vascular sinus**.

The red pulp receives a significant blood supply. Antigens enter the spleen from the blood. This differs from the lymph node, where antigens enter through the afferent lymphatic vessels. Although the white pulp mimics the lymphatic nodules of the lymph node cortex, the central arteriole is a distinctive feature.

Capsule   Corona   Germinal center   Central arteriole surrounded by T cells (PALS)

Spleen

The spleen is the largest secondary lymphoid organ of the body. The spleen **lacks a cortex and a medulla**.

The spleen has two major components with distinct functions (Figure 10-25):

1. The **white pulp**.
2. The **red pulp**.

The **white pulp is the immune component of the spleen**. The cell components of the white pulp are similar to those of the lymph node, except that antigens enter the spleen from the blood rather than from the lymph.

The **red pulp** is a filter that removes aged and damaged red blood cells and microorganisms from

Figure 10-26. **Vascularization of the spleen**

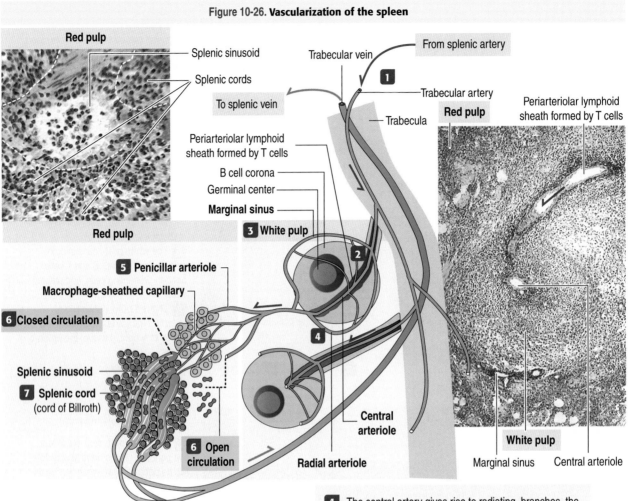

Red pulp

Splenic sinusoid

Splenic cords

To splenic vein

From splenic artery

Trabecular vein

Trabecular artery

Trabecula

Red pulp

Periarteriolar lymphoid sheath formed by T cells

Periarteriolar lymphoid sheath formed by T cells

B cell corona

Germinal center

Marginal sinus

Red pulp

3 White pulp

5 Penicillar arteriole

Macrophage-sheathed capillary

6 Closed circulation

Splenic sinusoid

7 Splenic cord (cord of Billroth)

6 Open circulation

Radial arteriole

Central arteriole

White pulp

Marginal sinus   Central arteriole

1 The **trabecular artery** enters the spleen through the connective tissue trabecula (derived from the splenic capsule).

2 When the trabecular artery leaves the trabecula, it becomes invested within the white pulp by T cells forming the **periarteriolar lymphoid sheath** (PALS). The trabecular artery is now the **central artery/arteriole** of the white pulp.

3 The white pulp consists of four components: (1) the **central arteriole**; (2) the **PALS**; (3) the **corona** formed by B cells and antigen-presenting cells; and (4) the **germinal center**.
The white pulp has the structural characteristics of an immune component (B and T cells and antigen-presenting cells).

4 The central artery gives rise to radiating branches, the **radial arterioles**, ending in the **marginal sinus** surrounding the white pulp.

5 Blood from the marginal sinus and the central arteriole is transported into the **penicillar arterioles**, which end in a capillary network surrounded by macrophages. The capillary network is called **macrophage-sheathed capillaries**.

6 The macrophage-sheathed capillaries drain into the **splenic sinusoids (closed circulation)** or into the stroma of the red pulp (**open circulation**).

7 The red pulp is formed by (1) the **penicillar arteriole**; (2) the **macrophage-sheathed capillaries**; (3) the **splenic sinusoids**; (4) **reticular cells** forming the **stroma** of the splenic cords (also known as **cords of Billroth**); and (5) **all cell types of the circulating blood**.

circulating blood. It also is a **storage site for red blood cells.**

Bacteria can be recognized by macrophages of the red pulp and removed directly or after they are coated with complement proteins (produced in the liver) and immunoglobulins (produced in the white pulp). The clearance of complement–immu-noglobulin coated bacteria or viruses by macrophages is very rapid and prevents infections of kidneys, meninges and lungs.

Vascularization of the spleen
The spleen is covered by a **capsule** consisting of dense, irregular connective tissue with elastic and smooth

Figure 10-27. **White pulp**

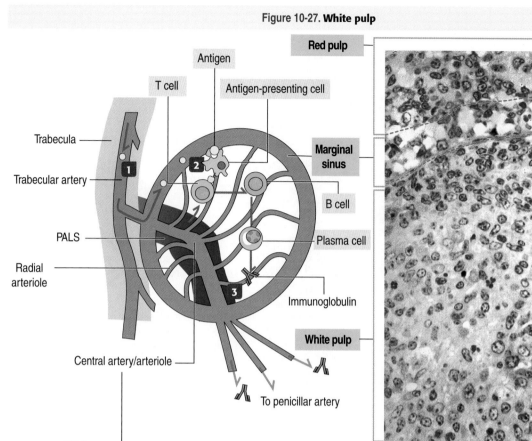

Red pulp

Antigen

T cell

Antigen-presenting cell

Trabecula

Trabecular artery

Marginal sinus

B cell

PALS

Plasma cell

Radial arteriole

Immunoglobulin

Central artery/arteriole

White pulp

To penicillar artery

PALS

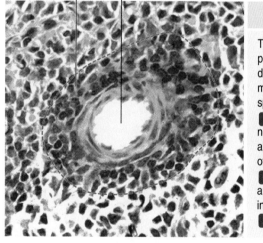

White pulp is a lymphoid follicle–like structure

The white pulp functions primarily as a lymph nodule producing B cell clones in the presence of T cells derived from the PALS. This function is particularly important during **bacteremia** (presence of viable bacteria in blood circulation) because macrophages can trap bacteria and present their antigens to lymphocytes in the spleen to stimulate a specific immune response.

1 Antigens enter the spleen from the blood (rather than from the lymph as in lymph nodes) and reach the white pulp through the trabecular artery into the central artery and the marginal sinus. The central artery and the marginal sinus are linked to each other by radial arterioles.

2 **Antigen-presenting cells** in the corona region detect blood-borne antigens that are sampled by **PALS-derived T cells**. T cells interact with **B cells** and from this interaction B cells proliferate and differentiate into **plasma cells**.

3 Plasma cells release immunoglobulins into the blood circulation.

muscle fibers (it varies with the species).

Trabeculae derived from the capsule carry blood vessels (**trabecular arteries** and **veins**) and nerves to and from the splenic red pulp (Figure 10-26). A brief review of vascularization of the spleen, which is similar to that of many organs with a significant blood supply such as the kidneys and lungs, provides a useful background for understanding the function and structure of this organ.

The **splenic artery** enters the hilum, giving rise to **trabecular arteries**, which are distributed to the splenic pulp along the connective tissue tra-

beculae. As an artery leaves the trabecula, it becomes invested by a sheath of T cells forming a **peri-arteriolar lymphoid sheath** (**PALS**) and penetrates a lymphatic nodule (the **white pulp**). The blood vessel is designated the **central artery** (also called the **follicular arteriole**, because of the nodular or follicular arrangement of the white pulp).

The **central artery** leaves the white pulp to become the **penicillar artery**.

Penicillar arteries end as **macrophage-sheathed capillaries**.

Terminal capillaries either drain directly into

Figure 10-28. **Red pulp**

Macrophage-sheathed capillary

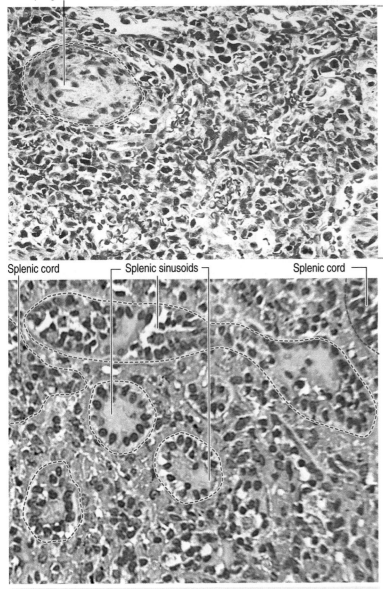

Splenic cord — Splenic sinusoids — Splenic cord —

Macrophage-sheathed capillaries

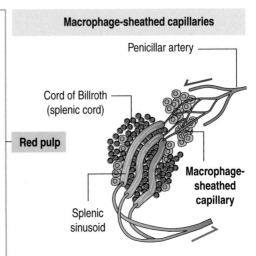

Penicillar artery

Cord of Billroth (splenic cord)

Red pulp

Macrophage-sheathed capillary

Splenic sinusoid

The branching of each **penicillar artery** gives rise to capillaries surrounded by macrophages and reticular cells. Many macrophages contain phagocytosed red blood cells.

Macrophages derive from monocytes entering the capillary sheath from the blood and differentiating into macrophages.

The major function of the macrophage sheath is to remove aged cells and particles from the blood.

Splenic sinusoids in the red pulp consist of **rod-shaped endothelial cells** arranged along the long axis of the vascular space. Endothelial cells are separated laterally by narrow slits but associated at their tapered ends by tight junctions. Ringlike strands of basal lamina material and reticular fibers surround the splenic sinusoid in a netlike fashion.

This netlike arrangement enables the passage of red blood cells through the wall of the sinus. **Plasma cells** are present. **Macrophages** surrounding the splenic sinusoids play roles in the uptake and destruction of particles and cellular debris present in the circulating blood.

The main function of the splenic sinusoid is blood filtration. Recall that Kupffer cells in liver sinusoids have a similar particulate blood cleaning function.

Splenic sinusoid

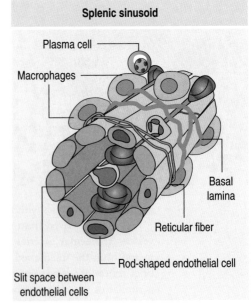

Plasma cell

Macrophages

Basal lamina

Reticular fiber

Rod-shaped endothelial cell

Slit space between endothelial cells

splenic sinusoids (**closed circulation**) or terminate as open-ended vessels within the **red pulp** (**open circulation**). Splenic sinusoids are drained by pulp veins, to trabecular veins, to splenic veins.

White pulp
This component of the spleen is nodular lymphoid tissue that **contains a central artery** or **arteriole**.

The white pulp includes (see Figure 10-26):

Figure 10-29. Sickle cell anemia and spleen

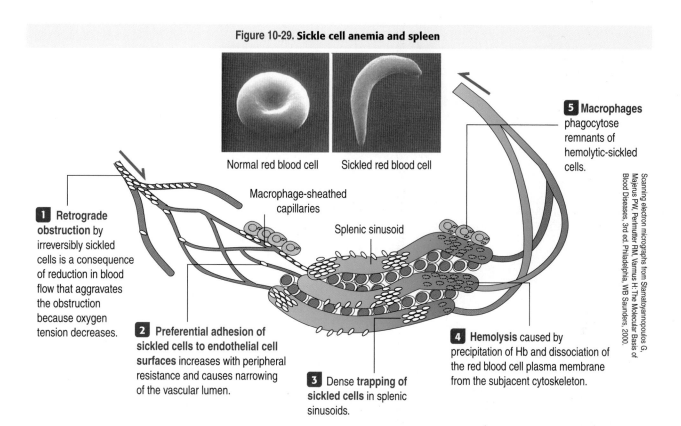

Normal red blood cell   Sickled red blood cell

Macrophage-sheathed capillaries

Splenic sinusoid

5 **Macrophages** phagocytose remnants of hemolytic-sickled cells.

1 **Retrograde obstruction** by irreversibly sickled cells is a consequence of reduction in blood flow that aggravates the obstruction because oxygen tension decreases.

2 **Preferential adhesion of sickled cells to endothelial cell surfaces** increases with peripheral resistance and causes narrowing of the vascular lumen.

3 Dense **trapping of sickled cells** in splenic sinusoids.

4 **Hemolysis** caused by precipitation of Hb and dissociation of the red blood cell plasma membrane from the subjacent cytoskeleton.

Scanning electron micrographs from Stamatoyannopoulos G, Majerus PW, Perlmutter RM, Varmus H: The Molecular Basis of Blood Diseases, 3rd ed. Philadelphia, WB Saunders, 2000.

Sickle cell anemia is determined by the substitution of normal hemoglobin (Hb A) by hemoglobin S (Hb S) caused by a point mutation (replacement of the nucleotide triplet CTC coding glutamic acid at the mRNA level [GAG] by the CAC triplet [GUG] coding for valine) that modifies the physicochemical properties of the β-globin chain of hemoglobin. All hemoglobin is abnormal in homozygous individuals for the mutant gene, and red blood cells show a sickling deformity and hemolytic anemia in the presence or absence of normal oxygen tension. Heterozygous individuals contain a mixture of Hb A and Hb S, and sickling and anemia are observed when the tension of oxygen decreases.

Irreversibly sickled red blood cells are trapped within the **splenic sinusoids** and are destroyed by adjacent macrophages. Hemolysis may also occur in the macrophage-sheathed capillaries of the red pulp.

1. The **central artery or arteriole** surrounded by a sheath of T cells (PALS).

2. The **lymphatic nodules**, consisting of B cells. Antigen-presenting cells and macrophages are also present in the white pulp.

There is a **marginal sinus zone** between the red and white pulps that receives **radial arterioles** from the central artery or arteriole (see Figure 10-26 and Figure 10-27).

This marginal sinus zone drains into **small sinusoids** located on the outer portion of the marginal zone. At the marginal zone, blood contacts the splenic parenchyma, which contains phagocytic macrophages and antigen-presenting cells. T and B cells enter the spleen and become segregated in their specific splenic location.

Red pulp

The red pulp contains an interconnected network of **splenic sinusoids** lined by elongated endothelial cells separated by narrow slits. **Splenic cords**, also known as the **cords of Billroth**, separate splenic sinusoids (see Figure 10-26 and Figure 10-27).

The **splenic cords** contain **plasma cells**, **macrophages**, and **blood cells**, all supported by a stroma of **reticular cells** and **fibers**.

Cytoplasmic processes of macrophages lie adjacent to the sinusoids and may project into the lumen of the sinusoids through the interendothelial cell slits to sample particulate material.

Splenic sinusoids are discontinuous vascular spaces lined by **rib-shaped endothelial cells** oriented in parallel along the long axis of the sinusoids (Figure 10-28). Junctional complexes can be found at the tapering ends of the endothelial cells.

Each splenic sinusoid is covered by a discontinuous **basal lamina** oriented like barrel hoops around the endothelial cells (see Figure 10-28). Adjacent hoops are cross-linked by strands of basal lamina material. In addition, a network of loose **reticular fibers** also encircles the splenic sinusoids. Consequently, blood cells have an unobstructed access to the sinusoids through the narrow slits between the fusiform endothelial cells and the loose basal lamina–reticular fiber network.

Two types of blood circulations have been described in the red pulp (see Figure 10-26):

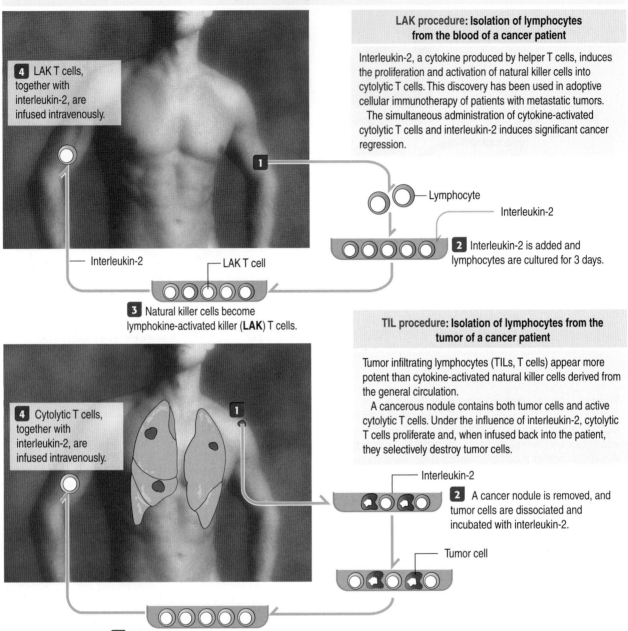

Figure 10-30. Adoptive cell transfer

LAK procedure: Isolation of lymphocytes from the blood of a cancer patient

Interleukin-2, a cytokine produced by helper T cells, induces the proliferation and activation of natural killer cells into cytolytic T cells. This discovery has been used in adoptive cellular immunotherapy of patients with metastatic tumors.

The simultaneous administration of cytokine-activated cytolytic T cells and interleukin-2 induces significant cancer regression.

4 LAK T cells, together with interleukin-2, are infused intravenously.

Lymphocyte

Interleukin-2

2 Interleukin-2 is added and lymphocytes are cultured for 3 days.

Interleukin-2

LAK T cell

3 Natural killer cells become lymphokine-activated killer (**LAK**) T cells.

TIL procedure: Isolation of lymphocytes from the tumor of a cancer patient

Tumor infiltrating lymphocytes (TILs, T cells) appear more potent than cytokine-activated natural killer cells derived from the general circulation.

A cancerous nodule contains both tumor cells and active cytolytic T cells. Under the influence of interleukin-2, cytolytic T cells proliferate and, when infused back into the patient, they selectively destroy tumor cells.

4 Cytolytic T cells, together with interleukin-2, are infused intravenously.

Interleukin-2

2 A cancer nodule is removed, and tumor cells are dissociated and incubated with interleukin-2.

Tumor cell

3 In the presence of interleukin-2, tumor cells die and tumor-infiltrating cytolytic T cells proliferate.

1. A **closed circulation**, in which arterial vessels connect directly to splenic sinusoids.

2. An **open circulation** with blood vessels opening directly into the red pulp spaces, blood flowing through these spaces and then entering the splenic sinusoids through the interendothelial cell slits.

Clinical significance: Sickle cell anemia

Sickle cell anemia is discussed briefly in Chapter 6, Blood and Hematopoiesis, within the context of the structure of the red blood cell. Here, we focus on the fate of irreversibly sickled red blood cells when they travel through the narrow passages of the red pulp. We also consider the function of macrophages associated with the splenic sinuses in the disposal of destroyed sickle cells.

When the oxygen tension decreases, sickle cells show preferential adhesion to postcapillary venules followed by trapping of irreversibly sickled cells and retrograde obstruction of the blood vessel (Figure 10-29).

An increased destruction of sickle cells leads to anemia and to an increase in the formation of bilirubin from the released hemoglobin (**chronic hyperbilirubinemia**). The **occlusion of splenic sinuses** by sickle cells is associated with **splenomegaly** (enlargement of the spleen), disrupted bacterial clearance function of the spleen in cases of bacteremia, and **painful crises** in the affected region. Similar vascular occlusions, causing infarctions, can also occur in the kidneys, liver, bones, and retinas.

Clinical significance: Asplenia

Asplenia, the lack of spleen, includes patients with:

1. **Surgical asplenia,** that may occur in healthy individuals after trauma or in patients with hematologic (for example, hereditary spherocytosis, β-thalassemia or sickle cell disease), immunologic (for example, immune thrombocytopenic purpura) or tumoral (spleen lymphoma)indication for splenectomy.

2. **Functional asplenia** is observed in patients with sickle cell anemia. Anatomic asplenia by autoinfarction starts to develop by about 1 year of age and is fully established after 6 to 8 years of age.

3. **Congenital asplenia,** isolated or associated with other abnormalities, in particular congenital heart disease (Ivemak syndrome).

Postsplenectomy sepsis is a clear demonstration of the function of the spleen in bacteremia, most commonly caused by *Streptococcus pneumoniae* (pneumococcus). Postsplenectomy sepsis, a life-threatening infection, is manifested in an asplenic patient by fever, chills, muscle aches, vomiting or diarrhea. Rapidly progressive septicemia is fatal in up to 50% of the cases.

Vaccinations against pneumococci, *Haemophhilus influenzae* type b, meningococci and influenza virus are recommended for asplenic patients. Adults who already have antibodies to microorganisms are less prone to bacteremia. Children who have not developed antibodies are more vulnerable and **prophylactic antimicrobial therapy** is recommended.

To a certain extent, the Kupffer cells of the liver sinusoids complement the role of the white pulp in the detection and removal of bacteria circulating in blood.

Clinical significance: Adoptive cell transfer

Surgery, cancer chemotherapy and radiotherapy are strategies for cancer treatment. Yet, it is known that the immune system contributes to tumor regression.

Strategies are being developed to enhance the immune response against tumor cells expressing tumor-related antigens. One strategy, called **adoptive cell transfer (ACT),** consists of the transfer of activated immune cells with antitumoral activity into a tumor-bearing host. ACT can also enhance antitumor and overall immunity; it has also been used for the treatment of viral infections.

Two procedures have been used for engineering immune cells of patients to recognize and attack their own tumor. (Figure 10-30):

1. The **LAK cell procedure** consists of the isolation of lymphokine-activated killer (LAK) cells from the blood of a cancerous patient and their treatment with the cytokine **interleukin-2 (IL-2)** to induce their proliferation in vitro. Activated LAK cells are infused into the patient, together with IL-2. A key issue in this procedure is the isolation of lymphocytes from the same patient, because the infusion of killer T cells from a second patient was not successful. The LAK procedure yields modest benefits when compared with the administration of IL-2 only.

2. The **TIL procedure,** which consists of the isolation of autologous tumor-infiltrating lymphocytes (TILs). In this procedure, a tumor nodule is removed and the cells are dissociated with enzymes. Dissociated cells are cultured with IL-2. This treatment results in the death of cancerous cells and the proliferation of TILs that have already been in contact with tumor cells. TILs are then returned to the patient by transfusion, together with IL-2. A preparative lymphocyte depletion treatment is administered to patients. About 34% of patients with advanced melanoma receiving TIL treatment had partial or complete tumor regression.

The limitations to ACT are:

1. The use an invasive procedure to obtain tissue for collecting TILs.

2. Tumors may not be readily accessible and the obtention of specimens can increase the risk of postoperative morbidity.

3. A difficulty of the TIL procedure is the isolation of sufficient number of TILs from all tumor specimens for ACT.

4. Another obstacle is the **cytokine release syndrome** following ACT, consisting in the sudden and massive secretion of IL-6 by T cells and macrophages into the blood circulation, that cause high fever and rapid drop in blood pressure.

These limitations have been confronted by modifying genes of any lymphocyte harvested from peripheral blood to induce the expression of required T cell receptors (TCR) or chimeric antigen receptors (CARs) that can recognize cancer cell antigens (thus bypassing the HLA-restriction encountered by TCRs in some patients).

A CAR is constructed by fusion of the intracellular signaling domain of TCR with an extracellular antigen-binding domain to enable cytolytic T cells to recognize and destroy the tumor cell bearing the intended tumor antigen.

• Organization of the immune-lymphatic system. The lymphatic system consists of primary and secondary lymphoid organs.

The primary lymphoid organs are the bone marrow and the thymus.

The secondary lymphoid organs include the lymph nodes, the spleen, the tonsils, and aggregates of lymphoid tissue in several organs, in particular Peyer's patches in the digestive tract (called gut-associated lymphoid tissue [GALT]) and in the lungs (called bronchial-associated lymphoid tissue [BALT]).

• The main function of the immune-lymphatic system is to protect the body against pathogens or antigens (bacteria, virus, and parasites). The basis for this defense mechanism, or immune response, is the ability to distinguish between self-antigens and non-self (foreign) antigens.

The two key cell components of the immune system are the lymphocytes and the accessory cells. Lymphocytes include two major groups:

(1) B cells, originated and differentiated in the bone marrow and responding to cell-bound or cell-free antigens.

(2) T cells, originated in the bone marrow, differentiated in the thymus, and responding to cell-bound antigens.

Accessory cells include the monocyte-derived cells: macrophages and dendritic cells. The follicular dendritic cells, present in lymphatic nodules in lymph nodes, do not derive from bone marrow.

• There are two types of immunity:

(1) Innate or natural immunity. This form of immunity, which does not require previous exposure to a pathogen or antigen, involves the epithelial barriers, phagocytic cells (macrophages and neutrophils), natural killer cells, and proteins of the complement system (synthesized by hepatocytes).

(2) Adaptive or acquired immunity. This form of immunity, which does require previous exposure to a pathogen or antigen, can be mediated by antibodies produced by plasma cells (humoral immunity), or requires the uptake of a pathogen by an antigen-presenting cell interacting with T cells and B cells (cell-mediated or cellular immunity).

Passive immunity is a temporary form of immunity provided by immunoglobulins produced by another individual in response to an exposure to a pathogen or antigen. Active immunity is a permanent form of immunity developed by an individual after direct exposure to a pathogen or antigen. Adaptive or acquired immunity has the following characteristics:

(1) It is specific for an antigen.

(2) It is diverse, because responding cells can detect several regions of the same antigen.

(3) It produces memory cells after the first encounter with the antigen. Memory cells can react more rapidly when the same antigen reappears.

(4) The immune response has a self-limitation; it stops when the antigen is neutralized or eliminated.

(5) The immune response has tolerance for self-antigens. A lack of tolerance results in autoimmune diseases.

• B cells originate and mature in the bone marrow. Under the influence of interleukin-7 (produced by stromal cells of the marrow), a pro–B cell gives rise to a pre–B cell. Pre–B cells give rise to immature B cells, which are released into the bloodstream as mature B cells. Maturation includes the expression of cell receptors with the purpose of recognizing and binding self-antigens. B cells that bind strongly to a self-antigen are eliminated by apoptosis. A less strong binding enables the B cell to survive, complete its maturation, and be released into the bloodstream.

• The presentation of antigens by macrophages (called antigen-presenting cells) to T cells is the basis of cell-mediated immunity, and the mechanism of clonal selection of immunocompetent T cells in the thymus. In the mouse, the presentation of antigens is carried out by a cell surface protein complex called major histocompatibility complex (MHC). The MHC-equivalent in humans is called human leukocyte antigen (HLA).

There are two types of MHC molecules:

(1) Class I MHC (formed by two polypeptide chains, α chain and β_2-microglobulin).

(2) Class II MHC (consisting of two polypeptide chains, α chain and β chain).

The coreceptor CD8, present on the surface of cytolytic T cells, binds to class I MHC; the coreceptor CD4, present on the surface of helper T cells, binds to class II MHC.

In humans, the class I MHC-equivalents consist of three variants, designated HLA-A, HLA-B, and HLA-C.

The class II MHC-equivalents also consist of three variants, designated HLA-DR, HLA-DQ, and HLA-DP.

• In addition to coreceptors, members of the immunoglobulin superfamily, T cells have a TCR (T cell receptor) complex on their surface.

Antigen recognition requires the participation of three components:

(1) Class I or II MHC.

(2) TCR.

(3) Coreceptor CD4 or CD8.

The TCR consists of two chains: α and β chains. Each chain has a variable domain (Vα and Vβ) and a constant domain (Cα and Cβ). The rearrangement at random of gene segments encoding the TCR enables recognition of different regions of a foreign (non-self) antigen.

• The maturation of bone marrow–derived thymocytes in the thymus requires recognition by maturing T cells of class I MHC and class II MHC, present on the surface of thymic epithelial cells, as well as an exposure to self-antigens and non-self (foreign) antigens.

Maturation requires the expression of TCR and coreceptors CD4 and CD8 on the surface of the maturing T cells undergoing a selection process. These molecule are the bases of clonal selection and clonal deletion.

During the maturation process, thymocytes arrive at the thymus without coreceptors or TCR on their surface (they are "double-negative" cells). As the maturation process advances, they express TCR and CD4 and CD8 coreceptors ("double-positive" cells). Finally, they become "single-positive" cells (CD4+ or CD8+).

During the maturation process, T cells must be MHC-restricted, tolerant to self-antigens, and bind to non-self antigens to undergo clonal selection.

T cells that do not bind to MHC or bind to a self-antigen undergo clonal deletion (they are discarded by apoptosis).

The final test takes place in the medullary region of the thymus, where thymic epithelial cells, regulated by the transcription factor aire, express a number of self-antigens that are sampled by the maturing T cells.

Mutations of the aire gene are associated with the human autosomal disorder autoimmune polyendocrinopathy–candidiasis–ectodermal dystrophy (APECED), also known as polyendocrine syndrome type-1, (APS-1). Autoreactive T cells are exported to the periphery and determine a number of autoimmune diseases.

• CD4+ Helper T cells, CD8+ cytolytic T cells, and CD56+ natural killer cells.

There are two subsets of helper T cells:

(1) TH1 cells, involved in reactions caused by intracellular pathogens.

(2) TH2 cells, involved in reactions caused by parasites.

After exposure to a fragment of an antigen presented by an antigen-presenting cell, the population of T cells expands by mitosis and recruits B cells. The population of B cells, under the influence of T cells, expands by mitosis.

Some of the B cells become memory cells; others differentiate into plasma cells, which secrete immunoglobulins to neutralize an extracellular antigen.

Helper T cells are targets of HIV-type 1 infection and the cause of the acquired immunodeficiency syndrome (AIDS).

An antigen-presenting cell can recruit a CD8+ cytolytic T cell (CTL), which undergoes mitotic expansion. The cytolytic T cell can bind to an antigen-presenting cell (for example, infected with a virus) and cause its destruction by the release of the pore-forming protein perforin, granzyme proteases, and Fas ligand to induce apoptosis of the affected cell.

CD8+ natural killer (NK) cells, which do not belong to the T cell and B cell types, are not activated by antigens—as helper and cytolytic cells are—and lack TCR. NK cells are activated in response to interferons or macrophage-derived cytokines.

NK cells express CD56, inhibitory and activating surface receptors, and abundant cytoplasmic granules containing perforin. NK cells are activated when the inhibitory receptor fails to be neutralized by class I MHC not expressed by tumor cells or virus infected cells. Activated NK cells respond by releasing perforin toward the target cell and secreting cytokines to activate macrophages.

• **Hypersensitivity** is a distinct immune response causing harmful host reactions rather than protection against a pathogen. There are four types of hypersensitivity reactions:

(1) Type 1 hypersensitivity, involving IgE and allergens leading to the degranulation of mast cells or basophils.

(2) Type 2 hypersensitivity reactions are caused by antibodies directed against plasma membrane-bound antigens resulting in cytolysis. Examples are autoimmune hemolytic anemia and Rh incompatibility leading to erythroblastosis fetalis.

(3) Type 3 hypersensitivity is determined by the formation of soluble antigen-antibody complexes that activate the complement system. An example is the Arthus reaction in response to intradermal injection of antigen.

(4) Type 4 hypersensitivity, also called delayed hypersensitivity, involves antigen–T cell–macrophage interactions determining the formation of a granuloma. The Mantoux reaction in the tuberculin skin test is a classic delayed hypersensitivity reaction.

• The **complement system** enables the destruction of pathogens by a mechanism known as opsonization. Proteins of the complement system, most of them produced by hepatocytes, "complement" the effect of antibodies, mannose-binding lectin, and spontaneous activation of C3. A number of complement proteins construct a membrane attack complex (MAC) to induce the lysis of infected cells.

Complement regulators (CRegs) modulate the activity of the complement cascade to protect unintended bystanders. The CReg CD59 is particularly important because it prevents the final assembly of MAC.

Paroxysmal nocturnal hemoglobinuria is caused by the destruction of red blood cells lacking CD59. Unprotected red blood cells are destroyed by the complement cascade.

• **Acute inflammation** is the initial non-specific reaction to tissue damage. If the damage persists and the destruction of the tissue (necrosis) continues, an immune response develops with the characteristics of chronic inflammation.

Two events define the pathogenesis of acute inflammation:

(1) **Responses of the microvasculature to injury.** Vasodilation allows increased blood flow into the damaged tissue (a condition called **hyperemia**).

Enhanced vascular permeability of capillar-

ies and venules results in the accumulation of fluid, or **exudate**, in the interstitial space, leading to tissue swelling.

An exudate is interstitial fluid with high protein content, in particular fibrin. Fibrin derives from fibrinogen. Fibrinogen is cleaved by thrombin into fibrinopeptides and fibrin monomers that are then assembled to form a fibrin meshwork.

A **transudate** is interstitial fluid with low protein content. An **effusion** is excess of fluid in body cavities (peritoneum, pleura and pericardium).

These microvasculature events are represented by the four classical clinical signs:

(1) Rubor (redness).
(2) Tumor (swelling).
(3) Calor (heat).
(4) Dolor (pain).

Hyperemia is responsible for the first three signs. Pain is determined by released specific local mediators and fluid compression of nerve endings.

(2) **Recruitment of neutrophils to the injury site.** Chemotactic factors produced by resident macrophages recruit neutrophils from circulating blood into the injured tissue. Neutrophils can eliminate pathogens by several mechanisms:

(1) Phagocytosis, involving antibacterial proteins released from cytoplasmic granules into phagosomes.

(2) Release of neutrophil extracellular traps (NETs), to trap pathogens to prevent spreading and facilitate subsequent phagocytosis. A NET consists of a core of DNA-histones and attached enzymes released from azurophilic and specific granules.

(3) Degranulation, to kill pathogens directly. Protease-like proteins and enzymes responsible for the production of reactive oxygen species, contained in cytoplasmic granules, have the capacity of direct killing or incapacitate microorganisms.

The resolution of acute inflammation pursues two objectives:

(1) The protection of the host from excessive tissue damage.

(2) To prevent amplification of acute inflammatory responses toward chronic inflammation.

Resolution of acute inflammation encompasses an anti-inflammatory phase and a pro-resolving phase.

(1) Anti-inflammatory phase: anti-inflammatory mediators (such as IL-10), are released. In addition, the pro-inflammatory activity of the nuclear factor (NF)-κB pathway is down regulated.

(2) Pro-resolving phase: It involves a switch of the pro-inflammatory activities of neutrophils and macrophages to anti-inflammatory activities. Neutrophils produce pro-resolving mediators, including protectins; macrophages secrete maresins (from macrophage mediator in resolving inflammation).

Healing and tissue repair are stimulated by combining the effects of the anti-inflammatory and pro-resolving phases.

Healing involves the formation of granulation tissue. The damaged tissue is replaced new capillaries (angiogenesis), macrophages and fibroblasts resulting in the organization of fibrovascular granulation tissue.

The bottom line: the fibrin-containing exudate is being replaced first by granulation tissue and subsequently by a fibrous scar by a process called fibrous repair.

There are three types of acute inflammation, based on the type of exudate or effusion:

(1) Suppurative acute inflammation, when neutrophils and debris of dead cells predominate and the affected tissue is liquefied by neutrophil-derived proteolytic enzymes to produce pus. Specific bacteria produce suppurative acute inflammation that can evolve into a pustule (at the skin surface) or an abscess, an enclosed collection of purulent tissue. Bacteria producing localized suppuration are called pyogenic (pus-producing).

(2) Fibrinous acute inflammation, when fibrin is the predominate component of the fluid or effusion deposited on the surface of the meninges, peritoneum, pleura and pericardium.

(3) Serous acute inflammation, when plasma-derived fluid has a low protein content.

The persistence of tissue damage caused by a pathogen can determine **chronic inflammation**, a process in which tissue necrosis and repair are simultaneous and persistent for many years.

In certain diseases, the granuloma is the hallmark of chronic inflammation, a structural pattern that defines granulomatous inflammation. As part of granulomas, macrophages acquire an epithelial-like pattern and fuse to form multinucleated giant cells.

A **granuloma** consists of a typical central necrotic zone surrounded by a la zone of activated epithelial-like macrophages coexisting with multinucleated giant cells. Surrounding the macrophage-containing zone are lymphocytes (CD4+ T cells) and then a limiting fibroblast-collagen zone establishing a capsule-like boundary with the surrounding tissue.

The characteristics of the central zone of a granuloma depends on the pathogen. For example, the tuberculous granuloma has a central caseation soft cheese-like mass zone surrounded by scattered multinucleated giant cells called Langhans' cells. The sarcoidosis granuloma, displays a fibrosis center and the multinucleated giant cells may contain calcified spherical deposits, called Schaumann bodies.

• **Lymph nodes**. The main function of lymph nodes is the filtration of the lymph. A lymph node is surrounded by a connective tissue capsule that sends partitions (trabeculae) inside the lymph node. The stroma of the lymph node consists of a three-dimensional network of reticular fibers (type III collagen). The convex side of the lymph node is the

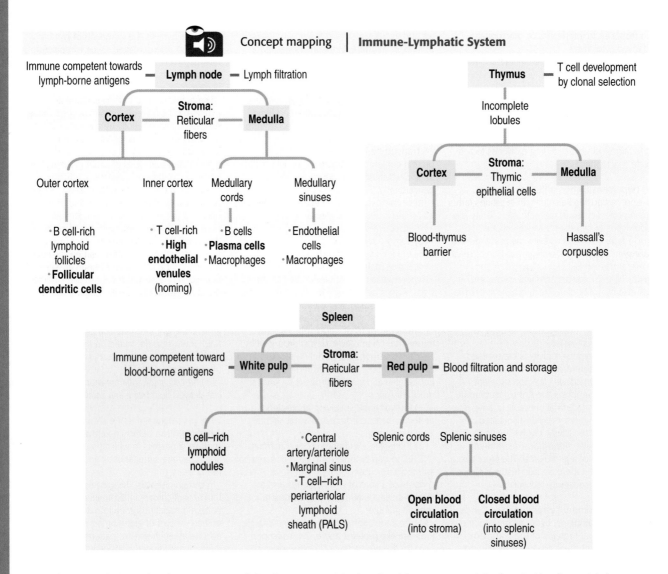

Immune competent towards lymph-borne antigens — **Lymph node** — Lymph filtration

Cortex — **Stroma:** Reticular fibers — **Medulla**

Outer cortex — Inner cortex — Medullary cords — Medullary sinuses

- B cell-rich lymphoid follicles
- **Follicular dendritic cells**

- T cell-rich
- **High endothelial venules** (homing)

- B cells
- **Plasma cells**
- Macrophages

- Endothelial cells
- Macrophages

Thymus — T cell development by clonal selection

Incomplete lobules

Cortex — **Stroma:** Thymic epithelial cells — **Medulla**

Blood-thymus barrier

Hassall's corpuscles

Spleen

Immune competent toward blood-borne antigens — **White pulp** — **Stroma:** Reticular fibers — **Red pulp** — Blood filtration and storage

B cell–rich lymphoid nodules

- Central artery/arteriole
- Marginal sinus
- T cell–rich periarteriolar lymphoid sheath (PALS)

Splenic cords Splenic sinuses

Open blood circulation (into stroma) **Closed blood circulation** (into splenic sinuses)

entry side of several afferent lymphatic vessels with valves. Lymph percolates through the subcapsular sinus and the paratrabecular sinus. The concave side of the lymph node is the hilum, the site where an artery enters the lymph node and vein and efferent lymphatic vessel drain the structure.

The lymph node consists of:
(1) A cortex.
(2) A medulla.

The cortex is subdivided into an outer cortex, where B cell–containing lymphatic nodules are present, and a deep cortex, where T cells (CD4[+]) predominate.

A lymphatic nodule or follicle consists of a mantle (facing the capsule) and a germinal center, containing proliferating B cells interacting with follicular dendritic cells (FDCs). Macrophages are also present. Macrophages take up particulate matter from the lymph as well as opsonized antigens and also phagocytose apoptotic B cells. FDCs have an antigen-presenting function. B and T cells reach the lymph node through the postcapillary venules present in the inner cortex.

The medulla contains medullary cords, housing B cells, plasma cells, and macrophages, separated by medullary sinuses, endothelial

cell–lined spaces containing lymph arriving from the cortical region of the node. Large blood vessels are present in the medulla close to the hilum.

Acute lymphadenitis is seen when an acute immune reaction occurs in response to locally drained bacteria. Local lymph nodes enlarge and become painful because of the distention of the capsule by cellular proliferation and edema.

Lymphomas are tumors of the lymphoid tissue. Most of the lymphomas are of B cell origin (80%); the remainder are of T cell origin. Lymphomas include Hodgkin's lymphoma and non-Hodgkin's lymphomas.

• **Thymus.** The main function of the thymus is the production of T cells from thymocytes derived from bone marrow.

The thymus derives from the endodermic third pharyngeal pouch (also the site of origin of the inferior parathyroid gland). The thymus is surrounded by a connective tissue capsule projecting trabeculae inside the tissue. Blood vessels are present in the trabeculae and capsule.

The thymus consists of several incomplete lobules. Each lobule has a complete cortex and

a medulla shared with adjacent lobules. Two important features are:
(1) The lack of lymphatic nodules in the cortex.
(2) The presence of Hassall's corpuscles in the medulla.

Two relevant functional characteristics are the blood-thymus barrier, present in the cortex of the thymus, and postcapillary venules at the corticomedullary junction.

The stroma of the thymus consists of a three-dimensional network of thymic epithelial cells (TECs) interconnected by desmosomes. TECs derive from a common precursor, which gives rise to thymic cortical and medullary epithelial cells when the transcription factor Foxn1 is active. Inactivation of the *Foxn1* gene prevents the development of the thymus, resulting in the failure of T cell development leading to a **congenital immunodeficiency**.

Cortical TECs express on their surface MHC molecules required for clonal selection. Medullary TECs, activated by the *aire* gene, express self-proteins necessary for clonal deletion of autoreactive T cells. Mutations in the *aire* gene cause a number of autoimmune diseases (including autoimmune polyendocrinopathy–candidiasis–ectodermal dystrophy [APECED], also known as autoimmune polyendocrine type-1 [APS-1]) because autoreactive T cells can reach several organs and tissues.

• **Spleen**. The spleen has a dual function:

(1) The **white pulp** is the immune component of the spleen; components of the white pulp detect and react to blood-borne antigens.

(2) The **red pulp** is a filter that removes aged and damaged red blood cells and microorganisms from circulating blood.

The spleen is covered by a capsule consisting of dense, irregular connective tissue with elastic and smooth muscle fibers.

The capsule gives raise to trabeculae that carry blood vessels (trabecular arteries and veins) and nerves.

The splenic artery enters the hilum, giving rise to trabecular arteries. As an artery leaves the trabecula, it becomes invested by a sheath of T cells forming a periarteriolar lymphoid sheath (PALS) and penetrates a lymphatic nodule (the white pulp). The blood vessel is designated central artery or follicular arteriole, because of the follicular-like arrangement of the white pulp.

A marginal sinus zone, between the red and white pulps, receives radial arterioles from the central artery or arteriole.

The central artery leaves the white pulp to become the penicillar artery. Penicillar arteries end as macrophage-sheathed capillaries. Terminal capillaries either drain directly into splenic sinusoids (closed circulation) or terminate as open-ended vessels within the red pulp (open circulation). Splenic sinusoids are drained by pulp veins, to trabecular veins, to splenic veins.

As you can see, there are two types of blood circulation in spleen:

(1) Open circulation, in which red blood cells enter the red pulp spaces.

(2) Closed circulation, in which arterial vessels are continuous with the splenic sinusoids.

• The spleen has distinctive structural features that you should remember:

(1) It lacks a cortex and a medulla.

(2) Similar to the lymph node, the white pulp is a lymphatic nodule-like equivalent: it has a germinal center, a mantle populated by B cells, and antigen-presenting cells. Contrary to the lymphatic nodule that handles lymph, the white pulp has an artery/arteriole surrounded by T cells, the PALS. Consequently, the white pulp is populated by the immune cells required to trap and process blood-borne antigens.

(3) The red pulp has two components involved in blood filtration and clearance of aged red blood cells:

The splenic sinuses are formed by rod-shaped endothelial cells separated by narrow slits that allow the passage of cells.

They are surrounded by an incomplete basal lamina and loose reticular fibers. Therefore, blood cell inside-out trafficking is facilitated by the interendothelial cell slits and the loose stroma.

The splenic cords separate splenic sinuses. They contain macrophages, plasma cells, and blood cells. In fact, macrophages in spleen start the recycling of hemoglobin of scavenged red blood cells resulting in the production of bilirubin.

Asplenia, the lack of spleen, includes patients with:

(1) Surgical asplenia, performed in healthy individuals after trauma or in patients with hematologic (for example, hereditary spherocytosis, β-thalassemia, and sickle cell disease), immunologic (for example, immune thrombocytopenic purpura) or tumoral (spleen lymphoma) conditions.

(2) Functional asplenia, observed in patients with sickle cell anemia following multiple episodes of spleen autoinfarction.

(3) Congenital asplenia, a rare observation that can be isolated or associated with other abnormalities such as congenital heart disease (Ivemak syndrome).

11. Integumentary System

The skin is the primary barrier between the body and the environment. It provides a line of defense against microbial pathogens and physical and chemicals agents. Skin integrity requires active defense mechanisms provided by dendritic cells, members of the immune system, and the resident keratinocytes, to discriminate between harmless commensal organisms and harmful pathogens. Many infectious and immunologic diseases produce characteristic skin changes leading to a correct diagnosis. In addition, the skin has diseases peculiar to itself. The skin is of particular significance in clinical physical examination. For example, the color of the skin may indicate the existence of a pathologic condition: a yellow color indicates jaundice; a blue-gray color may indicate cyanosis, reflecting a pathologic condition of cardiovascular and respiratory function; a pale color is indicative of anemia; lack of skin pigmentation suggests albinism. This chapter describes the organization of the skin and epidermal derivatives as well inflammatory and tumoral conditions.

General organization and types of skin

The integument is the largest organ of the body. It consists of two components:

1. The **skin**.
2. The **epidermal derivatives**, such as nails, hair, and glands (sweat and sebaceous glands and the mammary gland).

The skin has several **functions**:

1. **Protection from injury** (mechanical function).
2. As a **water barrier** to prevent dehydration.
3. **Regulation of body temperature** (conservation and dissipation of heat).
4. **Nonspecific defense** (barrier to microorganisms and housing of immunocompetent dendritic cells).
5. **Excretion of salts.**
6. **Synthesis of vitamin D.**
7. As a **sensory organ.**
8. **Sexual signaling.**

The skin consists of three layers firmly attached to one another:

1. The outer **epidermis**, derived from ectoderm.
2. The deeper **dermis**, derived from mesoderm.
3. The **hypodermis** or **subcutaneous layer**, corresponding to the **superficial fascia** of gross anatomy.

Skin is generally classified into two types:

1. **Thick skin.**
2. **Thin skin.**

Thick skin (more than 5 mm thick) covers the palms of the hands and the soles of the feet and has a thick epidermis and dermis. Thin skin (1 to 2 mm in thickness) lines the rest of the body; the epidermis is thin.

The surface of the skin of the palms and soles and digits of the hands and feet has narrow **epidermal ridges** separated by **furrows** (Figure 11-1). Impressions of the ridges create **fingerprint** patterns, useful for forensic identification.

Each epidermal ridge follows the outline of an underlying **dermal ridge**. A downgrowth of the epidermal ridge splits the **dermal ridge** into two **secondary dermal ridges or dermal papillae**. Consequently, the epidermal ridge downgrowth is designated **interpapillary peg**. As discussed later, the excretory ducts of the sweat glands in the skin open through the top of the interpapillary pegs.

Through this arrangement, the epidermis and dermis have a tight fit interface at the dermal-epidermal junction, stabilized by hemidesmosomes anchored to the basal lamina.

Epidermis

We start by presenting an outline of the general organization of the epidermis and its major cell components that serves as an orientation for a more detailed discussion.

The **stratified squamous epithelial layer** of the epidermis consists of four distinct cell types (Figures 11-2 and 11-3):

1. **Keratinocytes** are the predominant cell type, so called because its major product is **keratin**, an intermediate filament protein.
2. **Melanocytes** are neural crest–derived cells responsible for the production of **melanin** (see Figure 11-3).
3. **Langerhans cells** are resident dendritic cells derived from a bone marrow precursor, acting as antigen-trapping cells interacting with CD8+ T cells.
4. **Merkel cells** are neural crest–derived cells involved in tactile sensation.

Keratinocytes are arranged in **five layers** or **strata**:

1. The **stratum basale** (basal cell layer).
2. The **stratum spinosum** (spinous or prickle cell layer).
3. The **stratum granulosum** (granular cell layer).
4. The **stratum lucidum** (clear cell layer).
5. The **stratum corneum** (cornified cell layer).

The first cell layers consist of metabolically active cells. The cells of the last two layers undergo kera-

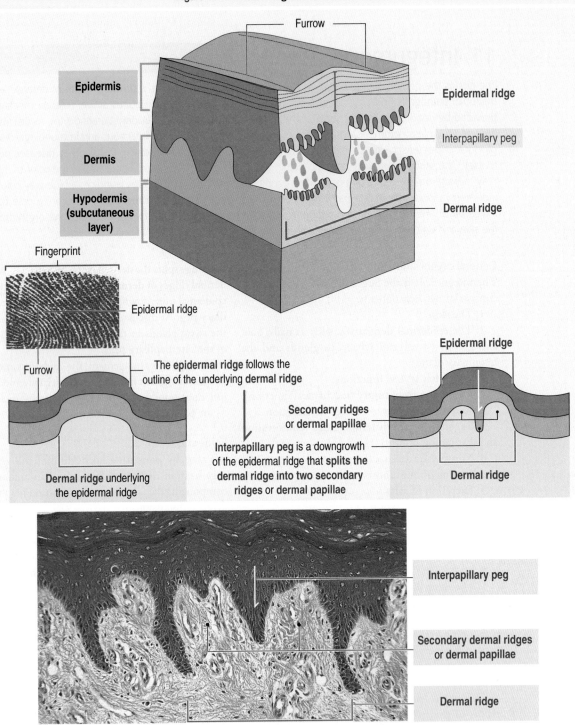

Figure 11-1. **General organization of the skin**

Furrow

Epidermis

Epidermal ridge

Interpapillary peg

Dermis

Hypodermis (subcutaneous layer)

Dermal ridge

Fingerprint

Epidermal ridge

Furrow

The **epidermal ridge** follows the outline of the underlying **dermal ridge**

Epidermal ridge

Secondary ridges or **dermal papillae**

Dermal ridge underlying the epidermal ridge

Interpapillary peg is a downgrowth of the epidermal ridge that splits the dermal ridge into two secondary ridges or dermal papillae

Dermal ridge

Interpapillary peg

Secondary dermal ridges or dermal papillae

Dermal ridge

tinization, or **cornification**, a process that involves cellular and intercellular molecular changes. The stratum basale and stratum spinosum form the **stratum of Malpighi**.

The **stratum basale** (or **stratum germinativum**) consists of a single layer of columnar or high cuboidal keratinocytes resting on a basement membrane. **Hemidesmosomes** and associated intermediate filaments anchor the basal domain of basal cells to the

basement membrane.

The cells of the stratum basale maintain the equilibrium between cell differentiation and mitotic cell division as well as the repair of damage. While some of the dividing cells add to the population of **stem cells** of the stratum basale, others migrate into the stratum spinosum, change from columnar or high cuboidal to become polygonal in shape and initiate the differentiation process by starting the synthesis of keratins

Figure 11-2. Layers of the epidermis of thick skin

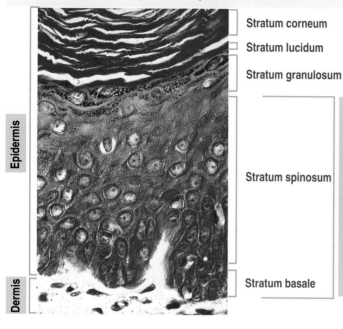

- Stratum corneum
- Stratum lucidum
- Stratum granulosum
- Stratum spinosum — Stratum of Malpighi
- Stratum basale

Epidermis

Dermis

that are distinct from the basal cells. The cytoplasm contains intermediate filaments associated with **desmosomes**. Bundles of intermediate filaments, visible under the light microscope, are called **tonofilaments**.

Keratinocytes in the stratum granulosum display dark clusters of cytoplasmic material, keratins and lipids. The stratum corneum, consisting terminally maturing keratinocytes, is the outermost layer of the epidermis and responsible for the barrier function of the skin. The barrier excludes many toxic agents and prevents dehydration.

General Pathology: Wound healing

Skin is an efficient protective barrier against external aggressions. If a portion of epidermis is damaged or destroyed, it must be repaired rapidly by a sequential mechanism called **wound healing** (Figure 11-4).

A damage recognition and repair mechanism consist of four stages:

1. **Coagulation** (the formation of a fibrin-platelet clot).

Figure 11-3. Immigrant cells in the epidermis

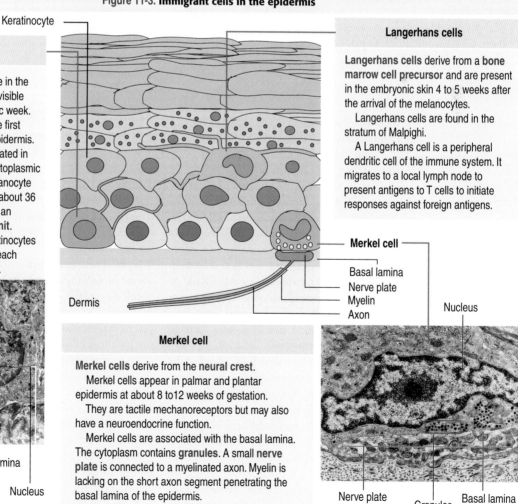

Keratinocyte

Melanocyte

Melanocytes originate in the **neural crest** and are visible from the 8th embryonic week.

Melanocytes are the first cells to arrive in the epidermis.

The cell body is located in the stratum basale. Cytoplasmic extensions of one melanocyte establish contact with about 36 keratinocytes, forming an **epidermal-melanin unit**. Melanocytes and keratinocytes are not associated to each other by desmosomes.

Langerhans cells

Langerhans cells derive from a **bone marrow cell precursor** and are present in the embryonic skin 4 to 5 weeks after the arrival of the melanocytes.

Langerhans cells are found in the stratum of Malpighi.

A Langerhans cell is a peripheral dendritic cell of the immune system. It migrates to a local lymph node to present antigens to T cells to initiate responses against foreign antigens.

Merkel cell
- Basal lamina
- Nerve plate
- Myelin
- Axon

Dermis

Merkel cell

Merkel cells derive from the **neural crest**.

Merkel cells appear in palmar and plantar epidermis at about 8 to 12 weeks of gestation.

They are tactile mechanoreceptors but may also have a neuroendocrine function.

Merkel cells are associated with the basal lamina. The cytoplasm contains **granules**. A small **nerve plate** is connected to a myelinated axon. Myelin is lacking on the short axon segment penetrating the basal lamina of the epidermis.

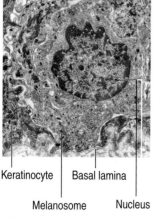

Keratinocyte   Basal lamina

Melanosome   Nucleus

Electron micrograph from Gray's Anatomy, 38th edition, New York, Churchill Livingstone, 1995.

Nucleus

Nerve plate   Granules   Basal lamina

Electron micrograph courtesy of Patricia C. Cross, Stanford, CA

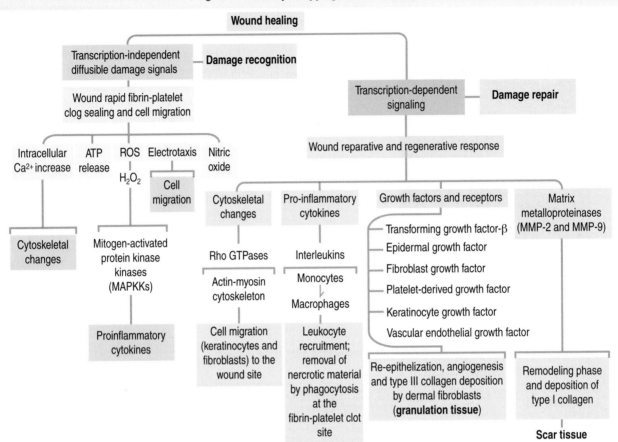

Figure 11-4. **Concept Mapping: Wound healing**

2. **Inflammation** (leukocyte recruitment).

3. **Proliferation** (neovascularization and formation of granulation tissue).

4. **Remodeling and resolution.**

Immediately following injury, **transcription-independent diffusible damage signals** are in place in the form of intracellular **Ca²⁺ increases, ATP release, H₂O₂, electrotaxis** (cell migration toward injury site triggered by electric stimuli) **and nitric oxide production** to induce cytoskeletal changes and activation of mitogen-activated kinase kinases (MAPKKs) to activate the release of proinflammatory cytokines (see Figure 11-4). Although fast and strong, immediate transcription-independent signaling, as a **damage recognition step**, is not precise.

Transcription-dependent signaling, aimed at the formation of temporary **granulation tissue**, initiates the **damage repair step**. Wound healing starts with the formation of a **blood clot** covering temporarily the open wound. As you recall, the blood clot consists of platelets embedded in a fibrous mesh of cross-linked fibrin molecules formed when thrombin cleaves fibrinogen.

Platelets contain platelet-derived growth factor (PDGF) stored in alpha granules. PDGF and other growth factors are released when platelets degranulate

before leukocytes arrive at the wound site. At the same time, vessel constriction occurs to limit blood loss.

While clot formation takes place, keratinocytes and endothelial cells start **transcription-dependent damage signaling** by expressing **cytokine CXC** (for cysteine-x-cysteine) and **CXC receptor**, which recruit neutrophils and monocytes to the wound site. A deletion of *CXC receptor* gene results in **delayed wound healing**.

Neutrophils arrive within minutes of injury and release proinflammatory cytokines to activate local fibroblasts in the dermis and keratinocytes in the epidermis. Next, monocytes are recruited and become **macrophages**, that produce cytokines and phagocytize pathogens and necrotic material.

Re-epithelialization starts when keratinocytes of the stratum basale layer migrate from the edges of the wound by the formation of F-actin–containing lamellopodia. This cell migratory response requires the activation and increased expression of **wound response genes**, including several cytoskeletal regulators (Rho GTPases) and calcium voltage channels to increase calcium influx to promote changes in the actin cytoskeleton.

As part of the wound response gene machinery, fibroblasts migrate from the adjacent tissue and lay

Figure 11-5. **Psoriasis**

Psoriasis is a chronic, immune-mediated inflammatory epidermal-dermal disease characterized by:
1. Persistent hyperplasia of the epidermis by abnormal cell proliferation and differentiation. Keratinocytes move from the basal layer to the superficial layer in 3 to 5 days, instead of the 28 to 30 days in normal skin. The stratum granulosum may be absent.
2. Abnormal angiogenesis in the dermis capillary plexus. Blood vessels are dilated and convoluted.
3. Infiltration of inflammatory cells in the epidermis and dermis, in particular activated TH17 cells. Neutrophils migrate to the epidermis and form microabscesses.

Thickening of the stratum corneum

Microabscess in the epidermis

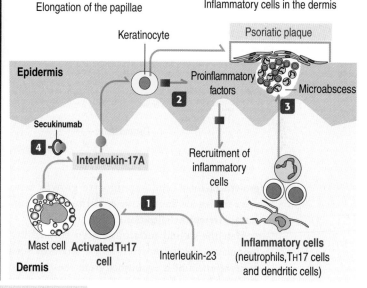

Elongation of the papillae

Inflammatory cells in the dermis

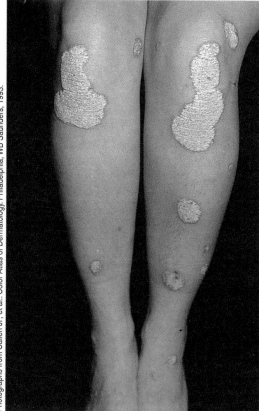

Photographs from Callen JP, et al.: Color Atlas of Dermatology. Philadelphia, WB Saunders, 1993.

Pathogenesis of psoriatic plaques

1 **Type 17 helper (TH17) cells** in the presence of interleukin-23, become activated and produce interleukin-17A (**IL-17A**). **Mast cells** also produce IL-17A.
2 IL-17A stimulates keratinocytes to modify their cell differentiation program (resulting in psoriatic plaques) and produce proinflammatory factors including antimicrobial peptides and chemokines (including CCL20), that recruit inflammatory cells (neutrophils, TH17 cells and dendritic cells).
3 Inflammatory cells produce chronically developing microabscesses and psoriatic plaques and secrete cytokines at sites of cutaneous inflammation.
4 **Secukinumab**, a human immunoglobulin G1κ monoclonal antibody, binds and neutralizes IL-17A, breaking the pathogenic cycle.

down type III collagen and other extracellular matrix proteins. New blood vessels develop (**angiogenic response** marked by vascular endothelial growth factor) and organize **granulation tissue**. The pink granular appearance of the granulation tissue is determined by

the formation of numerous blood capillaries.

Leading edge keratinocytes facilitate their displacement by disrupting hemidesmosome attachment to the basal lamina and by dissolving the fibrin clot barrier. To accomplish the dissolution of the fibrin clot, keratinocytes up-regulate the expression of **plasminogen activator** to convert **plasminogen** within the clot into the fibrinolytic enzyme **plasmin**.

Keratinocytes become free from hemidesmosome anchorage with the help of members of the **matrix metalloproteinase family** (MMP-2 and MMP-9) and downregulation of the tissue inhibitors of metalloproteinases, TIMP-1 and TIMP-2, produced by fibroblasts in the dermis. We discuss MMPs and TIMPs in Chapter 4, Connective Tissue.

Members of the **epidermal growth factor family** (including epidermal growth factor, transforming

Figure 11-6. Differentiation of keratinocytes: Expression of keratins

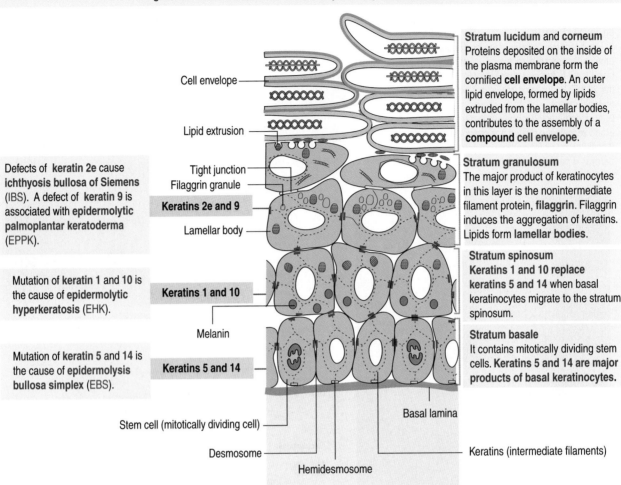

Stratum lucidum and **corneum**
Proteins deposited on the inside of the plasma membrane form the cornified **cell envelope**. An outer lipid envelope, formed by lipids extruded from the lamellar bodies, contributes to the assembly of a **compound** cell envelope.

Stratum granulosum
The major product of keratinocytes in this layer is the nonintermediate filament protein, **filaggrin**. Filaggrin induces the aggregation of keratins. Lipids form **lamellar bodies**.

Stratum spinosum
Keratins 1 and 10 replace keratins 5 and 14 when basal keratinocytes migrate to the stratum spinosum.

Stratum basale
It contains mitotically dividing stem cells. Keratins 5 and 14 are major products of basal keratinocytes.

Defects of **keratin 2e** cause **ichthyosis bullosa of Siemens** (IBS). A defect of **keratin 9** is associated with **epidermolytic palmoplantar keratoderma** (EPPK).

Mutation of **keratin 1 and 10** is the cause of **epidermolytic hyperkeratosis** (EHK).

Mutation of **keratin 5 and 14** is the cause of **epidermolysis bullosa simplex** (EBS).

Cell envelope
Lipid extrusion
Tight junction
Filaggrin granule
Keratins 2e and 9
Lamellar body
Keratins 1 and 10
Melanin
Keratins 5 and 14
Stem cell (mitotically dividing cell)
Desmosome
Hemidesmosome
Basal lamina
Keratins (intermediate filaments)

---

growth factor-β, and **keratinocyte growth factor** drive the regeneration of the epidermis on a wound surface (**re-epithelialization**).

After the wound surface has been covered by a monolayer of keratinocytes, a new stratified squamous epithelium is established from the margin of the wound toward the center. New hemidesmosomes are formed with the inactivation of matrix metalloproteinases.

Remodeling and resolution start within 3 to 4 days after the wound injury. The underlying connective tissue of the dermis contracts, bringing the wound margins toward one another. Macrophages, together with matrix metalloproteinases produced by fibroblasts, remove the granulation tissue and the alignment of type I collagen fibers promote the formation of **scar tissue**.

Stimulated by local levels of PDGF, fibroblast growth factor and transforming growth factor–β, dermal fibroblasts begin to proliferate, infiltrate the granulation tissue, and deposit type III collagen and extracellular matrix. About 1 week after wounding, a number of fibroblasts change into **myofibroblasts** (resembling smooth muscle cells), wound contraction

takes place, and healing with a scar occurs.

Retinol (**vitamin A**) is a precursor of **retinoic acid**, a hormone-like agent required for the differentiation of epithelia, including epidermis. Retinoids have a proliferative effect on the epidermis of normal skin. This effect is mediated at the messenger RNA (mRNA) level by inhibiting cell differentiation and stimulating cell proliferation.

Retinoic acid binds to **cellular retinoic acid binding** (**CRAB**) proteins, presumably involved in the regulation of the intracellular concentration of retinoic acid. Similar to steroid and thyroid hormones, retinoic acid binds to two types of nuclear receptors: **retinoic acid receptors** (**RARs**), and **rexinoid receptors** (**RXRs**).

The RAR/RXR heterodimer complex has binding affinity for **retinoic acid–responsive elements** (**RAREs**) on DNA and controls the expression of retinoic acid responsive genes. Retinoids are used in the prevention of acne scarring, psoriasis, and other scaling diseases of the skin.

Pathology: Psoriasis
Psoriasis is a chronic, immune-mediated inflammatory skin disorder. It is characterized by sharply

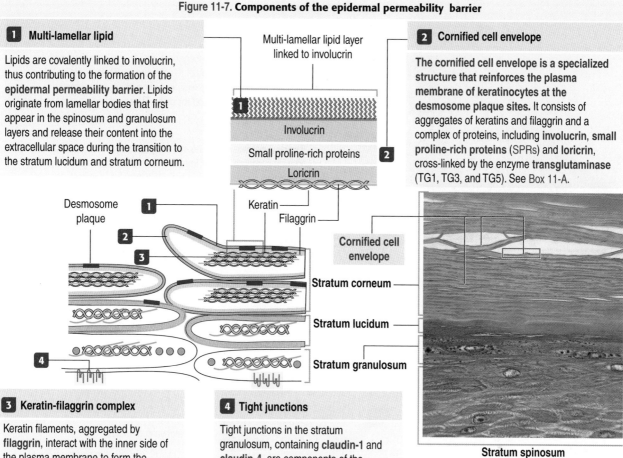

Figure 11-7. Components of the epidermal permeability barrier

1 Multi-lamellar lipid

Lipids are covalently linked to involucrin, thus contributing to the formation of the **epidermal permeability barrier**. Lipids originate from lamellar bodies that first appear in the spinosum and granulosum layers and release their content into the extracellular space during the transition to the stratum lucidum and stratum corneum.

Multi-lamellar lipid layer linked to involucrin

Involucrin

Small proline-rich proteins

Loricrin

Keratin

Filaggrin

Cornified cell envelope

2 Cornified cell envelope

The cornified cell envelope is a specialized structure that reinforces the plasma membrane of keratinocytes at the desmosome plaque sites. It consists of aggregates of keratins and filaggrin and a complex of proteins, including **involucrin, small proline-rich proteins** (SPRs) and **loricrin**, cross-linked by the enzyme **transglutaminase** (TG1, TG3, and TG5). See Box 11-A.

Desmosome plaque

Stratum corneum

Stratum lucidum

Stratum granulosum

Stratum spinosum

3 Keratin-filaggrin complex

Keratin filaments, aggregated by **filaggrin**, interact with the inner side of the plasma membrane to form the cornified cell envelope.

4 Tight junctions

Tight junctions in the stratum granulosum, containing **claudin-1** and **claudin-4**, are components of the permeability barrier.

---

demarcated plaques, called **psoriatic plaques**, covered by white scales commonly seen on the elbows, knees, scalp, umbilicus, and lumbar region. Physical trauma may produce psoriatic plaques at the sites of injury.

The histologic characteristics of the psoriatic plaque include (Figure 11-5):

1. **Excessive proliferation of epidermal keratinocytes** (caused by an accelerated migration of keratinocytes from the stratum basale to the stratum corneum).

2. Presence of inflammatory cells (in particular **type 17 helper T cells** [TH17], dendritic cells, and neutrophils) in the dermis and epidermis (**microabscesses**).

3. Elongation of epidermic papillae, and prominent **angiogenesis**.

Interleukin-23 activates TH17 **cells**. TH17 cells are distinct from the classic TH1 and TH2 subsets.

The proinflammatory cytokine **interleukin-17A (IL-17A)** is the primary effector of TH17 cells. IL-17A stimulates keratinocytes to secrete antimicrobial peptides, chemokines (including CCL20) and other proinflammatory proteins that recruit inflammatory cells, including TH17 cells, neutrophils and dendritic cells.

In addition, keratinocytes stimulated by IL-17A undergo persistent hyperplasia by abnormal cell proliferation and differentiation. Keratinocytes move from the basal layer to the superficial layer in 3 to 5 days, instead of the 28 to 30 days in normal skin. The stratum granulosum may be absent.

Treatment of psoriasis is targeted to the therapeutic inhibition of IL-17A. Secukinumab (Novartis Phar-

---

Box 11-A | Cornified cell envelope disorders

• About 50% of patients with lamellar **ichthyosis** (Greek *ichthys*, fish; *osis*, condition) carry mutations in the *transglutaminase-1* gene. Affected individuals display a collodion membrane (dryness and scaling of the skin seen at birth). This condition is caused by defective cross-linking of cornified cell envelope proteins.

• **Vohwinkel's syndrome** and progressive symmetric erythrokeratodermia are caused by defects in loricrin. Hyperkeratosis (increase in the thickness of the stratum corneum) of the palms and soles is observed.

• **X-linked ichthyosis** is an autosomal recessive disease associated with a lipid metabolic defect. Thick dark scales on the palms and soles, and corneal opacities, are caused by a defect in the enzyme steroid sulfatase. Accumulation of cholesterol sulfate in the extracellular space of the stratum corneum prevents desquamation and cross-linking of involucrin to the extracellular lipid layer. Cholesterol sulfate inhibits proteases involved in desquamation.

Figure 11-8. **Keratinocytes**

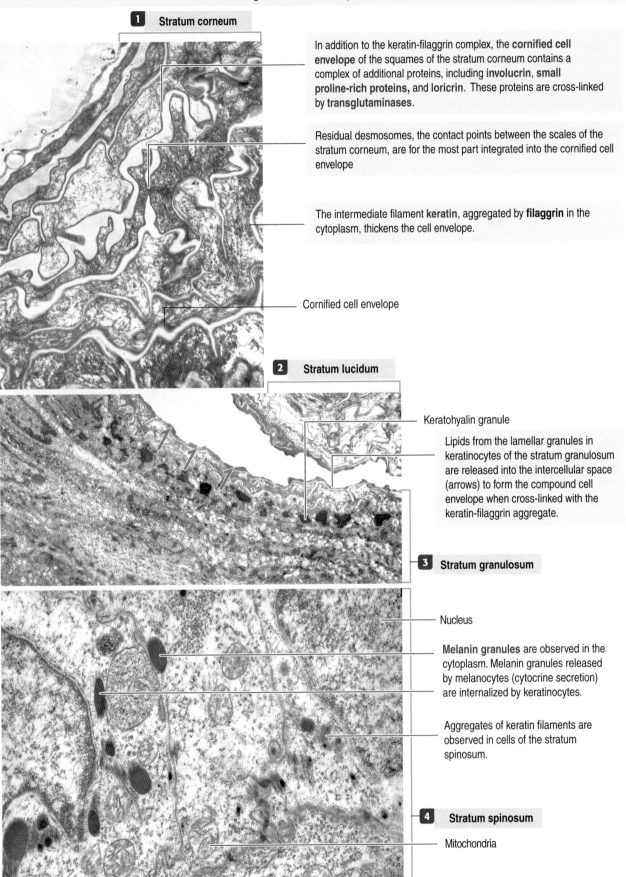

1 **Stratum corneum**

In addition to the keratin-filaggrin complex, the **cornified cell envelope** of the squames of the stratum corneum contains a complex of additional proteins, including **involucrin, small proline-rich proteins,** and **loricrin.** These proteins are cross-linked by **transglutaminases.**

Residual desmosomes, the contact points between the scales of the stratum corneum, are for the most part integrated into the cornified cell envelope

The intermediate filament **keratin**, aggregated by **filaggrin** in the cytoplasm, thickens the cell envelope.

Cornified cell envelope

2 **Stratum lucidum**

Keratohyalin granule

Lipids from the lamellar granules in keratinocytes of the stratum granulosum are released into the intercellular space (arrows) to form the compound cell envelope when cross-linked with the keratin-filaggrin aggregate.

3 **Stratum granulosum**

Nucleus

Melanin granules are observed in the cytoplasm. Melanin granules released by melanocytes (cytocrine secretion) are internalized by keratinocytes.

Aggregates of keratin filaments are observed in cells of the stratum spinosum.

4 **Stratum spinosum**

Mitochondria

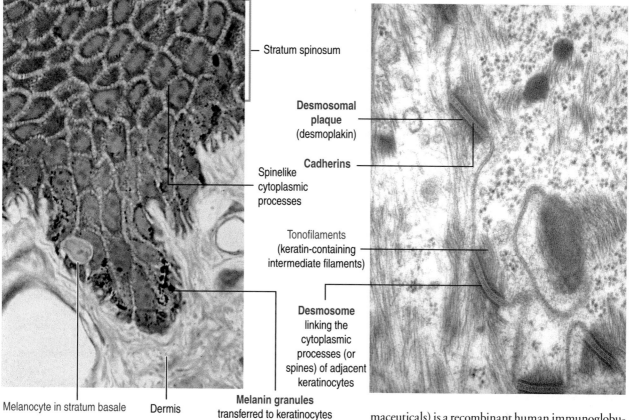

Figure 11-9. Melanocytes. Desmosomes in stratum spinosum

Stratum spinosum

Desmosomal plaque (desmoplakin)

Cadherins

Spinelike cytoplasmic processes

Tonofilaments (keratin-containing intermediate filaments)

Desmosome linking the cytoplasmic processes (or spines) of adjacent keratinocytes

Melanocyte in stratum basale   Dermis   **Melanin granules** transferred to keratinocytes

A **melanocyte** is seen in the stratum basale. Melanin granules are present in the cytoplasm of adjacent keratinocytes. Keratinocytes in the stratum spinosum are seen in a tangential section of the epidermis. Note the **spinelike cytoplasmic processes** of the keratinocytes. These processes contain bundles of **intermediate filament keratins** inserted in the plaques of desmosomes linking cell processes from adjacent keratinocytes.

Box 11-B | Disorders of keratinization

- **Stratum basale**
  Predominant keratins: Keratins 5 and 14
  Disorder: Epidermolysis bullosa simplex

- **Stratum spinosum**
  Predominant keratins: Keratins 1 and 10
  Disorder: Epidermolytic hyperkeratosis

- **Stratum granulosum/stratum corneum**
  Predominant keratin: Keratin 9 (palms and soles)
  Disorder: Epidermolytic plantopalmar keratoderma

- **Desmosomal defects**
  Desmoplakins; cadherins
  Disorder: Striate palmoplantar keratoderma

- **Cornified cell envelope (CCE)**
  Loricrin and transglutaminase-1 (TGA-1)
  Disorder: Vohwinkel's syndrome (loricrin) and congenital ichthyosiform erythroderma (TGA-1)

- **Abnormal lipid metabolism affecting the CCE**
  Disorder: Sjögren-Larsson syndrome

---

maceuticals) is a recombinant human immunoglobulin G1κ monoclonal antibody that specifically binds and neutralizes IL-17A to disrupt the pathogenic epidermis-dermis sequence.

Differentiation of a keratinocyte

Keratinocytes of the **stratum spinosum** have a flattened polygonal shape with a distinct ovoid nucleus. The cytoplasm displays small granules with a lamellar core, called **membrane-coating granules**, or **lamellar bodies**. Bundles of keratin intermediate filaments extend into the cytoplasmic spinous-like processes and attach to the **dense plaque** of a desmosome.

The **stratum granulosum** consists of a multilayered assembly of flattened nucleated keratinocytes with characteristic, irregularly shaped **keratohyalin granules** (containing **profilaggrin**) without a limiting membrane and associated with keratin intermediate filaments. The **lamellar bodies**, which first appear in keratinocytes of the stratum spinosum, increase in number in the stratum granulosum, and the lamellar product, the **glycolipid acylglucosylceramide**, is released into the intercellular spaces (Figure 11-6).

Tight junctions, containing **claudin-1** and **claudin-4**, are found in the stratum granulosum (Figure 11-7).

In the intercellular space, the lamellar lipid material forms a multilayered structure arranged in wide sheets, coating the surface of keratinocytes of the

Figure 11-10. Synthesis and transport of melanin from melanocytes to keratinocytes

Melanosome biogenesis

1 Premelanosomes, derived from the early endosomal compartment, contain **vesicles** and **melanofilaments**. Melanofilaments consist of Mα fragments. Mα fragments derive from **PMEL fibrils** cleaved to Mα and Mβ fragments by **proprotein convertase** (PC). **AP-3** and **AP-1 coating proteins** initiate the endosome-to-melanosome pathway.

2 **Melanosomes** contain melanin deposited on the Mα-containing melanofilaments that gradually increase in thickness. Melanin is a pigment resulting from the oxidation of tyrosine to DOPA (1,3,4-dihydroxy-phenylalanine), to melanin.

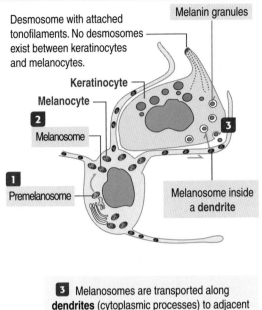

Desmosome with attached tonofilaments. No desmosomes exist between keratinocytes and melanocytes.

Melanin granules

Keratinocyte

Melanocyte

2

Melanosome

1

Premelanosome

3

Melanosome inside a **dendrite**

Golgi   Endosome

Adaptor protein-3 (AP-3)
Fibrils (PMEL)
Vesicle

AP-1

Fibril (PMEL)

PC

Mα   ✂   Mβ

Mα

Tyrosinase
Tyrosinase-related protein-1
DOPAchrome tautomerase

1

Melanin deposition on PMLEs increases the thickness of the melanofilaments

2

Alignment of Mα fragments to form **melanofilaments**

3 Melanosomes are transported along **dendrites** (cytoplasmic processes) to adjacent keratinocytes of the stratum spinosum. **Melanin granules** are internalized by adjacent keratinocytes. Melanin granules form a nuclear protective shield against ultraviolet radiation.

---

upper layer, the stratum lucidum. The glycolipid coating provides the water barrier of the epidermis.

The **stratum lucidum** is recognized by some histologists as an intermediate layer above the stratum granulosum and beneath the **stratum corneum**. However, no distinctive cytologic features are significantly apparent (Figure 11-8).

The stratum lucidum and stratum corneum consist of several layers of keratinocytes without nuclei and a cytoplasm containing aggregated intermediate filaments of keratin cross-linked with **filaggrin** (see Figure 11-7) by a process catalyzed by **transglutaminases**. Filaggrin aggregates keratin intermediate filaments into tight bundles, leading to cell flattening, a characteristic of the stratum corneum.

The keratin-filaggrin complex is deposited on the inside of the plasma membrane forming a structure called the **cornified cell envelope** (see Figure 11-7). Additional proteins, **involucrin**, **small proline–rich proteins (SPRs)**, **trichohyalin (THH)** and **loricrin**, are cross-linked by several **transglutaminases** (T1, T3 and T5)and reinforce the cornified cell envelope just beneath the plasma membrane at the desmosome location sites. On the outside of the cell, a complex of insoluble lipids (ceramides, fatty acids and cholesterol) extruded from lamellar bodies cross-link with proteins of the cell envelope, forming the **compound cornified cell envelope**.

In summary, the plasma membrane of keratinocytes of the stratum corneum consists of a cornified cell envelope containing a keratin-filaggrin matrix associated to a reinforcing involucrin–SPRs–loricrin–THH complex whose development is catalyzed by transglutaminases. Extracellular insoluble lipids, cross-linked to involucrin, make the cell membrane impermeable to fluids (permeability barrier). The cornified cell envelope provides elasticity and mechanical resistance to dead cell remnants in the uppermost layer of the epidermis. See Box 11-A for cornified cell envelope disorders.

The terminally differentiated keratinocytes of the stratum corneum consist of flattened squames with

Box 11-C | Melanocyte differentiation

• The process of melanocyte differentiation is regulated by **MITF**. MITF has two major roles: (1) melanocyte cell cycle arrest and (2) to stimulate the expression of genes encoding proteins involved in melanin production.

• Binding of α-MSH to MC1R stimulates cAMP production, which activates the gene expression of MITF after binding to CREB. MITF translocates to the cytoplasm of the melanocyte, is phosphorylated by the ERK pathway, returns to the cell nucleus, and increases the expression of proteins to arrest the melanocyte cell cycle, extend cell survival, and produce melanin.

• **MITF overexpression occurs in patients with melanoma.** Melanoma accounts for 4% of skin malignant tumors and is responsible for 80% of deaths from skin cancer. Patients with MITF overexpression have a negative clinical prognosis and are usually chemotherapy resistant. Inhibition of MITF function is a desirable target for the treatment of melanoma.

Figure 11-11. Melanocyte differentiation and melanosome transport

Figure 11-11. **Melanocyte differentiation and melanosome transport**

Melanocyte differentiation

1 Melanocytes undergo cell cycle arrest and express proteins required for the synthesis of melanin.

The **microphthalmia-associated transcription factor (MITF)** maintains the pool of melanocyte progenitors in adults and **regulates the differentiation of melanocytes**.

The expression of MITF occurs after α-**melanocyte-stimulating hormone** (α-MSH) binds to **melanocortin receptor 1 (MC1R)** on melanocytes.

Transport of melanosomes

3 Melanosomes move inside a dendrite along microtubules through an interaction with **kinesin**. Once at the periphery, melanosomes detach from microtubules and bind to **F-actin** (located at the subcortical region of dendrites) through an interaction with the molecular motor **myosin Va** recruited to the melanosome by **melanophilin** (an adapter) bound to **Rab27a** (present on the membrane of the melanosome). Melanosomes are transferred to surrounding keratinocytes.

Griscelli syndrome, associated with partial albinism of hair and skin, results from mutations in the *myosin Va* gene. A subset of Griscelli syndrome patients also have mutations in the *Rab27a* and *melanophilin* genes.

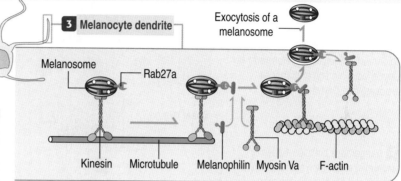

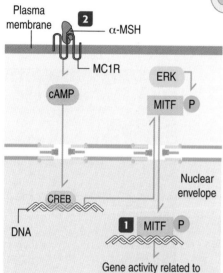

2 Binding of α-MSH to MC1R results in cyclic adenosine monophosphate (cAMP) production, activation of the cAMP response-element binding (CREB) protein on DNA, and increased expression of MITF.

MITF is released into the cytoplasm, where it is phosphorylated by the extracellular-related kinase (ERK) pathway.

Phosphorylated MITF translocates to the nucleus and stimulates the expression of enzymes (for example, tyrosinase) involved in melanin synthesis, cell cycle arrest, and melanocyte survival.

A lack of functional MITF produces albinism or premature graying. Excess of MITF production occurs in melanoma.

---

a highly resistant compound cell envelope. Squames are sloughed from the surface of the epidermis and are replaced by keratinocytes of the inner strata.

Two additional characteristics of the epidermis are:

1. The cell layer–specific expression of keratins observed during differentiation of keratinocytes (see Figure 11-6).

2. The presence of three types of junctions responsible for intercellular adhesion and cohesion of the epidermal cell layer: **tight junctions**, containing F-actin, and **desmosomes** and **hemidesmosomes**, containing keratin intermediate filaments.

A significant change at the transition between cells of the stratum granulosum and the stratum corneum is **the integration of the desmosomal cytoplasmic plaques into the cornified cell envelope** (see Figure 11-8). These modified desmosomes, called **corneodesmosomes**, contain in the extracellular space **desmoglein-1** and **desmocollin-1**, members of the Ca²⁺-dependent cadherin family, and another constituent, **corneodesmosin**. A proteolytic process in the upper stratum corneum, presumably involving cathepsin and calpain enzymes, disrupts corneodesmosin, thus allowing desquamation. Keep in mind that the loss of nuclei and mitochondria during the stratum granulosum-stratum corneum transition requires proteolytic processing.

Deregulation of cell adhesion in the epidermis is observed in blistering, epidermolytic, and proliferative diseases (see Box 11-B).

Melanocytes

Melanocytes are branching cells located in the stratum basale of the epidermis (Figure 11-9; see Figure 11-3). Melanocytes derive from **melanoblasts**, a cell precursor migrating from the **neural crest**.

The development of the melanoblast into melanocytes is under the control of the ligand **stem cell factor** interacting with the **c-kit receptor**, a membrane-bound tyrosine kinase.

The development of mast cells, primordial germinal cells, and hematopoietic stem cells is also dependent

Figure 11-12. Langerhans cell, an antigen-presenting dendritic cell of the epidermis

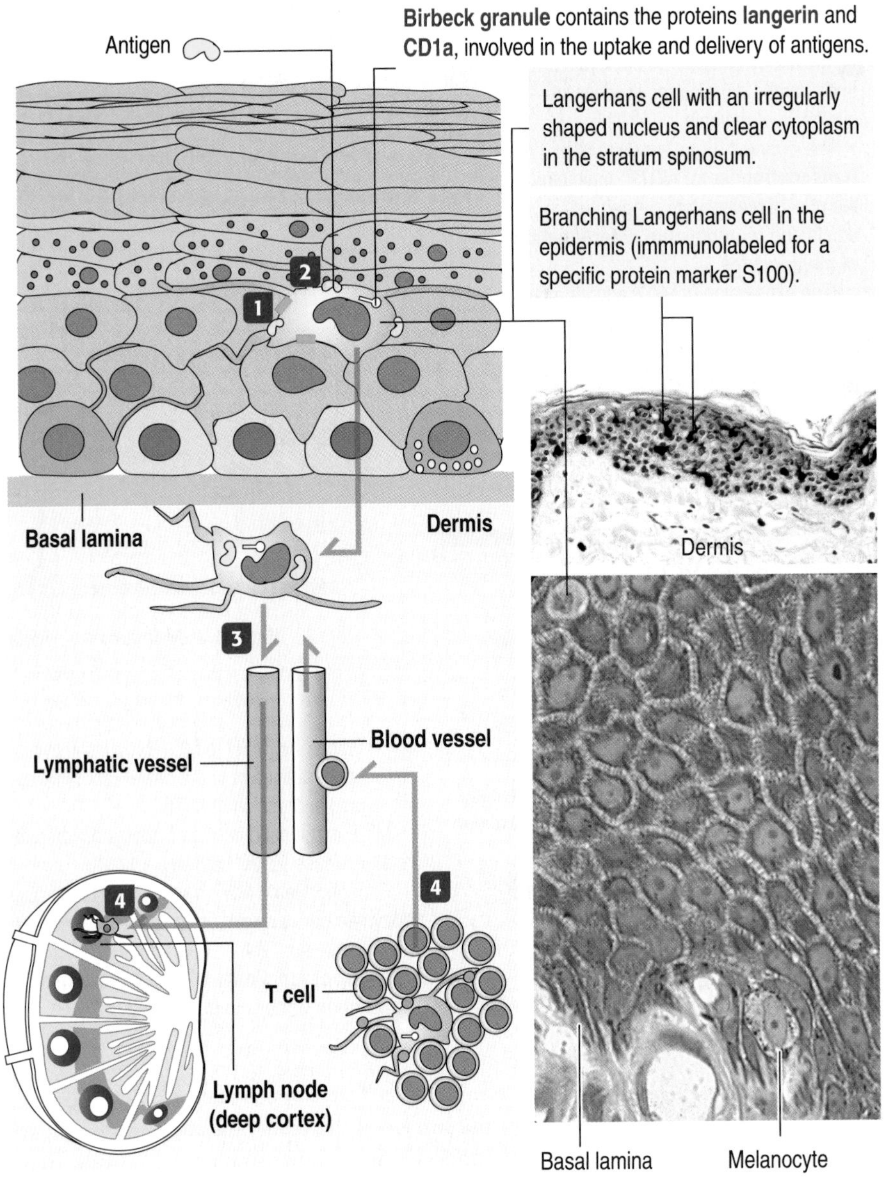

1 The Langerhans cell derives from a **monocyte precursor** of the bone marrow. Monocytes in the epidermis become **Langerhans cells** (**dendritic cells**) and interact with keratinocytes through **E-cadherins** on their surface.

As antigen-presenting cells, Langerhans cells monitor foreign antigens coming in contact with the epidermis. Dendritic cells are also present in the dermis.

2 Langerhans cells take up an epidermal antigen through **langerin** (a C-type lectin binding to mannose residues) and **CD1a**.

3 Langerhans cells leave the epidermis, enter the lymphatic system, and are transported to a regional lymph node.

4 In the lymph node, Langerhans cells interact with T cells in the deep cortex.

T cells, activated by the epidermal antigen, re-enter the blood circulation, extravasate at the site where the epidermal antigen is present, and secrete proinflammatory cytokines.

Antigen

Birbeck granule contains the proteins **langerin** and **CD1a**, involved in the uptake and delivery of antigens.

Langerhans cell with an irregularly shaped nucleus and clear cytoplasm in the stratum spinosum.

Branching Langerhans cell in the epidermis (immmunolabeled for a specific protein marker S100).

Basal lamina

Dermis

Dermis

Lymphatic vessel

Blood vessel

T cell

Lymph node (deep cortex)

Basal lamina

Melanocyte

Immunohistochemistry from Gray's Anatomy, 40th edition, London, Churchill Livingstone, 2008.

on the interaction of stem cell factor with the c-kit receptor.

Melanocytes enter the developing epidermis and remain as independent cells without desmosome attachment to the differentiating keratinocytes. The turnover of melanocytes is slower than that of keratinocytes.

Melanocytes produce **melanin**, contained in **melanosomes**, which are transferred to neighboring keratinocytes through their branching cell processes, called **melanocyte dendrites**, and released by **cytocrine** secretion (Figure 11-10; see Box 11-C).

Melanins are pigments that provide the skin and hairs (by cell transfer) and eyes (for storage in pigmented epithelia of the retina and ciliary body and iris) with color and photoprotection against

ionizing radiation. Melanins consist of copolymers of black and brown **eumelanins** and red and yellow **pheomelanins**.

Melanosomes develop and mature in melanocytes through four distinct stages:

1. During the first and second stages, **premelanosomes**, derived from the early endosome compartment by a sorting mechanism driven by membrane-bound **adaptor proteins-3 and -1** (AP-3 and AP-1), contain **PMEL fibrils** but lack melanin pigment. PMEL fibrils are cleaved to Mα and Mβ fragments by the enzyme **proprotein convertase**. Mα fragments begin to form **melanofilaments**, the scaffold for melanin deposition. Protein AP-3–depending premelanosome sorting is defective in the genetic disease **Hermansky–Pudlack syndrome** (HPS),

Figure 11-13. Hemidesmosomes

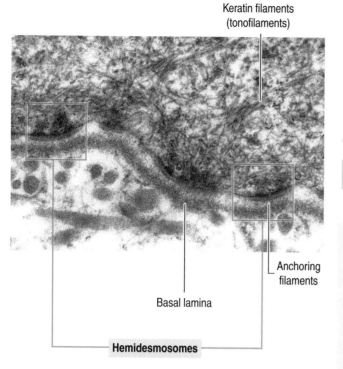

Keratin filaments (tonofilaments)

Anchoring filaments

Basal lamina

Hemidesmosomes

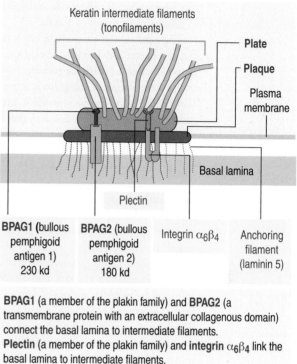

Keratin intermediate filaments (tonofilaments)

Plate

Plaque

Plasma membrane

Basal lamina

Plectin

BPAG1 (bullous pemphigoid antigen 1) 230 kd	**BPAG2 (bullous pemphigoid antigen 2) 180 kd**	**Integrin** $\alpha_6\beta_4$	**Anchoring filament (laminin 5)**

BPAG1 (a member of the plakin family) and **BPAG2** (a transmembrane protein with an extracellular collagenous domain) connect the basal lamina to intermediate filaments.
Plectin (a member of the plakin family) and **integrin** $\alpha_6\beta_4$ link the basal lamina to intermediate filaments.

characterized by oculocutaneous albinism, bleeding caused by a deficiency or absence of platelet stored granules and, in some cases, pulmonary fibrosis or granulomatous colitis.

2. The third stage starts once the melanofilaments are fully formed and the synthesis of melanin starts within the premelanosome by the activity of melanin biosynthetic enzymes tyrosinase, tyrosinase-related protein-1 and DOPAchrome tautomerase, also sorted as cargo from AP-3–coated endosomal buds to premelanosomes.

Melanin is produced by oxidation of **tyrosine** to **3,4-dihydroxyphenylalanine (DOPA)**. Oxidation is catalyzed by tyrosinase, whose activity is modulated by tyrosinase-related protein-1. DOPA is then transformed to eumelanin, which accumulates on the pre-assembled Mα-containing melanofilament scaffold.

3. The fourth stage is completed when the internal fibrillar structure of the premelanosome is masked by deposits of melanin and melanosomes are transported along microtubules by the motor protein **kinesin**. to actin-containing melanocyte dendritic tips to be transferred to adjacent keratinocytes,

Melanosome transfer occurs when **melanophilin**, an adapter protein, binds to **Rab27a**, a protein inserted in the melanosome membrane (Figure 11-11). The F-actin–based molecular motor **myosin Va** binds to the Rab27a-melanophilin complex and transports the melanosome to the plasma membrane. Extruded melanin by exocytosis is captured by ad-

jacent keratinocytes and internalized by endocytosis. The molecular characteristics of the unconventional myosin V are discussed in Chapter 1, Epithelium.

Albinism results from the inability of cells to form melanin. **Griscelli syndrome** is determined by mutations of the *myosin Va* gene. Patients with Griscelli syndrome have silvery hair, partial albinism, occasional neurologic defects, and immunodeficiency (due to a defective vesicular transport and secretion in cytolytic T cells). Similar pigmentation disorders are determined by mutations in the *Rab27a* and *melanophilin* genes.

Langerhans cells (dendritic cells)

Langerhans cells are bone marrow–derived cells present in the epidermis as immunologic sentinels, involved in immune responses, in particular the presentation of antigens to T cells (Figure 11-12).

Langerhans cells, containing an epidermal antigen, enter a lymphatic vessel in the dermis and migrate to a regional lymph node where they interact with T cells in the deep cortex (T cell zone). T cells, activated by the epidermal antigen, reenter the blood circulation, reach the site where the epidermal antigen is present, and release proinflammatory cytokines in an attempt to neutralize the antigen.

Similar to melanocytes, Langerhans cells have cytoplasmic processes (dendritic cells) extending among keratinocytes of the stratum spinosum without establishing desmosomal contact but associating with keratinocytes through **E-cadherin**. Langerhans cells express **CD1a**, a cell surface marker. CD1a mediates the presentation of nonpeptide antigens (for example, α-galactosylceramide) to T cells.

The nucleus of a Langerhans cell is indented, and the cytoplasm contains characteristic tennis racket–shaped inclusions (**Birbeck granules**) associated with the protein **langerin**. Langerin is a transmembrane C-type lectin (calcium-dependent protein with a carbohydrate-recognition domain) that facilitates the uptake of mannose-containing microbial fragments for their delivery to the endosomal compartment.

Langerhans cells use CD1a and langerin to trigger cellular immune responses to *Mycobacterium leprae*, the causative agent of **leprosy**, also known as **Hansen's disease**, a neurologic disease affecting the extremities.

Myelin-producing Schwann cells are the primary target. In the early stages, infected individuals have skin nodules (**chronic granulomas with multinucleated giant cells**) on the face and all over the body, followed by paralysis or loss of sensation in the affected areas, and eventually loss of fingers and toes. Blindness occurs in advanced stages of the disease. Multidrug therapy, consisting of rifampicin, clofazimine, and dapsone, is used to treat all cases of leprosy.

Merkel cells

Merkel cells resemble modified keratinocytes, are found in the stratum basale, and are numerous in the fingertips and lips. Merkel cells are **mechanoreceptor cells** linked to adjacent keratinocytes by desmosomes and in contact with an afferent myelinated nerve fiber projecting from the dermis into the epidermis. The nerve fiber becomes unmyelinated after passing through the basal lamina of the epidermis and expands into a platelike sensory ending, the **nerve plate**, in contact with the Merkel cell (see Figure 11-3).

The nucleus is irregularly shaped and the cytoplasm contains abundant **granules**, presumably neurotransmitters. We come back to Merkel cells when we discuss innervation of the skin.

Pathology: Tumors of the epidermis

A localized proliferation of keratinocytes results in diverse group of tumors of the epidermis. They include **hamartomas** (epidermal nevi), **reactive hyperplasias** (pseudoepitheliomatous hyperplasia), **benign tumors** (acanthomas), and **premalignant dysplasias**, **in situ**, and **invasive malignant tumors** (see Box 11-D).

Epidermal nevi are developmental deformations of the epidermis, in which excess keratinocytes undergo abnormal maturation (hyperkeratosis) and papillomatosis (an epidermal surface elevation). They localize in the neck, trunk, and extremities.

Pseudoepitheliomatous hyperplasia is a reaction in response to chronic irritation, such as around colostomy sites and to various inflammatory processes in the subjacent dermis (for example, mycoses).

Acanthomas are benign tumors characterized by abnormal keratinization, such as hyperkeratosis, dyskeratosis, or acantholysis (loss of cell-cell adhesion). An example is the **seborrheic keratosis**, gray-brown lesions of the skin that appear in middle life.

Premalignant epidermal dysplasias have the potential for malignant transformation. This group includes **solar keratosis** on the sun- or tanning bed-exposed skin of the face, ears, scalp, hands, and forearms of older individuals. The epidermis is thinner than normal and the normal cytologic features and stratified arrangement of keratinocytes are lost.

Bowen's disease is an in situ squamous cell carcinoma of the skin. It is characterized by a disorderly arrangement of keratinocytes displaying atypical nuclear features. The underlying dermis usually shows increased vascularity and inflammatory cell infiltrates. **Erythroplasia of Queyrat** is a carcinoma in situ of the penis, commonly found on the glans penis of uncircumcised individuals.

Invasive malignant tumors include **basal cell carcinoma** (the most common tumor) and **squamous cell carcinoma**. **Melanomas** are the most dangerous form of skin cancer.

Basal cell carcinoma (BCC) predominates on areas of the skin exposed to sun: head and neck. They arise from the basal layer of the epidermis and also from the external root sheath of the hair, or pilosebaceous unit (see below). A remarkable aspect of BCC is its stromal growth dependency, a possible explanation for the low frequency of metastasis of this tumor.

Genetic factors also have a role in the susceptibility to BCC. An often mutated gene in BCC is the *patched*

Box 11-D | Concept Map: Tumors of the epidermis

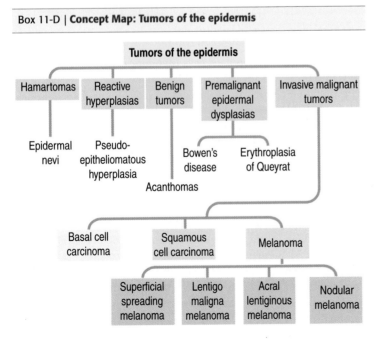

(*PTCH*) gene, a **tumor suppressor gene** that is part of the **Hedgehog signaling pathway** (see Chapter 3, Cell Signaling). For example, the accumulation of the transcription factor **GliI** (glioma I) contributes to the development of BCC.

Squamous cell carcinoma (SCC) is the second most common form of skin cancer. Like BSC, SCC affects areas of the skin directly exposed to the sun. Infection with high-risk types of **human papilloma virus (HPV)**.

For example, HPV-16 is responsible for a subgroup of SCC of the head and neck. SCC can arise from the hair follicle, in particular from cells of the hair follicle bulge (see Figure 11-16).

The typical SCC consists of abnormal keratin-containing squamous epithelial cells extending into the dermis. Keratinization and formation of horn pearl formations are often seen.

Melanomas originate in the melanin-producing melanocytes in the basal layer of the epidermis. The presence and number of large congenital nevi and atypical nevi are regarded as precursor lesions.

A mutation in the *BRAF* (**proto-oncogene B-Raf**) gene is observed in a large number of melanomas. *Raf* genes code for cytoplasmic serine/threonine kinases that are regulated by binding the GTPase Ras (see Figure 3-21 in Chapter 3, Cell Signaling). All mutations are within the kinase domain of the kinase, accounting for the elevated kinase activity of the mutated BRAF proteins.

Figure 3-19 in Chapter 3 illustrates the histopathology of a nodular melanoma.

The clinical features of melanoma are defined by the **mnemonic ABCD**: Asymmetry, Border irregularity, Color variation, and Diameter greater than 6 mm.

There are four types of melanomas:

1. **Superficial spreading melanoma** is the most frequent. It develops at any age on the trunk (men) and lower extremities (women), and is superficially invasive.

2. **Lentigo maligna melanoma** is similar to the superficial spreading type. It it preceded by the in situ form called lentigo maligna (an irregular freckle that progresses slowly) and, when it becomes invasive, it is called lentigo maligna melanoma. It occurs most frequently on the face and sun-exposed upper extremities of elderly people.

3. **Acral lentiginous melanoma** also spreads superficially before becoming invasive. It is the least common melanoma among Caucasians but most common in African-Americans and Asians.

4. **Nodular melanoma** is commonly invasive at the time it is first diagnosed. This type of melanoma displays vertical growth, in contrast to the three previous types that show radial growth (superficial spreading) before invasive or vertical growth takes place.

Dermis

The dermis is formed by two layers without distinct boundaries:

1. The **papillary layer**, consisting of numerous dermal papillae split by interpapillary pegs, form the dermal-epidermal junction (review Figure 11-1).

The junctional interface is stabilized by hemidesmosomes anchoring basal keratinocyte cells to the basal lamina. Loose connective tissue (fibroblasts, collagen fibers, and thin elastic fibers) provides mechanical anchorage and nutrients to the overlying epidermis.

2. The **reticular layer**, containing thick bundles of collagen fibers and coarse elastic fibers.

Hemidesmosomes on the basal domain of keratinocytes of the stratum basale attach the epidermis to the basement membrane and the papillary layer of the dermis by a **plate/plaque–anchoring filament complex** summarized in Figure 11-13. The molecular and structural components of the hemidesmosome are of considerable importance for understanding the cause of **blistering diseases** of the skin. We discuss in Chapter 1, Epithelium, the clinical significance of hemidesmosomes and intermediate filaments (see Figures 1-36 and 1-37).

Hair follicles and **sweat** and **sebaceous glands** are epidermal derivatives present at various levels of the dermis.

Pathology: Epithelial antimicrobial proteins

As a surface tissue of the body, the skin (of about 2 m² of surface area) is continuously exposed to bacteria, fungi, viruses and parasites that could act as pathogens.

Epithelial antimicrobial proteins (AMPs) are produced by keratinocytes and sweat and sebaceous glands to kill or inactivate microorganisms. AMPs are released quickly in response to a disruption of the skin barrier and provide a transient protection against infection. AMPs include:

1. **β-Defensins**.
2. **Cathelicidins**.

Keratinocytes of the hair follicle constitutively produce high levels of β-defensin and cathelicidins when compared to epidermic keratinocytes. In addition, secretory cells of the sweat and sebaceous glands produce additional AMPs and antimicrobial lipids (see later in this chapter). Mast cells in the dermis store large amounts of cathelicidins in their cytoplasmic granules, released top resist infections after skin injury.

Defensins and cathelicidins carry out a nonenzymatic disruption the integrity of cell wall or cell membrane structures to promote lysis of microorganisms. In addition, defensins and cathelicidins can by-pass the capacity of microorganisms to develop

Figure 11-14. **Blood supply to the skin**

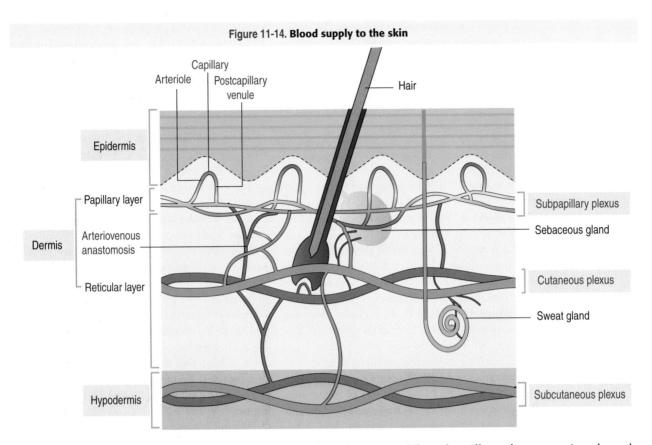

resistance to AMPs by signaling through **chemokine receptors** (to recruit leukocytes to elicit an acute inflammatory response) and also involving **Toll-like receptor (TLRs) signaling** (activated by microbial lipopolysaccharide to trigger the production of pro-inflammatory cytokines) to activate or inhibit inflammatory responses. We discuss details of TLRs in Chapter 10, Immune-Lymphatic System).

Atopic dermatitis, rosacea and psoriasis have been associated in part to the deficient production of AMPs. For example, infection with *Staphylococcus aureus* increases the production of AMPs in the skin. However, the expression of AMPs is partially suppressed in patients with atopic dermatitis during skin inflammation, triggered by cytokines produced by TH2 cells. In contrast, patients with rosacea and psoriasis are not susceptible to infection. Keratinocytes in these patients produce excessive cathelicidin, leading to inappropriate inflammatory reactions of the skin.

Blood and lymphatic supply

The cutaneous vascular supply has a primary function: **thermoregulation**. The secondary function is nutrition of the skin and appendages. The arrangement of blood vessels permits rapid modification of blood flow according to the required loss or conservation of heat.

Three interconnected networks are recognized in the skin (Figure 11-14):

1. The **subpapillary plexus**, running along the papillary layer of the dermis.
2. The **cutaneous plexus**, observed at the boundary of the papillary and reticular layers of the dermis.
3. The **hypodermic** or **subcutaneous plexus**, present in the hypodermis or subcutaneous adipose tissue.

The subpapillary plexus gives rise to single loops of capillaries within each dermal papilla. Venous blood from the subpapillary plexus drains into veins of the cutaneous plexus.

Branches of the hypodermic and cutaneous plexuses nourish the adipose tissue of the hypodermis, the sweat glands, and the deeper segment of the hair follicle.

Arteriovenous anastomoses (shunts) between the arterial and venous circulation bypass the capillary network. They are common in the reticular and hypodermic regions of the extremities (hands, feet, ears, lips, nose) and play a role in thermoregulation of the body. The vascular shunts, under autonomic vasomotor control, restrict flow through the superficial plexuses to reduce heat loss, ensuring deep cutaneous blood circulation. In some areas of the body (for example, the face), cutaneous blood circulation is also affected by an emotional state.

A special form of arteriovenous shunt is the **glomus apparatus**. It is found in the dermis of the fingertips, under the fingernails and toes and is involved in temperature regulation. The glomus consists of an endothelial-lined channel surrounded by cuboidal pericyte-like glomus cells and a rich nerve supply. **Glomus tumors** are benign, usually very small (about 1 cm in diameter) red-blue nodules, associated with sensitivity to cold and severe intermittent focal pain. Surgical excision provides immediate pain relief.

Lymphatic vessels are blind endothelial cell–lined spaces located below the papillary layer of the dermis, collecting interstitial fluid for return to the blood circulation. They also transport Langerhans cells to regional lymph nodes.

Pathology: Vascular disorders of the skin

Vascular abnormalities of the skin are common. Some vascular lesions derive from pre-existing vessels rather than the proliferation of new vessels (angiogenesis).

There are **vascular malformations** (vascular hamartomas and hemangiomas), **vascular dilatations** (telangiectases) and **tumors** (angiomas, Kaposi's sarcoma, and angiosarcomas).

Local and generalized vascular diseases affect the cutaneous vascular network (see Chapter 12, Cardiovascular System). **Vasculitis** includes a group of disorders in which there is inflammation of and damage to blood vessel walls. Most cases of cutaneous vasculitis affect small vessels, predominantly venules.

Noninflammatory **purpuras** (extravasation of blood in the dermis from small vessels) can be small (**petechiae**; less than 3 mm in diameter), or large (**ecchymoses**). Coagulation disorders, red blood cell diseases (sickle cell disease), and trauma are common causes.

Acute **urticaria** is a transient reaction caused by increased vascular permeability associated with edema in the dermis. In Chapter 4, Connective Tissue, we discussed the mechanism of degranulation of mast cells and release of histamine as determinants.

Sensory receptors of the skin

Sensory receptors are specialized neurons and epithelial-like cells that receive and convert a physical stimulus into an electrical signal transmitted to the central nervous system.

There are three general categories of sensory receptors:

1. **Exteroceptors**, that provide information about the external environment.

2. **Proprioceptors**, located in muscles (such as the muscle spindle), tendons, and joint capsules and provide information about the position and movement of the body.

3. **Interoceptors**, that provide sensory information from the internal organs of the body.

The classification of sensory receptors of the skin is based on the **type of stimulus**:

1. **Mechanoreceptors** respond to mechanical deformation of the tissue or the receptor itself (for example, stretch, vibration, pressure, and touch).

There are four primary mechanoreceptors in human skin (Figure 11-15):

1. **Merkel disk**.
2. **Meissner corpuscle**.
3. **Ruffini ending**.
4. **Pacinian corpuscle**.

The first two are located at the epidermal-dermal junction; the other two are located in the deep dermis and hypodermis.

Meissner corpuscle, Ruffini ending, pacinian corpuscle, and Krause end bulb are **encapsulated receptors**. **Krause end bulb** is a **thermoreceptor** found only in specialized regions.

The nerve ending of the **Merkel disk** mechanoreceptor discriminates fine touch and forms a flattened discoid structure attached to the Merkel cell. Merkel cells are found in the stratum basale of the epidermis of the fingertips and lips (see Figure 11-3).

The **Meissner corpuscle**, or tactile corpuscle, is found in the upper dermis, bulging into the epidermis (see Figure 11-15). They are found primarily in the fingertips and eyelids. This receptor is well suited for the detection of shape and texture during active touch.

The **Ruffini ending**, or bulbous corpuscle, is located in the deep dermis. It detects skin stretch and deformations within joints. They also provide feedback when gripping objects and controlling finger position and movement (for example, when we use the computer keyboard).

The **pacinian corpuscle** is found in the deep dermis and hypodermis. It responds to stimuli of deep, transient pressure and high-frequency vibration. They are found in the bone periosteum, joint capsules, pancreas, breast, and genitals.

2. **Thermoreceptors** respond to a temperature stimulus, either warmth or cold. The **Krause end bulb** is encapsulated but is not a mechanoreceptor. It is a **thermoreceptor** that detects **cold**. Krause end bulbs are found in the conjunctiva of the eye, in the mucosa of the lips and tongue, and in the epineurium of nerves. They are also found in the penis and the clitoris (hence, the name of genital corpuscle).

3. **Nociceptors** respond to pain stimuli. The simplest form of a pain detector are the **free nerve endings**. They derive from the **dermal nerve plexus**, supplied by **cutaneous branches** of the spinal nerves. Sensory nerve fibers extending toward the skin surface, shed their myelin sheaths before branching as naked axons between collagen fibers, forming **dermal nerve endings**, or within the epidermis, as **epidermal nerve endings** (see Figure 11-15).

The very sensitive **peritrichial nerve endings** are wrapped around the hair follicle just under the sebaceous glands. The myelinated portions of the nerve endings form a palisade of naked terminals along the

Figure 11-15. Sensory receptors of the skin

The **cutaneous nerve** branches of the spinal nerves give raise to fine nerve fibers of the **dermal nerve plexus** located in the dermis. Indiviual nerve fibers of the dermal plexus supply the sensory terminals.

1 Meissner corpuscle

Present in dermal papilla
Encapsulated tactile mechanoreceptor

Present in fingers of hand and foot, lips, and tongue

2 Merkel disk

Neural crest–derived cell located in the basal layer of the epidermis
Nonencapsulated high resolution tactile receptor
Present in fingertips and lips

3 Ruffini end organ

Responds to stretching and also to warmth

4 Pacinian corpuscle

Sensitive to pressure

Ruffini end organ

Present in skin and joint capsule

Pacinian corpuscle

Found in hypodermis and deep fascia

5 Free nerve endings

Lack myelin or Schwann cells
Respond to pain and temperature

Found in epidermis and corneal epithelium

6 Peritrichial nerve ending

Nerve fibers wrapped around the base of the hair follicle; stimulated by hair movement

7 Krause end bulb

Encapsulated thermoreceptor; it detects cold
Found in the conjunctiva of the eye, the mucosa of the lips and tongue, and the epineurium

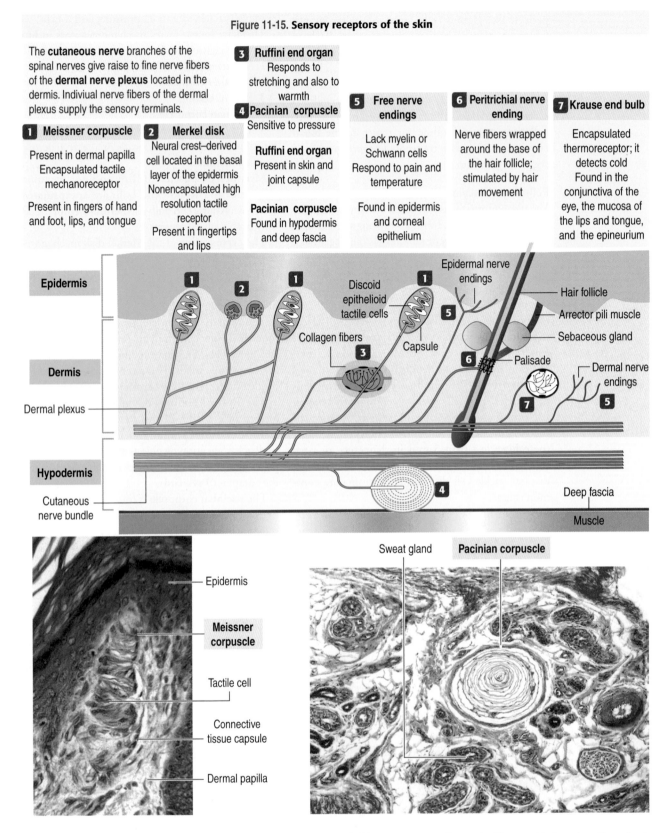

external root sheath of the hair follicle, surrounded by circumferential terminals. Peritrichial nerve endings are stimulated when the hairs bend.

The perception of pain is associated to **acute inflammation**, one of the classical responses to tissue in-

jury as we discuss in Chapter 10, Immune-Lymphatic System. Injured cells release chemical mediators, including **substance P**, acting on local blood vessels and nerve endings. Substance P triggers the degranulation of mast cells, histamine in particular, that enhances

Figure 11-16. Migratory pathways of bulge stem cells

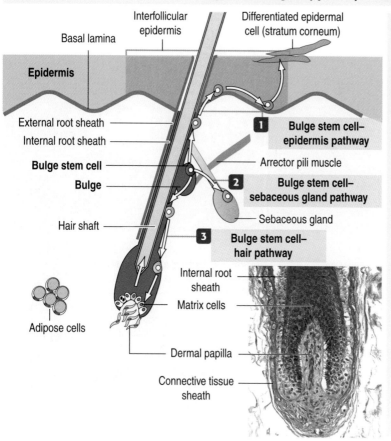

Bulge stem cells in the bulge region (located at the external root sheath of the hair follicle) can follow independent cell migration pathways:

1 In the **bulge stem cell–epidermis pathway**, bulge stem cells migrate upward into the **interfollicular epidermis** along the basal lamina. Bulge stem cells proliferate within the stratum basale and differentiate vertically into the keratin-rich cells of the stratum corneum. **Squamous cell carcinoma, basal cell carcinoma**, and **hair-follicle tumors** can originate from cells exiting the bulge following activation of specific genetic pathways.

2 In the **bulge stem cell–sebaceous gland pathway**, bulge stem cells respond to morphogenetic signals to generate **sebaceous glands**.

3 In the **bulge stem cell–hair pathway**, bulge stem cells migrate downward and give rise to a population of **matrix cells** located at the apex of the **dermal papilla**. These cells are responsible for producing new hair. Regulatory factors (**bone morphogenetic proteins and Wnt/β-catenin signaling**) released by cells of the dermal papilla and neighboring adipose cells, are essential for maintaining the proliferative potential of the matrix and their differentiation into the various hair cell lineages.

---

vascular dilation and plasma leakage, thereby causing edema in the injury surrounding area.

Hyperemia accounts for the **triple response of Lewis** when a line is made on the skin with a pointed object: **flush** (capillary dilation), **flare** (redness spreading because of arteriolar dilation), and **wheal** (localized edema). The triple response develops between 1 to 3 minutes.

In **summary**, the nociceptive receptors (the pain detectors) are found near the skin surface. Merkel disks and Meissner corpuscles, fine mechanoreceptor, are located at the epidermal-dermal junction so they can detect gentle touch. Pacinian corpuscles and Ruffini endings, the large encapsulated mechanoreceptors, are found in the deep dermis and hypodermis and respond to transient deeper touch.

Pathology: Leprosy

Leprosy (lepra) is a chronic infection of the skin, nasal mucosa, and peripheral nerves. It is caused by *Mycobacterium leprae*, an intracellular bacillus found in Schwann cells, endothelial cells and macrophages of the skin. Nerve lesions result in anesthesia in the extremities, claw hand, and foot drop. Acute episodes appear during the typical chronic clinical course of leprosy.

There are two histologic types of leprosy:

1. The **lepromatous reaction**, characterized by numerous macrophages in the dermis with intracellular acid-fast bacilli.

2. The **tuberculoid reaction**, identified by non-caseating granulomas consisting of macrophages, multinucleated giant cells, and lymphocytes (T cells). Bacilli are difficult to find. Granulomas tend to extend into the bundles of the cutaneous nerve, destroy the sweat glands, and erode the superficial dermis.

Hypodermis (superficial fascia)

The hypodermis, or subcutaneous layer of the skin, is a deeper continuation of the dermis. It consists of loose connective tissue and adipose cells forming a layer of variable thickness depending on its location in the body.

The hypodermis facilitates mobility of the skin, and the adipose tissue contributes to thermal insulation and storage of metabolic energy and acts as a shock absorber. The hypodermis contains muscles in the head and neck (for example, platysma). No adipose tissue is found in the subcutaneous portion of the eyelids, clitoris, or penis.

Epidermal derivatives: Hair (pilosebaceous unit)

Scattered in the epidermis are the hair follicles. During development, the epidermis and dermis interact

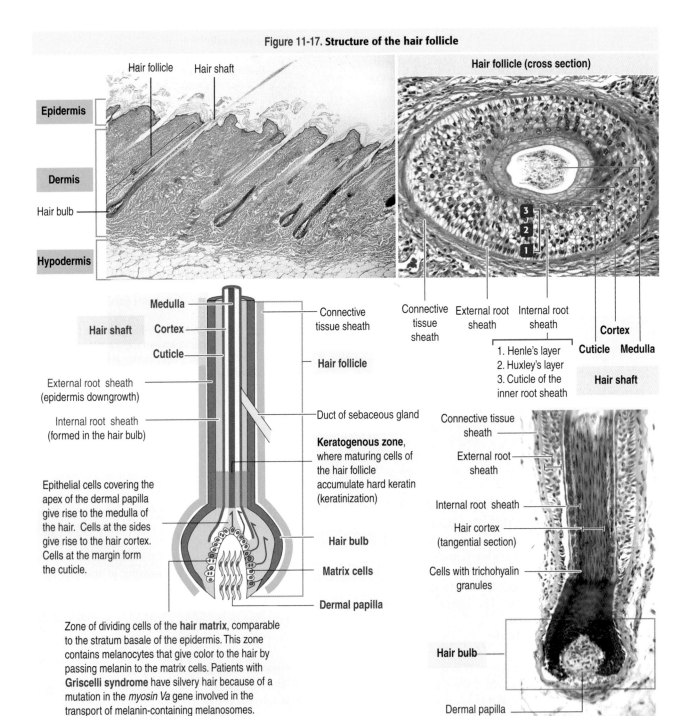

Figure 11-17. Structure of the hair follicle

Hair follicle   Hair shaft

Epidermis

Dermis

Hair bulb

Hypodermis

Hair follicle (cross section)

Connective tissue sheath

External root sheath

Internal root sheath

3
2
1

Connective tissue sheath

External root sheath

Internal root sheath

1. Henle's layer
2. Huxley's layer
3. Cuticle of the inner root sheath

Cortex

Cuticle Medulla

Hair shaft

Hair shaft

Medulla

Cortex

Cuticle

External root sheath (epidermis downgrowth)

Internal root sheath (formed in the hair bulb)

Connective tissue sheath

Hair follicle

Duct of sebaceous gland

Keratogenous zone, where maturing cells of the hair follicle accumulate hard keratin (keratinization)

Epithelial cells covering the apex of the dermal papilla give rise to the medulla of the hair. Cells at the sides give rise to the hair cortex. Cells at the margin form the cuticle.

Hair bulb

Matrix cells

Dermal papilla

Zone of dividing cells of the **hair matrix**, comparable to the stratum basale of the epidermis. This zone contains melanocytes that give color to the hair by passing melanin to the matrix cells. Patients with **Griscelli syndrome** have silvery hair because of a mutation in the *myosin Va* gene involved in the transport of melanin-containing melanosomes.

Connective tissue sheath

External root sheath

Internal root sheath

Hair cortex (tangential section)

Cells with trichohyalin granules

Hair bulb

Dermal papilla

to develop sweat glands and hair follicles.

A hair follicle primordium (called the **hair germ**) forms as a cell aggregate in the basal layer of the epidermis, induced by signaling molecules derived from fibroblasts of the dermal mesoderm. As basal epidermal cell clusters extend into the dermis, dermal fibroblasts form a small nodule (called a **dermal papilla**) under the hair germ.

The dermal papilla pushes into the core of the hair germ, whose cells divide and differentiate to form the keratinized hair shaft. Melanocytes present in the hair

germ produce and transfer melanin into the shaft.

A bulbous swelling (called the **follicular bulge**) on the side of the hair germ contains stem cells, **clonogenic keratinocytes**, that can migrate and regenerate the hair shaft, the epidermis, and sebaceous gland, forming **pilosebaceous units** (Figure 11-16), in response to morphogenetic signals.

The first adult hair follicle cycle starts once morphogenesis is completed about 18 days after birth, The first hair in the human embryo is thin, unpigmented, and spaced, and is called **lanugo**. Lanugo is shed before birth and replaced by short colorless hair called **vellus**. Terminal hair replaces vellus, which remains in the so-called hairless parts of the skin (such as the forehead of the adult and armpits of infants).

Hair follicles are tubular invaginations of the epidermis responsible for the growth of hair.

Hair follicles are constantly cycling between:

1. Growth (**anagen**) phase.
2. Regression (**catagen**) phase.
3. Resting (**telogen**) phase.

During the first 28 days of the telogen phase, hair follicles become quiescent because of growth inhibitory signals from the dermis (mainly from bone morphogenetic proteins). Increased Wnt/β-catenin signaling promotes stem cell activation to initiate the growth of new hair during the transition from telogen to anagen. Anagen, catagen and telogen will sequentially continue during the life of the individual.

Each **hair follicle** consists of two parts (Figure 11-17):

1. The **hair shaft**.
2. The **hair bulb**.

The hair shaft is a filamentous keratinized structure present almost all over the body surface, except on the thick skin of the palms and soles, the sides of the fingers and toes, the nipples, and the glans penis and the clitoris, among others.

A cross section of the hair shaft of thick hair reveals three concentric zones containing keratinized cells:

1. The **cuticle**.
2. The **cortex**.
3. The **medulla** (the last is absent in thin hair).

The hair shaft consists of **hard keratin**.

The **hair bulb** is the expanded end portion of the invaginated hair follicle. A vascularized connective tissue core (**dermal papilla**) projects into the hair bulb, in close proximity to **matrix cells**.

The hair shaft is surrounded by:

1. The **external root sheath**, a downgrowth of the epidermis.

2. The **internal root sheath**, generated by the hair bulb (the **hair matrix cells**), is made up of three layers of **soft keratin** (which from the outside to the inside are the Henle's layer, the Huxley's layer, and the cuticle of the inner root sheath, adjacent to the cuticle of the hair shaft).

The keratinization of the hair and internal root sheath occurs in a region called the **keratogenous zone**, the transition zone between maturing epidermal cells and hard keratin. The external root sheath is not derived from the hair bulb.

The hair follicle is surrounded by a connective tissue layer and associated with the **arrector pili muscle**, a bundle of smooth muscle fibers aligned at an oblique angle to the connective tissue sheath and the epidermis (see Figures 11-16 and 11-18). The

autonomic nervous system controls the arrector pili muscle, which contracts during fear, strong emotions, and cold temperature. The hairs stand up and the attachment site of the muscle bundle at the epidermis forms a small groove, the so called goose flesh.

The hair follicle is associated with **sebaceous glands** with their excretory duct connected to the lumen of the hair follicle. When the arrector pili muscle contracts and the hair stands up, sebum is forced out of the sebaceous gland into the lumen of the hair follicle.

The color of the hair depends on the amount and distribution of melanin in the hair shaft. Few melanosomes are seen in blond hair. Few melanocytes and melanin are seen in gray hair. Red hair has a chemically distinct melanin, and melanosomes are round rather than ellipsoid.

A structure that is not recognized in routine histologic sections of hairs is the **peritrichial nerve endings** wrapped around the base of the hair follicle. The nerve is stimulated by hair movement (see Figure 11-15).

We discussed earlier in this chapter the participation of myosin Va in the transport of melanin-containing melanosomes to keratinocytes (called **matrix cells** in the hair bulb) and the lack of hair pigmentation in patients with **Griscelli syndrome** caused by mutations of *myosin Va*, *Rab27a*, and *melanophilin* genes.

Bulge stem cell pathways

The **interfollicular epidermis** is contiguous with the external root sheath of the hair follicle, a structure responsible for developing the hair shaft. When the epidermis is lost in severely burned patients, stem cells migrate upward from the **follicular bulge** to reestablish the **epidermis** by populating the highly proliferative and self-renewing cells of the stratum basale (see Figure 11-16). These **bulge stem cells** can also give raise to **hair follicles** and **sebaceous glands**.

Different activated oncogenes expressed in cells exiting the bulge can give raise to specific tumor types: **squamous cell carcinoma** (Ras oncogene activation), **basal cell carcinoma** ((PTCH/Gli1/2 activation of the Hedgehog signaling pathway), and **hair-follicle tumors** (Wnt/β-catening signaling pathway).

There are two signaling pathways that stimulate stem cells to enter the epidermal differentiation pathway:

1. The **bone morphogenetic protein (BMP) signaling pathway** stimulates stem cell quiescence during the resting stage (telogen).

2. The **Wingless (Wnt)/β-catenin signaling pathway** is required to stimulate the activation of matrix stem cells and initiate hair growth during the transition from resting to growing stage (anagen). During this transition, the levels of BMPs decrease and the BMP inhibitor **noggin** increases, thus resulting in an inhibition of BMP signaling and consequent activa-

Figure 11-18. Sebaceous gland: Holocrine secretion

Sebaceous glands are appendages of the hair follicle. Their short ducts, lined by a stratified squamous epithelium continuous with the external root sheath of the hair, open into the hair canal (see arrow), Hair-independent sebaceous glands can be found on the lips, areolae of the nipples, the labia minora, and the inner surface of the prepuce.

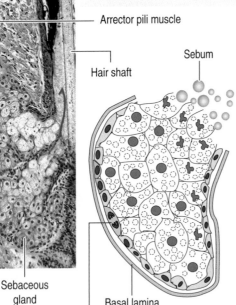

Arrector pili muscle

Hair shaft

Sebum

Sebaceous gland

Basal lamina

Basal cells divide by mitosis and accumulate lipids as they move into the central part of the acinus.

Sebum is the oily secretion of sebaceous cells. Sebum is released by a **holocrine mechanism**, resulting in the destruction of entire cells that become part of the secretion.

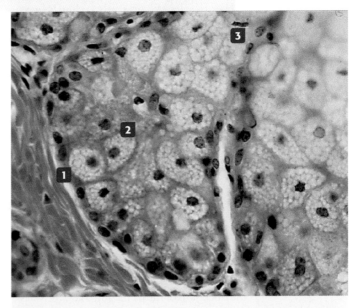

1 **Basal cells** regenerate sebum-producing cells lost during the **holocrine** secretory process.

2 Sebum-secreting cells on top of the basal cells begin to store the oily secretion within cytoplasmic droplets.

3 In proximity to the acinar duct, the nuclei of the sebum-secreting cells shrink and degenerate, and coalescing droplets of sebum are released into the short duct. The acini lack a proper lumen.

tion of matrix stem cells. You may like to review BMP and Wnt/β-catenin signaling pathways in Chapter 3, Cell Signaling.

Epidermal derivatives: Sebaceous glands

The glands of the skin are:

1. The **sebaceous glands** (see Figure 11-18).

2. The **sweat glands** (eccrine and apocrine sweat glands) (Figures 11-19 and 11-20).

3. The **mammary glands**. The mammary gland is discussed in Chapter 23, Fertilization, Placentation, and Lactation.

The **sebaceous gland** is a **holocrine simple saccular gland** extending over the entire skin except for the palms and soles. The **secretory portion** of the sebaceous gland lies in the **dermis**, and the **excretory duct opens into the neck of the hair follicle**. Sebaceous glands can be independent of the hairs and open directly on the surface of the skin of the lips, the corner of the mouth, the glans penis, the labia minora, and the mammary nipple.

The secretory portion of the sebaceous gland consists of groups of alveoli connected to the excretory duct by a short ductule.

Each alveolus is lined by cells resembling multilocular adipocytes with numerous small lipid droplets. The excretory duct is lined by stratified squamous epithelium continuous with the external root sheath of the hair and the epidermis (the malpighian layer).

The oily secretion of the gland (**sebum**) is released on the surface of the hair and the epidermis. In addition, sebaceous glands produce **cathelicidin** and human β-defensins (BD1, BD2, and BD3), endogenous AMPs that enhance the aqueous–lipid protective barrier of the epidermal surface.

Epidermal derivatives: Sweat glands

There are two types of sweat glands:

1. **Eccrine (merocrine) sweat glands** (see Figure 11-19).

2. **Apocrine (merocrine) sweat glands** (see Figure 11-20).

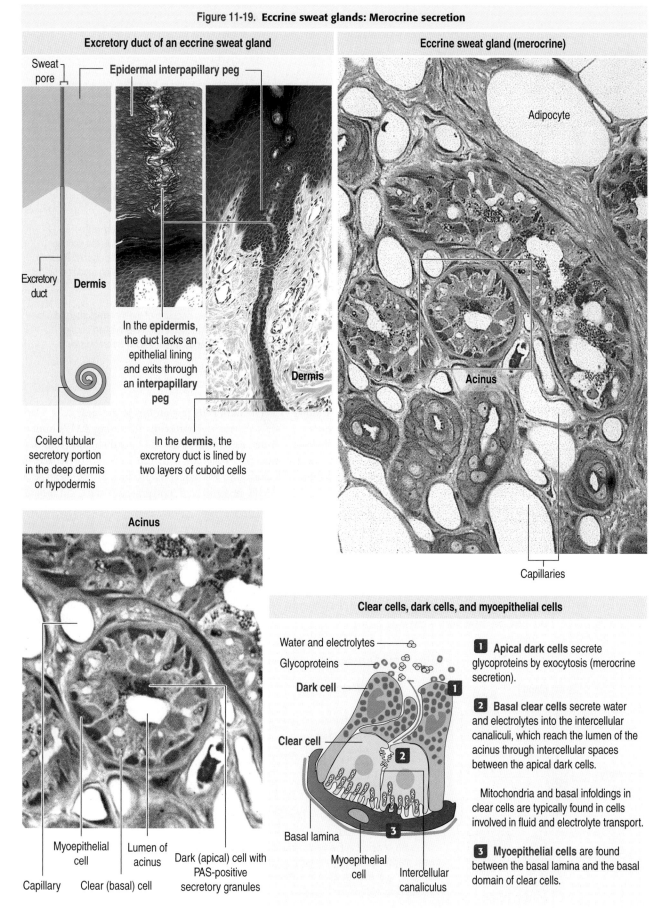

Figure 11-19. Eccrine sweat glands: Merocrine secretion

Excretory duct of an eccrine sweat gland

Sweat pore

Epidermal interpapillary peg

Dermis

Excretory duct

Coiled tubular secretory portion in the deep dermis or hypodermis

In the **epidermis**, the duct lacks an epithelial lining and exits through an **interpapillary peg**

Dermis

In the **dermis**, the excretory duct is lined by two layers of cuboid cells

Eccrine sweat gland (merocrine)

Adipocyte

Acinus

Capillaries

Acinus

Myoepithelial cell

Capillary

Clear (basal) cell

Lumen of acinus

Dark (apical) cell with PAS-positive secretory granules

Clear cells, dark cells, and myoepithelial cells

Water and electrolytes

Glycoproteins

Dark cell

Clear cell

Basal lamina

Myoepithelial cell

Intercellular canaliculus

1 Apical **dark cells** secrete glycoproteins by exocytosis (merocrine secretion).

2 Basal **clear cells** secrete water and electrolytes into the intercellular canaliculi, which reach the lumen of the acinus through intercellular spaces between the apical dark cells.

Mitochondria and basal infoldings in clear cells are typically found in cells involved in fluid and electrolyte transport.

3 **Myoepithelial cells** are found between the basal lamina and the basal domain of clear cells.

Figure 11-20. Apocrine sweat glands: Merocrine secretion

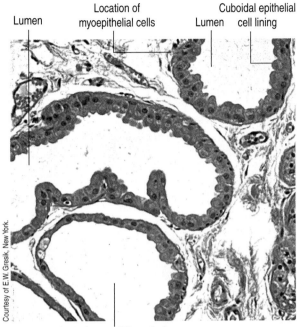

Lumen
Location of myoepithelial cells
Cuboidal epithelial cell lining
Lumen

Courtesy of E.W. Gresik, New York.

Large lumen of the coiled secretory portion

Apocrine sweat gland

Apocrine sweat glands are found in the **axilla, circumanal region, and mons pubis.**

The **coiled region of apocrine glands is larger** (~ 3 mm in diameter) than that of the eccrine sweat glands (~0.4 mm in diameter).

Apocrine sweat glands are located in the dermis, and the **excretory duct opens into the canal of the hair follicle.**

The secretory cells are cuboid and **associated with myoepithelial cells at their basal surface,** as in the eccrine sweat glands. The **secretory activity starts at puberty.** Their secretion acquires a conspicuous odor after being modified by local bacteria.

Although called apocrine, because of the incorrect interpretation that the apical domain of the secretory cells is shed during secretion, these sweat glands **release their secretion by a merocrine process.**

The **eccrine sweat glands** are **simple coiled tubular glands** with a role in the **control of body temperature.** Eccrine sweat glands are innervated by **cholinergic nerves.** The **secretory portion** of the eccrine sweat gland (see Figure 11-19) is a convoluted tube composed of three cell types:

1. **Clear cells.**
2. **Dark cells.**
3. **Myoepithelial cells.**

The **clear cells** are separated from each other by **intercellular canaliculi,** show an infolded basal domain with abundant mitochondria, rest on a basal lamina, and secrete most of the water and electrolytes (mainly Na$^+$ and Cl$^-$) of sweat.

The **dark cells** rest on top of the clear cells. Dark cells secrete glycoproteins, including AMPs human β-**defensins** (BD1 and BD2), **cathelicidin,** and **dermicidin.** Together with the secretion of sebaceous glands and the aqueous product of the clear cells, AMPs are produced under steady–state and inflammatory conditions.

Myoepithelial cells are found between the basal lamina and the clear cells. Their contractile activity assists in the release of secretion into the glandular lumen.

The **excretory portion** of the eccrine sweat gland is lined by a **bilayer of cuboid cells** that partially reabsorb NaCl and water under the influence of

Figure 11-21. Cystic fibrosis and sweat glands

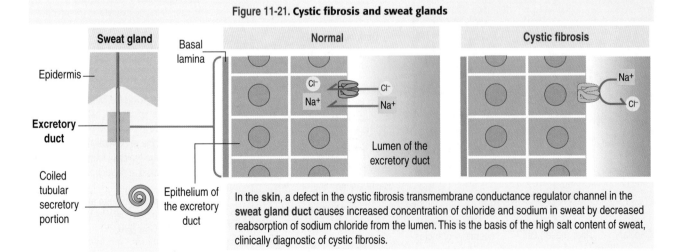

Sweat gland
Basal lamina
Epidermis
Excretory duct
Coiled tubular secretory portion
Epithelium of the excretory duct

Normal
Cl$^-$
Na$^+$
Cl$^-$
Na$^+$
Lumen of the excretory duct

Cystic fibrosis
Na$^+$
Cl$^-$

In the **skin,** a defect in the cystic fibrosis transmembrane conductance regulator channel in the **sweat gland duct** causes increased concentration of chloride and sodium in sweat by decreased reabsorption of sodium chloride from the lumen. This is the basis of the high salt content of sweat, clinically diagnostic of cystic fibrosis.

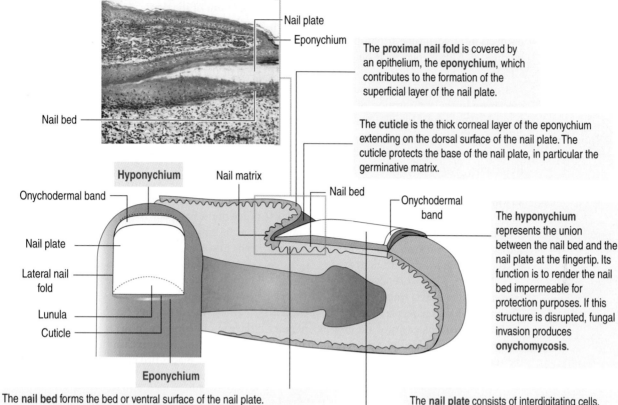

Figure 11-22. Structure and formation of the fingernail

Nail plate
Eponychium
Nail bed

The **proximal nail fold** is covered by an epithelium, the **eponychium**, which contributes to the formation of the superficial layer of the nail plate.

The **cuticle** is the thick corneal layer of the eponychium extending on the dorsal surface of the nail plate. The cuticle protects the base of the nail plate, in particular the germinative matrix.

Hyponychium   Nail matrix

Nail bed

Onychodermal band
Nail plate
Lateral nail fold
Lunula
Cuticle

Onychodermal band

The **hyponychium** represents the union between the nail bed and the nail plate at the fingertip. Its function is to render the nail bed impermeable for protection purposes. If this structure is disrupted, fungal invasion produces **onychomycosis**.

Eponychium

The **nail bed** forms the bed or ventral surface of the nail plate.

The **nail plate** is formed by the flattening of the epidermal cells, nuclear fragmentation, and condensation of the cytoplasm to form horny flat cells. The stratum granulosum is not present.

Normal nail growth is about 0.1 to 1.2 mm per day. Fingernails grow faster than toenails.

Nail growth is altered in several diseases (for example, hyperthyroidism).

The **nail plate** consists of interdigitating cells, corneocytes, lacking nuclei or organelles.

Calcium salts are important components of the nail plate. In addition, fibrillar and globular proteins containing sulfur are also found.

The hardness of the nail is due to high sulfur matrix proteins.

---

aldosterone. The reabsorption of NaCl by the excretory duct is deficient in patients with cystic fibrosis (see next section). The duct follows a **helical path** when it approaches the epidermis and opens on its surface at a **sweat pore** (see Figure 11-19). Within the epidermis, the excretory duct loses its epithelial wall and is surrounded by keratinocytes.

Apocrine sweat glands (see Figure 11-20) are coiled and occur in the axilla, mons pubis, and circumanal area. Apocrine sweat glands contain secretory acini larger than those in the eccrine sweat glands.

The secretory portion is located in the dermis and hypodermis. The **excretory duct opens into the hair follicle** (instead of into the epidermis as in the eccrine sweat glands). Apocrine sweat glands are functional after puberty and are supplied by **adrenergic nerves**.

Two special examples of apocrine sweat glands are the **ceruminous glands** in the external auditory meatus and the **glands of Moll** of the margins of the eyelids.

The ceruminous glands produce **cerumen**, a pig-mented lipid; the excretory duct opens, together with the ducts of sebaceous glands, into the hair follicles of the external auditory meatus.

The excretory duct of the glands of Moll opens into the free surface of the epidermis of the eyelid, or the eyelashes.

Clinical significance: Sweat glands and cystic fibrosis

Cystic fibrosis is a genetic disorder of epithelial transport of Cl^- by the channel protein **CFTR** (**cystic fibrosis transmembrane conductance regulator**), encoded by the *cystic fibrosis* gene located on chromosome 7.

Exocrine glands and the epithelial lining of the respiratory, gastrointestinal, and reproductive tracts are affected by a mutation of CFTR. Recurrent pulmonary infections, pancreatic insufficiency, steatorrhea, hepatic cirrhosis, intestinal obstruction, and male infertility are clinical features of cystic fibrosis.

The **excretory ducts of sweat glands** are lined by epithelial cells containing CFTR involved in the transport of Cl⁻ (Figure 11-21). The CFTR channel opens when an agonist, such as acetylcholine, induces an increase in cyclic adenosine monophosphate (cAMP), followed by activation of protein kinase A, production of adenosine triphosphate (ATP), and binding of ATP to two ATP-binding domains of CFTR.

A defect in CFTR in sweat gland ducts leads to a **decrease in the reabsorption of sodium chloride from the lumen**, resulting in **increased concentrations of chloride in sweat.**

In the respiratory epithelium (see Chapter 13, Respiratory System), a defect in CFTR results in a **reduction or loss of chloride secretion into the airways**, active reabsorption of sodium and water, and a consequent decrease in the water content of the protective mucus blanket. Dehydrated mucus causes defective mucociliary action and predisposes to recurrent pulmonary infections.

Epidermal derivatives: Fingernails

The nails are hard keratin plates on the dorsal surfaces of the terminal phalanges of the fingers and toes (Figure 11-22). The **nail plate** covers the **nail bed**, the surface of the skin that consists of the stratum basale and stratum spinosum only.

The body of the plate is surrounded by lateral **nail folds** with a structure similar to that of the adjacent epidermis of the skin.

When the lateral nail folds break down, an inflammatory process develops. This process is called **onychocryptosis** and is frequently observed in the nail of the first toe (ingrown nail).

The proximal edge of the plate is the **root** or **matrix** of the nail, where the whitish crescent-shaped **lunula** is located. The **nail matrix** is a region of the epidermis responsible for the formation of the nail substance. The distal portion of the plate is the free edge of the nail.

The nail plate consists of compact scales corresponding to cornified epithelial cells. The proximal edge of the nail plate is covered by the **eponychium**, a projecting fold of the stratum corneum of the skin, the **cuticle.**

A loss of the cuticle facilitates inflammatory and infective processes of the nail matrix, leading to **nail plate dystrophies.**

Under the distal and free edge of the nail plate, the stratum corneum of the epidermis forms a thick structure, the **hyponychium**. The hyponychium protects the matrix bed of the nail from bacterial and fungal invasion.

Essential concepts | **Integumentary System**

• Skin consists of three layers:
(1) Epidermis.
(2) Dermis.
(3) Hypodermis or subcutaneous layer.
There are two types of skin:
(1) Thick skin.
(2) Thin skin.
The epidermis and dermis are tightly interlocked. Epidermal ridges interact with dermal ridges. An epithelial-derived interpapillary peg divides the dermal ridge into secondary dermal ridges or papillae. Numerous dermal papillae interlock with the epidermal region. The dermal-epidermal interface is stabilized by hemidesmosomes.

• The epidermis is a stratified squamous epithelium consisting of four different cell types:
(1) Keratinocytes (ectoderm-derived cells).
(2) Melanocytes (neural crest–derived cells).
(3) Langerhans cells (bone marrow–derived dendritic cells).
(4) Merkel cells (neural crest–derived cells).
Keratinocytes are distributed in five strata or layers:
(1) Stratum basale (basal layer, which contains stem cells).
(2) Stratum spinosum (spinous or prickle cell layer).
(3) Stratum granulosum (granular cell layer).
(4) Stratum lucidum (clear cell layer), predominant in thick skin.
(5) Stratum corneum (cornified cell layer).

Keratinocytes are associated with each other by desmosomes and tight junctions.

• **Wound healing**. Skin is repaired rapidly to maintain an efficient protective barrier. Wound healing consists of four stages:
(1) Formation of a fibrin-platelet clot at the site of injury.
(2) Recruitment of leukocytes to protect the site from infection. Keratinocytes and endothelial cells express **cytokine CXC** (cysteine-x-cysteine) and its receptor to recruit leukocytes. Monocytes recruited to the injury site become macrophages.
(3) Neovascularization and cellular proliferation. **Granulation tissue**, rich in blood capillaries, is seen.
(4) Tissue remodeling. Keratinocytes express plasminogen activator to convert plasminogen within the fibrin clot into plasmin. Plasmin and matrix metalloproteinases (produced by fibroblasts in the dermis) free basal keratinocytes from their basal lamina anchorage site and re-epithelialization starts.
Epidermal growth factor and keratinocyte growth factor stimulate re-epithelialization. Fibroblasts in the dermis, stimulated by platelet-derived growth factor (PDGF) and transforming growth factor-β, start to proliferate. A number of fibroblasts change into myofibroblasts, and contraction of the dermis occurs (healing with a scar).

• **Psoriasis** is an inflammatory skin disorder producing a characteristic **psoriatic plaque**, commonly seen on the elbows, knees, scalp, umbilicus, and lumbar region. Persistent hyperplasia of the epidermis caused by abnormal cell proliferation and differentiation is observed. Keratinocytes move from the basal layer to the superficial layer in 3 to 5 days (instead of 28 to 30 days in normal skin).
The histologic characteristics of the psoriatic plaque are:
(1) Excessive proliferation of epidermal keratinocytes, caused by an accelerated migration of keratinocytes from the stratum basale to the stratum corneum.
(2) Presence of inflammatory cells, in particular type 17 helper T cells (TH17), dendritic cells, and neutrophils in the dermis and epidermis causing microabscesses. The proinflammatory cytokine interleukin-17A (IL-17A) is the primary effector of TH17 cells.
(3) Elongation of epidermic papillae, and prominent angiogenesis.
Keratinocytes stimulated by IL-17A undergo persistent hyperplasia by abnormal cell proliferation and differentiation. Treatment of psoriasis is targeted to the therapeutic inhibition of IL-17A.

• The differentiation of keratinocytes is characterized by:
(1) The expression of specific keratin pairs in each layer: keratins 5 and 14 in the stratum

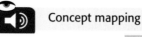
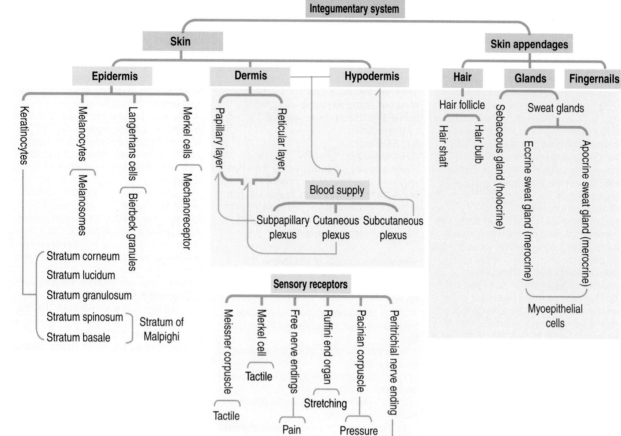

basale; keratins 1 and 10 in the stratum spinosum, and keratins 2e and 9 in the stratum granulosum.

(2) The presence in the stratum granulosum of lamellar bodies, containing the glycolipid acetylglucosylceramide extruded into the extracellular space to form a multilamellar lipid layer, and keratohyalin granules.

(3) The presence in the stratum corneum of the cornified cell envelope, an involucrin–small proline-rich–loricrin protein complex associated with keratin-filaggrin aggregates inside the cell. The extracellular multilamellar lipid layer is anchored to involucrin.

(4) The presence of desmosomes and tight junctions (containing claudin-1 and claudin-4).

• Melanocytes are branching cells located in the stratum basale. They migrate from the neural crest under control of c-kit receptor, a tyrosine kinase, and its ligand, stem cell factor.

Melanocytes produce melanin contained in melanosomes. Melanin is produced by oxidation of tyrosine to DOPA (1,3,4-dihydroxyphenylalanine) by tyrosinase. DOPA is transformed into melanin.

Melanosomes are transported along melanocyte dendritic processes. Kinesin transports melanosomes along microtubules toward

F-actin filaments located under the plasma membrane.

The microtubule–F-actin switch involves the attachment of the adapter melanophilin to Rab27a, a receptor on the melanosome membrane. Myosin Va recruits the melanosome–Rab27a–melanophilin complex, which is transported along F-actin tracks and released into the intercellular space by an exocrine mechanism (cytocrine secretion).

Keratinocytes of the stratum spinosum take up the melanin-containing melanosomes by endocytosis.

A genetic defect in myosin Va, melanophilin, and Rab27a disrupts the transport of melanin. **Griscelli syndrome** and its variants determine partial albinism, occasional neurologic defects, and immunodeficiency.

Microphthalmia-associated transcription factor (MITF) regulates the differentiation of melanocytes (cell cycle arrest, melanin production, and cell survival).

• **Langerhans cells** are dendritic cells of the epidermis derived from the bone marrow. Similar to melanocytes, Langerhans cells have dendritic processes in contact with keratinocytes through E-cadherin.

A characteristic landmark of Langerhans cells

is the Birbeck granule. Birbeck granule contains the proteins langerin and CD1a, involved in the uptake and delivery of antigens.

Langerhans cells take up antigens in the epidermis and migrate to regional lymph nodes, where they interact in the deep cortex with T cells. T cells, activated by the epidermal antigen, re-enter the blood circulation, extravasate at the site where the epidermal antigen is present, and secrete proinflammatory cytokines that produce an epidermic reaction.

• **Merkel cells** are found in the stratum basale. They are mechanoreceptors linked to adjacent keratinocytes by desmosomes.

• **Tumors of the epidermis.** They include hamartomas (epidermal nevi), reactive hyperplasias (pseudoepitheliomatous hyperplasia), benign tumors (acanthomas), and premalignant dysplasias, in situ, and invasive carcinomas.

Epidermal nevi are developmental deformations of the epidermis, in which excess keratinocytes undergo abnormal maturation (hyperkeratosis) and papillomatosis.

Pseudoepitheliomatous hyperplasia is a reaction in response to chronic irritation, such as around colostomy sites and to various inflammatory processes in the subjacent dermis (for example, mycoses).

Acanthomas are benign tumors characterized by abnormal keratinization , such as hyperkeratosis, dyskeratosis, or acantholysis (loss of cell-cell adhesion). An example is the seborrheic keratosis of the elderly.

Premalignant epidermal dysplasias have the potential for malignant transformation. This group includes solar keratosis on the sun- or tanning bed-exposed skin of the face, ears, scalp, hands, and forearms of older individuals.

Bowen's disease is an in situ squamous cell carcinoma of the skin characterized by a disorderly arrangement of keratinocytes displaying atypical nuclear features. Erythroplasia of Queyrat is a carcinoma in situ of the penis, commonly found on the glans penis of uncircumcised individuals.

Invasive malignant tumors include basal cell carcinoma (the most common tumor) and squamous cell carcinoma. Melanomas are the most dangerous form of skin cancer.

Basal cell carcinoma predominates on areas of the skin exposed to sun: head and neck. They arise from the basal layer of the epidermis and also from the external root sheath of the hair, or pilosebaceous unit. An often mutated gene in basal cell carcinomas is the *patched* (*PTCH*) gene, a tumor suppressor gene that is part of the Hedgehog signaling pathway.

Squamous cell carcinoma is the second most common form of skin cancer. Like basal cell carcinoma, squamous cell carcinoma affects areas of the skin directly exposed to the sun. Infection with high-risk types of human papilloma virus (HPV). For example, HPV-16 is responsible for a subgroup of squamous cell carcinoma of the head and neck.

Melanomas originate in the melanin-producing melanocytes in the basal layer of the epidermis. The presence and number of large congenital nevi and atypical nevi are regarded as precursor lesions.

A mutation in the *BRAF* (proto-oncogene B-Raf) gene is observed in a large number of melanomas. *Raf* genes code for cytoplasmic serine/threonine kinases that are regulated by binding the GTPase Ras.

The clinical features of melanoma are defined by the mnemonic ABCD: Asymmetry, Border irregularity, Color variation, and Diameter greater than 6 mm.

There are four types of melanomas:

(1) Superficial spreading melanoma is the most frequent.

(2) Lentigo maligna melanoma is similar to the superficial spreading type. It it preceded by the in situ form called lentigo maligna (an irregular freckle that progresses slowly) and, when it becomes invasive, it is called lentigo maligna melanoma.

(3) Acral lentiginous melanoma also spreads superficially before becoming invasive. It is the least common melanoma among Caucasians but most common in African-Americans and Asians.

(4) Nodular melanoma is commonly invasive at the time it is first diagnosed. This type of melanoma displays vertical growth, in contrast to the three previous types that show radial growth (superficial spreading) before invasive or vertical growth takes place.

• **Epithelial antimicrobial proteins (AMPs)** are produced by keratinocytes and sweat and sebaceous glands to kill or inactivate microorganisms.

AMPs are released quickly in response to a disruption of the skin barrier and provide a transient protection against infection.

AMPs include:

(1) β-Defensins.

(2) Cathelicidins.

Defensins and cathelicidins carry out a non-enzymatic disruption of the integrity of cell wall or cell membrane structures to promote lysis of microorganisms. Atopic dermatitis, rosacea and psoriasis have been associated in part to the deficient production of AMPs.

• The **dermis** consists of two layers:

(1) The papillary layer (loose connective tissue with collagen bundles and thin elastic fibers).

(2) The reticular layer (dense connective tissue with collagen bundles and thick elastic fibers).

Three interconnected blood vessel plexuses are in the dermis:

(1) The subpapillary plexus (along the papillary layer).

(2) The cutaneous plexus (at the papillary-reticular layer interface).

(3) The hypodermic or subcutaneous plexus (in the hypodermis).

The primary function of the vascular network is thermoregulation; the secondary function is nutrition of the skin and appendages.

• **Vascular abnormalities** of the skin are common. There are:

(1) Vascular malformations: vascular hamartomas and hemangiomas.

(2) Vascular dilatations: telangiectases.

(3) Tumors: angiomas, Kaposi's sarcoma, and angiosarcomas.

Vasculitis includes a group of disorders in which there is inflammation of and damage to blood vessel walls. Most cases of cutaneous vasculitis affect small vessels, predominantly venules.

Noninflammatory purpuras, caused by extravasation of blood in the dermis from small vessels, can be small (petechiae; less than 3 mm in diameter), or large (ecchymoses). Coagulation disorders, red blood cell diseases (sickle cell disease), and trauma are common causes.

Acute urticaria is a transient reaction caused by increased vascular permeability associated with edema in the dermis.

• **Sensory receptors** are specialized neurons and epithelial-like cells that receive and convert a physical stimulus into an electrical signal transmitted to the central nervous system.

Sensory receptors in general can be classified as:

(1) Exteroceptors: provide information about the external environment.

(2) Proprioceptors: provide information about the position and movements of the body.

(3) Interoceptors: provide information from the internal organs of the body.

Based on the type of stimulus, sensory receptors of the skin can be classified as:

(1) Mechanoreceptors: respond to mechanical stimulation. There are four primary tactile mechanoreceptors in human skin:

Merkel disk: found in the stratum basale of the epidermis of the fingertips and lips. The nerve ending of the Merkel disk mechanoreceptor discriminates fine touch and forms a flattened discoid structure attached to the Merkel cell.

Meissner corpuscle: found in the upper dermis, bulging into the epidermis of the fingertips and eyelids. This receptor detects shape and texture during active touch.

Ruffini ending: located in the deep dermis. It detects skin stretch and deformations within joints.

Pacinian corpuscle: found in the deep dermis and hypodermis. It responds to transient pressure and high-frequency vibration. They are found in the bone periosteum, joint capsules, pancreas, breast, and genitals.

Meissner corpuscle, Ruffini ending, pacinian corpuscle, and Krause end bulb are encapsuated receptors. Krause end bulb is a thermoreceptor found in the conjunctiva of the eye, in the mucosa of the lips and tongue, and in the epineurium of nerves.

(2) Thermoreceptors: respond to temperature changes. Krause end bulb detects cold. Krause end-bulbs are found in the conjunctiva of the eye, in the mucosa of the lips and tongue, and in the epineurium of nerves.

(3) Nociceptors: respond to pain. The simplest form of pain detectors are the free nerve endings. They derive from the dermal nerve plexus, supplied by cutaneous branches of the spinal nerves.

The perception of pain is associated to acute inflammation, one of the classical responses to tissue injury. Injured cells release chemical mediators, including substance P, acting on local blood vessels and nerve endings. Substance P triggers the degranulation of mast cells, histamine in particular, that enhances vascular dilation and plasma leakage.

Hyperemia accounts for the **triple response of Lewis** when a line is made on the skin with a pointed object: flush (capillary dilation), flare (redness spreading because of arteriolar dilation), and wheal (localized edema). The triple response develops between 1 to 3 minutes.

Peritrichial nerve endings are wrapped around the hair follicle just under the sebaceous glands. They are stimulated when the hairs bend.

• **Leprosy** (lepra) is a chronic infection of the skin, nasal mucosa, and peripheral nerves caused by *Mycobacterium leprae*, an intracellular bacillus found in Schwann cells, endothelial cells and macrophages of the skin. Nerve lesions result in anesthesia in the extremities, claw hand, and foot drop.

There are two histologic types of leprosy:

(1) The lepromatous reaction, characterized by numerous macrophages in the dermis with intracellular acid-fast bacilli.

(2) The tuberculoid reaction, identified by non-caseating granulomas consisting of macrophages, multinucleated giant cells, and lymphocytes (T cells). Bacilli are difficult to find. Granulomas tend to extend into the bundles of the cutaneous nerve, destroy the sweat glands, and erode the superficial dermis.

• Skin appendages

Hair (or pilosebaceous unit). The first type of hair of the human embryo is called lanugo and is thin and unpigmented.

Lanugo is replaced by vellus before birth.

Terminal hair replaces vellus, which remains in the hairless regions of the skin (for example, the forehead).

Hair follicles are constantly cycling between:
(1) Growth (anagen) phase.
(2) Regression (catagen) phase.
(3) Resting (telogen) phase.

Hair follicles are tubular invaginations of the epidermis. Each hair follicle consists of two components:

(1) The hair shaft, which includes the medulla, cortex, and cuticule, the latter associated with the internal root sheath.

(2) The hair bulb, the expanded portion of the hair follicle.

The hair follicle is surrounded by connective tissue (associated with the external root sheath, a downgrowth of the epidermis).

The dermal papilla extends into the hair bulb.

Hair is generated from the base of the hair bulb.

The hair bulb has two layers: the matrix zone, where all mitotic activity occurs, and the keratogenous zone, where hair cells undergo keratinization.

Two structures are associated with the hair follicle:

(1) The arrector pili muscle, spanning from the external root sheath of the hair follicle to the epidermis.

(2) The sebaceous glands, with their excretory ducts connected to the lumen of the hair follicle.

• Development of the skin

There are two signaling pathways that stimulate stem cells to enter the epidermal differentiation pathway:

(1) The Wnt (wingless-related) signaling pathway.

(2) The Notch signaling pathway.

The Wnt signaling pathway is important for the morphogenesis of the hair follicle.

The Notch signaling pathway stimulates epidermal differentiation in the postnatal epidermis.

• Glands of the skin include:
(1) Sebaceous glands.
(2) Sweat glands (eccrine and apocrine; both are merocrine).
(3) Mammary glands (see Chapter 23).

Sebaceous glands are holocrine simple saccular glands. The secretory portion is located in the dermis; the excretory duct opens into the hair follicle. Cells of the secretory portion (alveoli) contain small lipid droplets (sebum).

Eccrine (merocrine) sweat glands are simple coiled tubular glands. Their primary function is control of body temperature. The secretory portion consists of three cell types:

(1) Basal clear cells, separated from each other by intercellular canaliculi; they secrete water and electrolytes.

(2) Apical dark cells, that secrete glycoproteins, including AMPs human β-defensins (BD1 and BD2), cathelicidin, and dermicidin.

(3) Myoepithelial cells, whose contractile activity assists in the release of secretion into the glandular lumen.

The excretory portion is lined by a stratified cuboidal epithelium (except in the epidermis, where keratinocytes of the interpapillary peg constitute the wall of the excretory duct).

• Cystic fibrosis is a genetic disorder of epithelial transport of chloride ions by the channel protein cystic fibrosis transmembrane conductance regulator (CFTR). The lining epithelium of the excretory duct of eccrine sweat glands contains CFTR.

A defect in CFTR causes a decrease in the reabsorption of sodium chloride from the lumen, resulting in increased concentrations of Cl^- in sweat (salty skin).

Apocrine sweat glands are coiled and occur in the axilla, mons pubis, and circumanal area. The secretory acini are larger than in eccrine sweat glands. The excretory duct opens into the hair follicle, instead of into the epidermis as in the eccrine sweat glands. Ceruminous glands in the external auditory meatus and glands of Moll of the margins of the eyelids, are examples of apocrine sweat glands.

• Fingernails. The nails are hard keratin plates covering the nail bed, the surface of the skin consisting of the stratum basale and stratum spinosum only.

Nail plates are formed by scales of cornified epithelial cells. The proximal edge of the plate is the root or matrix of the nail, where the whitish crescent-shaped lunula is located.

The stratum corneum of the epidermis forms the hyponychium, a thick structure, under the distal and free edge of the nail plate.

The proximal edge of the plate is covered by the eponychium, a projection of the stratum corneum of the skin.

12. Cardiovascular System

The cardiovascular system is a continuous, completely closed network of endothelial tubes. The general purpose of the cardiovascular system is the perfusion of capillary beds permeating all organs with fresh blood over a narrow range of hydrostatic pressures. Local functional demands determine the structural nature of the wall surrounding the endothelial tubes. The heart is the main driver of the circulatory system. It functions as a pump. The architecture of the urinary and respiratory systems is based on the organization of the vasculature. Pathologic conditions of the cardiovascular system have a major impact on the normal function of the kidneys and lungs. In this chapter, the structural features of the heart, blood and lymphatic vessels are described and integrated with key pathologic conditions, including edema, vasculitis, atherosclerosis, thrombosis, embolism, and infarction.

General characteristics of blood circulation

The circulation is divided into the **systemic or peripheral circulation** and the **pulmonary circulation**.

Arteries transport blood under high pressure and their muscular walls are thick (Figure 12-1). The veins are conduits for transport of blood from tissues back to the heart. The pressure in the venous system is very low and the walls of the veins are thin.

There are variations in blood pressure in various parts of the cardiovascular system (see Figure 12-1). Because the heart pumps blood continuously in a pulsatile fashion into the aorta, the pressure in the aorta is high (about 100 mm Hg) and the arterial pressure fluctuates between a **systolic level** of 120 mm Hg and a **diastolic level** of 80 mm Hg.

As the blood flows through the systemic circulation, its pressure reaches the lowest value when it returns to the right atrium of the heart through the terminal vena cava. In the capillaries, the pressure is about 35 mm Hg at the arteriolar end and lower (10 mm Hg) at the venous end. Although the pressure in the pulmonary arteries is pulsatile, as in the aorta, the systolic pressure is less (about 25 mm Hg), and the diastolic pressure is 8 mm Hg. The pressure in the pulmonary capillaries is only 7 mm Hg, as compared with an average pressure of 17 mm Hg in the capillary bed of the systemic circulation.

Heart

The heart is a folded endothelial tube whose wall is thickened to act as a regulated pump. The heart is the major determinant of systemic blood pressure.

The cardiac wall consists of three layers:

1. **Endocardium**, consisting of an **endothelial lining** and **subendothelial connective tissue**.

2. **Myocardium**, a functional syncytium of striated cardiac muscle fibers forming three major types of cardiac muscle: **atrial muscle**, **ventricular muscle**, and **specialized excitatory** and **conductive muscle fibers**.

3. **Pericardium**. The **epicardium**, the visceral layer of the pericardium, is a low-friction surface lined by a **mesothelium** in contact with the parietal pericardial space.

The heart is composed of two syncytia of muscle fibers:

1. The **atrial syncytium**, forming the walls of the two atria.

2. The **ventricular syncytium**, forming the wall of the two ventricles. Atria and ventricles are separated by **fibrous connective tissue** surrounding the valvular openings between the atria and the ventricles.

Conductive system of the heart

The heart has two specialized conductive systems:

1. The **sinus node**, or **sinoatrial** (S-A) **node**, which generates impulses to cause rhythmic contractions of the cardiac muscle.

2. A specialized **conductive system**, consisting of the **internodal pathway**, which conducts the impulse

Figure 12-1. Blood pressure and vascular anatomy

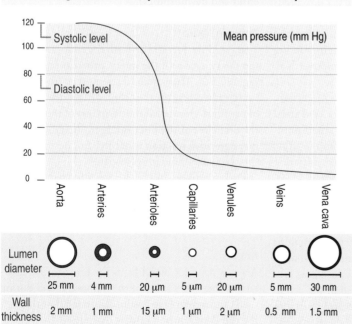

Mean pressure (mm Hg)

	Aorta	Arteries	Arterioles	Capillaries	Venules	Veins	Vena cava
Lumen diameter	25 mm	4 mm	20 μm	5 μm	20 μm	5 mm	30 mm
Wall thickness	2 mm	1 mm	15 μm	1 μm	2 μm	0.5 mm	1.5 mm

Figure 12-2. Heart: Purkinje fibers

Purkinje fibers are bundles of impulse-conducting cardiac fibers extending from the atrioventricular node. They can be found beneath the endocardium lining the interventricular septum.

Purkinje fibers can be distinguished from regular cardiocytes by their **location**, their **larger size**, and **lighter cytoplasmic staining** (glycogen content).

The **subendocardial connective tissue layer** consists of collagen and elastic fibers synthesized by fibroblasts.

This layer contains small blood vessels, nerves, and bundles of the conduction system (**Purkinje fibers**). The subendocardial layer is not present in papillary muscles and chordae tendineae inserted at the free edges of the mitral and tricuspid valves.

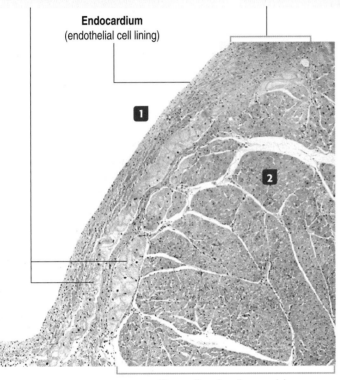

Endocardium
(endothelial cell lining)

Myocardium (cardiac muscle)

Heart

The wall of the heart consists of three layers:
1. **Endocardium**, homologous to the tunica intima of blood vessels.
2. **Myocardium**, continuous with the tunica media of blood vessels.
3. **Epicardium**, the visceral layer of the pericardium, similar to the tunica adventitia of blood vessels (not shown in the illustration).

The myocardium consists of three cell types:
1. **Contractile cardiocytes**, which contract to pump blood through the circulation.
2. **Myoendocrine cardiocytes**, producing atrial natriuretic factor.
3. **Nodal cardiocytes**, specialized to control the rhythmic contraction of the heart. These cells are located in (1) the **sinoatrial node**, at the superior vena cava–right atrium junction; and (2) the **atrioventricular node**, present under the endocardium of the interatrial and interventricular septa.

from the S-A node to the atrioventricular (A-V) node); the **A-V node**, in which the atrial impulse is delayed before reaching the ventricles; the **atrioventricular bundle**, which conducts the impulse from the atria to the ventricles; and the **left and right bundles of Purkinje fibers**, which conduct the impulse to all parts of the ventricles (Figure 12-2).

When stretched, cardiac muscle cells of the atrium, the atrial cardiocytes, secrete a hormone called **atrial natriuretic peptide** (ANP) (Figure 12-3) that stimulates both diuresis and excretion of sodium in urine (natriuresis) by increasing the glomerular filtration rate. By this mechanism, the blood volume is reduced.

Histologically (see Figure 7-18 in Chapter 7, Muscle Tissue), individual cardiac muscle cells have a central nucleus and are linked to each other by **intercalated disks**. The presence of **gap junctions** in the longitudinal segment of the intercalated disks between connected cardiac muscle cells allows free diffusion of ions and the rapid spread of the action potential from cell to cell. The electrical resistance is low because gap junctions bypass the **transverse**

components of the intercalated disk (**fasciae adherentes** and **desmosomes**).

Purkinje fibers
The **Purkinje fibers** lie **beneath the endocardium** lining the two sides of the interventricular septum (see Figure 12-2). They can be distinguished from cardiac muscle fibers because they contain a **reduced number of myofibrils located at the periphery of the fiber** and the **diameter of the fiber is larger**. In addition, they give a positive reaction for **acetylcholinesterase**, and they contain abundant **glycogen**.

Purkinje fibers lose these specific characteristics when they merge with cardiac muscle fibers. Like cardiac muscle fibers, Purkinje fibers are striated and are linked to each other by atypical intercalated disks.

Arteries
Arteries conduct blood from the heart to the capillaries. They store some of the pumped blood during each cardiac systole to ensure continued flow through the capillaries during cardiac diastole.

Figure 12-3. Atrial natriuretic peptide

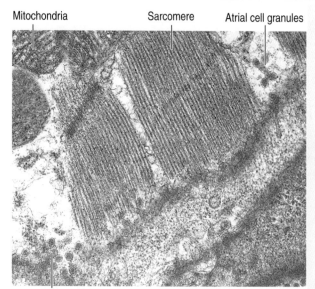

Mitochondria   Sarcomere   Atrial cell granules

Atrial cell granules

Atrial cardiocytes store membrane-bound granules whose density can be altered by varying the intake of salt and water.

Atrial cell granules contain the precursor of **atrial natriuretic peptide (ANP)**, a potent polypeptide hormone that stimulates **diuresis** (Greek *diourein*, to urinate) and **natriuresis** (Latin *natrium*, sodium + Greek *diourein*). Once outside the atrial cell, the ANP precursor undergoes a rapid enzymatic cleavage to produce circulating ANP.

ANP binding to **natriuretic peptide receptors NPR1, NPR2,** and **NPR3** (with guanylyl cyclase activity), causes the conversion of guanosine triphosphate (GTP) to cyclic guanosine monophosphate (cGMP). Then, cGMP activates a cGMP-dependent kinase that phosphorylates specific serine and threonine residues in target proteins.

ANP antagonizes the actions of **vasopressin**, a polypeptide released from the neurohypophysis, and **angiotensin II (ANG II)**. ANG II is a peptide derived from the **renin**-induced breakdown of **angiotensinogen (AGT)**, produced in liver and released into the systemic blood.

ANP prevents sodium and water reabsorption from causing **hypervolemia** (abnormal increase in the volume of circulating fluid in the body) and **hypertension** that can result in cardiac failure.

Arteries are organized in three major **tunics** or layers (Figure 12-4):

1. The **tunica intima** is the innermost coat. It consists of an **endothelial lining** continuous with the endocardium, the inner lining of the heart; an intermediate layer of loose connective tissue, the **subendothelium**; and an external layer of elastic fibers, the **internal elastic lamina**.

2. The **tunica media** is the middle coat. It consists mainly of smooth muscle cells surrounded by a variable number of collagen fibers, extracellular matrix, and elastic sheaths with irregular gaps (fenestrated elastic membranes).

Collagen fibers provide a supporting framework for smooth muscle cells and limit the distensibility of the wall of the vessel. Veins have a higher content of collagen than arteries.

3. The **tunica externa**, or **adventitia**, is the outer coat and consists mainly of connective tissue. An external elastic lamina can be seen separating the tunica media from the adventitia.

The adventitia of large vessels (arteries and veins) contains small vessels (**vasa vasorum**) that penetrate the outer portion of the tunica media to supply oxygen and nutrients.

From the heart to the capillaries, arteries can be classified into three major groups:

1. **Large-sized elastic arteries.**
2. **Medium-sized muscular arteries** (see Figure 12-4).
3. **Small-sized arteries** and **arterioles.**

Large elastic arteries are conducting vessels

The **aorta** and its largest branches (the **brachiocephal-ic, common carotid, subclavian,** and **common iliac** arteries) are **elastic arteries** (Figure 12-5). They are **conducting arteries** because they conduct blood from the heart to the medium-sized **distributing arteries**.

Large elastic arteries have two major characteristics:

1. They receive blood from the heart under high pressure.
2. They keep blood circulating continuously while the heart is pumping intermittently.

Because they distend during systole and recoil during diastole, elastic arteries can sustain a continuous blood flow despite the intermittent pumping action of the heart.

The **tunica intima** of the elastic arteries consists of the endothelium and the subendothelial connective tissue.

Large amounts of **fenestrated elastic sheaths** are found in the **tunica media**, with bundles of smooth muscle cells permeating the narrow gaps between the elastic lamellae. Collagen fibers are present in all tunics, but especially in the adventitia. We have seen in Chapter 4, Connective Tissue, that smooth muscle cells can synthesize **both elastic and collagen fibers**. Blood vessels (**vasa vasorum**), nerves (**nervi vasorum**), and **lymphatics** can be recognized in the tunica adventitia of large elastic arteries.

Pathology: Aortic aneurysms

Aneurysms are dilatations of arteries; the dilatations of veins are called varices.

The two major types of aortic aneurysms are the **syphilitic aneurysm** (relatively rare because syphilis is no longer common) and the **abdominal aneurysm**.

Syphilitic aneurysms are mostly localized in the

Figure 12-4. Structure of a muscular artery

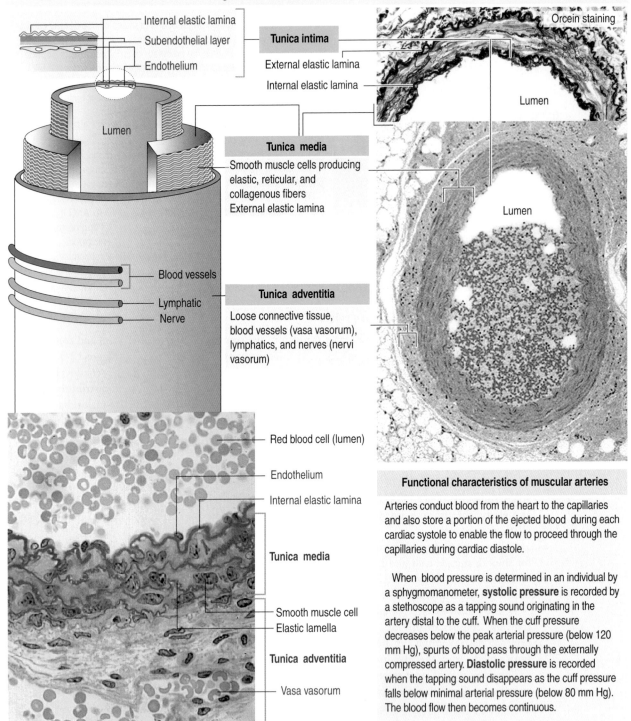

Internal elastic lamina
Subendothelial layer
Endothelium

Tunica intima

External elastic lamina
Internal elastic lamina

Orcein staining

Lumen

Lumen

Tunica media

Smooth muscle cells producing elastic, reticular, and collagenous fibers
External elastic lamina

Lumen

Blood vessels
Lymphatic
Nerve

Tunica adventitia

Loose connective tissue, blood vessels (vasa vasorum), lymphatics, and nerves (nervi vasorum)

Red blood cell (lumen)

Endothelium

Internal elastic lamina

Tunica media

Smooth muscle cell
Elastic lamella

Tunica adventitia

Vasa vasorum

Functional characteristics of muscular arteries

Arteries conduct blood from the heart to the capillaries and also store a portion of the ejected blood during each cardiac systole to enable the flow to proceed through the capillaries during cardiac diastole.

When blood pressure is determined in an individual by a sphygmomanometer, **systolic pressure** is recorded by a stethoscope as a tapping sound originating in the artery distal to the cuff. When the cuff pressure decreases below the peak arterial pressure (below 120 mm Hg), spurts of blood pass through the externally compressed artery. **Diastolic pressure** is recorded when the tapping sound disappears as the cuff pressure falls below minimal arterial pressure (below 80 mm Hg). The blood flow then becomes continuous.

ascending aorta and its arch. Abdominal aneurysms are caused by a weakening of the aortic wall produced by atherosclerosis.

Aortic aneurysms generate murmurs caused by blood turbulence in the dilated aortic segment. A severe complication of an aneurysm is aortic dissection caused by a tear in the tunica intima that enables blood to penetrate and form an intramural hematoma between the intima and the tunica media or the media and the tunica adventitia. Aortic dissection is associated with high mortality caused by exsanguination.

Marfan syndrome (see Chapter 4, Connective Tissue) is an autosomal dominant defect associated with aortic dissecting aneurysm and skeletal and ocular abnormalities due to mutations in the *fibrillin 1* gene. Fibrillins are major components of the elastic fibers found in the aorta, periosteum, and suspensory ligament of the lens.

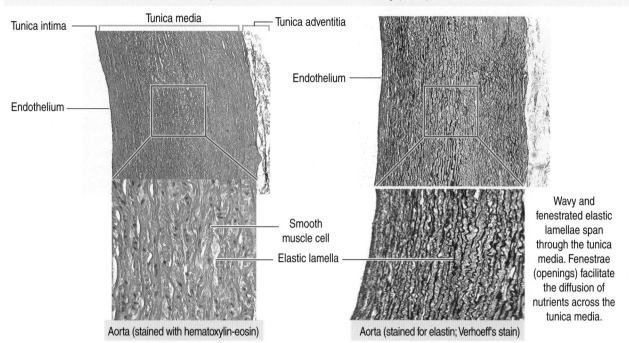

Figure 12-5. Structure of an elastic artery (aorta)

Tunica intima — Tunica media — Tunica adventitia

Endothelium

Endothelium

Smooth muscle cell

Elastic lamella

Wavy and fenestrated elastic lamellae span through the tunica media. Fenestrae (openings) facilitate the diffusion of nutrients across the tunica media.

Aorta (stained with hematoxylin-eosin)

Aorta (stained for elastin; Verhoeff's stain)

Medium-sized muscular arteries are distributing vessels

There is a gradual transition from large arteries, to medium-sized arteries, to small arteries and arterioles. Medium-sized arteries are **distributing vessels**, allowing a selective distribution of blood to different organs in response to functional needs. Examples of medium-sized arteries include the radial, tibial, popliteal, axillary, splenic, mesenteric, and intercostal arteries. The diameter of medium-sized muscular arteries is about 3 mm or greater.

The **tunica intima** consists of three layers:
1. The **endothelium**.
2. The **subendothelium**.
3. The **internal elastic lamina** (see Figure 12-4).

The internal elastic lamina is a fenestrated band of elastic fibers that often shows folds in sections of fixed tissue because of contraction of the smooth muscle cell layer (tunica media).

The **tunica media** shows a significant reduction in elastic components and an increase in smooth muscle fibers. In the larger vessels of this group, a fenestrated **external elastic lamina** can be seen at the junction of the tunica media and the adventitia.

Arterioles are resistance vessels

Arterioles are the final branches of the arterial system. Arterioles regulate the distribution of blood to different capillary beds by **vasoconstriction** and **vasodilation** in localized regions. Partial contraction (known as **tone**) of the vascular smooth muscle exists in arterioles. Arterioles are structurally adapted for vasoconstriction and vasodilation because their walls contain circularly arranged smooth muscle fibers. Arterioles are regarded as **resistance vessels** and are the major determinants of systemic blood pressure (Figure 12-6).

The diameter of arterioles and small arteries ranges from 20 to 130 μm. Because the lumen is small, these blood vessels can be closed down to generate high resistance to blood flow.

The **tunica intima** has an endothelium, subendothelium, and internal elastic lamina. The **tunica media** consists of two to five concentric layers of smooth muscle cells. The **tunica adventitia**, or **tunica externa**, contains slight collagenous tissue, binding the vessel to its surroundings.

The segment beyond the arteriole proper is the **metarteriole**, the terminal branch of the arterial system. It consists of one layer of muscle cells, often **discontinuous**, and represents an important local regulator of blood flow.

Capillaries are exchange vessels

Capillaries are extremely thin tubes formed by a single layer of highly permeable **endothelial cells** surrounded by a basal lamina. The diameter range of a capillary is about 5 to 10 μm, large enough to accommodate one red blood cell, and thin enough (0.5 μm) for gas diffusion.

The **microvascular bed**, the site of the **microcirculation** (Figure 12-7), is composed of the **terminal arteriole** (and **metarteriole**), the **capillary bed**, and the **postcapillary venules**. The capillary bed consists of slightly large capillaries (called **preferential** or **thoroughfare channels**), where blood flow is **continuous**,

Figure 12-6. Arterioles: Resistance vessels

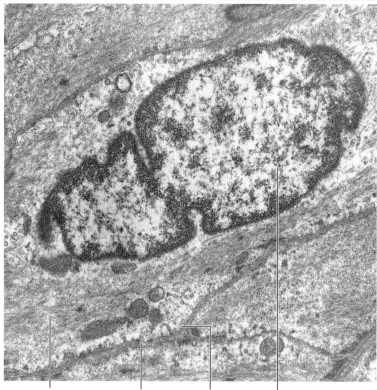

Actin-myosin bundle   Basal lamina   Pinocytosis   Nucleus

Vascular smooth muscle cells of arterioles

Vascular smooth muscle cells have a significant role in the control of total peripheral resistance, arterial and venous tone, and blood distribution throughout the body.

The cytoplasm of vascular smooth muscle cells contains actin and myosin filaments whose contraction is controlled by calcium. The increase in calcium concentration occurs through voltage-gated calcium channels (known as **electromechanical coupling**) and through receptor-mediated calcium channels (known as **pharmacomechanical coupling**). Both channels are present in the plasma membrane. Calcium can also be released from cytoplasmic storage sites (endoplasmic reticulum). Smooth muscle cells lack troponin.

The constant blood flow depends on a **myogenic mechanism**: arteriolar smooth muscle cells contract in response to increased transmural pressure and relax when the pressure decreases.

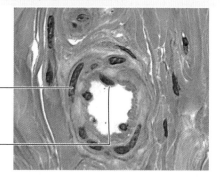

Vascular smooth muscle cell

Endothelial cell

and small capillaries, called the **true capillaries**, where blood flow is **intermittent**.

The amount of blood entering the microvascular bed is regulated by the contraction of smooth muscle fibers of the **precapillary sphincters** located where true capillaries arise from the arteriole or metarteriole. The capillary circulation can be bypassed by channels (**through channels**) connecting terminal arterioles to postcapillary venules.

When functional demands decrease, most precapillary sphincters are closed, forcing the flow of blood into thoroughfare channels. **Arteriovenous shunts**, or **anastomoses**, are direct connections between arterioles and postcapillary venules and bypass the microvascular bed.

The three-dimensional design of the microvasculature varies from organ to organ. The local conditions of the tissues (concentration of nutrients and metabolites and other substances) can control local blood flow in small portions of a tissue area.

Types of capillaries

Three morphologic types of capillaries are recognized (Figures 12-8 and 12-9):

1. **Continuous**.
2. **Fenestrated**.
3. **Discontinuous (sinusoids)**.

Continuous capillaries are lined by a complete simple squamous endothelium and a basal lamina. **Pericytes** can occur between the endothelium and the basal lamina. Pericytes are undifferentiated cells that resemble modified smooth muscle cells and are distributed at random intervals in close contact with the basal lamina. Endothelial cells are linked by tight junctions and transport fluids and solutes by **caveolae** and **pinocytotic vesicles**. Continuous capillaries occur in the brain, muscle, skin, thymus, and lungs.

Fenestrated capillaries have **pores**, or **fenestrae**, with or without **diaphragms**. Fenestrated capillaries with a diaphragm are found in intestines, endocrine glands, and around kidney tubules. Fenestrated capillaries without a diaphragm are characteristic of the renal glomerulus. In this particular case, the basal lamina constitutes an important permeability barrier, as we will analyze in detail in Chapter 14, Urinary System.

Discontinuous capillaries are characterized by an incomplete endothelial lining and basal lamina,

Figure 12-7. Microcirculation: Components and function

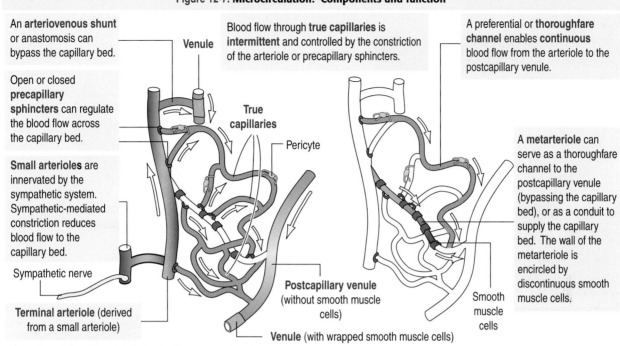

An **arteriovenous shunt** or anastomosis can bypass the capillary bed.

Open or closed **precapillary sphincters** can regulate the blood flow across the capillary bed.

Small arterioles are innervated by the sympathetic system. Sympathetic-mediated constriction reduces blood flow to the capillary bed.

Sympathetic nerve

Terminal arteriole (derived from a small arteriole)

Venule

Blood flow through **true capillaries** is **intermittent** and controlled by the constriction of the arteriole or precapillary sphincters.

True capillaries

Pericyte

Postcapillary venule (without smooth muscle cells)

Venule (with wrapped smooth muscle cells)

A preferential or **thoroughfare channel** enables **continuous** blood flow from the arteriole to the postcapillary venule.

A **metarteriole** can serve as a thoroughfare channel to the postcapillary venule (bypassing the capillary bed), or as a conduit to supply the capillary bed. The wall of the metarteriole is encircled by discontinuous smooth muscle cells.

Smooth muscle cells

Smooth muscle cell   Arteriole   Capillary   Venule

Arterioles have an endothelial lining, a thick smooth muscle layer, and a thin adventitial layer. Arterioles can give rise to capillaries or, in some tissues, to metarterioles, which then give rise to capillaries. Arterioles regulate blood flow through capillaries by constriction or dilation of the precapillary sphincters. However, most tissues lack metarterioles or precapillary sphincters.

Capillaries are numerous in metabolically active tissues (such as cardiac and skeletal muscle and glands). The diameter of the capillaries is variable (it can be less than the diameter of a red blood cell that is transiently deformed when passing through these capillaries).

The capillary bed provides for exchange of gases and solutes between blood and tissue (known as **nutritional flow**). Blood bypassing the capillaries, by a metarteriole or an arteriovenous shunt, is known as **non-nutritional** or **shunt flow**.

Endothelial cell   Pericyte   Smooth muscle cell   Collagen bundle

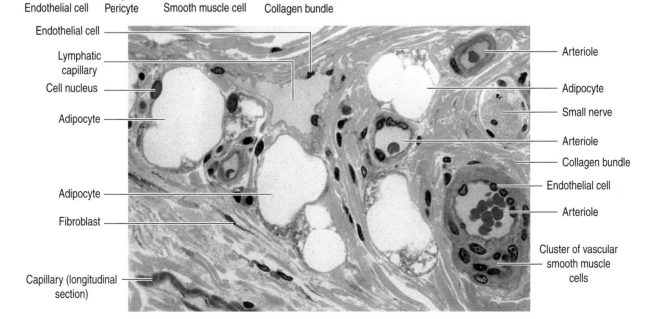

Endothelial cell

Lymphatic capillary

Cell nucleus

Adipocyte

Adipocyte

Fibroblast

Capillary (longitudinal section)

Arteriole

Adipocyte

Small nerve

Arteriole

Collagen bundle

Endothelial cell

Arteriole

Cluster of vascular smooth muscle cells

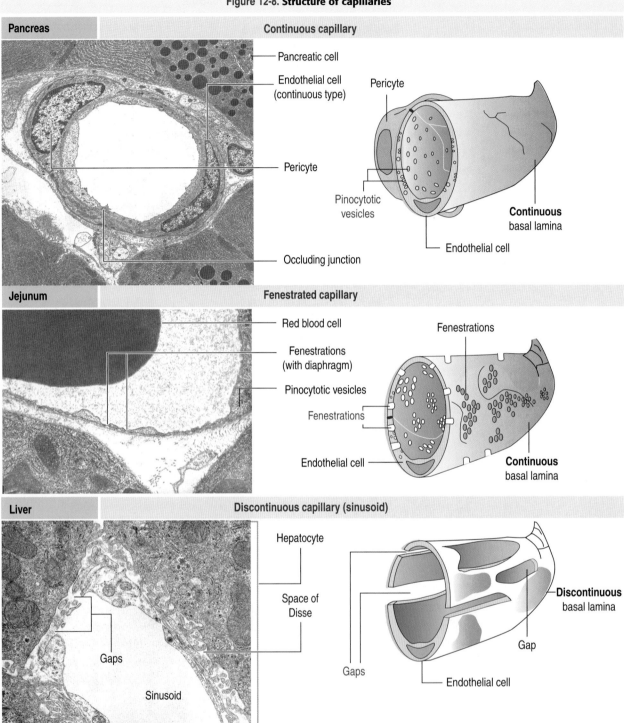

Figure 12-8. Structure of capillaries

Pancreas | **Continuous capillary**

- Pancreatic cell
- Endothelial cell (continuous type)
- Pericyte
- Occluding junction

- Pericyte
- Pinocytotic vesicles
- **Continuous** basal lamina
- Endothelial cell

Jejunum | **Fenestrated capillary**

- Red blood cell
- Fenestrations (with diaphragm)
- Pinocytotic vesicles
- Fenestrations
- Endothelial cell

- Fenestrations
- **Continuous** basal lamina

Liver | **Discontinuous capillary (sinusoid)**

- Hepatocyte
- Space of Disse
- Gaps
- Sinusoid

- **Discontinuous** basal lamina
- Gap
- Gaps
- Endothelial cell

with **gaps** or **holes** between and within endothelial cells. Discontinuous capillaries and sinusoids are found where an intimate relation is needed between blood and parenchyma (for example, in the liver and spleen).

Veins are capacitance, or reservoir, vessels

The venous system starts at the end of the capillary bed with a **postcapillary venule** that structurally resembles continuous capillaries but with a wider lumen.

Postcapillary venules, the preferred site of migration of blood cells into tissues by a mechanism called **diapedesis** (Greek *dia*, through; *pedan*, to leap), are tubes of endothelial cells supported by a basal lamina and an adventitia of collagen fibers and fibroblasts.

In lymphatic tissues, the endothelial cells are taller. **High endothelial venules are associated with the**

Figure 12-9. **Types of capillaries**

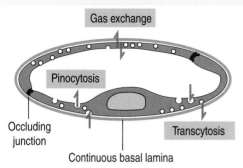

Continuous capillary

Endothelial cells have a complete (continuous) cytoplasm. This type is found in muscle, brain, thymus, bone, lung, and other tissues.

Caveolae and vesicles transport substances through the cytoplasm in a bidirectional pathway (**transcytosis**). The intracytoplasmic vesicles are coated by the protein **caveolin**.

The **basal lamina** is **continuous**. In the lung, the thin endothelial cell cytoplasm allows diffusion of gases from the alveolus into the blood (CO_2) and from the blood into the alveolus (O_2).

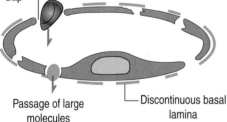

Fenestrated capillary

The endothelial cell has many fenestrae (10 to 100 nm in diameter) **with** or **without a thin diaphragm**. The **basal lamina** is **continuous**.

This type is present in tissues with substantial fluid transport (intestinal villi, choroid plexus, ciliary processes of the eyes).

A fenestrated endothelial cell is present in the glomerular capillaries of the kidneys supported by a significantly thicker basal lamina.

Discontinuous capillary (sinusoid)

The gaps in discontinuous capillaries are larger than in fenestrated capillaries. The **basal lamina** is **discontinuous**.

The gaps in venous sinusoids of the liver are wider than the discontinuous capillaries. The basal lamina is fragmented and often absent.

In the **spleen**, the endothelial cells are elongated and protrude into the lumen. The **basal lamina** is **incomplete** and surrounded by reticular fibers. Blood cells can pass readily through the walls of the splenic sinuses (see Chapter 10, Immune-Lymphatic System).

---

mechanism of homing of lymphocytes in lymphoid organs (see Chapter 10, Immune-Lymphatic System).

Postcapillary venules converge to form **muscular venules**, which converge into **collecting venules**, leading to a series of **veins** of progressively larger diameter.

Veins have a relatively thin wall in comparison with arteries of the same size (Figure 12-10). The high capacitance of veins is attributable to the distensibility of their wall (**compliance vessels**) and, therefore, the content of blood is large relative to the volume of the veins. A small increase in the intraluminal pressure results in a large increase in the volume of contained blood.

Similar to arteries, veins consist of tunics. However, the distinction of a tunica media from a tunica adventitia is often not clear. The lumen is lined by an endothelium and a subjacent basal lamina. **A distinct internal elastic lamina is not seen.**

The **muscular tunica media** is thinner than in arteries, and smooth muscle cells have an irregular orientation, approximately circular. A longitudinal

orientation is observed in the iliac vein, brachiocephalic vein, superior and inferior venae cavae, portal vein, and renal vein.

The **tunica adventitia** consists of collagen fibers and fibroblasts with few nerve fibers. In large veins, the vasa vasorum penetrate the wall.

A typical characteristic of veins is the presence of **valves** to prevent reflux of blood. A valve is a projection into the lumen of the tunica intima, covered by endothelial cells and strengthened by elastic and collagen fibers.

Examples of varices (dilatations of veins) are **hemorrhoids** (varices of the internal or external plexus of the rectum), **varicocele** (varices of the pampiniform plexus of the spermatic cord), **varicose veins of the legs** and **varices of the esophagus** (associated with portal hypertension and cirrhosis of the liver).

Pathology: Vasculitis

Vasculitis defines the acute and chronic inflammation of vessels. It can be caused by infectious and immu-

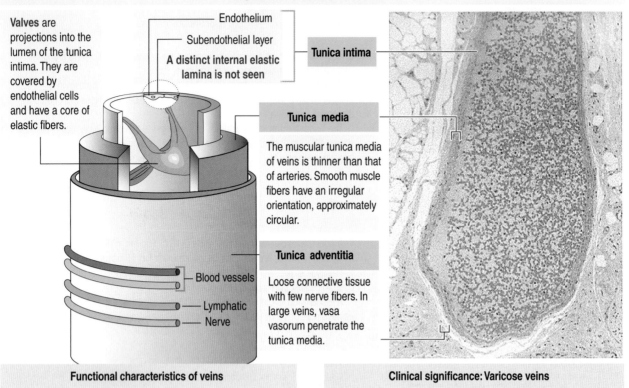

Figure 12-10. Structure of a vein

Valves are projections into the lumen of the tunica intima. They are covered by endothelial cells and have a core of elastic fibers.

Endothelium

Subendothelial layer

A distinct internal elastic lamina is not seen

Tunica intima

Tunica media

The muscular tunica media of veins is thinner than that of arteries. Smooth muscle fibers have an irregular orientation, approximately circular.

Tunica adventitia

Loose connective tissue with few nerve fibers. In large veins, vasa vasorum penetrate the tunica media.

Blood vessels

Lymphatic

Nerve

Functional characteristics of veins

Veins are high-capacitance vessels containing about 70% of the total blood volume.

In contrast to arteries, the tunica media contains fewer smooth muscle cell bundles associated with reticular and elastic fibers.

Although veins of the extremities have intrinsic vasomotor activity, the transport of blood back to the heart depends on external forces provided by the contraction of surrounding skeletal muscles and on valves that ensure one-way blood flow.

Clinical significance: Varicose veins

Varicose veins result from intrinsic weakness of the muscular tunica media caused by increased intraluminal pressure or from defects in the structure and function of the valves that hamper the flow of venous blood toward the heart.

Although varicose veins can be seen in any vein in the body, the most common are the saphenous veins of the legs, veins in the anorectal region (**hemorrhoids**), the veins of the lower esophagus (**esophageal varices**), and veins in the spermatic cord (**varicocele**).

---

nologic pathogens. Bacterial and rickettsial infection, syphilis and fungi cause vasculitis, thrombophlebitis (thrombosis and inflammation of the wall of a vein) and pseudoaneurysms (dilation of the wall of a blood vessel by the lytic activity of bacterial enzymes.

Most inflammatory conditions of the wall of arteries involve an immune-based pathogenesis.

Antigen-antibody complexes, accumulating in the wall of a blood vessel, can activate the complement cascade, as you have learned in Chapter 10, Immune-Lymphatic System. When neutrophils are attracted by chemotactic fragments released by the activated complement cascade and exposed to cytokines, they release **serine proteinase 3** and **myeloperoxidase**, capable of causing damage to the vascular wall.

Antibodies reacting with cytoplasmic components of neutrophils (**anti-neutrophil cytoplasmic antibody, ANCA**) release enzymes from the activated neutrophils, causing vascular wall injury.

Serine proteinase 3, a component of cytoplasmic granules in neutrophils, is the antigen that gener-

ates **C-ANCA (cytoplasmic ANCA); P-ANCA** are antibodies to myeloperoxidase showing a perinuclear pattern in neutrophils (**perinuclear ANCA**) by immunocytochemistry.

Vasculitis include (Figure 12-11):

1. **Giant cell arteritis** is a common form of vasculitis in adults (over the age of 50) that affects temporal, ophthalmic or vertebral arteries. Headache, pain in the shoulders, hips and jaw claudication as well as an elevated erythrocyte sedimentation rate are common findings. Blindness from giant cell arteritis of the ophthalmic artery is irreversible if the disease is not treated early with prednisone. A biopsy of the temporal artery, showing in most cases giant multinucleated cells (macrophages) and lymphocyte infiltrates in the wall, thickening of the tunica intima and thrombosis, confirms the nature of the disease.

2. **Buerger's disease** (thromboangitis obliterans, see Figure 12-11), involves medium-sized and small arteries of hands and feet of young males who are heavy cigarette smokers. Typical symptoms are

Figure 12-11. Vasculitis

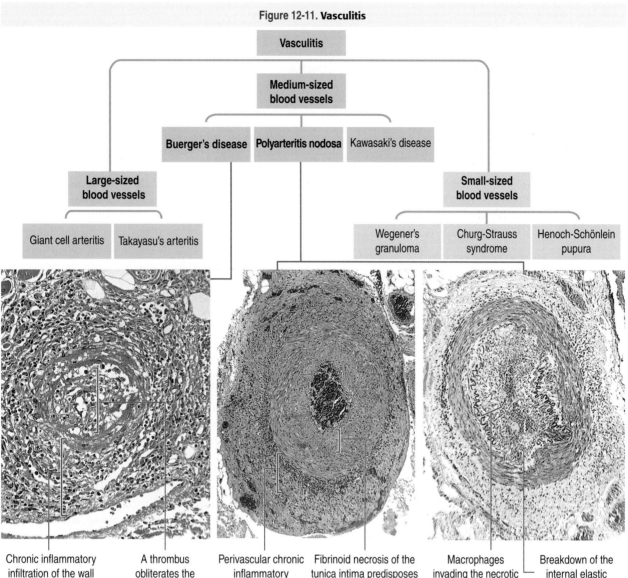

Chronic inflammatory infiltration of the wall of the artery

A thrombus obliterates the vascular lumen

Perivascular chronic inflammatory reaction

Fibrinoid necrosis of the tunica intima predisposes to thrombosis

Macrophages invading the necrotic tunica intima

Breakdown of the internal elastic lamina

claudication, pain in hands and feet caused by insufficient blood flow during exercise, and **Raynaud's phenomenon**, a condition in which fingers and toes turn white upon exposure to cold. Angiograms of the upper and lower extremities generally show blockage or narrowing segments. Stopping smoking is the most effective treatment.

3. **Polyarteritis nodosa** (PAN; see Figure 12-11) affects the wall of medium- to small-sized arteries of the skin, kidneys, liver, heart, and gastrointestinal tract. PAN has been associated with active hepatitis B and/or hepatitis C. The disease is more common in injection drug users. Immune complexes (immunoglobulin and viral antigens) circulating in the blood accumulate in the vascular wall. Prednisone is the effective treatment of PAN.

4. **Giant cell aortitis** (Takayasu's arteritis) is a rare disease that occurs with a high frequency in Asian women under the age of 40 and affects the aorta and its branches. It consists of an inflammatory phase followed by an occlusive phase, the narrowing and segmental dilation of the aorta and/or its branches, resulting in absent pulses. Takayasu's arteritis and giant cell arteritis are histologically similar: both show destruction of the blood vessel wall and giant multinucleated cells.

5. **Kaswasaki's disease** affects the coronary arteries as well as large, medium- and small-sized arteries of children. It is associated with fever, ulcerations of mouth, lips and throat mucosae and lymph node enlargement. The standard treatment includes intravenous immunoglobulin and aspirin. Affected children recover without serious complications.

6. **Churg-Strauss syndrome** (CSS) is a systemic vasculitis associated with asthma, rhinitis and eosinophilia. A biopsy of an affected blood vessel shows peri-

vascular eosinophils. The cause of CSS is unknown.

7. **Wegener's granulomatosis** is a necrotizing arteritis of the respiratory tract and kidneys. Although C-ANCAs are frequently present in patients with Wegener's granulomatosis, a lung biopsy is the most effective way of diagnosing this condition. The wall of blood vessels shows vasculitis, granulomas and extensive necrosis.

8. **Henoch-Schönlein purpura (HSP)** is the most common form of vasculitis in children. It is associated with purpura (purple-colored spots of the skin and mucosae), arthritis, nephritis and abdominal pain. In most cases, HSP follows upper respiratory tract infections. A typical finding in skin biopsies is the deposition of immunoglobulin A in the walls of affected blood vessels. HSP frequently resolves in a few weeks.

Lymphatic vessels

The functions of the lymphatic vascular system are to:

1. Conduct immune cells and lymph to lymph nodes.

2. Remove excess fluid accumulated in interstitial spaces.

3. Transport chylomicrons, lipid-containing particles, through lacteal lymphatic vessels inside the intestinal villi (see Chapter 16, Lower Digestive Segment).

The flow of lymph is under low pressure and unidirectional.

Lymphatic capillaries form networks in tissue spaces and begin as dilated tubes with closed ends (**blind tubes**) in proximity to blood capillaries. Lymphatic capillaries collect tissue fluid, the **lymph**.

The wall of a **lymphatic capillary** consists of a single layer of endothelial cells **lacking a complete basal lamina** (Figure 12-12). Bundles of **anchoring filaments** associated to the endothelium prevent the lymphatic capillaries from collapsing during changes in interstitial pressure and enable the uptake of soluble tissue components.

Lymphatic capillaries can be found in most tissues. Exceptions are cartilage, bone, epithelia, the central nervous system, bone marrow, and placenta.

The accumulation of fluid in the interstitial space is a normal event of circulation and blind-ended lymphatic capillaries take up the excess fluid. An increase in the intraluminal volume in the lymphatic capillary opens the overlapping cytoplasmic flaps drawing fluid in. When the lymphatic capillary fills, the overlapping flaps, acting as a primary valve opening, close, preventing fluid backflow into the interstitium.

Lymphatic capillaries converge into **precollecting lymphatic vessels** draining lymph into **collecting lymphatic vessels. The collecting vessels are surrounded by smooth muscle cells** (see Figure 12-12), **which provide intrinsic pumping activity.** Movement in the surrounding tissue provides a passive extrinsic pump.

The collecting vessels consist of bulblike segments separated by luminal valves. The sequential contraction of each segment, called **lymphangions**, propels the unidirectional flow of lymph (see Box 12-A).

A collecting lymphatic vessel gives rise to **terminal lymphatic vessels** in the proximity of a lymph node. These terminal lymphatic vessels branch and become lymphatic afferent vessels, which penetrate the lymph node capsule and release lymph and its contents into the subcapsular sinus. Lymph nodes are distributed along the pathway of the lymph vessels to filter the lymph before reaching the thoracic and right lymphatic ducts. A total of 2 to 3 L of lymph is produced each day.

Lymph is returned to the bloodstream via two main trunks:

1. The large **thoracic duct**.

2. The smaller **right lymphatic duct**.

Larger lymphatic vessels have three layers, similar to those of the small veins, but the lumen is larger.

The **tunica intima** consists of an endothelium and

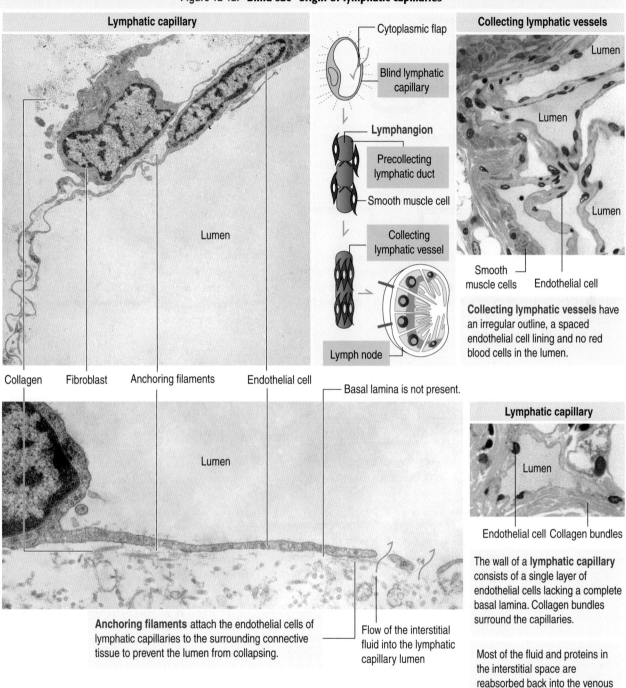

Figure 12-12. "Blind sac" origin of lymphatic capillaries

Lymphatic capillary

Lumen

Collagen   Fibroblast   Anchoring filaments   Endothelial cell

Lumen

Anchoring filaments attach the endothelial cells of lymphatic capillaries to the surrounding connective tissue to prevent the lumen from collapsing.

Cytoplasmic flap

Blind lymphatic capillary

Lymphangion

Precollecting lymphatic duct

Smooth muscle cell

Collecting lymphatic vessel

Lymph node

Basal lamina is not present.

Flow of the interstitial fluid into the lymphatic capillary lumen

Collecting lymphatic vessels

Lumen

Lumen

Lumen

Smooth muscle cells   Endothelial cell

Collecting lymphatic vessels have an irregular outline, a spaced endothelial cell lining and no red blood cells in the lumen.

Lymphatic capillary

Lumen

Endothelial cell Collagen bundles

The wall of a **lymphatic capillary** consists of a single layer of endothelial cells lacking a complete basal lamina. Collagen bundles surround the capillaries.

Most of the fluid and proteins in the interstitial space are reabsorbed back into the venous end of the capillary.
    About one tenth of this fluid enters the lymphatic capillaries, in particular large proteins.

a thin subendothelial layer of connective tissue.

The **tunica media** contains a few smooth muscle cells in a concentric arrangement separated by collagenous fibers.

The **tunica adventitia** is connective tissue with fibroelastic fibers.

Like veins, lymphatic vessels have **valves**, but their number is larger. The structure of the **thoracic duct** is similar to that of a medium-sized vein, but the muscular tunica media is more prominent.

Clinical significance: Edema
Edema occurs when the volume of interstitial fluid increases and exceeds the drainage capacity of the

Figure 12-13. Glomerulus and portal systems

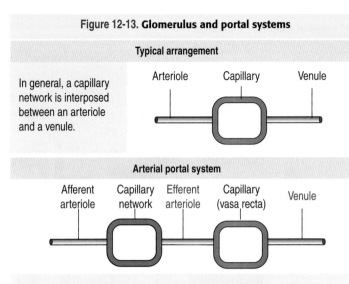

Typical arrangement

In general, a capillary network is interposed between an arteriole and a venule.

Arteriole — Capillary — Venule

Arterial portal system

Afferent arteriole — Capillary network — Efferent arteriole — Capillary (vasa recta) — Venule

In the kidneys, an arteriole is interposed between two capillary networks. An afferent arteriole gives rise to a mass of capillaries, the **glomerulus**. These capillaries coalesce to form an efferent arteriole, which gives rise to capillary networks (peritubular capillary network and the vasa recta) surrounding the nephrons.

Venous portal system

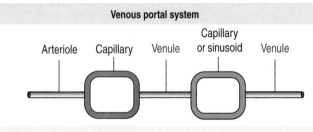

Arteriole — Capillary — Venule — Capillary or sinusoid — Venule

In the liver and hypophysis, venules feed into an extensive capillary or sinusoid network draining into a venule. This distribution is called the **venous portal system**.

lymphatics, or lymphatic vessels become blocked.

Subcutaneous tissue has the capacity to accumulate interstitial fluid and give rise to clinical edema (see Box 12-B). **Subcutaneous edema** is caused by an increase in hydrostatic pressure in the systemic venous system caused by a failure of the right–heart side.

In patients with extensive capillary injury (burns), both intravascular fluid and plasma proteins escape into the interstitial space. Proteins accumulating in the interstitial compartment increase the oncotic pressure, leading to additional fluid loss due to the greater osmotic force outside the capillary bed.

Edema can occur because of cardiac failure. **Pulmonary edema** is the accumulation of fluid in the lumen of the pulmonary alveoli. A failure of the left–heart side increases the hydrostatic pressure in the alveolar capillaries leading to the accumulation of fluid in the alveolar space.

Clinical significance: Hemorrhage

The rupture of a blood vessel, determined by trauma to a major artery or vein or the rupture of a blood vessel because of wall fragility, causes **hemorrhage**.

Significant blood loss can determine **hypovolemic shock**, manifested by a severe drop in blood pressure. Blood is diverted from the alimentary system and kidneys to maintain perfusion of the heart and brain.

Hematoma is a localized accumulation of blood in a tissue, usually following an injury. **Subdural hematoma** is an accumulation of blood on the brain surface, as the result of head injury or spontaneous blood vessel rupture in the elderly.

Petechiae (less than 3 mm in diameter), **purpura** (less than 10 mm in diameter) and **ecchymosis** (greater than 10 mm; a bruise) are small hemorrhages of the skin. With aging, the skin becomes less flexible and thinner as fat under the skin is reduced and blood vessels break easily when minor injuries occur.

Specific capillary arrangements: Glomerulus and portal systems

In general, blood from an arteriole flows into a capillary network and is drained by a venule. There are two specialized capillary systems that depart from this standard arrangement (Figure 12-13):

1. The **glomerulus**.
2. The **portal systems**.

In the kidneys, an **afferent arteriole** drains into a capillary network called the **glomerulus**. The glomerular capillaries coalesce to form an **efferent arteriole**, which branches into another capillary network called the **vasa recta**. The vasa recta surround the limbs of the loop of Henle and play a significant role in the formation of urine. The glomerulus system is essential for blood filtration in the renal corpuscle (see Chapter 14, Urinary System).

In the **portal system**, intestinal capillaries are drained by the portal vein to the liver. In the **liver**, the portal vein branches into venous sinusoids between cords of hepatocytes. Blood flows from the sinusoids into a collecting vein and then back to the heart via the inferior vena cava.

A similar portal system is observed in the hypophysis. Venules connect the primary sinusoidal plexus of the hypothalamus (median eminence) with the secondary plexus in the anterior lobe of the hypophysis, forming the **hypophyseal-portal system**. This system transports releasing factors from the hypothalamus to stimulate the secretion of hormones into the bloodstream by cells of the anterior hypophysis.

Endothelial cell–mediated regulation of blood flow

The general assumption that the endothelium is just an inert simple squamous epithelium lining blood vessels is no longer correct. In addition to enabling the passage of molecules and gases and retaining blood cells and large molecules, endothelial cells produce **vasoactive substances** that can induce contraction and relaxation of the smooth muscle vascular wall (Figure 12-14).

Figure 12-14. Endothelium

Endothelial cells control vascular cell growth

Angiogenesis occurs during normal wound healing and vascularization of tumors. Endothelial cells secrete factors that stimulate angiogenesis.

Some of these factors induce endothelial cell proliferation and migration; others activate endothelial cell differentiation or induce a secondary cell type to produce angiogenic factors.

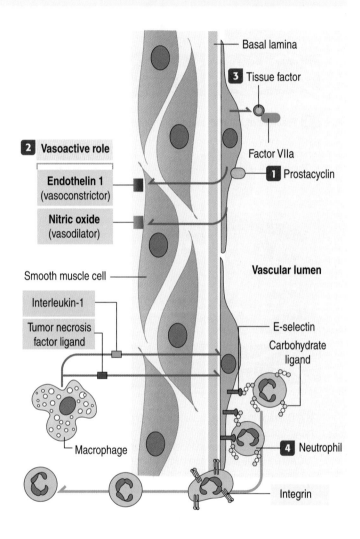

Basal lamina

3 Tissue factor

Factor VIIa

1 Prostacyclin

2 Vasoactive role

Endothelin 1 (vasoconstrictor)

Nitric oxide (vasodilator)

Smooth muscle cell

Vascular lumen

Interleukin-1

Tumor necrosis factor ligand

E-selectin

Carbohydrate ligand

Macrophage

4 Neutrophil

Integrin

Endothelial cells produce prostacyclin

1 Prostacyclin is formed by endothelial cells from arachidonic acid by a process catalyzed by prostacyclin synthase. Prostacyclin prevents the adhesion of platelets to the endothelium, and **avoids blood clot formation**. Prostacyclin is also a **vasodilator**.

Endothelial cells modulate smooth muscle activity

2 Endothelial cells secrete smooth muscle cell relaxing factors (such as **nitric oxide**), and smooth muscle cell contraction factors (such as **endothelin 1**).

Endothelial cells trigger blood coagulation

3 Endothelial cells release **tissue factor** that binds to factor VIIa to convert factor X into factor Xa and initiate the common pathway of blood clotting (see Blood Coagulation in Chapter 6, Blood and Hematopoiesis).

Thrombin (bound to its receptor on platelet surfaces) acts on fibrinogen to form fibrin monomers. **Fibrin monomers** self-aggregate to form a soft fibrin clot cross-linked by factor XIII.

Both platelets and fibrin form a hemostatic plug when there is an injury to the wall of a blood vessel.

Endothelial cells regulate the traffic of inflammatory cells

4 Endothelial cells facilitate transendothelial migration of cells involved in an inflammatory reaction (for example, **neutrophils**) in the surrounding extravascular connective tissue.

Activated macrophages secrete tumor necrosis factor ligand and interleukin-1, which induce the expression of **E-selectin** by endothelial cells.

Nitric oxide, synthesized by endothelial cells from L-arginine upon stimulation by acetylcholine or other agents, activates guanylyl cyclase and consequently cyclic guanosine monophosphate (cGMP) production, which induces **relaxation** of the smooth muscle cells of the vascular wall. **Endothelin 1** is a very potent **vasoconstrictor** peptide produced by endothelial cells.

Prostacyclin, synthesized from arachidonic acid by the action of cyclooxygenase and prostacyclin synthase in endothelial cells, determines the **relaxation** of vascular smooth muscle cells by the action of cyclic adenosine monophosphate (cAMP). Synthetic prostacyclin is used to produce vasodilation in severe

Raynaud's phenomenon (pain and discoloration of the fingers and toes produced by vasospasm), **ischemia**, and in the treatment of **pulmonary hypertension**. Prostacyclin also **prevents platelet adhesion and clumping leading to blood clotting**. We discuss later in this chapter how endothelial cell dysfunction can contribute to **thrombosis**, a mass of clotted blood formed inside a blood vessel due to the activation of the blood coagulation cascade.

The endothelium has a **passive role** in the transcapillary exchange of solvents and solutes by **diffusion**, **filtration**, and **pinocytosis**. The permeability of capillary endothelial cells is tissue-specific. Liver

Figure 12-15. Formation of an atherosclerotic plaque

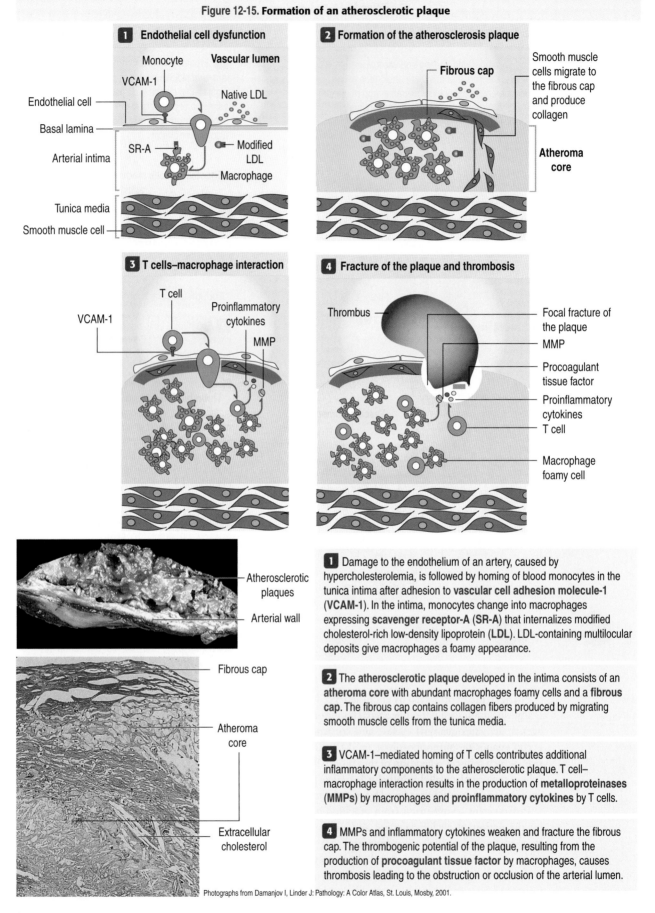

1 Endothelial cell dysfunction

Monocyte
VCAM-1
Native LDL
Vascular lumen
Endothelial cell
Basal lamina
SR-A
Modified LDL
Arterial intima
Macrophage
Tunica media
Smooth muscle cell

2 Formation of the atherosclerosis plaque

Fibrous cap
Smooth muscle cells migrate to the fibrous cap and produce collagen
Atheroma core

3 T cells–macrophage interaction

T cell
Proinflammatory cytokines
VCAM-1
MMP

4 Fracture of the plaque and thrombosis

Thrombus
Focal fracture of the plaque
MMP
Procoagulant tissue factor
Proinflammatory cytokines
T cell
Macrophage foamy cell

Atherosclerotic plaques
Arterial wall

Fibrous cap
Atheroma core
Extracellular cholesterol

1 Damage to the endothelium of an artery, caused by hypercholesterolemia, is followed by homing of blood monocytes in the tunica intima after adhesion to **vascular cell adhesion molecule-1 (VCAM-1)**. In the intima, monocytes change into macrophages expressing **scavenger receptor-A (SR-A)** that internalizes modified cholesterol-rich low-density lipoprotein (**LDL**). LDL-containing multilocular deposits give macrophages a foamy appearance.

2 The **atherosclerotic plaque** developed in the intima consists of an **atheroma core** with abundant macrophages foamy cells and a **fibrous cap**. The fibrous cap contains collagen fibers produced by migrating smooth muscle cells from the tunica media.

3 VCAM-1–mediated homing of T cells contributes additional inflammatory components to the atherosclerotic plaque. T cell–macrophage interaction results in the production of **metalloproteinases (MMPs)** by macrophages and **proinflammatory cytokines** by T cells.

4 MMPs and inflammatory cytokines weaken and fracture the fibrous cap. The thrombogenic potential of the plaque, resulting from the production of **procoagulant tissue factor** by macrophages, causes thrombosis leading to the obstruction or occlusion of the arterial lumen.

Photographs from Damanjov I, Linder J: Pathology: A Color Atlas, St. Louis, Mosby, 2001.

sinusoids are more permeable to albumin than are the capillaries of the renal glomerulus. In addition, there is a topographic permeability. The endothelial cells at the venous end are more permeable than those at the arterial end. Postcapillary venules have the greatest permeability to leukocytes.

Finally, recall the significance of endothelial cells in the process of **cell homing** and **inflammation**.

Pathology: Atherosclerosis

Atherosclerosis is the thickening and hardening of the walls of arteries caused by **atherosclerotic plaques** of lipids, cells, and connective tissue deposited in the **tunica intima**. Atherosclerosis is frequently seen in arteries sustaining high blood pressure, it does not affect veins and is the cause of myocardial infarction, stroke, and ischemic gangrene.

Atherosclerosis is a chronic inflammatory disease driven by the accumulation of cholesterol-laden macrophages in the artery wall. Atherosclerosis is characterized by features of inflammation at all stages of its development (Figure 12-15).

The atherosclerotic process is initiated when cholesterol-containing **low-density lipoproteins (LDLs)** accumulate in the intima as a consequence of endothelial cell dysfunction. A dysfunctional endothelium expresses **vascular cell adhesion molecule-1 (VCAM-1)** that enables **monocytes** to attach to the endothelial cell surface, cross the endothelium and penetrate the intima of the blood vessel.

Monocytes then differentiate into **macrophages** expressing on their surface **scavenger receptor-A (SR-A)**. SR-A uptakes a modified form of LDL (**oxidized LDL**) and the massive accumulation transforms macrophages into cholesterol-laden **foam cells**. Macrophage foam cells constitute the **atheroma core** of the atherosclerotic plaque. The atheroma core continues to enlarge and smooth muscle cells of the tunica muscularis migrate to the intima forming a collagen-containing **fibrous cap** overlying the atheroma core. The endothelium covers the fibrous cap.

The lipid core enlarges and triggers an inflamma-

tory response attracting T cells that stimulate macrophage foam cells to produce **metalloproteinases** that, together with **proinflammatory cytokines** produced by T cells, weaken the fibrous cap making it susceptible to fracture that predisposes to **thrombosis** in the presence of **procoagulant tissue factor**. An enlarging thrombus will eventually obstruct or occlude the lumen of the affected blood vessel.

As you can see, the clearance of lipoproteins by macrophages appears initially beneficial but, with time, the macrophage function is compromised and starts to contribute to the inflammatory response through the secretion of pro-inflammatory mediators and extracellular matrix proteases. With time, dying macrophages release their lipid contents, which leads to the enlargement of the atheroma core.

The major blood vessels involved are the **abdominal aorta** and the **coronary** and **cerebral arteries**. **Coronary arteriosclerosis** causes **ischemic heart disease** and **myocardial infarction** occurs when the arterial lesions are complicated by thrombosis.

Atherothrombosis of the cerebral vessels is the major cause of **brain infarct**, so-called **stroke**, one of the most common causes of neurologic disease. Arteriosclerosis of the abdominal aorta leads to **abdominal aortic aneurysm**, a dilation that sometimes ruptures to produce massive fatal hemorrhage.

Atherosclerosis correlates with the serum levels of cholesterol or **low-density lipoprotein (LDL)**. A genetic defect in lipoprotein metabolism (**familial hyper-cholesterolemia**) is associated with atherosclerosis and myocardial infarction before patients reach 20 years of age. We discuss in Chapter 2, Epithelial Glands, that familial hypercholesterolemia is caused by defects in the LDL receptor, resulting in increasing LDL circulating levels in blood. In contrast to LDL, **high-density lipoprotein (HDL)** transports cholesterol to the liver for excretion in the bile (see in the gallbladder section of Chapter 17, Digestive Glands).

Pathology: Vasculogenesis and angiogenesis
After birth, angiogenesis contributes to organ growth.

Box 12-C | Kaposi's sarcoma

• **Kaposi's sarcoma** is a tumor characterized by red or purple vascular nodules in the skin (face and legs), mucosa (nose, mouth and throat) lung, liver, spleen, and gastrointestinal tract, frequently found in AIDS patients.
• The vascular patches, plaques, or nodules consist of spindle-shaped tumor cells and highly developed vascular spaces (see the histopathology image). The spindle cells express blood and lymphatic endothelial cell markers.
• A severely weakened immune system in HIV infected individuals facilitates infection with human herpesvirus 8 (HHV8), also known as Kaposi's sarcoma-associated herpesvirus (KSHV).
• The classic, non-AIDS–related Kaposi's sarcoma develops slowly (over a period of 10 years or more) when compared to the more aggressive and extended nature of the lesions in HIV infected individuals.

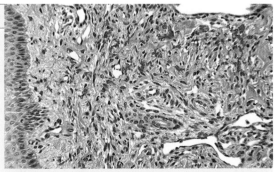

Proliferation in the dermis of jagged thin walled vascular channels lined by endothelial cells. Red blood cells can be seen within the vascular lumen or extravasated. The surrounding connective tissue displays bundles of fusiform cells.

Figure 12-16. **Angiogenesis**

Vasculogenesis (from angioblasts in the embryo)

In the embryo, blood vessels provide the necessary oxygen, nutrients, and trophic signals for organ morphgogenesis.

Development of an endothelial capillary tube

Angioblasts (endothelial cell precursors) proliferate and form endothelial capillary tubes.

Proliferation is regulated by the interaction of **vascular endothelial growth factor (VEGF)**, secreted by mesenchymal cells with **vascular endothelial growth factor receptor-2 (VEGF-R2)**.

Formation of capillary endothelial tubes is dependent on the interaction of **VEGF** with **VEGF-R1**.

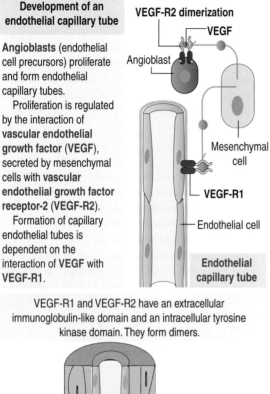

VEGF-R2 dimerization

VEGF

Angioblast

Mesenchymal cell

VEGF-R1

Endothelial cell

Endothelial capillary tube

VEGF-R1 and VEGF-R2 have an extracellular immunoglobulin-like domain and an intracellular tyrosine kinase domain. They form dimers.

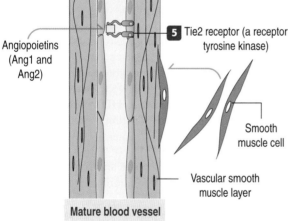

Angiopoietins (Ang1 and Ang2)

5 Tie2 receptor (a receptor tyrosine kinase)

Smooth muscle cell

Vascular smooth muscle layer

Mature blood vessel

Angiogenesis (from a preexisting vessel)

During angiogenesis, a vascular network expands by vessel sprouting and remodels into large and small vessels

Parental blood vessel

The following steps occur during angiogenesis:

1 Degradation of the basal lamina by lateral **podosomes** of the parental endothelial cell in the presence of **integrin** $\alpha_6\beta_1$, induced by **VEGF**, enables formation of lateral **sprouts**.

2 Migration and proliferation of endothelial cells, guided by a gradient of **angiogenic factors (VEGF, Ang1)**.

3 Maturation of endothelial cells into an **endothelial capillary tube**.

4 Assembly of a basal lamina and **recruitment of periendothelial cells** (smooth muscle cells).

Integrin $\alpha_6\beta_1$

Basal lamina breakdown

Lateral podosome

Capillary sprout

Smooth muscle cell

Basal lamina

Neovascularization during pathologic conditions

The formation of a blood vessel from a preexisting vessel, a process known as **neovascularization**, is relevant to chronic inflammation, development of collateral circulation, and tumor growth.

Formation of a mature blood vessel

5 Angiopoietin 1 (Ang1) interacts with the **endothelial cell receptor Tie2** (for tyrosine kinase with immunoglobulin-like and EGF-like domains) to recruit periendothelial smooth muscle cells to organize mature blood vessels.

Ang2, another angiopoietin, interacts with Tie2 to induce the loss of contact of endothelial cells with the extracellular matrix. This results in either the absence of growth or death of endothelial cells. **The role of Ang2 in tumor angiogenesis is emerging as a target for cancer treatment.**

In the adult, most blood vessels remain stable and angiogenesis occurs in the endometrium and ovaries during the menstrual cycle, and in the placenta during pregnancy. Under pathologic conditions, angiogenesis is excessive during malignant (see Box 12-C), ocular (age-related macular degeneration), and inflammatory conditions.

An understanding of vasculogenesis and angiogenesis is relevant to developing therapeutic strategies to produce revascularization of ischemic tissues or inhibit angiogenesis in cancer, ocular, joint, or skin disorders.

The vascular system is formed by two processes (Figure 12-16):

1. **Vasculogenesis**, a process initiated by the coalescence of free and migratory **vascular endothelial progenitors**, or **angioblasts**, during **embryogenesis** to form a **primitive vascular network in the yolk sac and trunk axial vessels**. Vasculogenesis is essential for embryonic survival.

2. **Angiogenesis**, a process initiated in a **preexisting vessel** and observed in the embryo and adult. Angiogenesis in the adult occurs during the uterine

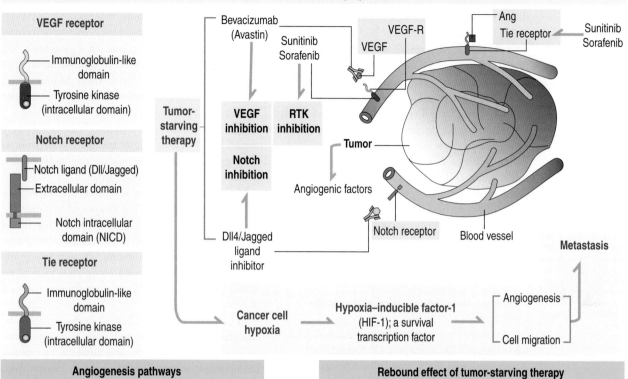

Figure 12-17. Tumor angiogenesis

VEGF receptor
- Immunoglobulin-like domain
- Tyrosine kinase (intracellular domain)

Notch receptor
- Notch ligand (Dll/Jagged)
- Extracellular domain
- Notch intracellular domain (NICD)

Tie receptor
- Immunoglobulin-like domain
- Tyrosine kinase (intracellular domain)

Bevacizumab (Avastin)
Sunitinib Sorafenib
VEGF-R
VEGF
Ang
Tie receptor
Sunitinib Sorafenib

Tumor-starving therapy

VEGF inhibition
RTK inhibition
Notch inhibition

Tumor
Angiogenic factors
Notch receptor
Blood vessel

Dll4/Jagged ligand inhibitor

Cancer cell hypoxia → Hypoxia–inducible factor-1 (HIF-1); a survival transcription factor

Metastasis
Angiogenesis
Cell migration

Angiogenesis pathways

The major key signaling pathways involved in angiogenesis are: (1) the vascular endothelial cell factor (**VEGF**)-VEGF receptor (**VEGF-R**) pathway; (2) the **Notch receptor** pathway; and (3) the **Tie** (for **t**yrosine kinase with **i**mmunoglobulin-like and **E**GF-like domains) receptor–angiopoietin (**Ang**) pathway.

The VEGF-R and Tie receptors have an intracellular tyrosine kinase domain. Ligand binding to VEGF-R and Tie receptors leads to their dimerization and subsequent autophosphorylation. The phosphorylated receptor interacts with a variety of cytoplasmic signaling molecules leading to angiogenesis involving the proliferation and differentiation of endothelial cells.

Activation of the Notch receptor by ligand (**Dll/Jagged**) binding results in the release of the **Notch intracellular cell domain** (**NICD**) that translocates into the cell nucleus to regulate gene expression involved in angiogenesis.

Rebound effect of tumor-starving therapy

Based on the importance of VEGF and its receptor in tumor angiogenesis, blocking tumor angiogenesis by suppressing the angiogenic pathways can provide maximal surviving benefits to cancer patients.

The monoclonal antibody to VEGF **bevacizumab** (Avastin) and receptor tyrosine kinase inhibitors (**RTKIs**) **sunitinib** and **sorafenib** have been developed. However, although tumor antiangiogenic targeted drugs inhibit primary tumor growth, they promote tumor invasion and metastasis.

The mechanism of **tumor hypoxia**, caused by oxygen deprivation resulting from blocking tumor angiogenesis, could explain the selective switch of tumor cells into an invasive and metastatic program. **Hypoxia–inducible factor-1** (**HIF-1**) acts as a transcription survival factor that activates genes involved in migration, invasion and angiogenesis. Hypoxia generated by tumor angiogenesis inhibition triggers pathways that make tumor cells aggressive and metastatic.

---

menstrual cycle, placental growth, wound healing, and inflammatory responses. We discuss below that **tumor angiogenesis** is a specific form of angiogenesis with important clinical implications.

Endothelial cells are involved in vasculogenesis and angiogenesis. Endothelial cells migrate, proliferate, and assemble into tubes to contain the blood. Periendothelial cells (smooth muscle cells, pericytes, and fibroblasts) are recruited to surround the newly formed endothelial tubes.

The following molecules are central to vascular morphogenesis:

1. **Vascular endothelial cell factors (VEGFs)**, with binding affinity to two different receptors, **VEGF-R1** and **VEGF-R2**, present on the surface of endothelial cells.

2. **Tie2**, a receptor tyrosine kinase that modulates a signaling cascade required for the induction or inhibition of endothelial cell proliferation. **Angiopoietins 1 and 2 (Ang1 and Ang2)** bind to the **Tie2** receptor (for tyrosine kinase with **i**mmunoglobulin-like and **E**GF-like domains). Ang1 binding to Tie2 has a stabilizing effect on blood vessels (proangiogenic), whereas Ang2 has a destabilizing effect (anti-angiogenic).

The extracellular region of VEGF-R and Tie receptors is an immunoglobulin-like domain; the intracellular domain has tyrosine kinase activity. Upon ligand binding, the receptors dimerize and the intracellular domain autophosphorylates.

3. The **Notch receptor** is a third pathway (Figure 12-17). Notch receptor signaling facilitates endothelial cell survival by activating the expression of a VEGF-R that protects endothelial cells from apoptosis. Notch receptor **Delta-like ligands** (Dll1, Dll3 and Dll4) and **Jagged** (Jagged 1 and Jagged 2) play significant roles in normal and tumoral angiogenesis by regulating the actions of VEGF.

Activation of Notch signaling is dependent on cell-cell interaction. It occurs when the extracellular domain of Notch receptor interacts with a ligand found on the surface of a nearby cell. Notch receptors participate in transcriptional regulation by a unique mechanism involving the cleavage of the Notch intracellular domain (**NICD**), which then translocates to the nucleus and regulates gene expression.

Pathology: Neovascularization and vascular co-option

All the three signaling pathways, VEGF-R–VEGF, Tie-Ang, and Notch receptor-Dll/Jagged, contribute synergistically to the process of neoangiogenesis.

Antineoangiogenic drugs exert therapeutic effects by blocking certain specific receptors of the VEGF-VEGF-R pathway, but none can fully block all the components. Thus, neoangiogenesis signaling can continue through the other signaling pathways.

In Chapter 4, Connective Tissue, we discuss the molecular biology of tumor invasion. We briefly mention that tumors secrete **angiogenic factors** that increase the vascularization and nutrition of an invading tumor. During inflammation, angiogenic factors stimulate the formation of the highly vascularized granulation tissue. The participating angiogenic factors are similar to those produced during normal wound healing. In addition, we indicate that newly formed blood vessels facilitate the dissemination of tumor cells to distant tissues (**metastasis**).

Based on the concept that oxygen and nutrients provided by the vasculature is essential for tumor growth and metastasis and on the role of VEGF and its receptor and receptor tyrosine kinase inhibitors (**RTKIs**) in angiogenesis, tumor antiangiogenic therapeutic approaches have been developed to provide cancer patients maximal survival time. Therapy with angiogenesis inhibitors reduce tumor growth but promote tumor invasiveness and metastasis (see Figure 12-17).

How can tumor invasiveness and metastasis be explained following VEGF-targeted therapy? A possible mechanism is **tumor hypoxia**. Following antiangiogenic tumor treatment, a lack of oxygen supply to the tumor selects for metastasis the less

sensitive cells to treatment. These cells escape the hypoxic environment leading to increasing metastasis by expressing **hypoxia-inducible factor-1** (**HIF-1**). HIF-1 is a survival factor of cancer cells by activating transcription of genes involved in angiogenesis. We discussed in Chapter 6, Blood and Hematopiesis, the role of hypoxia-inducible factor-1α in the production of erytropoietin, a regulator of erythropoiesis, under conditions of low oxygen tension.

The identification of biomarkers to monitor metastasis switch and resistance of cancer cells to antiangiogenic strategies could overcome the adverse effects of tumor-starving therapy.

However, some primary and metastatic tumors can develop and progress in the absence of angiogenesis by adapting, or co-opting, to a preexisting blood vessel. **Vascular co-option** is relevant to forthcoming tumor therapy by discriminating between angiogenic and nonangiogenic tumor growth, thus preventing tumor cells to attach and grow along the outer surface of blood vessels.

In Chapter 8, Nervous Tissue, we discuss the **perivascular** development of metastasis in brain. Metastatic tumor cells co-opt, or assimilate, to existing brain vessels by expressing the protein **neuroserpin**. Neuroserpin blocks plasmin and soluble Fas ligand, that prevent brain metastasis by inducing apoptosis of tumor cells entering the brain tissue.

Clinical significance: Hypertension

We already discussed atherosclerosis, a chronic inflammatory arterial disease. **Arteriosclerosis** describes the thickening and hardening of the arterial walls without any reference to the cause. The cause of atherosclerosis, the most common cause of arteriosclerosis, is the development of an **atheroma**. You have learned how atheromas affect large and medium-sized arteries and determine the thickening and hardening of the arterial wall.

You have also learned how defects of the vascular tunica media can determine an **aneurysm**, the abnormal regional dilation of the abdominal aorta or of a cerebral artery. If hereditary disorders such as **Marfan's syndrome** and a form of the **Ehlers-Danlos syndrome** result in degenerative changes in the tunica media of the aorta, **aortic dissection** is a likely outcome.

Hypertension (diastolic blood pressure greater than 90 mm Hg) is another condition that causes degenerative changes in the walls of the **small vessels** (arterioles). The vasculature of the brain, heart and kidneys and the aorta are the most affected.

There are two etiologic forms of hypertension (Figure 12-18):

1. **Primary (essential) hypertension**, without apparent cause, usually associated with genetic predisposition, obesity, alcohol consumption, and aging.

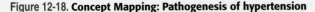

Figure 12-18. Concept Mapping: Pathogenesis of hypertension

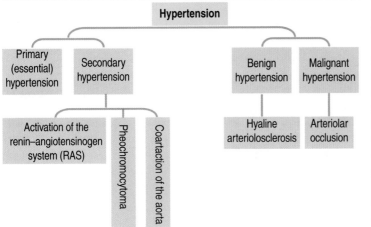

2. **Secondary hypertension**, related to an activation of the **renin-angiotensin system** (**RAS**), discussed in Chapter 14, Urinary System. Mutations in the genes involved in RAS, affecting Na^+ metabolism and blood volume, are important factors. Other factors include **pheochromocytoma** (epinephrine/norepinephrine–producing tumor of the adrenal medulla), congenital narrowing of the aorta (**coartaction of the aorta**) and **stenosis** (abnormal narrowing) by atherosclerosis of one renal artery.

There are two clinical forms of hypertension:

1. **Benign hypertension**, consisting in a gradual increase of blood pressure caused by hypertrophy of the muscular tunica media of **small arteries**, thickening of the intima and the internal elastic lamina and reduction in the diameter of the vascular lumen. The smooth muscle cells of the wall of the **arterioles** undergo hyaline degeneration and thickening (**hyaline arteriolosclerosis**), depriving the normal constriction and dilation of the vessel.

2. **Malignant hypertension**, consisting in acute degeneration and proliferative reparative events of the wall of small vessels causing substantial reduction of the vascular lumen.

Pathology: Thrombosis, embolism, and infarction

Thrombosis is the process of formation of a blood clot (**thrombus**) inside a blood vessel, obstructing blood flow.

One or more of the following three factors (**Virchow's triad**, Figure 12-19) can lead to thrombosis:

1. **Endothelial dysfunction** can occur by direct trauma or inflammation associated with an atheroma, a condition called **atherothrombosis**. Under normal conditions, the endothelial lining prevents thrombosis. As you recall, endothelial damage triggers the adhesion and aggregation of platelets, the starting point of thrombus formation (see Figure 12-14).

2. **Reduction in blood flow** can be caused by seden-

tary behavior (for example, sitting on a long airplane flight) or beyond a site of vascular injury, thus allowing platelets to contact the endothelial cell surface and activate components of the clotting cascade.

3. **Prone to blood clotting** (**hypercoagulability**), determined, among other causes, by an increase in the concentration of fibrinogen and prothrombin associated with estrogen-based therapy, autoantibodies to platelet phospholipids and a common mutation in factor V (**Leiden mutation**), a cofactor that allows factor Xa to activate thrombin. Remember that thrombin cleaves fibrinogen to form fibrin, which then organizes a dense meshwork, the substrate of a blood clot.

The mechanism of blood clotting, or hemostasis, the intrinsic, extrinsic and common pathways of blood clotting and the mechanism of fibrinolysis, to dissolve a thrombus, are described in Chapter 6, Blood and Hematopoiesis.

Note that a thrombus consists of layered components of the blood coagulation cascade (platelets, fibrin and entrapped blood cells) formed **inside** a blood vessel. In contrast, a blood clot, such as a hematoma, consists of similar unstructured components that have developed **outside** a blood vessel.

Obstruction of more of 75% of the lumen of an artery reduces blood flow and oxygen supply (**hypoxia**). An obstruction that exceeds 90% of the lumen of an artery causes **anoxia** (complete reduction of oxygen) and **infarction** (tissue necrosis). Details of the pathogenesis of cell and tissue injury and necrosis are discussed in Chapter 3, Cell Signaling.

There are two distinct forms of thrombosis:

1. **Venous thrombosis.**

2. **Arterial thrombosis.**

Venous thrombosis is the formation of a thrombus within a vein. This category includes:

1. **Deep vein thrombosis** (**DVT**). The iliac, femoral, popliteal and calf veins are the most commonly affected. Swelling, pain and redness of the affected area are characteristic indications of DVT.

2. **Portal vein thrombosis.** The hepatic portal vein is usually affected. It can determine portal hypertension and reduction of liver blood supply. It is associated with cirrhosis and pancreatitis.

3. **Budd-Chiari syndrome**, caused by the blockage of the hepatic vein or the inferior vena cava, this form of thrombosis is defined by abdominal pain, ascites, and hepatomegaly.

4. **Paget-Schroetter disease**, caused by the obstruction of an upper extremity vein (such as the axillary vein or subclavian vein) by a thrombus. It is seen after intense exercise in healthy and young individuals.

5. **Cerebral venous sinus thrombosis** (**CVST**), is a type of stroke resulting from the blockage of the dural venous sinuses by a thrombus.

Arterial thrombosis is the formation of a thrombus

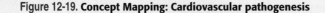

Figure 12-19. Concept Mapping: Cardiovascular pathogenesis

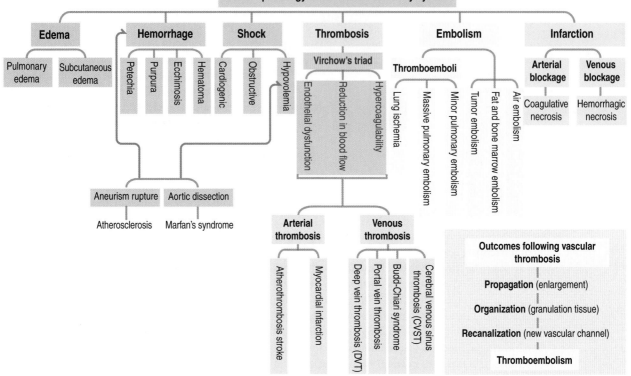

within an artery. This category includes:

1. **Stroke.** Atherothrombosis stroke originated in an atheroma located in large vessels (such as the internal carotids, vertebral and the circle of Willis) or in smaller vessels (such as the branches of the circle of Willis).

2. **Myocardial infarction.** We discuss in Chapter 3, Cell Signaling, and in Chapter 7, Muscle Tissue, several aspects of myocardial ischemia (produced by slow occlusion of a blood vessel) and infarction (determined by an abrupt vascular occlusion).

In general, arterial blockage causes **coagulative necrosis**, whereas the blockage of a vein determines **hemorrhagic necrosis**.

A thrombus can enlarge its size (**propagation**), **dissolved** by fibrinolysis, become **organized** by undergoing a granulation tissue transformation and reestablish blood flow by **recanalization**.

A potential outcome of a thrombus is **thromboembolism**, consisting in the fragmentation of the thrombus and migration of the fragments, called **emboli**, to other blood vessels. If the destination blood vessels have a small lumen, the **thromboemboli** cannot progress further, end up occluding the lumen and depriving local blood flow to produce **infarction**.

Thromboemboli can cause **pulmonary thrombo-**

embolism when emboli of systemic veins migrate to the heart and affect the pulmonary arterial tree.

Most emboli derive from DVT and, depending on the extent of vasculature blockage and size of the affected pulmonary arteries, thromboemboli can trigger an increase in pulmonary arterial pressure, Atherothrombosis stroke (causing in some cases lung **infarction**) and straining the right-side of the heart. A substantial sudden blockage (60% of the pulmonary vasculature; **massive pulmonary embolism**) produces a cardiovascular collapse leading to rapid death. **Minor pulmonary embolism** can result from the blockage of small peripheral lung vessels and cause pleuritic chest pain and dyspnea.

A **heart mural thrombus** can migrate through the aorta to the systemic arterial circulation and occlude an artery of the brain, kidneys, spleen, intestines and lower extremities.

Not all emboli originate from arterial and venous thromboembolism. **Tumor embolism** is the source of hematogenous metastasis. Severe bone fracture can cause **fat and bone marrow emboli** to enter the venous system and reach the pulmonary arteries through the right side of the heart. Accidental air pumping into the venous circulation can trigger **air embolism**.

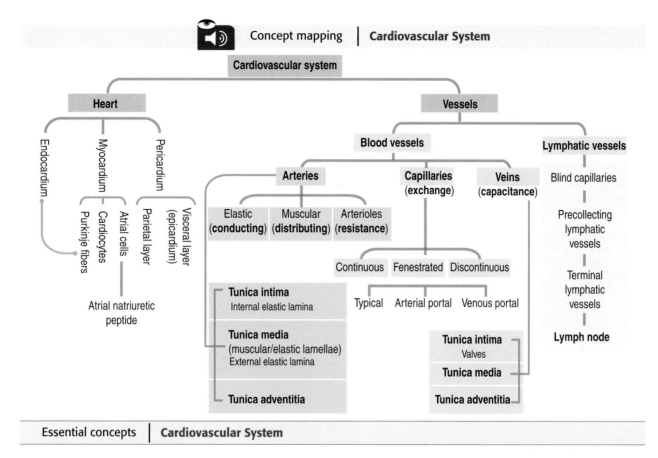

• **Heart**. The wall of the heart consists of three layers:

(1) Endocardium, formed by an endothelial lining and subendothelial connective tissues.

(2) Myocardium, formed by three types of cardiac muscle: atrial muscle, ventricular muscle, and conducting muscle fibers of Purkinje.

(3) Epicardium, lined by a mesothelium facing the serosal pericardial space. The epicardium is the visceral layer of the pericardium.

Cardiocytes of the atrium secrete atrial natriuretic factor, a protein that stimulates diuresis and natriuresis.

The conductive systems of the heart are the sinus node (or sinoatrial [S-A] node); the internodal pathway, linking the sinus node to the atrioventricular (A-V) node; the atrioventricular bundle, linking the atria to the ventricles; and the left and right bundles of Purkinje fibers.

Cardiocytes are striated cells with a central nucleus and are linked to each other by intercalated disks. The transverse components of the intercalated disk are fasciae adherentes and desmosomes; gap junctions are present in the longitudinal component. The cytoplasm contains myofibrils.

Purkinje cells lie beneath the endocardium along the two sides of the interventricular septum. Compared with cardiocytes, the number of myofibrils in Purkinje fibers is reduced, the diameter of the fibers is larger, and the cytoplasm contains abundant glycogen.

• **Circulation** is divided into:

(1) The systemic or peripheral circulation.

(2) The pulmonary circulation.

Remember that there are variations in blood pressure in various parts of the cardiovascular system. The construction of the blood vessels matches the blood pressure that they must sustain. As blood flows through the systemic circulation, its pressure reaches the lowest value when it returns to the right atrium of the heart through the terminal vena cava.

Arteries conduct blood from the heart to the capillaries. The wall of arteries consists of three layers:

(1) Tunica intima (endothelium, subendothelial connective tissue, and the internal elastic lamina).

(2) Tunica media (smooth muscle cells surrounded by collagen fibers, and elastic sheaths).

(3) Tunica externa or adventitia (connective tissue, vessels, and nerves).

There are three major groups of arteries:

(1) Large elastic arteries.

(2) Medium-sized arteries.

(3) Small arteries and arterioles.

Large elastic arteries are conducting vessels. The aorta is an example. Fenestrated elastic sheaths and elastic-producing smooth muscle cells are present in the tunica media. **Aortic aneurysms** are produced by atherosclerosis or defective synthesis and assembly of elastic fibers (**Marfan syndrome, dissecting aneurysm**).

Medium-sized arteries are distributing vessels. The tunica media shows a reduction in elastic fibers and an increase in smooth muscle fibers. An external elastic lamina is seen at the tunica media–adventitia junction.

Arterioles are resistance vessels. Arterioles regulate blood distribution to the microcirculation by vasoconstriction and vasodilation. Arterioles are the major determinants of systemic blood pressure. The tunica media consists of two to five layers of smooth muscle.

Capillaries are exchange vessels. The microvascular bed, the site of microcirculation, consists of the terminal arteriole, metarteriole, the capillary bed, and the postcapillary venules.

The capillary bed consists of slightly larger capillaries (called preferential or thoroughfare channels) characterized by continuous blood flow, and small capillaries (called true capillaries), where blood flow is intermittent. Precapillary sphincters (smooth muscle cells) are located at the origin site of true capillaries from the arteriole or metarteriole. Capillary circulation can be bypassed by through channels connecting terminal arterioles to postcapillary venules. Arteriovenous shunts, or anastomoses, connect arterioles to postcapillary venules, bypassing the microvascular bed.

There are three types of capillaries:

(1) Continuous capillaries.

(2) Fenestrated capillaries.

(3) Discontinuous (sinusoids).

Continuous capillaries are lined by a complete simple squamous endothelium and continuous basal lamina. Pericytes, smooth muscle cell–like, can be present between the endothelium and the basal lamina. Endothelial cells have two characteristics: they are linked by tight junctions, and the transport of solutes and fluids occurs by caveolae and pinocytotic vesicles.

Fenestrated capillaries have pores, or fenestrae, with or without diaphragms. The basal lamina is continuous.

Discontinuous capillaries have an incomplete endothelial cell lining and basal lamina. Gaps are seen between and within endothelial cells.

Veins are capacitance or reservoir vessels. The venous system starts with a postcapillary venule (the site of migration of blood cells into tissues by diapedesis), consisting of an endothelial tube surrounded by a basal lamina, and a loose connective tissue adventitia. In lymphatic tissues, endothelial cells of postcapillary venules are taller (high endothelial venules). Postcapillary venules converge to form muscular venules, which give rise to collecting venules, leading to veins of increasing diameter.

Veins have the following characteristics:

(1) Distinction of a tunica media from a tunica adventitia is often not discernible.

(2) A distinct internal elastic lamina is not visualized.

(3) Veins have valves, projections into the lumen of the tunica intima, to prevent blood reflux.

Lymphatic vessels conduct immune cells and lymph to lymph nodes, remove excess fluid accumulated in interstitial spaces, and transport chylomicrons collected by lacteal lymphatic vessels. Lymph flow is under low pressure and unidirectional.

Lymphatic capillaries begin as dilated, blind endothelial cell–lined tubes lacking a basal lamina and maintained open by bundles of anchoring filaments. Lymphatic vessels are not found in cartilage, bone, epithelia, the central nervous system, and placenta.

Lymphatic capillaries converge into precollecting lymphatic vessels draining lymph into collecting lymphatic vessels surrounded by smooth muscle cells, providing intrinsic pumping activity.

Lymphangions are bulblike segments separated by luminal valves.

Terminal lymphatic vessels are seen in the proximity of a lymph node. Lymph returns to the bloodstream through the large thoracic duct, and the smaller right lymphatic duct.

Lymphedema is caused by a defect in the transport of lymph determined by abnormal development or a damaged lymphatic vessel.

Filariasis (elephantiasis) is caused by a parasitic infection of lymphatic vessels. Chronic lymphedema of the legs and genitals is characteristic.

Chylous ascites and **chylothorax** is the accumulation of lymph with high fat content (chyle) in the abdomen and thorax, caused by trauma, obstruction, or abnormal development of lymphatic vessels.

• **Special capillary arrangements**:

(1) Arterial portal system: afferent arteriole followed by a capillary network draining into an efferent arteriole (instead of a venule).

(2) Venous portal system: capillary drained by a vein, which gives rise to venous capillaries or sinusoids and continues with a vein.

• **Endothelial cell functions**:

(1) Production of prostacyclin (from arachidonic acid) to avoid adhesion of platelets to the endothelium and intravascular blood clot formation, and to determine the relaxation of the smooth muscle cell wall.

(2) Production of angiogenic factors during normal wound healing and vascularization of tumors.

(3) Initiation of blood coagulation by releasing tissue factor to activate factor VIIa to convert factor X into factor Xa.

(4) Regulation of smooth muscle activity (nitric oxide produces vasodilation; endothelin 1 triggers vasoconstriction).

(5) Regulation of inflammatory cell trafficking. Macrophages in the connective tissue produce tumor necrosis factor ligand (TNFL) and interleukin-1 to accelerate homing of inflammatory cells to block the action of pathogens.

• **Arterial diseases**. Atherosclerosis is the thickening of the arterial walls caused by atherosclerotic plaques of lipids, cells, and connective tissue in the tunica intima.

Atherosclerosis is a chronic inflammatory disease involving the participation of monocytes that change into macrophages that internalize modified low-density lipoprotein (LDL).

There are four phases involving the development of an atheroma plaque.

(1) Endothelial cell dysfunction. Damage to the endothelium of an artery, caused by hypercholesterolemia, is followed by the recruitment of blood monocytes in the tunica intima. In the intima, monocytes change into macrophages expressing scavenger receptor-A (SR-A) that internalizes modified cholesterol-rich low-density lipoprotein (LDL). LDL-containing multilocular deposits give macrophages a foamy appearance.

(2) Formation of the atherosclerosis plaque. The atherosclerotic plaque developed in the intima consists of an atheroma core with abundant macrophages foamy cells and a fibrous cap. The fibrous cap contains collagen fibers produced by migrating smooth muscle cells from the tunica media.

(3) T cells–macrophage interaction. Recruited T cells contribute additional inflammatory components to the atherosclerotic plaque. T cell– macrophage interaction results in the production of metalloproteinases (MMPs) by macrophages and proinflammatory cytokines by T cells.

(4) Fracture of the plaque and thrombosis. MMPs and inflammatory cytokines weaken and fracture the fibrous cap. The thrombogenic potential of the plaque, resulting from the production of procoagulant tissue factor

by macrophages, causes thrombosis leading to the obstruction or occlusion of the arterial lumen.

The abdominal aorta, and the coronary and cerebral arteries are the major blood vessels involved. Abdominal aortic aneurysm, myocardial infarction, and brain infarct (stroke) are complications.

Familial hypercholesterolemia is a genetic defect in the lipoprotein metabolism caused by a defect in the receptor that internalizes LDL.

• **Vasculitis.** Vasculitis is the acute and chronic inflammation of vessels. It can be caused by infectious and immunologic pathogens.

The lytic activity of bacterial enzymes following bacterial infections cause vasculitis, thrombophlebitis (thrombosis and inflammation of the wall of a vein), and pseudoaneurysms (dilation of the wall of a blood vessel).

Most inflammatory conditions of the wall of arteries involve an immune-based pathogenesis:

(1) Antigen-antibody complexes, accumulating in the wall of a blood vessel, can activate the complement cascade.

(2) When neutrophils attracted by chemotactic fragments released by the activated complement cascade and cytokines, release serine proteinase 3 and myeloperoxidase, causing damage to the vascular wall.

(3) Antibodies reacting with cytoplasmic components of neutrophils (anti-neutrophil cytoplasmic antibody, ANCA) release enzymes from the activated neutrophils, causing vascular wall injury.

(4) Serine proteinase 3 generates C-ANCA (cytoplasmic ANCA); P-ANCA are antibodies to myeloperoxidase showing a perinuclear pattern in neutrophils (perinuclear ANCA) by immunocytochemistry.

Vasculitis types include:

(1) Giant cell arteritis, a common form of vasculitis in adults (over the age of 50) that affects temporal, ophthalmic or vertebral arteries.

(2) Buerger's disease (thromboangitis obliterans), involves medium-sized and small arteries of hands and feet of young males, who are heavy cigarette smokers.

(3) Polyarteritis nodosa (PAN) affects the wall of medium- to small-sized arteries of the skin, kidneys, liver, heart and gastrointestinal tract. PAN has been associated with active hepatitis B and/or hepatitis C.

(4) Giant cell aortitis (Takayasu's arteritis) is a rare disease that occurs with a high frequency in Asian women under the age of 40 and affects the aorta and its branches.

(5) Kaswasaki's disease affects the coronary arteries as well as large, medium- and small-sized arteries of children.

(6) Churg-Strauss syndrome (CSS) is a systemic vasculitis associated with asthma, rhinitis and eosinophilia.

(7) Wegener's granulomatosis is a necrotizing arteritis of the respiratory tract and kidneys.

(8) Henoch-Schönlein purpura (HSP) is the most common form of vasculitis in children.

• **Hemorrhage** is caused by the rupture of a blood vessel, determined by trauma to a major artery or vein or the rupture of a blood vessel because of wall fragility. Significant blood loss can determine hypovolemic shock, manifested by a severe drop in blood pressure.

Hematoma is a localized accumulation of blood in a tissue, usually following an injury.
Small hemorrhages of the skin are:
(1) Petechiae (less than 3 mm in diameter).
(2) Purpura (less than 10 mm in diameter).
(3) Ecchymosis (greater than 10 mm).

• **Vasculogenesis and angiogenesis**. Vasculogenesis is the process initiated by vascular endothelial progenitors (called angioblasts) during embryogenesis.

Angiogenesis is a process of vessel formation initiated from a preexisting vessel, and it is observed in the embryo and adult. Endothelial cells are involved in vasculogenesis and angiogenesis.

During vasculogenesis, angioblasts proliferate and assemble into tubes containing blood. Periendothelial cells (smooth muscle cells, pericytes, and fibroblasts) are recruited to complete the formation of the vessel. Endothelial proliferation is regulated by vascular endothelial growth factor (VEGF), secreted by mesenchymal cells, bound to its receptor VEGF-R1. Angiopoietin interacts with the endothelial cell receptor Tie2 to recruit periendothelial cells (pericytes and smooth muscle cells). During angiogenesis, a capillary sprout is formed from podosomes of a preexisting endothelial cell. Endothelial cells, stimulated by VEGF and angiopoietin, form an endothelial tube. The recruitment of periendothelial smooth muscle cells follows.

The Notch receptor pathway contributes, together with the VEGF-VEGF-R and the Tie1-angiopoietin pathways, to the process of angiogenesis.

• **Tumor angiogenesis**. Blocking blood supply starves tumors. Tumor antiangiogenic therapeutic approaches disrupting angiogenic pathways have been developed. Tumor hypoxia reduces the tumor size but also cancerous cells, less sensitive to hypoxia, escape the tumor site and establish metastatic tumor growth by expressing hypoxia-inducible factor-1, a transcription factor that activates the genes involved in angiogenesis.

However, some primary and metastatic tumors can develop and progress in the absence of angiogenesis by adapting, or co-opting, to a preexisting blood vessel.

Vascular co-option is relevant to forthcoming tumor therapy by discriminating between angiogenic and nonangiogenic tumor growth. The goal is to prevent tumor cells to attach and grow along the outer surface of blood vessels.

• **Hypertension** (diastolic blood pressure greater than 90 mm of Hg) is another condition that causes degenerative changes in the walls of the small vessels (arterioles). The vasculature of the brain, heart and kidneys and the aorta are the most affected.

There are two causes of hypertension:
(1) Primary (essential) hypertension, without apparent cause, usually associated with genetic predisposition, obesity, alcohol consumption and aging.
(2) Secondary hypertension, related to an activation of the renin-angiotensin system (RAS).
There are two clinical forms of hypertension:
(1) Benign hypertension, consisting in a gradual increase of blood pressure caused by hypertrophy of the muscular tunica media of small arteries, thickening of the intima and the internal elastic lamina and reduction in the diameter of the vascular lumen.
(2) Malignant hypertension, consisting in acute degeneration and proliferation of the wall of small vessels causing reduction of the vascular lumen.

• **Thrombosis** is the process of formation of a blood clot (thrombus) inside a blood vessel, obstructing blood flow.

One or more of the following three factors (Virchow's triad) can lead to thrombosis:
(1) Endothelial dysfunction can occur by direct trauma or inflammation associated with an atheroma, a condition called atherothrombosis.
(2) Reduction in blood flow can be caused by sedentary behavior (for example, sitting on a long airplane flight) or beyond a site of vascular injury.
(3) Prone to blood clotting (hypercoagulability).

A thrombus consists of layered components of the blood coagulation cascade (platelets, fibrin and entrapped blood cells) formed inside a blood vessel. In contrast, a blood clot, such as a hematoma, consists of similar unstructured components that have developed outside a blood vessel.

Obstruction of more of 75% of the lumen of an artery reduces blood flow and oxygen supply (hypoxia). An obstruction that exceeds 90% of the lumen of an artery causes anoxia (complete reduction of oxygen) and infarction (tissue necrosis).

There are two distinct forms of thrombosis:
(1) Venous thrombosis.
(2) Arterial thrombosis.

• **Venous thrombosis** is the formation of a thrombus within a vein. This category includes:
(1) Deep vein thrombosis (DVT). The iliac, femoral, popliteal and calf veins are the most commonly affected.
(2) Portal vein thrombosis. The hepatic portal vein is usually affected. It can determine portal hypertension and reduction of liver

blood supply. It is associated with cirrhosis and pancreatitis.
(3) Budd-Chiari syndrome, caused by the blockage of the hepatic vein or the inferior vena cava. This form of thrombosis is associated with abdominal pain, ascites, and hepatomegaly.
(4) Paget-Schroetter disease, caused by the obstruction of an upper extremity vein (such as the axillary vein or subclavian vein) by a thrombus. It is seen after intense exercise in healthy and young individuals.
(5) Cerebral venous sinus thrombosis (CVST), is a type of stroke resulting from the blockage of the dural venous sinuses by a thrombus.

• **Arterial thrombosis** is the formation of a thrombus within an artery. This category includes:
(1) Stroke. Atherothrombosis stroke originated in an atheroma located in large vessels (such as the internal carotids, vertebral and the circle of Willis) or in smaller vessels (such as the branches of the circle of Willis).
(2) Myocardial ischemia, produced by slow occlusion of a blood vessel and myocardial infarction (determined by an abrupt vascular occlusion).

In general, arterial blockage causes coagulative necrosis, whereas the blockage of a vein determines hemorrhagic necrosis.

A thrombus can enlarge its size (propagation), dissolved by fibrinolysis, become organized by undergoing a granulation tissue transformation and reestablish blood flow by recanalization.

A potential outcome of a thrombus is thromboembolism, consisting in the fragmentation of the thrombus and migration of the fragments, called emboli, to other blood vessels.

If the destination blood vessels have a small lumen, the thromboemboli cannot progress further, end up occluding the lumen and depriving local blood flow to produce infarction.

Thromboemboli can cause pulmonary thromboembolism when emboli of systemic veins migrate to the heart and affect the pulmonary arterial tree. A substantial sudden blockage (60% of the pulmonary vasculature; massive pulmonary embolism) produces a cardiovascular collapse leading to rapid death. Minor pulmonary embolism can result from the blockage of small peripheral lung vessels and cause pleuritic chest pain and dyspnea.

A heart mural thrombus can migrate through the aorta to the systemic arterial circulation and occlude an artery of the brain, kidneys, spleen, intestines and lower extremities. Severe bone fracture can cause fat and bone marrow emboli to enter the venous system and reach the pulmonary arteries through the right side of the heart.

13. Respiratory System

The respiratory system consists of three main portions with distinct functions: (1) An air-conducting portion. (2) A respiratory portion for gas exchange between blood and air. (3) A mechanism for ventilation, driven by the inspiratory and expiratory movements of the thoracic cage. The air-conducting portion consists, sequentially, of the nasal cavities and associated sinuses, the nasopharynx, the oropharynx, the larynx, the trachea, the bronchi, and the bronchioles. The oropharynx also participates in food transport. The conducting portion provides a passage for inhaled and exhaled air in and out of the respiratory portion. The respiratory portion is composed, in sequence, of the respiratory bronchioles, alveolar ducts, alveolar sacs, and alveoli. The main function is the exchange of gases between air and blood. Respiration involves the participation of a ventilation mechanism. The inflow (inspiration) and outflow (expiration) of air occur with the aid of four elements: (1) The thoracic or rib cage. (2) Associated intercostal muscles. (3) The diaphragm muscle. (4) The elastic connective tissue of the lungs. This chapter addresses the structure and function of the respiratory system leading to an understanding of pathologic abnormalities.

Nasal cavities and paranasal sinuses

The nasal cavities and paranasal sinuses provide an extensive surface area for:

1. Warming and moistening air.
2. Filtering dust particles present in the inspired air.

In addition, the roof of each nasal cavity and part of the superior concha contain the specialized **olfactory mucosa**.

Each nasal cavity, separated from the other by the **septum**, consists of the **vestibule**, the **respiratory portion**, and the **olfactory area** (Figure 13-1).

Air enters through the **nostril**, or **naris**, whose external surface is lined by **keratinized squamous epithelium**. At the **vestibule**, the epithelium becomes **nonkeratinized**.

The **respiratory portion** is lined by a **pseudostratified ciliated epithelium with goblet cells** supported by the lamina propria, which consists of connective tissue with **seromucous glands**. The lamina propria has a **rich superficial venous plexus**, known as **cavernous** or **erectile tissue**. The lamina propria is continuous with the periosteum or perichondrium of bone or cartilage, respectively, forming the wall of the nasal cavities.

Projecting into each nasal cavity from the lateral wall are three curved plates of bone covered by a mucosa: the **superior**, **middle**, and **inferior turbinate bones**, or **conchae** (Latin *concha*, shell).

Secretions from goblet cells and seromucous glands maintain the turbinate mucosal surface moist and humidify the inspired air.

Incoming air is warmed by blood in the venous plexus, which flows in a direction opposite to that of the inspired air (**countercurrent flow**). The highly vascular nature of the nasal mucosa, in particular of the anterior septum, accounts for common bleed-

Figure 13-1. Nasal cavities

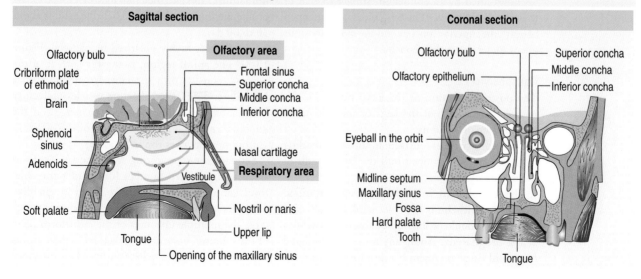

Sagittal section	Coronal section

Sagittal section labels:
- Olfactory bulb
- Cribriform plate of ethmoid
- Brain
- Sphenoid sinus
- Adenoids
- Soft palate
- Tongue
- Olfactory area
- Frontal sinus
- Superior concha
- Middle concha
- Inferior concha
- Nasal cartilage
- Respiratory area
- Vestibule
- Nostril or naris
- Upper lip
- Opening of the maxillary sinus

Coronal section labels:
- Olfactory bulb
- Olfactory epithelium
- Superior concha
- Middle concha
- Inferior concha
- Eyeball in the orbit
- Midline septum
- Maxillary sinus
- Fossa
- Hard palate
- Tooth
- Tongue

Figure 13-2. Olfactory mucosa

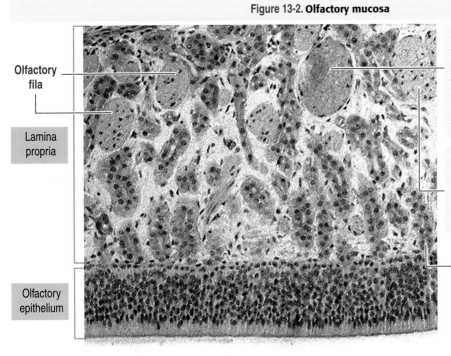

Olfactory
fila

Lamina
propria

Olfactory
epithelium

**Venous sinusoid of the cavernous
vascular tissue**
Local vascular changes controlled by
vasomotor autonomic innervation can
modify the thickness of the mucosa,
resulting in changes in the rate of airflow
through the nasal passages.

Groups of unmyelinated axons form
nerve fascicles (called **olfactory fila**) that
pass through the cribriform plate of the
ethmoid bone to terminate in the
glomeruli of the **olfactory bulb**.

Olfactory gland of Bowman

ing (**epistaxis**) after trauma or acute inflammation (**rhinitis**).

Conchae cause airflow turbulence, thus facilitating contact between the air and the mucus blanket covering the respiratory region of each nasal cavity. The mucus blanket traps particulates in the air that are transported posteriorly by ciliary action to the nasopharynx, where they are swallowed with the saliva.

Paranasal sinuses are air-containing cavities within the bones of the skull. They are the **maxillary, frontal, ethmoidal**, and **sphenoid sinuses**. The sinuses are lined by a thin **pseudostratified columnar ciliated epithelium**, with fewer goblet cells and glands in the lamina propria. No erectile tissue is present in the paranasal sinuses.

Sinuses communicate with the nasal cavity by openings lined by an epithelium similar to that of the main nasal cavity. The ethmoidal sinuses open beneath the superior conchae and the maxillary sinus opens under the middle concha.

Nasopharynx

The posterior portion of the nasal cavities is the nasopharynx, which at the level of the soft palate becomes the oropharynx.

The **auditory tubes** (**eustachian tubes**), extending from the middle ear, open into the lateral walls of the nasopharynx.

The **nasopharynx** is lined by a **pseudostratified columnar epithelium** like the nasal cavities, and changes into **nonkeratinizing squamous epithelium** at the oropharynx. Abundant **mucosa-associated lymphoid tissue** is present beneath the nasopharyn-

geal epithelium, forming the **Waldeyer's ring** (formed by the two palatine tonsils, the nasopharyngeal tonsils, the lingual tonsils and mucosa-associated lymphoid tissue, MALT). The **nasopharyngeal tonsils** (called **adenoids** when enlarged by inflammation) are present at the posterior and upper regions of the nasopharynx.

Olfactory epithelium

The olfactory epithelium contains three major types of cells (Figures 13-2; see Box 13-A):

1. **Basal cells**.
2. **Olfactory sensory neurons** (OSNs).
3. **Supporting or sustentacular cells**.

The **basal cells** are mitotically active stem cells, producing daughter cells that differentiate first into **immature OSNs** and then into **mature OSNs**. OSNs proliferate during adult life. Their life span is about 30 to 60 days.

The **OSN** is highly polarized bipolar cell (Figure 13-3). The **apical region**, facing the surface of the mucosa, consists of a specialized dendrite with a **knoblike ending** (called **olfactory vesicle** or **olfactory knob**). About 10 to 20 modified cilia emerge from the knoblike ending. The **basal region** of the olfactory sensory neuron gives rise to an **axon**.

Several axons, projecting from the OSNs, form small unmyelinated bundles (called **olfactory fila**; from Latin *filum*, thread), surrounded by glial-like cells. Nerve bundles, forming the first cranial nerve, cross the multiple openings of the **cribriform plate of the ethmoid bone** and contact in the **glomerulus** the dendrites of **mitral cells** (neurons of the **olfactory** bulb) to establish appropriate synaptic connections (see Figure 13-3 and Box 13-A).

The **supporting** or **sustentacular cells** are non-sensory epithelial cells with numerous apical microvilli and secretory granules releasing their contents onto the mucosal surface.

Olfactory serous glands, called **glands of Bowman**, are present under the epithelium and secrete a serous fluid in which odoriferous substances are dissolved. The secretory fluid contains the odorant-binding protein (**OBP**) with high binding affinity for a large number of **odorant molecules**.

OBP carries odorants to receptors present on the surface of the modified cilia and removes them after they have been sensed. In addition, the secretory product of the glands of Bowman contains protective substances such as **lysozyme** and immunoglobulin A (**IgA**) secreted by plasma cells.

The **odorant transduction pathway** involves:

1. G protein and activation of adenylyl cyclase 3, which produces cyclic adenosine monophosphate (cAMP) (see Figure 13-3).

2. cAMP regulates the phosphorylation of proteins and the transcription of genes involved in the growth and survival of OSNs.

3. cAMP binds to a cyclic nucleotide-gated (CNG) ion channel, allowing the influx of Ca^{2+} and Na^+ and efflux of intracellular Cl^-.

4. The ion flow depolarizes the cell membrane of the modified cilia and generates action potentials propagated down the axon of the OSNs to the synapses in the glomeruli, located in the olfactory bulb.

5. The glomerulus behave as a functional unit to which sensory input signals converge and become activated before transmission to the corticomedial amygdala portion of the brain.

Box 13-A | Olfactory epithelium: Highlights to remember

• The olfactory epithelium consists of **olfactory sensory neurons (OSNs)**, **basal cells** (a stem cell that differentiates into OSNs), and **sustentacular** or **supporting cells**. These cells can be identified on the basis of the position and shape of their nuclei (see Figure 13-3).
• An OSN is a bipolar neuron. It has two portions: an apical dendrite with a knob bearing about 10 to 20 olfactory nonmotile modified cilia and a basal axon, forming bundles that pass through the cribriform plate of the ethmoid bone.
• Cilia contain the **odorant receptor (OR)**. There are about 1000 genes expressing ORs, but each OSN expresses only one *OR* gene.
• Secretions of the serous glands of Bowman contain odorant-binding protein.
• Axons from OSNs with the same OR terminate in one to three glomeruli present in the olfactory bulb. Dendritic endings of predominantly mitral cells extend into the glomeruli. Axons of mitral cells form the olfactory tract.
• OSNs have a life span of 30 to 60 days and can regenerate from basal cells.
• Temporary or permanent damage to the olfactory epithelium causes **anosmia** (Greek *an*, not; *osme*, sense of smell).

Larynx

The two main functions of the larynx are:

1. To produce sound.

2. To close the trachea during swallowing to prevent food and saliva from entering the airway.

The **wall of the larynx** is made up of the **thyroid** and **cricoid hyaline cartilage** and the **elastic cartilage core of the epiglottis** extending over the lumen of the larynx (Figure 13-4).

Extrinsic laryngeal muscles attach the larynx to the **hyoid bone** to raise the larynx during swallowing.

Intrinsic laryngeal muscles (**abductor**, **adductors**, and **tensors**), innervated by the recurrent laryngeal nerve, link the thyroid and cricoid cartilages. When intrinsic muscles contract, the tension on the vocal cords changes to modulate phonation. The middle and lower laryngeal arteries (derived from the superior and inferior thyroid artery) supply the larynx. Lymphatic plexuses drain to the upper cervical lymph nodes and to the nodes along the trachea.

The larynx can be subdivided into three regions:

1. The **supraglottis**, which includes the epiglottis, false vocal cords (or folds), and laryngeal ventricles.

2. The **glottis**, consisting of the true vocal cords (or folds) and the anterior and posterior commissures.

3. The **subglottis**, the region below the true vocal cords, extending down to the lower border of the cricoid cartilage.

Upper respiratory tract infections caused by viruses and bacteria usually involve the supraglottis and glottis regions. Hoarseness and transient voice loss are typical symptoms.

During forced inspiration, vocal cords are **abducted**, and the space between the vocal cords widens.

During phonation, the vocal cords are **adducted** and the space between the vocal cords changes into a linear slit. The vibration of the free edges of the cords during passage of air between them produces sound. The contraction of the intrinsic muscles of the larynx, forming the body of the cords, increases tension on the vocal cords, changing the pitch of the produced sound (see Box 13-B).

The mucosa of the larynx is continuous with that of the pharynx and the trachea. A **stratified squamous epithelium** covers the **lingual surface** and a small extension of the pharyngeal surface of the epiglottis and the **true vocal cords**. Elsewhere, the epithelium is **pseudostratified ciliated, with goblet cells**.

Laryngeal seromucous glands are found throughout the lamina propria, except at the level of the true vocal cords. The lamina propria of the **true vocal cords** consists of three layers (see Figure 13-4):

1. A superficial layer containing extracellular matrix and few elastic fibers. This layer is known as **Reinke's space**.

2. An intermediate layer with elastic fibers.

Figure 13-3. Olfactory epithelium

1 Axons from olfactory sensory neurons are bundled in groups of 10 to 100 and penetrate the cribriform plate of the ethmoid bone reaching the **olfactory bulb**. In the olfactory bulb, the axon terminals connect with synaptic terminals of **mitral cells** forming synaptic structures called **glomeruli**.

2 The olfactory signal is sent by **mitral cells**, through the **olfactory nerve tract**, to the **corticomedial amygdala portion of the brain**.

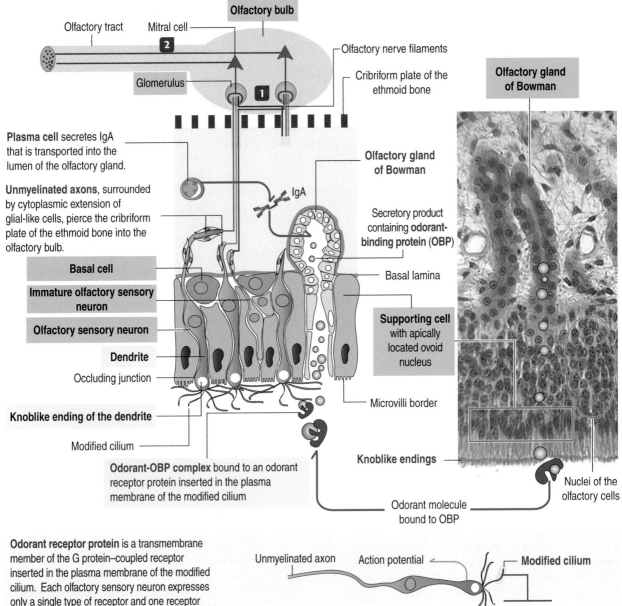

Olfactory tract

Mitral cell

2

Glomerulus

Olfactory bulb

1

Olfactory nerve filaments

Cribriform plate of the ethmoid bone

Olfactory gland of Bowman

Plasma cell secretes IgA that is transported into the lumen of the olfactory gland.

IgA

Olfactory gland of Bowman

Secretory product containing **odorant-binding protein (OBP)**

Unmyelinated axons, surrounded by cytoplasmic extension of glial-like cells, pierce the cribriform plate of the ethmoid bone into the olfactory bulb.

Basal cell

Basal lamina

Immature olfactory sensory neuron

Olfactory sensory neuron

Supporting cell with apically located ovoid nucleus

Dendrite

Occluding junction

Microvilli border

Knoblike ending of the dendrite

Modified cilium

Knoblike endings

Nuclei of the olfactory cells

Odorant-OBP complex bound to an odorant receptor protein inserted in the plasma membrane of the modified cilium

Odorant molecule bound to OBP

Odorant receptor protein is a transmembrane member of the G protein–coupled receptor inserted in the plasma membrane of the modified cilium. Each olfactory sensory neuron expresses only a single type of receptor and one receptor may bind to several different odorants.

Odorant-OBP complex binding to **type 1 receptor (TR1)** activates $G\alpha$ protein coupled to the receptor on its intracytoplasmic side. $G\alpha$ protein–activated adenylyl cyclase 3 catalyzes the conversion of adenosine triphosphate (ATP) to cyclic adenosine monophosphate (cAMP) which opens CNG channels to facilitate the **influx** of Na^+ and Ca^{2+}. Ca^{2+} activates the **efflux** of Cl^-. An action potential is generated and conducted down the axon of the olfactory sensory neurons to the **glomerulus** and along the olfactory nerve to the brain.

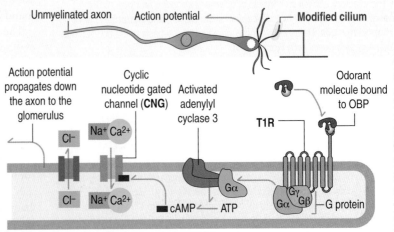

Unmyelinated axon

Action potential

Modified cilium

Action potential propagates down the axon to the glomerulus

Cyclic nucleotide gated channel (**CNG**)

Activated adenylyl cyclase 3

Odorant molecule bound to OBP

Cl^-

Na^+ Ca^{2+}

T1R

Cl^-

Na^+ Ca^{2+}

$G\alpha$

$G\gamma$

$G\alpha$ $G\beta$

G protein

cAMP ← ATP

Modified cilium of an olfactory sensory neuron

3. A deep layer with abundant elastic and collagen fibers.

The intermediate and deep layer of the lamina propria constitute the **vocal ligament**. Reinke's space and the epithelial covering are responsible for vocal cord vibration.

Reinke's edema results when viral infection or severe coughing spells cause fluid to accumulate in the superficial layer of the lamina propria.

Singer's nodules are small fibrosis clusters in the lamina propria covered by epithelium, where the margins of the true vocal cords contact each other.

The lamina propria is usually rich in **mast cells**. Mast cells participate in hypersensitivity reactions leading to edema and laryngeal obstruction, a potential medical emergency.

Croup designates a laryngotracheobronchitis in children, in which an inflammatory process narrows the airway and produces **inspiratory stridor**.

Trachea

The trachea, the major segment of the **conducting region** of the respiratory system, is the continuation of the larynx.

At the tracheal carina, the trachea branches into the right and left primary bronchi entering the hilum of each lung. The **hilum** is the region where the primary bronchus, **pulmonary artery**, **pulmonary vein**, **nerves**, and **lymphatics** enter and leave the lung. Secondary divisions of the bronchi and accompanying connective tissue septa divide each lung into lobes.

The right lung has three lobes, whereas the left lung has two lobes.

Subsequent bronchial divisions further subdivide each lobe into bronchopulmonary segments. **The bronchopulmonary segment is the gross anatomic unit of the lung that can be resected surgically.** Successive bronchial branching gives rise to several generations of **bronchopulmonary subsegments**.

The trachea and main bronchi are lined by **pseudostratified columnar ciliated epithelium** resting on a distinct basal lamina. Several types of cells can be identified (Figure 13-5):

1. **Columnar ciliated cells** are the predominant cell population, extending from the lumen to the basal lamina.

2. **Goblet cells** are abundant nonciliated cells, also in contact with the lumen and the basal lamina. They produce mucin polymers MUC5AC and MUC5B (see Figure 13-5).

3. **Basal cells** rest on the basal lamina but do not extend to the lumen.

4. **Cells of Kulchitsky** are neuroendocrine cells also resting on the basal lamina and are predominantly found at the bifurcation of lobar bronchi. They give rise to **small cell lung cancer** (SCLC; also called **oat-cell carcinoma**). These cells secrete peptide hormones such as serotonin, calcitonin, antidiuretic hormone (ADH), and adrenocorticotropic hormone (ACTH).

The lamina propria contains elastic fibers. The **submucosa** displays **mucous** and **serous glands** that, together with goblet cells, produce components of the airways mucus (see Box 13-C).

The framework of the trachea and extrapulmonary bronchi consists of a stack of **C-shaped hyaline cartilages**, each surrounded by a **fibroelastic layer** blending with the perichondrium.

In the **trachea** and **primary bronchi**, the open ends of the cartilage rings point posteriorly to the esophagus. The lowest tracheal cartilage is the **carinal cartilage**. Transverse fibers of the **trachealis muscle** attach to the inner ends of the cartilage. In branching bronchi, cartilage **rings** (see Figure 13-5) are replaced by irregularly shaped cartilage **plates** (Figure 13-6), surrounded by smooth muscle bundles in a spiral arrangement.

Figure 13-4. **Structure of the larynx**

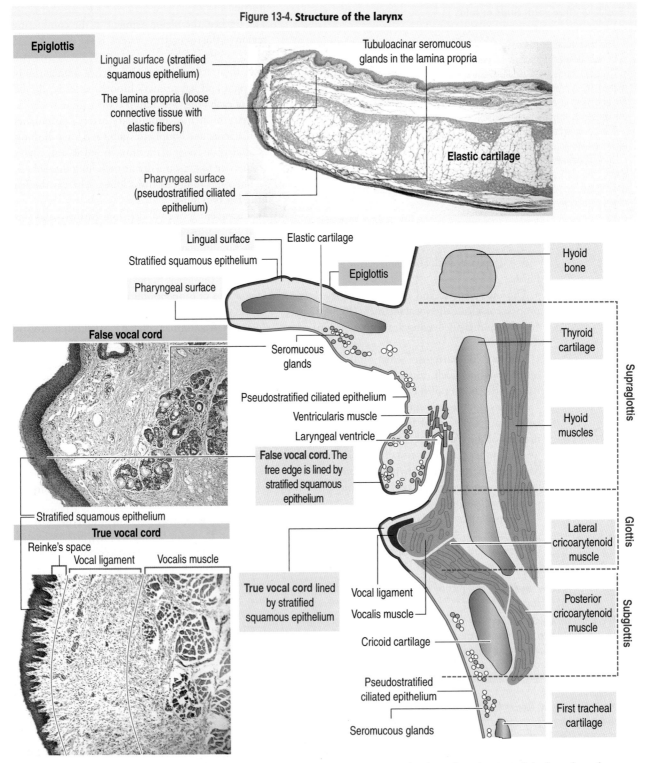

Epiglottis

Lingual surface (stratified squamous epithelium)

The lamina propria (loose connective tissue with elastic fibers)

Pharyngeal surface (pseudostratified ciliated epithelium)

Tubuloacinar seromucous glands in the lamina propria

Elastic cartilage

Lingual surface

Stratified squamous epithelium

Pharyngeal surface

Elastic cartilage

Epiglottis

Hyoid bone

Thyroid cartilage

Hyoid muscles

Supraglottis

False vocal cord

Seromucous glands

Pseudostratified ciliated epithelium

Ventricularis muscle

Laryngeal ventricle

False vocal cord. The free edge is lined by stratified squamous epithelium

Stratified squamous epithelium

True vocal cord

Reinke's space

Vocal ligament

Vocalis muscle

True vocal cord lined by stratified squamous epithelium

Vocal ligament

Vocalis muscle

Cricoid cartilage

Pseudostratified ciliated epithelium

Seromucous glands

Lateral cricoarytenoid muscle

Glottis

Posterior cricoarytenoid muscle

Subglottis

First tracheal cartilage

Segmentation of the bronchial tree

Within the pulmonary parenchyma, a segmental bronchus gives rise to large and small subsegmental bronchi. A small subsegmental bronchus is continuous with a bronchiole.

This transition involves **the loss of cartilage plates in the bronchiole and a progressive increase in the number of elastic fibers.**

The intrapulmonary segmentation results in the organization of a **pulmonary lobule** and a **pulmonary acinus** (Figure 13-7; see also Figure 13-6).

Pulmonary lobule and pulmonary acinus

A terminal bronchiole and the associated region of pulmonary tissues that it supplies constitute a **pulmonary lobule** (Figure 13-8). A pulmonary lobule includes the respiratory bronchioles, alveolar ducts, alveolar sacs, and alveoli.

Figure 13-5. Structure of the trachea

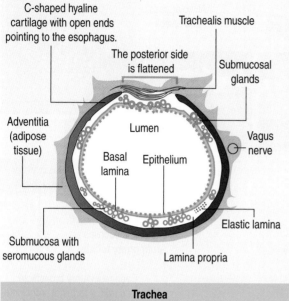

C-shaped hyaline cartilage with open ends pointing to the esophagus.

The posterior side is flattened

Trachealis muscle

Submucosal glands

Lumen

Adventitia (adipose tissue)

Basal lamina

Epithelium

Vagus nerve

Submucosa with seromucous glands

Lamina propria

Elastic lamina

Trachea

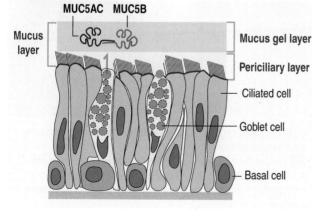

— Luminal surface

— Cross section of a hyaline cartilage ring

— Seromucous glands

— Respiratory epithelium

Epithelial lining of the trachea

1 Columnar ciliated cell
The apical density represents the linear alignment of basal bodies that give rise to cilia extending into the lumen. Columnar ciliated cells are about 30% of the total cell population.

2 Goblet cell
The apical portion of the cell contains mucus secretion that is released by exocytosis into the lumen, forming part of a protective mucus gel layer. Goblet cells are about 30% of the total cell population.

3 Basal cell
This cell does not extend to the free surface and functions as a stem cell population for the epithelium. Basal cells are about 30% of the total cell population.

Bronchial endocrine cells (of Kulchitsky; not shown)
Neuroendocrine cells with small granules can be observed in the basal region of the epithelium. They are predominant at the bifurcation of the lobar bronchi.

They are members of the **diffuse endocrine system** (previously known as **APUD, or amine precursor uptake and decarboxylation system**).

These cells resemble the enteroendocrine cells found in the digestive system. They may synthesize antidiuretic hormone, serotonin, calcitonin, somatostatin, and other small peptides of defined pharmacologic action.

Bronchial endocrine cells give rise to **small cell lung cancer (SCLC)**, that displays endobronchial growth and metastasizes rapidly to regional lymph nodes.

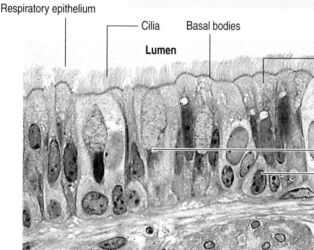

Cilia

Basal bodies

Lumen

1 Columnar ciliated cell

Respiratory epithelium: pseudostratified columnar epithelium with ciliated cells, goblet and basal cells

2 Goblet cell

3 Basal cell

Basal lamina with subjacent elastic lamina

Lamina propria

MUC5AC MUC5B

Mucus layer

Mucus gel layer

Periciliary layer

Ciliated cell

Goblet cell

Basal cell

Composition and function of airway mucus

Airway mucus traps pathogens, particles, and toxic chemicals in inhaled air. It is an extracellular gel containing water and glycoproteins (mucins) produced by goblet cells, submucosal glands, and club (Clara) cells. Airways mucus consists of two layers: (1) a **periciliary layer**, and (2) a **mucus gel layer**. MUC5AC and MUC5B are cross-linking glycoprotein monomers binding large amounts of fluid, which allows mucus to act as lubricant and maintain its viscous and elastic properties. Low viscosity and elasticity determine effective mucus clearance by cilia beating velocity and cough. MUC5AC is produced by goblet cells and MUC5B is secreted by goblet cells and submucosal glands (not shown in the diagram).

Figure 13-6. Segmentation of the intrapulmonary bronchial tree

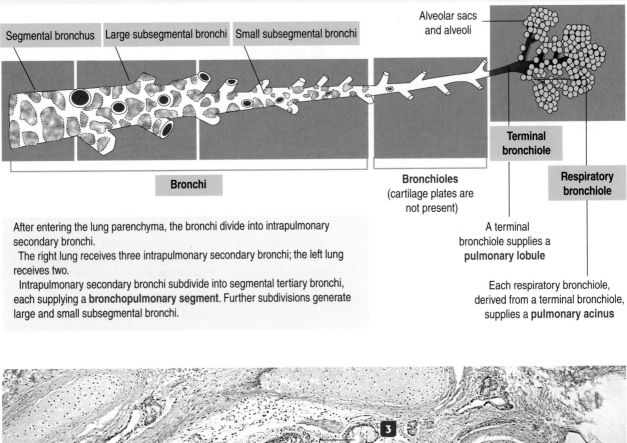

Segmental bronchus | Large subsegmental bronchi | Small subsegmental bronchi

Alveolar sacs and alveoli

Bronchi

Bronchioles (cartilage plates are not present)

Terminal bronchiole

Respiratory bronchiole

After entering the lung parenchyma, the bronchi divide into intrapulmonary secondary bronchi.

The right lung receives three intrapulmonary secondary bronchi; the left lung receives two.

Intrapulmonary secondary bronchi subdivide into segmental tertiary bronchi, each supplying a **bronchopulmonary segment**. Further subdivisions generate large and small subsegmental bronchi.

A terminal bronchiole supplies a **pulmonary lobule**

Each respiratory bronchiole, derived from a terminal bronchiole, supplies a **pulmonary acinus**

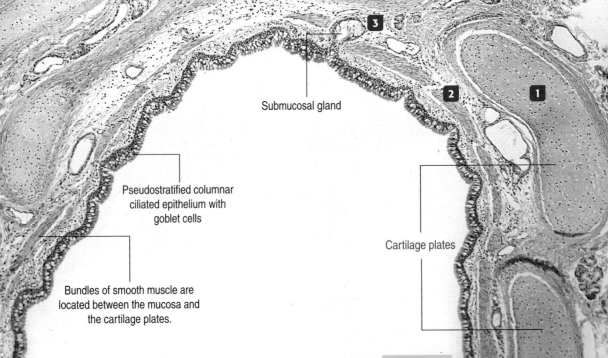

Submucosal gland

Pseudostratified columnar ciliated epithelium with goblet cells

Cartilage plates

Bundles of smooth muscle are located between the mucosa and the cartilage plates.

Bronchus

1 As bronchi become smaller, irregular **cartilage plates** are observed. Each cartilage plate, consisting of hyaline cartilage, is surrounded by a bundle of connective tissue fibers blending with the perichondrium.

2 Bundles of smooth muscle fibers are observed between the cartilage plates and the bronchial mucosa. The mucosa is lined by the typical respiratory epithelium.

3 Seromucous glands are observed in the lamina propria with the secretory acini projecting beyond the layer of smooth muscle cell bundles. The excretory ducts open into the bronchial lumen.

Figure 13-7. **Histology of the intrapulmonary bronchial tree**

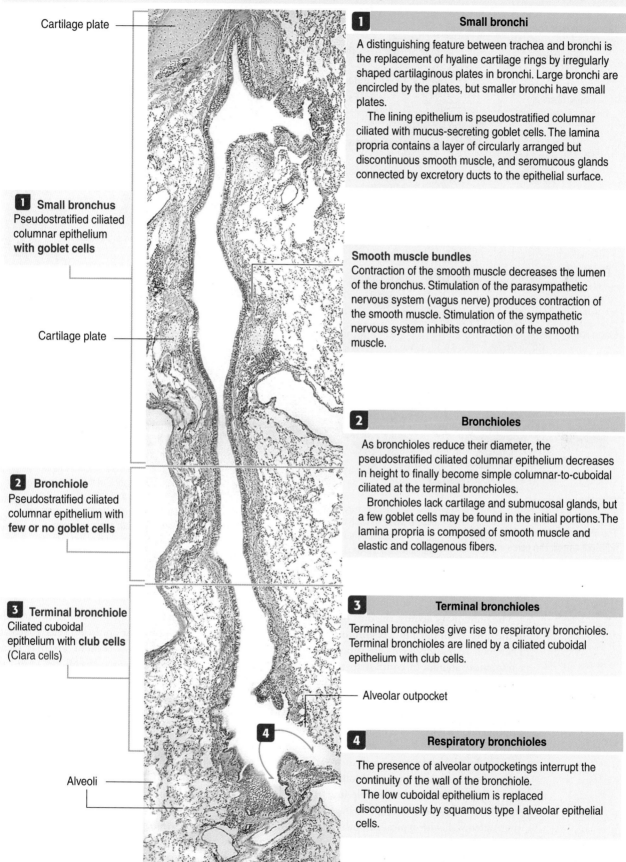

Cartilage plate

1 **Small bronchus**
Pseudostratified ciliated columnar epithelium **with goblet cells**

Cartilage plate

2 **Bronchiole**
Pseudostratified ciliated columnar epithelium with **few or no goblet cells**

3 **Terminal bronchiole**
Ciliated cuboidal epithelium with **club cells** (Clara cells)

Alveoli

1 **Small bronchi**

A distinguishing feature between trachea and bronchi is the replacement of hyaline cartilage rings by irregularly shaped cartilaginous plates in bronchi. Large bronchi are encircled by the plates, but smaller bronchi have small plates.

The lining epithelium is pseudostratified columnar ciliated with mucus-secreting goblet cells. The lamina propria contains a layer of circularly arranged but discontinuous smooth muscle, and seromucous glands connected by excretory ducts to the epithelial surface.

Smooth muscle bundles
Contraction of the smooth muscle decreases the lumen of the bronchus. Stimulation of the parasympathetic nervous system (vagus nerve) produces contraction of the smooth muscle. Stimulation of the sympathetic nervous system inhibits contraction of the smooth muscle.

2 **Bronchioles**

As bronchioles reduce their diameter, the pseudostratified ciliated columnar epithelium decreases in height to finally become simple columnar-to-cuboidal ciliated at the terminal bronchioles.

Bronchioles lack cartilage and submucosal glands, but a few goblet cells may be found in the initial portions. The lamina propria is composed of smooth muscle and elastic and collagenous fibers.

3 **Terminal bronchioles**

Terminal bronchioles give rise to respiratory bronchioles. Terminal bronchioles are lined by a ciliated cuboidal epithelium with club cells.

Alveolar outpocket

4 **Respiratory bronchioles**

The presence of alveolar outpocketings interrupt the continuity of the wall of the bronchiole.

The low cuboidal epithelium is replaced discontinuously by squamous type I alveolar epithelial cells.

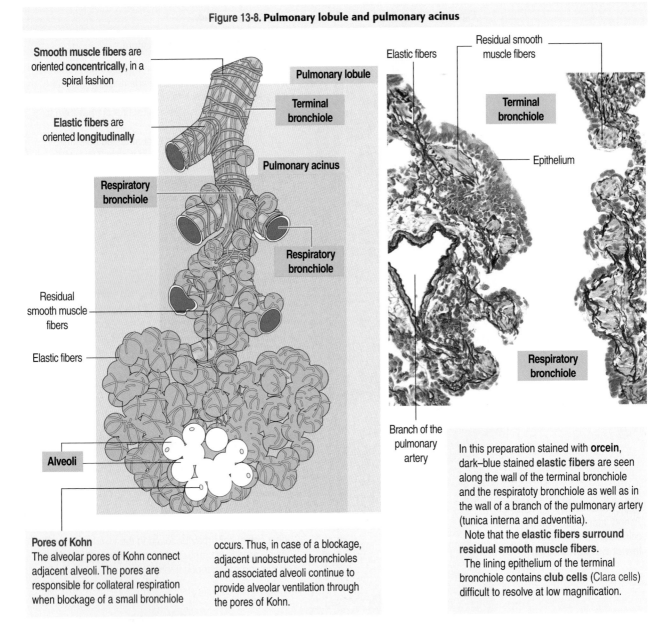

Figure 13-8. Pulmonary lobule and pulmonary acinus

Smooth muscle fibers are oriented **concentrically**, in a spiral fashion

Elastic fibers are oriented **longitudinally**

Respiratory bronchiole

Residual smooth muscle fibers

Elastic fibers

Alveoli

Pulmonary lobule

Terminal bronchiole

Pulmonary acinus

Respiratory bronchiole

Elastic fibers

Residual smooth muscle fibers

Terminal bronchiole

Epithelium

Respiratory bronchiole

Branch of the pulmonary artery

Pores of Kohn
The alveolar pores of Kohn connect adjacent alveoli. The pores are responsible for collateral respiration when blockage of a small bronchiole

occurs. Thus, in case of a blockage, adjacent unobstructed bronchioles and associated alveoli continue to provide alveolar ventilation through the pores of Kohn.

In this preparation stained with **orcein**, dark–blue stained **elastic fibers** are seen along the wall of the terminal bronchiole and the respiratoty bronchiole as well as in the wall of a branch of the pulmonary artery (tunica interna and adventitia).
Note that the **elastic fibers surround residual smooth muscle fibers**.
The lining epithelium of the terminal bronchiole contains **club cells** (Clara cells) difficult to resolve at low magnification.

The pulmonary acinus, the unit of gas exchange of the lung, is supplied by a respiratory bronchiole. Therefore, respiratory acini are subcomponents of a respiratory lobule. In contrast to the acinus, the pulmonary lobule includes the terminal bronchiole.

The pulmonary lobule–pulmonary acinus concept is important for understanding the types of emphysema. Emphysema is permanent enlargement of the air spaces distal to the terminal bronchioles, associated with the destruction of their walls.

Distal to the respiratory bronchiole is the **alveolar duct**. The respiratory bronchiole and the initial portion of the alveolar duct are characterized by an interrupted wall with typical **smooth muscle knobs and associated scattered elastic fibers** bulging into the lumen (Figure 13-9).

At the distal end of the alveolar duct, the smooth muscle knobs disappear and the lining epithelium is primarily **type I alveolar epithelial cells**. Alveolar ducts branch to form two or more **alveolar sacs**. Alveolar sacs are formed by the **alveoli**, the terminal part of the airway.

Pathology: Chronic obstructive pulmonary disease
Chronic obstructive pulmonary disease (COPD) is characterized by progressive and often irreversible airflow limitations. COPD includes **chronic bronchitis** and **emphysema**.

Chronic bronchitis develops in smokers and in response to inhalation of toxic fumes and long-standing exposure to high levels of air pollutants. It is characterized by hyperplasia and long-term hypersecretion of the seromucous glands causing airways obstruction and mucus plugging. As a result, a reduction in

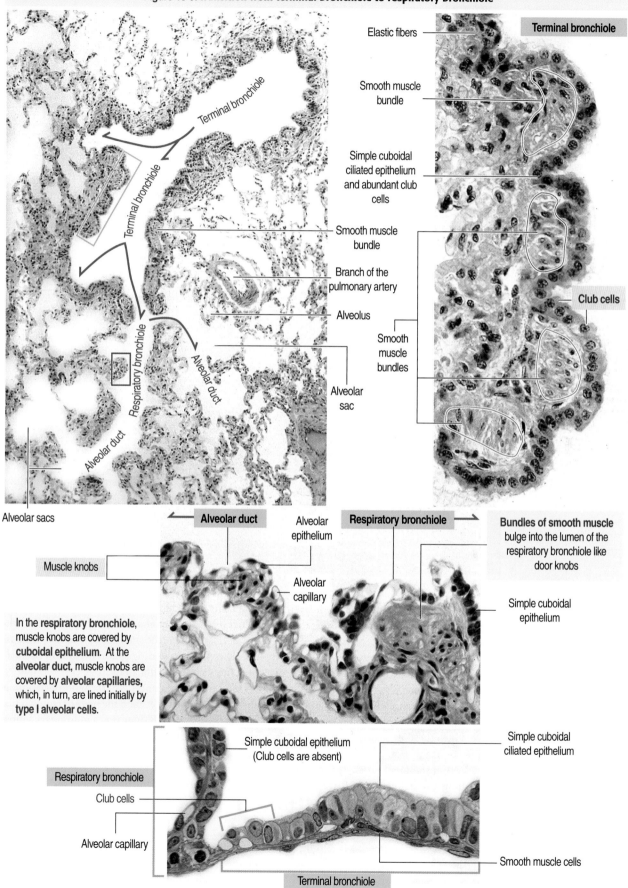

Figure 13-9. **Transition from terminal bronchiole to respiratory bronchiole**

Terminal bronchiole

Terminal bronchiole

Terminal bronchiole

Respiratory bronchiole

Alveolar duct

Alveolar duct

Alveolar sacs

Elastic fibers

Smooth muscle bundle

Simple cuboidal ciliated epithelium and abundant club cells

Smooth muscle bundle

Branch of the pulmonary artery

Alveolus

Alveolar sac

Terminal bronchiole

Club cells

Smooth muscle bundles

Alveolar duct

Alveolar epithelium

Muscle knobs

Alveolar capillary

Respiratory bronchiole

Bundles of smooth muscle bulge into the lumen of the respiratory bronchiole like door knobs

Simple cuboidal epithelium

In the **respiratory bronchiole,** muscle knobs are covered by **cuboidal epithelium.** At the **alveolar duct,** muscle knobs are covered by **alveolar capillaries,** which, in turn, are lined initially by **type I alveolar cells.**

Respiratory bronchiole

Club cells

Alveolar capillary

Simple cuboidal epithelium (Club cells are absent)

Simple cuboidal ciliated epithelium

Smooth muscle cells

Terminal bronchiole

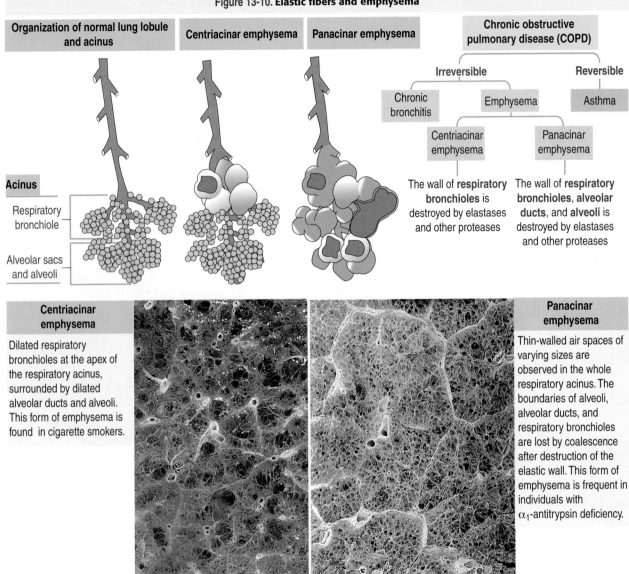

Figure 13-10. Elastic fibers and emphysema

Organization of normal lung lobule and acinus

Centriacinar emphysema

Panacinar emphysema

Chronic obstructive pulmonary disease (COPD)

Irreversible — Reversible

Chronic bronchitis — Emphysema — Asthma

Centriacinar emphysema — Panacinar emphysema

Acinus

Respiratory bronchiole

Alveolar sacs and alveoli

The wall of **respiratory bronchioles** is destroyed by elastases and other proteases

The wall of **respiratory bronchioles, alveolar ducts**, and **alveoli** is destroyed by elastases and other proteases

Centriacinar emphysema

Dilated respiratory bronchioles at the apex of the respiratory acinus, surrounded by dilated alveolar ducts and alveoli. This form of emphysema is found in cigarette smokers.

Panacinar emphysema

Thin-walled air spaces of varying sizes are observed in the whole respiratory acinus. The boundaries of alveoli, alveolar ducts, and respiratory bronchioles are lost by coalescence after destruction of the elastic wall. This form of emphysema is frequent in individuals with α_1-antitrypsin deficiency.

Photographs from Damjanov I, Linder J: Pathology: A Color Atlas. St. Louis, Mosby, 2000.

alveolar ventilation leads to **hypoxemia** (low levels of oxygen in blood) and **hypercapnia** (increased level of carbon dioxide in blood).

Hypoxemia can cause secondary pulmonary hypertension and eventual right heart failure (cor pulmonale). Hypercapnia results in cyanosis (Greek *kyanos*, a dark blue substance) but no significant dyspnea (Greek, *dys*, difficult; *pnoe,* breathing). Cyanosis is a bluish color to the skin or mucosae membranes usually caused by a reduction of oxygen in the blood.

COPD occurs in the **small-airways**, the bronchioles, and in **lung parenchyma**. You have seen that **elastic fibers** are important components of bronchioles and alveolar walls. A loss of elasticity and breakdown of elastic fibers give rise to **emphysema**, characterized by chronic airflow obstruction. As a result, adjacent alveoli become confluent, creating large **air spaces**, or **blebs** (Figure 13-10).

Terminal and respiratory bronchioles are also affected by the loss of elastic tissue. As a result of the loss of elastic fibers, the small airways tend to collapse during expiration, leading to chronic airflow obstruction and secondary infections.

Let us review the concepts of the pulmonary lobule and the acinus to understand the types of emphysema. Figures 13-6 and 13-8 show that a **pulmonary lobule includes the terminal bronchiole and the first to third generations of derived respiratory bronchioles.** Each respiratory bronchiole gives rise to alveolar ducts and alveoli, an arrangement known as the **acinus**, so called because aggregates of alveoli cluster like acini in connection with the ductlike respiratory bronchiole. Because a pulmonary lobule generates several respiratory bronchioles, each resolved into an acinus, a pulmonary lobule is made up of several acini.

Centriacinar (or centrilobular) **emphysema** origi-

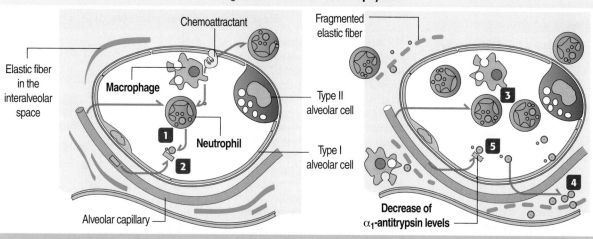

Figure 13-11. Elastase and emphysema

Chemoattractant

Fragmented elastic fiber

Elastic fiber in the interalveolar space

Macrophage

Type II alveolar cell

1

Neutrophil

Type I alveolar cell

2

3

5

4

Decrease of α₁-antitrypsin levels

Alveolar capillary

Pathogenesis of emphysema

A stimulus (for example, smoking) increases the number of macrophages, which secrete **chemoattractants** for neutrophils. Neutrophils accumulate in the alveolar lumen and interstitium.

1 Neutrophils release elastase into the alveolar lumen.

2 Serum α₁-**antitrypsin** neutralizes elastase and prevents its destructive effect on the alveolar wall.

3 A persistent stimulus continues to increase the number of neutrophils and macrophages in the alveolar lumen and interstitium.

4 Neutrophils release elastase into the alveolar lumen and interalveolar space.

5 Serum α₁-**antitrypsin levels decrease** and elastase starts the destruction of elastic fibers, leading to the development of emphysema. **Damaged elastic fibers cannot recoil when stretched.**

nates when the **respiratory bronchioles** are affected. The more distal alveolar duct and alveoli are intact. Thus, emphysematous and normal air spaces coexist within the same lobule and acini.

In **panacinar** (or panlobular) **emphysema**, blebs are observed from the respiratory bronchiole down to the alveolar sacs. This type of emphysema is more common in patients with a **deficiency in the α₁-antitrypsin gene** encoding a serum protein.

Protein α₁-antitrypsin is a major inhibitor of proteases, in particular **elastase**, secreted by neutrophils during inflammation (Figure 13-11). Under the influence of a stimulus, such as cigarette smoke, **macrophages** in the alveolar wall and alveolar lumen secrete proteases and chemoattractants (mainly leukotriene B₄) to recruit **neutrophils**.

Chemoattracted neutrophils appear in the alveolar lumen and wall and release **elastase**, normally neutralized by α₁-**antitrypsin**. Chronic smokers have low serum levels of α₁-antitrypsin, and elastase continues the unopposed destruction of elastic fibers present in the alveolar wall. This process develops in 10% to 15% of smokers and leads to emphysema.

Asthma is a chronic inflammatory process characterized by the **reversible narrowing of the airways (bronchoconstriction)** in response to various stimuli. The classic **symptoms of asthma** are **wheezing**, **cough**, and **shortness of breath** (**dyspnea**).

Emphysema differs from asthma in that the abnormalities limiting airflow are **irreversible** and a **destructive process** targets the lung parenchyma.

Pathology: Asthma

Asthma consists in **airway hyperresponsiveness**, defined by three salient features (Figure 13-12):

1. Airway wall inflammation, involving **neutrophils**, **T cells** (CD8⁺), **alveolar dendritic cells**, and **macrophages**. Asthma is characterized by the recruitment of **T cells** (CD4⁺) by dendritic cells in the alveolar air spaces, and of **eosinophils** in bronchioles (see Figure 13-12).

2. Luminal obstruction of airways by mucus, caused by hypersecretion of bronchial mucous glands, along with infiltration by inflammatory cells.

3. Vasodilation of the bronchial microvasculature with increased vascular permeability and edema.

Asthma can be triggered by repeated antigen exposure (**allergic asthma**) or by an abnormal autonomic neural regulation of airway function (**nonallergic asthma**).

The pathophysiologic aspects of asthma appear to result from the aberrant proliferation of CD4⁺ helper TH2 cells producing three cytokines: **interleukin (IL)-4**, IL-5, and IL-13. IL-4 stimulates immature T cells to develop into the TH2 cell type, which produces IL-13 to precipitate an asthma attack.

Club cells (Clara cells)

Club cells, formerly called Clara cells, are epithelial cells with a dome-shaped apical domain lacking cilia. They represent **80% of the epithelial cell population** of the **terminal bronchiole** (Figure 13-13). Their function is to protect the bronchiolar epithelium.

Figure 13-12. Pathogenesis of asthma

Synthesis of MUC5AC by goblet cells

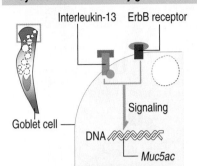

Upon ligand binding, interleukin-13 and Erb-receptor signaling increase the expression of the *Muc5ac* gene

Secretion of MUC5AC by goblet cells

ATP, acting on apical membrane **P2Y₂** purinergic receptors, stimulates the secretion of **polymeric Muc5AC**. P2Y₂ receptor is coupled to **Gq**, activating phospholipase C (**PLC**), which produces diacylglycerol (**DAG**) and inositol triphosphate (**IP₃**). DAG activates **Munc13** to prepare plasma membrane-bound **syntaxin** to facilitate Rab-mediated docking and fusion of the MUC5AC-containing vesicle with the plasma membrane for exocytosis. Calcium-activated **synaptotagmin** and vesicle-associated membrane protein (**VAMP**) draw together the vesicle and plasma membrane.

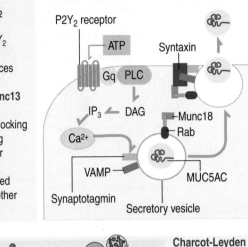

Mucus dysfunction in disease: Asthma

1 An inhaled allergen crosses the bronchial epithelium.

2 The allergen interacts with **IgE receptors** on the surface of mast cells and induces **degranulation.** Released mediators (histamine, leukotrienes, eosinophil chemotactic factor, and others) induce:
1. Chemoattraction of **eosinophils.**
2. Increased permeability of blood vessels (**edema**).
3. Constriction of smooth muscle (**bronchoconstriction**).
4. Hypersecretion of mucus by goblet cells.

3 In the presence of an allergen, TH2 cells secrete **interleukin-13,** which causes airway tightening and increase in mucus production. TH2 cells secrete **interleukin-5,** essential for the maturation of eosinophils.

4 Inflammatory cells and **Charcot-Leyden crystals** in the bronchial lumen.

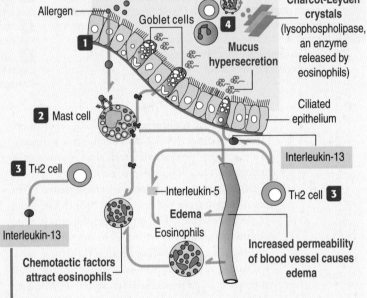

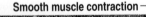

Smooth muscle contraction

Visceral pleura

The lumen of the bronchioles is occupied by thick mucus plugs

Airway mucus in severe asthma is highly viscous and contributes to impaired clearance and plug formation. Plugs contain high concentrations of MUC5AC and MUC5B and plasma proteins, preventing protease digestion of MUC5AC and MUC5B by neutrophil elastase. This airflow obstructive condition causes cough and dyspnea, accompanied by bronchial breath sounds and wheezes.

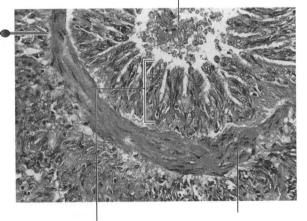

Mucus plug

Abnormal increase in the number and size of cells of the respiratory epithelium (**hyperplastic epithelium**)

Smooth muscle (**hypertrophy**)

Macroscopy (detail) from Cooke RA, Stewart B: Colour Atlas of Anatomical Pathology. New York, Churchill Livingstone, 1995. Microscopy from Damjanov I, Linder J: Pathology. A Color Atlas. St.Louis, Mosby, 2000.

Figure 13-13. **Structure and function of club cells**

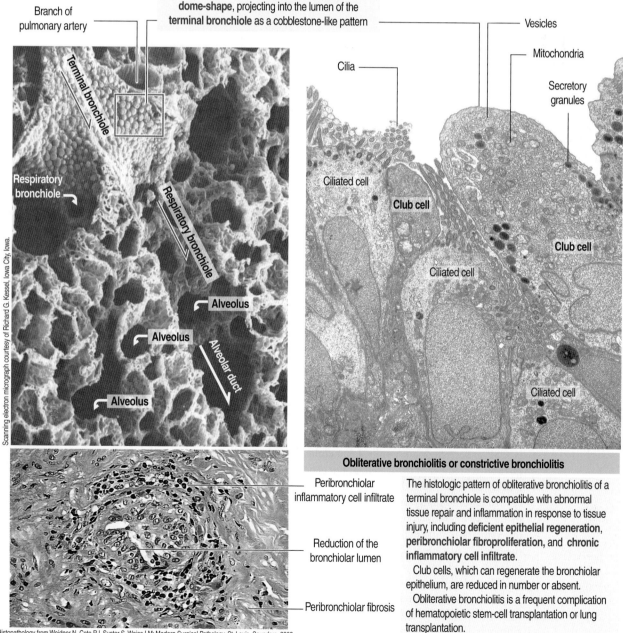

Club cells (Clara cells)

Nonciliated club cells coexist in terminal bronchioles with a single layer of ciliated cuboidal cells. After airway injury, club cells can proliferate to regenerate the bronchiolar epithelium and even migrate to replenish alveolar epithelial cells. This process is known as **alveolar bronchiolization.**

Club cells produce: (1) **Surfactant proteins** SP-A and SP-D, coating the surface of the bronchiolar epithelium and presumably also regulating the transport of **chloride ions.**
(2) Mucin **MUC5AC** and **MUC5B** monomers, present as polymers in the airway mucus.
(3) Anti-inflammatory **club cell secretory protein (CCSP)**, involved in protecting airway homeostasis against injury or infection.

At the electron microscope level, the apical dome-shaped region of club cells contains cytoplasmic dense **secretory granules**, **mitochondria**, and numerous **vesicles**.

MUC5AC
CCSP   MUC5B
Surfactant proteins   Cl⁻
(SP-A and SP-D)

Cuboidal ciliated cell   **Club cell**   Basal lamina

Branch of pulmonary artery

Club cells are recognized by their **apical dome-shape**, projecting into the lumen of the **terminal bronchiole** as a cobblestone-like pattern

Vesicles
Mitochondria
Cilia
Secretory granules

Terminal bronchiole

Respiratory bronchiole

Respiratory bronchiole

Ciliated cell
Club cell
Ciliated cell
Club cell

Alveolus
Alveolus
Ciliated cell
Alveolar duct
Alveolus

Scanning electron micrograph courtesy of Richard G. Kessel, Iowa City, Iowa.

Obliterative bronchiolitis or constrictive bronchiolitis

Peribronchiolar inflammatory cell infiltrate

Reduction of the bronchiolar lumen

Peribronchiolar fibrosis

The histologic pattern of obliterative bronchiolitis of a terminal bronchiole is compatible with abnormal tissue repair and inflammation in response to tissue injury, including **deficient epithelial regeneration, peribronchiolar fibroproliferation,** and **chronic inflammatory cell infiltrate.**

Club cells, which can regenerate the bronchiolar epithelium, are reduced in number or absent.

Obliterative bronchiolitis is a frequent complication of hematopoietic stem-cell transplantation or lung transplantation.

Histopathology from Weidner N, Cote RJ, Suster S, Weiss LM: Modern Surgical Pathology, St. Louis, Saunders, 2003.

Figure 13-14. **Cystic fibrosis**

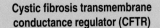

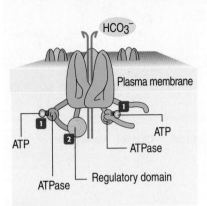

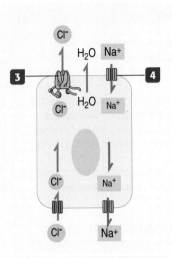

Three cytoplasmic domains regulate the chloride-permeable CFTR channel:

1 Two ATP–binding domains (ATPase)

2 A regulatory domain

The channel becomes permeable to Cl⁻ when ATP is bound and **the regulatory domain is phosphorylated.** The CFTR channel also transports HCO_3^-.

In **normal individuals**: Epithelial cells lining the airways display two types of channels:

3 The CFTR channel releases Cl⁻

4 The other channel takes up Na⁺. Water follows the movement of Cl⁻ by osmosis.

This mechanism maintains the mucus made by goblet cells and mucus-secreting glands to remain wet and less viscous.

In **patients with cystic fibrosis:**

5 A defective or absent CFTR channel prevents Cl⁻ movement

6 The cell takes up extra Na⁺

Reduced Cl⁻ secretion and increased Na⁺ absorption results in insufficient fluid in the mucus. The mucus, containing entangled mucin polymers, becomes thick and traps bacteria and neutrophils. Cell destruction occurs.

Following airway injury, club cells proliferate and migrate to replenish alveolar epithelial cells. This process is known as **alveolar bronchiolization**. In addition, proliferative club cells can produce ciliated cells and additional club cells.

Club cells produce:

1. **Surfactant proteins** **SP-A** and **SP-D**, coating the surface of the bronchiolar epithelium and also regulating the transport of **chloride ions** across a cystic fibrosis transmembrane conductance regulator channel. Chloride transport is controlled by a cyclic guanosine monophosphate (cGMP)–guanylyl cyclase C mechanism.

2. **Mucin MUC5AC** and **MUC5B monomers**, present as polymers in the airway mucus.

3. Anti-inflammatory **club cell secretory protein (CCSP or secretoglobin family 1A member 1 [Scgb1a1])**, a member of the secretoglobin gene family, is involved in the protection of the airway epithelium against chronic injury or infection. Chronic injury to the airway inhibits normal epithelial repair and differentiation and is characterized by a decline in the number of club cells and in the levels of CCSP in lungs and serum.

Obliterative bronchiolitis (OB) or **constrictive bronchiolitis** is characterized by progressive airflow obstruction. OB, attributed to a defective function of club cells, shows significant peribronchiolar inflam-

mation and obstructive fibrosis, causing a reduction in the diameter of the terminal bronchioles (see Figure 13-13). OB affects most hematopoietic stem-cell transplantation or lung transplant recipients. Bone marrow stem cells administered to experimental animals by transtracheal delivery can express CCSP, cytokeratins, and chloride channels in the lung.

Clinical significance: Cystic fibrosis

Cystic fibrosis is a recessive genetic disease affecting children and young adults. Cystic fibrosis is caused by mutations in the gene encoding **cystic fibrosis transmembrane conductance regulator (CFTR)**, which results in **reduced chloride secretion, increased sodium absorption, and insufficient airway luminal fluid** (see Box 13-D and Figure 13-14).

These alterations in the respiratory and gastrointestinal tracts result in:

1. **Deficient mucus clearance**, which determines a chronic cycle of infection, inflammation, and injury.

2. The **formation of a mucus gel matrix with reduced pore size**, which consists of highly entangled polymeric MUC5AC and MUC5B molecules infiltrated with pathogens and immobilized neutrophils that might otherwise clear the infection.

Respiratory disease results from the obstruction of the pulmonary airways by thick mucus plugs, followed by bacterial infections. Cough, chronic

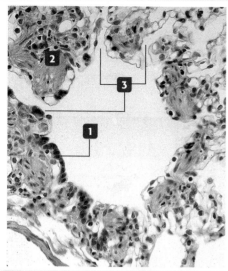

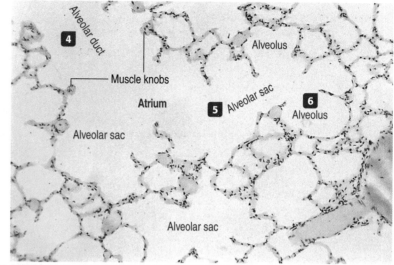

1 The lining epithelium of the **terminal bronchiole** consists of a **few ciliated** and **nonciliated cuboidal epithelial cells (club cells)**. **Goblet cells are no longer present**. Bundles of smooth muscle cells and elastic fibers are observed in the wall. There are no cartilaginous plates in the wall and no glands in the lamina propria.

2 Smooth muscle cell bundles (**muscle knobs**), innervated by **parasympathetic nerve fibers**, contract to constrict the lumen of the bronchiole. In **asthma**, muscle contraction, triggered by histamine release from mast cells, is persistent. Elastic fibers are seen in the knobs.

3 The wall of the **respiratory bronchiole** is interrupted at intervals by saccular outpocketings, the **alveoli**.

4 Several **alveolar ducts** result from the division of a single bronchiole. The wall of an alveolar sac consists of alveolar openings. Remnants of the muscle knobs lined by a low cuboidal-to-squamous simple epithelium can be seen at the alveolar openings.

5 An **alveolar sac** is continuous with a cluster of alveoli sharing a wider space called the alveolar sac. The alveolar duct–alveolar sac junction is called the **atrium**.

6 Several **alveoli** open into an alveolar sac.

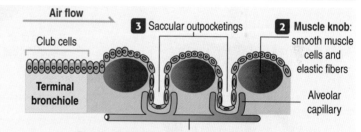

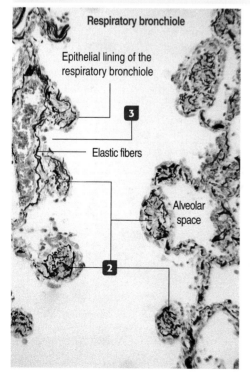

Respiratory bronchiole

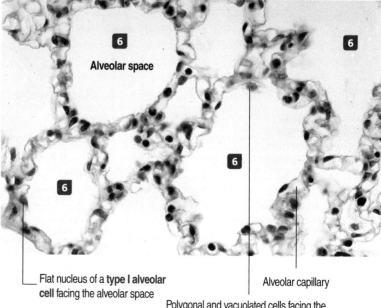

Flat nucleus of a **type I alveolar cell** facing the alveolar space

Alveolar capillary

Polygonal and vacuolated cells facing the alveolar space are **type II alveolar cells**

Figure 13-16. **Structure of the alveolus**

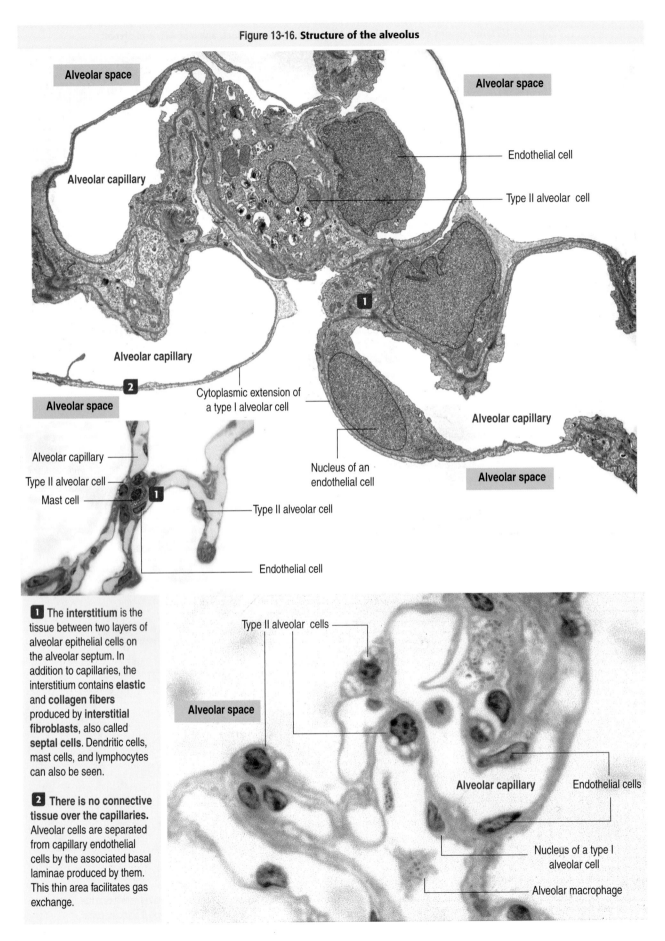

Alveolar space

Alveolar space

Endothelial cell

Alveolar capillary

Type II alveolar cell

Alveolar capillary

2

Alveolar space

Cytoplasmic extension of
a type I alveolar cell

Alveolar capillary

Alveolar space

Alveolar capillary

Nucleus of an
endothelial cell

Type II alveolar cell

Mast cell

Type II alveolar cell

Endothelial cell

1 The **interstitium** is the
tissue between two layers of
alveolar epithelial cells on
the alveolar septum. In
addition to capillaries, the
interstitium contains **elastic**
and **collagen fibers**
produced by **interstitial
fibroblasts**, also called
septal cells. Dendritic cells,
mast cells, and lymphocytes
can also be seen.

2 There is no connective
tissue over the capillaries.
Alveolar cells are separated
from capillary endothelial
cells by the associated basal
laminae produced by them.
This thin area facilitates gas
exchange.

Type II alveolar cells

Alveolar space

Alveolar capillary

Endothelial cells

Nucleus of a type I
alveolar cell

Alveolar macrophage

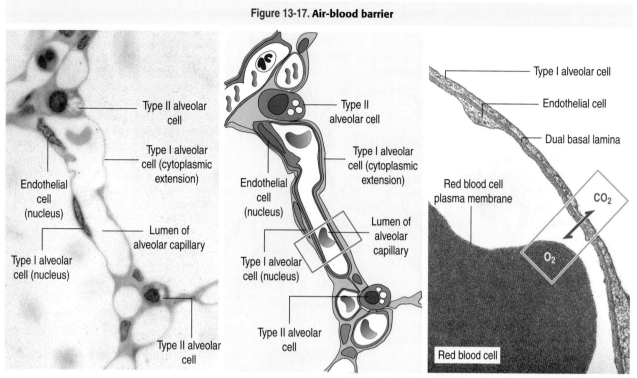

Figure 13-17. Air-blood barrier

Labels in figure:
- Type II alveolar cell
- Type I alveolar cell (cytoplasmic extension)
- Endothelial cell (nucleus)
- Lumen of alveolar capillary
- Type I alveolar cell (nucleus)
- Type II alveolar cell
- Type I alveolar cell
- Endothelial cell
- Dual basal lamina
- Red blood cell plasma membrane
- CO_2
- O_2
- Red blood cell

The lung is a gas-exchanging organ for the provision of O_2 to the blood and removal of CO_2 from the blood. Alveolar capillaries are closely apposed to the alveolar lumen.

Gas exchange by **passive diffusion** occurs across the **air-blood barrier** consisting of (1) cytoplasmic extensions of **type I alveolar cells**; (2) a **dual basal lamina**, synthesized by type I alveolar cells and endothelial cells; (3) cytoplasmic extensions of continuous **endothelial cells**; and (4) the plasma membrane of **red blood cells**.

Type II alveolar cells contribute indirectly to the gas-exchange process by secreting **surfactant**, a lipid-protein complex that reduces the surface tension of the alveolus and prevents alveolar collapsing.

Clinical significance: Alveolar gas exchange and acid-base balance

Changes in **partial pressure of CO_2** (designated P_{CO_2}) caused by inadequate ventilation leads to **acid-base balance** disturbances and, consequently, to an alteration in **blood pH**.

An increase in P_{CO_2} decreases blood pH; a decrease of P_{CO_2} increases pH. An increase in ventilation decreases P_{CO_2}. P_{CO_2} increases as ventilation decreases.

Both blood pH and P_{CO_2} are critical regulators of the ventilation rate sensed by **chemoreceptors**, located in the brain (medulla) and carotid and aortic bodies.

---

purulent secretions, increased numbers of mucin-secreting cells in the submucosal glands, and dyspnea are typical symptoms of this COPD. These events are manifested radiographically as **bronchiectasis** (localized widening of bronchi).

Box 13-D | Cystic fibrosis gene

The cystic fibrosis gene encodes the protein **CFTR**, belonging to the ABC transporter family, so called because it contains adenosine triphosphate (ATP)–binding domains, or ATP-binding cassettes, and requires ATP hydrolysis to transport ions, sugars, and amino acids. In 70% of patients with cystic fibrosis, the amino acid 508, of a total of 1480 amino acids in CFTR protein, is missing.

As a member of the ABC transporter family, CFTR is rather unusual because it appears to require both ATP hydrolysis and cyclic adenosine monophosphate (cAMP)–dependent phosphorylation to function as a Cl⁻ channel.

Inherited mutations of CFTR in patients with cystic fibrosis result in defective chloride transport and increased sodium absorption. The CFTR channel also transports bicarbonate ions. Inherited mutations of CFTR are associated with reduced bicarbonate transport, resulting in excessive mucin cross-linking by calcium.

In most patients, the blockage of pancreatic ducts by mucus causes pancreatic dysfunction. Pancreatic ductules release a bicarbonate-rich fluid under regulation of secretin. Secretin is produced by enteroendocrine cells in response to acidic gastric contents entering the duodenum (see Chapter 17, Digestive Glands). In the skin, the excessive presence of salt secretion by sweat glands is diagnostic of cystic fibrosis (see Chapter 11, Integumentary System).

Treatment of the disease consists of physical therapy to facilitate bronchial drainage, antibiotic treatment of infections, and pancreatic enzyme replacement.

Respiratory portion of the lung

Terminal bronchioles give rise to three generations of **respiratory bronchioles** (0.5 to 0.2 mm in diameter).

Respiratory bronchioles are the transition from the conducting to the respiratory portion of the lung (Figure 13-15).

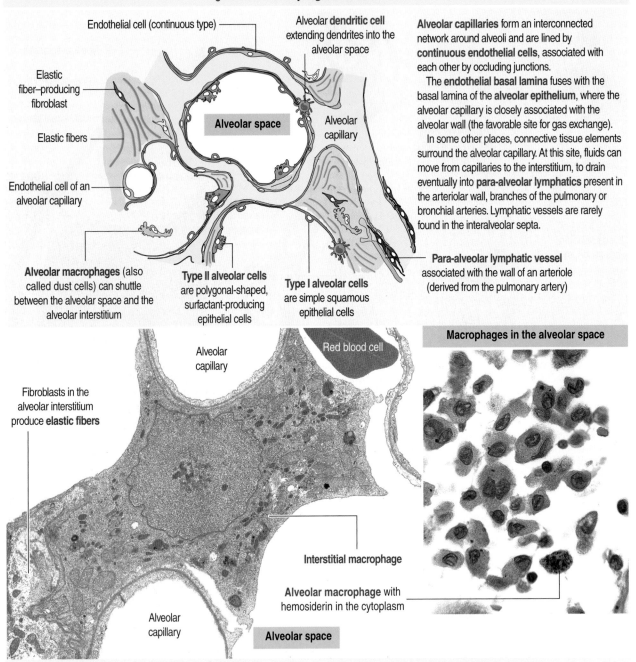

Figure 13-18. Macrophages and dendritic cells

Endothelial cell (continuous type)

Alveolar **dendritic cell** extending dendrites into the alveolar space

Elastic fiber–producing fibroblast

Elastic fibers

Endothelial cell of an alveolar capillary

Alveolar space

Alveolar capillary

Alveolar capillaries form an interconnected network around alveoli and are lined by **continuous endothelial cells**, associated with each other by occluding junctions.

The **endothelial basal lamina** fuses with the basal lamina of the **alveolar epithelium**, where the alveolar capillary is closely associated with the alveolar wall (the favorable site for gas exchange).

In some other places, connective tissue elements surround the alveolar capillary. At this site, fluids can move from capillaries to the interstitium, to drain eventually into **para-alveolar lymphatics** present in the arteriolar wall, branches of the pulmonary or bronchial arteries. Lymphatic vessels are rarely found in the interalveolar septa.

Alveolar macrophages (also called dust cells) can shuttle between the alveolar space and the alveolar interstitium

Type II alveolar cells are polygonal-shaped, surfactant-producing epithelial cells

Type I alveolar cells are simple squamous epithelial cells

Para-alveolar lymphatic vessel associated with the wall of an arteriole (derived from the pulmonary artery)

Alveolar capillary

Red blood cell

Fibroblasts in the alveolar interstitium produce **elastic fibers**

Macrophages in the alveolar space

Interstitial macrophage

Alveolar macrophage with hemosiderin in the cytoplasm

Alveolar capillary

Alveolar space

Alveolar macrophages are sentinel cells migrating over the luminal surface of the alveolus. These cells monitor any inhaled dust or bacteria that may have escaped entrapment by the mucous lining in the airway.

When stimulated by metabolic products of bacteria, macrophages release chemotactic factors that induce transendothelial migration of leukocytes, which join macrophages to neutralize invading microorganisms. **Alveolar dendritic cells** scan and take up antigens

from the alveolar air space for presentation to T cells.

In patients with heart disease, alveolar macrophages contain many vacuoles filled with **hemosiderin**, resulting from phagocytosis of red blood cells and degradation of their hemoglobin.

Alveolar macrophages migrate from the alveoli to the surface of the bronchi and are transported by ciliary action to the upper airway to the pharynx where they are swallowed with the saliva.

They are lined initially by **simple cuboidal epithelial cells**. The epithelium becomes **low cuboidal** and **nonciliated** in subsequent branches.

The respiratory bronchiole subdivides to give rise to an **alveolar duct** that is continuous with the **alveolar sac**. Several alveoli open into an alveolar sac.

The alveolus

About 300 million air sacs, or **alveoli,** in each lung provide a total surface area of 75 m² for oxygen and carbon dioxide exchange.

Each alveolus has a thin wall with capillaries lined by **simple squamous epithelial cells** (Figure 13-16)

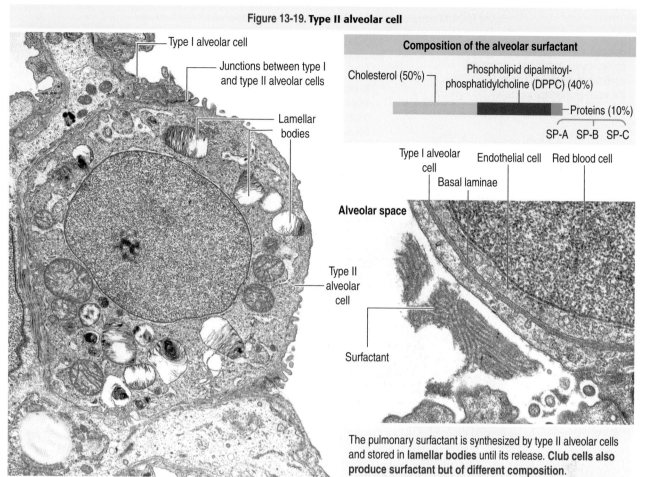

Figure 13-19. Type II alveolar cell

Type I alveolar cell

Junctions between type I and type II alveolar cells

Lamellar bodies

Type II alveolar cell

Composition of the alveolar surfactant

Cholesterol (50%)

Phospholipid dipalmitoyl-phosphatidylcholine (DPPC) (40%)

Proteins (10%)

SP-A   SP-B   SP-C

Alveolar space

Type I alveolar cell

Basal laminae

Endothelial cell

Red blood cell

Surfactant

The pulmonary surfactant is synthesized by type II alveolar cells and stored in **lamellar bodies** until its release. **Club cells also produce surfactant but of different composition.**

The surfactant contains three major components: **phospholipid DPPC, cholesterol,** and **surfactant proteins (SPs)**. **SP-A and SP-B combine with DPPC within the lamellar bodies.** In the alveolar space, SP-B and SP-C stabilize the surfactant coat.

forming part of the **air-blood barrier** (Figure 13-17).

The **alveolar epithelium** consists of two cell types (see Figures 13-16 and 13-17):

1. **Type I alveolar cells,** representing about **40%** of the epithelial cell population but lining **90%** of the alveolar surface.

2. **Type II alveolar cells,** approximately **60%** of the cells, covering only **10%** of the alveolar surface area.

Each alveolus opens into an alveolar sac. However, a few of them open directly into the respiratory bronchiole (see Figure 13-15). **This particular feature distinguishes the respiratory bronchiole from the terminal bronchiole, whose wall is not associated with alveolar outpocketings.**

The low cuboidal epithelium of the respiratory bronchiole is continuous with the squamous type I alveolar cells of the alveolus (see Figure 13-9).

Additional cells of the alveolar septa are:

1. The **alveolar macrophages** (Figure 13-18), also called **dust cells.** They derive from bone-marrow monocytes and are frequently seen in the alveolar lumen and interstitium.

2. **Alveolar dendritic cells,** actively monitor for antigens the alveolar air space and take them up for presentation to T cells. Dendritic processes extend into the surfactant layer (see Figure 13-18).

Alveolar capillaries are lined by continuous endothelial cells juxtaposed to type I alveolar cells through a dual basal lamina produced by these two cells.

Lymphatic vessels are rarely present in the interalveolar space. Instead, they are observed associated to the wall of the arterioles and branches from the pulmonary artery and bronchial artery. Multiple small perivascular lymphatics are responsible for maintaining fluid balance in the alveolar interstitium.

Alveolar endothelial cells contain **angiotensin-converting enzyme (ACE)** for the conversion of angiotensin I (ANG I) to angiotensin II (ANG II) (see Figure 14-19 in Chapter 14, Urinary System).

Type II alveolar cells

Type II alveolar cells are predominantly located at the **angles formed by adjacent alveolar septa.** Contrasting with the more squamous type I alveolar cells, type II

Figure 13-20. **Macrophages: degradation of alveolar surfactant and asbestosis**

Surfactant proteins and polyunsaturated phospholipids spread and stabilize the dipalmitoylphosphatidylcholine (DPPC) layer at the water-air interface on the alveolar surface.

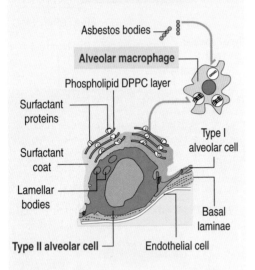

Asbestos bodies

Alveolar macrophage

Phospholipid DPPC layer

Surfactant proteins

Surfactant coat

Lamellar bodies

Type II alveolar cell

Type I alveolar cell

Basal laminae

Endothelial cell

Abundant collagen bundles, asbestos and macrophages in the pulmonary interstitium

Alveolar macrophages remove degraded surfactant. Surfactant degradation is by oxidation of polyunsaturated phospholipids associated with DPPC. The oxidation process is triggered by air pollutants.

Asbetosis is an interstitial pulmonary fibrosis caused by inhaled asbestos dust. An excess of asbestos (composed of silica, iron, sodium, magnesium and other metals) causes macrophages to release chemical agents producing **alveolitis** and eventual **fibrosis of the lung**. The alveolar spaces are not affected.

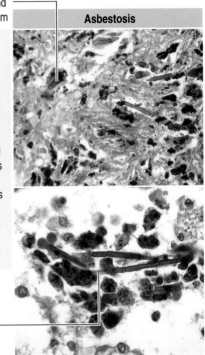

Asbestosis

Asbestos bodies and macrophages in the alveolar lumen

---

alveolar cells are polygonal-shaped, vacuolated and bulge beyond the level of the surrounding epithelium.

The free surface of type II alveolar cells is covered by short microvilli. The cytoplasm displays dense membrane-bound **lamellar bodies**, representing secretory granules containing **pulmonary surfactant** (Figure 13-19).

Surfactant is released by exocytosis and spreads over a thin layer of fluid that normally coats the alveolar surface. By this mechanism, the **pulmonary surfactant lowers the surface tension at the air-fluid interface and thus reduces the tendency of the alveolus to collapse at the end of expiration.** As previously indicated, club cells, located in terminal bronchioles, also secrete pulmonary surfactant.

The pulmonary surfactant contains (see Figure 13-19):

1. **Phospholipids.**
2. **Cholesterol.**
3. **Proteins.**

Specific surfactant proteins (SPs) consist of one hydrophilic glycoprotein (**SP-A**) and two **hydrophobic proteins (SP-B and SP-C)**.

Within the lamellar bodies, SP-A and SP-B transform the **phospholipid dipalmitoylphosphatidylcholine (DPPC)** into a mature surfactant molecule.

In the alveolar space, SP-B and SP-C **stabilize** the phospholipid layer and enhance the surfactant action of the phospholipid DPPC–protein complex (Figure 13-20).

Surfactant turnover is facilitated by the phagocytic function of alveolar macrophages (see Figures 13-18 and 13-20).

Macrophages can also take up inhaled asbestos and trigger interstitial pulmonary fibrosis, **asbestosis,** characterized by extensive deposition of collagen and **asbestos bodies** (asbestos fibers coated by iron particles, see Figure 13-20).

The alveolar spaces may be involved and type II alveolar cells increase in number (hyperplasia). An additional function of type II alveolar cells is the **maintenance and repair of the alveolar epithelium when injury occurs.**

When type I alveolar cells are damaged, type II alveolar cells increase in number and differentiate into type I alveolar-like cells (see Figure 13-20).

As already discussed, club cells also have a reparative function during injury of the bronchiolar and alveolar epithelium (**alveolar bronchiolization**).

Pathology: Acute respiratory distress syndrome

The significance of the cell components of the alveolus becomes clear when we analyze the relevant aspects of the **acute respiratory distress syndrome (ARDS)**.

ARDS results from a disruption of the normal barrier that prevents leakage of fluid of the alveolar capillaries into the interstitium and alveolar spaces.

Two mechanisms can alter the alveolar barrier:

1. An **increase in hydrostatic pressure in the alveolar capillaries,** caused, for example, by failure of the left ventricle or stenosis of the mitral valve, This determines increased fluid and proteins in the alveolar

Figure 13-21. Acute respiratory distress syndrome (ARDS) and pulmonary edema

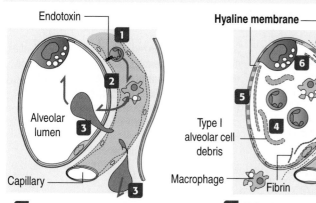

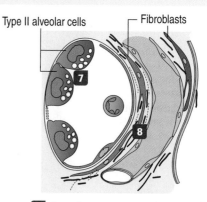

1 Endotoxin induces the release of proinflammatory substances that cause the attachment of neutrophils to endothelial cells.

2 Neutrophils release proteolytic enzymes and, together with endotoxin, damage the endothelial cells. Macrophages are activated by inflammatory cytokines and contribute to the endothelial cell damage.

3 The alveolar-capillary barrier becomes permeable and cells and fluid enter the interstitium and alveolar space.

Edema, intra-alveolar hemorrhage and fibrin deposition result from an increase in pulmnary microvascular permeability to plasma proteins. **Hyaline membranes**, eosinophilic deposits lining the alveoli, develop. Remnants of hyaline membranes can remain in the alveolar septa.

4 Following the endothelial cell injury, type I alveolar cells die, denuding the alveolar side of the barrier. Neutrophils and macrophages are seen in the alveolar lumen and interstitium.

5 Fibrin and cell debris accumulated in the alveolar lumen form a **hyaline membrane**.

6 Fibrin inhibits the synthesis of surfactant by type II alveolar cells.

7 A repair process can restore normal function or cause progressive fibrosis. Type II alveolar cells proliferate, reestablish the production of surfactant, and differentiate into type I alveolar cells.

8 If the initial damage is severe, interstitial fibroblasts proliferate, progressive interstitial and intra-alveolar fibrosis develops, and gas exchange is seriously affected.

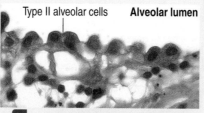

7 Proliferation of type II alveolar cells

Cardiogenic pulmonary edema

A dysfunction of the left ventricle is the main cause of this type of pulmonary edema.

Pulmonary capillaries are dilated and an increase in hydrostatic pressure leads to interstitial and alveolar edema. Abundant leukocytes and red blood cells and protein-rich fluid are visualized in the lumen of dilated alveoli.

spaces. The resulting edema is called **cardiogenic** or **hydrostatic pulmonary edema**.

2. The hydrostatic pressure is normal, but the **endothelial lining of the alveolar capillaries or the epithelial lining of the alveoli is damaged.** Inhalation of agents such as smoke, water (near drowning), or bacterial endotoxins (resulting from sepsis), or trauma can cause a defect in **permeability**. A cardiac component may or may not be involved. Although the resulting edema is called **noncardiogenic**, it can coexist with a **cardiogenic** condition.

A **common pathologic pattern** of diffuse alveolar damage (Figure 13-21) can be observed in cardiogenic and noncardiogenic ARDS.

The **first phase** of ARDS is an **acute exudative process** defined by interstitial and alveolar edema, neutrophil infiltration, hemorrhage, and deposits of fibrin. Cellular debris, resulting from dead type I alveolar cells, and fibrin deposit in the alveolar space and form **hyaline membranes**.

Neonatal respiratory distress syndrome (RDS) in premature infants is characterized by a protein-rich, fibrin-rich exudation into the alveolar space, forming a hyaline membrane that leads to CO_2 retention (Figure 13-22). In the newborn, surfactant deficiency causes the lungs to collapse (**atelectatic lung**) with each successive breath.

The **second phase** is a **proliferative process** in which alveolar cells proliferate and differentiate to restore the epithelial alveolar lining, returning gas exchange to normal in most cases. In other cases, the interstitium displays inflammatory cells and fibroblasts. Fibroblasts proliferate and invade the alveolar spaces through gaps of the basal lamina. Hyaline membranes are either removed by phagocytosis by macrophages or invaded by fibroblasts.

The **third phase** is **chronic fibrosis** and occlusion of blood vessels. Because ARDS is part of a systemic inflammatory response, the outcome of the lung process depends on improvement of the systemic condition. The prognosis for return to normal lung function is good. The diagnosis of ARDS is based on clinical (dyspnea, cyanosis, and tachypnea) and radiologic examination.

Figure 13-22. **Neonatal respiratory distress syndrome (RDS)**

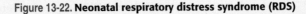

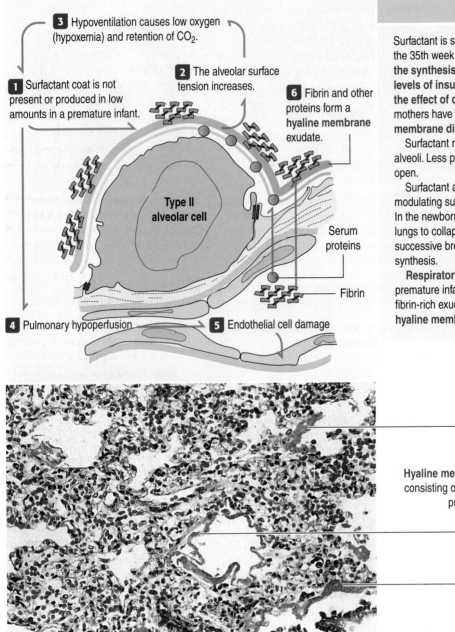

3 Hypoventilation causes low oxygen (hypoxemia) and retention of CO_2.

2 The alveolar surface tension increases.

1 Surfactant coat is not present or produced in low amounts in a premature infant.

6 Fibrin and other proteins form a **hyaline membrane** exudate.

Type II alveolar cell

Serum proteins

Fibrin

4 Pulmonary hypoperfusion

5 Endothelial cell damage

Hyaline membrane exudate consisting of fibrin and other proteins

Photograph from Damjanov I, Linder J: Pathology: A Color Atlas. St. Louis, Mosby, 2000.

Surfactant deficiency

Surfactant is synthesized by type II alveolar cells after the 35th week of gestation. **Corticosteroids induce the synthesis of surfactant in the fetus. High levels of insulin (diabetic mothers) can antagonize the effect of corticosteroids.** Infants of diabetic mothers have a higher risk of developing **hyaline membrane disease.**

Surfactant reduces surface tension within the alveoli. Less pressure is required to keep alveoli open.

Surfactant also maintains alveolar expansion by modulating surface tension with alveolar size. In the newborn, **surfactant deficiency** causes the lungs to collapse (**atelectatic lung**) with each successive breath. A lack of O_2 impairs surfactant synthesis.

Respiratory distress syndrome (RDS) in premature infants is characterized by a protein-rich, fibrin-rich exudation into the alveolar space, forming a **hyaline membrane** that leads to CO_2 retention.

Treatment is focused on neutralizing the disorder causing ARDS and providing support of gas exchange until the condition improves.

Pathology: Lung cancer

Most lung tumors are malignant. They can be **primary tumors**, originated in the lung, or **secondary** or **metastatic**, spreading from other tumors.

Local intrathoracic spread include:

1. Invasion of the **cervical sympathetic chain**, represented by the **Horner's syndrome**, usually affecting only one side of the face. The common signs and symptoms include **miosis** (persistently small pupil), **anisocoria** (difference in pupil size between the two eyes), reduced or delayed dilation of the affected pupil in dim light, and **ptosis** (drooping of the upper eyelid).

2. Invasion of the recurrent laryngeal nerve and brachial plexus.

Hematogenous spreading to bones, central nervous system, and liver are the most common.

Based on the type of cells, primary lung cancer can be classified into two major groups:

1. **Small cell lung cancer** (SCLC; also called **oat-**

Figure 13-23. **Blood supply and lymph drainage of the pulmonary lobule**

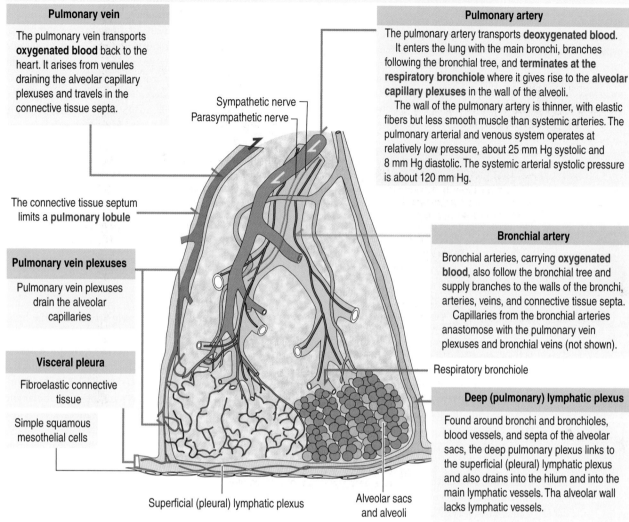

Pulmonary vein

The pulmonary vein transports **oxygenated blood** back to the heart. It arises from venules draining the alveolar capillary plexuses and travels in the connective tissue septa.

The connective tissue septum limits a **pulmonary lobule**

Pulmonary vein plexuses

Pulmonary vein plexuses drain the alveolar capillaries

Visceral pleura

Fibroelastic connective tissue

Simple squamous mesothelial cells

Sympathetic nerve
Parasympathetic nerve

Superficial (pleural) lymphatic plexus

Alveolar sacs and alveoli

Respiratory bronchiole

Pulmonary artery

The pulmonary artery transports **deoxygenated blood**.
It enters the lung with the main bronchi, branches following the bronchial tree, and **terminates at the respiratory bronchiole** where it gives rise to the **alveolar capillary plexuses** in the wall of the alveoli.
The wall of the pulmonary artery is thinner, with elastic fibers but less smooth muscle than systemic arteries. The pulmonary arterial and venous system operates at relatively low pressure, about 25 mm Hg systolic and 8 mm Hg diastolic. The systemic arterial systolic pressure is about 120 mm Hg.

Bronchial artery

Bronchial arteries, carrying **oxygenated blood**, also follow the bronchial tree and supply branches to the walls of the bronchi, arteries, veins, and connective tissue septa.
Capillaries from the bronchial arteries anastomose with the pulmonary vein plexuses and bronchial veins (not shown).

Deep (pulmonary) lymphatic plexus

Found around bronchi and bronchioles, blood vessels, and septa of the alveolar sacs, the deep pulmonary plexus links to the superficial (pleural) lymphatic plexus and also drains into the hilum and into the main lymphatic vessels. Tha alveolar wall lacks lymphatic vessels.

Disorders of the pleura

Pleuritic chest pain: A symptom resulting from inflammation of the pleural surfaces. The pain originates in the parietal pleura, innervated by the intercostal nerves.
Pleural effusion: Abnormal accumulation of liquid in the pleural space. Large pleural effusion restricts pulmonary function because air spaces and pulmonary circulation are compressed.
Hydrothorax: Accumulation of water may be an early sign of congestive heart failure. It is also observed in cirrhosis, malignant disease, and pulmonary embolism.
Hemothorax: Direct hemorrhage into the pleural space resulting from trauma to the thorax (rib fracture or penetrating object).
Chylothorax: Accumulation of chyle, a lipid-rich liquid transported from intestinal lacteals to systemic veins in the thorax through the thoracic duct. Obstruction or disruption of the thoracic duct by mediastinal tumors are the most common cause of chylothorax.
Pneumothorax: Accumulation of air in the pleural space indicates disruption of the visceral or parietal pleura after tracheobronchial rupture or focal pulmonary destructive processes (e.g., AIDS).

Visceral pleura

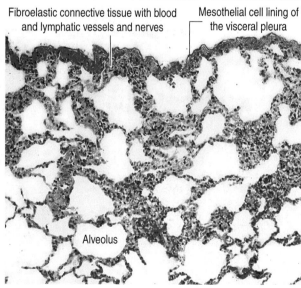

Fibroelastic connective tissue with blood and lymphatic vessels and nerves

Mesothelial cell lining of the visceral pleura

Alveolus

Figure 13-24. **Pleuresy**

Inflammation of the pleura, **pleuresy**, is often secondary to an inflammatory disease in the lungs. The differential diagnosis of **reactive mesothelial hyperplasia** includes **malignant mesothelioma**. The linear arrangement of the hyperplastic mesothelial lining, reflecting the mesothelial surface, differs with the invasion nature of malignant mesothelioma. The illustration shows a fibrinous exudate covering a reactive mesothelial hyperplastic layer of the visceral pleura. The submesothelial space depicts intense vascularization and fibrosis, indicators of a chronic inflammatory process of the pleura.

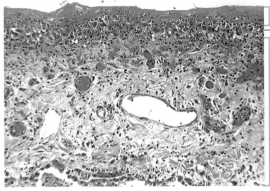

Fibrinous exudate

Reactive mesothelial hyperplasia

Fibrosis and vascularization of the submesothelial layer of the visceral pleura

cell carcinoma). Although less frequent (about 15% of all lung cancers), SCLC is highly malignant and spreads very rapidly. In fact, metastases are found when a diagnosis is made.

2. **Non-small cell lung cancer** (**NSCLC**), the most frequent tumor (about 85% of all lung cancers).

The NSCLC group includes two major subtypes of tumors:

1. **Squamous cell carcinoma**, a tumor derived from the transformation of the respiratory epithelium into a squamous metaplastic epithelium.

2. **Adenocarcinoma**, a tumor originated from the bronchial epithelium and the bronchiolar and

alveolar epithelium (**bronchioalveolar carcinoma**). Adenocarcinoma is the most common type of lung cancer in women who have never smoked.

Molecular screening of lung cancer samples is widely used for determining lung-cancer types and subtypes, estimating prognosis, and predicting the response to therapy. For example, translocations of the *anaplastic lymphoma kinase* (*ALK*) gene, present in approximately 5% of NSCLC, and mutations in the kinase domain of the **epidermal growth factor receptor** (**EGFR**), observed in 10% to 15% of NSCLC, are common in pulmonary adenocarcinomas.

Tyrosine kinase inhibitors, which target the intracellular tyrosine kinase domain of EGFR, have shown efficacy in the treatment of advanced-stage NSCLC when compared to conventional chemotherapy.

Pleura
The pleura consists of two layers:
1. A **visceral layer**.
2. A **parietal layer**.

The **visceral layer** is closely attached to the lung. It is lined by a **simple squamous epithelium**, called **mesothelium**, and consists of cells with **apical microvilli** resting on a basal lamina applied to a connective tissue rich in **elastic fibers** (Figure 13-23). This connective tissue is continuous with the interlobular and interlobar septa of the lung. The parietal layer is also lined by the mesothelium.

The **visceral layer** seals the lung surface, preventing leakage of air into the thoracic cavity. The **parietal layer** is thicker and lines the inner surface of the thoracic cavity. A very thin liquid film in between the visceral and parietal layers permits the smooth gliding of one layer against the other.

Blood vessels to the visceral pleura derive from pulmonary and bronchial blood vessels (see Figure 13-23). The vascular supply to the parietal pleura derives from the systemic blood vessels. Branches of the phrenic and intercostal nerves are found in the parietal pleura; the visceral pleura receives branches of the vagus and sympathetic nerves supplying the bronchi.

Pathology: Disorders of the pleura
Under **normal conditions**, the visceral pleura glides smoothly on the parietal pleura during respiration. However, during an **inflammatory process**, characteristic friction sounds can be detected during the physical examination.

If fluid accumulates in the pleural cavity (**hydrothorax**), the lung collapses gradually and the mediastinum is displaced toward the opposite site. The presence of air in the pleural cavity (**pneumothorax**), caused by a penetrating wound, rupture of the lung, or injections for therapeutic reasons (to immobilize

Figure 13-25. **Mesothelioma**

The pleural mesothelioma (yellowish mass) has invaded the pericardium and enclosed the heart

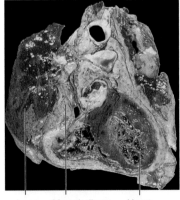

Lung   Mesothelioma   Heart

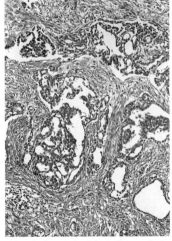

Mesothelioma: glandulopapillary variant

Macroscopy and microscopy from Damjanov I, Linder J: Pathology. A Color Atlas. St. Louis, Mosby, 2000.

the lung in the treatment of tuberculosis), also collapses the lung.

Collapse of the lung is caused by the recoil properties of its elastic fibers. In the normal lung, such a recoil is prevented by negative intrapleural pressure and the close association of the parietal and visceral layers of the pleura.

Acute and chronic inflammation of the pleura is secondary to a bacterial or viral inflammatory disease in the lungs. A fibrinous exudate covers the mesothelial layer that may show reactive hyperplasia (Figure 13-24).

Mesothelioma is a tumor that originates in the mesothelial cell lining of the pleura, the peritoneum, and the pericardium.

Mesothelioma is associated with previous long exposure (15 to 40 years) to asbestos, a fibrous silicate mineral (see Figure 13-20).

Pleural mesothelioma spreads within the thoracic cavity (pericardium or diaphragm, Figure 13-25) and metastasis can involve any organ, including the brain. Symptoms include pleural effusion, chest pain, and dyspnea. Organ imaging studies of the thorax can detect thickening of the pleura (**asbestos plaques**) and fluid containing tumoral cells.

In general, the most frequent cause of neoplasm in the pleura are metastatic tumors from breast and lung causing pleural effusion containing cancerous cells detected by cytology.

Essential concepts | Respiratory System

• The respiratory system consists of three portions:
(1) An air-conducting portion.
(2) A respiratory portion for gas exchange between blood and air.
(3) A mechanism of ventilation, controlled by the inspiratory and expiratory movements of the thoracic cage.

• The **air-conducting portion** consists of:
(1) The nasal cavities and associated sinuses.
(2) The nasopharynx.
(3) The oropharynx.
(4) The larynx.
(5) The trachea.
(6) The bronchi.
(7) The bronchioles.
The **respiratory portion** includes:
(1) The respiratory bronchioles.
(2) The alveolar ducts, alveolar sacs, and alveoli.
The **ventilation mechanism** involves:
(1) The thoracic or rib cage.
(2) The intercostal muscles.
(3) The diaphragm muscle.
(4) The elastic connective tissue of the lungs.

• The functions of the nasal cavity and paranasal sinuses are warming and moistening air and filtering dust particles present in the inspired air.
The respiratory portion is lined by pseudostratified ciliated epithelium with goblet cells supported by a lamina propria consisting of connective tissue, seromucous glands, and a rich superficial venous plexus (called cavernous or erectile tissue).
Incoming air is warmed by blood in the venous plexus and moistened by secretions of the seromucous glands and goblet cells. The superior, middle, and inferior turbinate bones, or conchae, determine airflow disturbance to facilitate warming and moistening of air.

Paranasal sinuses (maxillary, frontal, ethmoidal, and sphenoidal sinuses) are lined by a thin pseudostratified columnar ciliated epithelium with few goblet cells.

• The nasopharynx is lined by a pseudostratified columnar epithelium that changes to nonkeratinizing squamous epithelium at the oropharynx. Aggregates of mucosa-associated lymphoid tissue, forming part of Waldeyer's ring, are present at the nasopharynx.

• The **olfactory area** is present on the roof of the nasal cavity. The mucosa of the olfactory area consists of pseudostratified ciliated columnar epithelium with goblet cells flanking the olfactory epithelium.
The olfactory epithelium consists of three cell types:
(1) Olfactory cells (bipolar neurons).
(2) Basal cells (stem cells that differentiate into olfactory cells).
(3) Sustentacular or supporting cells.
The underlying lamina propria contains the superficial venous plexus, the glands of Bowman, and nerve bundles (called fila olfactoria).
The olfactory cell has an apical region (the dendrite) characterized by a knob bearing nonmotile olfactory cilia.
Olfactory cilia contain odorant receptors that bind to odorant-binding proteins (produced by the gland of Bowman) carrying an inhaled odorant particle.
On the opposite site of the ciliary dendritic region, olfactory cells form small fascicles of unmyelinated axons surrounded by ensheathing glial cells.
Axons penetrate the cribriform plate of the ethmoid bone and synapse with neurons in the olfactory bulb. The axons of the olfactory cells converge to one or more glomeruli and interact predominantly with dendrites of mitral cells.
The olfactory bulb also contains interneurons

called granule cells and tufted cells. Axons from mitral cells and tufted cells form the olfactory tract (olfactory nerve, or cranial nerve I), which carries olfactory information to the olfactory cortex.
The odorant–odorant binding protein complex attaches to receptors on cilia. Binding of the odorant receptor activates G protein coupled to the receptor. G protein activates adenylyl cyclase, which catalyzes the production of cAMP from ATP. Ligand-gated Na^+ channels are opened by cAMP to facilitate the diffusion of Na^+ into the cell. The influx of Na^+ across the plasma membrane generates an action potential conducted to the brain along the olfactory nerve.
Anosmia refers to deprivation of the sense of smell by disease or injury.
Olfactory cells have a life span of about 1 to 2 months and are replaced throughout life by undifferentiated basal cells. Sensory endings of the trigeminal nerve, found in the olfactory epithelium, are responsible for the harmful sensation caused by irritants such as ammonia.

• The **larynx** consists of:
(1) Cartilages (epiglottis, thyroid cartilage, cricoid cartilage, and arytenoid cartilage).
(2) Intrinsic muscles (abductor, adductors, and tensors involved in phonation).
(3) Extrinsic muscles (involved in swallowing).
A nonkeratinizing stratified squamous epithelium covers the lingual surface of the epiglottis and the false and true vocal cords (also called folds). The rest is lined by a pseudostratified ciliated epithelium with goblet cells and seromucous glands in the lamina propria.
The lamina propria of the true vocal cords has special characteristics of clinical significance:
(1) The superficial layer (under the stratified

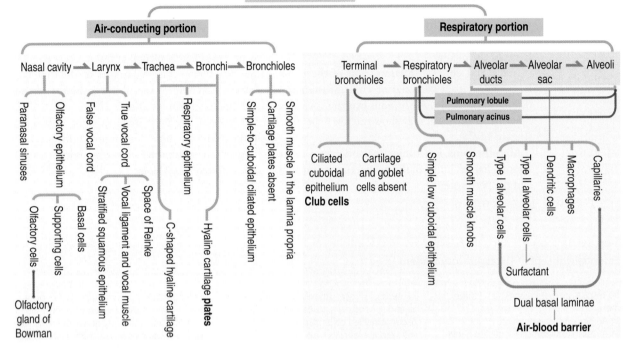

squamous epithelium) consists of extracellular matrix and very few elastic fibers and fibroblasts. This layer, called Reinke's space, can accumulate fluid (Reinke's edema).

(2) The subjacent layers contain elastic and collagen fibers corresponding to the vocal ligament.

(3) Deep in the lamina propria is the vocalis (thyroarytenoid) muscle.

There are no seromucous glands in the lamina propria of the true vocal cord.

• The **trachea** is lined by pseudostratified columnar ciliated epithelium with goblet cells. Basal cells and cells of Kulchitsky (neuroendocrine cells) rest on the basal lamina but do not extend to the lumen. The lamina propria contains elastic fibers. Seromucous glands are observed in the submucosa.

Goblet cells, serous cells of the submucosa glands, and club cells of the terminal bronchioles secrete MUC5AC and MUC5B, two hygroscopic and lubricant glycoproteins, called mucins. They form a polymer in the mucus.

The mucus consists of:

(1) A periciliary layer, in contact with the apical domain of the ciliated columnar cells.

(2) A mucus gel layer atop the periciliary layer.

In addition to mucins, the mucus contains antimicrobial agents, immunomodulatory proteins, and protective molecules.

A stack of C-shaped hyaline cartilage forms the framework of the trachea. The trachealis muscle (smooth muscle) connects the free ends of the C-shaped hyaline cartilage.

Bronchial carcinoid tumors arise from cells of Kulchitsky. These small cells secrete peptide hormones (serotonin, somatostatin, calcitonin,

antidiuretic hormone [ADH], adrenocorticotropic hormone [ACTH], and others). Bronchial carcinoid tumors (including small cell lung carcinoma) can invade locally and metastasize to regional lymph nodes.

• As **bronchi** divide into intrapulmonary bronchi, the tracheal C-shaped rings break down into cartilage plates (distributed around the lumen) and smooth muscle bundles shift between the mucosa and the cartilage plates.

Aggregates of lymphoid tissue are observed in the wall of intrapulmonary bronchi (known collectively as BALT, bronchial-associated lymphoid tissue).

Further subdivisions give rise to **terminal bronchioles**, each supplying a **pulmonary lobule**.

Each **respiratory bronchiole**, subdivisions of a terminal bronchiole, gives rise to a **pulmonary acinus**. Essentially, a pulmonary lobule consists of several pulmonary acini.

Relevant features of the wall of the terminal and respiratory bronchioles are the spiral-like arrangement of smooth muscle fibers and the longitudinal distribution of elastic fibers.

Branches of the pulmonary artery, transporting deoxygenated blood, run parallel to the bronchial tree. Branches of the bronchial artery provide nutrients to the walls of the bronchial tree. Recall that the pulmonary vein, carrying oxygenated blood, travels in the connective tissue septa limiting pulmonary lobules.

Asthma is characterized by:

(1) Reversible bronchoconstriction of the smooth muscle bundles encircling the bronchiolar lumen.

(2) Mucus hypersecretion by goblet cells

triggered by allergens or autonomic neural factors.

The consequence is a reduction in the lumen of the airways. Wheezing, cough, and shortness of breath (dyspnea) are classic symptoms.

• **Terminal bronchioles** lack cartilage and submucosal glands. The pseudostratified columnar ciliated epithelium decreases in height to finally become low columnar-to-cuboidal with few ciliated cells. Surfactant-, protein-, and mucin-secreting **club cells** (formerly called Clara cells) predominate in the terminal bronchiole. Remember that the terminal bronchiole is the initiation site of a pulmonary lobule.

Club cells produce:

(1) Surfactant proteins SP-A and SP-D.

(2) Mucin MUC5AC and MUC5B monomers, present as polymers in the airway mucus.

(3) Anti-inflammatory club cell secretory protein (CCSP), involved in the protection of the airway epithelium against chronic injury or infection.

Obliterative bronchiolitis (OB), or constrictive bronchiolitis, is characterized by progressive airflow obstruction. OB, attributed to a defective function of club cells, shows significant peribronchiolar inflammation and obstructive fibrosis, causing a reduction in the diameter of the terminal bronchioles.

• **Cystic fibrosis** results in the production of abnormally thick mucus by glands lining the respiratory and gastrointestinal tracts.

Inherited mutations of cystic fibrosis transmembrane conductance regulator (CFTR) result in defective Cl⁻ transport and increased Na⁺ absorption. Bacterial infections are associated with the thick mucus plugs consisting of entangled MUC5AC and MUC5B polymers and dehydrated mucus. Cough, purulent secretions, and dyspnea are typical symptoms.

• The wall of a **respiratory bronchiole** is discontinuous, interrupted by the saccular outpocketing of alveoli. Note that the wall of terminal bronchioles is not associated with alveoli.

Bundles of smooth muscle fibers form knobs bulging into the lumen and the lining epithelium is cuboidal-to-simple squamous. Elastic fibers are important components of the bronchioles and alveolar walls.

Emphysema is caused by a permanent enlargement of the air spaces distal to the terminal bronchioles due to the progressive and irreversible destruction of elastic tissue of the alveolar walls.

Elastic tissue in the interalveolar wall can be destroyed by elastase released by neutrophils present in the alveolar lumen. Serum α₁-antitrypsin neutralizes elastase. A persistent stimulus increases the number of neutrophils in the alveolar lumen, the source of elastase.

Serum levels of α₁-antitrypsin decrease and elastase starts the destruction of elastic fibers. Damaged elastic fibers cannot recoil when stretched and, as a result, adjacent alveoli become confluent, producing large air spaces, or blebs, the structural landmark of emphysema. The loss of elastic tissue also affects terminal and respiratory bronchioles.

Chronic obstructive pulmonary disease (COPD) includes emphysema and asthma.

• The **respiratory bronchiole** represents the interface between the conducting and respiratory portions of the respiratory tract. The respiratory bronchiole is regarded as the beginning of the respiratory portion. Remember that the respiratory bronchiole is the initiation site of a pulmonary or lung acinus.

Each respiratory bronchiole gives rise to alveolar ducts, alveolar sacs, and alveoli.

The **alveolar epithelium** consists of two cell types lining the surface of the capillaries (terminal branches of the pulmonary artery), and the alveolar wall.

(1) Type I alveolar cells represent about 40% of the alveolar epithelial cell population and cover 90% of the alveolar surface.

(2) Type II alveolar cells, about 60% of the cells, cover only 10% of the alveolar surface and are preferentially located at the angles formed by adjacent alveolar septa. Type II alveolar cells produce surfactant.

Pulmonary surfactant contains:
(1) Cholesterol (50%).
(2) Phospholipids (40%).
(3) SP (surfactant protein) SP-A, SP-B, and SP-C (10%).

Club cells also produce surfactant. Surfactant maintains alveolar expansion by modulating surface tension.

Additional components of the alveolus include:
(1) Endothelial cells (lining the alveolar capillaries).
(2) Macrophages (alveolar phagocytes, or dust cells).
(3) Alveolar dendritic cells.
(4) Fibroblasts in the interalveolar septum (producing elastic fibers).
(5) Mast cells.

Neonatal respiratory distress syndrome (RDS) in premature infants is caused by surfactant deficiency leading to the collapse of the alveolar walls. The development of a fibrin-rich exudation, covering with a hyaline membrane the alveolar surface, complicates the RDS condition. Corticosteroids induce the synthesis of surfactant in the fetus. High levels of insulin in diabetic mothers antagonize the effect of corticosteroids.

• The **air-blood barrier** consists of:
(1) The thin cytoplasmic extensions of type I alveolar cells.
(2) A dual basal lamina produced by type I alveolar cells and subjacent endothelial cells lining the alveolar capillaries.
(3) Cytoplasmic extensions of endothelial cells.
(4) The plasma membrane of red blood cells.

Keep in mind that the biconcave shape of red blood cells favors the rapid O_2-CO_2 exchange in the alveolar capillaries. Also note that surfactant contributes indirectly to an effective gas exchange by preventing alveolar collapse.

• **Acute respiratory distress syndrome (ARDS)** results from an increase in the hydrostatic pressure in the alveolar capillaries (cardiogenic) or damage to the alveolar epithelial lining caused by bacterial endotoxins or trauma (noncardiogenic). These mechanisms result in increases in fluid and proteins in the alveolar spaces (pulmonary edema).

• **Lung cancer**. Most lung tumors are malignant. They can be primary tumors, originated in the lung, or secondary, or metastatic, spreading from other tumors.

According to the cell types, primary lung cancer can be classified into two major groups:
(1) Small cell lung cancer (SCLC; also called oat-cell carcinoma). SCLC is highly malignant and spreads very rapidly. About 15% of all lung cancers are SCLC.
(2) Non-small cell lung cancer (NSCLC) is the most frequent tumor (about 85% of all lung cancers).

The NSCLC group includes:
(1) Squamous cell carcinoma, a tumor derived from the transformation of the respiratory epithelium into a squamous metaplastic epithelium.
(2) Adenocarcinoma, a tumor originated from the bronchial epithelium and the bronchioalveolar epithelium (bronchioalveolar carcinoma).

Molecular screening of lung cancer samples is widely used for determining lung-cancer types and subtypes. For example, *anaplastic lymphoma kinase* (*ALK*) gene rearrangements, present in approximately 5% of NSCLC, and mutations in the kinase domain of the epidermal growth factor receptor (EGFR), observed in 10% to 15% of NSCLC, are common in lung adenocarcinomas.

• The **pleura** consists of two layers:
(1) The visceral layer closely attached to the lung and lined by a simple squamous epithelium (mesothelium).
(2) The parietal layer also lined by mesothelial cells and supported by connective tissue rich in fat. The visceral pleura glides on the parietal pleura during respiration.

Disorders of the pleura include:
(1) Inflammatory processes causing pleural effusion (abnormal accumulation of liquid in the pleural space).
(2) Accumulation of fluid (hydrothorax).
(3) Accumulation of blood (hemothorax).
(4) Accumulation of chyle, a lipid-rich liquid transported from intestinal lacteals to systemic veins in the thorax through the thoracic duct (chylothorax).
(5) Accumulation of air (pneumothorax).

Mesothelioma is a localized or diffuse malignant tumor of the pleura associated with asbestos exposure for long periods of time. Symptoms include pleural effusion, chest pain, and dyspnea. Mesothelioma can also affect the peritoneum and pericardium.

14. Urinary System

The urinary system has several essential functions: (1) to clear the blood of nitrogenous and other waste metabolic products by filtration and excretion; (2) to balance the concentration of body fluids and electrolytes, also by filtration and excretion; (3) to recover by reabsorption small molecules (amino acids, glucose, and peptides), ions (Na^+, Cl^-, Ca^{2+}, PO^{3-}), and water, in order to maintain blood homeostasis; (4) to regulate blood pressure by producing the enzyme renin, that initiates the conversion of angiotensinogen (a plasma protein produced in liver) to the active component angiotensin II; (5) to produces erythropoietin, a stimulant of red blood cell production in bone marrow; and (6) to activate 1,25-hydroxycholecalciferol, a vitamin D derivative involved in the control of calcium metabolism. This chapter correlates structure and function, highlighted by relevant renal physiologic and pathologic conditions.

The kidneys

The urinary system consists of paired kidneys and ureters and a single urinary bladder and urethra. Each kidneys has a **cortex** (subdivided into **outer cortex** and **juxtamedullary cortex**) and a **medulla** (subdivided into **outer medulla** and **inner medulla**).

The medulla is formed by conical masses, the **renal medullary pyramids**, with their bases located at the corticomedullary junction. A renal medullary pyramid, together with the associated covering cortical region, constitutes a **renal lobe**. The base of the renal lobe is the renal capsule. The lateral boundaries of each renal lobe are the **renal columns** (of Bertin), residual structures representing the fusion of primitive lobes within the metanephric blastema. The apex of each renal lobe terminates in a conic-shaped **papilla** surfaced by the **area cribrosa** (perforated area; the opening site of the papillary ducts). The papilla is surrounded by a **minor calyx**. Each minor calyx collects the urine from a papilla dripping from the area cribrosa. Minor calyces converge to form the **major calyces** which, in turn, form the **pelvis**.

Organization of the renal vascular system

The main function of the kidneys is to **filter the blood** supplied by the renal arteries branching from the descending aorta.

The kidneys receive about 20% of the cardiac output per minute and filter about 1.25 L of blood per minute. Essentially, all the blood of the body passes through the kidneys every 5 minutes.

About 90% of the cardiac output goes to the renal cortex; 10% of the blood goes to the medulla. Approximately 125 mL of filtrate is produced per minute, but 124 mL of this amount is reabsorbed.

About 180 L of fluid ultrafiltrate is produced in 24 hours and transported through the uriniferous tubules. Of this amount, 178.5 L is recovered by the tubular cells and returned to the blood circulation, whereas only 1.5 L is excreted as **urine**.

We start our discussion by focusing on the vascularization of the kidneys (Figure 14-1).

Oxygenated blood is supplied by the **renal artery**. The renal artery gives rise to several **interlobar arteries**, running across the medulla through the renal columns along the sides of the pyramids.

At the corticomedullary junction, interlobar arteries give off several branches at right angles, changing their vertical path to a horizontal direction to form the **arcuate arteries**, running along the corticomedullary boundary.

The renal arterial architecture is **terminal**. There are no anastomoses between interlobular arteries. This is an important concept in renal pathology for understanding **focal necrosis** as a consequence of an arterial obstruction. For example, **renal infarct** can be caused by atherosclerotic plaques in the renal artery or embolization of atherosclerotic plaques in the aorta.

Vertical branches emerging from the arcuate arteries, the **interlobular arteries**, penetrate the cortex. As interlobular arteries ascend toward the outer cortex, they branch several times to form the **afferent glomerular arterioles** (see Figure 14-1).

The afferent glomerular arteriole, in turn, forms the **glomerular capillary network**, enveloped by the two-layered **capsule of Bowman**, and continues as the **efferent glomerular arteriole**. This particular arrangement, a capillary network flanked by two arterioles (instead of an arteriole and a venule) is called the **glomerulus** or **arterial portal system** (Figure 14-2). As discussed in Chapter 12, Cardiovascular System, the glomerular **arterial portal system** is structurally and functionally distinct from the **venous portal system** of the liver.

Both the glomerulus and the surrounding capsule of Bowman form the **renal corpuscle**

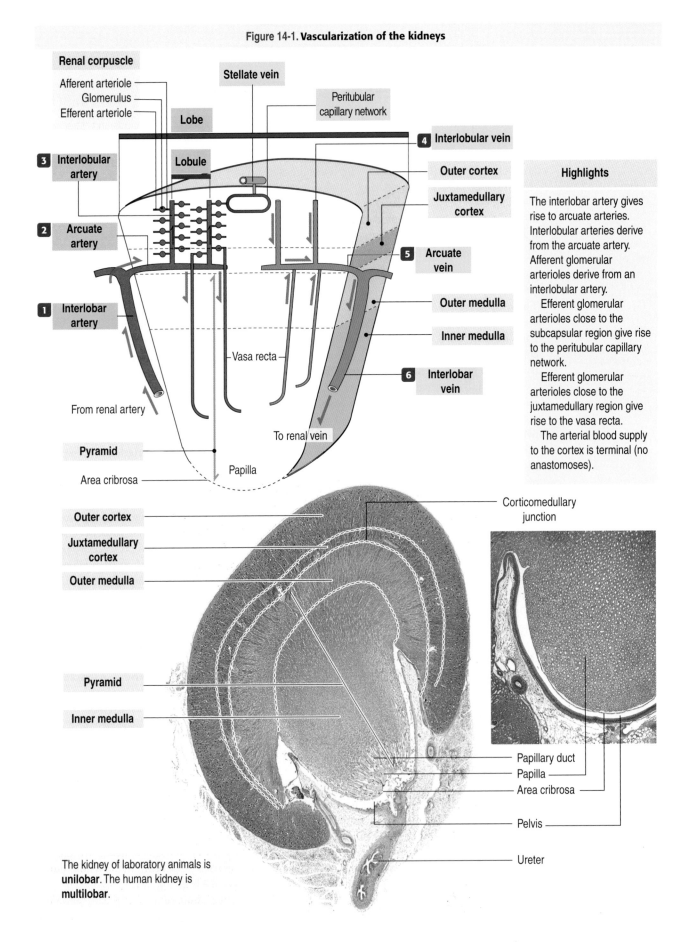

Figure 14-1. **Vascularization of the kidneys**

Renal corpuscle
Afferent arteriole
Glomerulus
Efferent arteriole
Stellate vein
Peritubular capillary network
Lobe
3 **Interlobular artery**
Lobule
4 **Interlobular vein**
Outer cortex
Juxtamedullary cortex
2 **Arcuate artery**
5 **Arcuate vein**
1 **Interlobar artery**
Outer medulla
Inner medulla
Vasa recta
6 **Interlobar vein**
From renal artery
To renal vein
Pyramid
Area cribrosa
Papilla

Highlights

The interlobar artery gives rise to arcuate arteries. Interlobular arteries derive from the arcuate artery. Afferent glomerular arterioles derive from an interlobular artery.

Efferent glomerular arterioles close to the subcapsular region give rise to the peritubular capillary network.

Efferent glomerular arterioles close to the juxtamedullary region give rise to the vasa recta.

The arterial blood supply to the cortex is terminal (no anastomoses).

Outer cortex
Juxtamedullary cortex
Outer medulla
Corticomedullary junction

Pyramid
Inner medulla

Papillary duct
Papilla
Area cribrosa

Pelvis

Ureter

The kidney of laboratory animals is **unilobar**. The human kidney is **multilobar**.

Figure 14-2. Arterial and venous portal systems

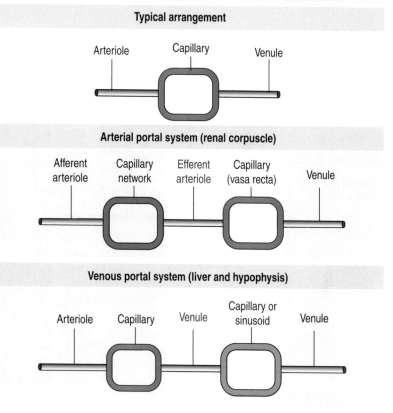

In general, a capillary network is interposed between an arteriole and a venule.

Typical arrangement

Arteriole   Capillary   Venule

In the kidneys, an arteriole is interposed between two capillary networks. An afferent arteriole gives rise to a mass of capillaries, the **glomerulus**. These capillaries coalesce to form an efferent arteriole, which gives rise to capillary networks (peritubular capillary network and the vasa recta) surrounding the nephrons.

Arterial portal system (renal corpuscle)

Afferent   Capillary   Efferent   Capillary   Venule
arteriole   network   arteriole   (vasa recta)

In the **liver** and **hypophysis**, veins feed into an extensive capillary or sinusoid network draining into a vein. This distribution is called the **venous portal system**.

Venous portal system (liver and hypophysis)

Arteriole   Capillary   Venule   Capillary or   Venule
sinusoid

(also called the **malpighian corpuscle**). The smooth muscle cell wall of the **afferent glomerular arteriole** displays epithelial-like cells, called **juxtaglomerular cells**, with secretory granules containing renin. A few juxtaglomerular cells may be found in the wall of the efferent glomerular arteriole.

Vasa recta

Depending on the location of the renal corpuscle in the outer cortex or juxtamedullary cortex, the efferent glomerular arteriole gives rise to two different capillary networks:

1. A **peritubular capillary network,** derived from afferent arterioles of renal corpuscles located in the outer cortex.

The peritubular capillary network, lined by fenestrated endothelial cells, drains into the **interlobular vein** converging to the **arcuate vein**. Arcuate veins drain into the **interlobar veins**, which are continuous with the **renal vein.**

2. The **vasa recta** (**straight vessels**), formed by multiple branching of the efferent arterioles located close to the corticomedullary junction. The **descending** components of the vasa recta (**arterial capillaries lined by continuous endothelial cells**) extend into the **medulla**, parallel to the medullary segments of the uriniferous tubules, make a hairpin turn, and return to the corticomedullary junction

as **ascending venous capillaries lined by fenestrated endothelial cells.**

Note that the vascular supply to the renal medulla is largely derived from the efferent glomerular arterioles. The descending vasa recta bundles penetrate to varying depths of the renal medulla, alongside the **descending** and **ascending limbs** of the **loop of Henle** and the **collecting ducts**. Side branches connect the returning ascending vasa recta to the **interlobular** and **arcuate veins**. Remember the close relationship of the vasa recta with each other and adjacent tubules and ducts. This is the structural basis of the countercurrent exchange and multiplier mechanism of urine formation as we discuss later.

Renal medullary pyramid, renal lobe, and renal lobule

A **renal medullary pyramid** is a **medullary** structure limited by interlobar arteries at the sides. The corticomedullary junction is the base and the papilla is the apex of the pyramid.

A **renal lobe** is a combined cortical-medullary structure. It consists of a renal medullary pyramid, together with the associated covering renal cortical region.

A **renal lobule** is a cortical structure that can be defined in two different ways (see Figure 14-1):

1. The renal lobule is a portion of the cortex **flanked by two adjacent ascending interlobular arter-**

Figure 14-3. **Medullary ray**

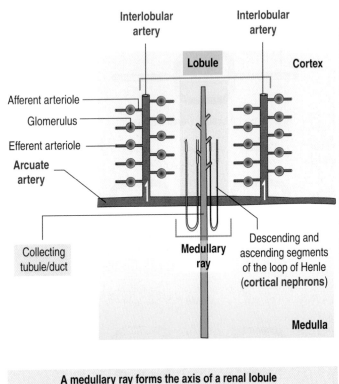

Interlobular artery

Interlobular artery

Lobule

Cortex

Afferent arteriole

Glomerulus

Efferent arteriole

Arcuate artery

Collecting tubule/duct

Medullary ray

Descending and ascending segments of the loop of Henle (cortical nephrons)

Medulla

A medullary ray forms the axis of a renal lobule

The descending and ascending segments of cortical nephrons and a collecting tubule/duct are closely aggregated at the middle of the renal lobule. This group of straight tubules forms a **medullary ray** within the cortex.

A medullary ray is the axis of the lobule, a cortical structure. Nephrons of the same lobule drain into the collecting duct.

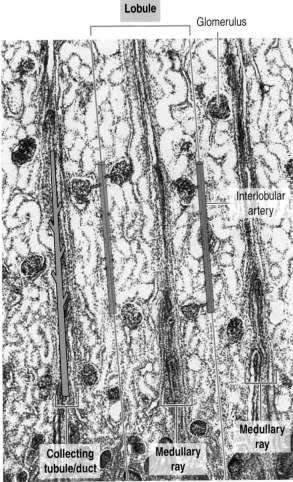

Lobule

Glomerulus

Interlobular artery

Collecting tubule/duct

Medullary ray

Medullary ray

ies. Each interlobular artery gives rise to a series of glomeruli, each consisting of an afferent glomerular arteriole, a capillary network, and the efferent glomerular arteriole.

2. The renal lobule consists of a single **collecting duct** (of Bellini) and the surrounding cortical nephrons that drain into it. The ascending and descending segments of cortical nephrons, together with the single collecting duct, are components of a **medullary ray** (of Ferrein). A medullary ray is the **axis of the lobule** (Figure 14-3).

Note that the **cortex has many lobules** and that **each lobule has a single medullary ray.**

The uriniferous tubule: Nephron and collecting duct
Each kidney has about 1.3 million uriniferous tubules surrounded by a stroma containing loose connective tissue, blood vessels, lymphatics, and nerves.

Each uriniferous tubule consists of two embryologically distinct segments (Figure 14-4):
1. The **nephron.**
2. The **collecting duct.**
The **nephron** consists of two components:

1. The **renal corpuscle** (300 μm in diameter).
2. A long **renal tubule** (5 to 7 mm long).
The **renal tubule** consists of:
1. The **proximal convoluted tubule.**
2. The **loop of Henle.**
3. The **distal convoluted tubule**, which empties into the **collecting tubule.**

Collecting tubules have three distinct topographic distributions:
1. A **cortical collecting tubule**, found in the renal cortex as the centerpiece of the medullary ray.
2. An **outer medullary collecting tubule**, present in the outer medulla.
3. An **inner medullary** segment, located in the inner medulla.

Depending on the distribution of renal corpuscles, nephrons can be either **cortical** or **juxtamedullary.**

Renal tubules derived from **cortical nephrons** have a **short** loop of Henle that penetrates just up to the outer medulla.

Renal tubules from **juxtamedullary nephrons** have a **long** loop of Henle projecting deep into the inner medulla (Figure 14-5).

Figure 14-4. **Uriniferous tubule**

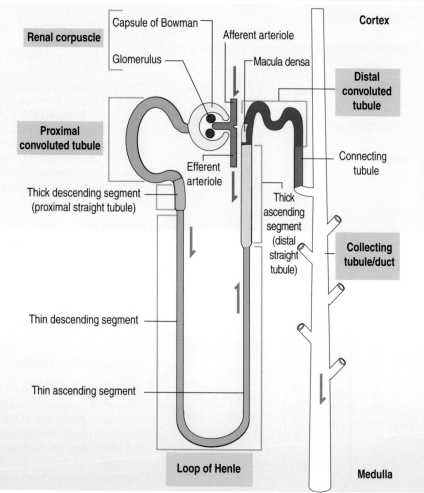

Renal corpuscle

Capsule of Bowman

Glomerulus

Afferent arteriole

Macula densa

Cortex

Distal convoluted tubule

Proximal convoluted tubule

Efferent arteriole

Connecting tubule

Thick descending segment (proximal straight tubule)

Thick ascending segment (distal straight tubule)

Collecting tubule/duct

Thin descending segment

Thin ascending segment

Loop of Henle

Medulla

The **uriniferous tubule** consists of two components of different embryologic origin: the **nephron** and the **collecting tubule/duct**.

The **nephron** comprises the **renal corpuscle**, the **proximal convoluted tubule**, the **loop of Henle** and the **distal convoluted tubule**.

Note that the macula densa is located at the initial portion of the distal convoluted tubule and that the proximal and convoluted tubules are adjacent to the renal corpuscle.

The renal corpuscle

The **renal corpuscle**, or **malpighian corpuscle** (Figure 14-6), consists of the **capsule of Bowman** investing a capillary tuft, the **glomerulus**.

The **capsule of Bowman** has two layers:

1. The **visceral layer**, attached to the capillary glomerulus.

2. The **parietal layer**, facing the connective tissue stroma.

The visceral layer is lined by epithelial cells called **podocytes** supported by a basal lamina. The parietal layer consists of a **simple squamous epithelium** continuous with the **simple cuboidal epithelium** of the proximal convoluted tubule (Figure 14-6).

A **urinary space** (**Bowman's space or capsular space**), containing the **plasma ultrafiltrate** (primary urine), exists between the visceral and parietal layers of the capsule.

The urinary space is continuous with the lumen of the proximal convoluted tubule at the **urinary pole**, the gate through which the plasma ultrafiltrate flows into the proximal convoluted tubule. The opposite

pole, the site of entry and exit of the afferent and efferent glomerular arterioles, is called the **vascular pole**.

The **glomerulus** consists of three cell components (Figure 14-7):

1. The **podocytes**, the visceral layer of the capsule of Bowman.

2. The fenestrated **endothelial cells, lining the glomerular capillaries**.

3. The **mesangial cells,** embedded in the **mesangial matrix**. **Mesangium** designates the combined mesangial cells-mesangial matrix complex.

Glomerular filtration barrier

The podocytes are mesenchymal-derived postmitotic cells. They are polarized cells with their nucleus-containing cell body bulging into the glomerular urinary space. Long primary processes, arising from the cell body, branch and give rise to multiple endings, called **foot processes** or **pedicels**. Pedicels encircle and attach to the surface of the glomerular capillary, except at the endothelial cell-mesangial matrix interface (see Figure 14-6).

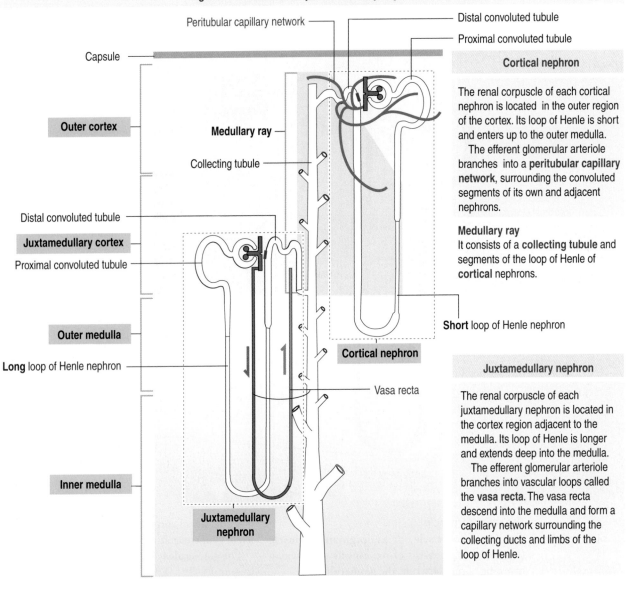

Figure 14-5. Cortical and juxtamedullary nephrons

Peritubular capillary network

Distal convoluted tubule

Proximal convoluted tubule

Capsule

Cortical nephron

The renal corpuscle of each cortical nephron is located in the outer region of the cortex. Its loop of Henle is short and enters up to the outer medulla.

The efferent glomerular arteriole branches into a **peritubular capillary network**, surrounding the convoluted segments of its own and adjacent nephrons.

Outer cortex

Medullary ray

Collecting tubule

Medullary ray
It consists of a **collecting tubule** and segments of the loop of Henle of **cortical** nephrons.

Distal convoluted tubule

Juxtamedullary cortex

Proximal convoluted tubule

Short loop of Henle nephron

Cortical nephron

Outer medulla

Long loop of Henle nephron

Juxtamedullary nephron

The renal corpuscle of each juxtamedullary nephron is located in the cortex region adjacent to the medulla. Its loop of Henle is longer and extends deep into the medulla.

The efferent glomerular arteriole branches into vascular loops called the **vasa recta**. The vasa recta descend into the medulla and form a capillary network surrounding the collecting ducts and limbs of the loop of Henle.

Vasa recta

Inner medulla

Juxtamedullary nephron

Podocytes and fenestrated endothelial cells each produce a basal lamina that, when combined, constitute the **glomerular basement membrane (GBM)**, a member of the **glomerular filtration barrier**. The major components of the GBM are type IV collagen, laminin, fibronectin, and heparan sulfate-containing proteoglycan.

The **pedicels**, derived from the same podocyte or from adjacent podocytes, interdigitate to cover the GBM. Pedicels are separated from each other by gaps, called **filtration slits**. Filtration slits are bridged by a membranous material, the **filtration slit diaphragm** (Figure 14-8). The filtration slit diaphragm is the major size barrier to protein leakage.

Pedicels are attached to the basal lamina by dystroglycans and $\alpha_3\beta_1$ **integrin**. Podocyte injury causes the detachment of pedicels from the GBM, a condition known as **foot process effacement**.

The podocyte filtration slit diaphragm consists of nephrin molecules interacting in a homophilic manner, and with the nephrin-related transmembrane proteins **Neph1** and **Neph2** (not shown in Figure 14-8). **Nephrin** is anchored to bundles of actin filaments (forming the core of the pedicel) which interact with the proteins **podocin** and CD2-associated protein (**CD2AP**).

The nephrin dimers create a structure retarding the passage of molecules that have crossed the endothelial fenestrations and the GBM.

In addition to the components of the glomerular filtration barrier, other limiting factors controlling the passage of molecules in the plasma ultrafiltrate are **molecular size** and **electric charge**. Molecules with a size less than 3.5 nm and positively charged or neutral are filtered more readily. Albumin (3.6 nm and anionic) filters poorly.

Figure 14-6. Renal corpuscle

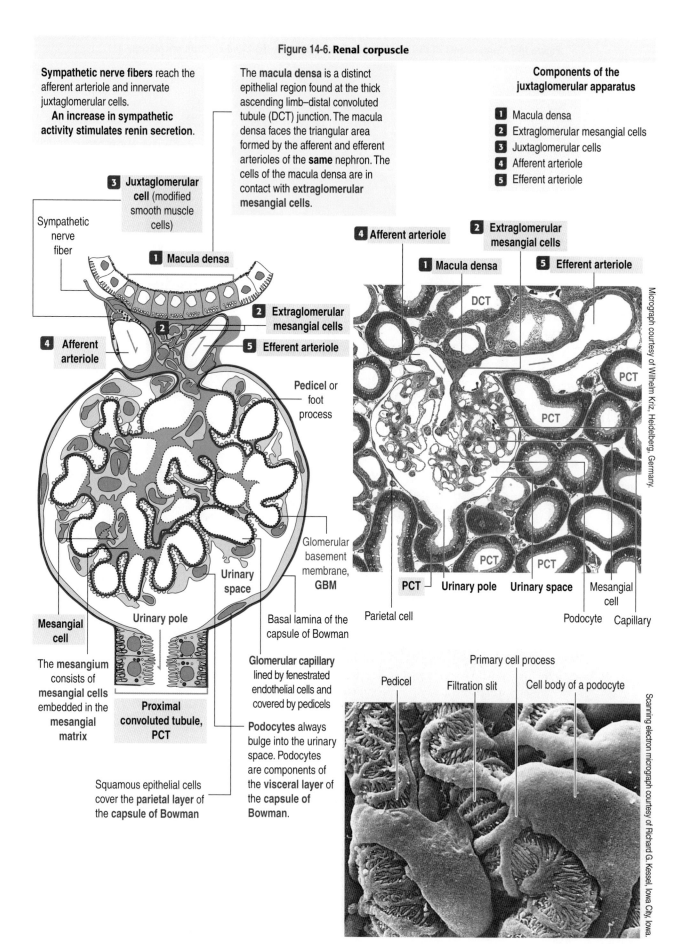

Sympathetic nerve fibers reach the afferent arteriole and innervate juxtaglomerular cells.

An increase in sympathetic activity stimulates renin secretion.

The **macula densa** is a distinct epithelial region found at the thick ascending limb–distal convoluted tubule (DCT) junction. The macula densa faces the triangular area formed by the afferent and efferent arterioles of the **same** nephron. The cells of the macula densa are in contact with **extraglomerular mesangial cells**.

Components of the juxtaglomerular apparatus

1 Macula densa
2 Extraglomerular mesangial cells
3 Juxtaglomerular cells
4 Afferent arteriole
5 Efferent arteriole

3 **Juxtaglomerular cell** (modified smooth muscle cells)

Sympathetic nerve fiber

1 **Macula densa**

4 **Afferent arteriole**

2 **Extraglomerular mesangial cells**

5 **Efferent arteriole**

Pedicel or foot process

Glomerular basement membrane, GBM

Urinary space

Basal lamina of the capsule of Bowman

Mesangial cell

Urinary pole

The **mesangium** consists of **mesangial cells** embedded in the **mesangial matrix**

Proximal convoluted tubule, PCT

Squamous epithelial cells cover the **parietal layer** of the **capsule of Bowman**

Glomerular capillary lined by fenestrated endothelial cells and covered by pedicels

Podocytes always bulge into the urinary space. Podocytes are components of the **visceral layer** of the **capsule of Bowman**.

4 **Afferent arteriole**
2 **Extraglomerular mesangial cells**
1 **Macula densa**
5 **Efferent arteriole**

DCT

PCT

PCT

PCT

PCT

PCT **Urinary pole** **Urinary space** Mesangial cell

Parietal cell

Podocyte   Capillary

Micrograph courtesy of Wilhelm Kriz, Heidelberg, Germany.

Primary cell process

Pedicel   Filtration slit   Cell body of a podocyte

Scanning electron micrograph courtesy of Richard G. Kessel, Iowa City, Iowa.

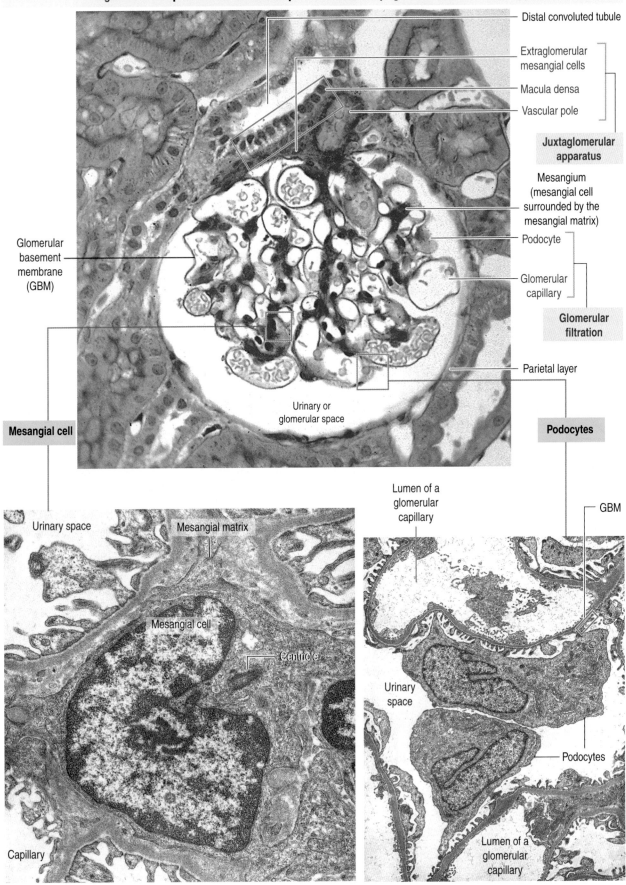

Figure 14-7. **Components of the renal corpuscle visualized by light and electron microscopy**

Distal convoluted tubule

Extraglomerular mesangial cells

Macula densa

Vascular pole

Juxtaglomerular apparatus

Mesangium (mesangial cell surrounded by the mesangial matrix)

Podocyte

Glomerular capillary

Glomerular filtration

Parietal layer

Urinary or glomerular space

Glomerular basement membrane (GBM)

Mesangial cell

Podocytes

Lumen of a glomerular capillary

GBM

Urinary space

Mesangial matrix

Mesangial cell

Centriole

Urinary space

Capillary

Podocytes

Lumen of a glomerular capillary

Figure 14-8. Glomerular filtration barrier

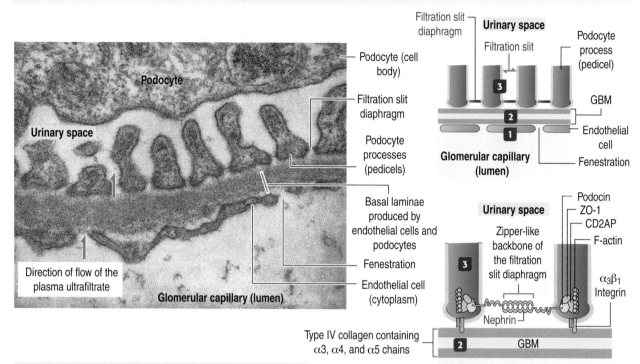

Filtration slit diaphragm

Urinary space

Filtration slit

Podocyte process (pedicel)

Podocyte (cell body)

Filtration slit diaphragm

Podocyte processes (pedicels)

GBM

Endothelial cell

Fenestration

Glomerular capillary (lumen)

Podocyte

Urinary space

Direction of flow of the plasma ultrafiltrate

Glomerular capillary (lumen)

Basal laminae produced by endothelial cells and podocytes

Fenestration

Endothelial cell (cytoplasm)

Urinary space

Zipper-like backbone of the filtration slit diaphragm

Podocin
ZO-1
CD2AP
F-actin

$\alpha_3\beta_1$ Integrin

Nephrin

Type IV collagen containing α_3, α_4, and α_5 chains

GBM

Components of the filtration barrier

1 The **endothelium** of the glomerular capillaries is **fenestrated** and permeable to water, sodium, urea, glucose, and small proteins. Endothelial cells are coated by **negatively charged glycoproteins** (heparan sulfate), which slow down the filtration of large anionic proteins.

2 The **glomerular basement membrane (GBM)**, a product of endothelial cells and podocytes, contains type IV collagen, laminin, fibronectin, and proteoglycans rich in the glycosaminoglycan heparan sulfate, which also slows down the filtration of anionic proteins.

3 The pedicels are interdigitating cell processes of podocytes covering the GBM and coated by a negatively charged glycoprotein coat. The space between adjacent pedicels is called the **filtration slit**. A **filtration slit diaphragm** bridges adjacent pedicels. $\alpha_3\beta_1$ integrin anchors the pedicel to the basal lamina.

The diaphragm consists of **nephrin**, a cell adhesion molecule of the immunoglobulin superfamily, anchored to actin filaments within the pedicel by the proteins CD2AP, zonula occludens (ZO)-1, and podocin.

A mutation of the gene encoding nephrin causes **congenital nephrotic syndrome**, characterized by massive proteinuria (leakage of albumin in urine) and edema.

Pathology: Defects of the GBM

The **fenestrated endothelial cells** of the glomerular capillaries are covered by the GBM to which the foot processes of the podocytes attach (see Figure 14-8). Podocytes produce **glomerular endothelial growth factor** to stimulate the development of the endothelium and maintenance of its fenestrations.

The endothelium is permeable to water, urea, glucose, and small proteins. The surface of the endothelial cells is coated with negatively charged polyanionic proteoglycans blocking the passage of large anionic proteins.

The GBM contains **type IV collagen, fibronectin, laminin**, and **heparan sulfate** as major proteins. Type IV collagen of the GBM consists of three α chains, α3, α4 and α5, forming a triple helix. Most other basal laminae contain α1 and α2 chains and α5 and α6 chains. A correctly assembled flexible non-fibrillar network, that also includes laminin 11, is critical for

maintaining the integrity of the GBM and its permeability function.

Type IV collagens are directly involved in the pathogenesis of three renal diseases:

1. **Goodpasture syndrome**, an autoimmune disorder consisting in progressive glomerulonephritis and pulmonary hemorrhage, caused by α3 autoantibodies binding to the glomerular and lung alveolar basal laminae.

2. **Alport's syndrome**, a progressive inherited nephropathy, characterized by irregular thinning, thickening, and splitting of the GBM. Alport's syndrome is transmitted by an **X-linked recessive** trait, is predominant in **males**, and involves mutations of the α5 chain gene. Patients with Alport's syndrome, often associated with hearing loss (defective function of the stria vascularis of the cochlea) and ocular symptoms (defect of the lens capsule), have **hematuria** (blood in the urine) and **progressive glomerulonephritis** lead-

Figure 14-9. **Juxtaglomerular apparatus**

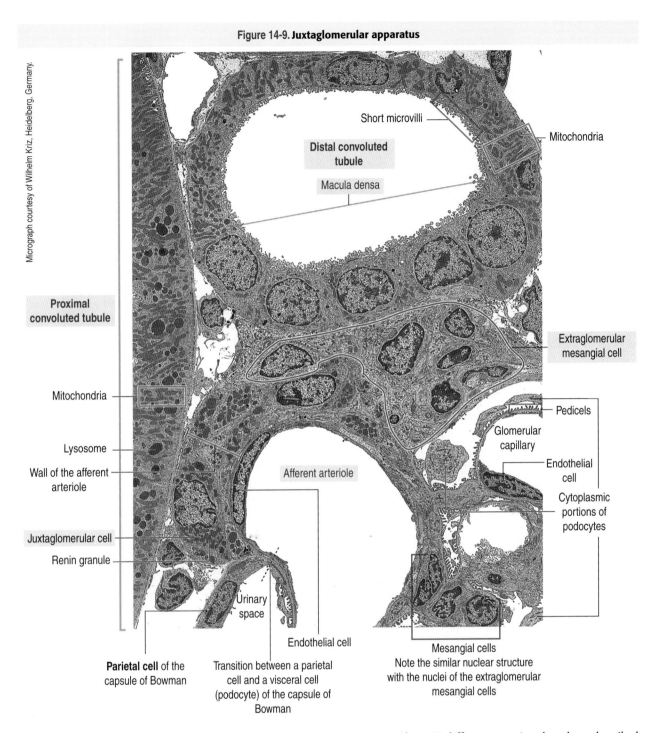

Short microvilli

Mitochondria

Distal convoluted tubule

Macula densa

Proximal convoluted tubule

Extraglomerular mesangial cell

Mitochondria

Pedicels

Glomerular capillary

Lysosome

Endothelial cell

Wall of the afferent arteriole

Afferent arteriole

Cytoplasmic portions of podocytes

Juxtaglomerular cell

Renin granule

Urinary space

Endothelial cell

Parietal cell of the capsule of Bowman

Transition between a parietal cell and a visceral cell (podocyte) of the capsule of Bowman

Mesangial cells
Note the similar nuclear structure with the nuclei of the extraglomerular mesangial cells

ing to renal failure (**end-stage renal disease, ESRD**). The abnormal glomerular filtration membrane enables the passage of red blood cells and proteins.

3. **Benign familial hematuria**, caused by a dominant inherited mutation of the *α4 chain* gene, which does not lead to renal failure as seen in ESRD.

Clinical significance: Slit filtration diaphragm

Congenital nephrotic syndrome is caused by a mutation in the *nephrin* gene leading to the absence or malfunction of the podocyte's slit filtration diaphragm.

About 70 different mutations have been described. Affected children have massive proteinuria even in utero and the nephrotic syndrome develops soon after birth. Infants display abdominal distention, hypoalbuminemia, hyperlipidemia, and edema. Congenital nephrotic syndrome, particularly common in Finland, is lethal.

Mesangium

The mesangium (Greek *mesos*, middle; *angeion*, vessel) is an **intraglomerular** structure interposed between the glomerular capillaries.

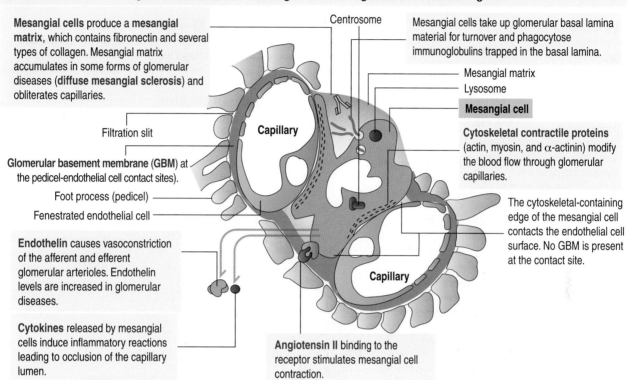

Figure 14-10. Functions of mesangial cells and organization of the mesangium

Centrosome

Mesangial cells produce a **mesangial matrix**, which contains fibronectin and several types of collagen. Mesangial matrix accumulates in some forms of glomerular diseases (**diffuse mesangial sclerosis**) and obliterates capillaries.

Mesangial cells take up glomerular basal lamina material for turnover and phagocytose immunoglobulins trapped in the basal lamina.

Mesangial matrix

Lysosome

Capillary

Mesangial cell

Filtration slit

Cytoskeletal contractile proteins (actin, myosin, and α-actinin) modify the blood flow through glomerular capillaries.

Glomerular basement membrane (GBM) at the pedicel-endothelial cell contact sites).

Foot process (pedicel)

Fenestrated endothelial cell

The cytoskeletal-containing edge of the mesangial cell contacts the endothelial cell surface. No GBM is present at the contact site.

Endothelin causes vasoconstriction of the afferent and efferent glomerular arterioles. Endothelin levels are increased in glomerular diseases.

Capillary

Cytokines released by mesangial cells induce inflammatory reactions leading to occlusion of the capillary lumen.

Angiotensin II binding to the receptor stimulates mesangial cell contraction.

It consists of two components:

1. The **mesangial cell.**
2. The **mesangial matrix.**

In addition, mesangial cells aggregate outside the glomerulus (**extraglomerular mesangial cells**; Figure 14-9; see Figures 14-6 and 14-7) in a space limited by the macula densa and the afferent and efferent glomerular arterioles. Intraglomerular mesangial cells are continuous with **extraglomerular mesangial cells**.

Mesangial cells are specialized **pericytes** with characteristics of smooth muscle cells and macrophages.

Mesangial cells are:

1. **Contractile cells.**
2. **Phagocytic cells.**
3. Capable of **proliferation.**

They synthesize **matrix (fibronectin) and several types of collagen** (types IV, V, and VI), and secrete **biologically active substances** (prostaglandins and endothelins). **Endothelins** induce the constriction of afferent and efferent glomerular arterioles (Figure 14-10).

Mesangial cells participate indirectly in the glomerular filtration process by:

1. **Providing mechanical support for the glomerular capillaries.**
2. **Controlling the turnover of the GBM material** by their phagocytic activity.
3. **Regulating blood flow** by their contractile activity.
4. **Secreting prostaglandins and endothelins.**

5. **Responding to angiotensin II.**

The mesangial cell-matrix complex is in direct contact with endothelial cells. Note that the GBM is not present at the mesangium site (see Figure 14-10). Instead, cytoplasmic margins of mesangial cells, containing cytoskeletal contractile proteins, are closely associated to the endothelial cell surface.

Immunoglobulins and complement molecules, unable to cross the filtration barrier remain in the mesangial matrix. The accumulation of immunoglobulin complexes in the matrix induces the production of cytokines by mesangial cells that trigger an immune response leading to the eventual occlusion of the glomerular capillaries.

Pathology: Podocyte injury

Podocyte injury of **congenital, hereditary,** and **acquired** origin can cause glomerular diseases. Acquired glomerular diseases can be of immune and non-immune origin.

Congenital nephrotic syndrome is an example of a congenital cause of podocyte injury (see Figure 14-8). Hereditary causes of podocyte injury include mutations in genes expressing podocyte-specific proteins (such as podocin and β1 integrin subunit). The most characteristic feature is the loss of interdigitating pedicels contacting the GBM, a condition known as **foot process effacement** (Figure 14-11).

Most glomerular diseases caused by podocyte injury are acquired. The damage to the glomerulus can be

Figure 14-11. Podocyte injury and pathology of the mesangium

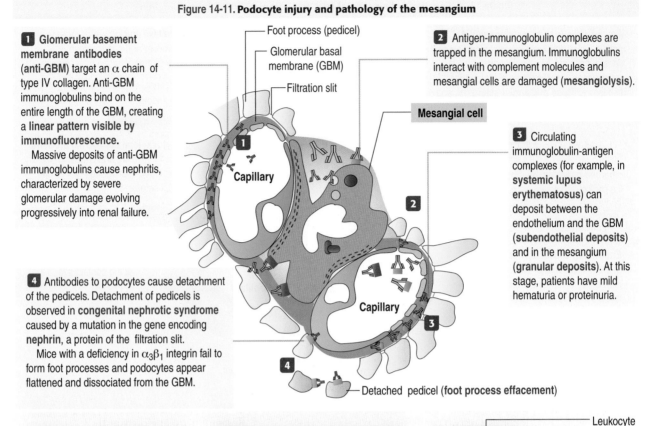

1 Glomerular basement membrane antibodies (**anti-GBM**) target an α chain of type IV collagen. Anti-GBM immunoglobulins bind on the entire length of the GBM, creating a **linear pattern visible by immunofluorescence.**

Massive deposits of anti-GBM immunoglobulins cause nephritis, characterized by severe glomerular damage evolving progressively into renal failure.

Foot process (pedicel)
Glomerular basal membrane (GBM)
Filtration slit
Capillary

2 Antigen-immunoglobulin complexes are trapped in the mesangium. Immunoglobulins interact with complement molecules and mesangial cells are damaged (**mesangiolysis**).

Mesangial cell

3 Circulating immunoglobulin-antigen complexes (for example, in **systemic lupus erythematosus**) can deposit between the endothelium and the GBM (**subendothelial deposits**) and in the mesangium (**granular deposits**). At this stage, patients have mild hematuria or proteinuria.

Capillary

4 Antibodies to podocytes cause detachment of the pedicels. Detachment of pedicels is observed in **congenital nephrotic syndrome** caused by a mutation in the gene encoding **nephrin**, a protein of the filtration slit.

Mice with a deficiency in $\alpha_3\beta_1$ integrin fail to form foot processes and podocytes appear flattened and dissociated from the GBM.

Detached pedicel (**foot process effacement**)

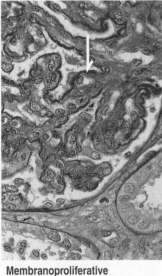

Photographs from Damjanov I, Linder J: Pathology: A Color Atlas, St. Louis, Mosby, 2000.

Membranoproliferative glomerulonephritis caused by deposition of immunoglobulins and complement proteins in the mesangial matrix and GBM. Note the increased thickness of the GBM (arrow).

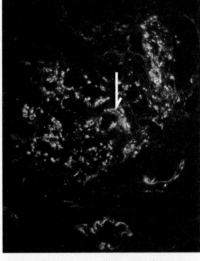

Immunofluorescence microscopy shows a **granular pattern** (arrow) of complement proteins deposited in the mesangial matrix.

Leukocyte
Capillary lumen
Podocyte
Urinary space

Electron microscopy shows dense deposits of proteins along the GBM (arrows).

initiated by immune mechanisms. **Antibodies against glomerular components** (podocytes, mesangial cells, and GBM) and **antibody-complement complexes circulating in blood** in patients with systemic autoimmune diseases can cause **membranoproliferative glomerulonephritis** (see Figure 14-11) and **immunoglobulin A nephropathy** (Berger's disease).

Antibody-antigen complexes are not immunologically targeted to glomerular components. They are trapped in the glomerulus because of the filtration

Figure 14-12. **Pathology of the renal corpuscle: Glomerulonephritis**

Acute proliferative diffuse glomerulonephritis

The deposition of immune complexes in the **glomerular basement membrane** (resulting from a bacterial, viral, or protozoal infection) triggers the **proliferation of endothelial and mesangial cells**. In the presence of complement proteins, neutrophils accumulate in the lumen of the capillaries, which become occluded.

A **nephritic syndrome**, characterized by hematuria, oliguria, hypertension, and edema, is diagnosed. Children are predominantly affected.

The nephritic syndrome is **reversible**: Immune complexes are removed from the GBM, endothelial cells are shed, and the population of proliferative mesangial cells returns to normal. The renal function is reestablished.

Rapidly progressive (crescentic) glomerulonephritis

The proliferation of the epithelial cells of the capsule of Bowman and infiltration of macrophages produce a crescent-like mass in most glomeruli. The crescent enlarges and compresses the glomerular capillaries, which are displaced and stop functioning. This condition progresses rapidly to renal failure.

The accumulation of fibrin and other serum proteins and the necrosis of the glomerular capillaries stimulate the proliferative process.

Rapidly progressive glomerulonephritis is an immune-mediated process and is detected in a number of conditions, such as **Goodpasture's syndrome** (caused by antibodies binding to the 7S domain of type IV collagen of the GBM), **systemic lupus erythematosus**, or of unknown cause (**idiopathic**).

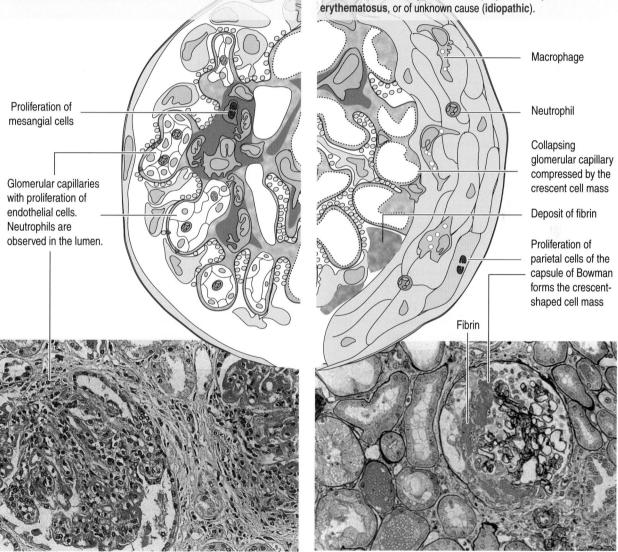

Proliferation of mesangial cells

Glomerular capillaries with proliferation of endothelial cells. Neutrophils are observed in the lumen.

Macrophage

Neutrophil

Collapsing glomerular capillary compressed by the crescent cell mass

Deposit of fibrin

Proliferation of parietal cells of the capsule of Bowman forms the crescent-shaped cell mass

Fibrin

Photographs from Damjanov I, Linder J: Pathology: A Color Atlas, St. Louis, Mosby, 2000.

properties of the glomerular filtration barrier. A complicating factor is that trapped antibody-antigen complexes provide binding sites to complement proteins, which also contribute to the glomerular damage (see Chapter 10, Immune-Lymphatic System, for a review of the complement cascade).

As we have seen, autoantibodies can target specific chains of type IV collagen, a component of the glomerular filtration barrier. In addition, the deposit of complement proteins in the mesangial matrix produces a **granular pattern** (see Figure 14-11). Systemic lupus erythematosus and bacterial (streptococci) and viral (hepatitis B virus) infections generate antibody-antigen complexes circulating in blood and trapped in the glomerular filtration barrier.

Immune complexes can deposit between the endothelial cells of the glomerular capillaries and the basal lamina (**subendothelial deposits**, see Figure 14-11), in the mesangium, and less frequently between the basal lamina and the foot processes of podocytes.

Immune complexes produced after bacterial infection can cause the proliferation of glomerular cells (endothelial and mesangial cells) and attract neutrophils and monocytes. This condition, known as **acute proliferative glomerulonephritis**, is observed in children and is generally reversible with treatment. This disease is more severe in adults: it can evolve into **rapidly progressive (crescentic) glomerulonephritis** (Figure 14-12).

A typical feature of crescentic glomerulonephritis is the presence of glomerular cell debris and fibrin, causing severe glomerular injury. The proliferation of parietal cells of the capsule of Bowman and migrating neutrophils and lymphocytes into the space of Bowman occur. Both the cellular crescents and deposits of fibrin compress the glomerular capillaries.

Juxtaglomerular apparatus

The juxtaglomerular apparatus is a well defined endocrine structure consisting of:

1. The **macula densa** (see Figures 14-6, 14-7, and 14-9), a distinct region of the initial portion of the distal convoluted tubule.

2. The **extraglomerular mesangial cells** (see Figure 14-9), a space outlined by the macula densa and the afferent and efferent glomerular arterioles.

3. The **renin-producing cells (juxtaglomerular cells)** of the afferent glomerular arteriole (see Figures 14-7 and 14-9) and, to a lesser extent, the efferent glomerular arteriole.

The macula densa is sensitive to changes in NaCl concentration and affects renin release by juxtaglomerular cells. Renin is secreted when the NaCl concentration in the filtrate decreases. Extraglomerular mesangial cells (also called **lacis cells**) are connected to each other and to juxtaglomerular cells by gap junctions.

The juxtaglomerular apparatus is one of the components of the **tubuloglomerular feedback mechanism** involved in the autoregulation of **renal blood flow** and **glomerular filtration**.

The other component is the **sympathetic nerve fibers** (adrenergic) innervating the juxtaglomerular cells. Renin secretion is enhanced by **norepinephrine** and **dopamine** secreted by adrenergic nerve fibers. Norepinephrine binds to α_1-adrenergic receptors in the afferent glomerular arteriole to cause vasoconstriction. There is no parasympathetic innervation.

We come back to the tubuloglomerular feedback mechanism when we discuss the renin-angiotensin regulatory mechanism.

Proximal convoluted tubule

Cuboidal epithelial cells, held together by apical **tight junctions**, line the proximal convoluted tubule (PCT) and have structural characteristics for reabsorption. They display the following features (Figure 14-13):

1. An apical domain with a well-developed **brush border** consisting of **microvilli**.

2. A basolateral domain with extensive plasma membrane **infoldings** and **interdigitations**.

3. Long mitochondria located between the plasma membrane folds provide adenosine triphosphate (ATP) for active transport of ions mediated by an **Na$^+$, K$^+$-ATPase activated pump**.

4. Apical **tubulovesicles** and **lysosomes** provide a mechanism for endocytosis and breakdown of small proteins into amino acids. The movement of **glucose** and Na$^+$ across the plasma membrane is mediated by a **symport transport protein**.

The plasma ultrafiltrate in the glomerular urinary space is transported by **active** and **passive** mechanisms along the PCT, where about 70% of filtered water, glucose, Na$^+$, Cl$^-$, and K$^+$, and other solutes are reabsorbed.

The driving force for water reabsorption is the electrochemical gradient produced by the reabsorption of solutes, such as NaCl and glucose. Because of the higher water permeability of the PCT, water passes by osmosis across tight junctions (**paracellular pathway**) into the lateral intercellular space. An increase in the hydrostatic pressure in the intercellular compartment forces fluids and solutes to move into the capillary network.

Epithelial cells lining the PCT are involved in the production of **calcitriol**, the active form of vitamin D. We discuss in Chapter 19, Endocrine System, details of the metabolism of vitamin D and calcium absorption.

The **Fanconi syndrome** is a renal hereditary (primary) or acquired (secondary) disease in which PCTs fail to reabsorb amino acids and glucose. Consequently, these substances are excreted in urine. The cause is a defective cellular energy metabolism resulting from impaired mitochondrial ATP levels or abnormal activity of the Na$^+$ K$^+$ ATPase pump. **Aminoaciduria** (an abnormal amount of amino acids in the urine) is the prominent feature of Fanconi syndrome.

Pathology: Acute kidney injury

Acute kidney injury is defined by a **sudden increase in the concentration of creatinine in serum** and **a decrease in urinary output**. It is caused by glomerulonephritis, renal vascular disease, prerenal

Figure 14-13. **Proximal convoluted tubule (PCT)**

Proximal convoluted tubule (PCT)

The PCT reabsorbs about 70% of filtered water and the bulk of solutes. The osmotic gradient established by reabsorbed glucose and NaCl is the driving force for water reabsorption across tight junctions and the PCT epithelial cells. **Aquaporin 1** is a channel protein found in the apical and basolateral domains of the plasma membrane of epithelial cells lining the PCT. It is also present in the thin descending segment of the loop of Henle. It is involved in water transport.

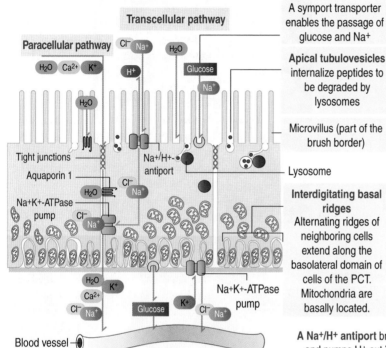

Transcellular pathway

Paracellular pathway

Tight junctions
Aquaporin 1
Na+K+-ATPase pump
Blood vessel

A symport transporter enables the passage of glucose and Na+

Apical tubulovesicles internalize peptides to be degraded by lysosomes

Microvillus (part of the brush border)

Na+/H+-antiport

Lysosome

Interdigitating basal ridges
Alternating ridges of neighboring cells extend along the basolateral domain of cells of the PCT. Mitochondria are basally located.

Na+K+-ATPase pump

A Na+/H+ antiport brings Na+ into the cell and pumps H+ out into the tubular fluid

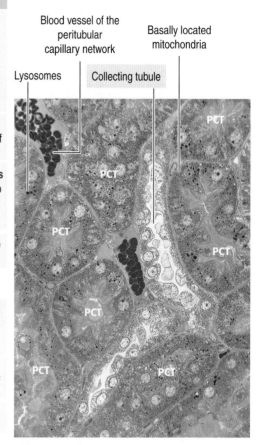

Blood vessel of the peritubular capillary network
Basally located mitochondria
Lysosomes
Collecting tubule

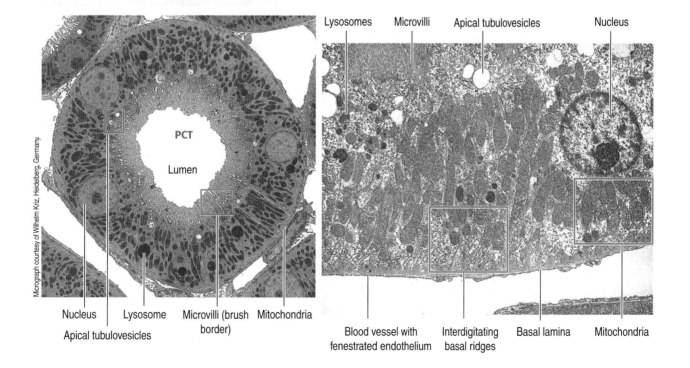

Micrograph courtesy of Wilhelm Kriz, Heidelberg, Germany.

PCT
Lumen

Nucleus   Lysosome   Microvilli (brush border)   Mitochondria
Apical tubulovesicles

Lysosomes   Microvilli   Apical tubulovesicles   Nucleus

Blood vessel with fenestrated endothelium   Interdigitating basal ridges   Basal lamina   Mitochondria

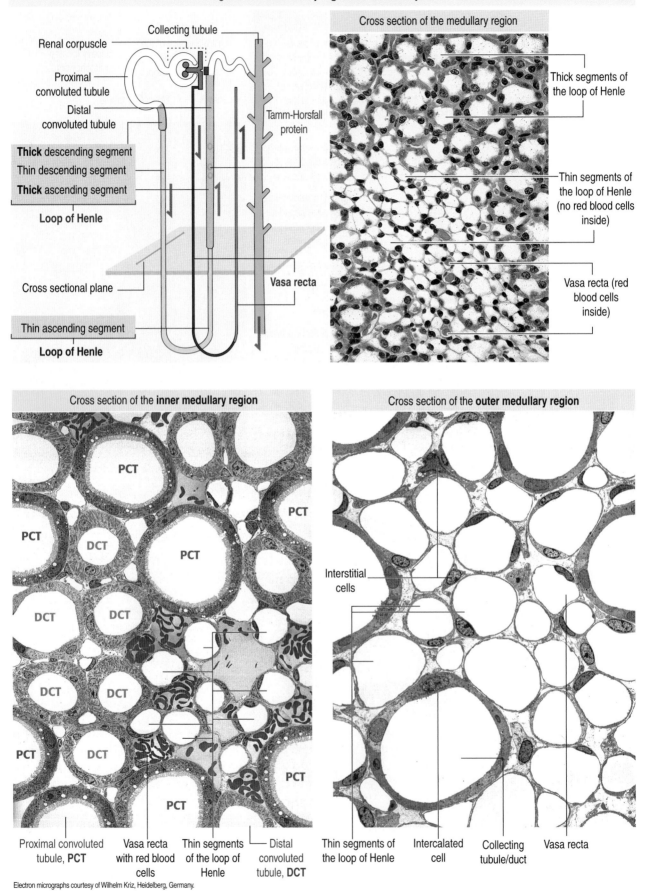

Figure 14-14. **Medullary region of the kidneys**

Cross section of the medullary region

Thick segments of the loop of Henle

Thin segments of the loop of Henle (no red blood cells inside)

Vasa recta (red blood cells inside)

Collecting tubule

Renal corpuscle

Proximal convoluted tubule

Distal convoluted tubule

Tamm-Horsfall protein

Thick descending segment
Thin descending segment
Thick ascending segment

Loop of Henle

Cross sectional plane

Vasa recta

Thin ascending segment

Loop of Henle

Cross section of the inner medullary region

PCT
PCT
PCT
DCT
PCT
DCT
DCT
DCT
DCT
PCT
DCT
PCT
PCT

Proximal convoluted tubule, **PCT**

Vasa recta with red blood cells

Thin segments of the loop of Henle

Distal convoluted tubule, **DCT**

Cross section of the outer medullary region

Interstitial cells

Thin segments of the loop of Henle

Intercalated cell

Collecting tubule/duct

Vasa recta

Electron micrographs courtesy of Wilhelm Kriz, Heidelberg, Germany.

Figure 14-15. Medullary region of the kidneys

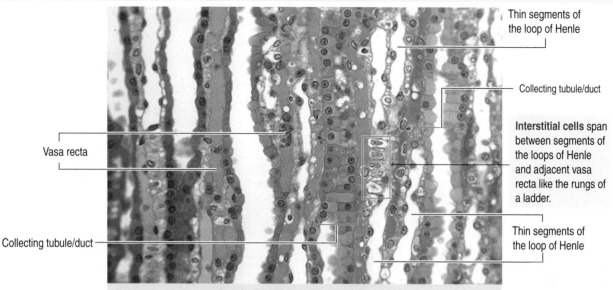

Thin segments of the loop of Henle

Collecting tubule/duct

Interstitial cells span between segments of the loops of Henle and adjacent vasa recta like the rungs of a ladder.

Thin segments of the loop of Henle

Vasa recta

Collecting tubule/duct

Longitudinal section of the medullary region

azotemia (abnormally high level of nitrogen waste products in the blood), acute tubular necrosis, and acute interstitial nephritis.

The epithelial lining of the PCT loses the brush border and the connective tissue of the intertubular space is infiltrated by inflammatory cells (lymphocytes and macrophages). Activated fibroblasts produce collagen causing interstitial fibrosis. Tubulointerstitial damage and endothelial injury affect renal cellular function and increase the risk of the development of cardiovascular disease.

An episode of acute kidney injury may progress to subsequent **chronic kidney disease,** regardless the cause of acute kidney injury, and an enhanced risk of ESRD and mortality resulting from complications of cardiovascular disease.

Loop of Henle
The loop of Henle consists of a **descending limb** and an **ascending limb**. Each limb is formed by a **thick segment** and a **thin segment** (Figure 14-14).

The thick descending segment (proximal straight tubule) is a continuation of the PCT. The thick ascending segment (distal straight tubule) is continuous with the distal convoluted tubule.

The length of the thin segments varies in cortical and juxtamedullary nephrons. Like the PCT, **the thin descending segment harbors aquaporin 1 channels and is highly permeable to water. The thin ascending segment is impermeable to water but reabsorbs salts.**

Salt moves into the interstitium of the medulla; water is transported towards the outer medulla and juxtamedullary cortex where it returns to the systemic blood circulation.

The loop of Henle reabsorbs about 15% of the filtered water and 25% of the filtered NaCl, K^+, Ca^{2+}, and HCO_3^-. As in the PCT, an **Na^+, K^+-ATPase pump** in the ascending limb is a key element in the reabsorption of salts. Inhibition of this pump by **diuretics** such as **furosemide** (Lasix) inhibits the reabsorption of NaCl and increases urinary excretion of both NaCl and water by reducing the osmolality of the interstitial fluid in the medulla.

The thick segments of the limbs are lined by a low cuboidal epithelium in transition with the epithelial lining of the convoluted tubules.

Epithelial cells in this segment synthesize the **Tamm-Horsfall protein,** the most abundant protein present in urine. The thin segments are lined by a squamous simple epithelium (Figure 14-15, see Figure 14-14).

Distal convoluted tubule
The cuboidal epithelial cell lining of the distal convoluted tubule (DCT) has the following characteristics (Figure 14-16; see also Figure 14-9):

1. **Cuboidal cells are shorter** than those in the PCT and **lack a prominent brush border.**

2. As in the PCT, the plasma membrane of the basolateral domain is infolded and lodges mitochondria.

3. The cells of the **macula densa** display **reversed polarity**: the nucleus occupies an apical position and the basal domain faces the juxtaglomerular cells and extraglomerular mesangial cells (see Figure 14-9). The macula densa, located at the junction of the ascending thick segment of the loop of Henle with the DCT, senses changes in Na^+ concentration in the tubular fluid.

The DCT and the collecting duct reabsorb approxi-

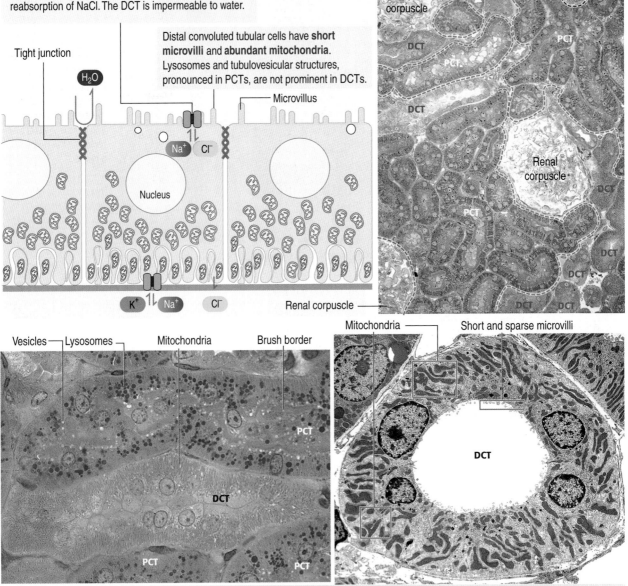

Figure 14-16. Distal convoluted tubule (DCT)

A **symport mechanism** (coupled transport of two or more solutes in the same direction) enables the reabsorption of NaCl. The DCT is impermeable to water.

Tight junction

Distal convoluted tubular cells have **short microvilli** and **abundant mitochondria**. Lysosomes and tubulovesicular structures, pronounced in PCTs, are not prominent in DCTs.

Microvillus

H_2O

Na^+ Cl^-

Nucleus

K^+ Na^+ Cl^-

Renal corpuscle

Renal corpuscle

Renal corpuscle

Mitochondria   Short and sparse microvilli

Vesicles — Lysosomes   Mitochondria   Brush border

PCT

DCT

PCT   PCT

DCT

Identification parameters of PCTs and DCTs

The identification of proximal convoluted tubules (PCTs) and DCTs is facilitated by the following parameters:
1. Both are adjacent to renal corpuscles.
2. PCTs contain cells with abundant **lysosomes** (stained dark in both light microscope illustrations).

3. The **apical domain** of PCTs has a prominent **brush border (microvilli)** and **vesicles**. In contrast, the apical domain of DCTs has sparse microvilli and vesicles.
4. Cells lining the PCTs and DCTs contain abundant **mitochondria**.

Electron micrograph courtesy of Wilhelm Kriz, Heidelberg, Germany.

mately 7% of the filtered NaCl. The **distal portion of the DCT** and the **collecting ducts** are permeable to water in the presence of **antidiuretic hormone** (ADH, or vasopressin).

NaCl enters the cell across the apical domain and leaves the cell by an **Na⁺, K⁺-ATPase pump** (Figure 14-16). The reabsorption of NaCl is reduced by **thiazide diuretics** that inhibit the apical domain

transporting mechanism (discussed later).

The active dilution of the tubular fluid initiated in the ascending segments of the loop of Henle continues in the DCT. Because the ascending segment of the loop of Henle is the major site where water and solutes are separated, the excretion of both dilute and concentrated urine requires the normal function of this segment of the loop of Henle.

Figure 14-17. Collecting tubule/duct

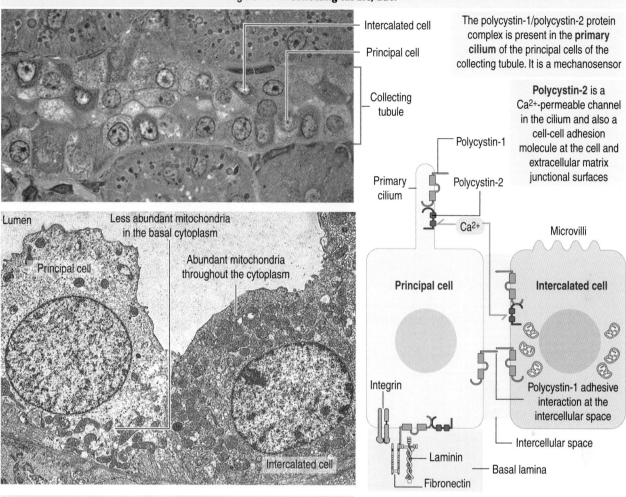

Intercalated cell

Principal cell

Collecting tubule

The polycystin-1/polycystin-2 protein complex is present in the **primary cilium** of the principal cells of the collecting tubule. It is a mechanosensor

Polycystin-2 is a Ca^{2+}-permeable channel in the cilium and also a cell-cell adhesion molecule at the cell and extracellular matrix junctional surfaces

Polycystin-1

Primary cilium

Polycystin-2

Ca^{2+}

Microvilli

Principal cell

Intercalated cell

Integrin

Polycystin-1 adhesive interaction at the intercellular space

Intercellular space

Laminin

Basal lamina

Fibronectin

Lumen

Less abundant mitochondria in the basal cytoplasm

Principal cell

Abundant mitochondria throughout the cytoplasm

Intercalated cell

Collecting tubule

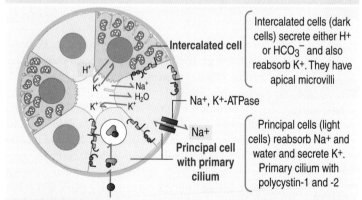

Intercalated cell

Intercalated cells (dark cells) secrete either H+ or HCO_3^- and also reabsorb K+. They have apical microvilli

H^+
K^+
Na^+
H_2O
K^+
K^+

Na+, K+-ATPase

Na+

Principal cell with primary cilium

Principal cells (light cells) reabsorb Na+ and water and secrete K+. Primary cilium with polycystin-1 and -2

Aldosterone (from the zona glomerulosa of the adrenal gland cortex) stimulates the reabsorption of Na+ at the collecting tubule. Retention of Na+ results in water retention, helping to correct hypovolemia (decrease in total body water) and hyponatremia (decrease in total body Na+).

Autosomal dominant polycystic kidney disease (ADPKD) results from mutations in either two genes: *PKD1* and *PKD2,* encoding polycystin-1 and polycystin-2 proteins, which occur predominantly in the cilium of principal cells lining the collecting tubules.

Polycystin-1 is a membrane receptor interacting with proteins, carbohydrates, and lipids. **Polycystin-2** acts as a Ca^{2+}-permeable channel.

Mutations of the *PKD1* gene account for 85% to 90% of cases of ADPKD mutations; mutations of the *PKD2* gene account for 10% of cases. A complete loss of *PKD1* or *PKD2* gene expression results in extensive cystic enlargement of both kidneys. Cysts are derived from the dilation of the collecting tubules and remain connected to the nephron of origin. Nephron segments also show cystic dilations.

Hypertension and renal failure are clinical manifestations.

Collecting tubule/duct

The DCT is linked to the collecting tubule by a **connecting tubule**. The connecting tubule and the collecting tubule (called duct as it increases in diameter) are lined by a cuboidal epithelium composed of two cell types (Figure 14-17):

1. **Principal cells.**
2. **Intercalated cells.**

Principal cells have an apical **primary cilium** and a basolateral domain with moderate infoldings and mitochondria. They reabsorb Na+ and water and secrete K+ in an Na+,K+-ATPase pump-dependent manner.

Figure 14-18. **Urinary bladder and ureter**

Urinary bladder

The **mucosa** of the urinary bladder is folded and lined by the urothelium. Fibroelastic connective tissue of the lamina propria extends into the folds.

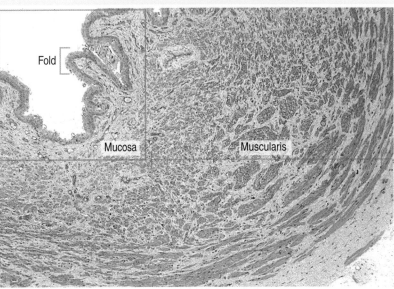

Fold

Mucosa

Muscularis

Urothelium of an **empty urinary bladder**

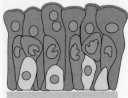

Urothelium of a **urinary bladder filled with urine**

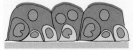

The **muscularis** contains numerous bundles of smooth muscle cells arranged irregularly as outer and inner longitudinal layers and a middle circular layer.

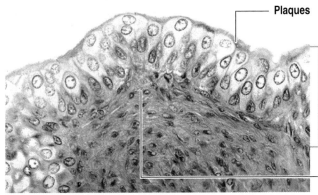

Plaques

Interplaque region
Apical plaque
Cytoskeleton

Urothelium

The transitional nature of the urothelium is determined by its ability to stretch and contract when urine is present or not in the urinary bladder.
Apical plaques generate thickened domains able to adjust to large changes in surface area.

Fibroelastic connective tissue

Plaques are formed by the aggregation of hexagonal intramembranous proteins, called **uroplakins**, to which cytoskeletal proteins are anchored on the cytoplasmic side.

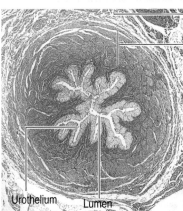

Adventitia

Muscularis

Ureter

The mucosa of the ureter is lined by the urothelium. The mucosa is surrounded by a fibroelastic lamina propria and a muscularis with two to three helical layers of smooth muscle. The ureter is surrounded by an adventitia containing loose connective tissue and adipose tissue.

Urothelium   Lumen

Intercalated cells have apical microvilli and abundant mitochondria and secrete either H^+ or HCO_3^-. Therefore, they are important regulators of acid-base balance. They also reabsorb K^+.

The primary cilium of principal cells is a **mechanosensor** of fluid flow and contents. The ciliary plasma membrane contains membrane-associated proteins **polycystin-1** and **polycystin-2**. Polycystin-1 is regarded as a cell-cell and cell-extracellular matrix adhesive protein. Polycystin-2 acts as a Ca^{2+}-permeable channel.

A mutation of either the gene *PKD1*, encoding polycystin-1, or *PKD2*, encoding polycystin-2, results in **autosomal dominant polycystic kidneys disease** (**ADPKD**). A complete loss of *PKD1* or *PKD2* gene expression results in the formation of massive renal cysts derived from dilated collecting ducts. Blood hypertension and progressive renal failure after the third decade of life are characteristic findings in patients with ADPKD. Renal dialysis and renal transplantation can extend the life span of patients.

Renal interstitium

We noted in Figure 14-15 the presence of vertical stacks of **resident fibroblasts** extending from the loops of Henle to adjacent vasa recta like the rungs of a ladder. **Dendritic cells**, migrating cells of the immune system, are also seen in the renal interstitium.

There are two populations of interstitial cells:
1. **Renal cortical fibroblasts.**
2. **Renal medullary fibroblasts.**

Cortical fibroblasts predominate in the juxtamedullary cortex and produce **erythropoietin**. Synthetic erythropoietin is used in the treatment of anemia resulting from chronic renal failure or cancer chemotherapy. We discussed in Chapter 6, Blood and Hematopoiesis, the mechanism by which erythropoietin stimulates the production of red blood cells.

Medullary fibroblasts, within the inner medulla, are arranged in a ladder-like fashion (see Figure 14-15) and contain lipid droplets in the cytoplasm. They produce glycosaminoglycans and vasoactive prostaglandin E2 that may regulate papillary blood flow.

Activated dendritic cells, expressing class II major histocompatibility antigen, and inflammatory cells (macrophages and lymphocytes) participate in **interstitial nephritis** (tubulointerstitial disease) caused by nephrotoxic drugs (such as heavy metals or hypersensitivity to penicillin) or by an immunologic mechanism (for example, lupus erythematosus).

Excretory passages of urine

The urine released at the openings of the papillary ducts flows from the calyces and pelvis into the ureters and enters the urinary bladder. Peristaltic waves, spreading from the calyces along the ureter, force the urine toward the bladder.

The walls of the ureter and urinary bladder (Figure 14-18) contain folds (rugae). As the bladder fills with urine, the folds flatten and the volume of the bladder increases with minimal rise in intravesical pressure.

The renal calyces, pelvis, ureter, and urinary bladder are lined by the **urothelium**, a pseudotratified epithelium with a transitional configuration in response to distension and contraction. The urothelium is composed of basal cells, intermediate cells and dome-shaped superficial cells, all of them contacting the basal lamina. The epithelium and the subjacent fibroelastic lamina propria are surrounded by **combined helical and longitudinal layers of smooth muscle fibers.**

In the bladder, a mixture of randomly arranged smooth muscle cells form the syncytial **detrusor muscle**. At the neck of the urinary bladder, the muscle fibers form a three-layer (inner longitudinal, middle circular, and outer longitudinal) internal functional sphincter.

Micturition, the process of emptying the urinary bladder, involves the micturition reflex, an automatic spinal cord reflex, and the stimulation of the detrusor muscle by parasympathetic fibers to contract.

Nephrolithiasis is a condition in which kidneys stones, composed of calcium salts, uric acid, or magnesium-ammonium acetate, form by crystallization when urine is concentrated. When the ureter is blocked by a stone, the contraction of the smooth muscle generates severe pain in the flank.

The **male urethra** is 20 cm long and consists of three segments. Upon leaving the urinary bladder, the **prostatic urethra**, lined by transitional epithelium, crosses the prostate gland, continues as a short **membranous urethra** segment, and ends as the **penile urethra**, which is enclosed by the corpus spongiosum of the penis (see Figure 21-12 in Chapter 21, Sperm Transport and Maturation). Both the membranous and penile urethra are lined by pseudostratified or stratified columnar epithelium.

The **female urethra** is 4 cm long and its longitudinally microfolded mucosa is covered by a pseudostratified columnar to stratified squamous epithelium that becomes moderately keratinized stratified squamous epithelium near the urethral meatus. The lamina propria contains elastic fibers and a venous plexus. An **inner smooth muscle layer** and an **external striated muscle layer** (continuous with the internal sphincter) are present in the wall. Additional structural details of the male and female urethra can be found in Chapter 21, Sperm Transport and Maturation, and Chapter 22, Follicle Development and The Menstrual Cycle, respectively.

Regulation of water and NaCl absorption

Several hormones and factors regulate the absorption of water and NaCl (see Box 14-A for a review of terminology related to **osmoregulation**):

1. **Angiotensin II** stimulates NaCl and water reabsorption in the PCT. A decrease in the extracellular fluid volume activates the renin-angiotensin-aldosterone system and increases the concentration of plasma angiotensin II.

2. **Aldosterone**, synthesized by the glomerulosa cells of the adrenal cortex, stimulates the reabsorption of NaCl at the ascending segment of the loop of Henle, the DCT, and the collecting tubule. An increase in the plasma concentration of angiotensin II and K^+ stimulates aldosterone secretion.

3. **Atrial natriuretic peptide**, a 28-amino-acid peptide secreted by atrial cardiocytes (see Figure 12-3 in Chapter 12, Cardiovascular System), has two main functions:

(1) It increases the urinary excretion of NaCl and water.

(2) It inhibits NaCl reabsorption.

The atrial-renal reflex pursues an enhancement of sodium and water excretion by sensing a distended left atrium resulting in a reduction in the secretion of renin and aldosterone.

4. **Antidiuretic hormone**, or **vasopressin**, is the most important hormone in the regulation of water balance. ADH is a small peptide (nine amino acids in

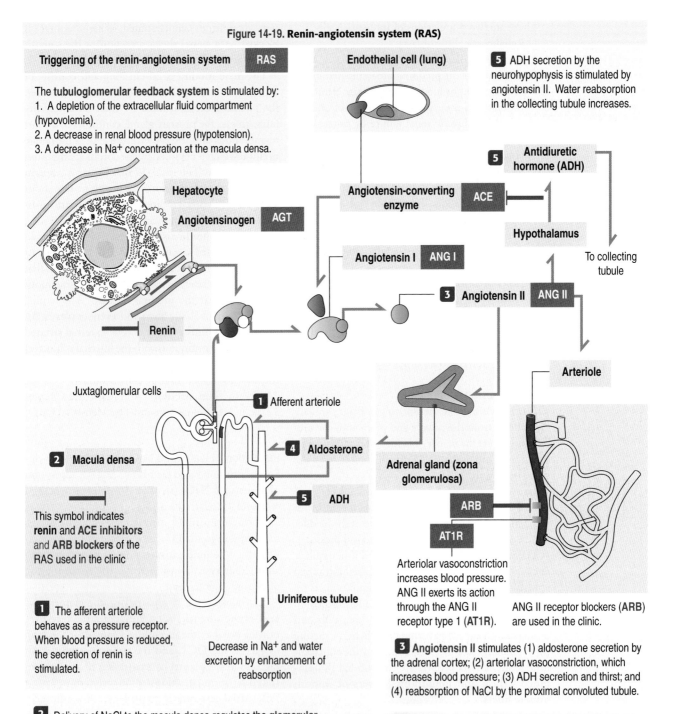

Figure 14-19. Renin-angiotensin system (RAS)

Triggering of the renin-angiotensin system [RAS]

The **tubuloglomerular feedback system** is stimulated by:
1. A depletion of the extracellular fluid compartment (hypovolemia).
2. A decrease in renal blood pressure (hypotension).
3. A decrease in Na^+ concentration at the macula densa.

Hepatocyte

Angiotensinogen [AGT]

Renin

Juxtaglomerular cells

[1] Afferent arteriole

[2] Macula densa

[4] Aldosterone

[5] ADH

This symbol indicates **renin** and **ACE inhibitors** and **ARB blockers** of the RAS used in the clinic

[1] The afferent arteriole behaves as a pressure receptor. When blood pressure is reduced, the secretion of renin is stimulated.

Uriniferous tubule

Decrease in Na^+ and water excretion by enhancement of reabsorption

[2] Delivery of NaCl to the macula densa regulates the **glomerular filtration rate (GFR)** by a process known as tubuloglomerular feedback.
The tubuloglomerular feedback mechanism links changes in NaCl concentration (sensed by the macula densa) with the control of afferent and efferent arteriolar resistance to autoregulate renal blood flow and the GFR.

Endothelial cell (lung)

Angiotensin-converting enzyme [ACE]

Angiotensin I [ANG I]

[3] **Angiotensin II** [ANG II]

Adrenal gland (zona glomerulosa)

[ARB]

[AT1R]

Arteriolar vasoconstriction increases blood pressure. ANG II exerts its action through the ANG II receptor type 1 (**AT1R**).

ANG II receptor blockers (**ARB**) are used in the clinic.

[5] ADH secretion by the neurohypophysis is stimulated by angiotensin II. Water reabsorption in the collecting tubule increases.

[5] **Antidiuretic hormone (ADH)**

Hypothalamus

To collecting tubule

Arteriole

[3] Angiotensin II stimulates (1) aldosterone secretion by the adrenal cortex; (2) arteriolar vasoconstriction, which increases blood pressure; (3) ADH secretion and thirst; and (4) reabsorption of NaCl by the proximal convoluted tubule.

[4] **Aldosterone**, a steroid hormone secreted by the zona glomerulosa of the adrenal cortex, reduces the excretion of NaCl by stimulating its reabsorption by the thick ascending limb of the loop of Henle, the distal convoluted tubule, and the collecting tubule.

length) synthesized by neuroendocrine cells located within the **supraoptic** and **paraventricular nuclei** of the **hypothalamus**.

When the extracellular fluid volume decreases (hypovolemia), ADH increases the permeability of the collecting tubule to water, thereby increasing water reabsorption. When ADH is not present, the collecting tubule is impermeable to water. ADH has little effect on the urinary excretion of NaCl.

Diabetes insipidus is a disorder associated with a low production of ADH (central diabetes insipidus) or a failure of the kidneys to respond to circulating ADH (nephrogenic diabetes insipidus). In the absence of ADH, water cannot be reabsorbed normally

• **Osmolality** is the concentration of solutes in body fluids. Alterations in osmolality depend on the gain or loss of water or on the loss or gain of osmoles (for example, glucose, urea, and salts). Plasma osmolality is kept normalized by the excretion of excess water, recovery of lost water, or by normalization of solute levels in the body.

• **Molarity** and **molality** refer to the concentration of a solute in a solution. The units of molarity are mol solute/L solution. The units of molality are mol solute/kg solvent. Osmolality and osmolarity represent the number of moles of solute particles in a solution (for example, Na^+ and Cl^- separately) instead of moles of compound in solution (for example, $NaCl$).

• **Osmosis** is the passive diffusion of water (the solvent) across a membrane from an area of low solute concentration to an area of high solute concentration. Osmotic equilibrium is reached when the amount of solute is equal on both sides of a membrane and the influx of water stops. Osmosis depends on the number of free dissolved particles without distinction between different molecular species (for example, Na^+ and Cl^-).

• **Osmotic pressure** is an indicator of how much water a compartment will draw into it through osmosis. Osmolarity and osmolality of the compartments on either side of a membrane determine the osmotic pressure of a compartment.

• **Plasma membrane pumps and channels** ensure that solutes are not distributed evenly on either side of a membrane as water does. If solutes distributed evenly, a concentration gradient would not exist to drive osmosis.

• **Effective osmoles**. A solute such as urea is not an effective osmole because it does not create osmotic pressure. Solutes such as Na^+, K^+, and Cl^- are effective osmoles. Pumps and channels keep Na^+ outside of cells and K^+ inside of cells as effective osmoles.

• **Aquaporins**. The permeability of cells to water is facilitated by plasma membrane water channels called aquaporins. Different tissues have variable amounts of aquaporins and the cells may be more or less permeable to water than others. Antidiuretic hormone determines the insertion of aquaporins in the collecting duct, increasing its permeability to water.

to correct hyperosmolality, and **hypernatremia** (high levels of Na^+ in plasma), **polyuria** (excessive volume of urine and frequency of urination), and **polydipsia** (thirst and increasing drinking) occur.

In **diabetes mellitus,** the concentration of glucose in plasma is abnormally elevated. Glucose overwhelms the reabsorptive capacity of the PCT, and intratubular glucose levels increase. Acting as an effective osmole, intratubular glucose hampers water reabsorption even in the presence of ADH.

Osmotic diuresis is responsible for **glucosuria** (presence of glucose in urine), polyuria, and polydipsia in the diabetic patient.

No glucosuria is observed in patients with diabetes insipidus.

Renin-angiotensin system (RAS)

The RAS is a significant component of the **tubuloglomerular feedback system**, essential for the maintenance of systemic arterial blood pressure when there is a reduction in the vascular volume.

A reduction in vascular volume results in a decrease in the rate of glomerular filtration and the amount of filtered NaCl. A reduction in filtered NaCl is sensed

by the macula densa, which triggers renin secretion and the production of angiotensin II, a potent vasoconstrictor.

The **tubuloglomerular feedback system** consists of:

1. A **glomerular component**: The **juxtaglomerular cells** predominate in the muscle cell wall of the afferent glomerular arteriole but are also present in smaller number in the efferent glomerular arteriole. Juxtaglomerular cells synthesize, store, and release **renin**. Activation of sympathetic nerve fibers results in the increased secretion of renin.

2. A **tubular component**: The **macula densa** mediates renin secretion after sensing the NaCl content in the incoming urine from the thick ascending segment of the limb of Henle. When the delivery of NaCl to the macula densa decreases, renin secretion is enhanced. Conversely, when NaCl increases, renin secretion decreases.

The **RAS** consists of the following components (Figure 14-19):

1. **Angiotensinogen (AGT)**, a circulating protein in plasma produced by the liver.

2. The **juxtaglomerular cells**, the source of the proteolytic enzyme **renin**, which converts **angiotensinogen** to **angiotensin I (ANG I)**, a decapeptide with no known physiologic function.

3. The **angiotensin-converting enzyme (ACE)**, a product of pulmonary and renal **endothelial cells**, which converts **angiotensin I** to the octapeptide **angiotensin II (ANG II)**.

ANG II has several important functions:

1. It stimulates the secretion of aldosterone by the adrenal cortex.

2. It causes vasoconstriction, which, in turn, increases blood pressure. ANG II binds to **ANG II receptor type 1 (AT1R)**. ANG II receptor blockers (ARB) are extensively used in the clinic to regulate elevated blood pressure.

3. It enhances the reabsorption of NaCl by the PCT of the nephron.

4. It stimulates ADH release.

Aldosterone acts primarily on **principal cells of the collecting tubule** and secondarily on the thick ascending segment of the loop of Henle to increase the entry of NaCl across the apical membrane. As with all steroid hormones, aldosterone enters the cell and binds to a cytosolic receptor. The aldosterone-receptor complex enters the nucleus and stimulates gene activity required for the reabsorption of NaCl.

An activated RAS is a major risk factor of cardiovascular and renal disease. **Inhibitors of RAS (renin and ACE inhibitors and ARB)** are extensively used in the clinic. The RAS is also closely associated to metabolic diseases. Inhibitors of RAS have shown to prevent the onset of type 2 diabetes in high risk populations.

Figure 14–20. Countercurrent multiplier and exchanger

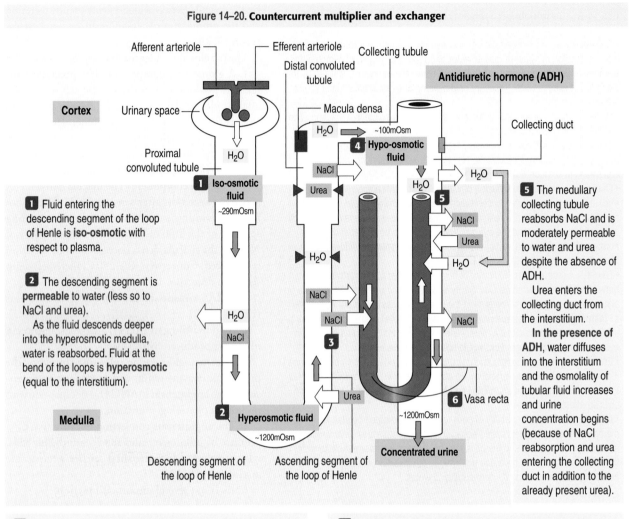

1 Fluid entering the descending segment of the loop of Henle is **iso-osmotic** with respect to plasma.

2 The descending segment is **permeable** to water (less so to NaCl and urea).
As the fluid descends deeper into the hyperosmotic medulla, water is reabsorbed. Fluid at the bend of the loops is **hyperosmotic** (equal to the interstitium).

3 The ascending segment is **impermeable** to water but permeable to NaCl and urea.
NaCl is passively reabsorbed (the concentration of luminal NaCl is greater than the interstitial NaCl concentration) and urea diffuses into the tubular fluid (urea concentration in the lumen is less than that in the interstitium).
Dilution of the tubular fluid occurs and urine becomes gradually **hypo-osmotic** with respect to plasma.
Note that NaCl and urea (and other solutes) in the interstitial fluid provide the driving force for reabsorption.
Urea is produced in the liver as a product of protein metabolism and enters the nephron by glomerular filtration.

4 The distal convoluted tubule and part of the collecting tubule reabsorb NaCl (under the influence of **aldosterone**) but are impermeable to urea.
In the absence of ADH, the collecting duct is impermeable to water (NaCl is reabsorbed without water) and the osmolality is reduced. The fluid entering the collecting ducts is **hypo-osmotic with respect to plasma**.

6 The **vasa recta** are a capillary network that removes, in a flow-dependent manner, excess of water and solutes continuously added to the interstitium by the nephron segments.

5 The medullary collecting tubule reabsorbs NaCl and is moderately permeable to water and urea despite the absence of ADH.
Urea enters the collecting duct from the interstitium.
In the presence of ADH, water diffuses into the interstitium and the osmolality of tubular fluid increases and urine concentration begins (because of NaCl reabsorption and urea entering the collecting duct in addition to the already present urea).

Countercurrent multiplier and exchanger

The kidneys regulate water balance and are the major site for the release of water from the body. Water is also lost by evaporation from the skin and the respiratory tract and from the gastrointestinal tract (fecal water and diarrhea).

Water excretion by the kidneys occurs independently of other substances, such as Na^+, Cl^-, K^+, H^+, and urea. The kidneys excrete either **concentrated** (hyperosmotic) or **diluted** (hypo-osmotic) urine.

ADH regulates the volume and osmolality of the urine without modifying the excretion of other solutes. The primary action of ADH is to increase the permeability of the collecting tubule to water. An additional action is to increase the permeability of the collecting ducts at the medullary region to urea.

Figure 14-20 summarizes the essential steps of urine formation and excretion. Briefly:

1. The fluid from the proximal convoluted tubules entering the loop of Henle is **iso-osmotic** with respect to plasma.

2. The **descending segment of the loop of Henle is highly permeable to water and, to a lesser extent, to NaCl.** As the fluid descends into the hyperosmotic

Figure 14-21. **Diuretics: Mechanism of action**

Diuretics are drugs that increase the output of urine (**diuresis**) by acting on specific membrane transport proteins. The common effect of diuretics is the inhibition of Na$^+$ reabsorption by the nephron leading to an increase in the excretion of Na$^+$ (**natriuresis**).

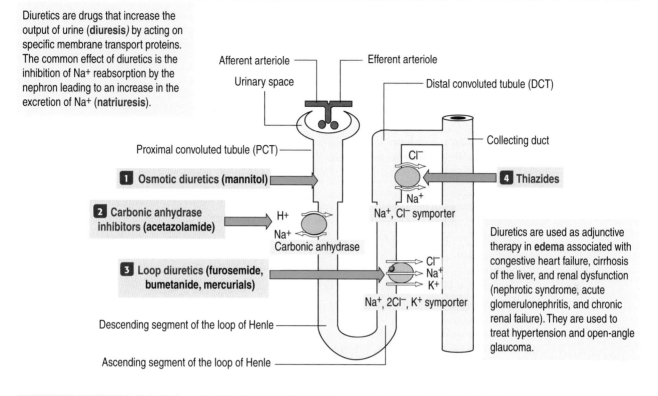

Diuretics are used as adjunctive therapy in **edema** associated with congestive heart failure, cirrhosis of the liver, and renal dysfunction (nephrotic syndrome, acute glomerulonephritis, and chronic renal failure). They are used to treat hypertension and open-angle glaucoma.

1 Osmotic diuretics (mannitol)

Osmotic diuresis affects the transport of water across the epithelial cells lining the **PCT and thin descending segment of the loop of Henle**. Osmotic diuretics enter the nephron by glomerular filtration and generate an osmotic pressure gradient.

Osmotic diuretics do not inhibit a specific membrane transport protein. When urea and glucose are present in abnormally high concentrations (diabetes mellitus or renal diseases), they can behave as osmotic diuretics.

2 Carbonic anhydrase inhibitors (acetazolamide)

Carbonic acid inhibitors reduce Na$^+$ reabsorption by their effects on carbonic anhydrase, present mainly in the PCT. The Na$^+$,H$^+$ antiporter in the apical membrane of PCT cells depends on H$^+$ for Na$^+$ exchange.

H$^+$ is secreted in the tubular fluid where it combines with filtered HCO$_3^-$ to form H$_2$CO$_3$. H$_2$CO$_3$ is hydrolyzed to CO$_2$ and H$_2$O by carbonic anhydrase located on the apical membrane of the PCT to facilitate CO$_2$ and H$_2$O reabsorption. Carbonic anhydrase inhibitors reduce the reabsorption of HCO$_3^-$. Because the amount of secreted H$^+$ depends on Na$^+$, inhibition of carbonic anhydrase causes a decrease in Na$^+$, H$_2$O, and HCO$_3^-$ reabsorption, leading to natriuresis.

3 Loop diuretics (furosemide, bumetanide, mercurials)

Loop diuretics are the most potent diuretics available to inhibit Na$^+$ reabsorption by the **thick ascending segment of the loop of Henle** by blocking the Na$^+$, 2Cl$^-$, K$^+$ symporter located in the apical membrane of the epithelial cells. Loop diuretics also perturb the process of countercurrent multiplication (the ability to dilute or concentrate urine).

4 Thiazides (chlorothiazide)

Thiazide diuretics inhibit Na$^+$ reabsorption in the **initial portion of the DCT** by blocking the Na$^+$, Cl$^-$ symporter present in the apical cell membrane. Because water cannot cross this portion of the nephron and this is the site of urine dilution, thiazides reduce the ability to dilute the urine by inhibition of NaCl reabsorption.

interstitium, water and NaCl equilibrate and the tubular fluid becomes **hyperosmotic**.

3. When the fluid reaches the **bend of the loop**, its composition is **hyperosmotic**.

4. The **ascending limb of the loop of Henle is impermeable to water**. The concentration of NaCl in the lumen, greater than in the interstitium, is reabsorbed and enters the descending (arterial) portion of the vasa recta. Therefore, the fluid leaving this

tubular segment is **hypo-osmotic**. This segment of the nephron is called the **diluting segment**.

5. The distal convoluted tubule and cortical portions of the collecting tubule reabsorb NaCl. In the **absence** of ADH, water permeability is low. In the **presence** of ADH, water diffuses out of the collecting tubule into the interstitium and enters the ascending (venous) segment of the vasa recta. The process of urine concentration starts.

6. The **medullary regions** of the collecting tubule reabsorb urea. A small amount of water is reabsorbed and the urine is concentrated.

A relevant function of the loop of Henle is to produce and maintain and interstitial osmotic gradient that increases from the renal cortex (~290 mOsm/kg) to the tip of the medulla (~1200 mOsm/kg). The mechanism by which the loop of Henle generates the hypertonic medullary osmotic gradient is known as **countercurrent multiplication**.

This designation is based on:

1. The **flow of fluid in opposite directions (countercurrent flow)** within the two parallel limbs of the loop of Henle.

2. The **differences in permeability** of sodium and water in the descending and ascending segments.

3. The **active reabsorption of sodium** in the thick ascending segment.

Note that:

1. The fluid flows **into the medulla** in the descending segment and **out of the medulla** in the ascending segment.

2. The countercurrent flow within the descending and ascending segments of the loop of Henle "multiplies" the osmotic gradient between the tubular fluid in the descending and ascending segments.

3. A **hyperosmotic interstitium** is generated by the reabsorption of NaCl in the **ascending segment** of the loop of Henle. This is an important step for the uriniferous tubule to excrete hyperosmotic urine with respect to plasma.

4. The concentration of NaCl increases progressively with increasing depth into the medulla. The highest concentration of NaCl is at the level of the papilla. This **medullary gradient** results from the accumulation of NaCl reabsorbed by the process of countercurrent multiplication.

5. The **vasa recta** transport nutrients and oxygen to the uriniferous tubules. They also remove excess water and solutes, continuously added by the countercurrent multiplication process. An increase in blood flow through the vasa recta dissipates the medullary gradient.

Clinical significance: Mechanism of action of diuretics

The main function of diuretics is to increase the excretion of Na^+ by inhibiting Na^+ reabsorption by the nephron. By this mechanism, Na^+ excretion takes water that is eliminated in urine.

The effect of diuretics depends on the volume of the extracellular fluid (ECF) compartment and the effective circulating volume (ECV). If the ECV decreases, the glomerular filtration rate (GFR) decreases, the load of filtered Na^+ is reduced, and the reabsorption of Na^+ by the PCT increases.

With these events in mind, you realize that the action of diuretics acting on the DCT can be compromised by the presence of lower concentrations of Na^+ when the ECV is reduced.

Figure 14-21 provides a summary of the mechanism of action of osmotic diuretics, carbonic anhydrase inhibitors, loop diuretics, and thiazide diuretics.

Osmotic diuretics inhibit the reabsorption of water and solutes in the PCT and descending thin limb of the loop of Henle.

Carbonic anhydrase inhibitors inhibit Na^+, HCO_3^-, and water reabsorption in the PCT.

Loop diuretics inhibit the reabsorption of NaCl in the thick ascending limb of the loop of Henle. About 25% of the filtered load of Na^+ can be excreted by the action of loop diuretics.

Thiazide diuretics inhibit the reabsorption of NaCl in the DCT.

Essential concepts | **Urinary System**

• Functions of the urinary system:

(1) Filtration of the blood and excretion of waste metabolic products (from proteins, urea; from nucleic acids, uric acid; from muscle, creatinine; from hemoglobin metabolism, urobilin, which gives urine its color).

(2) Regulation of water and electrolyte balance.

(3) Regulation of arterial blood pressure (by maintaining blood volume and producing renin, a key initiator of the angiotensin-aldosterone cascade).

(4) Regulation of erythropoiesis (through erythropoietin, produced by renal interstitial cells). Chronic renal diseases are associated with anemia because of a decrease in the production of erythropoietin.

(5) Production of active vitamin D.

• Each kidneys consists of a cortex and a medulla.

The cortex is subdivided into outer cortex and juxtamedullary cortex.

The medulla is subdivided into outer medulla and inner medulla.

• The organization of the renal vascular system is key for understanding the structure and function of the kidneys.

After entering the kidneys, the renal artery divides into interlobar arteries, running through the renal columns along the sides of the renal pyramids. At the corticomedullary junction, interlobar arteries change from a vertical to a horizontal direction to form the arcuate arteries. Vertical branches of the arcuate arteries enter the renal cortex and become interlobular

arteries. You are now ready to visualize the boundaries of a renal lobe and a renal lobule.

A **renal lobe** is a combined cortical- medullary structure: It has a triangular shape, the medullary pyramid, formed by the outer and inner medullary regions. The triangle is capped by the corresponding cortex.

The base of the triangle is the renal capsule; the apex of the triangle is the papilla; the lateral boundaries are the renal columns (of Bertin), the site where interlobar arteries reside. A minor calyx collects urine dripping from the area cribrosa (perforated area) of each papilla. The area cribrosa is the opening site of multiple papillary ducts.

A **renal lobule** resides in the cortex. It is defined as the portion of the cortex between two adjacent interlobular arteries. The axis

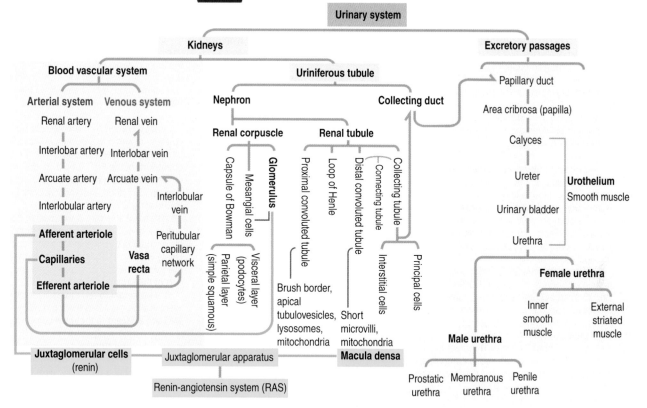

of the lobule is occupied by a medullary ray (of Ferrein) consisting of a single collecting duct (of Bellini) receiving the fluid of the correponding intralobular nephrons. As you can see, renal lobules are subcomponents of the renal lobes.

We continue our discussion with the renal vascular system. The vertical interlobular arteries that entered the cortex branch several times to form afferent arterioles. Each afferent arteriole forms a glomerular capillary that continues not as a venule, but as an efferent arteriole. This arteriolar-capillary-arteriolar arrangement is called the glomerular or arterial portal system.

One last and important point: The glomerular efferent arterioles give rise to two different vascular networks:

(1) A peritubular capillary network, derived from the efferent arterioles of cortical nephrons.

(2) The vasa recta (straight vessels), derived from the efferent arterioles of juxtamedullary nephrons. The vasa recta consists of a descending arteriolar-capillary component and an ascending capillary-venous component, alongside the descending and ascending limbs of the loops of Henle, respectively. This vascular-tubular arrangement is essential for understanding the countercurrent multiplier and exchange mechanism of urine formation.

• The **uriniferous tubule** consists of two com-

ponents of different embryologic origin:
(1) The nephron.
(2) The collecting tubule/duct.
The nephron consists of two components:
(1) The renal corpuscle.
(2) The renal tubule.
The renal corpuscle (of Malpighi) is formed by the capsule of Bowman investing the glomerular capillaries (the glomerulus).
The renal tubule consists of:
(1) The proximal convoluted tubule (PCT).
(2) The loop of Henle.
(3) The distal convoluted tubule (DCT), which drains into the collecting tubule.

The collecting tubule can be found in the cortex (cortical collecting tubules), the outer medulla (outer medullary collecting tubule), and inner medulla (inner medullary collecting tubule).

Depending on the distribution of renal corpuscles, nephrons can be either cortical nephrons (with short loops of Henle) or juxtamedullary nephrons (with long loops of Henle).

The capsule of Bowman has two layers:
(1) A parietal layer (simple squamous epithelium supported by a basement membrane).
(2) A visceral layer attached to the wall of the glomerular capillaries. The visceral layer consists of branched epithelial cells, the podocytes.
The space between the parietal and visceral

layers of the capsule of Bowman is the urinary space or Bowman's space. The urinary space is continuous with the lumen of the PCT, the initial segment of the renal tubule. At this region, the urinary pole, the simple squamous epithelium of the parietal layer of the capsule of Bowman, becomes simple cuboidal with apical microvilli (brush border). This is the lining of the PCT.

The glomerulus consists of three components:
(1) The glomerular capillaries, lined by fenestrated endothelial cells.
(2) The mesangium, consisting of mesangial cells producing the mesangial matrix.
(3) The podocytes.
Note that renal corpuscle and glomerulus are not synonyms: A renal corpuscle includes the capsule of Bowman and the glomerulus. The designation glomerulus does not include the capsule of Bowman.

Mesangial cells are embedded in an extracellular matrix present between glomerular capillaries. Aggregates of mesangial cells can be seen outside the glomerulus (extraglomerular mesangial cells). Mesangial cells are pericyte-like cells with contractile and phagocytic properties.

Mesangial cells participate indirectly in glomerular filtration by providing mechanical support to glomerular capillaries, turning over glomerular basal lamina components, and secreting vasoactive substances (prostaglandins and endothelins).

- An understanding of the structure of the **glomerular filtration barrier** is essential for grasping the clinical characteristics of proteinuria syndromes.

The filtration barrier has three components:
(1) The fenestrated endothelial cells of the glomerular capillaries.
(2) The dual glomerular basal lamina (produced by endothelial cells and podocytes). It is known as glomerular basement membrane (GBM).
(3) The podocytes, including a filtration slit diaphragm between the interdigitating foot processes of podocytes.

- The **podocyte filtration slit diaphragm** has a relevant role in glomerular filtration. Defects in some of its protein components lead to **hereditary proteinuria syndromes.**

The filtration slit diaphragm is supported by intracellular F-actin present in pedicels, small podocyte cytoplasmic processes anchored to the dual basal lamina.

The C-terminal intracellular segment of the protein **nephrin** is attached to F-actin by podocin, ZO-1, and CD2AP proteins. The N-terminal extracellular segment of nephrin interacts with another nephrin molecule (homophilic interaction) extending from an adjacent pedicel to form the backbone of the slit diaphragm.

The *nephrin* gene is mutated in **congenital nephrotic syndrome**. Affected children display massive proteinuria and edema.

Podocyte injury of congenital, hereditary, and acquired origin can cause glomerular diseases. Acquired glomerular diseases can be of immune and non-immune origin.

Congenital nephrotic syndrome is an example of a congenital cause of podocyte injury.

Hereditary causes of podocyte injury include mutations in genes expressing podocyte-specific proteins (such as podocin and β1 integrin subunit). The most characteristic feature is foot process effacement, the loss of interdigitating pedicels contacting the GBM.

Most glomerular diseases caused by podocyte injury are acquired, initiated by immune mechanisms (such as deposits of antibodies against glomerular components). Examples are membranoproliferative glomerulonephritis and immunoglobulin A nephropathy (Berger's disease).

- The GBM contains type IV collagen, a molecule directly involved in the pathogenesis of three renal diseases:
(1) **Goodpasture's syndrome**, an autoimmune disorder consisting in progressive glomerulonephritis and pulmonary hemorrhage caused by α3 autoantibodies targeting the glomerular and alveolar basal lamina.
(2) **Alport's syndrome,** an inherited X-linked recessive nephropathy, predominant in males, and involving mutations of the *α5 chain* gene. Alport's syndrome is associated with deafness and ocular symptoms, hematuria and progressive glomerulonephritis leading to renal failure (end-stage renal disease, ESRD).
(3) **Benign familial hematuria**, caused by a dominant inherited mutation of the *α4 chain* gene, which does not lead to renal failure as seen in ESRD.

- **Glomerulonephritis** defines an inflammatory process of the renal corpuscle.

Antibody-antigen complexes circulating in blood trapped in the glomerular filtration barrier contribute to glomerular damage. Antibody-antigen complexes are produced by autoimmune diseases (systemic lupus erythematosus) or bacterial and viral infections (streptococci and hepatitis B virus).

Acute proliferative glomerulonephritis observed in children is reversible. It is caused by proliferation of endothelial and mesangial cells in the presence of neutrophils.

Rapid progressive (crescentic) glomerulonephritis consists in proliferation of parietal cells of the capsule of Bowman and infiltration of macrophages forming a crescent-like mass within the glomerulus. This form of glomerulonephritis is observed in Goodpasture syndrome.

- The **juxtaglomerular apparatus** consists of:
(1) The macula densa, an Na⁺ sensor present in the initial portion of the DCT.
(2) The extraglomerular mesangial cells, a supporting cushion of the macula densa located at the vascular pole of the renal corpuscle.
(3) The renin-producing juxtaglomerular cells, modified smooth muscle cells of the wall of the afferent arteriole.

The juxtaglomerular apparatus is one of the components of the tubuloglomerular feedback mechanism participating in the autoregulation of renal blood flow and glomerular filtration.

- The **PCT**, a continuation of the urinary space (or Bowman's capsular space), is the major reabsorption component of the nephron.

The PCT is lined by a simple cuboidal epithelium with well-developed apical microvilli (brush border) and tubulovesicles and lysosomes involved in the endocytosis and breakdown of peptides into amino acids.

A basolateral domain displays plasma membrane infoldings and interdigitations that lodge numerous mitochondria. Mitichondria provide adenosine triphosphate (ATP) for active ion transport mediated by an Na⁺, K⁺–activated ATPase pump.

A paracellular transport pathway (across tight junctions) mobilizes, by osmosis, water into the lateral intercellular space. A transcellular transport pathway is involved in the reabsorption of solutes such as NaCl, peptides, and glucose.

Fanconi syndrome is a renal hereditary (primary) or acquired (secondary) disease in which amino acids and glucose are not reabsorbed and are found in urine. The cause appears to be a defect in the cellular energy metabolism decreasing the levels of ATP by the impaired activity of the Na⁺, K⁺–ATPase pump.

- The **loop of Henle** consists of a descending limb and an ascending limb.

Each limb is formed by a thick segment (lined by simple cuboidal epithelium) and a thin segment (lined by simple squamous epithelium).

The descending thick segment is a continuation of the proximal convoluted tubule. The ascending thick segment is continuous with the distal convoluted tubule.

The U-shaped thin segment forms most of the loop in juxtamedullary nephrons deep in the medulla. Recall that the loop of Henle of cortical nephrons penetrates up to the outer medulla.

- The **DCT** is lined by a simple cuboidal epithelium with a less developed apical brush border when compared with the lining epithelium of the PCT. Tubulovesicles and lysosomes are less prominent. The basolateral domain is infolded and mitochondria are abundant at this location.

A distinctive structure is the macula densa, a cluster of cells located at the junction of the ascending thick segment of the loop of Henle with the DCT. The macula densa faces the extraglomerular mesangial cells and is part of the juxtaglomerular apparatus.

It is important to remember for histologic identification purposes that both PCT and DCT are adjacent to the renal corpuscle.

- The **collecting tubules** (also called ducts) originate in the cortical medullary rays. Remember that a medullary ray is the axis of a renal lobule, a cortical subdivision bordered laterally by adjacent interlobular arteries, branches of the arcuate artery. Cortical medullary rays join others to form wider papillary ducts in the papilla. Papillary ducts open on the surface of the papilla forming a perforated area cribrosa.

The lining epithelium is simple cuboidal. The outline of the epithelial cells is very distinct. The epithelium consists of two cell types:
(1) Principal cells, light cells with an apical nonmotile primary cilium.
(2) Intercalated cells, dark cells with apical microvilli and abundant mitochondria.

Principal cells respond to aldosterone, a mineralocorticoid produced by cells of the zona glomerulosa of the adrenal cortex.

The apical nonmotile primary cilium of principal cells is a mechanosensor receiving signals from the fluid contents in the tubular lumen. Ciliary bending by fluid flow or mechanical stimulation induce Ca²⁺ release from intracellular storage sites. The ciliary plasma membrane contains the polycystin-1/polycystin-2 protein complex. Polycystin-2 acts as a Ca²⁺-permeable channel.

Autosomal dominant polycystic kidneys disease (ADPKD) results from mutations in either two genes: *PKD1*, encoding polycystin-1, or *PKD2,* encoding polycystin-2. Extensive cystic enlargement of both kidneys results from a complete loss of *PKD1* or *PKD2* gene expression. Blood hypertension preceding progressive renal failure is observed in patients with ADPKD. Renal dialysis and renal transplantation are the indicated treatments.

- Renal interstitial cells, mainly fibroblasts and dendritic cells, can be found in the renal cortex and medulla.
There are two populations of interstitial cells:
  (1) Renal cortical fibroblasts.
  (2) Renal medullary fibroblasts.
Cortical fibroblasts predominate in the juxtamedullary cortex and produce erythropoietin. Synthetic erythropoietin is used in the treatment of anemia resulting from chronic renal failure or cancer chemotherapy.
Medullary fibroblasts are arranged in a ladder-like fashion and contain lipid droplets in the cytoplasm. They produce glycosaminoglycans and vasoactive prostaglandin E2 that may regulate papillary blood flow.
Activated dendritic cells, expressing class II major histocompatibility antigen, and inflammatory cells (macrophages and lymphocytes) participate in interstitial nephritis (tubulointerstitial disease) caused by nephrotoxic drugs (such as heavy metals or hypersensitivity to penicillin) or by an immunologic mechanism (for example, lupus erythematosus).

- The **excretory passages of urine** include:
  (1) The renal calyces and pelvis.
  (2) Ureters.
  (3) Urinary bladder, lined by a transitional epithelium (urothelium) supported by a lamina propria and surrounded by spiral and longitudinally arranged layers of smooth muscle.
  (4) The male urethra consists of three segments: prostatic urethra (lined by transitional epithelium), membranous urethra, and penile urethra (both lined by pseudostratified-to-stratified columnar epithelium. The penile urethra is surrounded by the corpus spongiosum.
The female urethra is lined sequentially by a columnar pseudostratified to stratified squamous epithelium to low keratinized stratified squamous epithelium. The wall of the female urethra consists of an inner smooth muscle layer surrounded by an external striated muscle layer.

- The **renin-angiotensin system (RAS)** is essential for the maintenance of systemic blood pressure when there is a reduction in the blood volume or pressure. The system is triggered by a tubuloglomerular feedback mechanism originating in the juxtaglomerular apparatus:
  (1) The tubular component is the Na^+-sensing macula densa.
  (2) The glomerular component is the renin-producing juxtaglomerular cells.
The immediate objectives of the tubuloglomerular feedback mechanism are the regulation of the glomerular filtration rate (by controlling afferent and efferent arteriolar resistance; remember the glomerular arterial portal arrangement already discussed) and the release of renin from juxtaglomerular cells to produce angiotensin II.
The major steps leading to the production of angiotensin II and its activities are:
  (1) Renin converts angiotensinogen (AGT, produced in hepatocytes) to angiotensin I (ANGI).
  (2) Angotensin-converting enzyme (ACE, produced by pulmonary and renal endothelial cells) converts angiotensin I to angiotensin II (ANGII).
  (3) ANG II has several important functions:
  - It stimulates the secretion of aldosterone by the adrenal cortex.
  - It causes vasoconstriction, which, in turn, increases blood pressure. ANG II binds to ANG II receptor type 1 (AT1R). ANG II receptor blockers (ARB) are extensively used in the clinic to regulate elevated blood pressure.
  - It enhances the reabsorption of NaCl by the PCT of the nephron.
  - It stimulates ADH release.
An activated RAS is a major risk factor of cardiovascular and renal disease. Inhibitors of RAS (renin and ACE inhibitors and ARB) are extensively used in the clinic.

- The loop of Henle creates an osmotic gradient causing water to flow out the collecting tubule into the surrounding interstitial tissue.
A **countercurrent multiplication** in the loop of Henle maintains high solute concentration in the renal medulla.
Countercurrent multiplication occurs because:
  (1) The thin descending segment of the loop of Henle is permeable to water but has low permeability to salt.
  (2) The thin ascending segment is permeable to salt but not to water.
  (3) The thick ascending segment reabsorbs salt by active transport and is impermeable to water.
As you can see, countercurrent multiplication results in increasing salt concentration in the medullary interstitium with the descent of the loop of Henle segment. When ADH increases water permeability of the collecting duct, water can flow down its osmotic gradient into the salty medullary interstitium. Water and some salt must find their way back from the salty interstitium to the bloodstream to reduce plasma osmolality.
The parallel arrangement of the vasa recta with the U-shaped loop of Henle enables the absorption of solute and water by **countercurrent exchange**:
  (1) The arterial descending segment of the vasa recta absorbs some salt.
  (2) The venous ascending segment of the vasa recta reabsorbs water.
In this way, the loop of Henle–dependent countercurrent multiplication does not accumulate salt and water indefinitely in the interstitium with the help of the vasa recta–dependent countercurrent exchange.

- **Diuretics** are drugs that increase the output of urine (diuresis) by acting on specific membrane transport proteins. Inhibition of Na^+ resorption by the nephron leads to an increase in the excretion of Na^+ (natriuresis) and water.
Diuretics are used as adjunctive therapy in edema associated with congestive heart failure, cirrhosis of the liver, and renal dysfunction (nephrotic syndrome, acute glomerulonephritis, and chronic renal failure). They are used to treat hypertension and open-angle glaucoma.
There are different types of diuretics:
  (1) Osmotic diuretics inhibit the reabsorption of water and solutes in the PCT and descending thin limb of the loop of Henle.
  (2) Carbonic anhydrase inhibitors prevent Na^+, $HCO3^-$, and water reabsorption in the PCT.
  (3) Loop diuretics inhibit the reabsorption of NaCl in the thick ascending limb of the loop of Henle. About 25% of the filtered load of Na^+ can be excreted by the action of loop diuretics.
  (4) Thiazide diuretics inhibit the reabsorption of NaCl in the DCT.

15. Upper Digestive Segment

Swallowing, digestion, and absorption take place through the digestive or alimentary tube, a 7- to 10-meter hollow muscular conduit. The digestive process converts food material into a soluble form easy to absorb by the small intestine. The elimination of insoluble residues and other materials is the function of the large intestine. Histologically, the digestive tube consists of four major layers: (1) an inner mucosal layer encircling the lumen, (2) a submucosal layer, (3) a muscularis externa layer, and (4) a serosal/adventitial layer. The inner mucosal layer shows significant variations along the digestive tube. It is subdivided into three components: (1) an epithelial layer, (2) a connective tissue lamina propria, and (3) a smooth muscle muscularis mucosae. This chapter focuses on the histologic features of the oral cavity, the esophagus, and the stomach with a particular emphasis on the mechanisms that affect the function of these specific segments of the alimentary system.

Mouth, or oral cavity

The oral cavity is the entrance to the digestive tube and the oral epithelium, including aggregates of lymphoid tissue. It represents the primary barrier to pathogens. **Ingestion**, **partial digestion**, and **lubrication** of the food, or **bolus**, are the main functions of the mouth and its associated **salivary glands**. We study the salivary glands in Chapter 17, Digestive Glands.

The **mouth**, or **oral cavity**, includes the lips, cheeks, teeth, gums (gingivae), tongue, uvula, and palate. The various regions of the oral cavity are lined by three types of mucosae with structural variations:

1. **Lining mucosa** (lips, cheeks, ventral surface of the tongue, soft palate, mouth floor, and alveolar mucosa).

2. **Masticatory mucosa** (gingiva and hard palate).

3. **Specialized mucosa** (dorsal surface of the tongue).

There are three transition sites of the oral mucosa:

1. The **mucocutaneous junction** (between the skin and the mucosa of the lips).

2. The **mucogingival junction** (between the gingiva and alveolar mucosa), involving a transition from the keratinized stratified squamous epithelium of the gingiva, firmly attached to the periosteum by collagen bundles, to the nonkeratinized epithelium of the alveolar mucosa, supported by a loose lamina propria with elastic fibers.

3. The **dentogingival junction** (between the mucosa of the gingiva and the enamel of the tooth), a

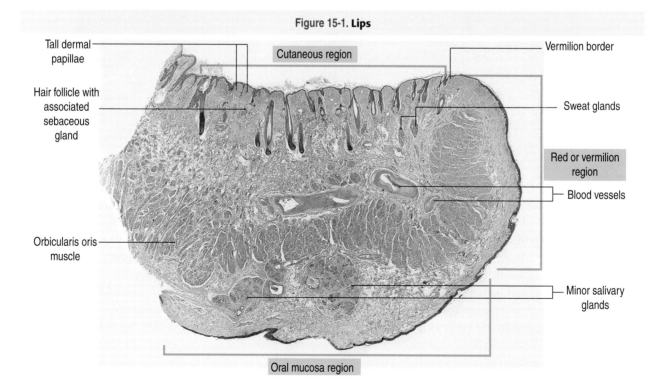

Figure 15-1. Lips

Tall dermal papillae

Cutaneous region

Vermilion border

Hair follicle with associated sebaceous gland

Sweat glands

Red or vermilion region

Blood vessels

Orbicularis oris muscle

Minor salivary glands

Oral mucosa region

Figure 15-2. Tongue

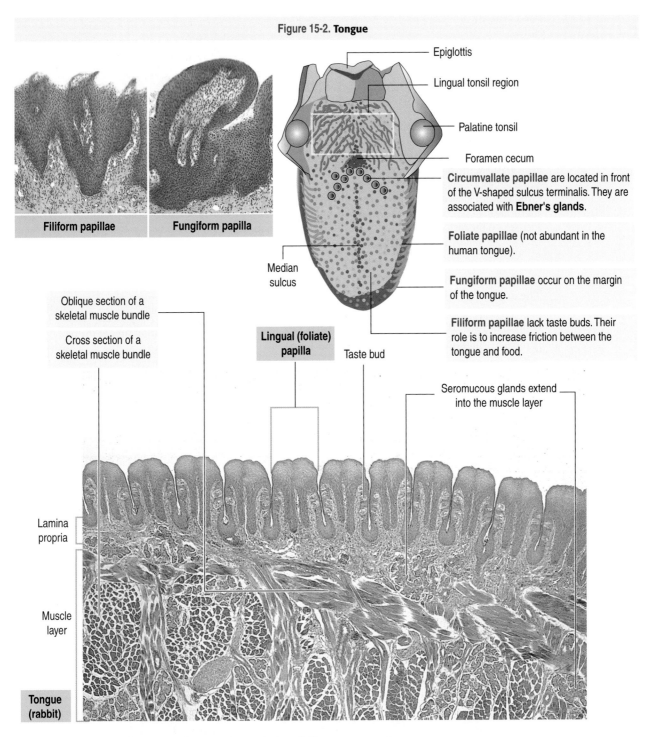

Filiform papillae

Fungiform papilla

Epiglottis

Lingual tonsil region

Palatine tonsil

Foramen cecum

Circumvallate papillae are located in front of the V-shaped sulcus terminalis. They are associated with **Ebner's glands.**

Foliate papillae (not abundant in the human tongue).

Fungiform papillae occur on the margin of the tongue.

Filiform papillae lack taste buds. Their role is to increase friction between the tongue and food.

Median sulcus

Oblique section of a skeletal muscle bundle

Cross section of a skeletal muscle bundle

Lingual (foliate) papilla

Taste bud

Seromucous glands extend into the muscle layer

Lamina propria

Muscle layer

Tongue (rabbit)

sealing point that prevents periodontal diseases.

Except for the teeth, the mouth is lined by a **stratified squamous epithelium**, with a submucosa, consisting of loose connective tissue, blood vessels and nerves, present only in certain regions (cheeks, lips and part of the hard palate). In some regions, such as the gingiva and parts of the hard palate, the oral mucosa is firmly attached to the periosteum of the subjacent bone, an arrangement called **mucoperiosteum**. The oral mucosa lacks a muscularis mucosa.

Lips

The **lips** consist of three regions:

1. The **cutaneous region.**
2. The **red or vermilion region.**
3. The **oral mucosa region.**

The cutaneous region is covered by thin skin with tall dermal papillae (**keratinized stratified squamous epithelium with hair follicles and sebaceous and sweat glands**). The red or vermilion region is lined by a stratified squamous epithelium supported by connective tissue containing blood vessels responsible for the red color of this region.

Note in Figure 15-1 that no salivary glands are present in the mucosa of the vermilion region. This region drys out and becomes cracked in cold weather. A sharp vermilion border separates the skin from the vermilion region.

The oral mucosa region, that is continuous with the mucosa of the cheeks and gums, displays minor salivary glands. The muscle tissue seen in Figure 15-1 is the orbicularis oris.

The stratified squamous epithelium covering the inner surface of the lips and cheeks is nonkeratinized and supported by a dense lamina propria (**lining mucosa**) and a submucosa, closely bound by connective tissue fibers to the underlying skeletal muscles.

Gingiva, hard, and soft palate

Masticatory mucosa covers the hard palate and gingivae and sustains abrasion during food mastication. The **gums**, or **gingivae**, are similar to the red region of the lips, except on the free margin, where significant keratinization is seen. The lamina propria of the gums binds tightly to the periosteum of the alveolar processes of the maxillae and mandible and to the periodontal membrane. The gums lack submucosa or glands.

The **hard palate** is lined by a keratinizing stratified squamous epithelium similar to that of the free margins of the gums. A submucosa is present in the midline but absent in the area adjacent to the gums. Collagenous fibers in the submucosa bind the mucosa to the periosteum of the hard palate, enabling the mucosa to resists shear forces and compression. Areas of fat and glandular tissue cushion the mucosa to protect nerves and blood vessels of the hard palate.

The **soft palate** and **uvula** are lined by a nonkeratinized stratified squamous epithelium extending into the oropharynx where it becomes continuous with the pseudostratified ciliated columnar epithelium of the upper respiratory tract. The submucosa is loose and contains abundant mucous and serous glands. Skeletal muscle fibers are present in the soft palate and uvula.

Tongue

The anterior two thirds of the tongue consist of a core mass of **skeletal muscle** oriented in three directions: **longitudinal**, **transverse**, and **oblique**. The posterior one third displays aggregations of lymphatic tissue, the **lingual tonsils**.

The dorsal surface of the tongue is covered by a **specialized mucosa** consisting of a **nonkeratinized stratified squamous epithelium** supported by a lamina propria associated with the muscle core of the tongue. **Serous** and **mucous glands** extend across the lamina propria and the muscle. Their ducts open into the **crypts** and **furrows** of the **lingual tonsils** and **circumvallate papillae**, respectively.

The dorsal surface of the tongue contains numerous mucosal projections called **lingual papillae** (Figure 15-2). Each **lingual papilla** is formed by a highly vascular connective tissue core and a covering layer of stratified squamous epithelium.

According to their shape, lingual papillae can be divided into four types:

1. **Filiform papillae** (narrow conical), the most abundant.
2. **Fungiform papillae** (mushroom-shaped).
3. **Circumvallate papillae** (wall-like).
4. **Foliate papillae** (leaf-shaped), rudimentary in humans but well developed in rabbits and monkeys.

Taste buds are found in all lingual papillae except the filiform papillae. Taste buds are barrel-shaped epithelial structures containing chemosensory cells called **gustatory receptor cells**. Gustatory receptor cells are in synaptic contact with the terminals of the gustatory nerves.

Circumvallate papillae are located in the posterior part of the tongue, aligned **in front of the sulcus terminalis**. The circumvallate papilla occupies a recess in the mucosa and, therefore, it is surrounded by a **circular furrow** or **trench**.

Serous glands, or **Ebner's glands**, in the connective tissue, in contact with the underlying muscle, are associated with the circumvallate papilla. **The ducts of Ebner's glands open into the floor of the circular furrow.**

The sides of the circumvallate papilla and the facing wall of furrow contain several taste buds. Each **taste bud**, depending on the species, consists of 50 to 150 cells, with its narrow apical ends extending into a **taste pore**.

A taste bud has three cell components (Figure 15-3):

1. **Taste receptor cells.**
2. **Supporting cells** (or immature taste cells).
3. **Precursor cells** (or basal cells).

Taste receptor cells have a life span of 10 to 14 days. **Precursor cells give rise to supporting cells (or immature taste cells) which, in turn, become mature taste receptor cells.** The basal portion of a taste receptor cell makes contact with an **afferent nerve terminal** derived from neurons in the sensory ganglia of the **facial**, **glossopharyngeal**, and **vagus** nerves.

Sweet, **sour**, **bitter**, and **salty** are the four classic taste sensations. A fifth taste is **umami** (the taste enhanced by monosodium glutamate).

A specific taste sensation is generated by specific

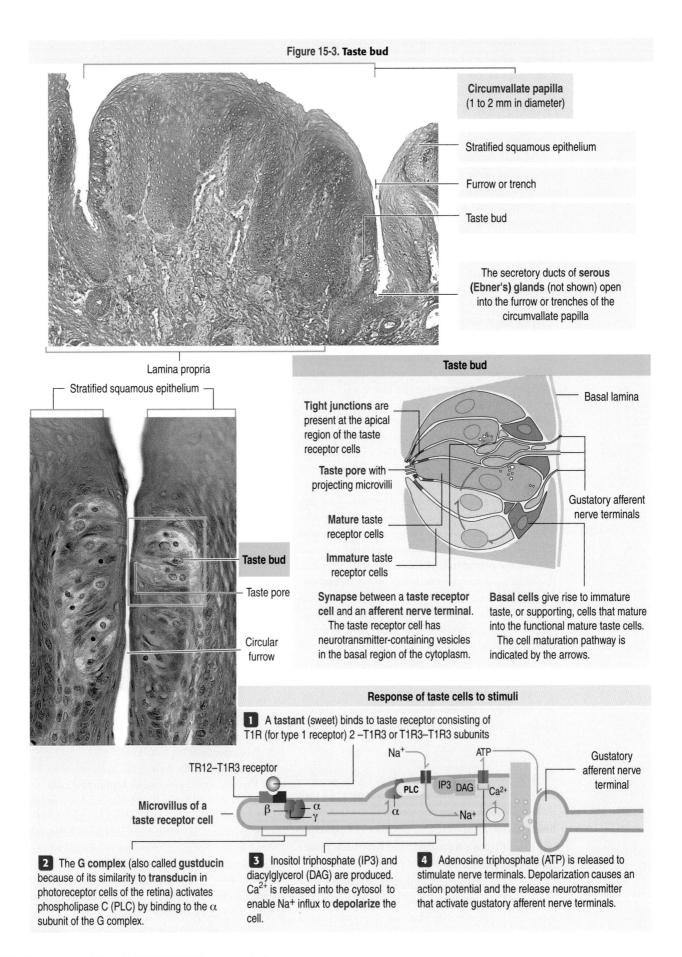

Figure 15-3. **Taste bud**

Circumvallate papilla (1 to 2 mm in diameter)

Stratified squamous epithelium

Furrow or trench

Taste bud

The secretory ducts of **serous (Ebner's) glands** (not shown) open into the furrow or trenches of the circumvallate papilla

Lamina propria

Stratified squamous epithelium

Taste bud

Taste pore

Circular furrow

Taste bud

Basal lamina

Tight junctions are present at the apical region of the taste receptor cells

Taste pore with projecting microvilli

Mature taste receptor cells

Immature taste receptor cells

Gustatory afferent nerve terminals

Synapse between a **taste receptor cell** and an **afferent nerve terminal**. The taste receptor cell has neurotransmitter-containing vesicles in the basal region of the cytoplasm.

Basal cells give rise to immature taste, or supporting, cells that mature into the functional mature taste cells. The cell maturation pathway is indicated by the arrows.

Response of taste cells to stimuli

1 A **tastant** (sweet) binds to taste receptor consisting of T1R (for type 1 receptor) 2 –T1R3 or T1R3–T1R3 subunits

TR12–T1R3 receptor

Na^+

ATP

Gustatory afferent nerve terminal

Microvillus of a taste receptor cell

PLC

IP3   DAG

Ca^{2+}

β   α
γ
α

Na^+

2 The **G complex** (also called **gustducin** because of its similarity to **transducin** in photoreceptor cells of the retina) activates phospholipase C (PLC) by binding to the α subunit of the G complex.

3 Inositol triphosphate (IP3) and diacylglycerol (DAG) are produced. Ca^{2+} is released into the cytosol to enable Na^+ influx to **depolarize** the cell.

4 Adenosine triphosphate (ATP) is released to stimulate nerve terminals. Depolarization causes an action potential and the release neurotransmitter that activate gustatory afferent nerve terminals.

taste receptor cells. The **facial nerve** carries the five taste sensations; the **glossopharyngeal nerve** carries sweet and bitter sensations.

When a sweet **tastant** diffuses through the taste pore of a taste bud, it interacts with **type 1 receptors** (designated **T1R**) present in the **apical microvilli** of the **taste receptor cells**. Taste receptors can form heterodimers (T1R2+T1R3) or homodimers (T1R3+T1R3).

T1Rs are linked to the G-protein α, β, and γ subunit complex, called **gustducin** (see Figure 15-3). Binding of the α subunit of the G-protein complex to **phospholipase C (PLC)** triggers the production of the second messengers **inositol triphosphate (IP3)** and **diacylglycerol (DAG)** that activate ion channels in the taste receptor cells.

An influx of Na+ within taste cells causes depolarization of the taste receptor cells. An increase in intracellular Ca2+, released from intracellular storage sites, triggers the release into the **extracellular space** of **adenosine triphosphate (ATP)** and **neurotransmitters** at the synapses with gustatory afferent nerve terminals.

In **summary**, taste receptor cells can detect and discriminate sweet, bitter or umami tastants by cell depolarization, gustducin–dependent Ca2+ and Na+ signaling and release of ATP and neurotransmitters.

The salty taste of Na+ is detected by direct influx of Na+ through membrane ion channels to depolarize the plasma membrane. Some taste receptor cells respond to only one of the basic taste substances. Others are sensitive to more than one taste substance.

Tooth

In the adult human, dentition consists of 32 permanent teeth. The 16 upper teeth are embedded in **alveolar processes** of the maxilla. The lower 16 teeth are embedded in similar alveolar processes of the mandible.

The permanent dentition is preceded by a set of 20 **deciduous teeth**, also called **milk** or **baby teeth**. Deciduous teeth appear at about 6 months of age and the entire set is present by age 6 to 8 years. The deciduous teeth are replaced between ages 10 and 12 by the 32 permanent teeth. This replacement process ends at about age 18.

Each of the several types of teeth has a distinctive shape and function: **incisors** are specialized for cutting; **canines,** for puncturing and holding; and **molars,** for crushing.

Each tooth consists of a **crown** and either single or multiple **roots** (Figure 15-4). The crown is covered by highly calcified layers of **enamel** and **dentin**. The outer surface of the root is covered by another calcified tissue called **cementum**.

The dentin forms the bulk of the tooth and contains a central chamber filled with soft tissue, the **pulp**. The pulp chamber opens at the **apical foramen** into the bony alveolar process by the **root canal**. Blood vessels, nerves, and lymphatics enter and leave the pulp chamber through the apical foramen. Myelinated nerve fibers run along with the blood vessels.

Tooth development

The ectoderm, cranial neural crest, and mesenchyme contribute to the development of the tooth (Figure 15-5). **Ameloblasts** derive from the **ectoderm**. **Odontoblasts** derive from the **cranial neural crest**. **Cementocytes** derive from the **mesenchyme**.

Secreted signaling molecules, **activin βA**, **fibroblast growth factor**, and **bone morphogenetic proteins**, mediate the interaction between the dental epithelium and the mesenchyme during tooth morphogenesis. Figure 15-5 illustrates the relevant steps of tooth development.

Odontoblasts

Odontoblasts differentiate from mesenchymal cells of the dental papilla under the control of the inner enamel epithelium. The dental papilla becomes the dental pulp (see Figure 15-5).

A layer of odontoblasts is present at the periphery of the dental pulp in the adult tooth (Figure 15-6). Odontoblasts are active secretory cells that synthesize and secrete type I collagen and noncollagenous material, the organic components of the **dentin**.

The **odontoblast** is a columnar epithelial-like cell located at the **inner side** of the dentin, in the pulp cavity (see Figure 15-6).

The apical cell domain is embedded in **predentin**, a nonmineralized layer of dentin-like material. The apical domain projects a main **apical cell process** that becomes enclosed within a canalicular system just above the **junctional complexes** linking adjacent odontoblasts.

A well-developed **rough endoplasmic reticulum** and **Golgi apparatus** as well as **secretory granules** are found in the apical region of the odontoblast. The secretory granules contain **procollagen**. When procollagen is released from the odontoblast, it is enzymatically processed to **tropocollagen**, which aggregates into **type I collagen** fibrils.

Predentin is the layer of dentin adjacent to the odontoblast cell body and processes. Predentin is **nonmineralized** and consists mainly of collagen fibrils that will become covered (mineralized) by hydroxyapatite crystals in the dentin region. A demarcation **mineralization front** separates predentin from dentin.

Dentin consists of 20% organic material, mainly type I collagen; 70% inorganic material, mainly crystals of hydroxyapatite and fluoroapatite; and 10% water.

Figure 15-4. **Longitudinal section of the tooth**

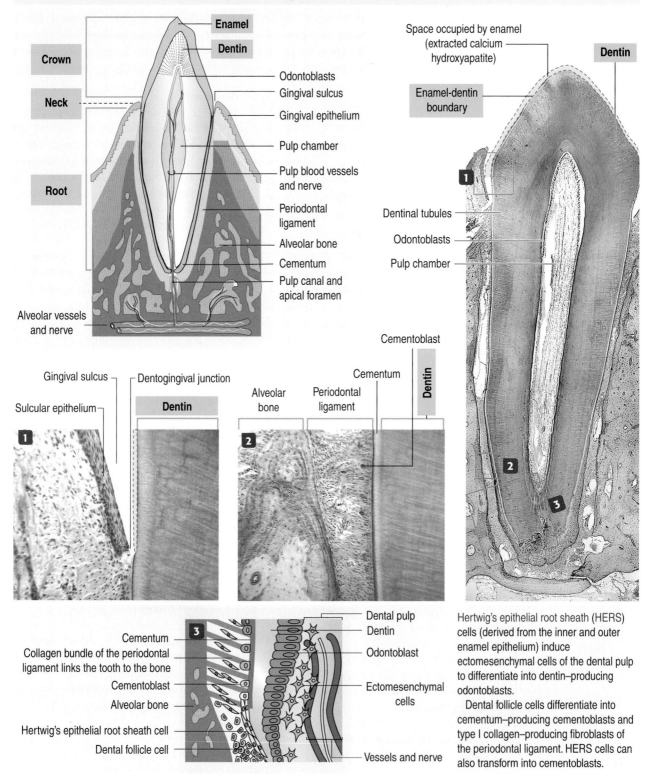

Hertwig's epithelial root sheath (HERS) cells (derived from the inner and outer enamel epithelium) induce ectomesenchymal cells of the dental pulp to differentiate into dentin–producing odontoblasts.

Dental follicle cells differentiate into cementum–producing cementoblasts and type I collagen–producing fibroblasts of the periodontal ligament. HERS cells can also transform into cementoblasts.

Coronal dentin dysplasia (also known as **dentin dysplasia, type II**) is a rare inherited autosomal defect characterized by abnormal development of dentin, extremely short roots (rootless teeth), and obliterated pulp chambers.

Dental pulp

The dental **pulp** consists of blood vessels, nerves, and lymphatics surrounded by fibroblasts and mesenchyme-like extracellular elements. Blood vessels (arterioles) branch into a capillary network that,

Figure 15-5. Stages of tooth development

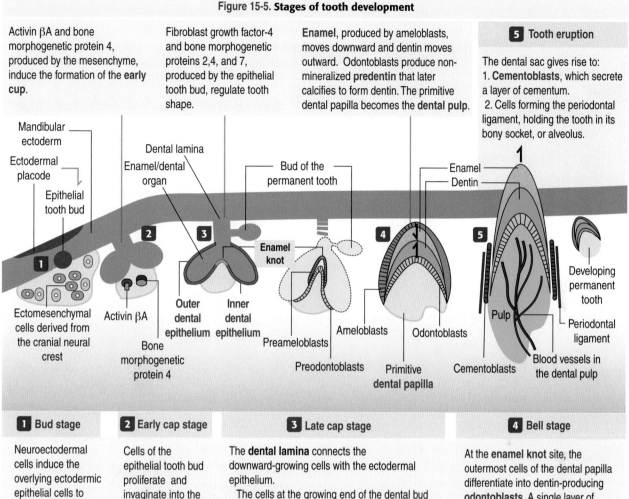

Activin βA and bone morphogenetic protein 4, produced by the mesenchyme, induce the formation of the **early cup**.

Fibroblast growth factor-4 and bone morphogenetic proteins 2,4, and 7, produced by the epithelial tooth bud, regulate tooth shape.

Enamel, produced by ameloblasts, moves downward and dentin moves outward. Odontoblasts produce non-mineralized **predentin** that later calcifies to form dentin. The primitive dental papilla becomes the **dental pulp**.

5 **Tooth eruption**

The dental sac gives rise to:
1. **Cementoblasts**, which secrete a layer of cementum.
2. Cells forming the periodontal ligament, holding the tooth in its bony socket, or alveolus.

Mandibular ectoderm
Ectodermal placode
Epithelial tooth bud
Dental lamina
Enamel/dental organ
Bud of the permanent tooth
Enamel
Dentin

Ectomesenchymal cells derived from the cranial neural crest
Activin βA
Bone morphogenetic protein 4
Outer dental epithelium
Inner dental epithelium
Enamel knot
Preameloblasts
Preodontoblasts
Ameloblasts
Primitive dental papilla
Odontoblasts
Pulp
Cementoblasts
Blood vessels in the dental pulp
Developing permanent tooth
Periodontal ligament

1 Bud stage	**2** Early cap stage	**3** Late cap stage	**4** Bell stage
Neuroectodermal cells induce the overlying ectodermic epithelial cells to proliferate and form the epithelial tooth bud. There are 20 buds, one for each of the deciduous teeth.	Cells of the epithelial tooth bud proliferate and invaginate into the underlying mesoderm.	The **dental lamina** connects the downward-growing cells with the ectodermal epithelium. The cells at the growing end of the dental bud form a caplike structure. The epithelial tooth bud is lined by an **outer** and **inner dental epithelium**. The bud of the permanent tooth develops from the dental lamina and remains dormant. The **enamel knot** signals tooth development.	At the **enamel knot** site, the outermost cells of the dental papilla differentiate into dentin-producing **odontoblasts**. A single layer of enamel-secreting **ameloblasts** develops in the inner dental epithelium portion of the enamel knot.

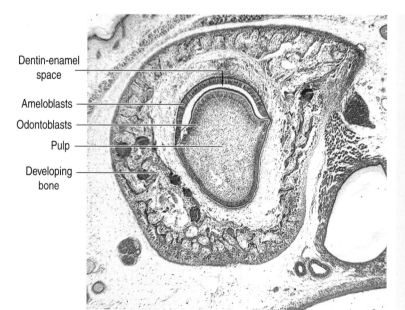

Dentin-enamel space
Ameloblasts
Odontoblasts
Pulp
Developing bone

Tooth development proceeds in three morphologic stages: **bud**, **cup**, and **bell**. The primordium is called **dental** or **enamel organ**.

The earliest indication of tooth development is at day 11 of embryogenesis. The formation of **ectodermal placodes** (local thickenings of the oral epithelium of the first branchial arch) marks the initiation site. Neural crest and mesenchymal cells, forming the **ectomesenchyme**, have odontogenic potential.

The first genes to be expressed in the oral epithelium encode the **transcription factors Lhx-6** and **Lhx-7** (Lim-homeobox domain genes). Expression of several genes in the ectomesenchyme marks the sites of tooth initiation.

Ectodermal dysplasias, affecting the development of ectodermal placodes, cause multiple missing teeth (**oligodontia**) and small misshapen teeth.

Figure 15-6. **Odontoblasts**

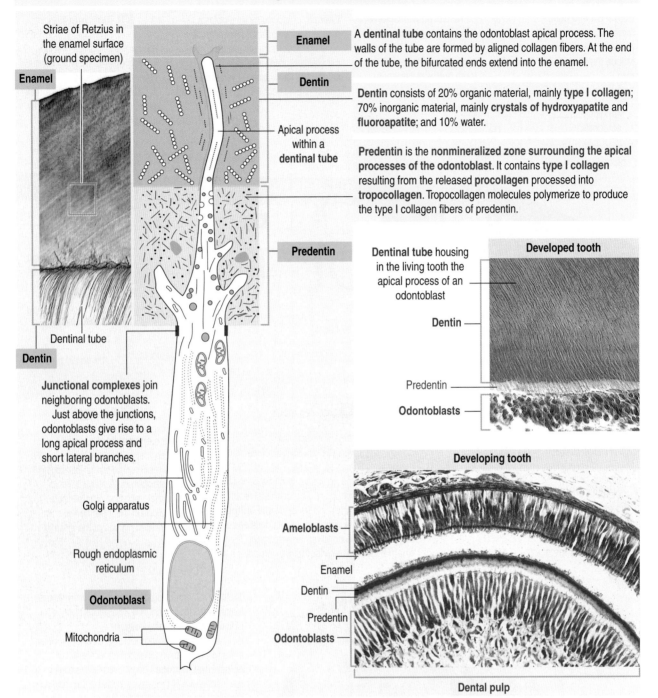

Striae of Retzius in the enamel surface (ground specimen)

Enamel

Dentin

Dentinal tube

Enamel

A **dentinal tube** contains the odontoblast apical process. The walls of the tube are formed by aligned collagen fibers. At the end of the tube, the bifurcated ends extend into the enamel.

Dentin

Dentin consists of 20% organic material, mainly **type I collagen**; 70% inorganic material, mainly **crystals of hydroxyapatite** and **fluoroapatite**; and 10% water.

Apical process within a **dentinal tube**

Predentin is the **nonmineralized zone surrounding the apical processes of the odontoblast**. It contains **type I collagen** resulting from the released **procollagen** processed into **tropocollagen**. Tropocollagen molecules polymerize to produce the type I collagen fibers of predentin.

Predentin

Dentinal tube housing in the living tooth the apical process of an odontoblast

Developed tooth

Dentin

Predentin

Odontoblasts

Junctional complexes join neighboring odontoblasts. Just above the junctions, odontoblasts give rise to a long apical process and short lateral branches.

Golgi apparatus

Rough endoplasmic reticulum

Odontoblast

Mitochondria

Developing tooth

Ameloblasts

Enamel

Dentin

Predentin

Odontoblasts

Dental pulp

together with nerves, form a neurovascular bundle beneath the basal cell domain of the odontoblasts in a cell-free zone (of Weil) of the dental pulp.

An inflammation in the pulp causes swelling and pain. Because there is no space for swelling in the pulp cavity, the blood supply is suppressed by compression, leading rapidly to the death of the pulp cells.

Pulp stones are single or multiple calcified deposits found in the dental pulp, close to the orifice of the pulp chamber or within the root canals. Pulp stones reduce the number of cells within the dental pulp

and interfere with the enlargement of the root canal during endodontic treatment.

Periodontium

The periodontium supports and surrounds the tooth. It consists of the following components:
1. Cementum.
2. Periodontal ligament.
3. Bone of the alveolus or socket.
4. The sulcus epithelium, part of the gingiva facing the tooth.

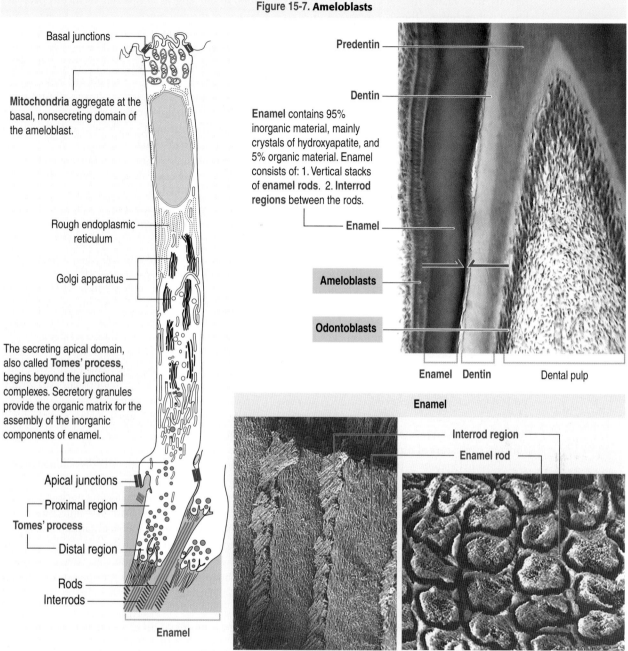

Figure 15-7. **Ameloblasts**

Basal junctions

Mitochondria aggregate at the basal, nonsecreting domain of the ameloblast.

Rough endoplasmic reticulum

Golgi apparatus

The secreting apical domain, also called **Tomes' process**, begins beyond the junctional complexes. Secretory granules provide the organic matrix for the assembly of the inorganic components of enamel.

Apical junctions

Proximal region

Tomes' process

Distal region

Rods

Interrods

Enamel

Predentin

Dentin

Enamel contains 95% inorganic material, mainly crystals of hydroxyapatite, and 5% organic material. Enamel consists of: 1. Vertical stacks of **enamel rods**. 2. **Interrod regions** between the rods.

Enamel

Ameloblasts

Odontoblasts

Enamel   Dentin   Dental pulp

Enamel

Interrod region

Enamel rod

Scanning electron micrographs from Nanci A: Oral Histology, 7th edition, St. Louis, Mosby, 2008.

The **cementum** is an avascular bonelike mineralized tissue covering the outer surface of the root. Like bone, the cementum consists of calcified collagenous fibrils and trapped osteocyte-like cells called **cementocytes**. Note that the tooth has three mineralized components: enamel, dentin and cementum.

The cementum meets the enamel at the **cementoenamel junction** and separates the crown from the root at the **neck region** of the tooth. The outermost layer of the cementum is uncalcified and is produced by **cementoblasts** in contact with the **periodontal ligament**, a collagen- and fibroblast-rich and vascularized suspensory ligament holding the tooth in the sockets of the alveolar bone (see Figure 15-4). The

strength of the periodontal ligament fibers gives teeth mobility and strong bone attachment, both useful in orthodontic treatment.

Ameloblasts

Ameloblasts are enamel-producing cells present only during tooth development. Ameloblasts are no longer present following tooth eruption.

The ameloblast (Figure 15-7) is a polarized columnar cell with mitochondria and a nucleus present in the basal region of the cell. The supranuclear region contains numerous cisternae of rough endoplasmic reticulum and Golgi apparatus.

Beyond apical junctional complexes joining contiguous ameloblasts, the apical domain displays a broad cell extension, **Tomes' process**, in proximity to the calcified enamel matrix. Tomes' processes are fully developed during the secretory stage of the ameloblast. They have abundant secretory granules containing glycoproteins that regulate the nucleation of carbonated apatite crystals, growth and organization of the enamel.

Electron microscopic examination shows that the basic building units of the enamel matrix are thin undulated **enamel rods** separated by an **interrod region** with a structure similar to that of the enamel rods but with its crystals oriented in a different direction. Each rod is coated with a thin layer of organic matrix, called the **rod sheath** (see Figure 15-7).

The **enamel** is the hardest substance found in the body. About 95% of the enamel is composed of crystals of hydroxyapatite (carbonated hydroxyapatite); less than 5% is protein and water. The high mineral content is responsible for the extreme hardness of enamel, a property that enables enamel to withstand mechanical force during mastication. The underlying layer of dentin is more resilient and protects the structural integrity of enamel.

The newly secreted enamel has a high content of protein (about 30%), whose concentration decreases to 1% during enamel mineralization. The extracellular matrix of the developing enamel (**amelogenesis**) contains two classes of proteins: **amelogenin** (90%) and **nonamelogenins** (10%), including **enamelin** and **ameloblastin**.

Amelogenin (25 kd) is the major constituent, unique to the developing enamel. It controls the calcification of the enamel. Enamelin and ameloblastin are minor components. A 32 kd proteolytic fragment of enamelin (186 kd) has strong affinity to adsorb enamel crystals. Ameloblastin (70 kd) has calcium–binding properties.

Dental caries develop when the supportive layer of dentin is destroyed and hydroxyapatite of the enamel dissolves.

Amelogenesis imperfecta is an X chromosome–linked inherited disease affecting the synthesis of amelogenin required for the formation of the tooth enamel; affected enamel does not attain its normal thickness, hardness, and color. **Autosomal-dominant amelogenesis imperfecta** is caused by a mutation of the *enamelin* gene.

Pathology: Non-neoplastic and neoplastic lesions of the oral mucosa

Non-neoplastic lesions of the oral mucosa include:

1. **Reactive fibroepithelial hyperplasia** following traumatic injury or irritation of the gingiva and palate caused by dentures.

2. **Herpes simplex viral infection** can cause ulceration of the gingiva and palate. **Verrucous papillary lesions** of the oral mucosa are seen in human papillomavirus infection.

3. **Hairy** (papillate) **leukoplakia** in the lateral margins of the tongue occurs in HIV-positive patients and in individual with immuno-suppressed conditions as opportunistic Epstein-Barr viral infection. Koilocytosis (perinuclear halo) in cells of the stratum spinosum of the stratified squamous epithelium and intranuclear viral inclusions are characteristic.

Neoplastic lesions of the oral mucosa include:

1. **Squamous cell carcinoma** represents the predominant oral malignant condition seen in adults with predominant localizations in the lateral tongue and the floor of the mouth. Squamous cell carcinoma generally starts from a dysplasia, in situ carcinoma or a proliferative verrucous leukoplakia (a white patch or plaque that cannot be rubbed off).

2. **Oral melanomas** are generally localized in palate and gingiva and can be in situ or multiple invasive lesions with irregular borders and ulcerated. Most melanomas are detected in advanced stages.

3. **Non-Hodgkin's lymphomas** are observed in the mucosa-associated lymphoid tissue (Waldeyer's ring) in patients with HIV-infection. Epstein-Barr virus is frequently detected in the lesions.

4. **Kaposi's sarcoma** is seen in palate and gingiva in the form of macular or nodular lesions, in association with cutaneous localization. The lesion consists in the proliferation of endothelial cells of blood vessels. Vascular spaces are lined by elongated cells expressing CD34 antigen and with moderate nuclear atypia. A clinical correlation exists with HIV infection.

5. **Neural tumors** include schwannoma, an encapsulated tumor containing Schwann cells; single or multiple neurofibromas, also consisting of Schwann cells but not limited by a capsule; and traumatic neuroma, usually present in the tongue.

General organization of the digestive tube

Although we study each segment of the digestive or alimentary tube separately, it is important to discuss first the general organization of the tube to understand that each segment does not function as an independent unit.

We start with the general histologic features of the digestive tube by indicating that, except for the oral cavity, the digestive tube has a uniform histologic organization.

This organization is characterized by distinct and significant structural variations reflecting changes in functional activity.

After the oral cavity, the digestive tube is differentiated into four major organs: **esophagus**, **stomach**, **small intestine**, and **large intestine**. Each of these

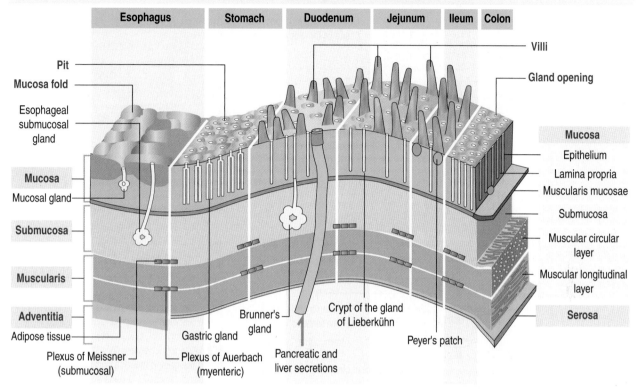

Figure 15-8. Overall histologic organization of the digestive tube

organs is made up of four concentric layers (Figure 15-8):

1. The **mucosa**.
2. The **submucosa**.
3. The **muscularis**.
4. The **adventitia**, or **serosa**.

The mucosa has three components:

1. A **lining epithelium**.
2. An underlying **lamina propria** consisting of a vascularized loose connective tissue.
3. A thin layer of smooth muscle, the **muscularis mucosae**.

Lymphatic nodules and scattered immunocompetent cells (lymphocytes, plasma cells, and macrophages) are present in the lamina propria. The lamina propria of the small and large intestines is a relevant site of immune responses (see Chapter 16, Lower Digestive Segment).

The lining epithelium invaginates to form **glands**, extending into the **lamina propria** (**mucosal glands**) or **submucosa** (**submucosal glands**), and **ducts**, transporting secretions from the liver and pancreas through the wall of the digestive tube (duodenum) into its lumen.

In the stomach and small intestine, both the mucosa and submucosa extend into the lumen as folds, called **rugae** and **plicae**, respectively. In other instances, the mucosa alone extends into the lumen

as finger-like projections, or **villi. Mucosal glands increase the secretory capacity**, whereas **villi increase the absorptive capacity of the digestive tube.**

The **mucosa** shows significant variations from segment to segment of the digestive tract. The submucosa consists of a dense irregular connective tissue with large blood vessels, lymphatics, and nerves branching into the mucosa and muscularis. Glands are present in the submucosa of the esophagus and duodenum.

The **muscularis** contains two layers of smooth muscle: the smooth muscle fibers of the inner layer are arranged around the tube lumen (circular layer); fibers of the outer layer are disposed along the tube (longitudinal layer). **Contraction of the smooth fibers of the circular layer reduces the lumen; contraction of the fibers of the longitudinal layer shortens the tube.** Skeletal muscle fibers are present in the upper esophagus and the anal sphincter.

The **adventitia** of the digestive tube consists of loose connective tissue. When the digestive tube is suspended by the mesentery or peritoneal fold, the adventitia is covered by a **mesothelium** (**simple squamous epithelium**) forming a **serosa**, or serous membrane. An exception is the esophagus, surrounded by the adipose tissue of the mediastinum.

Microvasculature of the digestive tube

We start our discussion with the **microvasculature of the stomach. The microcirculation of the small**

Figure 15-9. **Gastric microvasculature**

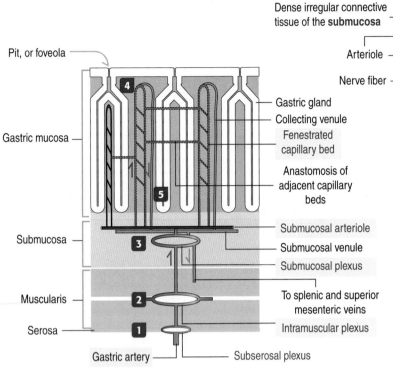

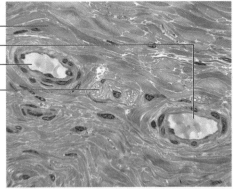

Dense irregular connective tissue of the **submucosa**

Arteriole

Nerve fiber

Pit, or foveola

Gastric mucosa

Gastric gland
Collecting venule
Fenestrated capillary bed
Anastomosis of adjacent capillary beds

Submucosa

Submucosal arteriole
Submucosal venule
Submucosal plexus

Muscularis

To splenic and superior mesenteric veins

Serosa

Intramuscular plexus

Gastric artery — Subserosal plexus

1 Gastric arteries form a subserosal plexus that links to the intramuscular plexus.

2 The highly developed intramuscular plexus supplies branches to the submucosal plexus and the layers of the muscularis.

3 The submucosal plexus supplies arterioles to the mucosa.

4 Arterioles become fenestrated capillaries within the gastric mucosa and around the glands. Periglandular capillary beds anastomose with each other.

5 Collecting venules drain the capillaries into submucosal venules of the submucosal venous plexus.

Clinical significance
Gastric microcirculation is relevant to the pathogenesis of **peptic ulcer disease** (PUD) and the protection of the gastric mucosa from the action of hydrochloric acid and pepsin.

---

intestine and differences from the gastric microcirculation are discussed in Chapter 16, Lower Digestive Segment (see Figure 16-3).

Blood and lymphatic vessels and nerves reach the walls of the digestive tube through the supporting mesentery or the surrounding tissues. After entering the walls of the stomach, arteries organize three arterial networks (Figure 15-9):

1. The **subserosal plexus.**
2. The **intramuscularis plexus.**
3. The **submucosal plexus.**

Some branches from the plexuses run longitudinally in the muscularis and submucosa; other branches extend perpendicularly into the mucosa and muscularis.

In the mucosa, **arterioles** derived from the submucosal plexus supply a bed of **fenestrated capillaries** around the gastric glands and anastomose laterally with each other. As discussed later, the fenestrated nature of the capillaries facilitates bicarbonate delivery to protect the surface epithelial cells against hydrochloric acid damage (see Figure 15-18).

Collecting venules descend from the mucosa into the submucosa as veins, leave the digestive tube

through the mesentery, and drain into the splenic and superior mesenteric veins. Mesenteric veins drain into the portal vein, leading to the liver (see Chapter 17, Digestive Glands).

Pathology: Gastric microcirculation and gastric ulcers

Gastric microcirculation plays a significant role in the protection of the integrity of the gastric mucosa. A breakdown in this protective mechanism, including mucus and bicarbonate secretion, allows the destructive action of hydrochloric acid and pepsin and bacterial infection, leading to **peptic ulcer disease** (PUD). PUD includes a group of disorders characterized by a partial or total loss of the mucosal surface of the stomach or duodenum or both.

The rich blood supply to the gastric mucosa is of considerable significance in understanding bleeding associated with **stress ulcers**. Stress ulcers are superficial gastric mucosal erosions observed after severe trauma or severe illness and after the long-term use of aspirin and corticosteroids. In most cases, stress ulcers are clinically asymptomatic and are detected only when they cause severe bleeding.

Figure 15-10. Innervation of the digestive tube

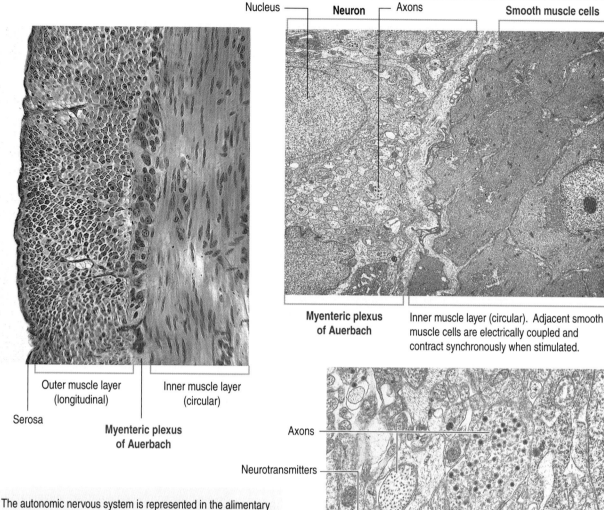

Nucleus — Neuron — Axons — Smooth muscle cells

Myenteric plexus of Auerbach

Inner muscle layer (circular). Adjacent smooth muscle cells are electrically coupled and contract synchronously when stimulated.

Outer muscle layer (longitudinal)

Inner muscle layer (circular)

Serosa

Myenteric plexus of Auerbach

Axons

Neurotransmitters

The autonomic nervous system is represented in the alimentary tube by two distinct interconnected neuronal networks: the **myenteric plexus of Auerbach** (located between the circular and longitudinal muscle layers and innervating the muscle fibers) and the **submucosal plexus of Meissner** (found between the muscularis and the mucosa and innervating the secretory glands).

The two plexuses are linked by axons and consist of sensory and motor neurons connected by interneurons. Although they can function independently of the central nervous system (CNS), they are regulated by preganglionic fibers of parasympathetic neurons of the vagus and pelvic nerves and postganglionic fibers of sympathetic neurons of the spinal cord and prevertebral ganglia.

Some of the chemical neurotransmitters found in the enteric nerves are **acetylcholine** (excitatory); the two major inhibitory neurotransmitters **nitric oxide** and **vasoactive intestinal peptide** (VIP); and **tachykinins** (such as substance P). **Serotonin** and **somatostatin** are products of interneurons.

Nerve supply of the digestive tube

The digestive tube is innervated by the autonomic nervous system (ANS). The ANS consists of an **extrinsic component** (the parasympathetic and sympathetic innervation) and an **intrinsic**, or **enteric**, **component**.

Sympathetic nerve fibers derive from the thoracic and lumbar spinal cord. **Parasympathetic** nerve fibers derive from the vagal dorsal motor nucleus of the medulla oblongata. **Visceral sensory** fibers originate in the spinal dorsal root ganglia.

The **intrinsic** or **enteric innervation** is represented by two distinct interconnected neuronal circuits formed by sensory and motor neurons linked by interneurons:

1. The **submucosal plexus of Meissner**, present in the **submucosa**.

2. The **myenteric plexus of Auerbach** (Figure 15-10), located **between the inner circular and outer longitudinal layers of the muscularis**.

Neurons and interneurons of the plexuses give off axons that branch to form the networks. The plexuses are connected to the extrinsic sympathetic and parasympathetic ANS: the plexuses of Auerbach and Meissner receive **preganglionic axons** of the **parasympathetic neurons** and **postganglionic axons** of **sympathetic neurons**.

The intrinsic or enteric nervous system enables the digestive tube to respond to both local stimuli and input from extrinsic nerves of the ANS. The integrated extrinsic and intrinsic (enteric) networks regulate and control the following functions:

1. Peristaltic contractions of the muscularis and movements of the muscularis mucosae.

2. Secretory activities of the mucosal and submucosal glands.

Stimulation of **preganglionic parasympathetic nerve fibers (cholinergic terminals)** of the muscularis causes **increased motility** as well as glandular secretory activity. Stimulation of **postganglionic sympathetic nerve fibers (adrenergic terminals)** on the smooth muscle cells causes **decreased motility**.

Esophagus

The esophagus is a muscular tube linking the pharynx to the stomach. It runs through the thorax, crosses the diaphragm, and enters the stomach. Contractions of the muscularis propel the food down the esophagus in about 2 seconds. At this velocity, changes of pressure and volume within the thorax are minimal. No disruption of respiration and cardiopulmonary circulation takes place.

The esophageal **mucosa** consists of a **stratified squamous epithelium** overlying a lamina propria with numerous connective tissue papillae (Figure 15-11). The **muscularis mucosae** is not present in the upper portion of the esophagus, but it becomes organized near the stomach.

The mucosa and the submucosa in the undistended esophagus form **longitudinal folds** that give the lumen an irregular outline. As the bolus of food moves down the esophagus, the folds disappear transiently and then are restored by the recoil of the elastic fibers of the submucosa.

The **submucosa** contains a network of collagen and elastic fibers and many small blood vessels. At the lower end of the esophagus, **submucosal venous plexuses** drain into both the systemic venous system and the portal venous system. An increase in pressure in the portal venous system, caused by chronic liver disease, results in dilation of the submucosal venous sinuses and the formation of **esophageal varices**. Rupture of the varices or ulceration of the overlying mucosa can produce hemorrhage into the esophagus

and stomach, often causing vomiting (**hematemesis**).

Mucosal and **submucosal glands** are found in the esophagus. Their function is to produce continuously a thin layer of mucus that lubricates the surface of the epithelium.

The **mucosal tubular glands**, residing in the lamina propria, resemble the cardiac glands of the stomach and are called **cardiac esophageal glands**.

The **submucosal tubuloacinar glands**, found in the submucosa just beneath the muscularis mucosae, are organized into small lobules drained by a single duct (see Figure 15-11). The acini are lined by two secretory cell types: a **mucous** and a **serous** cell type, the latter with secretory granules containing lysozyme.

The composition of the inner circumferential (or circular) and outer longitudinal layers of the **muscularis** shows **segment-dependent variations**. In the **upper third** of the esophagus, both layers consist of **striated muscle**. In the **middle third, smooth muscle fibers can be seen deep to the striated muscle**. In the **lower third**, both layers of the muscularis contain **smooth muscle cells**.

Clinical significance: Barrett's metaplasia

The esophagus has **two sphincters**:

1. The anatomically defined **upper esophageal sphincter (UES)**, or **cricopharyngeal sphincter**.

2. The functionally defined **lower esophageal sphincter (LES)**, or **gastroesophageal sphincter**.

The **UES participates in the initiation of swallowing**. The **LES prevents reflux of gastric contents into the esophagus**.

Because the esophageal stratified squamous lining epithelium at the **epithelial transformation zone** may be replaced at the lower end by a poorly resistant columnar epithelium (a process called **Barrett's esophagus** or **metaplasia**). Gastroesophageal reflux disease, (GERD) causes chronic inflammation or ulceration and difficulty in swallowing (**dysphagia**).

When the esophageal hiatus in the diaphragm does not close entirely during development, a **hiatus hernia** enables a portion of the stomach to move into the thoracic cavity. In **sliding hiatus hernia**, the stomach protrudes through the diaphragmatic hiatus, normally occupied by the lower esophagus.

GERD and peptic ulceration in the intrathoracic portion of the stomach and lower esophagus leads to difficulty in swallowing and the feeling of a lump in the throat. This condition, commonly seen in family practice patients, affects young and middle-aged women in particular.

The movements involved in swallowing are coordinated by nerves from the cervical and thoracic sympathetic trunks, forming plexuses in the submucosa and in between the inner and outer layers of the muscularis.

Figure 15-11. Esophagus

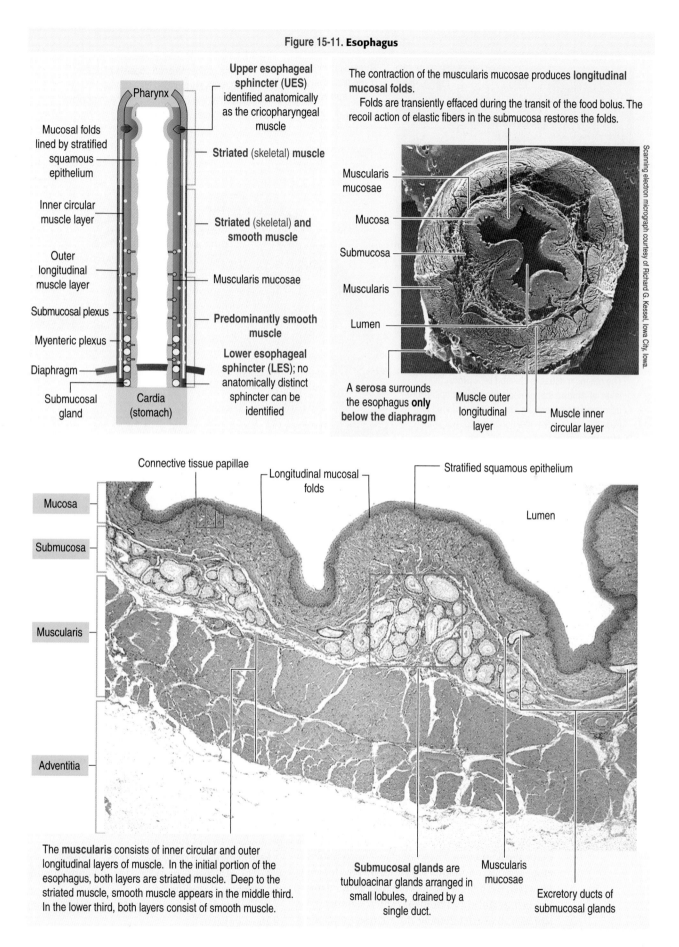

Mucosal folds lined by stratified squamous epithelium

Inner circular muscle layer

Outer longitudinal muscle layer

Submucosal plexus

Myenteric plexus

Diaphragm

Submucosal gland

Pharynx

Cardia (stomach)

Upper esophageal sphincter (UES) identified anatomically as the cricopharyngeal muscle

Striated (skeletal) **muscle**

Striated (skeletal) **and smooth muscle**

Muscularis mucosae

Predominantly smooth muscle

Lower esophageal sphincter (LES); no anatomically distinct sphincter can be identified

The contraction of the muscularis mucosae produces **longitudinal mucosal folds**.

Folds are transiently effaced during the transit of the food bolus. The recoil action of elastic fibers in the submucosa restores the folds.

Muscularis mucosae

Mucosa

Submucosa

Muscularis

Lumen

Scanning electron micrograph courtesy of Richard G. Kessel, Iowa City, Iowa.

A **serosa** surrounds the esophagus **only below the diaphragm**

Muscle outer longitudinal layer

Muscle inner circular layer

Connective tissue papillae

Longitudinal mucosal folds

Stratified squamous epithelium

Mucosa

Submucosa

Muscularis

Adventitia

Lumen

The **muscularis** consists of inner circular and outer longitudinal layers of muscle. In the initial portion of the esophagus, both layers are striated muscle. Deep to the striated muscle, smooth muscle appears in the middle third. In the lower third, both layers consist of smooth muscle.

Submucosal glands are tubuloacinar glands arranged in small lobules, drained by a single duct.

Muscularis mucosae

Excretory ducts of submucosal glands

Figure 15-12. Stomach: Ruga

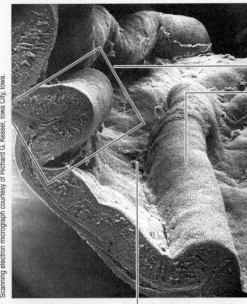

Ruga is a longitudinal fold of the gastric **mucosa** and **submucosa**

The gastric mucosa consists of gastric glands, surrounded by a lamina propria containing capillaries, and the muscularis mucosae.

Pits

Scanning electron micrograph courtesy of Richard G. Kessel, Iowa City, Iowa.

The gastric mucosa is covered by a **protective layer of mucus** that protects the surface epithelium from mechanical erosion by the ingested food and from the destructive effect of acid and hydrolytic enzymes present in the gastric juice.

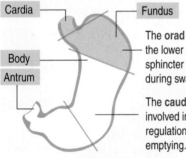

Cardia

Fundus

Body

Antrum

The **orad area** and the lower esophageal sphincter (LES) relax during swallowing.

The **caudad area** is involved in the regulation of gastric emptying.

The stomach is usually divided into the **cardia, fundus, body,** and **antrum**. Based on the **motility patterns** of the stomach, it can be divided into an **orad area**, consisting of the fundus, and a portion of the body, and a **caudad area**, consisting of the distal body and the antrum.

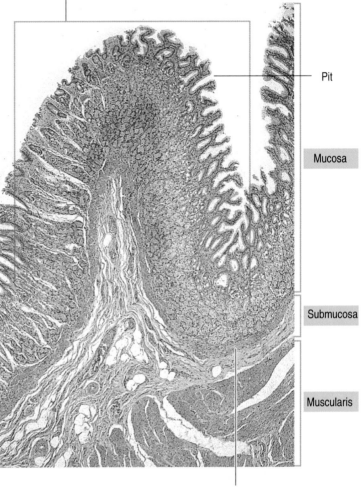

Pit

Mucosa

Submucosa

Muscularis

Muscularis mucosae

Diseases affecting this neuromuscular system may result in muscle spasm, difficulty in swallowing, and substernal pain.

Stomach

The stomach extends from the esophagus to the duodenum. The epithelium changes from stratified squamous to a simple columnar type at the **gastroesophageal junction.** The muscularis mucosae of the esophagus is continuous with that of the stomach. However, the submucosa does not have a clear demarcation line, and glands from the cardiac portion of the stomach may extend under the stratified squamous

epithelium and contact the esophageal cardiac glands.

The **function of the stomach is to homogenize and chemically process the swallowed semisolid food**. Both the contractions of the muscular wall of the stomach and the acid and enzymes secreted by the gastric mucosa contribute to this function. Once the food is transformed into a thick fluid, it is released gradually into the duodenum.

Four regions are recognized in the stomach:

1. The **cardia**, a 2- to 3-cm-wide zone surrounding the esophageal opening.

2. The **fundus**, projecting to the left of the opening of the esophagus.

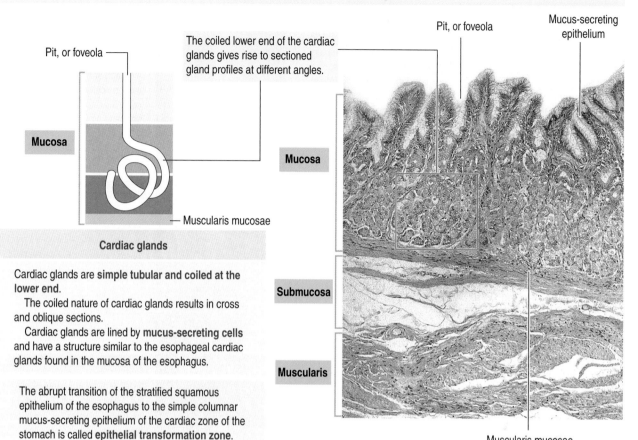

Figure 15-13. Stomach: Cardiac region

Pit, or foveola

The coiled lower end of the cardiac glands gives rise to sectioned gland profiles at different angles.

Pit, or foveola

Mucus-secreting epithelium

Mucosa

Mucosa

Muscularis mucosae

Submucosa

Cardiac glands

Muscularis

Cardiac glands are **simple tubular and coiled at the lower end.**

The coiled nature of cardiac glands results in cross and oblique sections.

Cardiac glands are lined by **mucus-secreting cells** and have a structure similar to the esophageal cardiac glands found in the mucosa of the esophagus.

The abrupt transition of the stratified squamous epithelium of the esophagus to the simple columnar mucus-secreting epithelium of the cardiac zone of the stomach is called **epithelial transformation zone.**

Muscularis mucosae

3. The **body**, an extensive central region.

4. The **pyloric antrum** (Greek *pyloros*, gatekeeper), ending at the gastroduodenal orifice.

Based on the **motility** characteristics of the stomach, the **orad area**, consisting of the fundus and the upper part of the body, relaxes during swallowing. The **caudad area**, consisting of the lower portion of the body and the antrum, participates in the regulation of gastric emptying.

The empty stomach shows gastric mucosal folds, or **rugae**, covered by **gastric pits** or **foveolae** (Figure 15-12). A **gastric mucosal barrier**, produced by **surface mucous cells**, protects the mucosal surface. The surface mucous cells contain apical periodic acid–Schiff (PAS)–positive granules and are linked to each other by apical tight junctions.

Cardia region

Glands of the cardia region are **tubular**, with a **coiled end** and an **opening continuous with the gastric pits** (Figure 15-13). A mucus-secreting epithelium lines the cardiac glands.

The gastric gland

Gastric glands of the fundus-body region are the major contributors to the gastric juice. About 15 million gastric glands open into 3.5 million gastric pits. From two to seven gastric glands open into a single gastric pit, or foveola.

A gastric gland consists of three regions:

1. The **pit**, or **foveola**, lined by surface mucous cells.

2. The **neck**, containing mucous neck cells, mitotically active stem cells, and parietal cells.

3. The **body**, representing the major length of the gland. The upper and lower portions of the body contain different proportions of cells lining the gastric gland.

The gastric glands proper house five major cell types (Figure 15-14; see also Figure 15-13):

1. **Mucous cells**, including the surface mucous cells and the mucous neck cells.

2. **Chief cells**, also called peptic cells.

3. **Parietal cells**, also called oxyntic cells.

4. **Stem cells.**

5. **Gastroenteroendocrine cells**, called enterochromaffin cells because of their staining affinity for chromic acid salts. We discuss them later in this chapter.

The upper portion of the main body of the gastric gland contains abundant parietal cells. Chief cells and gastroenteroendocrine cells predominate in the lower portion (see Figure 15-14).

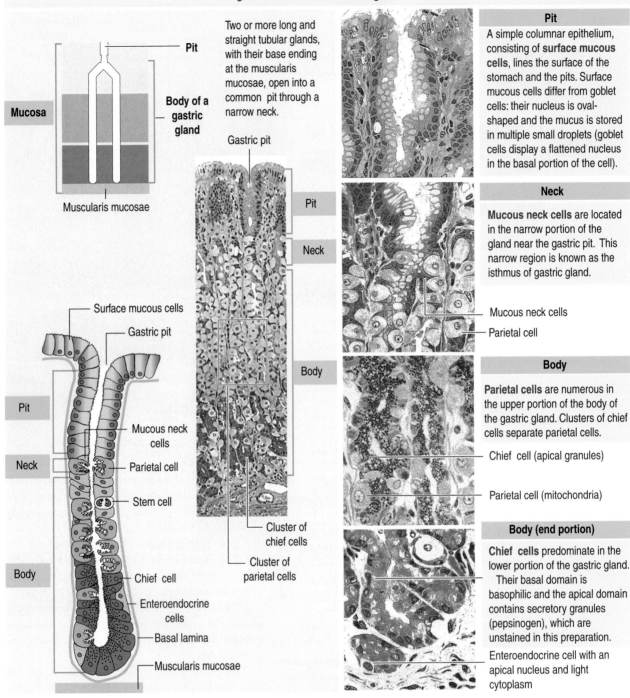

Figure 15-14. Stomach: Gastric gland

Two or more long and straight tubular glands, with their base ending at the muscularis mucosae, open into a common pit through a narrow neck.

Mucosa

Pit

Body of a gastric gland

Muscularis mucosae

Gastric pit

Pit

Neck

Body

Surface mucous cells

Gastric pit

Pit

Mucous neck cells

Neck

Parietal cell

Stem cell

Body

Chief cell

Enteroendocrine cells

Basal lamina

Muscularis mucosae

Cluster of chief cells

Cluster of parietal cells

Pit

A simple columnar epithelium, consisting of **surface mucous cells**, lines the surface of the stomach and the pits. Surface mucous cells differ from goblet cells: their nucleus is oval-shaped and the mucus is stored in multiple small droplets (goblet cells display a flattened nucleus in the basal portion of the cell).

Neck

Mucous neck cells are located in the narrow portion of the gland near the gastric pit. This narrow region is known as the isthmus of gastric gland.

Mucous neck cells

Parietal cell

Body

Parietal cells are numerous in the upper portion of the body of the gastric gland. Clusters of chief cells separate parietal cells.

Chief cell (apical granules)

Parietal cell (mitochondria)

Body (end portion)

Chief cells predominate in the lower portion of the gastric gland. Their basal domain is basophilic and the apical domain contains secretory granules (pepsinogen), which are unstained in this preparation.

Enteroendocrine cell with an apical nucleus and light cytoplasm

Mucous cells. The gastric mucosa of the fundus-body region has two classes of mucus-producing cells (see Figure 15-15):

1. The **surface mucous cells**, lining the pits.

2. The **mucous neck cells**, located at the opening of the gastric gland into the pit.

Both cells produce mucins, glycoproteins with high molecular mass. A mucus layer, containing 95% water and 5% mucins, forms an insoluble gel that attaches to the surface of the gastric mucosa, forming a 100-μm-thick protective mucosal barrier. This protective mucus blanket traps bicarbonate ions and neutralizes the microenvironment adjacent to the apical region of the surface mucous cells to an alkaline pH.

Na^+, K^+, and Cl^- are constituents of the protective mucosal barrier. Patients with chronic vomiting or undergoing continuous aspiration of gastric juice require intravenous replacement of NaCl, dextrose, and K^+ to prevent hypokalemic metabolic acidosis.

Figure 15-15. **Gastric gland: Surface and neck cells**

Surface mucous cells

Lamina propria

Surface mucous cells sectioned at different angles

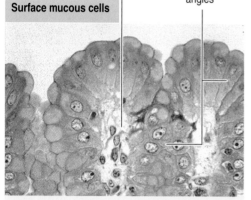

Mucous surface cells have **apical granules** containing glycoproteins (mucins). Mucins combine with water on the surface of the gastric mucosa to form a **protective gel**. In addition, abundant **mitochondria**, together with **carbonic anhydrase**, contribute to the formation of bicarbonate ions to increase the pH of the protective gel.

Apical mucus granules   Mitochondria   Surface mucous cell

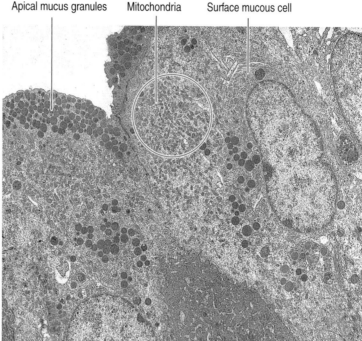

Mucous neck cells   Gastric pit

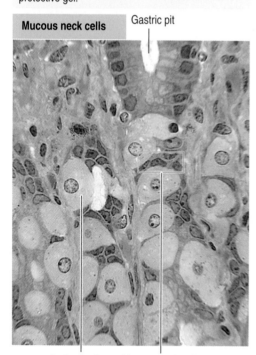

Parietal cells   Mucous neck cells

Lamina propria   Mucous neck cells   Chief cell   Parietal cell

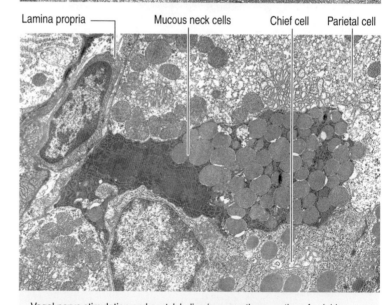

Vagal nerve stimulation and acetylcholine increase the secretion of soluble mucus by neck cells, located where the gland opens into the pit.

Similar to mucins produced by surface mucous cells, the soluble mucus mixes with the gastric chyme to lubricate the glandular and mucosal surfaces.

Ménétrier's disease is a condition associated with transforming growth factor-α (TGF-α)–induced **hyperplasia of surface mucous cells** in the gastric mucosa.

Clinical manifestations of the disease include nausea, vomiting, epigastric pain, gastrointestinal bleeding, diarrhea, and hypoalbuminemia. The diagnosis of Ménétrier's disease is established by endoscopy (presence of large gastric folds) and biopsy, showing significant gastric pit hyperplasia with glandular atrophy and

reduction in the numbers of parietal cells. Treatment includes medications to relieve nausea and gastric pain, as well as cetuximab, a monoclonal antibody that blocks TGF-α receptor signaling.

Chief cells (Figure 15-16) predominate in the lower third of the gastric gland. Chief cells are not **present in cardiac glands and are seldom found in the pyloric antrum**. Chief cells have a structural similarity to the zymogenic cells of the exocrine pancreas: the basal

Figure 15-16. Gastric gland: Chief and parietal cells

Chief cell

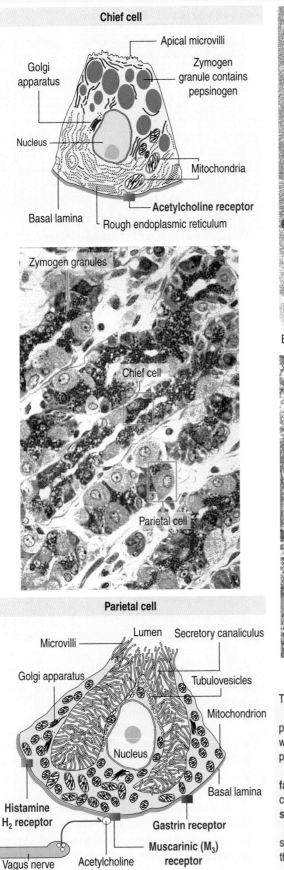

Chief cell

Golgi apparatus
Apical microvilli
Zymogen granule contains pepsinogen
Nucleus
Mitochondria
Acetylcholine receptor
Basal lamina
Rough endoplasmic reticulum

Zymogen granules
Chief cell
Parietal cell

Parietal cell

Microvilli
Lumen   Secretory canaliculus
Golgi apparatus
Tubulovesicles
Mitochondrion
Nucleus
Basal lamina
Histamine H$_2$ receptor
Gastrin receptor
Muscarinic (M$_3$) receptor
Vagus nerve   Acetylcholine

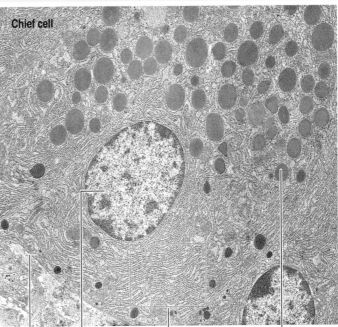

Chief cell

Basal lamina   Nucleus   Rough endoplasmic reticulum   Zymogen granule

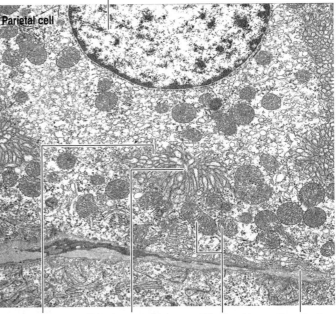

Parietal cell

Tubulovesicles   Secretory canaliculus   Mitochondria   Basal lamina

The gastric glands of the fundus-body region contain two major cell types:

1. **Chief** or **peptic cells**, which produce and secrete **pepsinogen** (42.5 kd), a precursor of the proteolytic enzyme **pepsin** (35 kd) produced in the gastric juice when the pH is below 5.0. Pepsin can catalyze the formation of additional pepsin from pepsinogen. **Acetylcholine** stimulates the secretion of pepsinogen.

2. **Parietal** or **oxyntic cells**, which secrete **hydrochloric acid** and **intrinsic factor** in humans (in some species, chief cells secrete intrinsic factor). The cytoplasm of parietal cells displays numerous **tubulovesicles** and an **secretory canaliculus** continuous with the lumen of the gastric gland.

After stimulation, the tubulovesicles fuse with the plasma membrane of the secretory canaliculus. **Carbonic anhydrase** and **H$^+$,K$^+$-ATPase** are localized in the microvilli projecting into the lumen of the secretory canaliculus.

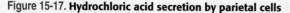

Figure 15-17. Hydrochloric acid secretion by parietal cells

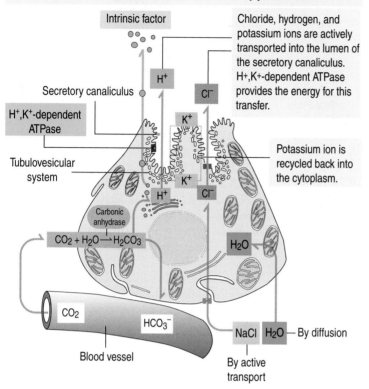

Intrinsic factor

Chloride, hydrogen, and potassium ions are actively transported into the lumen of the secretory canaliculus. H+,K+-dependent ATPase provides the energy for this transfer.

Secretory canaliculus

H^+

Cl^-

H^+,K^+-dependent ATPase

K^+

Tubulovesicular system

Potassium ion is recycled back into the cytoplasm.

K^+

H^+

Cl^-

Carbonic anhydrase

$CO_2 + H_2O \longrightarrow H_2CO_3$

H_2O

CO_2

HCO_3^-

Blood vessel

NaCl H_2O — By diffusion

By active transport

region of the cytoplasm contains an extensive rough endoplasmic reticulum. Pepsinogen-containing secretory granules (**zymogen granules**) are observed in the apical region of the cell.

Pepsinogen, a proenzyme stored in the zymogen granules, is released into the lumen of the gland and converted in the acid environment of the stomach to **pepsin**, a proteolytic enzyme capable of digesting most proteins. Exocytosis of pepsinogen is rapid and stimulated by feeding (after fasting).

Parietal cells predominate near the neck and in the upper segment of the gastric gland and are linked to chief cells by junctional complexes.

Parietal cells produce the **hydrochloric acid** of the gastric juice and **intrinsic factor**, a glycoprotein that binds to vitamin B_{12}.

Vitamin B_{12} binds in the stomach to the transporting binding protein intrinsic factor. In the small intestine, the vitamin B_{12}–intrinsic factor complex binds to intrinsic factor receptor on the surface of enterocytes in the ileum and is transported to the liver through the portal circulation.

Autoimmune gastritis is caused by autoantibodies to H^+,K^+-dependent ATPase, a parietal cell antigen, and intrinsic factor. Destruction of parietal cells causes a reduction in hydrochloric acid in the gastric juice (**achlorhydria**) and a lack of synthesis of intrinsic factor.

The resulting vitamin B_{12} deficiency disrupts the formation of red blood cells in the bone marrow,

leading to a condition known as pernicious anemia, identified by examination of peripheral blood as megaloblastic anemia characterized by macrocytic red blood cells and hypersegmented large neutrophils (see Chapter 6, Blood and Hematopoiesis).

Parietal cells have three distinctive features (see Figure 15-16):

1. **Abundant mitochondria**, which occupy about 40% of the cell volume and provide the adenosine triphosphate (ATP) required to pump H^+ **ions** into the lumen of the secretory canaliculus.

2. A **secretory or intracellular canaliculus**, formed by an invagination of the apical cell surface and continuous with the lumen of the gastric gland, which is lined by numerous microvilli.

3. An H^+,K^+-dependent ATPase-rich **tubulovesicular system**, which is distributed along the secretory canaliculus during the resting state of the parietal cell.

After stimulation, the tubulovesicular system fuses with the membrane of the secretory canaliculus, and numerous microvilli project into the canalicular space. Membrane fusion increases the amount of H^+,K^+-ATPase and expands the secretory canaliculus. H^+,K^+-ATPase represents about 80% of the protein content of the plasma membrane of the microvilli.

Secretion of hydrochloric acid

Parietal cells produce an acidic secretion (pH 0.9 to 2.0) rich in hydrochloric acid, with a concentration of H^+ ions one million times greater than that of blood (Figure 15-17). The release of H^+ ions and Cl^- by the parietal cell involves the membrane fusion of the tubulovesicular system with the secretory canaliculus.

The parasympathetic (vagus nerve) mediator **acetylcholine** (bound to a **muscarinic (M_3) receptor**) and the peptide gastrin, produced by enteroendocrine cells of the pyloric antrum, stimulate parietal cells to secrete HCl (see Figure 15-20).

Acetylcholine also stimulates the release of gastrin. Histamine potentiates the effects of acetylcholine and gastrin on parietal cell secretion after binding to the histamine H_2 receptor. Histamine is produced by enterochromaffin-like (ECL) cells within the lamina propria surrounding the gastric glands. Cimetidine is an H_2 receptor antagonist that inhibits histamine-dependent acid secretion.

H^+,K^+-dependent ATPase facilitates the exchange of H^+ and K^+. Cl^- and Na^+ (derived from the dissociation of NaCl) are actively transported into the lumen of the secretory canaliculus, leading to the production of HCl. K^+ and Na^+ are recycled back into the cell by separate pumps once H+ has taken their place.

Omeprazole, with binding affinity to H^+,K^+-dependent ATPase, inactivates acid secretion and is an effective agent in the treatment of peptic ulcer.

Water enters the cell by osmosis, because of the

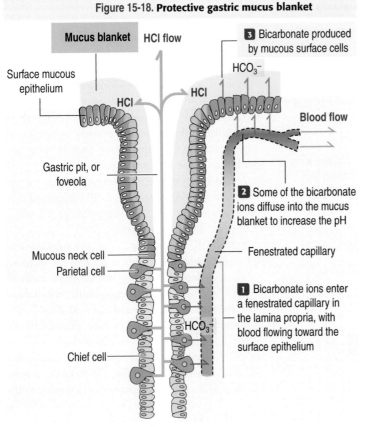

Figure 15-18. Protective gastric mucus blanket

Mucus blanket   HCl flow

Surface mucous epithelium

HCl

3 Bicarbonate produced by mucous surface cells

HCO_3^-

HCl

Blood flow

Gastric pit, or foveola

2 Some of the bicarbonate ions diffuse into the mucus blanket to increase the pH

Fenestrated capillary

Mucous neck cell
Parietal cell

HCO_3^-

1 Bicarbonate ions enter a fenestrated capillary in the lamina propria, with blood flowing toward the surface epithelium

Chief cell

---

secretion of ions into the canaliculus, and dissociates into H^+ and hydroxyl ions (HO^-). Carbon dioxide, entering the cell from the blood or formed during metabolism of the cell, combines with HO^- to form carbonic acid under the influence of carbonic anhydrase. Carbonic acid dissociates into bicarbonate ions (HCO_3^-) and hydrogen ions. HCO_3^- diffuses out of the cell into the blood and accounts for the increase in blood plasma pH during digestion.

Pathology: *Helicobacter pylori* infection

The gastric juice is a combination of two separate secretions:

1. An alkaline mucosal gel protective secretion, produced by surface mucous cells and mucous neck cells.

2. HCl and pepsin, two parietal cell–chief cell–derived potentially aggressive secretions. The protective secretion is constitutive; it is always present. The aggressive secretion is facultative because hydrochloric acid and pepsin levels increase above basal levels after food intake.

The viscous, highly glycosylated gastric mucus blanket, produced by surface mucous cells and mucous neck cells, maintains a neutral pH at the epithelial cell surfaces of the stomach. In addition, the mitochondrial-rich surface mucous cells (see Figure 15-15) produce HCO_3^- ions diffusing into the surface mucus gel. Recall the clinical significance

during chronic vomiting of Na^+, K^+, and Cl^- present in the protective mucosal barrier and gastric juice (see section on functions of the gastric gland).

HCO_3^- ions, produced by parietal cells, enter the fenestrated capillaries of the lamina propria. Some of the HCO_3^- ions diffuse into the mucus blanket and neutralize the low pH created by the HCl content of the gastric lumen at the vicinity of the surface mucous cells (Figure 15-18).

However, the mucus blanket lining the gastric epithelium, in particular in the pyloric antrum, is the site where the flagellated bacterium *Helicobacter pylori* resides in spite of the hostile environment.

H. pylori survives and replicates in the gastric lumen. Its presence has been associated with acid peptic ulcers and adenocarcinoma of the stomach.

Three phases define the pathogenesis of *H. pylori* (Figure 15-19):

1. An **active phase**, in which motile bacteria increase the gastric pH by producing ammonia through the action of urease.

2. A **stationary phase**, consisting in the bacterial attachment to fucose-containing receptors on the surface of mucous surface cells of the pyloric region. *H. pylori* attachment results in the production of cytotoxic proteases that ensure the bacteria a supply of nutrients from surface mucous cells and also attract leukocytes. Both ammonia production and cytotoxic proteases correlate with the development of peptic ulcers of the pyloric mucosa.

3. During the **colonization phase**, *H. pylori* detach from the fucose-containing receptors of the surface mucus epithelium, increase in number by replication within the mucus blanket, and remain attached to glycoproteins containing sialic acid. Despite the rapid turnover of the gastric mucus-secreting cells, *H. pylori* avoids being flushed away with dead epithelial cells by producing urease and displaying high motility.

About 20% of the population is infected with *H. pylori* by age 20 years. The incidence of the infection increases to about 60% by age 60. Most infected individuals do not have clinical symptoms. Intense, sudden, **persistent stomach pain** (relieved by eating and antacid medications), **hematemesis** (blood vomit), or **melena** (tarlike black stool) are clinical symptoms in some patients. Increasing evidence for the infectious origin of acid peptic disease and chronic gastritis led to the implementation of antibiotic therapy for all ulcer patients shown to be infected with *H. pylori*.

Blood tests to detect antibodies to *H. pylori* and urea breath tests are effective diagnostic methods. Treatment usually consists in a combination of antibiotics, suppressors of H^+,K^+-dependent ATPase, and stomach protectors.

More recently, attention has been directed to adhesins and fucose-containing receptors as potential

Figure 15-19. *Helicobacter pylori* and chronic gastric inflammation and ulcers

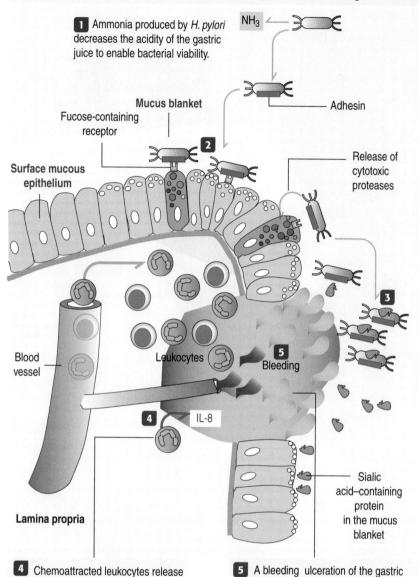

1 Ammonia produced by *H. pylori* decreases the acidity of the gastric juice to enable bacterial viability.

NH$_3$

Adhesin

Mucus blanket

Fucose-containing receptor

2

Surface mucous epithelium

Release of cytotoxic proteases

3

Blood vessel

Leukocytes

5 Bleeding

IL-8

4

Sialic acid–containing protein in the mucus blanket

Lamina propria

4 Chemoattracted leukocytes release interleukin-8 (IL-8), and the epithelial cell lining damaged by cytotoxic proteases released by *H. pylori* is destroyed.

5 A bleeding ulceration of the gastric mucosa with local inflammation in the lamina propria develops when cells of the surface epithelium are destroyed by *H. pylori*.

---

1   **Active phase**

During the active phase, *H. pylori* in the pyloric antrum are highly motile for a short period of time. About six flagella provide the motility. During this time, *H. pylori* decrease the acidity by producing **ammonia (NH$_3$)** by the action of the enzyme **urease**.

2   **Stationary phase**

H. pylori enter the mucus blanket, produce **adhesins**, adhesion molecules with binding affinity to **fucose-containing receptors**, and attach to the apical surfaces of the mucous epithelial cells containing fucose-binding sites. Cell attachment enables adherent *H. pylori* to obtain nutrients from epithelial cells, which later die.

3   **Colonization phase**

Well-nourished *H. pylori* detach from the apical surface of the mucus-secreting surface cells, replicate within the mucus blanket, and attach to **sialic acid–containing mucous proteins**. Bacteria reenter the active phase (motility and NH$_3$ production) and reinitiate their life cycle.

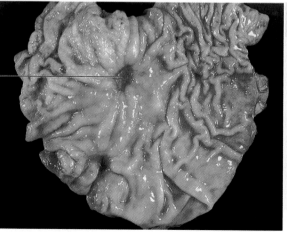

Chronic peptic ulcer of the stomach. Partial gastrectomy was carried out because of a bleeding vessel in the base of the ulcer caused hematemesis.

Regeneration of epithelial cells of the gastric mucosa

Stem cells are mitotic-dividing cells present adjacent to the neck region of the gastric gland and are responsible for the continuous renewal of the gastric mucosa. Daughter cells derived from the stem cell migrate either upward to replace surface mucous cells, or downward to differentiate into parietal cells, chief cells, and gastroenteroendocrine cells.

Surface mucous cells have a life span of about 3 days; parietal and chief cells have a life span of more than 190 days.

Photograph from Cooke RA, Stewart B: Anatomical Pathology. 2nd edition, Edinburgh, Churchill Livingstone, 1995.

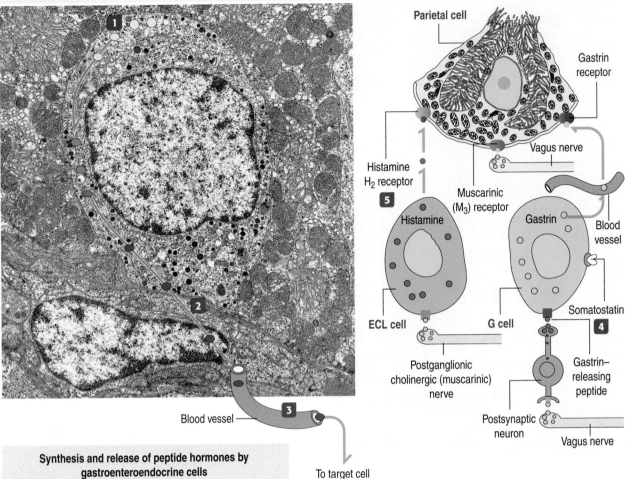

Figure 15-20. G cell (pyloric antrum)

Synthesis and release of peptide hormones by gastroenteroendocrine cells

1 Lipid-soluble amino acids enter a gastroenteroendocrine cell and are decarboxylated to form amines. Amines are part of polypeptide hormones that can stimulate or inhibit target cell function.

2 A polypeptide hormone is released from the gastroenteroendocrine cell into the surrounding lamina propria and reaches the blood capillaries.

3 Blood-borne peptides bind to target cells to stimulate or inhibit a cellular function.

4 Vagal stimulation of the pyloric antrum causes the release of **gastrin-releasing peptide** from postsynaptic neurons that stimulate directly the release of gastrin from G cells present in the antrum. Somatostatin released from adjacent **D cells** (not shown) inhibits gastrin release.

5 **Histamine**, released by **enterochromaffin-like** (ECL) **cells** in the lamina propria in response to acetylcholine released by postganglionic fibers, binds to the **H_2 receptor** on parietal cells.
Histamine **potentiates** the effect of acetylcholine and gastrin on the secretion of hydrochloric acid by parietal cells.

targets for drug action. The objective is to prevent binding of pathogenic bacteria without interfering with the endogenous bacterial flora by the use of antibiotics.

Gastroenteroendocrine cells

The function of the alimentary tube is regulated by peptide hormones, produced by gastroenteroendocrine cells, and **neuroendocrine mediators**, produced by neurons.

Peptide hormones are synthesized by gastroenteroendocrine cells dispersed throughout the mucosa from the stomach through the colon. The population of gastroenteroendocrine cells is so large that the gastrointestinal segment is regarded as the **largest endocrine organ in the body**.

Gastroenteroendocrine cells are members of the **APUD system**, so called because of the **amine precursor uptake and decarboxylation** property of amino acids (Figure 15-20).

Because not all the cells accumulate amine precursors, the designation APUD has been replaced by **DNES** (for **diffuse neuroendocrine system**).

Neuroendocrine mediators are released from nerve

terminals. **Acetylcholine** is released at the terminals of postganglionic cholinergic nerves. **Gastrin-releasing peptide** is released by postsynaptic neurons activated by stimulation of the vagus nerve (see Figure 15-20).

Peptide hormones produced by gastrointestinal endocrine cells have the following general functions:

1. Regulation of water, electrolyte metabolism, and enzyme secretion.

2. Regulation of gastrointestinal motility and mucosal growth.

3. Stimulation of the release of other peptide hormones.

We consider six major gastrointestinal peptide hormones: **secretin**, **gastrin**, **cholecystokinin (CCK)**, **glucose-dependent insulinotropic peptide**, **motilin**, and **ghrelin**.

Secretin was the first peptide hormone to be discovered (in 1902). Secretin is released by cells in the **duodenal glands of Lieberkühn** when the gastric contents enter the duodenum. Secretin stimulates **pancreatic and duodenal (Brunner's glands) bicarbonate and fluid release to control the gastric acid secretion** (antacid effect) and regulate the pH of the duodenal contents. Secretin, together with CCK, stimulates the growth of the exocrine pancreas. In addition, **secretin** (and acetylcholine) **stimulates chief cells to secrete pepsinogen**, and **inhibits gastrin** release to reduce HCl secretion in the stomach.

Gastrin is produced by **G cells** located in the pyloric antrum. Three forms of gastrin have been described: **little gastrin**, or G_{17} (which contains 17 amino acids), **big gastrin**, or G_{34} (which contains 34 amino acids), and **minigastrin**, or G_{14} (which consists of 14 amino acids). G cells produce primarily G_{17}. The duodenal mucosa in humans contains G cells producing mainly G_{34}. The neuroendocrine mediator **gastrin-releasing peptide** regulates the release of gastrin. **Somatostatin**, produced by adjacent **D cells**, inhibits the release of gastrin (see Figure 15-20).

The main function of gastrin is to stimulate the production of HCl by parietal cells. Low gastric pH inhibits further gastrin secretion.

Gastrin can also activate CCK to stimulate gallbladder contraction. **Gastrin has a trophic effect on the mucosa** of the small and large intestine and the fundic region of the stomach.

Gastrin stimulates the growth of **ECL cells** of the stomach. Continued hypersecretion of gastrin results in hyperplasia of ECL cells. ECL cells produce histamine by decarboxylation of histidine. Histamine binds to the **histamine H_2 receptor** on **parietal cells** to **potentiate the effect of gastrin and acetylcholine on HCl secretion** (see Figure 15-19). Histamine H_2 receptor blocking drugs (such as cimetidine [Tagamet] and ranitidine [Zantac]) are effective inhibitors of acid secretion.

CCK is produced in the duodenum. CCK stimulates **gallbladder contraction** and **relaxation of the sphincter of Oddi** when protein- and fat-rich chyme enters the duodenum.

Glucose-dependent insulinotropic peptide (GIP), formerly called **gastric-inhibitory peptide**, is produced in the duodenum. GIP stimulates insulin release (**insulinotropic effect**) when glucose is detected in the small intestine.

Motilin is released cyclically (every 90 minutes) during fasting from the upper small intestine and stimulates gastrointestinal motility. A **neural control mechanism** regulates the release of motilin.

Ghrelin is produced in the stomach (fundus). Ghrelin, binds to its receptor present in **growth hormone–secreting cells of the anterior hypophysis**, and stimulates the secretion of growth hormone. Ghrelin plasma levels increase during fasting triggering hunger by acting on hypothalamic feeding centers.

Plasma levels of ghrelin are high in patients with **Prader-Willi syndrome** (caused by abnormal gene imprinting; see section on epigenetics in Chapter 20, Spermatogenesis). Severe hypotonia and feeding difficulties in early infancy, followed by obesity and uncontrollable appetite, hypogonadism, and infertility are characteristics of Prader-Willi syndrome.

Clinical significance: Zollinger-Ellison syndrome

Patients with gastrin-secreting tumors (**gastrinomas**, or **Zollinger-Ellison syndrome**) display parietal cell hyperplasia, mucosal hypertrophy of the fundic region of the stomach, and high acid secretion independent of feeding. **The secretion of gastrin is not regulated by the low gastric pH feedback mechanism.**

Gastrinoma is a rare tumor of the pancreas and duodenum that causes ectopic hypersecretion of gastrin resulting in the hypersecretion of HCl by parietal cells, leading to severe peptic ulcer disease. Gastrinoma is more common in men than in women, and the age at onset is generally between 40 and 55 years of age.

The complications of gastrinomas are **fulminant stomach ulceration**, **diarrhea** (due to an inhibitory effect of water and sodium reabsorption by the small intestine due to excessive gastrin), **steatorrhea** (caused by inactivation of pancreatic lipase determined by the low pH), and **hypokalemia**.

Pyloric glands

Pyloric glands differ from the cardiac and gastric glands in the following layers:

1. The gastric pits, or foveolae, are deeper and extend halfway through the depth of the mucosa.

2. Pyloric glands have a larger lumen and are highly branched (Figure 15-20).

The predominant epithelial cell type of the pyloric

Figure 15-21. Pyloric region of the stomach

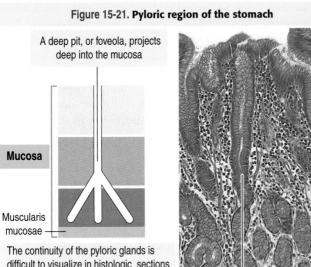

A deep pit, or foveola, projects deep into the mucosa

Mucosa

Muscularis mucosae

The continuity of the pyloric glands is difficult to visualize in histologic sections because of their tortuous path and highly branched nature.

Deep pit lined by mucus-secreting cells

Muscularis mucosae

Pyloric glands are **simple tubular and branched at the very lower end.**
The **pits are deeper** than in the cardiac glands and gastric glands of the fundus-body region.
Pyloric glands are lined by **mucus-secreting cells.**
At the distal end, the contents of the mucus-secreting cells displace and flatten the nuclei to the basal domain of the cell.

gland is a mucus-secreting cell that resembles the mucous neck cells of the gastric glands. Most of the cell contains large and pale secretory mucus and secretory granules containing **lysozyme,** a bacterial lytic enzyme. Occasionally, parietal cells can be found in the pyloric glands.

Enteroendocrine cells, **gastrin-secreting G cells** in particular, are abundant in the antrum pyloric region. Lymphoid nodules can be seen in the lamina propria.

Mucosa, submucosa, muscularis, and serosa of the stomach

We complete this discussion by pointing out additional structural and functional details of the mucosa, submucosa, muscularis, and serosa of the stomach.

The **mucosa** consists of loose connective tissue, called the **lamina propria,** surrounding cardiac, gastric, and pyloric glands.

Reticular and collagen fibers predominate in the lamina propria, and elastic fibers are rare. The cell components of the lamina propria include fibroblasts, lymphocytes, mast cells, eosinophils, and a few plasma cells. The muscularis mucosae can project thin strands of muscle cells into the mucosa to facilitate the release of secretions from the gastric glands.

The **submucosa** consists of dense irregular connective tissue in which collagenous and elastic fibers are abundant. A large number of arterioles, venous plexuses, and lymphatics are present in the submucosa. Also present are the cell bodies and nerve fibers of the **submucosal plexus of Meissner.**

The **muscularis** (or **muscularis externa**) of the stomach consists of three poorly defined layers of smooth muscle oriented in circular, oblique, and longitudinal directions. At the level of the distal pyloric antrum, the circular muscle layer thickens to form the annular **pyloric sphincter.**

Contraction of the muscularis is under control of the autonomic nerve plexuses located between the muscle layers (myenteric plexus of Auerbach).

Based on motility functions, the stomach can be divided into two major regions:

1. The **orad** (Latin *os* [plural *ora*], mouth; *ad*, to; toward the mouth) **portion,** consisting of the fundus and part of the body.

2. The **caudad** (Latin *cauda,* tail; *ad,* to; toward the tail) **portion,** comprising the distal body and the antrum (see Figure 15-11).

During swallowing, the orad region of the stomach and the LES relax to accommodate the ingested material. The tonus of the muscularis adjusts to the volume of the organ without increasing the pressure in the lumen.

Contraction of the caudad portion of the stomach mixes and propels the gastric contents toward the gastroduodenal junction. Most solid contents are propelled back (**retropulsion**) into the main body of the stomach because of the closure of the distal antrum. Liquids empty more rapidly. Retropulsion determines both mixing and mechanical dissociation of solid particles. When the gastric juice empties into the duodenum, peristaltic waves from the orad to the caudad portion of the stomach propel the contents in coordination with the relaxation of the pyloric sphincter.

The **serosa** consists of loose connective tissue and blood vessels of the subserosal plexus.

Concept mapping | **Upper Digestive Segment**

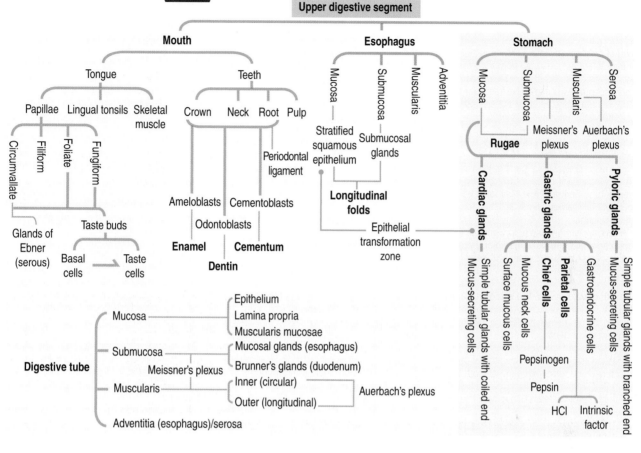

Essential concepts | **Upper Digestive Segment**

• **Mouth or oral cavity.** The mouth is the entry site to the digestive tube. Its functions are ingestion, partial digestion, and lubrication of the food, or bolus. The mouth includes the lips, cheeks, teeth, gums (or gingivae), tongue, uvula, and hard and soft palate.

The oral cavity are lined by three types of mucosae with structural variations:
  (1) Lining mucosa (lips, cheeks, ventral surface of the tongue, soft palate, floor of the mouth and alveolar mucosa).
  (2) Masticatory mucosa (gingiva and hard palate).
  (3) Specialized mucosa (dorsal surface of the tongue).

There are three transition sites of the oral mucosa:
  (1) The mucocutaneous junction (between the skin and the mucosa of the lips).
  (2) The mucogingival junction (between the gingiva and alveolar mucosa).
  (3) The dentogingival junction (between the mucosa of the gingiva and the enamel of the tooth), a sealing site that prevents from periodontal diseases.

Lips consist of three regions:
  (1) The cutaneous region (thin skin; keratinized stratified squamous epithelium with hair follicles, and sebaceous and sweat glands).
  (2) The red or vermilion region (lined by stratified squamous epithelium supported by a highly vascularized connective tissue and skeletal muscles). Salivary glands are not present in the mucosa of the vermilion region.
  (3) The oral mucosal region, continuous with the mucosa of the cheeks and gums.
  The epithelial lining of the gums is similar to the red region of the lips. The lamina propria binds to the periosteum of the alveolar processes of the maxilla and mandible. Submucosa or glands are not seen.
  The hard palate is lined by a keratinizing stratified squamous epithelium. Collagenous fibers in the submucosa bind the mucosa to the periosteum of the hard palate.
  The soft palate and uvula are lined by nonkeratinizing stratified squamous epithelium extending into the oropharynx.

• **Tongue.** The dorsal surface of the tongue is covered by nonkeratinizing stratified squamous epithelium supported by a lamina propria associated to a skeletal muscle core. The posterior one third displays aggregations of lymphatic tissue, the lingual tonsils.
  The dorsal surface of the tongue contains lingual papillae.
  They are of four types of lingual papillae:
  (1) Filiform papillae, the most abundant; the only type of papilla without taste buds.
  (2) Fungiform papillae.
  (3) Circumvallate papillae (with taste buds; associated with serous glands, or Ebner's glands).
  (4) Foliate papillae (poorly developed in humans).
  Serous and mucous glands extend across the lamina propria and the muscle. Their ducts open into the crypts and furrows of the lingual tonsils and circumvallate papillae, respectively.
  Taste buds consist of taste receptor cells, supporting cells (immature taste cells), and precursor taste cells (basal cells).
  Tastants (sweet, sour, bitter, salty, and umami) enter through the taste pore and bind to taste receptors (type 1 receptors, designated T1Rs) present in apical microvilli of taste receptor cells.
  T1Rs are linked to the G-protein α, β, and γ subunit complex (called gustducin). Binding

of the α subunit of the G-protein complex to phospholipase C (PLC) triggers the production of second messengers (inositol triphosphate, IP3, and diacylglycerol, DAG) that activate ion channels in the taste receptor cells. An influx of Na+ within taste cells causes depolarization of the taste receptor cells. An increase in intracellular Ca2+, released from intracellular storage sites, triggers the release of adenosine triphosphate (ATP) into the extracellular space and of neurotransmitters at the synapses with gustatory afferent nerve terminals.

• **Tooth.** It consists of a crown, neck, and a single or multiple roots.
   Enamel and dentin are parts of the crown. The outer surface of the root is covered by cementum. Cementum is associated with the periodontal ligament, firmly attached to the alveolar bone.
   A central chamber, the pulp, opens at the apical foramen, the site where blood vessels, nerves, and lymphatics enter and leave the pulp chamber.

   Tooth development. The ectoderm (amelo-blasts), cranial neural crest (odontoblasts), and mesenchyme (cementocytes) contribute to tooth development.
   The stages of tooth development are:
   (1) Bud stage: Ectodermic epithelial cells to proliferate and form the epithelial tooth bud.
   (2) Early cap stage: Cells of the epithelial tooth bud proliferate and invaginate into the underlying mesoderm.
   (3) Late cap stage: The cells at the growing end of the dental bud form a caplike structure. The epithelial tooth bud is lined by an outer and inner dental epithelium. The bud of the permanent tooth develops from the dental lamina and remains dormant. The enamel knot signals tooth development.
   (4) Bell stage: At the enamel knot site, the outermost cells of the dental papilla differentiate into dentin-producing odontoblasts. A single layer of enamel-secreting ameloblasts develops in the inner dental epithelium portion of the enamel knot.
   (5) Tooth eruption: The dental sac gives rise to cementoblasts, which secrete a layer of cementum, and cells forming the periodontal ligament, holding the tooth in its bony socket, or alveolus.

   Odontoblasts are present at the periphery of the pulp. Odontoblasts produce predentin (nonmineralized material surrounding the apical processes of the odontoblast) and dentin (consisting of 20% organic material, primarily type I collagen; 70% inorganic material; and 10% water).
   Mineralized dentin (crystals of hydroxyapatite and fluoroapatite) forms the dentinal tubes containing the odontoblast apical processes.

   Ameloblasts, present in the developing tooth only, face the dentin material and secrete enamel. The apical region of the ameloblast, Tomes' process, becomes surrounded

by enamel, the hardest substance found in the body (95% crystals of hydroxyapatite and a decreasing content of protein during mineralization).
   Enamel consists of enamel rods separated by an interrod region. The extracellular matrix of the developing enamel (amelogenesis) contains two classes of proteins: amelogenin (90%) and nonamelogenins (10%), including enamelin and ameloblastin.
   Amelogenesis imperfecta is an X chromosome–linked inherited disease affecting the synthesis of amelogenin required for the formation of the tooth enamel; affected enamel does not attain its normal thickness, hardness, and color. Autosomal-dominant amelogenesis imperfecta is caused by a mutation of the *enamelin* gene.

• **Non-neoplastic and neoplastic lesions** of the oral mucosa include:
   (1) Reactive fibroepithelial hyperplasia following traumatic injury or irritation of the gingiva and palate caused by dentures.
   (2) Viral infections: Herpes simplex viral infection can cause ulceration of the gingiva and palate. Verrucous papillary lesions of the oral mucosa are seen in human papillomavirus infection.
   (3) Hairy (papillate) leukoplakia in the lateral margins of the tongue occurs in HIV-positive patients and in individual with immuno-suppressed conditions as opportunistic Epstein-Barr viral infection.
   (4) Squamous cell carcinoma represents the predominant oral malignant condition seen in adults with predominant localizations in the lateral tongue and the floor of the mouth.
   (5) Oral melanomas are generally localized in palate and gingiva and can be in situ or multiple invasive lesions with irregular borders and ulcerated.
   (6) Non-Hodgkin's lymphomas are observed in the mucosa-associated lymphoid tissue (Waldeyer's ring) in patients with HIV-infection.
   (7) Kaposi's sarcoma is seen in palate and gingiva in the form of macular or nodular lesions, in association with cutaneous localization. The lesion consists in the proliferation of endothelial cells of blood vessels.
   (8) Neural tumors include schwannoma, an encapsulated tumor containing Schwann cells.

• **General organization of the digestive tube** (esophagus, stomach, small intestine, and large intestine).
   Digestive organs have four concentric layers:
   (1) Mucosa (epithelium, lamina propria, and muscularis mucosae).
   (2) Submucosa.
   (3) Muscularis (inner circular layer; outer longitudinal layer).
   (4) Adventitia, or serosa.

   Remember the following distinctions:
   (1) The mucosa of the esophagus has folds.
   (2) The mucosa of the stomach has gastric glands with opening pits or foveola.
   (3) The mucosa of the small intestine

(duodenum, jejunum, and ileum) displays evaginations (villi) of segment-specific shape and length, and invaginations called the crypts or glands of Lieberkühn.
   (4) The mucosa of the large intestine has tubular glands with openings.

   The digestive tube is innervated by the autonomic nervous system, consisting of an extrinsic component (parasympathetic and sympathetic innervation) and intrinsic components: the submucosal plexus of Meissner and the myenteric plexus of Auerbach.

• **Esophagus.** The esophagus is a muscular tube lined by a mucosa consisting of stratified squamous epithelium.
   The mucosa and submucosa form longitudinal folds. Mucosal and submucosal glands lubricate the surface of the esophageal epithelium.
   The muscularis has segment-dependent variations: the upper region consists of skeletal muscle; the middle region has a combination of skeletal and smooth muscle; and the lower region has predominantly smooth muscle. Contractions of the muscularis propel the food down the esophagus in about 2 seconds.
   An anatomically upper esophageal sphincter ([UES]; cricopharyngeal muscle) is involved in the initiation of swallowing; a functional lower esophageal sphincter (LES) prevents reflux of gastric juice into the esophagus.
   At the gastroesophageal junction (transformation zone), the esophageal epithelium changes from stratified squamous to a simple columnar type.
   Gastric juice reflux can produce an inflammatory reaction (**reflux esophagitis**) or ulceration and difficulty in swallowing (**dysphagia**). Persistent reflux replaces, at the gastroesophageal junction, the esophageal stratified columnar epithelium by a less resistant columnar epithelium.
   Hiatus hernia, caused by a failure of the diaphragm to close during development, enables a portion of the stomach to move into the thoracic cavity. A portion of the stomach can slide through the diaphragmatic hiatus causing a **sliding hiatus hernia**.

• **Stomach.** The function of the stomach is to homogenize and chemically process the swallowed semisolid food.
   The stomach is divided into:
   (1) The cardia.
   (2) The fundus.
   (3) The body.
   (4) The pyloric antrum.
   The glands of the cardia region are tubular with a coiled end. In the fundus and body, the gastric glands are simple tubular branched. In the pyloric antrum, glands have a deep pit and are simple tubular branched.
   Characteristic features of the stomach are:
   (1) The ruga, a fold of the gastric mucosa and submucosa.
   (2) A gastric mucosal blanket.

The gastric gland (present in the fundus and body) has a pit, a neck, and a body.

The cell types found in the gastric glands are:
(1) Surface mucous cells are found in the pit or foveola. Surface mucous cells have apical secretory granules containing glycoproteins (mucins) that, when combined with water on the surface of the gastric mucosa form a protective gel.
Mitochondria are abundant. Together with carbonic anhydrase, surface mucous cells produce bicarbonate ions to increase the pH of the protective gel.
Ménétrier's disease is associated with transforming growth factor-α (TGF-α)–induced hyperplasia of surface mucous cells in the gastric mucosa. The diagnosis of Ménétrier's disease is established by endoscopy (presence of large gastric folds) and biopsy, showing significant gastric pit hyperplasia in the folds, glandular atrophy, and reduction in the numbers of parietal cells.
(2) Mucous neck cells, located at the junction of the pit with the body, secrete mucus that is part of the protective gastric mucosal blanket.
(3) Chief cells secrete pepsinogen, a precursor of the proteolytic enzyme pepsin produced in the gastric juice when the pH is below 5.0.
(4) Parietal cells are seen in the upper region of the body of the gland and produce:
• HCl following stimulation by acetylcholine (bound to the muscarinic M_3 receptor), gastrin, and histamine (bound to histamine H_2 receptor).
• Intrinsic factor.
The cytoplasm of parietal cells shows numerous mitochondria, tubulovesicles and a secretory canaliculus continuous with the lumen of the gastric gland.
After stimulation, the tubulovesicles fuse with the plasma membrane of the secretory canaliculus. Carbonic anhydrase and H^+,K^+-ATPase are localized in the microvilli projecting into the lumen of the secretory canaliculus.
Autoantibodies to H^+,K^+-dependent ATPase and intrinsic factor cause autoimmune gastritis. Destruction of parietal cells reduces HCl in the gastric juice (achlorhydria) and intrinsic factor (required for the transport and uptake of vitamin B_{12} by enterocytes in the ileum).
Vitamin B_{12} deficiency causes pernicious anemia characterized by a decrease in the production of red blood cells and the release into the blood circulation of large red blood cells (megaloblastic anemia).
Two additional cell types are the stem cells (precursor cells of all glandular cells), and gastroenteroendocrine cells (enterochromaffin cells, see below).

Based on the motility pattern, the stomach can be divided into an orad area (consisting of the fundus and a portion of the body, which relax during swallowing), and a caudad area (consisting of the distal body and the antrum, which are involved in the regulation of gastric emptying).
Helicobacter pylori infection affects the integrity of the protective gastric mucus blanket, enables the aggressive action of pepsin and HCl, and of H. pylori–derived cytotoxic proteases on the unprotected gastric mucosa.
The stages of H. pylori infection are:
(1) Active phase. H. pylori are highly motile, propelled by about six flagella. During this time, H. pylori decrease the acidity by producing ammonia (NH_3) by the action of the enzyme urease.
(2) Stationary phase. H. pylori enter the mucus blanket, produce adhesins that attach to the apical surfaces of the surface mucous epithelial cells containing fucose-binding sites. Cell attachment enables adherent H. pylori to obtain nutrients from epithelial cells, which undergo necrosis.
(3) Colonization phase. Well-nourished H. pylori detach from the mucus-secreting surface cells, replicate within the mucus blanket, and attach to sialic acid– containing mucous proteins. Bacteria reenter the active phase (motility and NH_3 production) and reinitiate their life cycle.
Gastritis and peptic ulcer disease develop as a consequence of H. pylori infection. Hematemesis (blood vomit) or melena (tar-like black stool) are typical findings in patients with bleeding gastric ulcers.

• Gastroenteroendocrine cells, present in the mucosa from the stomach to the colon, synthesize peptide hormones, which regulate several functions of the digestive system and associated glands.
Originally, gastroenteroendocrine cells (called enterochromaffin cells) were regarded as members of the APUD system because of their property of amino precursor uptake and decarboxylation of amino acids.
The designation diffuse neuroendocrine system (DNES) has replaced the APUD designation because not all cells accumulate amine precursors.

Secretin is produced by cells in the duodenal glands of Lieberkühn when the gastric content enters the duodenum. Secretin stimulates the production of pancreatic and Brunner's gland bicarbonate to regulate the duodenal pH by buffering the entering gastric acid secretion.
Gastrin stimulates the production of HCl by parietal cells. It is produced by G cells in the glands of the pyloric antrum. The release of gastrin is regulated by gastrin-releasing peptide, a neuroendocrine mediator. Somatostatin, produced by D cells (adjacent to G cells) inhibits the release of gastrin. The low gastric pH inhibits further gastrin secretion.
Excessive production of gastrin is a characteristic of the Zollinger-Ellison syndrome (parietal cell hyperplasia).
A gastrinoma, a gastrin-producing tumor of the pyloric antrum or the pancreas, causes parietal cell hyperplasia resulting in excessive HCl production leading to the development of multiple gastric and duodenal ulcers. Low gastric pH does not inhibits gastrin secretion derived from a gastrinoma.

Cholecystokinin stimulates the contraction of the gallbladder and relaxes the sphincter of Oddi.
Glucose-dependent insulinotropic peptide, produced in the duodenum, stimulates insulin release (insulinotropic effect) when glucose is detected in the small intestine.
Motilin is released cyclically during fasting from the upper small intestine and stimulates gastrointestinal motility.
Ghrelin is produced in the stomach (fundus). Ghrelin stimulates the secretion of growth hormone. Ghrelin plasma levels increase during fasting, triggering hunger by acting on hypothalamic feeding centers. Plasma levels of ghrelin are high in patients with Prader-Willi syndrome.
Severe hypotonia and feeding difficulties in early infancy, followed by obesity and uncontrollable appetite, are characteristics of Prader-Willi syndrome.

16. Lower Digestive Segment

The main functions of the small intestine are (1) to continue in the duodenum the digestive process initiated in the stomach and (2) to absorb digested food after enzymes produced in the intestinal mucosa and the pancreas, together with the emulsifying bile produced in the liver, enable uptake of protein, carbohydrate, and lipid components. Bacteria, a component of the microbiota, reside preferentially in the intestinal tract and maintain a normal functional relationship with the gut-associated lymphoid tissue (GALT) to prevent the aggression of pathogens. This chapter describes the relevant histologic features of the three major segments of the small intestine, discusses details of the various mechanisms of defense of the intestinal mucosa, the pathologic and clinical consequences of an immune defense breakdown and relevant aspects of colorectal tumorigenesis.

Figure 16-1. **Small intestine**

Serosa

Muscularis

Submucosa

Muscularis mucosae

Villi

Villi are folds of the mucosa projecting into the lumen. Villi increase the absorptive surface of the mucosa.

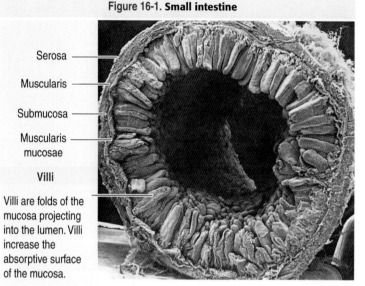

Scanning electron micrograph courtesy of Richard G. Kessel, Iowa City, Iowa.

Small intestine

The 4- to 7-meter-long small intestine is divided into three sequential segments:

1. Duodenum.
2. Jejunum,.
3. Ileum.

The duodenum is about 25 cm in length, is mainly retroperitoneal, and surrounds the head of the pancreas. At its distal end, the duodenum is continuous with the jejunum, a movable intestinal segment suspended by a mesentery. The ileum is the continuation of the jejunum.

The wall of the small intestine consists of four layers (Figures 16-1 to 16-3):

1. The mucosa.
2. The submucosa.
3. The muscularis.
4. The serosa, or **peritoneum**.

As you will see, histologic differences are seen in the mucosa and submucosa of the three major portions of the small intestine. The muscularis externa and serosa layers are similar.

The peritoneum

The peritoneum is a serous membrane consisting of a connective tissue stroma (containing elastic fibers, blood and lymphatic vessels, and nerves) lined by mesothelial cells. The **parietal peritoneum** lines the abdominal wall and reflects to cover the abdominal viscera as the **visceral peritoneum**.

The **mesentery** is a layer of loose connective tissue (areolar connective tissue) covered with peritoneum. We discuss the histology of the mesentery in Chapter 4, Connective Tissue. The mesentery attaches the abdominal viscera to the posterior abdominal wall and it serves as a conduit of blood and lymphatic vessels and nerves to these organs. The blood vessels are components of the subserosal plexus (see Figure 16-3). During digestion, the lymphatic vessels emerging from the walls of the small intestine carry a fluid rich in absorbed fat emulsion, or **chyle**. Numerous lymph nodes and adipose tissue are seen in the mesentery. The mesentery can be short to anchor certain viscera to the abdominal wall, or longer to enable visceral displacement. As indicated in Chapter 15, Upper Digestive Segment, the esophagus lacks a serosa. The duodenum and ascending and descending colon attach to the abdominal cavity by the **adventitia**, a loose connective tissue continuous with the surrounding stroma of the abdominal wall.

The **omenta** and **visceral ligaments** have a structure similar to the mesentery. The **greater omentum** has considerable adipose tissue.

Intestinal wall

The intestinal wall shows an increase in the total surface of the mucosa that reflects the absorptive function of the small intestine.

Four degrees of folding amplify the absorptive surface area of the mucosa (see Figure 16-2):

1. The **plicae circulares** (circular folds; also known as the **valves of Kerkring**).
2. The **intestinal villi**.
3. The **intestinal glands**.

Figure 16-2. Plica circularis, villi, glands of Lieberkühn, and microvilli

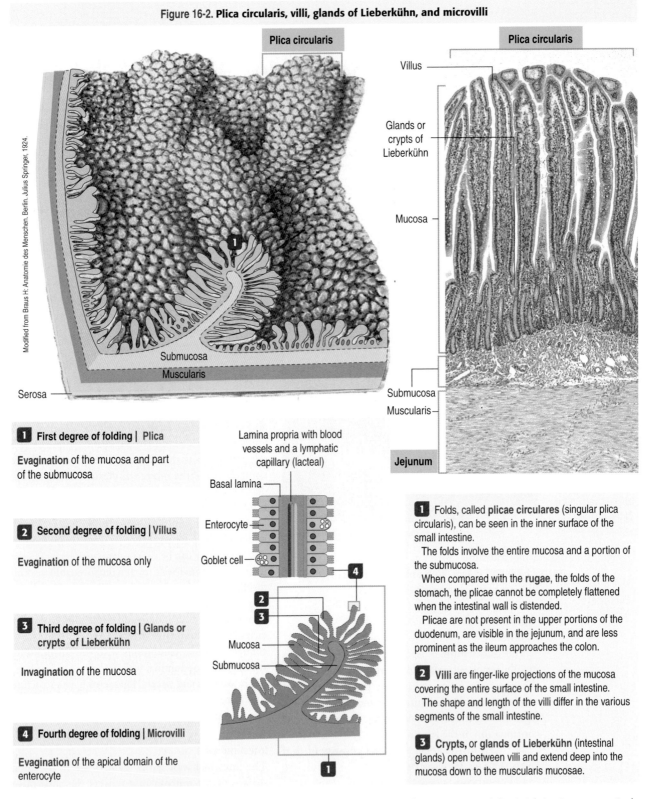

Modified from Braus H: Anatomie des Menschen. Berlin. Julius Springer, 1924.

Plica circularis

- Villus
- Glands or crypts of Lieberkühn
- Mucosa
- Submucosa
- Muscularis

Jejunum

Serosa

Submucosa

Muscularis

1 First degree of folding | Plica

Evagination of the mucosa and part of the submucosa

2 Second degree of folding | Villus

Evagination of the mucosa only

3 Third degree of folding | Glands or crypts of Lieberkühn

Invagination of the mucosa

4 Fourth degree of folding | Microvilli

Evagination of the apical domain of the enterocyte

Lamina propria with blood vessels and a lymphatic capillary (lacteal)

Basal lamina

Enterocyte

Goblet cell

Mucosa

Submucosa

1 Folds, called **plicae circulares** (singular plica circularis), can be seen in the inner surface of the small intestine.

The folds involve the entire mucosa and a portion of the submucosa.

When compared with the **rugae**, the folds of the stomach, the plicae cannot be completely flattened when the intestinal wall is distended.

Plicae are not present in the upper portions of the duodenum, are visible in the jejunum, and are less prominent as the ileum approaches the colon.

2 **Villi** are finger-like projections of the mucosa covering the entire surface of the small intestine.

The shape and length of the villi differ in the various segments of the small intestine.

3 **Crypts,** or **glands of Lieberkühn** (intestinal glands) open between villi and extend deep into the mucosa down to the muscularis mucosae.

4. The **microvilli** on the apical surface of the lining epithelium of the intestinal cells (enterocytes).

A **plica circularis** is a permanent fold of the **mucosa** and **submucosa** encircling the intestinal lumen.

Plicae appear about 5 cm distal to the pyloric outlet of the stomach, become distinct where the duodenum joins the jejunum, and diminish in size progressively to disappear halfway along the ileum.

The **intestinal villi** are finger-like projections of the **mucosa** covering the entire surface of the small intestine. Villi extend deep into the mucosa to form crypts ending at the muscularis mucosae. The length

Figure 16-3. Blood, lymphatic, and nerve supply to the small intestine

1 The microvascular system of the villus derives from two arteriolar systems. One system supplies the tip of the villus (**capillary villus plexus**). The second system forms the **pericryptal capillary plexus**. Both plexuses drain into the **submucosal venule**.

2 A single blind-ending **central lymphatic capillary**, called a **lacteal**, is present in the core or lamina propria of a villus. The lacteal is the initiation of a lymphatic vessel that, just above the muscularis mucosae, forms a lymphatic plexus whose branches surround a lymphoid nodule in the submucosa.

Efferent lymphatic vessels of the lymphoid nodule anastomose with the lacteal and exit the digestive tube together with the blood vessels.

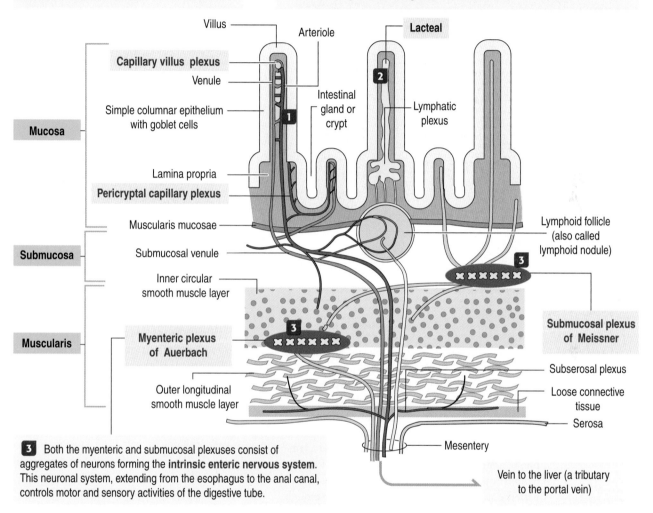

3 Both the myenteric and submucosal plexuses consist of aggregates of neurons forming the **intrinsic enteric nervous system**. This neuronal system, extending from the esophagus to the anal canal, controls motor and sensory activities of the digestive tube.

of the villi depends on the degree of distention of the intestinal wall and the contraction of smooth muscle fibers in the villus core.

Crypts of Lieberkühn, or **intestinal glands**, are **simple tubular glands** that increase the intestinal surface area. The crypts are formed by invaginations of the mucosa between adjacent intestinal villi.

The **muscularis mucosae** is the boundary between the mucosa and submucosa (see Figure 16-3).

The **muscularis** consists of inner circular smooth muscle and outer longitudinal smooth muscle. The muscularis is responsible for **segmentation** and **peristaltic movement** of the contents of the small intestine (Figure 16-4).

A thin layer of loose connective tissue is covered by the **visceral peritoneum**, a serosa layer lined by a

simple squamous epithelium, or **mesothelium**. The **parietal peritoneum** covers the inner surface of the abdominal wall.

Microcirculation of the small intestine

A difference from the microcirculation of the stomach (see Figure 15-9 in Chapter 15, Upper Digestive Segment) is that **the intestinal submucosa is the main distribution site of blood and lymphatic flow** (see Figure 16-3).

Branches of the submucosal plexus supply capillaries to the muscularis and intestinal mucosa. Arterioles derived from the **submucosal plexus** enter the mucosa of the small intestine and give rise to two capillary plexuses:

1. The **villus capillary plexus** supplies the intestinal

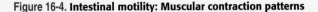

Figure 16-4. Intestinal motility: Muscular contraction patterns

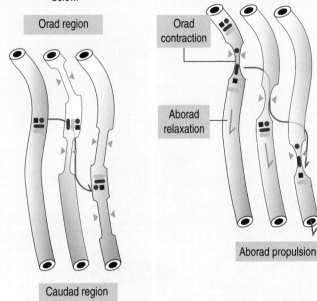

Segmentation	Peristalsis
Intestinal contents are mixed within an intestinal segment. This occurs when the contraction above is **not coordinated** with relaxation below.	Contents advance along the intestine when proximal contraction is **coordinated** with relaxation below.

Orad region

Caudad region

Orad contraction

Aborad relaxation

Aborad propulsion

villus and upper portion of the crypts of Lieberkühn.

2. The **pericryptal capillary plexus** supplies the lower half of the crypts of Lieberkühn.

A single blind-ending **central lymphatic capillary**, the **lacteal**, is present in the core or lamina propria of a villus. The lacteal is the initiation of a lymphatic vessel that, just above the muscularis mucosae, forms a **lymphatic plexus** whose branches surround a lymphoid nodule in the mucosa-submucosa. Efferent lymphatic vessels of the lymphoid nodule anastomose with the lacteal and leave the digestive tube through the mesentery, together with the blood vessels.

Innervation and motility of the small intestine

Motility of the small intestine is controlled by the autonomic nervous system. The intrinsic autonomic nervous system of the small intestine, consisting of the submucosal **plexus of Meissner** and **myenteric plexus of Auerbach**, is similar to that of the stomach (see Figure 15-9 in Chapter 15, Upper Digestive Segment).

Neurons of the plexuses receive **intrinsic input from the mucosa and muscle wall** of the small intestine and **extrinsic input from the central nervous system** through the **parasympathetic** (vagus nerve) **and sympathetic nerve trunks**.

Contraction of the muscularis is coordinated to achieve two objectives (see Figure 16-4):

1. To **mix and mobilize the contents within an intestinal segment**. This is accomplished when muscular contraction activity is not coordinated and the intestine becomes transiently divided into segments. This process is known as **segmentation**.

2. To **propel the intestinal contents** when there is a proximal (**orad**) contraction coordinated with a distal (**aborad**; Latin *ab*, from; *os*, mouth; away from the mouth) relaxation.

When coordinated contraction-relaxation occurs sequentially, the intestinal contents are propelled in an **aborad direction**. This process is known as **peristalsis** (Greek *peri*, around; *stalsis*, constriction).

Histologic differences between the duodenum, jejunum, and ileum

Each of the three major anatomic portions of the small intestine, the duodenum, jejunum, and ileum, has **distinctive features that allow recognition under the light microscope** (Figure 16-5).

The **duodenum** extends from the pyloric region of the stomach to the junction with the jejunum and has the following characteristics:

1. It has **Brunner's glands in the submucosa**. Brunner's glands are **tubuloacinar mucous glands** producing an **alkaline secretion** (pH 8.8 to 9.3) that neutralizes the acidic chyme coming from the stomach.

2. The **villi are broad and short** (leaflike shape).

3. The duodenum is surrounded by an incomplete serosa and an extensive adventitia rather than a serosa.

4. The duodenum collects bile and pancreatic secretions transported by the common bile duct and pancreatic duct, respectively. The **sphincter of Oddi** is present at the terminal ampullary portion of the two converging ducts.

5. The base of the crypts of Lieberkühn may contain **Paneth cells**.

The **jejunum** has the following characteristics:

1. It has long finger-like villi and a **well-developed lacteal in the core of the villus**.

2. The jejunum **does not contain Brunner's glands** in the submucosa.

3. Peyer's patches in the lamina propria may be present but they are not predominant in the jejunum. Peyer's patches are a characteristic feature of the ileum.

4. **Paneth cells** are found at the base of the crypts of Lieberkühn.

The **ileum** has a prominent diagnostic feature: **Peyer's patches**, lymphoid follicles (also called **nodules**) found in the mucosa and part of the submucosa. The lack of Brunner's glands and the presence of shorter finger-like villi, when compared with the jejunum, are additional landmarks of the ileum. As in the jejunum, **Paneth cells** are found at the base of the crypts of Lieberkühn.

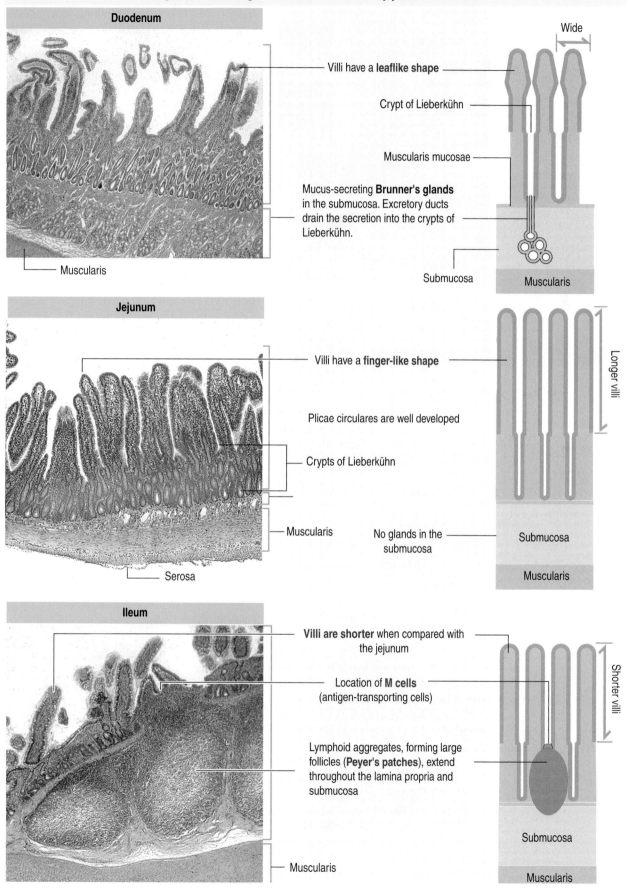

Figure 16-5. Histologic differences: Duodenum, jejunum, and ileum

Duodenum

Villi have a **leaflike shape**

Crypt of Lieberkühn

Muscularis mucosae

Mucus-secreting **Brunner's glands** in the submucosa. Excretory ducts drain the secretion into the crypts of Lieberkühn.

Muscularis

Submucosa

Muscularis

Wide

Jejunum

Villi have a **finger-like shape**

Plicae circulares are well developed

Crypts of Lieberkühn

Muscularis

No glands in the submucosa

Serosa

Longer villi

Submucosa

Muscularis

Ileum

Villi are shorter when compared with the jejunum

Location of **M cells** (antigen-transporting cells)

Lymphoid aggregates, forming large follicles (**Peyer's patches**), extend throughout the lamina propria and submucosa

Muscularis

Shorter villi

Submucosa

Muscularis

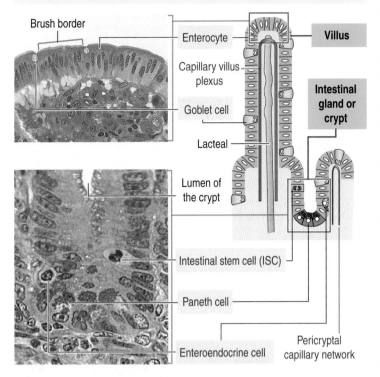

Figure 16-6. Epithelial cells of the villus and crypt of Lieberkühn

Brush border
Enterocyte
Villus
Capillary villus plexus
Goblet cell
Intestinal gland or crypt
Lacteal
Lumen of the crypt
Intestinal stem cell (ISC)
Paneth cell
Enteroendocrine cell
Pericryptal capillary network

Villi and crypts of Lieberkühn

The intestinal mucosa, including the crypts of Lieberkühn, are lined by a **simple columnar epithelium** containing five major cell types (Figure 16-6):

1. **Enterocytes or absorptive cells.**
2. **Goblet cells.**
3. **Enteroendocrine cells.**
4. **Paneth cells.**
5. **Intestinal stem cells.**

Enteroendocrine cells, Paneth cells, and intestinal stem cells are found in the crypts of Lieberkühn (see Figure 16-6). We discuss Paneth cells within the context of the protection mechanisms of the small intestine.

Enterocytes: Absorptive cells

The **absorptive intestinal cell** or **enterocyte** has an apical domain with a prominent **brush border** (also called a **striated border**), ending on a zone, called the **terminal web**, which contains transverse cytoskeletal filaments. The brush border of each absorptive cell contains about 3000 closely packed **microvilli**, which increase the surface luminal area 30-fold.

The length of a microvillus ranges from 0.5 to 1.0 μm. The core of a microvillus (Figure 16-7) contains a bundle of 20 to 40 parallel **actin filaments** cross-linked by **fimbrin** and **villin**. The actin bundle core is anchored to the plasma membrane by **formin** (protein of the cap), **myosin I**, and the calcium-binding protein **calmodulin**. Each actin bundle projects into the apical portion of the cell as a **rootlet**, which is

cross-linked by an **intestinal isoform of spectrin** to an adjacent rootlet. The end portion of the rootlet attaches to **cytokeratin-containing intermediate filaments**. Spectrin and cytokeratins form part of the **terminal web**. The terminal web is responsible for maintaining the upright position and shape of the microvillus and anchoring the actin rootlets.

A **surface coat** or **glycocalyx**, consisting of glycoproteins as integral components of the plasma membrane, covers each microvillus.

Trafficking of sugars and peptides in enterocytes

The **microvilli**, forming a **brush border**, contain intramembranous enzymes, including **lactase**, **maltase**, and **sucrase** (Figure 16-8). These oligosaccharides reduce carbohydrates to monosaccharides, which can be transported into the enterocyte by **carrier proteins**. Glucose and galactose cross the apical membrane with the help of a Na^+-dependent carrier system: involving the **sugar glucose/galactose transporter-1 (SGLT-1)**. Na^+-K^+ ATPase drives SGLT-1. Fructose (derived, together with glucose, from the breakdown of sucrose) enters and leaves the enterocyte by **passive diffusion**.

A **genetic defect in lactase** prevents the absorption of lactose-rich milk, causing diarrhea (**lactose intolerance**). Lactose is converted by intestinal bacteria to lactic acid, methane, and H_2 gas causing an osmotic diarrhea by drawing water into the intestinal lumen. A **lactose-H_2 breath test** is positive in individuals with lactase deficiency. H_2 enters the blood circulation and expired by the lungs.

Therefore, the brush border not only increases the absorptive surface of enterocytes but is also the site where enzymes are involved in the terminal digestion of carbohydrates and proteins.

Final breakdown of oligopeptides, initiated by the action of gastric pepsin, is extended by pancreatic trypsin, chymotrypsin, elastase, and carboxypeptidases A and B.

Enterokinase and **aminopeptidase**, localized in the microvilli, degrade oligopeptides into dipeptides, tripeptides, and amino acids before entering the enterocyte across **symporter channels** together with Na^+.

Cytoplasmic peptidases degrade dipeptides and tripeptides into amino acids, which then diffuse or are transported by a carrier-mediated process across the basolateral plasma membrane into the blood.

In **summary**, concerning carbohydrates, they can only be absorbed as monosaccharides. A two-step process enables the absorption of glucose and galactose monosaccharides: active transport across the apical membrane of the enterocyte involving SGLT-1, followed by transport across the basolateral membrane by facilitated diffusion.

Trafficking of lipids and cholesterol in enterocytes

The **absorption of lipids** involves the enzymatic

Figure 16-7. **Intestinal epithelium**

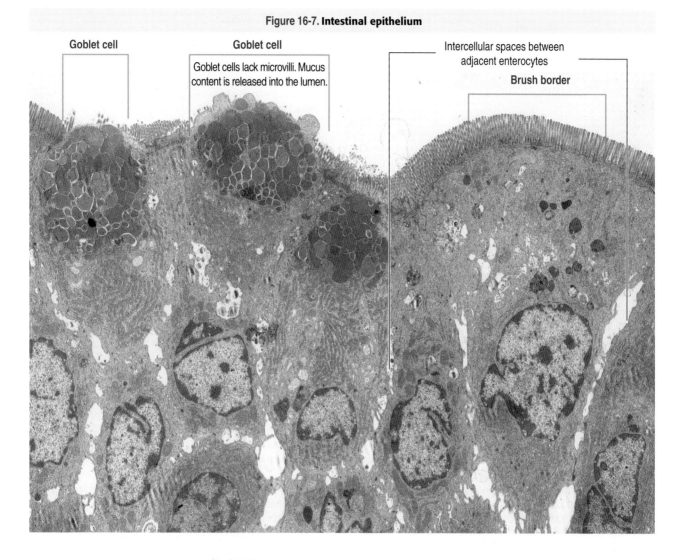

Goblet cell

Goblet cell

Goblet cells lack microvilli. Mucus content is released into the lumen.

Intercellular spaces between adjacent enterocytes

Brush border

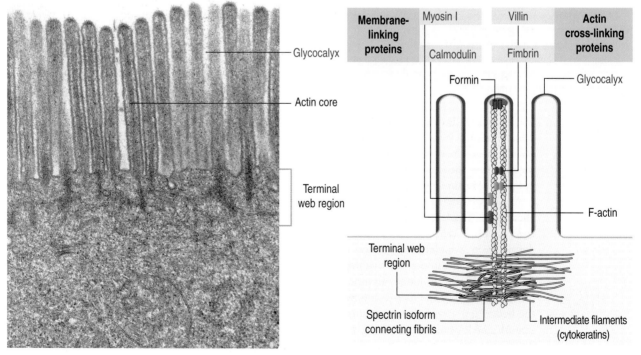

Glycocalyx

Actin core

Terminal web region

Membrane-linking proteins	Myosin I	Villin	**Actin cross-linking proteins**
	Calmodulin	Fimbrin	

Formin

Glycocalyx

F-actin

Terminal web region

Spectrin isoform connecting fibrils

Intermediate filaments (cytokeratins)

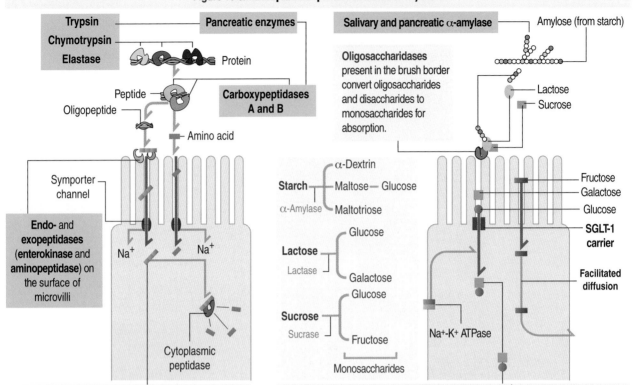

Figure 16-8. **Absorption of proteins and carbohydrates**

Trypsin
Chymotrypsin
Elastase
Pancreatic enzymes

Salivary and pancreatic α-amylase — Amylose (from starch)

Protein

Peptide

Oligopeptide

Carboxypeptidases A and B

Amino acid

Oligosaccharidases present in the brush border convert oligosaccharides and disaccharides to monosaccharides for absorption.

Lactose
Sucrose

Symporter channel

Endo- and **exopeptidases** (**enterokinase** and **aminopeptidase**) on the surface of microvilli

Na⁺   Na⁺

Cytoplasmic peptidase

α-Dextrin
Starch ─ Maltose — Glucose
α-Amylase ─ Maltotriose

Lactose ─ Glucose
Lactase ─ Galactose

Sucrose ─ Glucose
Sucrase ─ Fructose

Monosaccharides

Fructose
Galactose
Glucose

SGLT-1 carrier

Facilitated diffusion

Na⁺-K⁺ ATPase

The absorption of amino acids and di- and tripeptides occurs across **symporter channels** together with Na⁺. The transport is active.

Glucose and galactose enter the enterocyte using an Na⁺-dependent carrier system (**sugar glucose/galactose transporter-1 [SGLT-1]**) for glucose and galactose. The transport is active (driven by Na⁺-K⁺ ATPase). Fructose enters and leaves the enterocyte by facilitated diffusion.

Protein digestion starts in the stomach in the presence of pepsin derived from the precursor pepsinogen secreted by chief cells. Pepsin activity ends in the alkaline environment of the duodenum. Pancreatic proteases, **endopeptidases** and **exopeptidases**, continue proteolysis.

Trypsinogen is activated to **trypsin** by **enterokinase**, located on the microvilli. Active trypsin, in turn, activates the bulk of trypsinogen.

Chymotrypsinogen and **proelastase** are activated to chymotrypsin and elastase, respectively. Carboxypeptidases A and B derive from procarboxypeptidase A and B precursors.

Trypsin plays a significant role in the activation and inactivation of pancreatic proenzymes. Tripeptides in the cytosol are digested by cytoplasmic peptidases into amino acids.

Starch, sucrose, lactose, and **maltose** are the main dietary carbohydrates. Starch consists of amylose (a glucose polymer) and amylopectin (a plant starch). **Sucrose** is a glucose-fructose disaccharide. **Lactose** is a galactose-glucose disaccharide. **Maltose** is a glucose dimer. Salivary α-amylase initiates the digestion of starch in the mouth. Pancreatic α-amylase completes the digestion in the small intestine. Other major dietary sugars are hydrolyzed by **oligosaccharidases** (sucrase, lactase, isomaltase) present in the plasma membrane of the microvilli.

Cellulose is not digested in the human small intestine because cellulase is not present. Cellulose accounts for the undigested dietary fiber.

breakdown of dietary lipids into **fatty acids** and **monoglycerides**, which can diffuse across the plasma membrane of the microvilli and the apical plasma membrane of the enterocyte. Details of the **process of lipid absorption** are depicted in Figure 16-9.

We address now in detail how enterocytes handle cholesterol. **Cholesterol** is an essential structural component of cell membranes. Body cholesterol derives from two sources: diet and new synthesis from acetyl CoA through the mevalonate pathway. Dietary cholesterol is initially transported from the intestine to the liver and then distributed throughout the body. Newly synthesized cholesterol leaves the smooth endoplasmic reticulum by a non-vesicular transport mechanism bypassing the endoplasmic

reticulum-Golgi transport pathway and rapidly targeted to the plasma membrane. We discuss mitochondrial cholesterol transport in Chapter 19, Endocrine System, within the context of steroidogenesis in the adrenal cortex.

Enterocytes and hepatocytes package cholesterol, along with triglycerides, into **lipoproteins** (chylomicrons). **Chylomicrons** consist of triglycerides (85%), phospholipids (9%), cholesterol (4%) and proteins (2%, including the apolipoprotein APOB48).

Cholesterol is secreted from the liver into the bile as cholesterol or bile acids, entering the small intestine. Cholesterol and bile salts can be reabsorbed and return to the liver by the enterohepatic cycle or excreted into the feces.

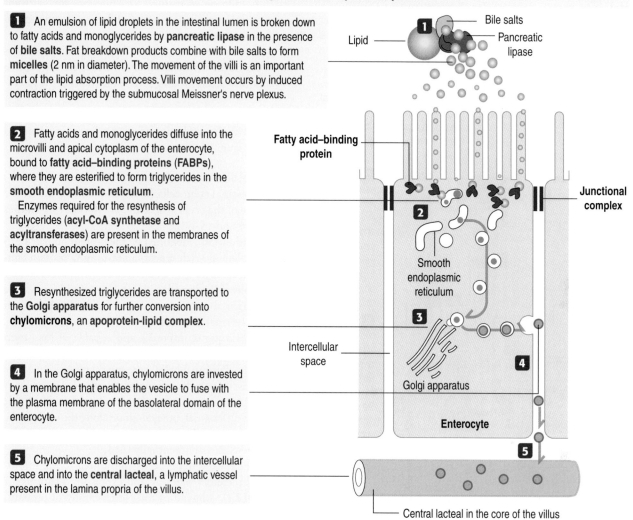

Figure 16-9. Absorption of lipids

1 An emulsion of lipid droplets in the intestinal lumen is broken down to fatty acids and monoglycerides by **pancreatic lipase** in the presence of **bile salts**. Fat breakdown products combine with bile salts to form **micelles** (2 nm in diameter). The movement of the villi is an important part of the lipid absorption process. Villi movement occurs by induced contraction triggered by the submucosal Meissner's nerve plexus.

2 Fatty acids and monoglycerides diffuse into the microvilli and apical cytoplasm of the enterocyte, bound to **fatty acid–binding proteins (FABPs)**, where they are esterified to form triglycerides in the **smooth endoplasmic reticulum**.

Enzymes required for the resynthesis of triglycerides (**acyl-CoA synthetase** and **acyltransferases**) are present in the membranes of the smooth endoplasmic reticulum.

3 Resynthesized triglycerides are transported to the **Golgi apparatus** for further conversion into **chylomicrons**, an **apoprotein-lipid complex**.

4 In the Golgi apparatus, chylomicrons are invested by a membrane that enables the vesicle to fuse with the plasma membrane of the basolateral domain of the enterocyte.

5 Chylomicrons are discharged into the intercellular space and into the **central lacteal**, a lymphatic vessel present in the lamina propria of the villus.

Figure 16-10 illustrates the relevant steps of **cholesterol trafficking** in enterocytes. As in the absorption of dietary lipids, cholesterol is solubilized in the intestinal lumen into micelles by bile acids to facilitate micellar movement through the diffusion barrier of the enterocytes.

Note in Figure 16-10 that the **ABCG5/ABCG8** (ATP-binding cassette, ABC) heterodimeric transporters at the apical domain of enterocytes export absorbed cholesterol back into the intestinal lumen, a step that facilitates the removal of cholesterol from the body. Mutations in *ABCG5* **or** *ABCG8* genes cause **sitosterolemia**, an autosomal recessive disorder in which cholesterol and plant sterols accumulate in the circulation leading to premature cardiovascular disease.

In contrast, the **NPC1L1** (Niemann-Pick C1-like-1) protein, located also at the apical domain, enables the uptake of cholesterol esterified by **ACAT2** (Acyl CoA cholesterol acyltransferase isoform 2).

Esterified cholesterol becomes part of **chylomicron particles**, assembled in the smooth endoplasmic

reticulum in the presence of **APOB48 apoprotein**, triglycerides and **MTP** (microsomal triglyceride protein), which transfers cholesterol esters from the smooth endoplasmic reticulum membranes to nascent APOB 48 apolipoproteins.

The newly assembled chylomicron leaves the endoplasmic reticulum in **COPII-coated vesicles** and released through the Golgi apparatus into the basolateral domain of the enterocyte to reach a lymphatic capillary in the lamina propria of the intestinal villus.

Knowledge of the cholesterol transport pathway can help you understand its regulation in patients with atherosclerotic cardiovascular disease. For example, the pharmacologic targeting of ACAT2 can decrease the esterification of cholesterol. About 70-80% of cholesterol entering the lymphatic system is esterified.

Goblet cells

Goblet cells are columnar mucus-secreting cells scattered among enterocytes of the intestinal epithelium (see Figure 16-7).

Figure 16-10. Cholesterol uptake and trafficking in enterocytes

2 NPC1L1 *(Niemann-Pick C1-like protein)* facilitates the uptake of cholesterol. Inhibitors of NPC1L1 prevent cholesterol uptake.

3 ABCG5/ABCGG8 heterodimer transporter is involved in the transfer of cholesterol into the intestinal lumen for disposal from the body

1 Cholesterol undergoes micellar solubilization by bile salts

4 ACAT2 (Acyl CoA cholesterol acyltransferase isoform 2*)* esterifies the absorbed cholesterol that relocates to the smooth endoplasmic reticulum

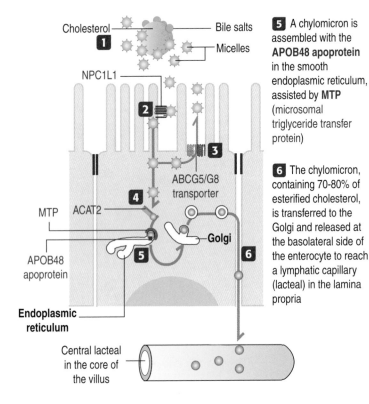

5 A chylomicron is assembled with the **APOB48 apoprotein** in the smooth endoplasmic reticulum, assisted by **MTP** (microsomal triglyceride transfer protein)

6 The chylomicron, containing 70-80% of esterified cholesterol, is transferred to the Golgi and released at the basolateral side of the enterocyte to reach a lymphatic capillary (lacteal) in the lamina propria

Goblet cells have two domains:

1. A cup- or goblet-shaped **apical domain** containing large mucus granules that are discharged on the surface of the epithelium.

2. A narrow **basal domain**, which attaches to the basal lamina. The basal domain houses the rough endoplasmic reticulum and Golgi apparatus, in which the protein portion of mucus is produced and transported, and the nucleus

The **Golgi apparatus**, which adds oligosaccharide groups to mucus, is prominent and situated above the basally located nucleus.

The secretory product of goblet cells contains **glycoproteins** (80% carbohydrate and 20% protein) released by **exocytosis**.

On the surface of the epithelium, **the mucus hydrates to form a protective gel coat to shield the epithelium from mechanical abrasion and bacterial invasion** by concentrating specific antimicrobial proteins, including defensins and cathelicidins.

Enteroendocrine cells

In addition to its digestive function, the gastrointestinal tract is the largest diffuse endocrine gland in the body.

As in the stomach (see Chapter 15, Upper Digestive Segment), enteroendocrine cells secrete peptide hormones controlling several functions of the gastrointestinal system.

The location and function of **gastrin-**, **secretin-**, and **cholecystokinin**-secreting cells are summarized in Figure 16-11.

Intestinal stem cells

Intestinal stem cells (**ISCs**) reside in a niche at the base of the crypts, close to Paneth cells (see Figures 16-6 and 16-17).

Adult ISC, identified by the protein marker **Lgr5** (for **leucine-rich repeat-containing G protein coupled receptor 5**), can differentiate into the secretory goblet cells, Paneth cells, and enteroendocrine cells and the absorptive enterocytes lining the epithelium of the small intestine.

ISCs are multipotent and capable of long-term self-renewal as long as they remain at the crypt niche. Presumably ISCs are subject to positional cues derived from the microenvironment of the niche.

As clusters of enterocytes and goblet cells divide and differentiate, they migrate along the walls of the crypts and villi until they reach the tip of the villus where they are eventually shed.

Following injury, cells committed to the intestinal secretory pathway and expressing **Delta-like 1** (**DLL1**), a ligand of the Notch family of proteins, can return to the stem cell compartment and revert into multipotent ISCs. At this point, you may like to take another look at Box 3-D in Chapter 3, Cell Signaling, to review the Notch signaling pathway.

Protection of the small intestine

The large surface area of the gastrointestinal tract, about 200 m² in humans, is vulnerable to resident microorganisms, called **microbiota**, and potentially harmful microorganisms and dietary antigens. Microbiota includes bacteria, fungi, parasites and viruses.

We discuss in Chapter 15, Upper Digestive Segment, the role of the mucus blanket in the protection of the surface of the stomach during *Helicobacter pylori* infection.

In the small and large intestines, **goblet cells** secrete mucin glycoproteins assembled into a viscous gel-like blanket limiting direct bacterial contact with enterocytes. When the blanket lacks one of its components, mucin glycoprotein 2 (MIC2), spontaneous intestinal inflammation occurs.

Several defensive mechanisms operate in the alimentary tube to limit tissue invasion of pathogens and

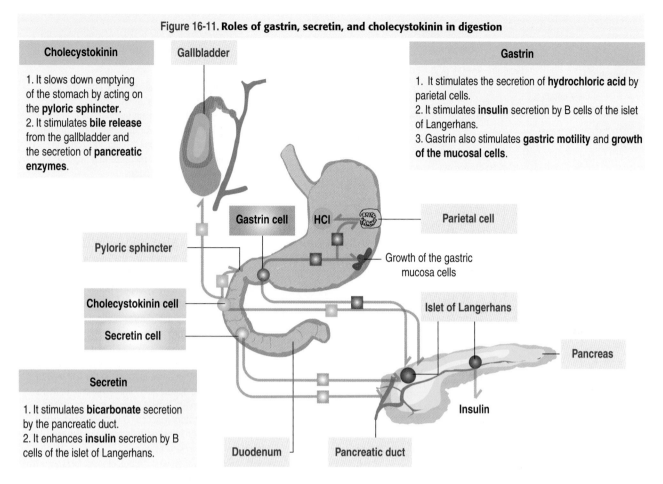

Figure 16-11. Roles of gastrin, secretin, and cholecystokinin in digestion

Cholecystokinin

1. It slows down emptying of the stomach by acting on the **pyloric sphincter**.
2. It stimulates **bile release** from the gallbladder and the secretion of **pancreatic enzymes**.

Gastrin

1. It stimulates the secretion of **hydrochloric acid** by parietal cells.
2. It stimulates **insulin** secretion by B cells of the islet of Langerhans.
3. Gastrin also stimulates **gastric motility** and **growth of the mucosal cells**.

Secretin

1. It stimulates **bicarbonate** secretion by the pancreatic duct.
2. It enhances **insulin** secretion by B cells of the islet of Langerhans.

Gallbladder · Gastrin cell · HCl · Parietal cell · Pyloric sphincter · Growth of the gastric mucosa cells · Cholecystokinin cell · Secretin cell · Islet of Langerhans · Pancreas · Insulin · Duodenum · Pancreatic duct

avoid potentially harmful overreactions that could damage intestinal tissues. The defensive mechanisms include:

1. The **intestinal tight junction barrier**, formed by apical **tight junctions** linking enterocytes. The barrier of pathogens is monitored by the immune–competent cells residing in the subjacent **lamina propria**.

2. **Peyer's patches** and associated **M cells,** regarded as the immune sensors of the small intestine.

3. **Polymeric immunoglobulin A (IgA)**, a secretory product of **plasma cells** located in the lamina propria, reaching the intestinal lumen by the mechanism of **transcytosis**.

4. **Paneth cells,** whose bacteriostatic secretions control the resident microbiota of the small intestine.

In addition, we need to keep in mind the defensive roles of the acidity of the **gastric juice**, that inactivates ingested microorganism, and the propulsive intestinal motility (**peristalsis**), that prevents bacterial colonization.

Intestinal tight junction barrier

Intestinal tight junctions link adjacent enterocytes and provide a barrier function impermeable to most hydrophilic solutes in absence of specific transporters.

Tight junctions establish a separation between the intestinal luminal content and the mucosal immune function that occurs within the lamina propria. Plasma cells, lymphocytes, eosinophils, mast cells and macrophages are present in the intestinal lamina propria.

Claudin and **occludin** are two transmembrane proteins of tight junctions that regulate solute permeability of the transcellular pathway. Flux of dietary proteins and bacterial lipopolysaccharides across leaky tight junctions can increase in the presence of **tumor necrosis factor ligand** and **interferon-γ**, two proinflammatory cytokines that affect tight junction integrity.

Many diseases associated with intestinal epithelial dysfunction, including **inflammatory bowel disease** and **intestinal ischemia**, are associated with increased levels of tumor necrosis factor ligand.

A minor defect of the tight junction barrier can allow bacterial products or dietary antigens to cross the epithelium and enter the lamina propria. Antigens can bind to **Toll-like receptor (TLR)** on the surface of dendritic cells. We discuss TLR in Chapter 10, Immune-Lymphatic System (see Box 10-A).

Dendritic cells migrate to a local mesentery lymph node and the antigen is presented to naïve T cells by the major histocompatibility complex to determine their differentiation into T helper 1 (TH1) and T

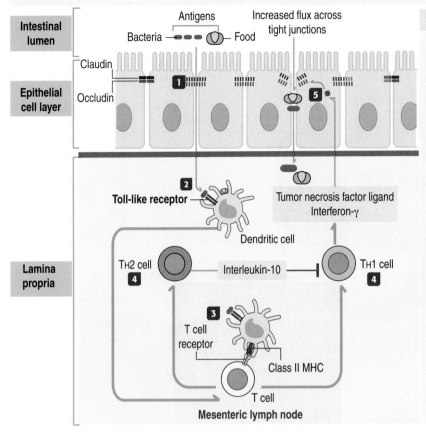

Figure 16-12. Intestinal tight junction barrier

Intestinal lumen

Antigens

Bacteria — Food

Increased flux across tight junctions

Epithelial cell layer

Claudin

Occludin

1

5

Lamina propria

Toll-like receptor

2

Dendritic cell

Tumor necrosis factor ligand Interferon-γ

TH2 cell **4**

Interleukin-10

TH1 cell **4**

3

T cell receptor

Class II MHC

T cell

Mesenteric lymph node

Intestinal tight junction barrier

1 A defect in the intestinal tight junction barrier enables the unrestricted passage of antigens to the lamina propria.

2 In the lamina propria, antigens are taken up by a dendritic cell through the **Toll-like receptor** that then migrates to a regional mesenteric lymph node.

3 In the node, naïve T cells interacts with the dendritic cell. The antigen is presented to the T cell receptor by the class II major histocompatibility complex (class II MHC). T cells differentiate into T helper 1 (TH1) and T helper 2 (TH2) cells that translocate to the lamina propria.

4 In the lamina propria, a TH1 cell expresses proinflammatory cytokines **tumor necrosis factor ligand** and **interferon-γ**. A regulatory TH2 cell expresses interleukin-10 to block the release of proinflammatory cytokines by the TH1 cell.

5 Unregulated proinflammatory cytokines signal enterocytes to increase the passage of antigens across leaky tight junctions, from the lumen to the lamina propria, thus amplifying the inflammatory reaction. This mechanism can lead to an intestinal inflammatory disease.

helper 2 (TH2) cells that relocate to the lamina propria (Figure 16-12).

TH1 cells produce the proinflammatory cytokines tumor necrosis factor ligand and interferon-γ. TH2 cells downregulate the proinflammatory activity of TH1 cells by secreting **interleukin-10**. If the mucosa immune cell activation response proceeds unchecked, proinflammatory cytokines will continue enhancing further leakage across the tight junction barrier, a condition leading to intestinal chronic inflammatory diseases.

Peyer's patches

Peyer's patches, the main component of the **gut-associated lymphoid tissue (GALT)**, are specialized lymphoid follicles found predominantly in the intestinal mucosa and part of the submucosa of the **ileum** (see Box 16-A). GALTs participate in the uptake of antigens and their exposure to antigen-presenting cells. Therefore, these structures serve important functions that can lead to inflammation or tolerance.

The microbiota is involved in the normal development and maturation of GALTs. In the fetus, lymphoid tissue inducer cells stimulate the development of Peyer's patches in the absence of microbiota.

Peyer's patches consist of cells able to take up and transport luminal antigens and bacteria to antigen-presenting cells leading to immune tolerance or an inflammatory reaction against pathogens.

Peyer's patches are regarded the **immune sensors of the small intestine**. An equivalent to Peyer's patches in the large intestine are the **isolated lymphoid follicles (ILFs)**, requiring TLRs and **nucleotide-binding oligomerization domain 2 (NOD2)** to become activated. TLRs are **extracellular** sensors and NODs are **cytoplasmic** sensors. We come back to NOD2 in our discussion of the bacteriostatic Paneth cells.

Box 16-A | Development of Peyer's patches

• Hematopoietic cells aggregate in the small intestine to form the primordia of Peyer's patches. A subset of hematopoietic cells expresses receptor tyrosine kinase (**RET**), which is also essential for the development of the enteric nervous system (submucosal plexus of Meissner and myenteric plexus of Auerbach).

• The protooncogene *Ret* encodes RET, expressed in tissues and tumors derived from the neural crest and neuroectoderm.

• The RET ligand artemin (**ARTN**), a member of the glial cell line–derived neurotrophic factor (GDNF) family ligands, regulates the development of the nervous and lymphoid system of the intestine. However, a failure to develop Peyer's patches in *Ret* mutant mice is **independent** of the development of the enteric nervous system.

• As discussed later in this chapter, a deficiency in the Ret/ligand signaling pathway is the cause of distal colonic aganglionosis (Hirschsprung's disease). This pathway is also critical for the formation of the enteric hematopoietic Peyer's patches system.

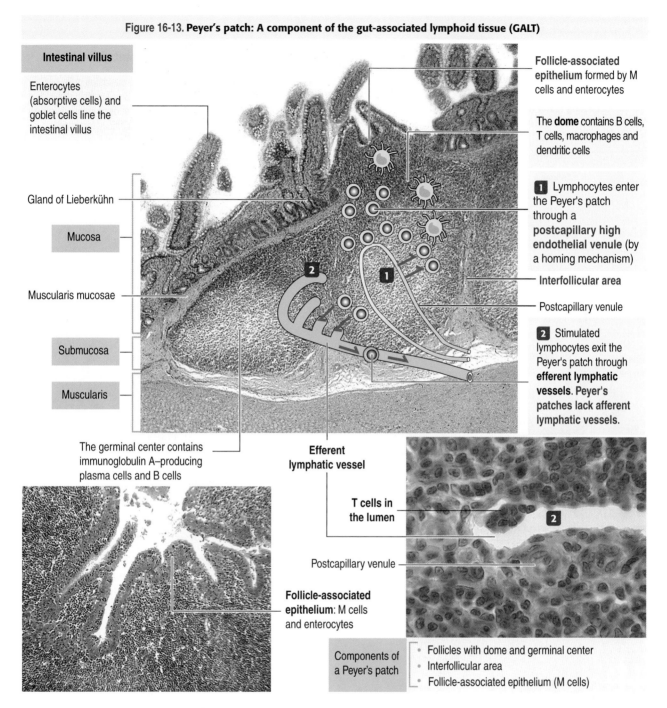

Figure 16-13. Peyer's patch: A component of the gut-associated lymphoid tissue (GALT)

Intestinal villus

Enterocytes (absorptive cells) and goblet cells line the intestinal villus

Gland of Lieberkühn

Mucosa

Muscularis mucosae

Submucosa

Muscularis

The germinal center contains immunoglobulin A–producing plasma cells and B cells

Follicle-associated epithelium formed by M cells and enterocytes

The **dome** contains B cells, T cells, macrophages and dendritic cells

1 Lymphocytes enter the Peyer's patch through a **postcapillary high endothelial venule** (by a homing mechanism)

Interfollicular area

Postcapillary venule

2 Stimulated lymphocytes exit the Peyer's patch through **efferent lymphatic vessels**. Peyer's patches lack afferent lymphatic vessels.

Efferent lymphatic vessel

T cells in the lumen

Postcapillary venule

Follicle-associated epithelium: M cells and enterocytes

Components of a Peyer's patch
- Follicles with dome and germinal center
- Interfollicular area
- Follicle-associated epithelium (M cells)

A Peyer's patch displays three main components (Figure 16-13):

1. The **follicle-associated epithelium (FAE)**, consisting of **M cells and enterocytes**.

2. The **lymphoid follicles**, each showing a germinal center and a subepithelial dome area.

3. The **interfollicular area,** with blood vessels and efferent lymphatic vessels connecting Peyer's patches to the mesenteric lymph nodes.

High endothelial venules, enabling the immigration of lymphocytes, are present in the lymphoid follicles. Activated lymphocytes leave the Peyer's patches through the lymphatic vessels (see Figure 16-13).

The main components of the FAE are **M cells** and **dendritic cells:**

1. **M cells** (Figure 16-14), forming an enterocyte specialized cell layer that takes up antigens and replaced the brush border by short **microfolds** (hence the name M cell). M cells differentiate from enterocytes when stimulated by membrane-bound lymphotoxin (LTα1β2) present on local B cells.

M cells form **intraepithelial pockets**, where a subpopulation of intraepithelial B cells resides and express **IgA receptors** allowing the capture and phagocytosis of IgA-bound bacteria.

Antigens are transported by M cell and presented

Figure 16-14. Peyer's patch: Cellular immune surveillance system of the intestinal tract

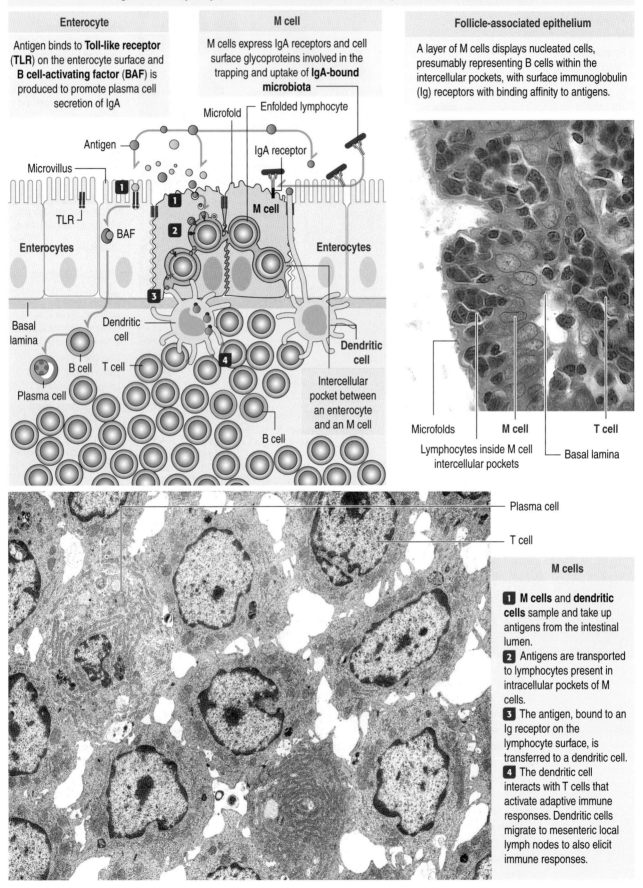

Enterocyte

Antigen binds to **Toll-like receptor** (**TLR**) on the enterocyte surface and **B cell-activating factor** (**BAF**) is produced to promote plasma cell secretion of IgA

M cell

M cells express IgA receptors and cell surface glycoproteins involved in the trapping and uptake of **IgA-bound microbiota**

Follicle-associated epithelium

A layer of M cells displays nucleated cells, presumably representing B cells within the intercellular pockets, with surface immunoglobulin (Ig) receptors with binding affinity to antigens.

Microfold — Enfolded lymphocyte

IgA receptor

Antigen

Microvillus

M cell

TLR

Enterocytes

BAF

Enterocytes

Basal lamina

Dendritic cell

Dendritic cell

B cell   T cell

Plasma cell

Intercellular pocket between an enterocyte and an M cell

B cell

Microfolds

M cell

T cell

Lymphocytes inside M cell intercellular pockets

Basal lamina

Plasma cell

T cell

M cells

1 **M cells** and **dendritic cells** sample and take up antigens from the intestinal lumen.

2 Antigens are transported to lymphocytes present in intracellular pockets of M cells.

3 The antigen, bound to an Ig receptor on the lymphocyte surface, is transferred to a dendritic cell.

4 The dendritic cell interacts with T cells that activate adaptive immune responses. Dendritic cells migrate to mesenteric local lymph nodes to also elicit immune responses.

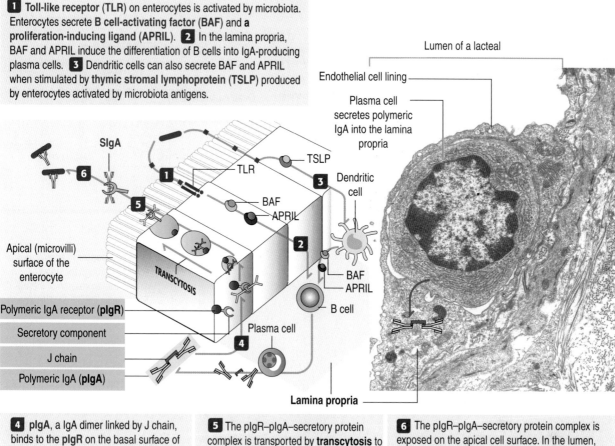

Figure 16-15. Polymeric IgA: Immune surveillance of the intestinal tract

1 Toll-like receptor (TLR) on enterocytes is activated by microbiota. Enterocytes secrete B cell-activating factor (BAF) and a proliferation-inducing ligand (APRIL). **2** In the lamina propria, BAF and APRIL induce the differentiation of B cells into IgA-producing plasma cells. **3** Dendritic cells can also secrete BAF and APRIL when stimulated by thymic stromal lymphoprotein (TSLP) produced by enterocytes activated by microbiota antigens.

4 pIgA, a IgA dimer linked by J chain, binds to the pIgR on the basal surface of an enterocyte. A secretory component is part of pIgR.

5 The pIgR–pIgA–secretory protein complex is transported by transcytosis to the apical domain of the enterocyte.

6 The pIgR–pIgA–secretory protein complex is exposed on the apical cell surface. In the lumen, the secretory component is cleaved from its transmembrane anchorage. The IgA–secretory component complex SIgA is released into the intestinal lumen. IgAs bind to bacteria then presented to M cells (see Figure 16-14).

to the immunocompetent B cells residing in the intraepithelial pockets.

The population of M cells increases rapidly in the presence of pathogenic bacteria in the intestinal lumen (for example, *Salmonella typhimurium*). When confronting *Salmonella*, the microfolds of M cells change into large ruffles and, within 30 to 60 minutes, M cells undergo necrosis and the population of M cells is depleted. **Poliovirus**, the pathogen of poliomyelitis, uses the Peyer's patches to replicate.

2. **Dendritic cell**, extending cytoplasmic processes between tight junctions linking enterocytes (see Figure 16-14).

Lymphoid follicles have a **germinal center** that contains IgA-positive B cells, CD4$^+$ T cells, antigen-presenting cells and follicular dendritic cells. A few plasma cells are present in the Peyer's patches. The **subepithelial dome** contains B cells, T cells, macrophages, and dendritic cells.

Antigens in the intestinal lumen activate TLRs

expressed by enterocytes (see Figure 16-14). TLR-antigen interaction stimulates the production of **B cell-activating factor** (**BAF**) and cytokines to activate the production of immunoglobulin (Ig) A by plasma cells located in the lamina propria and Peyer's patches.

Intestinal antigens, bound to immunoglobulin receptors on the surface of B cells, interact with **antigen-presenting cells** at the subepithelial dome region. Antigens are presented to **follicular dendritic cells** and CD4$^+$ T cells to initiate an immune reaction.

In **summary**, Peyer's patches have the ability to transport luminal antigens and microorganisms and respond to them by inducing immune tolerance or a systemic immune defense response. An example of the functional deficiency of Peyer's patches is **Crohn's disease**, an inflammatory bowel disease characterized by chronic or relapsing inflammation.

Polymeric IgA

Plasma cells secrete **polymeric IgA** into the intestinal

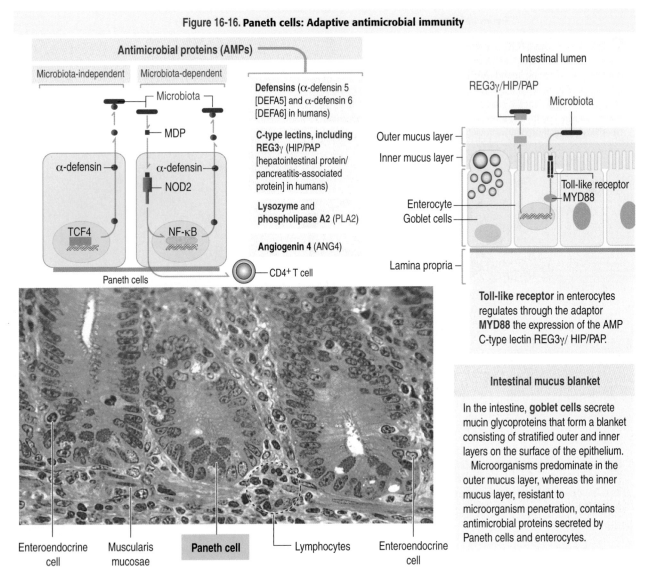

Figure 16-16. Paneth cells: Adaptive antimicrobial immunity

Antimicrobial proteins (AMPs)

Microbiota-independent

Microbiota-dependent

Microbiota

MDP

α-defensin

α-defensin

NOD2

TCF4

NF-κB

Paneth cells

CD4⁺ T cell

Defensins (α-defensin 5 [DEFA5] and α-defensin 6 [DEFA6] in humans)

C-type lectins, including REG3γ (HIP/PAP [hepatointestinal protein/ pancreatitis-associated protein] in humans)

Lysozyme and **phospholipase A2** (PLA2)

Angiogenin 4 (ANG4)

Intestinal lumen

REG3γ/HIP/PAP

Microbiota

Outer mucus layer

Inner mucus layer

Enterocyte

Goblet cells

Toll-like receptor

MYD88

Lamina propria

Toll-like receptor in enterocytes regulates through the adaptor **MYD88** the expression of the AMP C-type lectin REG3γ/ HIP/PAP.

Intestinal mucus blanket

In the intestine, **goblet cells** secrete mucin glycoproteins that form a blanket consisting of stratified outer and inner layers on the surface of the epithelium.

Microorganisms predominate in the outer mucus layer, whereas the inner mucus layer, resistant to microorganism penetration, contains antimicrobial proteins secreted by Paneth cells and enterocytes.

Enteroendocrine cell

Muscularis mucosae

Paneth cell

Lymphocytes

Enteroendocrine cell

lumen, the respiratory epithelium, the lactating mammary gland, and salivary glands. Most plasma cells are present in the **lamina propria** of the intestinal villi, together with **lymphocytes, eosinophils, mast cells,** and **macrophages.**

Polymeric IgA molecules secreted by plasma cells are transported from the lamina propria to the intestinal lumen by a **transcytosis mechanism** consisting of the following steps (Figure 16-15):

1. **Polymeric** IgA is secreted as a dimeric molecule joined by a peptide called the **J chain.**

2. Polymeric IgA binds to a specific receptor, called the **polymeric immunoglobulin receptor (pIgR),** available on the basal surfaces of the enterocytes. The pIgR has an attached **secretory component.**

3. The polymeric **IgA–pIgR–secretory component complex is internalized and transported across the cell to the apical surface** of the epithelial cell.

4. At the apical surface, the complex is cleaved enzymatically and the polymeric IgA-secretory component complex is released into the intestinal lumen

as **secreted IgA (SIgA).** The secretory component protects the dimeric IgA from proteolytic degradation.

5. IgA attaches to bacteria and soluble antigens, preventing a direct damaging effect to intestinal cells and penetration into the lamina propria.

How are plasma cells induced to produce polymeric IgA?

When TLR on enterocytes is activated by microbiota, they secrete **B cell-activating factor (BAF)** and **a proliferation-inducing ligand (APRIL).**

In the lamina propria, BAF and APRIL induce the differentiation of B cells into IgA-producing plasma cells (see Figure 16-15).

In addition, the microbiota instructs enterocytes through **thymic stromal lymphoprotein (TSLP)** to engage **dendritic cells** in the lamina propria to secrete BAF and APRIL and induce the differentiation of B cells into plasma cells.

One last point: IgA regulates the composition and the function of the intestinal microbiota by affecting **bacterial gene expression.** By this mechanism, IgA

Figure 16-17. **Lower half of an intestinal gland (crypt of Lieberkühn)**

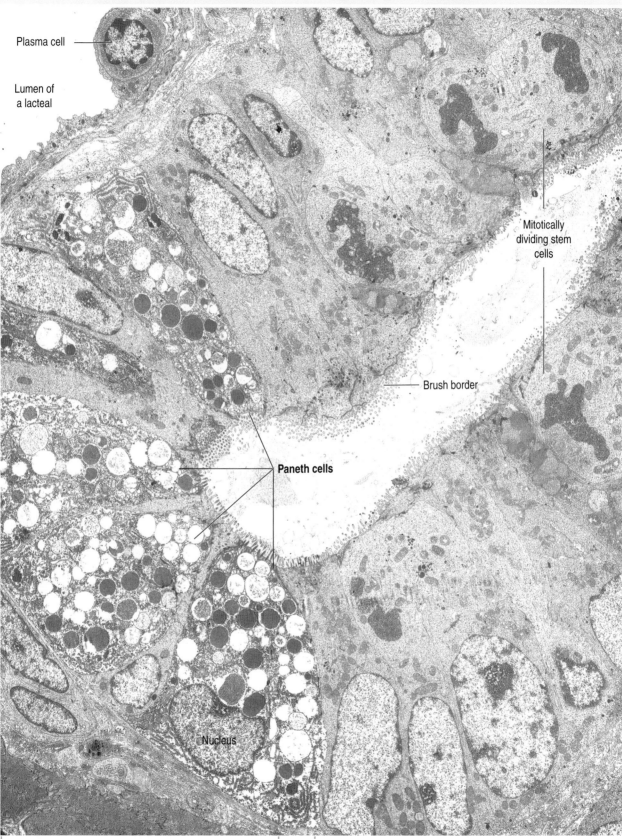

Plasma cell

Lumen of
a lacteal

Mitotically
dividing stem
cells

Brush border

Paneth cells

Nucleus

Muscularis mucosae

Enterocytes

Figure 16-18. **Crohn's disease**

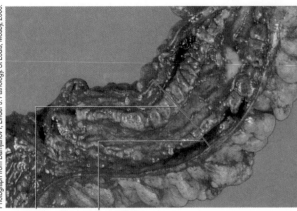

Thick wall   Narrow lumen

Patients with defects in NOD2 (for nucleotide-binding oligomerization domain-containing protein 2) have lower expression of α-defensins by Paneth cells and severe intestinal inflammation. Low levels of α-defensin proteins allow increased association of microorganisms with the epithelial cell surface and may contribute to Crohn's disease, a chronic inflammatory bowel disease.

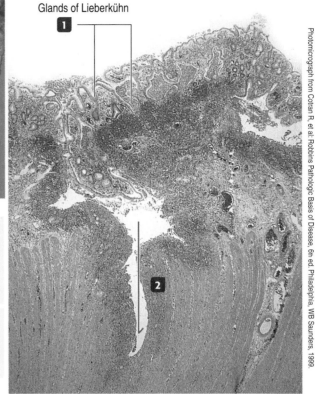

Glands of Lieberkühn
1

1 Crypts of Lieberkühn are invaded by inflammatory cells. This process results in occlusion and atrophy of the intestinal gland.

2 Chronic granulomas invade and destroy the muscularis, which is replaced by connective tissue.

keeps a congenial relationship between the host and the microbiota.

In our discussion of Peyer's patches, we indicated that M cells express IgA receptors allowing the uptake of IgA–bound bacteria. As you realize, luminal SIgA not only immobilize bacteria but also redirects them to the M cells for internalization and disposal.

Paneth cells

Enterocytes and **Paneth cells** in particular secrete proteins to limit bacteria pathogenic challenges. We discuss in Chapter 11. Integumentary System, how epithelial **antimicrobial proteins** (**AMPs**) protect skin surfaces against microorganisms. We continue the discussion within the context of the antimicrobial defense of the intestinal mucosa involving Paneth cells and enterocytes.

Most AMPs inactivate or kill bacteria directly by enzymatic degradation of the bacterial wall or by disrupting the bacterial inner membrane. A group of AMPs deprive bacteria of essential heavy metal such as iron.

AMPs produced by Paneth cells and enterocytes are retained in the **intestinal mucus blanket produced by goblet cells**. Therefore, the mucus layer protects the intestinal mucosa by two mechanisms:

1. By creating a barrier that limits direct access of luminal bacteria to the epithelium.

2. By concentrating AMPs near the enterocyte surface. AMPs are virtually absent from the luminal content.

Paneth cells are present at the base of the crypts of Lieberkühn and have a lifetime of about 20 days. The pyramid-shaped Paneth cells have a basal domain containing the rough endoplasmic reticulum. The apical region shows numerous protein granules representing a diverse array of AMPs, an indication of the microbial diversity and impending threats (Figures 16-16 and 16-17).

Paneth cells produce several AMPs:

1. **Defensins** (α-defensin 5 [DEFA5] and α-defensin 6 [DEFA6] in humans)

2. C-type lectins, including regenerating islet-derived protein 3γ (**REG3γ**), also known as hepatointestinal protein/pancreatitis-associated protein (**HIP/PAP**).

3. **Lysozyme** and **phospholipase A2** (**PLA2**).

4. **Angiogenin 4** (**ANG4**).

α-Defensins (2–3 kd) target Gram-positive and Gram-negative bacteria, fungi, viruses, and protozoa to produce membrane disruption by the formation of defensin pores. Pores cause swelling and membrane rupture enabling the entrance of water into the pathogen. Defensins can also be chemotactic to CD4+ T cells, CD8+ T cells, monocytes, and macrophages and modulate an inflammatory response. Defensins enhance the recruitment of dendritic cells to the site of infection and facilitate the uptake of antigens by forming defensin-antigen complexes.

Like all C-type lectins, the carbohydrate-recognition domain of **REG3γ/HIP/PAP** (15 kd) binds to the glycan chain of peptidoglycan present in the bacterial cell wall of Gram-positive bacteria and causes wall disruption. Peptidoglycan is present in bacteria but not in human cells.

Recall that selectins, a member of the group of Ca^{2+}-dependent cell adhesion molecules, belong to the C-type lectin family that have carbohydrate-recognition domains.

Lysozyme is a proteolytic enzyme that cleaves glycosidic linkages that maintain the integrity of cell wall peptidoglycan. **PLA2** kills bacteria by hydrolysis of phospholipids in the bacterial membrane.

Paneth cells secrete **ANG4**, an RNAse with bactericidal properties.

It is important to emphasize that the expression and function of AMPs are highly regulated by the presence or absence of the microbiota (see Figure 16-16).

In the presence of microorganisms:

1. **TLR** in enterocytes controls the expression of REG3γ/HIP/PAP through the TLR-signaling adaptor myeloid-differentiation primary response protein 88 (**MYD88**).

2. Cytoplasmic **NOD2**, expressed by Paneth cells, controls the expression of α-defensins when it binds to an internalized peptidoglycan peptide fragment (muramyl dipeptide, MDP) and activates the transcription factor NF-κB.

Note that NOD2 is in a strategic position to contribute to immunogenic tolerance toward the microbiota when confronting MDP: NOD2 can also limit the development of a CD4+ T cell-initiated immune response. However, α-defensins can be expressed independently of the microbiota by activation of the transcription factor TCF4.

Defensins are produced continuously or in response to microbial products or proinflammatory cytokines (for example, TNF ligand). As mentioned in our discussion on the intestinal tight junction barrier, TNF ligand is a proinflammatory cytokine produced in response to diverse infectious agents and tissue injury.

In summary, enterocytes and Paneth cells produce a diverse group of AMPs that directly kill or inhibit the growth of pathogenic microorganisms that can contribute to inflammatory bowel diseases.

Pathology: Inflammatory bowel diseases

Inflammatory bowel disease includes **ulcerative colitis** and **Crohn's disease**. Both are clinically characterized by diarrhea, pain, and periodic relapses.

Ulcerative colitis affects the mucosa of the large intestine. Crohn's disease affects any segment of the intestinal tract.

Crohn's disease is a chronic inflammatory process involving the terminal ileum but is also observed in the large intestine. Inflammatory cells (neutrophils, lymphocytes, and macrophages) produce cytokines that cause damage to the intestinal mucosa (Figure 16-18).

The initial alteration of the intestinal mucosa consists in the infiltration of **neutrophils into the crypts of Lieberkühn**. This process results in the destruction of the intestinal glands by the formation of **crypt abscesses** and the progressive **atrophy** and **ulceration** of the mucosa.

The chronic inflammatory process infiltrates the submucosa and muscularis. Abundant accumulation of lymphocytes forms aggregates of cells, or **granulomas**, a typical feature of Crohn's disease.

Major complications of the disease are **occlusion of the intestinal lumen by fibrosis** and the **formation of fistulas** in other segments of the small intestine, and **intestinal perforation**. Segments affected by Crohn's disease are separated by normal stretches of intestinal segments.

The cause of Crohn's disease is unknown. There is increasing evidence suggesting that the disease arises from dysregulated interactions between microorganisms and the intestinal epithelium involving NOD2.

Patients with intestinal bowel disease have an increased number of bacteria associated with the epithelial cell surface, suggesting a failure of mechanisms limiting direct contact between microorganisms and the epithelium.

A contributing factor is the reactive immune response of the intestinal mucosa determined by an abnormal signaling exchange with the resident bacteria (**microbiota**). In genetically susceptible individuals, inflammatory bowel disease occurs when the mucosal immune machinery regards the microbiota present in normal and healthy individuals as pathogenic and triggers an immune response.

As discussed (see Figure 16-12), cytokines produced by helper T cells within the intestinal mucosa cause a proinflammatory response that characterizes inflammatory bowel disease. In Crohn's disease, **type 1 helper cells** (TH1 cells) produce TNF ligand and interferon-γ. Because TNF ligand is a proinflammatory cytokine, antibodies to this cytokine are being administered to patients with Crohn's disease to attenuate proinflammatory activity.

Clinical significance: Malabsorption syndromes

Malabsorption syndromes are characterized by a deficit in the absorption of fats, proteins, carbohydrates, salts, and water by the mucosa of the small intestine.

Malabsorption syndromes can be caused by:

Figure 16-19. **Large intestine**

Large intestine

The layers of the large intestine are the same as those in the small intestine: mucosa, submucosa, muscularis, and serosa.

The **main function of the mucosa** is the absorption of water, sodium, vitamins, and minerals. The transport of sodium is active (energy-dependent), causing water to move along an osmotic gradient. As a result, the fluid chyme entering the colon is concentrated into semisolid feces. Potassium and bicarbonate are secreted into the lumen of the colon.

The absorptive capacity of the colon favors the uptake of many substances, including sedatives, anesthetics, and steroids. This property is of considerable therapeutic importance when medication cannot be administered through the mouth (for example, because of vomiting).

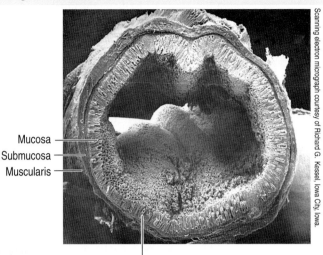

Mucosa
Submucosa
Muscularis

Scanning electron micrograph courtesy of Richard G. Kessel, Iowa City, Iowa.

Tubular glands, or crypts of Lieberkühn, are oriented perpendicular to the long axis of the colon, are much deeper than in the small intestine, and have a higher proportion of goblet cells.

— Mucosa

— Muscularis mucosae

Mucosa of the large intestine

The mucosa of the colon is free of folds and villi.

Four cell types are present in the surface epithelium and tubular glands:

1. Simple columnar absorptive cells with apical microvilli (striated apical border).
2. Predominant goblet cells.
3. Stem cells at the base of the tubular glands of Lieberkühn, which give rise to absorptive and goblet cells.
4. Enteroendocrine cells.

The intestinal tubular glands are longer than in the small intestine (0.4 to 0.6 mm).

Lymphatic follicles can be seen in the lamina propria just under the muscularis mucosae, extending into the submucosa.

— Submucosa

— Muscularis

1. **Abnormal digestion of fats and proteins** by pancreatic diseases (pancreatitis or cystic fibrosis) or **lack of solubilization of fats by defective bile secretion** (hepatic disease or obstruction of the flow of bile into the duodenum).

2. **Enzymatic abnormalities at the brush border**, where disaccharidases and peptidases cannot hydro-

lyze carbohydrates (lactose intolerance) and proteins, respectively.

3. A **defect in the transepithelial transport by enterocytes.**

Malabsorption syndromes affect many organ systems. **Anemia** occurs when vitamin B_{12}, iron, and other cofactors cannot be absorbed. Disturbances of

Figure 16-20. Large intestine

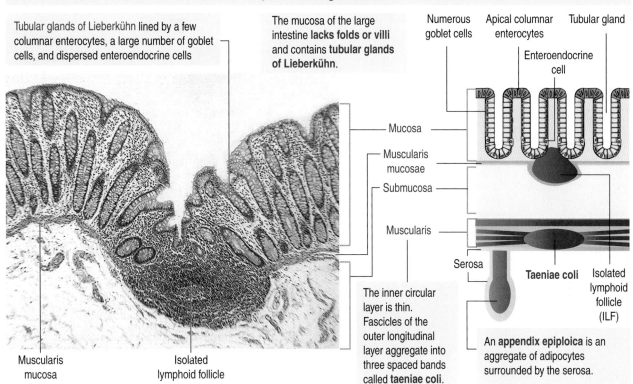

Tubular glands of Lieberkühn lined by a few columnar enterocytes, a large number of goblet cells, and dispersed enteroendocrine cells

The mucosa of the large intestine **lacks folds or villi** and contains **tubular glands of Lieberkühn.**

Numerous goblet cells

Apical columnar enterocytes

Tubular gland

Enteroendocrine cell

Mucosa

Muscularis mucosae

Submucosa

Muscularis

Serosa

Taeniae coli

Isolated lymphoid follicle (ILF)

Muscularis mucosa

Isolated lymphoid follicle

The inner circular layer is thin. Fascicles of the outer longitudinal layer aggregate into three spaced bands called **taeniae coli.**

An **appendix epiploica** is an aggregate of adipocytes surrounded by the serosa.

---

the musculoskeletal system are observed when proteins, calcium, and vitamin D fail to be absorbed. A typical clinical feature of malabsorption syndromes is **diarrhea**.

Large intestine

The large intestine is formed by several successive segments:

1. The **cecum**, projecting from which is the **appendix**.

2. The **ascending, transverse,** and **descending colon**.

3. The **sigmoid colon**.

4. The **rectum**.

5. The **anus**.

Plicae circulares and intestinal villi are not found beyond the ileocecal valve. Numerous openings of the straight **tubular glands** or **crypts of Lieberkühn** are characteristic of the mucosa of the colon (Figure 16-19).

The lining of the tubular glands of the colon consists of the following (Figures 16-20 and 16-21):

1. A **surface simple columnar epithelium** formed by absorptive **enterocytes** and **goblet cells**. Enterocytes have **short apical microvilli**, and the cells participate in the **transport of ions and water**. All regions of the colon absorb Na⁺ and Cl⁻ ions facilitated by plasma membrane channels that are regulated by mineralocorticoids. Aldosterone increases the number of Na⁺ channels and increases the absorption of

Na⁺. Na⁺ ions entering the absorptive enterocytes are extruded by an Na⁺ pump. Goblet cells secrete mucus to lubricate the mucosal surface and serve as a protective barrier.

2. A **glandular epithelium**, lining the glands or crypts of Lierberkühn, consists of enterocytes and predominant goblet cells, stem cells, and dispersed **enteroendocrine cells**. Paneth cells may be present in the cecum.

A lamina propria and a muscularis mucosae are present, as are **isolated lymphoid follicles (ILFs)** penetrating the submucosa. Glands are not present in the submucosa. Unlike Peyer's patches, ILFs are not associated with M cells.

The muscularis has a particular feature: The bundles of its outer longitudinal layer fuse to form the **taeniae coli**. The taeniae coli consist of three longitudinally oriented ribbon-like bands, each 1 cm wide. The contraction of the taeniae coli and circular muscle layer draws the colon into sacculations called **haustra**.

The serosa has scattered sacs of adipose tissue, the **appendices epiploicae**, which is a unique feature, together with the haustra, of the colon.

The appendix

The **appendix** (Figure 16-22) is a diverticulum of the cecum and has layers similar to those of the large intestine. The characteristic features of the appendix are the **lymphoid tissue**, represented by multiple

Figure 16-21. **Cell types of the glands of the large intestine**

Brush border   Terminal web   Enterocyte

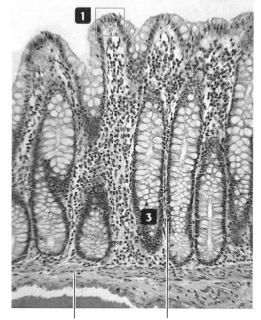

Muscularis mucosa   Enteroendocrine cell

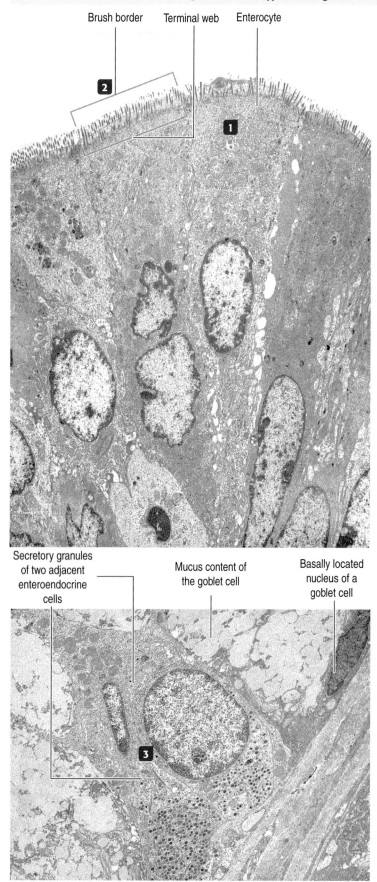

Secretory granules of two adjacent enteroendocrine cells

Mucus content of the goblet cell

Basally located nucleus of a goblet cell

Bundle of actin filaments forming the core of the short microvilli

Interdigitation of adjacent enterocytes

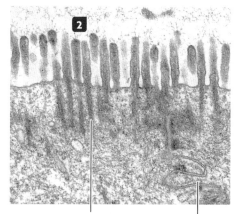

Mucosa of the large intestine: Cell types

The mucosa of the large intestine consists of straight tubular glands longer than in the small intestine. **Neither plicae nor villi are seen in the large intestine.**

1 The glands are lined by **columnar absorptive enterocytes** located in the upper portion of the gland. **Goblet cells** are the predominant cell type and increase in number in the distal segments of the large intestine.

2 The apical domain of the columnar absorptive cells has **microvilli shorter** than those seen in the enterocytes of the small intestine.

3 Scattered **enteroendocrine cells** are present. **Paneth cells are not present in the large intestine.**

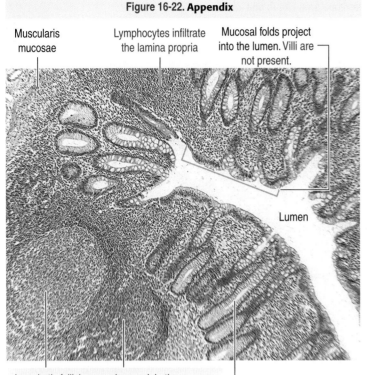

Figure 16-22. Appendix

Muscularis mucosae

Lymphocytes infiltrate the lamina propria

Mucosal folds project into the lumen. Villi are not present.

Lumen

Lymphatic follicles are observed in the mucosa and submucosa. The follicles resemble the lymphatic follicles surrounding the crypts of the palatine tonsils. A clear difference is that the tubular glands lined by predominant goblet cells are not seen in the tonsils.

Tubular glands are lined by abundant goblet cells

lymphatic follicles, and **lymphocytes** infiltrating the lamina propria. Lymphatic follicles extend into the mucosa and submucosa and disrupt the continuity of the muscularis mucosae. The submucosa contains adipocytes and dense irregular connective tissue. The inner circular layers of the muscularis is well developed in contrast with the outer longitudinal layer covered by the serosa.

The rectum

The **rectum**, the terminal portion of the intestinal tract, is a continuation of the sigmoid colon. The rectum consists of two parts (Figure 16-23):

1. The **upper part**, or **rectum proper**.
2. The **lower part**, or **anal canal**.

The mucosa is thicker, with prominent veins, and the crypts of Lieberkühn are longer (0.7 mm) than in the small intestine and lined predominantly by goblet cells. At the level of the anal canal, the crypts gradually disappear and the serosa is replaced by an adventitia.

A characteristic feature of the mucosa of the anal canal are 8 to 10 longitudinal **anal columns**. The base of the anal columns is the **pectinate line**. The anal columns are connected at their base by **valves**, corresponding to transverse folds of the mucosa.

Small pockets, called **anal sinuses**, or crypts, are found behind the valves. **Anal mucous glands** open into each sinus.

The valves and sinuses prevent leakage from the anus. When the canal is distended with feces, the columns, sinuses, and valves flatten, and mucus is discharged from the sinuses to lubricate the passage of the feces.

Beyond the pectinate line, the simple columnar epithelium of the rectal mucosa is replaced by a **stratified squamous epithelium**. This **epithelial transformation zone** has clinical significance in pathology: colorectal adenocarcinoma (gland-like) originates above the transformation zone; epidermoid (epidermis-like) carcinoma originates below the transformation zone (anal canal).

At the level of the anus, **the inner circular layer of smooth muscle thickens to form the internal anal sphincter**. The longitudinal smooth muscle layer extends over the sphincter and attaches to the connective tissue. Below this zone, the mucosa consists of stratified squamous epithelium with a few sebaceous and sweat glands in the submucosa (**circumanal glands** similar to the axillary sweat glands). The **external anal sphincter** is formed by **skeletal muscle** and lies inside the levator ani muscle, also with a sphincter function.

Pathology: Hirschsprung's disease

We discussed in Chapter 8, Nervous Tissue, that during formation of the neural tube, neural crest cells migrate from the neuroepithelium along defined pathways to tissues, where they differentiate into various cell types.

One destination of neural crest cells is the alimentary tube, where they develop the **enteric nervous system**. The enteric nervous system partially controls and coordinates the normal movements of the alimentary tube that facilitate digestion and transport of bowel contents.

The large intestine, like the rest of the alimentary tube, is innervated by the enteric nervous system receiving impulses from extrinsic parasympathetic and sympathetic nerves and from receptors within the large intestine.

The transit of contents from the small intestine to the large intestine is intermittent and regulated at the ileocecal junction by a sphincter mechanism: When the sphincter relaxes, ileal contractions propel the contents into the large intestine.

Segmental contractions in an orad-to-aboral direction move the contents over short distances. The material changes from a liquid to a semisolid state when it reaches the descending and sigmoid colon. The rectum is usually empty.

Contraction of the inner anal sphincter closes the anal canal. Defecation occurs when the sphincter re-

Figure 16-23. **Rectum, anal canal, and anus**

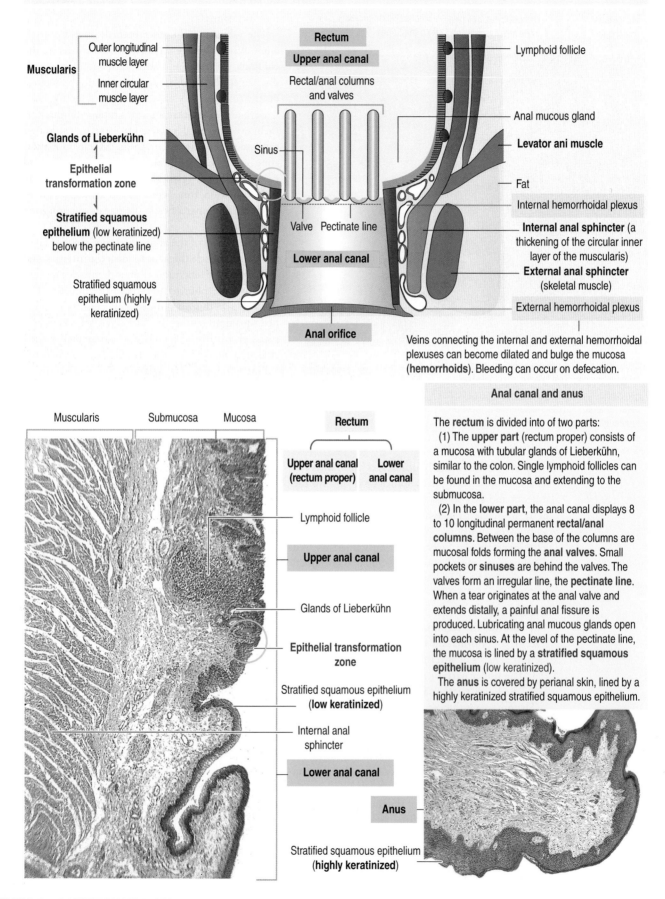

Muscularis
- Outer longitudinal muscle layer
- Inner circular muscle layer

Rectum

Upper anal canal

Rectal/anal columns and valves

Glands of Lieberkühn

↕

Epithelial transformation zone

↓

Stratified squamous epithelium (low keratinized) below the pectinate line

Sinus

Stratified squamous epithelium (highly keratinized)

Valve   Pectinate line

Lower anal canal

Anal orifice

Lymphoid follicle

Anal mucous gland

Levator ani muscle

Fat

Internal hemorrhoidal plexus

Internal anal sphincter (a thickening of the circular inner layer of the muscularis)

External anal sphincter (skeletal muscle)

External hemorrhoidal plexus

Veins connecting the internal and external hemorrhoidal plexuses can become dilated and bulge the mucosa (**hemorrhoids**). Bleeding can occur on defecation.

Anal canal and anus

The **rectum** is divided into of two parts:
  (1) The **upper part** (rectum proper) consists of a mucosa with tubular glands of Lieberkühn, similar to the colon. Single lymphoid follicles can be found in the mucosa and extending to the submucosa.
  (2) In the **lower part**, the anal canal displays 8 to 10 longitudinal permanent **rectal/anal columns**. Between the base of the columns are mucosal folds forming the **anal valves**. Small pockets or **sinuses** are behind the valves. The valves form an irregular line, the **pectinate line**. When a tear originates at the anal valve and extends distally, a painful anal fissure is produced. Lubricating anal mucous glands open into each sinus. At the level of the pectinate line, the mucosa is lined by a **stratified squamous epithelium** (low keratinized).
  The **anus** is covered by perianal skin, lined by a highly keratinized stratified squamous epithelium.

Muscularis   Submucosa   Mucosa

Rectum

Upper anal canal (rectum proper)   **Lower anal canal**

Lymphoid follicle

Upper anal canal

Glands of Lieberkühn

Epithelial transformation zone

Stratified squamous epithelium (**low keratinized**)

Internal anal sphincter

Lower anal canal

Anus

Stratified squamous epithelium (**highly keratinized**)

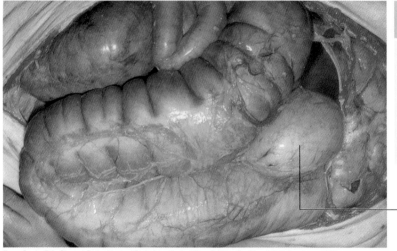

Figure 16-24. Hirschsprung's disease (congenital megacolon)

Defects of neural crest cell migration and development: Hirschsprung's disease

Hirschsprung's disease (congenital aganglionic megacolon) is caused by mutations of the **RET** (**receptor tyrosine kinase**) gene that prevents the migration and differentiation of neural crest cells into neurons of the enteric nervous system.

Aganglionosis may result from defects in the migration, proliferation, differentiation and survival of the neural crest cell precursor population.

Megacolon

From Cooke RA, Stewart B: Anatomical Pathology. 2nd edition, Edinburgh, Churchill Livingstone, 1995.

laxes as part of the **rectosphincteric reflex** stimulated by distention of the rectum.

Delayed transit through the colon leads to severe **constipation**. An abnormal form of constipation is seen in **Hirschsprung's disease (congenital megacolon)** caused by the **absence of the enteric nervous system in a segment of the distal colon** (Figure 16-24).

This condition, called **aganglionosis**, results from an **arrest in the migration of cells from the neural crest**, the precursors of the intramural ganglion cells of the plexuses of Meissner and Auerbach. Aganglionosis is caused by mutations of the **RET** gene encoding a receptor tyrosine kinase.

RET signaling is required for:

1. The formation of Peyer's patches (see Box 16-A).

2. The migration of neural crest cells into the distal portions of the large intestine.

3. The differentiation of neural crest cells into neurons of the enteric nervous system.

The permanently contracted aganglionic segment does not allow the entry of the contents. An increase in muscular tone in the orad segment results in its dilation, thus generating a megacolon or megarectum.

This condition is apparent shortly after birth when the abdomen of the infant becomes distended and little meconium is eliminated.

The diagnosis is confirmed by a biopsy of the mucosa and submucosa of the rectum showing thick and irregular nerve bundles, abundant acetylcholinesterase detected by immunohistochemistry and a lack of ganglion cells.

Surgical removal of the affected colon segment is the treatment of choice but intestinal dysfunction may persist after surgery.

Pathology: Colorectal tumorigenesis

Colorectal tumors develop from a **polyp**, a tumoral mass that protrudes into the lumen of the intestine. Some polyps are non-neoplastic and are relatively common in persons 60 years and older. Polyps can be present in large number (100 or more) in **familial polyposis syndromes** such as **familial adenomatous polyposis (FAP)** and the **Peutz-Jeghers syndrome**.

FAP is determined by autosomal dominant mutations, in particular in the *APC* (**adenomatous polyposis coli**) **gene**. FAP patients develop multiple polyps in the colon in their teenage years, increase in number with age and later become cancerous.

Mutations in the *APC* gene have been detected in 85% of colon tumors, indicating that, as with the retinoblastoma (*Rb*) gene, the inherited gene is also important in the development of the sporadic form of the cancer.

The *APC* gene encodes **APC protein** with binding affinity to β-catenin, a molecule associated with a catenin complex linked to E-cadherin (discussed in Chapter 1, Epithelium) and also a transcriptional coactivator.

Mutations in the APC gene have also been found in people with **desmoid tumors**, a benign tumor of the connective tissue. Mutations in the APC gene are also observed in **Turcot syndrome**, characterized by an association of colorectal cancer with medulloblastoma, a brain tumor. The *APC* gene is located on the long (q) arm of chromosome 5.

When β-catenin is not part of the catenin complex:

1. Free cytoplasmic β-catenin can be phosphorylated by glycogen synthase kinase 3β (GSK3β) (coassembled with proteins APC, axin and casein kinase Iα, CKIα) and targeted for proteasomal degradation (Figure 16-25).

Phosphorylated β-catenin is recognized by a **ubiquitin ligase complex** that catalyzes the attachment of polyubiquitin chains to phosphorylated β-catenin.

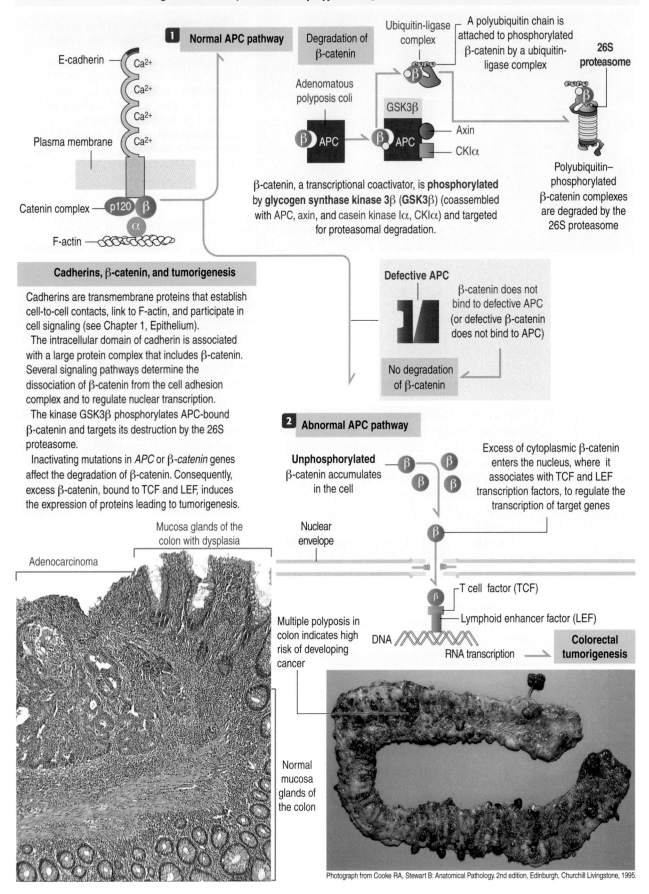

Figure 16-25. APC (adenomatous polyposis coli) and cancer of the colon

1 Normal APC pathway

E-cadherin

Ca^{2+}
Ca^{2+}
Ca^{2+}
Ca^{2+}

Plasma membrane

Catenin complex — p120 β

α

F-actin

Degradation of β-catenin

Adenomatous polyposis coli

Ubiquitin-ligase complex

A polyubiquitin chain is attached to phosphorylated β-catenin by a ubiquitin-ligase complex

26S proteasome

GSK3β

β APC → β APC — Axin
— CKIα

β-catenin, a transcriptional coactivator, is **phosphorylated** by **glycogen synthase kinase 3β (GSK3β)** (coassembled with APC, axin, and casein kinase Iα, CKIα) and targeted for proteasomal degradation.

Polyubiquitin–phosphorylated β-catenin complexes are degraded by the 26S proteasome

Cadherins, β-catenin, and tumorigenesis

Cadherins are transmembrane proteins that establish cell-to-cell contacts, link to F-actin, and participate in cell signaling (see Chapter 1, Epithelium).

The intracellular domain of cadherin is associated with a large protein complex that includes β-catenin. Several signaling pathways determine the dissociation of β-catenin from the cell adhesion complex and to regulate nuclear transcription.

The kinase GSK3β phosphorylates APC-bound β-catenin and targets its destruction by the 26S proteasome.

Inactivating mutations in *APC* or *β-catenin* genes affect the degradation of β-catenin. Consequently, excess β-catenin, bound to TCF and LEF, induces the expression of proteins leading to tumorigenesis.

Defective APC

β-catenin does not bind to defective APC (or defective β-catenin does not bind to APC)

No degradation of β-catenin

2 Abnormal APC pathway

Unphosphorylated β-catenin accumulates in the cell

Excess of cytoplasmic β-catenin enters the nucleus, where it associates with TCF and LEF transcription factors, to regulate the transcription of target genes

Nuclear envelope

— T cell factor (TCF)
— Lymphoid enhancer factor (LEF)

DNA

RNA transcription →

Colorectal tumorigenesis

Multiple polyposis in colon indicates high risk of developing cancer

Adenocarcinoma

Mucosa glands of the colon with dysplasia

Normal mucosa glands of the colon

Photograph from Cooke RA, Stewart B: Anatomical Pathology. 2nd edition, Edinburgh, Churchill Livingstone, 1995.

Polyubiquitin conjugates of β-catenin are rapidly degraded by the **26S proteasome**.

2. Alternatively, free cytoplasmic β-catenin can enter the nucleus and interact with the transcription factors **TCF (T cell factor)** and **LEF (lymphoid enhancer factor)** to stimulates transcription of target genes (see Figure 16-25).

A mutation in the *APC* gene results in a truncated nonfunctional protein unable to interact with β-catenin and initiate its disposal when is no longer needed. Essentially, *APC* behaves as a tumor suppressor gene.

The *APC* gene is also a major regulator of the **Wnt pathway**, a signaling system expressed during early development and embryogenesis (see Chapter 3, Cell Signaling). Wnt proteins can inactivate GSK3β, prevent the phosphorylation of β-catenin, and abrogate its destruction by the 26S proteasome. Consequently, an excess of β-catenin translocates to the cell nucleus to affect gene transcription.

A defective β-catenin pathway can overexpress the **microphthalmia-associated transcription factor (MITF)**. We discussed in Chapter 11, Integumentary System, the significance of MITF in the survival and proliferation of melanoma cells.

Hereditary nonpolyposis colon cancer (HNPCC; Lynch syndrome) is an inherited form of colorectal cancer caused by mutations in DNA *mismatch repair, MMR,* genes, involved in the repair of DNA defects.

Mutation analysis of *MMR* genes (including *MLH1, MSH2, MSH6, PMS2,* and *EPCAM* genes) by **microsatellite instability (MIS)** screening testing using colon tumor tissue removed by colonoscopy or surgery, is carried out when there is evidence of a DNA repair defect in a tumor. Note that not all individuals who carry these mutations develop cancerous tumors.

DNA repair defects increase the frequency of somatic mutations leading to malignant transformation. HNPCC is an example of a cancer syndrome caused by **mutations in DNA repair proteins**.

Patients with the HNPCC syndrome do not show the very large number of colon polyps typical of the familial polyposis syndrome, but a small number of polyps occur frequently among gene carriers.

| Essential concepts | **Lower Digestive Segment** |

• **Small intestine**. The main functions of the small intestine are to continue in the duodenum the digestive process initiated in the stomach, and to absorb digested food after enzymatic breakdown.

The intestinal wall is constructed to perform absorptive functions and propel the intestinal contents to the next segment of the small intestine.

There are four degrees of folding to amplify the absorptive intestinal surface:

(1) The plicae circulares, permanent evaginations or folds of the mucosa and part of the submucosa.

(2) The intestinal villi, finger-like evaginations of the mucosa only; a typical feature of the small intestine.

(3) The glands or crypts of Lieberkühn, invaginations of the mucosa between adjacent villi, extending down to the muscularis mucosae.

(4) Microvilli, apical differentiation of the enterocyte, the absorptive cell of the small intestine.

The muscularis mucosae is a component of the mucosa. Together with the lining epithelium of the villi and intestinal glands and the connective tissue lamina propria, is the boundary between the mucosa and submucosa.

The muscularis consists of inner circular smooth muscle fibers and outer longitudinal smooth muscle fibers. It is responsible for mixing the intestinal contents and for peristaltic movements from a proximal (orad) to a distal (aborad) direction.

Loose connective tissue adjacent to the muscularis is covered by the peritoneum.

• The **peritoneum** is a serous membrane consisting of a connective tissue stroma (containing elastic fibers, blood and lymphatic vessels, and nerves) lined by mesothelial cells. The parietal peritoneum lines the abdominal wall and reflects to cover the abdominal viscera as the visceral peritoneum.

The mesentery is a layer of loose connective tissue (areolar connective tissue) covered with peritoneum.

The mesentery attaches the abdominal viscera to the posterior abdominal wall and it serves as a conduit of blood and lymphatic vessels and nerves to these organs. The blood vessels are components of the subserosal plexus. During digestion, the lymphatic vessels emerging from the walls of the small intestine carry a fluid rich in absorbed fat emulsion, or chyle.

The esophagus lacks a serosa. The duodenum and ascending and descending colon attach to the abdominal cavity by the adventitia, loose connective tissue continuous with the surrounding stroma of the wall.

The omenta and visceral ligaments have a structure similar to the mesentery. The greater omentum has considerable adipose tissue.

• The intestinal wall is supplied by a rich blood, lymphatic, and nerve supply. The nerve supply derives from the submucosal plexus of Meissner and myenteric plexus of Auerbach, components of the autonomic nervous system.

A central lymphatic vessel (lacteal) is present in the lamina propria of the intestinal villus. A capillary villus plexus supplies the intestinal villus; a pericryptal capillary plexus supplies the glands of Lieberkühn.

• The three major sequential segments of the small intestine are:
(1) The duodenum.
(2) The jejunum.
(3) The ileum.

Remember the following:
• The **duodenum** has Brunner's glands in the submucosa, and the villi are broad and short (leaflike).
• The **jejunum** has long villi (finger-like), each with a prominent lacteal. Brunner's glands are not present in the submucosa.
• The **ileum** has shorter finger-like villi. A relevant feature are the **Peyer's patches**.
• **Paneth cells** are found at the base of the glands of Lieberkühn in the jejunum and ileum.

• The intestinal villus and glands of Lieberkühn are lined by a simple columnar epithelium consisting of:
(1) Absorptive enterocytes, columnar cells with apical microvilli, the brush border.
(2) Goblet cells, a mucus-secreting cell forming a double layer protective gel coat to

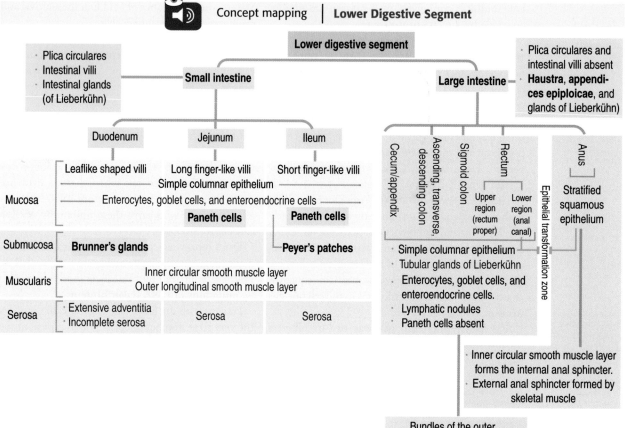

Lower digestive segment

Small intestine
- Plica circulares
- Intestinal villi
- Intestinal glands (of Lieberkühn)

Large intestine
- Plica circulares and intestinal villi absent
- **Haustra, appendices epiploicae**, and glands of Lieberkühn)

	Duodenum	Jejunum	Ileum
Mucosa	Leaflike shaped villi	Long finger-like villi	Short finger-like villi
	Simple columnar epithelium		
	Enterocytes, goblet cells, and enteroendocrine cells		
		Paneth cells	**Paneth cells**
Submucosa	**Brunner's glands**		**Peyer's patches**
Muscularis	Inner circular smooth muscle layer		
	Outer longitudinal smooth muscle layer		
Serosa	· Extensive adventitia · Incomplete serosa	Serosa	Serosa

Cecum/appendix · Ascending, transverse, descending colon · Sigmoid colon · Rectum (Upper region (rectum proper) / Lower region (anal canal)) · Anus

Epithelial transformation zone

Stratified squamous epithelium

- Simple columnar epithelium
- Tubular glands of Lieberkühn
- Enterocytes, goblet cells, and enteroendocrine cells.
- Lymphatic nodules
- Paneth cells absent

- Inner circular smooth muscle layer forms the internal anal sphincter.
- External anal sphincter formed by skeletal muscle

Bundles of the outer longitudinal smooth muscle fuse to form the taeniae coli

shield the epithelium from mechanical abrasion and bacterial invasion.

(3) Paneth cells (reviewed below).

(4) Enteroendocrine cells, produce gastrin, secretin, and cholecystokinin. The distribution and function of enteroendocrine cells are summarized in Essential Concepts in Chapter 15, Upper Digestive Segment.

(5) Intestinal stem cell (ISCs) reside in a niche at the base of the crypts, close to Paneth cells.

Adult ISCs, identified by the protein marker Lgr5 (for leucine-rich repeat-containing G protein coupled receptor 5), can differentiate into the secretory goblet cells, Paneth cells, and enteroendocrine cells and the absorptive enterocytes, lining the epithelium of the small intestine.

ISCs are multipotent and capable of long-term self-renewal as long as they remain at the crypt niche.

Following injury, cells committed to the intestinal secretory pathway and expressing Delta-like 1 (DLL1), a ligand of the Notch family of proteins, can return to the stem cell compartment and revert into multipotent ISCs.

The surface of the epithelium is coated by the **glycocalyx**, consisting of glycoproteins representing enzymes involved in the digestive process: absorption of proteins, carbohydrates, and lipids.

• Enterocytes are involved in the absorption of proteins, carbohydrate, lipids, cholesterol, calcium, and other substances.

Absorption of proteins and carbohydrates: Pancreatic proteolytic enzymes break down proteins into peptides and amino acids. Once absorbed, peptides are broken down by cytoplasmic peptidases into amino acids.

Salivary and pancreatic amylase, and enzymes (oligosaccharidases) present in the plasma membrane of the intestinal villi convert sugars into monosaccharides (galactose and glucose), which are transported inside the enterocyte by an Na$^+$-dependent carrier system, the sugar glucose transporter-1 (SGLT-1) driven by a Na$^+$,K$^+$-ATPase.

Absorption of lipids. Lipids are emulsified in the intestinal lumen by bile salts and pancreatic lipase to form micelles (fatty acids and monoglycerides). Micelles diffuse into the cytoplasm of the enterocyte bound to fatty acid–binding protein, and esterified into triglycerides in the smooth endoplasmic reticulum. Tryglycerides are transported to the Golgi apparatus and converted into chylomicrons (apoprotein-lipid complex). Chylomicrons are released into the enterocyte intercellular space and into the central lacteal.

Absorption of cholesterol. Similar to the absorption of dietary lipids, cholesterol is solu-

bilized in the intestinal lumen into micelles by bile acids to facilitate micellar movement through the diffusion barrier of the enterocytes.

Two cholesterol pathways are important to remember: the uptake and export pathways.

(1) The NPC1L1 (Niemann-Pick C1-like-1) protein, located also at the apical domain, facilitates the **uptake** of cholesterol that is esterified by ACAT2 (Acyl CoA cholesterol acyltransferase isoform 2). Esterified cholesterol becomes part of chylomicron particles, assembled in the smooth endoplasmic reticulum.

(2) The ABCG5/ABCG8 (ATP-binding cassette, ABC) heterodimeric transporters at the apical domain of enterocytes **export** absorbed cholesterol back into the intestinal lumen. This step facilitates the removal of cholesterol from the body. Mutations in ABCG5 or ABCG8 genes cause sitosterolemia, an autosomal recessive disorder in which cholesterol accumulates in the circulation leading to premature cardiovascular disease.

Malabsorption syndromes can be caused by abnormal digestion of fats and proteins by pancreatic diseases (pancreatitis or cystic fibrosis), or lack of solubilization of fats by defective bile secretion (hepatic disease or obstruction of bile flow to the duodenum).

Enzymatic abnormalities in the brush border hamper protein and carbohydrate (lactose intolerance) absorption. An abnormal transport mechanism across enterocytes can cause malabsorption syndromes.

Anemia can occur when the **intrinsic factor–vitamin B_{12} complex**, iron, and other cofactors fail to be absorbed. **Functional alterations of the musculoskeletal system** occur when proteins, calcium, and vitamin D are not absorbed.

• The small intestine is protected from pathogens by:

(1) An **intestinal tight junction barrier** linking adjacent enterocytes. Claudin and occludin are two transmembrane proteins of tight junctions that regulate solute permeability of the transcellular pathway. A defect of the tight junction barrier can allow bacterial products or dietary antigens to cross the epithelium and enter the lamina propria.

(2) **Peyer's patches** participate in the cellular surveillance and processing of antigens. Peyer's patches have the ability to transport luminal antigens and microorganisms and respond to them by inducing immune tolerance or a systemic immune defense response. An example of the functional deficiency of Peyer's patches is Crohn's disease, an inflammatory bowel disease characterized by chronic or relapsing inflammation.

Peyer's patches display three main components:

• The follicle-associated epithelium (FAE), consisting of M cells and enterocytes.

• Lymphoid follicles, each showing a germinal center and a subepithelial dome area.

• The interfollicular area, with blood vessels and efferent lymphatic vessels.

The main components of the FAE are M cells and dendritic cells.

M cells are specialized enterocytes that have replaced the brush border by short microfolds (hence the name M cell) and takes up antigens. M cells form intraepithelial pockets, where a subpopulation of intraepithelial B cells resides and express IgA receptors allowing the capture and phagocytosis of IgA-bound bacteria.

Dendritic cell extend cytoplasmic processes between tight junctions linking enterocytes to monitor antigens.

(3) The neutralization of antigens by **polymeric IgA**, produced by plasma cells in the lamina propria of the intestinal villus and transported to the intestinal lumen across the enterocyte by a mechanism called transcytosis.

• Polymeric IgA binds to a specific receptor, called the polymeric immunoglobulin receptor (pIgR), available on the basal surfaces of the enterocytes.

• The pIgR has an attached secretory component. The polymeric IgA–pIgR–secretory component complex is internalized and transported across the cell to the apical surface of the epithelial cell (transcytosis).

• At the apical surface, the complex is cleaved enzymatically and the polymeric IgA-secretory component complex is released into the intestinal lumen as secreted IgA (SIgA).

• IgA attaches to bacteria and soluble antigens, preventing a direct damaging effect to intestinal cells and penetration into the lamina propria.

Plasma cells are induced to produce polymeric IgA when Toll-like receptor (TLR) on enterocytes is activated by microbiota.

• Enterocytes secrete B cell-activating factor (BAF) and a proliferation-inducing ligand (APRIL).

• In the lamina propria, BAF and APRIL induce the differentiation of B cells into IgA-producing plasma cells..

• In addition, the microbiota instructs enterocytes through thymic stromal lymphoprotein (TSLP) to engage dendritic cells in the lamina propria to secrete BAF and APRIL and induce the differentiation of B cells into plasma cells.

(4) The inactivation of microbial pathogens by antimicrobial proteins (AMPs), products of **Paneth cells** and enterocytes retained in the intestinal mucus blanket produced by goblet cells. Therefore, the mucus layer protects the intestinal mucosa by two mechanisms:

• By creating a barrier that limits direct access of luminal bacteria to the epithelium.

• By concentrating AMPs near the enterocyte surface. AMPs are virtually absent from the luminal content.

Most AMPs inactivate or kill bacteria directly by enzymatic degradation of the bacterial wall or by disrupting the bacterial inner membrane.

Paneth cells produce several AMPs:

(1) Defensins (α-defensin 5 [DEFA5] and α-defensin 6 [DEFA6] in humans)

(2) C-type lectins, including regenerating islet-derived protein 3γ (REG3γ), also known as hepatointestinal protein/pancreatitis-associated protein (HIP/PAP).

(3) Lysozyme and phospholipase A2 (PLA2).

(4) Angiogenin 4 (ANG4).

The expression and function of AMPs is highly regulated by the presence or absence of the microbiota.

In the presence of microorganisms:

• TLR on enterocytes controls the expression of REG3γ/HIP/PAP through the TLR-signaling adaptor myeloid-differentiation primary response protein 88 (MYD88).

• Cytoplasmic NOD2 (nucleotide-binding oligomerization domain 2), expressed by Paneth cells, controls the expression of α-defensins when it binds to an internalized peptidoglycan peptide fragment (muramyl dipeptide, MDP) and activates the transcription factor NF-κB.

• NOD2 can also limit the development of a CD4+ T cell-initiated immune response, thus contributing to immunogenic tolerance toward the microbiota.

• A defect in the protective system accounts for inflammatory bowel diseases, including **ulcerative colitis** (large intestine) and **Crohn's disease** (involving the terminal ileum but also observed in the large intestine).

• The **large intestine** consists of:

(1) The cecum and associated appendix.

(2) The ascending, transverse, and descending colon.

(3) The sigmoid colon.

(4) The rectum.

(5) The anus.

Plicae circulares and intestinal villi are not observed beyond the ileocecal valve.

The mucosa of the large intestine is lined by a simple columnar epithelium formed by enterocytes and abundant goblet cells.

Enterocytes have short apical microvilli. A major function of enterocytes in the large intestine is the transport of ions and water. Secretory products of goblet cells lubricate the mucosal surface.

Glands of Lieberkühn are observed. They contain enteroendocrine cells and stem cells. Paneth cells are not observed (they may be present in the cecum).

Three characteristic features of the large intestine are:

(1) The taeniae coli, formed by fused bundles of the outer smooth muscle layer.

(2) The haustra, periodic saccular structures formed by the contraction of the taeniae coli and the inner circular smooth muscle layer.

(3) The appendix epiploica, aggregates of adipose tissue covered by the serosa (peritoneum).

The appendix is a diverticulum of the cecum. Prominent lymphoid follicles or nodules are seen in the mucosa and submucosa. M cells are not present.

The rectum, the terminal portion of the large intestine and a continuation of the sigmoid colon, consists of two regions:

(1) The upper region, or rectum proper.

(2) The lower region, or anal canal, which extends from the anorectal junction to the anus.

The mucosa of the rectum displays long glands of Lieberkühn; glands disappear at the level of the anal canal.

Anal columns are present in the anal canal. The anal columns are connected at their base by valves, corresponding to transverse folds of the mucosa. Small pockets, called anal sinuses, or crypts, are found behind the valves. Mucous glandular crypts behind the valves secrete lubricating mucus.

A tear originating at the anal valves and extending distally produces painful **anal fissures**.

The base of the anal columns forms the pectinate line. Beyond the pectinate line, the simple columnar epithelium of the rectal mucosa is replaced by a stratified squamous epithelium (**epithelial transformation zone**), and the inner circular layer of smooth muscle thickens to form the internal anal sphincter.

Beyond this region, the anal mucosa is lined by a keratinizing stratified squamous epithelium and the submucosa contains sebaceous and sweat glands (circumanal glands). The external anal sphincter, formed by skeletal muscle, is present.

• **Hirschsprung's disease** (congenital megacolon) is caused by a defect in the migration and differentiation of neural crest cells, which give rise to neurons of the enteric nervous system.

This condition, called aganglionosis, is caused by mutations of the *RET* gene encoding a receptor tyrosine kinase. RET signaling is required for the migration of neural crest cells into the distal portions of the large intestine and their differentiation into intramural ganglion cells of the plexuses of Meissner and Auerbach of the enteric nervous system.

Delayed transit through the colon leads to severe constipation resulting from the absence of the enteric nervous system in a segment of the distal colon.

The diagnosis is confirmed by a biopsy of the mucosa and submucosa of the rectum showing thick and irregular nerve bundles, abundant acetylcholinesterase detected by immunohistochemistry and a lack of ganglion cells.

Surgical removal of the affected colon segment is the treatment of choice but intestinal dysfunction may persist after surgery.

• **Colorectal tumors** develop from a polyp. Some polyps are non-neoplastic and are relatively common in persons 60 years and older. Polyps can be present in large number (100 or more) in familial polyposis syndromes such as familial adenomatous polyposis (FAP) and the Peutz-Jeghers syndrome.

FAP is determined by autosomal dominant mutations, in particular in the *APC* (adenomatous polyposis coli) gene. FAP patients develop multiple polyps in the colon in their teenage years, increase in number with age and later become cancerous.

The *APC* gene encodes APC protein with binding affinity to β-catenin, a molecule associated with a catenin complex linked to E-cadherin and also a transcriptional coactivator.

When β-catenin is not part of the catenin complex:

(1) Free cytoplasmic β-catenin can be phosphorylated by glycogen synthase kinase 3β (GSK3β) (coassembled with proteins APC,

axin and casein kinase Iα, CKIα) and targeted for proteasomal degradation.

(2) Alternatively, free cytoplasmic β-catenin can enter the nucleus and interact with the transcription factors TCF (T cell factor) and LEF (lymphoid enhancer factor) to stimulates transcription of target genes.

(3) A mutation in the APC gene results in a truncated nonfunctional protein unable to interact with β-catenin and initiate its disposal when is no longer needed.

(4) An excess of β-catenin translocates to the cell nucleus to affect gene transcription and trigger tumorigenesis.

Hereditary nonpolyposis colon cancer (HNPCC; Lynch syndrome) is an inherited form of colorectal cancer caused by mutations in DNA mismatch repair, *MMR*, genes, involved in the repair of DNA defects.

Mutation analysis of *MMR* genes (including *MLH1*, *MSH2*, *MSH6*, *PMS2*, and *EPCAM* genes) by microsatellite instability (MIS) screening testing using colon tumor tissue, is carried out when there is evidence of a DNA repair defect in a tumor.

17. Digestive Glands

Digestive glands have lubricative, protective, digestive, and absorptive functions mediated by their secretory products. The three main digestive glands are: (1) The major salivary glands (parotid, submandibular, and sublingual glands), associated with the oral cavity through independent excretory ducts. (2) The exocrine pancreas, that secretes its alkaline aqueous and enzymatic product into the duodenum. (3) The liver, an endocrine and exocrine gland with extensive access to the blood circulation. It releases bile into the duodenum. In this chapter, the structure and function of salivary glands, exocrine pancreas, and liver are described. Molecular aspects of the parotid gland, pancreas, and liver are presented to emphasize the role of specific structures and cell types in frequent medical and pathologic conditions.

General structure of a salivary gland

We start the discussion by reviewing the general organization and function of a salivary gland, in particular its branching ducts (see Box 17-A). An initial discussion concerning the general features of a compound or branched gland is included in Chapter 2, Epithelial Glands.

A salivary gland is surrounded by a connective tissue **capsule**. Partitions or **septa** extend from the capsule into the gland creating **lobes** as large divisions. **Interlobar septa** continue to branch as **interlobular septa**, subdividing lobes into several small **lobules**. The amount of connective tissue decreases from the interlobar septa to the interlobular septa. It is greatly reduced within each lobule.

Septa provide appropriate conduits for the main branches of a duct to extend from the interior of a gland to its exterior and for vessels and nerves to reach the interior of a gland.

Figures 17-1 and 17-2 summarize the pathway followed by a secretory product of a salivary gland to reach the exterior of a gland.

The basic histologic features of a salivary gland are the **secretory units**, the **acini**, and the **excretory ducts**. We start with the excretory ducts inside a lobule (see Figure 17-1):

1. An **intercalated duct**, lined by **low squamous-to-cuboidal epithelium**, is the smallest duct connecting an acinus to a striated duct. Its diameter is smaller than an acinus. Intercalated ducts are the longest in the parotid gland.

2. A **striated duct** is lined by **cuboidal-to-columnar epithelial cells** with **basal infoldings** containing numerous **mitochondria**. It is well developed in the submandibular gland. The intercalated and striated ducts are modestly developed in the sublingual gland.

3. A number of striated ducts leave the lobule to connect with an **interlobular duct**. An interlobular duct is initially lined by **cuboidal-to-columnar epithelium** and becomes **pseudostratified columnar**. Interlobular ducts are located in **interlobular septa**.

4. Several interlobular ducts converge to form a **lobar duct** present in **interlobar septa**. Lobar ducts are lined by **stratified columnar epithelium**, one of the few sites in the body with this type of epithelium.

5. Several lobar ducts, lined by **stratified squamous epithelium**, join the **main duct** that drains the entire gland near the opening into the oral cavity.

The **parotid**, **submandibular** (or **submaxillary**), and **sublingual glands** are classified as **branched tubuloalveolar glands**.

Saliva

Saliva, amounting to a half-liter daily, contains proteins, glycoproteins (mucus), ions, water, and polymeric immunoglobulin A (pIgA) attached to a secretory component (SIgA) (Figure 17-3).

The submandibular gland produces about 70% of the saliva. The parotid gland contributes 25% and secretes an amylase-rich saliva. The production of saliva is under the control of the autonomic nervous system. Upon stimulation, the parasympathetic system induces the secretion of a water-rich saliva; the sympathetic system stimulates the release of a protein-rich saliva.

The mucus and water in saliva **lubricate** the mucosa of the tongue, cheeks, and lips during speech and

---

Box 17-A | Classification of exocrine glands: Highlights to remember

- Depending on the **structure of the excretory duct**, glands can be divided into **simple** (unbranched duct) and **branched** or **compound** (branched duct).
- According to the **structure of the secretory units**, glands can be classified as **tubular** or **alveolar** (acinar).
- Considering the **secretory product**, glands are **serous** when they secrete a watery fluid, or **mucous** when the secretion is thick and rich in glycoproteins.
- Taking into account the **secretory mechanism**, glands can be **merocrine** when the product is released by exocytosis (for example, the pancreas). In **holocrine** glands, the whole cell is the secretory product (for example, the sebaceous glands of the skin). An **apocrine** gland releases its product together with a small amount of the apical cytoplasm of the secretory cell (for example, the mammary gland).

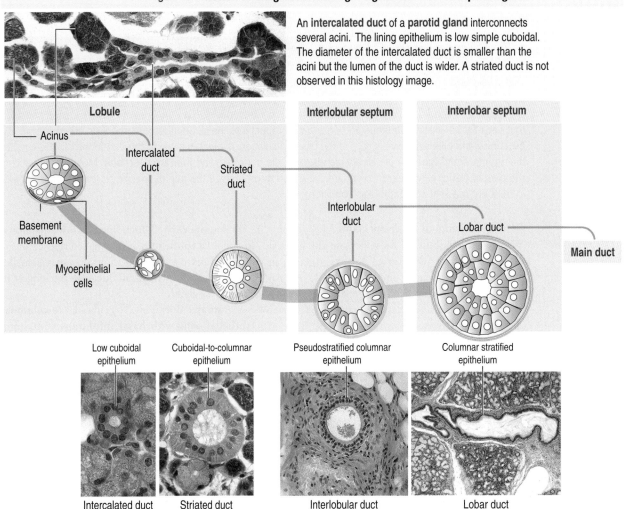

Figure 17-1. Review of the general histologic organization of a compound gland

An **intercalated duct** of a **parotid gland** interconnects several acini. The lining epithelium is low simple cuboidal. The diameter of the intercalated duct is smaller than the acini but the lumen of the duct is wider. A striated duct is not observed in this histology image.

Lobule

Interlobular septum

Interlobar septum

Acinus

Intercalated duct

Striated duct

Interlobular duct

Lobar duct

Main duct

Basement membrane

Myoepithelial cells

Low cuboidal epithelium

Cuboidal-to-columnar epithelium

Pseudostratified columnar epithelium

Columnar stratified epithelium

Intercalated duct

Striated duct

Interlobular duct

Lobar duct

swallowing, dissolve food for the function of the taste buds, and moisten food for easy swallowing.

The **protective** function of the saliva depends on the antibacterial function of three constituents:

1. **Lysozyme**, which attacks the walls of bacteria.

2. **Lactoferrin**, which chelates iron necessary for bacterial growth.

3. **SIgA**, which neutralizes bacteria and viruses.

The **digestive** function of saliva relies on:

1. **Amylase** (ptyalin), which initiates the digestion of carbohydrates (starch) in the oral cavity.

2. **Lingual lipase**, which participates in the hydrolysis of dietary lipids.

Parotid gland

The parotid gland is the largest salivary gland. It is a **branched tubuloalveolar gland** surrounded by a connective tissue capsule with **septa**, representing a component of the **stroma**, the supporting tissue of the gland. Adipose cells are frequently found in the stroma.

Septa divide the gland into lobes and lobules (see Figure 17-1). Septa also provide support to blood vessels, lymphatics, and nerves gaining access to the **acini**, the main components of the **parenchyma**, the functional constituent of the gland.

Acini are surrounded by reticular connective tissue, a rich capillary network, plasma cells, and lymphocytes. Acini consist mainly of **serous secretory cells** and, therefore, are classified as **serous acini**.

Each serous acinus is lined by pyramidal cells with a basally located nucleus. Similar to all protein-producing cells, a prominent rough endoplasmic reticulum system occupies the cell basal region. Secretory granules are visible in the apical region (Figure 17-4).

The lumen of the acinus collects the secretory products, which are transported by **long intercalated ducts to the less abundant striated ducts** (see Figure 17-1 and Figure 17-5).

The secretory product of the serous acini is modified by the secretion of the striated duct and then transported by interlobular ducts and lobar ducts to the oral cavity by a main excretory duct (**Stensen's duct**).

Figure 17-2. General organization of the salivary glands and pancreas

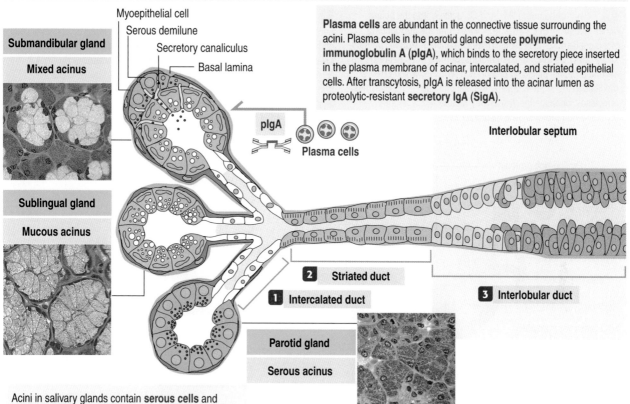

Submandibular gland

Mixed acinus

Myoepithelial cell

Serous demilune

Secretory canaliculus

Basal lamina

Sublingual gland

Mucous acinus

pIgA

Plasma cells

Plasma cells are abundant in the connective tissue surrounding the acini. Plasma cells in the parotid gland secrete **polymeric immunoglobulin A (pIgA)**, which binds to the secretory piece inserted in the plasma membrane of acinar, intercalated, and striated epithelial cells. After transcytosis, pIgA is released into the acinar lumen as proteolytic-resistant **secretory IgA (SigA)**.

Interlobular septum

2 **Striated duct**

1 **Intercalated duct**

3 **Interlobular duct**

Parotid gland

Serous acinus

Acini in salivary glands contain **serous cells** and **mucous cells**. The **parotid gland** consists solely of serous acini, whereas the **submandibular** and **sublingual glands** contain both cell types. In the submandibular gland, serous cells predominate. In the sublingual gland, mucous cells are more abundant.

Serous and mucous cells can coexist in the same acinus: The serous cells are located at the fundus of the acinus, forming a crescent-shaped structure (called the **serous demilune**) embracing the mucous cells located closer to the opening of the acinus into the intercalated duct.

In mixed acini, extensions of the acinar lumen project deeply between serous cells forming **intercellular secretory canaliculi** for the transport of serous secretions.

The outer surface of the acinus is surrounded by contractile **myoepithelial cells** in a basket-like fashion. Both myoepithelial cells and the acinus are enclosed by a basal lamina.

1 The secretion of the acinus enters the intercalated duct, lined by a low simple cuboidal epithelium. Myoepithelial cells are associated with acini and intercalated ducts.

Intercalated ducts are longest in the parotid gland. Several intercalated ducts join to form the **striated duct. Intercalated ducts and striated ducts are found within a lobule.**

2 The next segment is the **striated duct**, lined by cuboidal to columnar cells with basal striations created by vertically aligned **mitochondria** within deep infoldings of the basal plasma membrane. **This epithelium is involved in the transport of water and ions.** Striated ducts are well developed in the submandibular and parotid glands.

3 Following the striated duct is the **interlobular duct**, lined initially by columnar epithelium and then by a pseudostratified columnar epithelium. Interlobular ducts are located in **interlobular septa**.

Several interlobular ducts drain into a wider **lobar duct** located in the **interlobar septum**. Connective tissue, vessels, and nerves are seen in septa.

Pancreatic acinus

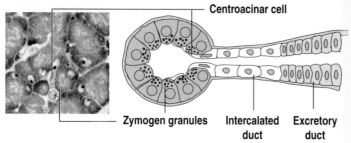

Centroacinar cell

Zymogen granules

Intercalated duct

Excretory duct

In the exocrine pancreas, only serous acini are present.

A unique feature of the pancreatic acinus is the presence of squamous-to-cuboidal epithelial **centroacinar cells**. Squamous centroacinar cells are inserted on one side of the acinar lumen. Centroacinar cells and striated ductal cells secrete HCO_3^-, Na^+, and water. The free apical domain of the serous acinar discharges zymogen granules between gaps of the centroacinar cell layer.

Striated ducts and myoepithelial cells are not present in the exocrine pancreas.

Figure 17-3. Functional aspects of a salivary gland

1 **Acinar cells** pump Na^+ and Cl^- actively into the acinar lumen and allow free passage of water from the surrounding blood capillaries. This results in the formation of isotonic primary saliva. **Mucous cells** release mucins. **Serous cells** secrete several proteins, including proline-rich proteins (which are modified in the striated duct by the enzyme kallikrein), enzymes (amylases, peroxidases, lysozyme), lactoferrin, cystatins (cysteine-rich proteins) and histatins (histidine-rich proteins).

2 In the **striated duct**, Na^+ and Cl^- are reabsorbed and the saliva becomes hypotonic. **Kallikrein**, a serine protease secreted by epithelial cells of the striated duct, processes the proline-rich proteins and cystatins in the saliva. In addition, plasma cells secrete **polymeric immunoglobulin A (pIgA)**, which reaches the lumen of the acinus and striated duct by transcytosis. The final saliva contains a complex of proteins with antimicrobial activity and with digestive function (amylase). **Bicarbonate**, the primary buffering agent of the saliva, is produced in the **striated duct**.

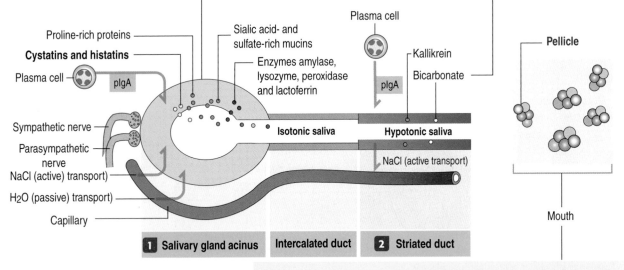

In the mouth, proteins in the saliva form protective films on the teeth called **pellicles**. The function of the pellicles is to provide a barrier against acids, retain moisture, and regulate the adherence and activity of bacteria and yeast in the oral cavity. Histatin inhibits the growth of *Candida albicans*. **Dysfunction of the salivary glands** causes tooth decay, yeast infections, and inflammation of the oral mucosa.

Pathology: Mumps, rabies, and tumors

In addition to its role in the production of saliva, the parotid gland is the primary target of the **rabies and mumps virus** transmitted in saliva containing the virus. The mumps virus causes transient swelling of the parotid gland and confers immunity.

Two complications of mumps are **viral orchitis** and **meningitis**. Bilateral orchitis caused by the mumps virus can result in sterility.

The parotid gland is the most frequent site for slow-growing **benign salivary gland mixed tumor (pleomorphic adenoma)**. It consists of myxochondroid zones with ductal epithelial and mesenchyme-like myoepithelial cells. Its surgical removal is complicated by the need to protect the facial nerve running through the parotid gland. Enucleation of mixed tumors results in a multifocal high recurrence rate.

Warthin tumor (papilloma cystoadenoma lymphomatosum), the second most common benign salivary gland tumor, occurs in the parotid gland with a high risk incidence in smokers.

The tumor stroma consist of a papillary arrangement of lymphoid tissue centers surrounded by squamous, mucous, and sebaceous epithelial cells. This tumor may develop from intraparotid or periparotid lymph nodes.

Submandibular (submaxillary) gland

The submandibular gland is a branched tubuloalveolar gland surrounded by a connective tissue capsule. Septa derived from the capsule divide the parenchyma of the gland into lobes and lobules.

Although both serous and mucous cells are present in the secretory units, the **serous cells are the predominant component** (see Figure 17-4). Mucous cell–containing acini are capped by **serous demilunes**.

The intercalated ducts are shorter and the striated ducts are longer than those in the parotid gland. Adipocytes are not frequently seen in the submandibular gland.

The main excretory duct of the submandibular gland (**Wharton's duct**) opens near the frenulum of the tongue.

Sublingual gland

Contrasting with the parotid and submandibular glands, which are surrounded by a dense connective tissue capsule, the sublingual gland does not have a

Figure 17-4. Histologic aspects of the major salivary glands

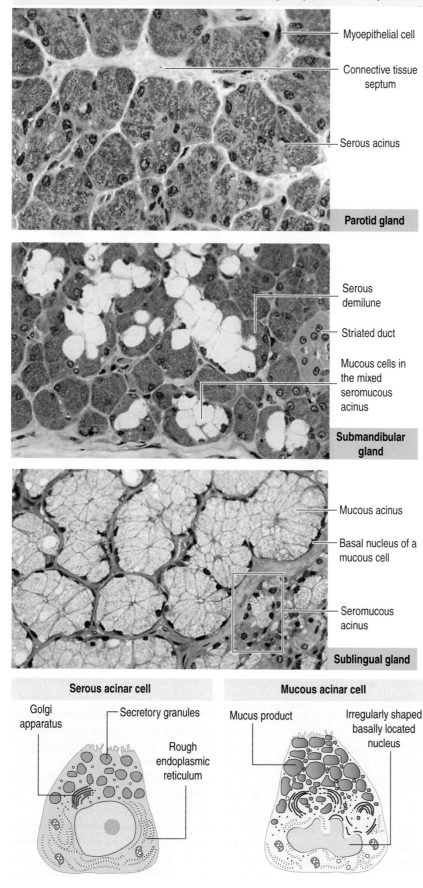

Myoepithelial cell

Connective tissue septum

Serous acinus

Parotid gland

Serous demilune

Striated duct

Mucous cells in the mixed seromucous acinus

Submandibular gland

Mucous acinus

Basal nucleus of a mucous cell

Seromucous acinus

Sublingual gland

The **parotid gland** is formed by acini containing exclusively serous cells with a basal nucleus and an apical cytoplasm with secretory granules. Granules are rich in proteins, including **proline-rich proteins, enzymes** (amylase, peroxidase, and lysozyme), and proteins with antimicrobial activity (**cystatins** and **histatins**). Although not visible in this image, **the parotid gland has the longest intercalated ducts**.

Connective tissue and blood vessels (not seen here) surround the serous acini.

Myoepithelial cells can be visualized at the periphery of each acinus.

Submandibular glands are mixed serous and mucous tubuloacinar glands. **Mixed seromucous and serous acini are readily found. Pure mucous acini are uncommon in the submandibular gland.** Striated ducts with basal infoldings, containing mitochondria, are observed within the lobule together with intercalated ducts (not seen here). Mucous cells secrete highly glycosylated mucins rich in sialic acid and sulfate that lubricate hard tissue surfaces, forming a thin protective film called a **pellicle**.

This film modulates the attachment of bacteria to oral surfaces and forms complexes with other proteins present in saliva.

Sublingual glands are mixed serous and mucous tubuloacinar glands in which mucous cells predominate. A few seromucous acini can be found. **The intercalated and striated ducts are poorly developed in the sublingual gland.** Mucous cells resemble goblet cells of the intestinal epithelium. The nucleus is flattened against the basal plasma membrane. The apical region of the mucous cells is occupied by mucin-filled secretory vesicles (unstained). The cell boundaries are sharp. Mucous cells secrete highly glycosylated mucins that contribute to the formation of the protective pellicle film.

Serous acinar cell	Mucous acinar cell	Striated duct cell
Golgi apparatus — Secretory granules — Rough endoplasmic reticulum	Mucus product — Irregularly shaped basally located nucleus	Kallikrein-containing vesicles

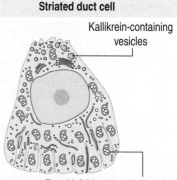

Basal infolds with mitochondria

Figure 17-5. **Structure of a mixed acinus and its striated duct**

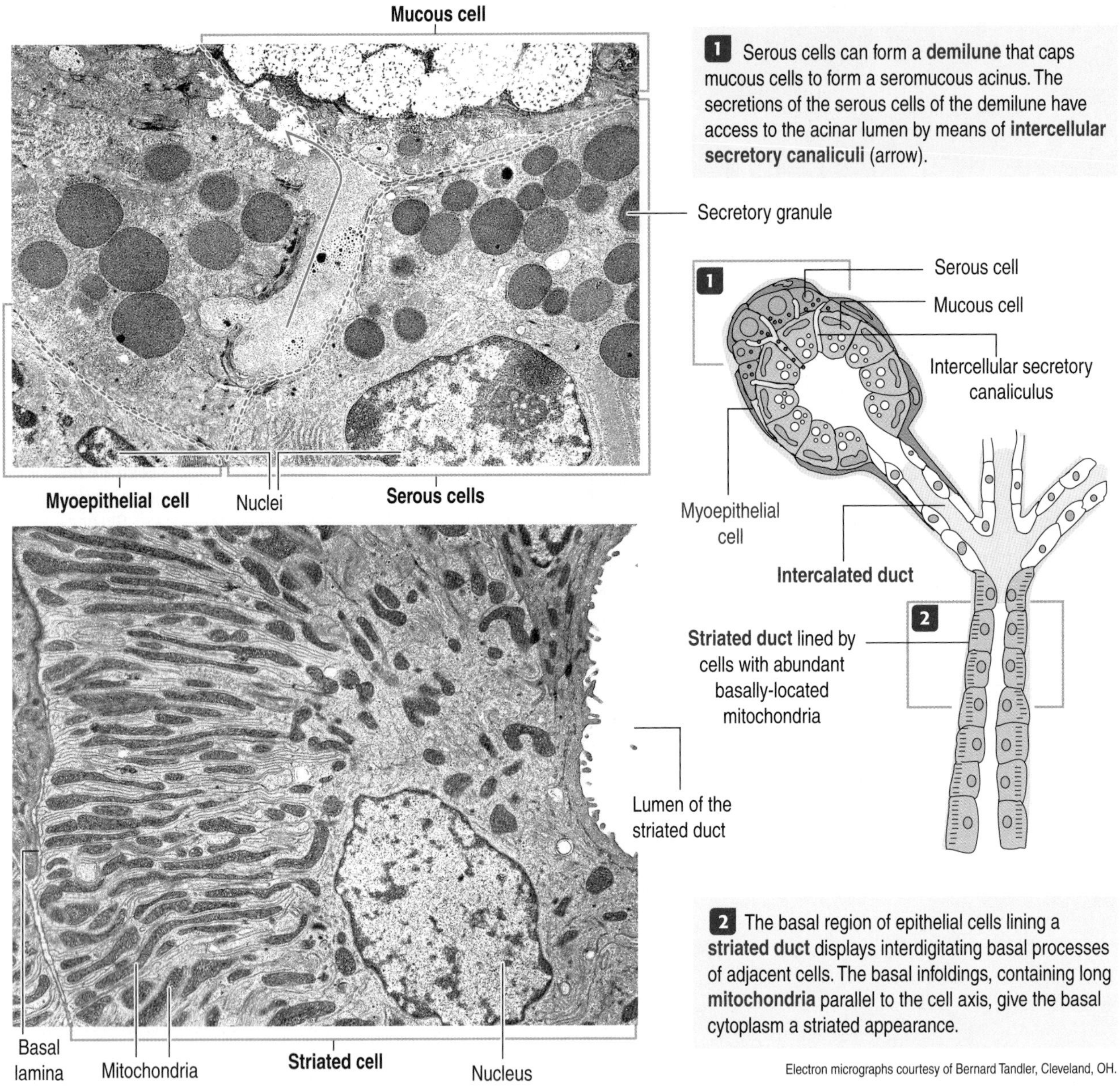

Mucous cell

1 Serous cells can form a **demilune** that caps mucous cells to form a seromucous acinus. The secretions of the serous cells of the demilune have access to the acinar lumen by means of **intercellular secretory canaliculi** (arrow).

Secretory granule

1

Serous cell

Mucous cell

Intercellular secretory canaliculus

Myoepithelial cell

Intercalated duct

2

Striated duct lined by cells with abundant basally-located mitochondria

Lumen of the striated duct

Myoepithelial cell   Nuclei   **Serous cells**

2 The basal region of epithelial cells lining a **striated duct** displays interdigitating basal processes of adjacent cells. The basal infoldings, containing long **mitochondria** parallel to the cell axis, give the basal cytoplasm a striated appearance.

Basal lamina   Mitochondria   **Striated cell**   Nucleus

Electron micrographs courtesy of Bernard Tandler, Cleveland, OH.

defined capsule. However, connective tissue septa divide the glandular parenchyma into small lobes.

The sublingual gland is a branched **tubuloalveolar gland with both serous and mucous cells** (see Figure 17-4), although most of the secretory units contain mucous cells.

The intercalated and striated ducts are poorly developed. Usually each lobe has its own excretory duct that opens beneath the tongue.

Exocrine pancreas

The pancreas is a combined **endocrine** and **exocrine gland**. The endocrine component is the **islet of Langerhans** and represents about 2% of the pancreas volume.

The main function of the endocrine pancreas is the **regulation of glucose metabolism** by hormones secreted into the bloodstream (see discussion of the islet of Langerhans in Chapter 19, Endocrine System).

The exocrine pancreas is a **branched tubuloacinar gland** organized into four anatomic components:

1. A **head**, lying in the concavity of the second and third parts of the duodenum.

2. A **neck**, in contact with the portal vein.

3. A **body**, placed anterior to the aorta.

4. A **tail**, ending near the hilum of the spleen.

The pancreas lies close to the posterior abdominal wall in the upper abdomen, and therefore it is protected from severe trauma.

Blood is provided by vessels derived from the celiac

Figure 17-6. Exocrine pancreas

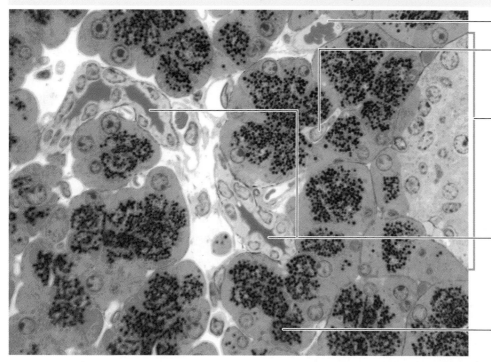

Capillary

Centroacinar cell
It is recognized by its location in the center of the pancreatic acinus and by its pale cytoplasm.

Islet of Langerhans
This endocrine component of the pancreas is surrounded by serous acini.

Intercalated duct
It is the continuation of the centroacinar cells into the connective tissue stroma.

Zymogen granules
They are present at the apical portion of the pancreatic acinar cell.

artery, the superior mesenteric artery, and the splenic artery. The venous drainage flows into the portal venous system and the splenic vein. Efferent innervation is through the vagus and splanchnic nerves.

The pancreas has structural similarities to the salivary glands:

1. It is surrounded by connective tissue but does not have a capsule proper.

2. Lobules are separated by connective tissue septa carrying blood and lymphatic vessels, nerves, and excretory ducts.

The functional histologic unit of the exocrine pancreas is the **acinus** (Figures 17-6 to 17-8). The lumen of the acinus is the initiation of the secretory-excretory duct system and contains **centroacinar cells that are unique to the pancreas**. Centroacinar cells are continuous with the **low cuboidal epithelial** lining of the **intercalated duct**. Centroacinar cells and the epithelial lining of the intercalated duct secrete HCO_3^-, Na^+, and water. The secretion of HCO_3^- is maintained by the cystic fibrosis transmembrane conductance regulator (CFTR) that also provides Cl^-.

The intercalated ducts merge into intralobular ducts. The intralobular ducts join to form the interlobular ducts, which drain into the main pancreatic duct.

The **main pancreatic duct (of Wirsung)** runs straight through the tail and the body, collecting secretions from ductal tributaries. It turns downward when it reaches the head of the pancreas and drains directly into the duodenum at the **ampulla of Vater**, after joining the **common bile duct**. A circular smooth **muscle sphincter (of Oddi)** is seen where the common pancreatic and bile duct cross the wall of the duodenum.

The exocrine pancreas lacks striated ducts and myoepithelial cells. Intercalated ducts converge to form **interlobular ducts** lined by a **columnar epithelium** with a few goblet cells and occasional enteroendocrine cells.

Pathology: Carcinoma of the pancreas

The pancreatic duct–bile duct anatomic relationship is of clinical significance in **carcinoma of the pancreas** localized in the **head region**, because compression of the bile duct causes **obstructive jaundice**.

Ductal adenocarcinoma is the most common primary malignant tumor of the pancreas. Most of them arise in the head of the pancreas. Tumoral masses obstruct and dilate the distal common bile and pancreatic ducts. Hyperplasia and carcinoma in situ of the duct epithelial lining are the precursor changes of the infiltrating ductal adenocarcinoma. Activation of the oncogene K-*ras* and inactivation of tumor suppressor genes, including *p53*, are molecular characteristics of the tumor.

The close association of the pancreas with large blood vessels, the extensive and diffuse abdominal drainage to lymph nodes, and the frequent spread of carcinoma cells to the liver via the portal vein are factors contributing to the ineffectiveness of surgical removal of pancreatic tumors.

Cystic tumors of the pancreas are not neoplastic. This category includes **serous cystoadenomas** (with

Figure 17-7. **Pancreatic acinus**

Pancreatic acinar cell

Inactive proenzymes are synthesized in the **1** **rough endoplasmic reticulum** of the pancreatic acinar cells and transferred to the **2** **Golgi apparatus** where they are concentrated in vesicles to form **3** **zymogen granules**.

3 Each zymogen granule contains several pancreatic enzymes whose relative concentration depends on changes in the diet.

The secretion of pancreatic enzymes is controlled by peptides released by enteroendocrine cells present in the duodenum and also by peptide hormones synthesized in the endocrine pancreas (**islets of Langerhans**).

Dual blood supply
Acinar and insuloacinar vascular systems

4 Each islet of Langerhans is supplied by afferent arterioles forming a network of capillaries lined by fenestrated endothelial cells. This network is called the **insuloacinar portal system**.

Venules leaving the islet supply blood to the pancreatic acini surrounding the islet. This vascular system enables a local action on the exocrine pancreas of hormones produced in the islet.

5 An independent arterial system, the **acinar vascular system**, supplies the pancreatic acini.

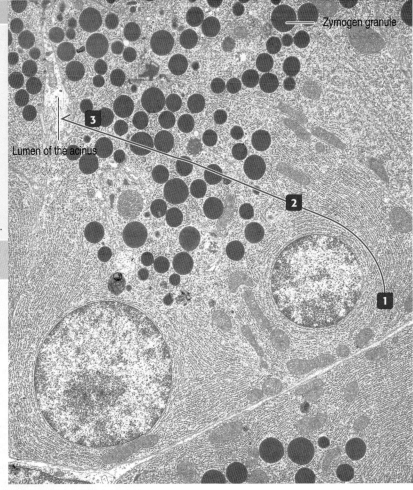

Zymogen granule

Lumen of the acinus

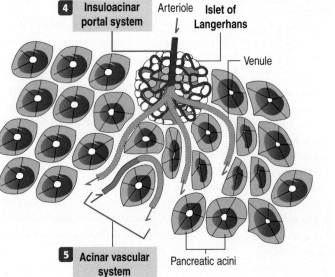

4 Insuloacinar portal system — Arteriole — **Islet of Langerhans**

Venule

5 Acinar vascular system — Pancreatic acini

cysts containing a clear fluid) and **mucinous cystoadenomas** (with cysts filled with a mucoid product). Untreated mucinous cystoadenomas evolve into an infiltrating tumor (mucinous cystoadenocarcinoma).

Less common are the **endocrine tumors** of the pancreas that can be detected as isolated pancreatic masses or a component of the multiple endocrine neoplasia syndrome, type 1 (MEN1).

MEN1 is an autosomal dominant hereditary endocrine cancer syndrome characterized primarily by tumors of the parathyroid glands, gastroenteroendocrine cells, and adenohypophysis. This tumor type does not show activation of the K-*ras* gene or *p53* gene inactivation.

Mutations in the *MEN1* (producing the tumor suppressor menin), *RET* (*Ret* protoncogene producing receptor tyrosine kinase), and *CDKN1B* (for cyclin-dependent kinase inhibitor 1B, encoding the tumor suppressor p27) genes can cause MENs.

You may remember that mutations of the *RET* gene causes Hirschsprung's disease (congenital aganglionic megacolon).

Endocrine tumors of the pancreas can be well differentiated (with structural evidences of endocrine function) or moderately differentiated. Gastrinomas, insulinomas, and glucagonomas are examples of endocrine tumors showing cytoplasmic secretory granules. This tumors belong to the category

Figure 17-8. Pancreatic acinus

Pathway of the pancreatic exocrine secretion

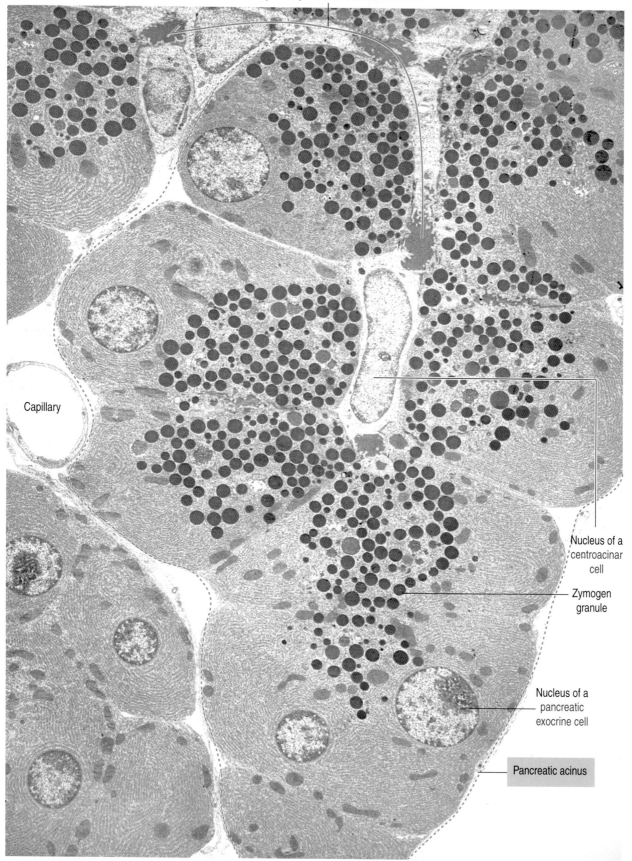

Capillary

Nucleus of a centroacinar cell

Zymogen granule

Nucleus of a pancreatic exocrine cell

Pancreatic acinus

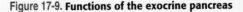

Figure 17-9. Functions of the exocrine pancreas

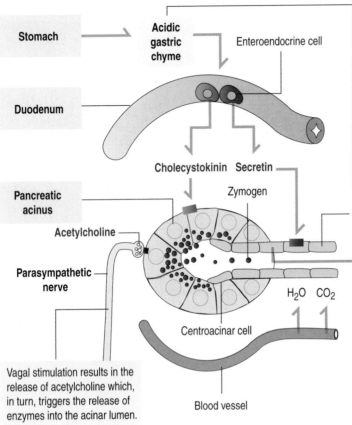

Stomach → **Acidic gastric chyme**

Enteroendocrine cell

Duodenum

Cholecystokinin   Secretin

Zymogen

Pancreatic acinus

Acetylcholine

Parasympathetic nerve

Centroacinar cell

Intercalated duct

HCO_3^- H_2O

H_2O CO_2

Blood vessel

Vagal stimulation results in the release of acetylcholine which, in turn, triggers the release of enzymes into the acinar lumen.

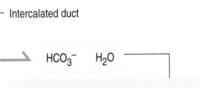

Secretin and **cholecystokinin** are secreted into the blood by enteroendocrine cells of the **duodenum** when chyme enters the small intestine.

Acinar pancreatic cells secrete the inactive forms of the enzymes **trypsin**, **chymotrypsin**, and **carboxylpeptidases**. Active **amylase**, **lipase**, **cholesterol esterase**, and **phospholipase** are also secreted.
   Acinar pancreatic cells secrete **trypsin inhibitor**, which prevents the activation of trypsin and other proteolytic enzymes within the acinar lumen and ducts.
   Epithelial cells of the **intercalated duct** secrete **water and bicarbonate ions**.

The **secretion of bicarbonate ions and water is regulated by secretin** and involves the following steps:
1. Diffusion of CO_2 from a blood vessel into intercalated duct epithelial cells.
2. CO_2 binds to water and forms carbonic acid under the influence of carbonic anhydrase.
3. Carbonic acid dissociates into HCO_3^- and H^+.
4. HCO_3^- is actively transported to the lumen of the duct.
5. H^+ and Na^+ are actively exchanged (cell-blood exchange) and Na^+ flows into the ductular lumen to achieve electrical neutrality.

of **syndromic functioning tumors** (associated with a syndrome). For example, gastrinomas produce the **Zollinger-Ellison syndrome**, that, as you remember from our discussion in Chapter 15, Upper Digestive Segment, is characterized by multiple peptic ulcers caused by continuous stimulation of HCl production by parietal cells in the stomach.

Functions of the pancreatic acinus

The pancreatic acinus is lined by pyramidal cells joined to each other by apical junctional complexes (see Figure 17-8), which prevent the reflux of secreted products from the ducts into the intercellular spaces.

The basal domain of an acinar pancreatic cell is associated with a basal lamina and contains the nucleus and a well-developed rough endoplasmic reticulum. The apical domain displays numerous **zymogen granules** (see Figure 17-8) and the Golgi apparatus.

The concentration of about 20 different pancreatic enzymes in the zymogen granules varies with the dietary intake. For example, an increase in the synthesis of **proteases** is associated with a **protein-rich diet**. A **carbohydrate-rich diet** results in the selective synthesis of **amylases** and a decrease in the synthesis of proteases. Amylase gene expression is regulated by

insulin, an event that stresses the significance of the **insuloacinar portal system**.

The administration of a cholinergic drug or of the gastrointestinal hormones cholecystokinin and secretin increases the flow of pancreatic fluid (about 1.5 to 3.0 L/day).

The polypeptide hormone **cholecystokinin**, produced in enteroendocrine cells of the duodenal mucosa, binds to specific receptors of **acinar cells** and **stimulates the release of zymogen** (Figure 17-9).

Secretin is released when acid chyme enters the duodenum. Secretin is produced in the duodenum, binds to receptors on the surface of **centroacinar cells** and **intercalated ductal cells**, and **triggers the release of water and HCO_3^- and Na^+, through a Na^+–HCO_3^- cotransporter** into the pancreatic ducts.

HCO_3^- ions and the alkaline secretion of Brunner's glands, present in the submucosa of the duodenum, neutralize the acidic gastric chyme in the duodenal lumen and activate the pancreatic digestive enzymes.

Pathology: Pancreatitis and cystic fibrosis

Zymogen granules contain **inactive proenzymes** that are activated within the duodenal environment. A premature activation of pancreatic enzymes, in par-

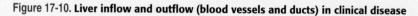

Figure 17-10. Liver inflow and outflow (blood vessels and ducts) in clinical disease

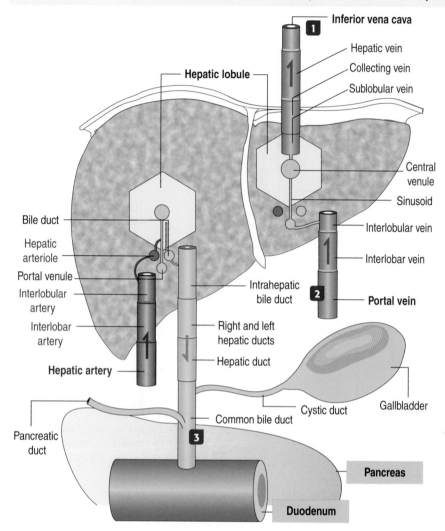

Inferior vena cava

1

Hepatic vein

Collecting vein

Sublobular vein

Hepatic lobule

Central venule

Sinusoid

Interlobular vein

Interlobar vein

2

Portal vein

Bile duct

Hepatic arteriole

Portal venule

Interlobular artery

Interlobar artery

Hepatic artery

Intrahepatic bile duct

Right and left hepatic ducts

Hepatic duct

Cystic duct

Gallbladder

Pancreatic duct

Common bile duct

3

Pancreas

Duodenum

1   **Congestive heart failure**

Valves are not present in the inferior vena cava and hepatic veins.
   An increase in central venous pressure (as in congestive heart failure) causes an enlargement of the liver due to blood engorgement.

2   **Portal hypertension**

An obstruction to blood flow in the liver during **cirrhosis**, together with failure of hepatocytes to produce plasma proteins, in particular albumin, result in **portal hypertension**.
   Portal hypertension increases the hydrostatic pressure in the portal vein and its intrahepatic branches and fluid accumulates in the peritoneal cavity (**ascites**). The loss of fluid is aggravated by reduced plasma oncotic pressure due to a reduction in plasma albumin.
   Cirrhosis may develop following chronic hepatitis or alcoholic liver disease.

3   **Carcinoma of the pancreas**

A carcinoma of the head of the pancreas (60% of pancreatic tumors) obstructs by compression the outflow of bile through the ampullary region.

ticular **trypsinogen** to **trypsin**, and the inactivation of **trypsin inhibitor** (tightly bound to the active site of trypsin), result in the autodigestion of the pancreatic gland following their release into the interstitium.

This condition, known to occur in **acute pancreatitis**, usually follows trauma, heavy meals or excessive alcohol ingestion or biliary tract disease.

The clinical features of acute pancreatitis are severe abdominal pain, nausea, and vomiting. A rapid elevation of amylase and lipase in serum (within 24 to 72 hours) are typical diagnostic features. The normal structure and function of the pancreas are normalized when the cause of pancreatitis is removed. However, acute pancreatitis can give rise to complications, such as **abscess formation** and **cysts**.

Chronic pancreatitis is characterized by fibrosis and partial or total destruction of the pancreatic tissue. Alcoholism is the major cause of chronic pancreatitis, leading to a permanent loss of pancreatic endocrine and exocrine functions.

Cystic fibrosis is an inherited, autosomal recessive disease affecting the function of mucus-secreting tissues of the respiratory (see Chapter 13, Respiratory System), intestinal, and reproductive systems; the sweat glands of the skin (see Chapter 11, Integumentary System); and the **exocrine pancreas** in children and young adults.

A thick sticky mucus obstructs the duct passages of the airways, pancreatic and biliary ducts, and intestine, followed by bacterial infections and damage of the functional tissues. Some affected babies have **meconium ileus**, a blockage of the intestine that occurs soon after birth.

A large number of patients (85%) have **chronic pancreatitis** characterized by a loss of acini and dilation of the pancreatic excretory ducts into cysts surrounded by extensive fibrosis (hence the designation **cystic fibrosis of the pancreas**).

Insufficient exocrine pancreatic secretions cause the malabsorption of fat and protein, reflected by bulky and fatty stools (**steatorrhea**).

The lack of transport of Cl⁻ ions across epithelia

Figure 17-11. **Portal space and the bile ducts**

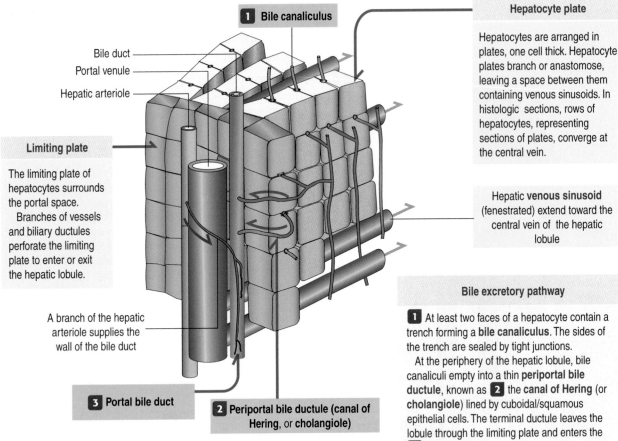

1 Bile canaliculus

Bile duct

Portal venule

Hepatic arteriole

Limiting plate

The limiting plate of hepatocytes surrounds the portal space.
   Branches of vessels and biliary ductules perforate the limiting plate to enter or exit the hepatic lobule.

A branch of the hepatic arteriole supplies the wall of the bile duct

3 Portal bile duct

2 Periportal bile ductule (canal of Hering, or cholangiole)

Hepatocyte plate

Hepatocytes are arranged in plates, one cell thick. Hepatocyte plates branch or anastomose, leaving a space between them containing venous sinusoids. In histologic sections, rows of hepatocytes, representing sections of plates, converge at the central vein.

Hepatic **venous sinusoid** (fenestrated) extend toward the central vein of the hepatic lobule

Bile excretory pathway

1 At least two faces of a hepatocyte contain a trench forming a **bile canaliculus**. The sides of the trench are sealed by tight junctions.
   At the periphery of the hepatic lobule, bile canaliculi empty into a thin **periportal bile ductule**, known as **2** the **canal of Hering** (or **cholangiole**) lined by cuboidal/squamous epithelial cells. The terminal ductule leaves the lobule through the limiting plate and enters the **3** **portal bile duct** in the portal space.

is associated with a defective secretion of Na⁺ ions and water.

A genetic defect in the chloride channel protein, **CFTR**, is responsible for cystic fibrosis.

The disease is detected by the demonstration of increased concentration of NaCl in sweat. Children with cystic fibrosis "taste salty" after copious sweating.

Liver

The liver, the largest gland in the human body, consists of four poorly defined **lobes**. The liver is surrounded by a collagen-elastic fiber–containing **capsule (of Glisson)** and is lined by the peritoneum.

Blood is supplied to the liver by two blood vessels (Figure 17-10):

1. The **portal vein** (75% to 80% of the afferent blood volume) transports blood from the digestive tract, spleen, and pancreas.

2. The **hepatic artery**, a branch of the celiac trunk, supplies 20% to 25% of oxygenated blood to the liver by the **interlobar artery** and **interlobular artery** pathway before reaching the **portal space**.

Blood from branches of the portal vein and the hepatic artery mixes in the **sinusoids** of the **liver lobules**, as we discuss in detail later.

Sinusoidal blood converges at the **central venule** of the liver lobule.

Central venules converge to form the **sublobular veins**, and blood returns to the **inferior vena cava** following the **collecting veins** and **hepatic veins** pathway.

The **right** and **left hepatic bile ducts** leave the liver and merge to form the **hepatic duct**. The hepatic duct becomes the **common bile duct** soon after giving rise to the **cystic duct**, a thin tube connecting the bile duct to the **gallbladder** (see Figure 17-10).

General organization of the hepatic lobule

The structural and functional unit of the liver is the **hepatic lobule**. The hepatic lobule consists of anastomosing **plates of hepatocytes** limiting blood **sinusoidal spaces** (Figure 17-11).

A **central venule** (or vein) in the core of the hepatic lobule collects the sinusoidal blood transporting a mixture of blood supplied by branches of the portal vein and the hepatic artery.

Branches of the hepatic artery and portal vein, together with a bile duct, form the classic **portal triad** found in the portal space surrounding the hexagonal-shaped hepatic lobule (Figure 17-12).

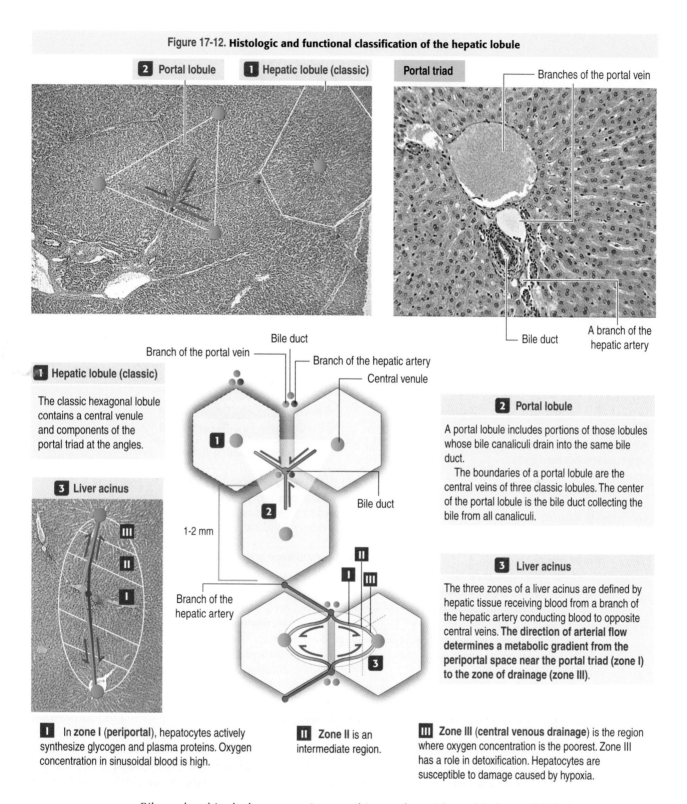

Figure 17-12. Histologic and functional classification of the hepatic lobule

2 Portal lobule   **1** Hepatic lobule (classic)

Portal triad

Branches of the portal vein

Bile duct — A branch of the hepatic artery

Bile duct
Branch of the portal vein
Branch of the hepatic artery
Central venule

1 Hepatic lobule (classic)

The classic hexagonal lobule contains a central venule and components of the portal triad at the angles.

3 Liver acinus

1-2 mm

Branch of the hepatic artery

Bile duct

2 Portal lobule

A portal lobule includes portions of those lobules whose bile canaliculi drain into the same bile duct.

The boundaries of a portal lobule are the central veins of three classic lobules. The center of the portal lobule is the bile duct collecting the bile from all canaliculi.

3 Liver acinus

The three zones of a liver acinus are defined by hepatic tissue receiving blood from a branch of the hepatic artery conducting blood to opposite central veins. **The direction of arterial flow determines a metabolic gradient from the periportal space near the portal triad (zone I) to the zone of drainage (zone III).**

I In **zone I (periportal)**, hepatocytes actively synthesize glycogen and plasma proteins. Oxygen concentration in sinusoidal blood is high.

II **Zone II** is an intermediate region.

III **Zone III (central venous drainage)** is the region where oxygen concentration is the poorest. Zone III has a role in detoxification. Hepatocytes are susceptible to damage caused by hypoxia.

Bile produced in the hepatocytes is secreted into narrow intercellular spaces, the **bile canaliculi**, located between the apposed surfaces of adjacent hepatocytes. **Bile flows in the opposite direction to the blood.** Bile flows from the **bile canaliculi** into **periportal bile ductules** (**cholangioles**, or **canals of Hering**), and then into the **bile ducts** (or ductules) of the portal space after crossing the **hepatic plate** at

the periphery of the hepatic lobule (see Figure 17-11). Bile ductules converge at the **intrahepatic bile ducts.**

Functional views of the hepatic lobule

There are three conceptual interpretations of the architecture of the liver lobule (see Figure 17-12):

1. The **classic concept** of the **hepatic lobule**, based on structural parameters.

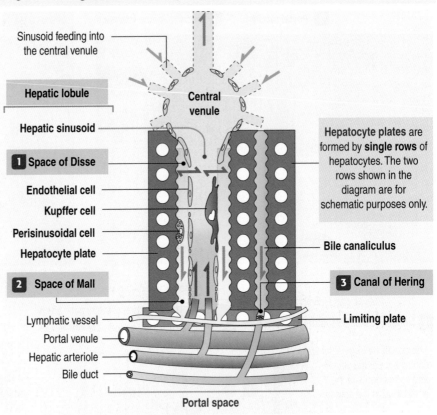

Figure 17-13. Organization of the hepatic lobule

1 The perisinusoidal **space of Disse** separates the basolateral domain of the hepatocyte from blood circulating in the hepatic sinusoid.

The space of Disse contains types I, III, and IV collagen fibers. Protein absorption and secretion take place across the narrow space of Disse (0.2 to 0.5 μm wide).

2 The **space of Mall**, found at the periphery of the hepatic lobule, is continuous with the space of Disse. The space of Mall is drained by lymphatic vessels piercing the **limiting plate**.

Lymphatic vessels surround the blood vessels and bile ductules in the portal space.

3 The **canal of Hering** (or cholangiole) is the terminal point of the network of bile canalicular trenches found on the hepatocyte surfaces.

The canal of Hering is located at the periphery of the hepatic lobule (periportal site), is lined by a squamous-to-cuboidal simple epithelium, and connects with the bile ductules in the portal space after perforating the limiting plate.

Sinusoid feeding into the central venule

Hepatic lobule

Hepatic sinusoid

1 Space of Disse

Endothelial cell

Kupffer cell

Perisinusoidal cell

Hepatocyte plate

2 Space of Mall

Lymphatic vessel

Portal venule

Hepatic arteriole

Bile duct

Central venule

Hepatocyte plates are formed by **single rows** of hepatocytes. The two rows shown in the diagram are for schematic purposes only.

Bile canaliculus

3 Canal of Hering

Limiting plate

Portal space

The connective tissue of the **portal space** provides support to the **portal triad** formed by branches of the **hepatic artery** (arteriole), **portal vein** (venule), and **bile duct** (ductule). In addition, lymphatic vessels and nerve fibers are present in the portal space (also designated portal canal, portal area, or portal tract).

Note that blood and bile and lymph flow in opposite directions

2. The **portal lobule concept**, based on the bile drainage pathway from adjacent lobules toward the same bile duct.

3. The **liver acinus concept**, based on the gradient distribution of oxygen along the venous sinusoids of adjacent lobules.

The **classic hepatic lobule** is customarily described as a polyhedral structure, usually depicted as a hexagon with a central venule to which blood sinusoids converge (see Figure 17-12).

Components of the **portal triad**, constituting a branch of the portal vein and hepatic artery and a bile duct, are usually found at the angles of the hexagon. This geometric organization is poorly defined in humans because the limiting perilobular connective tissue is not abundant. However, recognition of the components of the portal triad is helpful in determining the boundaries of the human hepatic lobule.

In the **portal lobule**, the portal triad is the central axis, draining bile from the surrounding hepatic parenchyma.

Functional considerations have modified the classic view and a **liver acinus** concept has gained ground in pathophysiology. In the liver acinus, **the boundaries are determined by a terminal branch of the hepatic artery**. The flow of arterial blood within the venous sinusoids creates gradients of oxygen and nutrients classified as **zones I, II, and III**.

Zone I is the richest in oxygen and nutrients. Zone III, closer to the central vein, is oxygen-poor. Zone II is intermediate in oxygen and nutrients (see Figure 17-12).

Although pathologic changes in the liver are usually described in relation to the classic lobule, the liver acinus concept is convenient for understanding liver regeneration patterns, liver metabolic activities, and the development of cirrhosis.

Hepatocyte

The hepatocyte is the functional **exocrine** and **endocrine** cell of the hepatic lobule. Hepatocytes form anastomosing **one-cell-thick plates** limiting the sinusoidal spaces.

The perisinusoidal **space of Disse** separates the

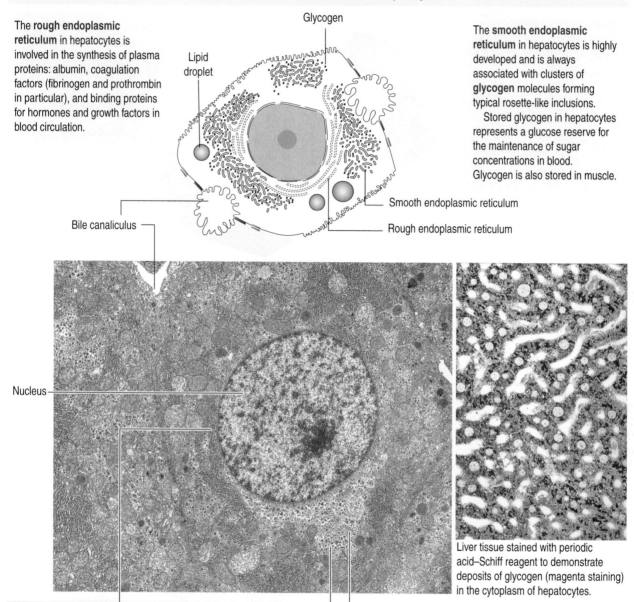

Figure 17-14. Endoplasmic reticulum in hepatocytes

The **rough endoplasmic reticulum** in hepatocytes is involved in the synthesis of plasma proteins: albumin, coagulation factors (fibrinogen and prothrombin in particular), and binding proteins for hormones and growth factors in blood circulation.

Glycogen

Lipid droplet

The **smooth endoplasmic reticulum** in hepatocytes is highly developed and is always associated with clusters of **glycogen** molecules forming typical rosette-like inclusions.

Stored glycogen in hepatocytes represents a glucose reserve for the maintenance of sugar concentrations in blood. Glycogen is also stored in muscle.

Smooth endoplasmic reticulum

Rough endoplasmic reticulum

Bile canaliculus

Nucleus

Liver tissue stained with periodic acid–Schiff reagent to demonstrate deposits of glycogen (magenta staining) in the cytoplasm of hepatocytes.

Rough endoplasmic reticulum

Albumin, a major product of the hepatocyte, maintains plasma oncotic pressure. A decrease of albumin in a liver disease causes **edema** and **ascites**.

Blood coagulation depends on **fibrinogen**, **prothrombin**, and **factor VIII** produced in the hepatocyte. **Bleeding** is associated with liver failure. **Complement proteins**, synthesized by hepatocytes, participate in the destruction of pathogens.

Glycogen

Smooth endoplasmic reticulum

The smooth endoplasmic reticulum has an important function in **detoxification**.

Enzymes necessary for the detoxification of drugs (barbiturates), steroids, alcohol, and other toxicants reside in the membrane of the smooth endoplasmic reticulum.

hepatocyte plates from the blood sinusoidal space (Figure 17-13).

The components of the portal triad, embedded in connective tissue, are separated from the hepatic lobule by a **limiting plate** of hepatocytes (see Figure 17-11). Blood from the portal vein and hepatic artery flows into the sinusoids and is drained by the central venule (no apparent smooth muscle cell wall).

Recall that bile and lymph flow in the opposite direction: from the hepatocytes to the bile duct and to lymphatic vessels in the portal space (see Figure 17-13).

A hepatocyte has two cellular domains:
1. A **basolateral domain**.
2. An **apical domain** (Figures 17-14 to 17-16):
The **basolateral domain** contains abundant **micro-**

Figure 17-15. **Apical and basolateral domains of hepatocytes**

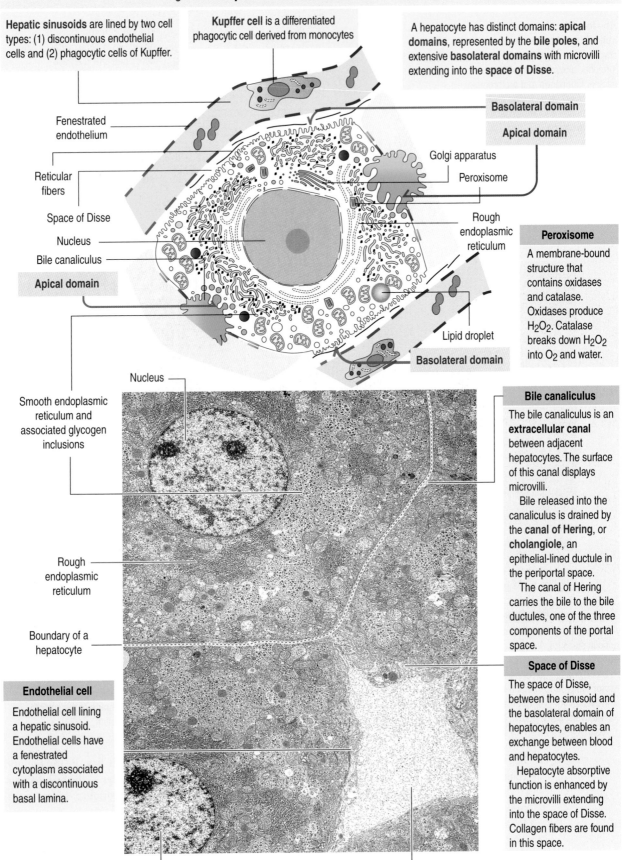

Hepatic sinusoids are lined by two cell types: (1) discontinuous endothelial cells and (2) phagocytic cells of Kupffer.

Kupffer cell is a differentiated phagocytic cell derived from monocytes

A hepatocyte has distinct domains: **apical domains**, represented by the **bile poles**, and extensive **basolateral domains** with microvilli extending into the **space of Disse**.

Fenestrated endothelium

Reticular fibers

Space of Disse

Nucleus

Bile canaliculus

Apical domain

Basolateral domain

Apical domain

Golgi apparatus

Peroxisome

Rough endoplasmic reticulum

Lipid droplet

Basolateral domain

Peroxisome

A membrane-bound structure that contains oxidases and catalase. Oxidases produce H_2O_2. Catalase breaks down H_2O_2 into O_2 and water.

Nucleus

Smooth endoplasmic reticulum and associated glycogen inclusions

Rough endoplasmic reticulum

Boundary of a hepatocyte

Endothelial cell

Endothelial cell lining a hepatic sinusoid. Endothelial cells have a fenestrated cytoplasm associated with a discontinuous basal lamina.

Bile canaliculus

The bile canaliculus is an **extracellular canal** between adjacent hepatocytes. The surface of this canal displays microvilli.

Bile released into the canaliculus is drained by the **canal of Hering**, or **cholangiole**, an epithelial-lined ductule in the periportal space.

The canal of Hering carries the bile to the bile ductules, one of the three components of the portal space.

Space of Disse

The space of Disse, between the sinusoid and the basolateral domain of hepatocytes, enables an exchange between blood and hepatocytes.

Hepatocyte absorptive function is enhanced by the microvilli extending into the space of Disse. Collagen fibers are found in this space.

Nucleus

Sinusoid

Figure 17-16. **Hepatic sinusoids and bile canaliculi**

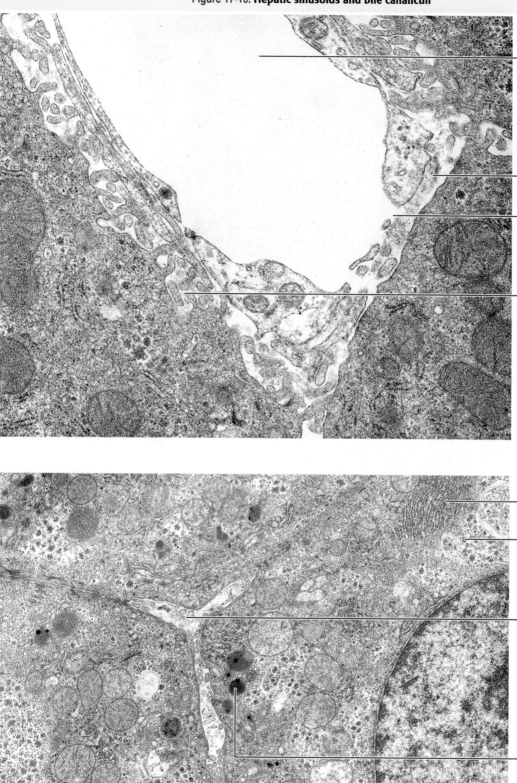

Lumen of a **hepatic sinusoid**

A **discontinuous basal lamina** supports the fenestrated endothelial cell lining of a hepatic sinusoid.

Fenestrated endothelial cell lining of a hepatic sinusoid

Microvilli of the basolateral domain of a hepatocyte extending into the **subendothelial space of Disse**

Rough endoplasmic reticulum

Glycogen

The **bile canaliculus** is a space limited by two or more hepatocytes. Small hepatocyte microvilli extend into the bile canaliculus. Tight junctions seal the intercellular space, thus preventing the leakage of bile.

Lysosomes are frequently seen surrounding the bile canaliculus.

Nucleus of a hepatocyte

Figure 17-17. **Ethanol metabolism in hepatocytes**

Alcohol dehydrogenase (ADH) pathway

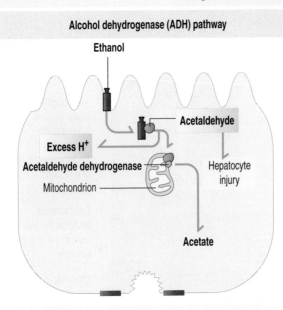

The ADH is the major pathway. **Alcohol is oxidized to acetaldehyde** in the cytoplasm and **acetaldehyde is converted to acetate** in mitochondria.

An excess of H+ and acetaldehyde causes mitochondrial damage, disrupts microtubules, and alters proteins that can induce autoimmune responses leading to hepatocyte injury.

Microsomal ethanol-oxidizing system (MEOS)

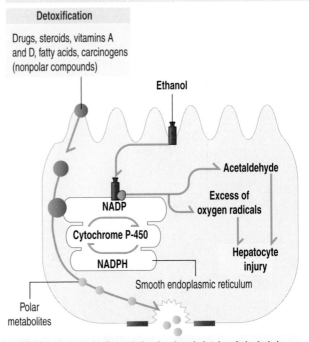

The MEOS pathway is significant during the **chronic intake of alcohol**. In contrast to the ADH pathway that produces acetaldehyde and excess H+, **the MEOS pathway produces acetaldehyde and an excess of oxygen radicals**.

Reactive oxygen produces injury to hepatocytes by causing lipid peroxidation, resulting in cell membrane damage. In addition, an up-regulated MEOS affects detoxification activities of the hepatocyte that require cytochrome P-450 for the oxidation of various drugs, toxins, vitamins A and D, and potential carcinogens. The accumulation of these products is often toxic.

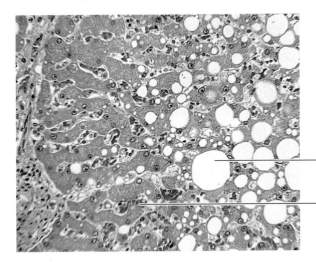

Large fat deposits in the cytoplasm of hepatocytes are observed in **fatty liver (steatosis)** following long-term consumption of alcohol.

— Sinusoid

---

villi and **faces the space of Disse**. Excess fluid in the space of Disse is collected in the **space of Mall**, located at the periphery of the hepatic lobule. Lymphatic vessels piercing the limiting plate drain the fluid of the space of Mall. **Gap junctions** on the lateral surfaces of adjacent hepatocytes enable intercellular functional coupling.

The basolateral domain participates in the **absorption of blood-borne substances** and in the **secretion of plasma proteins** (such as **albumin**, **fibrinogen**, **prothrombin**, and **coagulation factors V, VII**, and **IX**). Note that hepatocytes synthesize several plasma proteins required for blood clotting (see Chapter 6, Blood and Hematopoiesis). Blood coagulation disorders are associated with liver disease.

The **apical domain** borders the **bile canaliculus**, a trenchlike depression lined by microvilli and sealed at the sides by **occluding junctions** to prevent leakage of **bile**, the exocrine product of the hepatocyte (see Figure 17-15).

The hepatocyte contains **rough endoplasmic reticulum** (see Figure 17-14), involved in the synthesis of plasma proteins, and a highly developed **smooth endoplasmic reticulum**, associated with the synthesis of **glycogen**, **lipid**, and **detoxification mechanisms** (Figure 17-16). **Enzymes** inserted in the membrane of the **smooth endoplasmic reticulum** are involved in the following **functions**:

Figure 17-18. Perisinusoidal cell and chronic liver disease

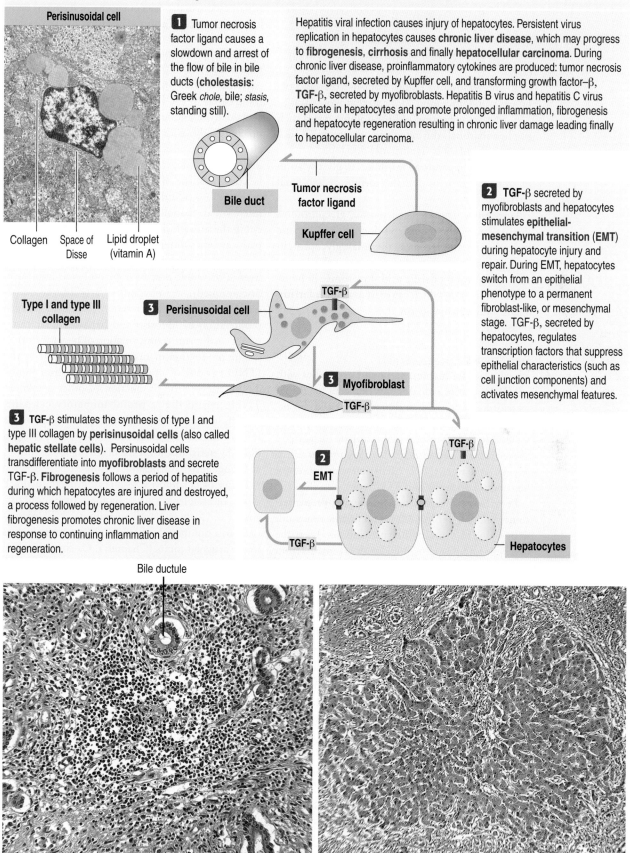

Perisinusoidal cell

Collagen Space of Disse Lipid droplet (vitamin A)

1 Tumor necrosis factor ligand causes a slowdown and arrest of the flow of bile in bile ducts (**cholestasis**: Greek *chole*, bile; *stasis*, standing still).

Bile duct

Hepatitis viral infection causes injury of hepatocytes. Persistent virus replication in hepatocytes causes **chronic liver disease**, which may progress to **fibrogenesis**, **cirrhosis** and finally **hepatocellular carcinoma**. During chronic liver disease, proinflammatory cytokines are produced: tumor necrosis factor ligand, secreted by Kupffer cell, and transforming growth factor–β, **TGF-β**, secreted by myofibroblasts. Hepatitis B virus and hepatitis C virus replicate in hepatocytes and promote prolonged inflammation, fibrogenesis and hepatocyte regeneration resulting in chronic liver damage leading finally to hepatocellular carcinoma.

Tumor necrosis factor ligand

Kupffer cell

2 TGF-β secreted by myofibroblasts and hepatocytes stimulates **epithelial-mesenchymal transition (EMT)** during hepatocyte injury and repair. During EMT, hepatocytes switch from an epithelial phenotype to a permanent fibroblast-like, or mesenchymal stage. TGF-β, secreted by hepatocytes, regulates transcription factors that suppress epithelial characteristics (such as cell junction components) and activates mesenchymal features.

Type I and type III collagen

TGF-β

3 **Perisinusoidal cell**

3 **Myofibroblast**

TGF-β

3 TGF-β stimulates the synthesis of type I and type III collagen by **perisinusoidal cells** (also called **hepatic stellate cells**). Perisinusoidal cells transdifferentiate into **myofibroblasts** and secrete TGF-β. **Fibrogenesis** follows a period of hepatitis during which hepatocytes are injured and destroyed, a process followed by regeneration. Liver fibrogenesis promotes chronic liver disease in response to continuing inflammation and regeneration.

2 EMT

TGF-β

TGF-β

Hepatocytes

Bile ductule

Chronic liver disease. Fibrosis and inflammatory cells, mainly lymphocytes and macrophages, are seen in the distorted portal space.

Cirrhosis. Regenerated hepatocyte nodule surrounded and infiltrated by connective tissue containing collagens and extracellular matrix material.

1. The synthesis of cholesterol and bile salts.

2. The glucuronide conjugation of bilirubin, steroids and drugs.

3. The breakdown of glycogen into glucose

4. The esterification of free fatty acids to triglycerides.

5. The removal of iodine from the thyroid hormones triiodothyronine (T_3) and thyroxine (T_4).

6. The **detoxification of lipid-soluble drugs** such as **phenobarbital**, during which the smooth endoplasmic reticulum is significantly developed.

The **Golgi apparatus** contributes to glycosylation of secretory proteins and the sorting of lysosomal enzymes.

Lysosomes degrade aged plasma glycoproteins internalized at the basolateral domain by a hepatic lectin membrane receptor, the **asialoglycoprotein receptor**, with binding affinity to terminal galactose after the removal of sialic acid. Lysosomes in hepatocytes store iron, which can exist as **soluble ferritin** and **insoluble hemosiderin**, the degradation product of ferritin.

Peroxisomes

Peroxisomes are **membrane-bound organelles** with a high content of **oxidases** and **catalases** for the β-oxidation of fatty acids and production and breakdown of **hydrogen peroxide**.

Because hydrogen peroxide is a toxic metabolite, the enzyme **catalase** degrades this product into **oxygen** and **water**. This catalytic event occurs in hepatocytes and cells of the kidneys.

Peroxisomes derive from preexisting preperoxisomes budding off from the endoplasmic reticulum or by fission from pre-existing peroxisomes. Then, the organelle imports peroxisomal matrix proteins from the cytosol, targeted to peroxisomes by peroxisome targeting signals.

Peroxisomes contain **peroxins**, proteins involved in peroxisome biogenesis. Some of the peroxins are defective and associated with peroxisome biogenesis disorders, including **Zellweger syndrome**.

The biogenesis of peroxisomes and their role in inherited disorders are outlined in Chapter 2, Epithelial Glands.

Pathology: Liver iron-overload disorders

Severe liver diseases can result from the excessive storage of iron and copper.

Hereditary hemochromatosis is an example of a disease characterized by increased iron absorption and accumulation in lysosomal hepatocytes. Cirrhosis and cancer of the liver are complications of hemochromatosis. We discuss in detail iron-overload disorders in Chapter 6, Blood and Hematopoiesis.

Wilson's disease (hepatolenticular degeneration) is a hereditary disorder of **copper** metabolism in which excessive deposits of copper in liver and brain lysosomes produce chronic hepatitis and cirrhosis.

Pathology: Alcoholism and fatty liver (alcoholic steatohepatitis)

After absorption in the stomach, most ethanol is transported to the liver, where it is metabolized to **acetaldehyde** and **acetate** in the hepatocytes. Ethanol is mainly oxidized by **alcohol dehydrogenase**, an NADH (reduced form of nicotinamide adenine dinucleotide)–dependent enzyme. This mechanism is known as the **alcohol dehydrogenase (ADH) pathway**. An additional metabolic pathway is the **microsomal ethanol-oxidizing system (MEOS)**, present in the smooth endoplasmic reticulum. The two pathways are summarized in Figure 17-17.

Long-term consumption of ethanol results in **fatty liver** (a reversible process if ethanol consumption is discontinued), **steatohepatitis** (fatty liver accompanied by an inflammatory reaction), **cirrhosis** (collagen proliferation or fibrosis), and **hepatocellular carcinoma** (malignant transformation of hepatocytes).

The production of **tumor necrosis factor ligand (TNFL)** is one of the initial events in liver injury. TNFL triggers the production of other cytokines. TNFL, regarded as a **proinflammatory cytokine**, recruits inflammatory cells that cause hepatocyte injury and promote the production of type I collagen fibers by **perisinusoidal cells of Ito** (a process known as **fibrogenesis**) as a healing response.

Injury of hepatocytes results in programmed cell death, or apoptosis, caused by the activation of caspases (see Chapter 3, Cell Signaling). TNFL participates in a number of inflammatory processes such as in the articular joints (Chapter 5, Osteogenesis) and the extravasation of inflammatory cells (Chapter 10, Immune-Lymphatic System).

Ethanol, viruses, or toxins induce Kupffer cells to synthesize TNFL as well as **transforming growth factor–β (TGF-β)** and **interleukin-6** (Figure 17-18). TGF-β stimulates the production of type I collagen by perisinusoidal cells, which increase in number. TNFL acts on biliary ducts to interfere with the flow of bile (cholestasis).

Pathology: Perisinusoidal cells

Perisinusoidal cells (of Ito; also called **hepatic stellate cells)** are found in the space of Disse in proximity to the hepatic sinusoids (see Figure 17-13).

These cells are of mesenchymal origin, contain fat, and are involved in:

1. The storage and release of retinoids.

2. The production and turnover of extracellular matrix.

3. The regulation of blood flow in the sinusoids.

Figure 17-19. **Bile canaliculus and the polarity of the hepatocyte**

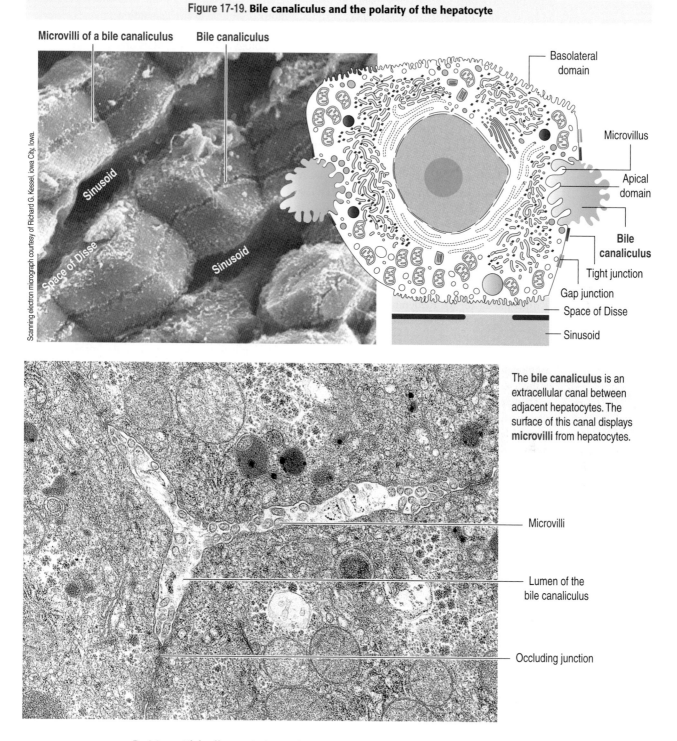

Microvilli of a bile canaliculus

Bile canaliculus

Sinusoid

Space of Disse

Sinusoid

Scanning electron micrograph courtesy of Richard G. Kessel, Iowa City, Iowa.

Basolateral domain

Microvillus

Apical domain

Bile canaliculus

Tight junction

Gap junction

Space of Disse

Sinusoid

The **bile canaliculus** is an extracellular canal between adjacent hepatocytes. The surface of this canal displays **microvilli** from hepatocytes.

Microvilli

Lumen of the bile canaliculus

Occluding junction

Perisinusoidal cells remain in a quiescent, nonproliferative state, but can proliferate when activated by Kupffer cells and hepatocytes. Activation occurs after partial hepatectomy (see Box 17-B), focal hepatic lesions, and in different conditions that lead to fibrosis (Figure 17-18).

In pathologic conditions, perisinusoidal cells change into **myofibroblasts** and contribute to fibrogenesis during chronic liver disease by producing type I and type II collagens and extracellular matrix proteins. Fibrogenesis compromises regeneration.

Once activated, myofibroblasts secrete **transforming growth factor-β (TGF-β) to** stimulate, by an autocrine mechanism, their own activity and promote type 2 **epithelial-mesenchymal transition (EMT)** of hepatocytes.

EMT comprises the switch of epithelial cell characteristics into a fibroblast-like or mesenchymal phenotype. It involves the suppression E-cadherin gene expression to disrupt cell-cell adhesion and the activation of Wnt/β-catenin cell signaling pathways and others, that are not active in normal hepatocytes.

In Chapter 3, Cell Signaling, we point to three types of EMT:

1. Type 1 EMT occurs during embryonic development.

2. Type 2 EMT takes place during the repair of tissue injury and inflammation. Liver fibrogenesis is an example of type 2 EMT. It requires fibroblasts and mesenchymal cells to repair acute and chronic hepatitis.

3. Type 3 EMT occurs in cancer and metastasis. A possible progression of cirrhosis into hepatocellular cancer occurs when **hepatitis Bx (HBx) antigen**, a regulatory protein of the hepatitis B virus, stimulates **cancer stem cells** into hepatocellular cancer pathogenesis.

Cancer stem cells express **stemness-associated genes**, such as *Nanog, Oct4, Myc, Sox2* and *Klf4* (Krüpel-like factor 4). Remember that stemness is the characteristic gene expression pattern of different stem cells not observed in ordinary, non-stem cells.

The deposit of collagen and extracellular matrix components increases, leading to a progressive fibrosis of the liver, a typical feature of **cirrhosis**.

An increased deposit of collagen fibers and extracellular matrix within the space of Disse is followed by a **loss of fenestrations and gaps of sinusoidal endothelial cells**. As the fibrotic process advances, myofibroblasts constrict the lumen of the sinusoids and increase vascular resistance. **An increase in resistance to the flow of portal venous blood in the hepatic sinusoids leads to portal hypertension in cirrhosis.**

In summary, hepatocytes have regenerative capability in response to damage and macrophages secrete matrix metalloproteases that breakdown scar tissue and enhance hepatocyte proliferation. However, the liver extracellular matrix controls the epithelial regenerative responses. In chronic liver injury, progressive fibrosis inhibits liver regeneration.

Pathology: Chronic hepatitis and cirrhosis

Hepatitis is an inflammatory condition of the liver determined predominantly by viruses but also by bacteria (of intestinal origin or hematogenous) and parasites (amebiasis and schistosomiasis).

Viral hepatitis can be caused by **hepatotropic viruses,** in particular **hepatitis virus A (HAV), B (HBV) and C (HCV),** the most common. Each type of virus belongs to different groups.

HAV causes acute hepatitis that rarely becomes chronic. HAV infections are caused by spread through the ingestion of contaminated food or water.

HBV infection can be determined by sexual contact and the transfer of blood or serum through shared needles in drug abusers. About 10% of the infected individuals develop chronic hepatitis.

HCV is caused in about 90% of the cases by blood transfusion and about 50-70% of the affected individuals develop chronic hepatitis. Therapy of HCV infection is based in the oral administration of combined **direct-acting antiviral agents**.

Other types of viral hepatitis includes virus types D, E, and G. Immunity determined by one type of virus does not protect against infection caused by other viruses.

Patients with chronic forms of viral hepatitis, lasting more than 6 months, can transmit the infection to others with blood or body fluids, and evolve over time to cirrhosis or lead to the development of hepatocellular cancer (liver cancer).

Typical clinical manifestations of **acute hepatitis** are loss of appetite, nausea, vomiting, and jaundice. Biochemical abnormalities include:

1. An elevation in serum of **liver aminotransferases (aspartate aminotransferase,** AST, and **alanine aminotrasferase,** ALT), resulting from the enzyme leakage of injured hepatocytes into blood.

2. **Viral antibodies** detected in blood within weeks of infection.

The histopathologic features of **acute hepatitis** are hepatocyte injury (necrosis) and apoptosis and accumulation of bile within hepatocytes. Inflammatory cells, including neutrophils, lymphocytes and macrophages, are seen in the sinusoids around the central venule (zone III of the liver acinus) and portal spaces.

Chronic hepatitis is defined by the presence of fibrosis, together with hepatocyte necrosis and inflammatory lymphocytic activity (see Figure 17-18).

Disruption of the limiting plate (zone I of liver acinus), progression of fibrosis into the portal spaces, nodular regeneration of hepatocytes and proliferation of bile ductules (cholangiolar proliferation) are indications of a progression to cirrhosis (see Figure 17-18).

Box 17-B | Liver regeneration

- The liver has an excellent regenerative potential following acute necrosis determined by viral infections or toxins. However, it undergoes fibrosis after chronic injury.
- After extensive hepatectomy (about 70%), human hepatocytes leave their quiescent state and initiate the cell cycle sequence to regenerate the original liver mass within a 6-8 week period.
- The **early phases** of the regenerative process involve **perisinusoidal cells, macrophages,** and **endothelial cells** lining the hepatic sinusoids. Endothelial cells synthesize **vascular endothelial growth factor receptor 2 (VEGFR2),** the initial step of a molecular program leading to the production of **hepatocyte growth factor (HGF)** to stimulate hepatocyte proliferation.
- During **prolonged liver injury** (such as chronic viral hepatitis or excessive alcohol intake), **perisinusoidal cells change into myofibroblasts** and contribute to **fibrogenesis** by depositing extracellular matrix. Fibrogenesis disrupts the regenerative potential of hepatocytes and biliary epithelial cells to the point that liver regeneration is compromised. The vascular structures become abnormal, collagen bundles surround hepatocytes, and cirrhosis develops.

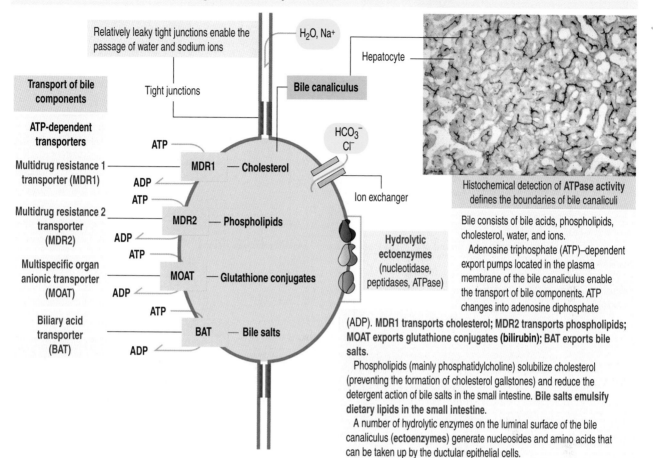

Figure 17-20. Transport of bile into the bile canaliculus

Relatively leaky tight junctions enable the passage of water and sodium ions

H_2O, Na^+

Hepatocyte

Tight junctions

Bile canaliculus

Transport of bile components

HCO_3^-
Cl^-

ATP-dependent transporters

ATP

Multidrug resistance 1 transporter (MDR1)

MDR1 — Cholesterol

ADP

Ion exchanger

ATP

Multidrug resistance 2 transporter (MDR2)

MDR2 — Phospholipids

ADP

Hydrolytic ectoenzymes (nucleotidase, peptidases, ATPase)

ATP

Multispecific organ anionic transporter (MOAT)

MOAT — Glutathione conjugates

ADP

ATP

Biliary acid transporter (BAT)

BAT — Bile salts

ADP

Histochemical detection of **ATPase activity** defines the boundaries of bile canaliculi

Bile consists of bile acids, phospholipids, cholesterol, water, and ions.

Adenosine triphosphate (ATP)–dependent export pumps located in the plasma membrane of the bile canaliculus enable the transport of bile components. ATP changes into adenosine diphosphate (ADP). MDR1 transports cholesterol; MDR2 transports phospholipids; MOAT exports glutathione conjugates (**bilirubin**); BAT exports bile salts.

Phospholipids (mainly phosphatidylcholine) solubilize cholesterol (preventing the formation of cholesterol gallstones) and reduce the detergent action of bile salts in the small intestine. **Bile salts emulsify dietary lipids in the small intestine.**

A number of hydrolytic enzymes on the luminal surface of the bile canaliculus (**ectoenzymes**) generate nucleosides and amino acids that can be taken up by the ductular epithelial cells.

Preparation courtesy of Tibor Barka, New York.

Bile: Mechanism of secretion

Bile is a complex mixture of organic and inorganic substances produced by the hepatocyte, transported by the bile canaliculus, an extracellular canal between adjacent hepatocytes. The bile canaliculus defines the **apical domain** of the hepatocyte. The **basolateral domain** faces the sinusoidal space. **Tight junctions** between adjacent hepatocytes seal the biliary canalicular compartment (Figure 17-19).

The primary organic components of bile are conjugated bile acids (called bile salts), glycine, and taurine *N*-acylamidated derivatives of bile acids derived from cholesterol.

Bile has five major functions:

1. The excretion of **cholesterol, phospholipids, bile salts, conjugated bilirubin**, and **electrolytes**.

2. Contributes to **fat absorption in the intestinal lumen** (see Chapter 16, Lower Digestive Segment).

3. Transports polymeric **IgA** to the intestinal mucosa by the enterohepatic circulation.

4. The excretion of metabolic products of drugs and heavy metals processed in the hepatocyte.

5. Conjugated bile acids inhibit the growth of bacteria in the small intestine.

The transport of bile and other organic substances from the hepatocyte to the lumen of the bile canaliculus is an adenosine triphosphate (ATP)–mediated process. Four ATP-dependent transporters, present in the canalicular plasma membrane, participate in transport mechanisms of the bile (Figure 17-20).

1. **Multidrug resistance 1** transporter (**MDR1**), which mobilizes cholesterol across the plasma membrane.

2. **Multidrug resistance 2** transporter (**MDR2**), which transports phospholipids.

3. **Multispecific organ anionic transporter** (**MOAT**), which exports bilirubin glucuronide and glutathione conjugates.

4. **Biliary acid transporter** (**BAT**), which transports bile salts.

These ATP transporters belong to the family of **ABC transporters** characterized by highly conserved ATP-binding domains, or ATP binding cassettes. The first ABC transporter was discovered as the product of the gene *mdr* (for multiple drug resistance). The *mdr* gene is highly expressed in cancer cells and the encoded product, MDR transporter, pumps drugs out of cells, making cancer cells resistant to cancer treatment with chemotherapeutic agents.

The secretion of bile acids generates the osmotic

Figure 17-21. **Metabolism of bilirubin**

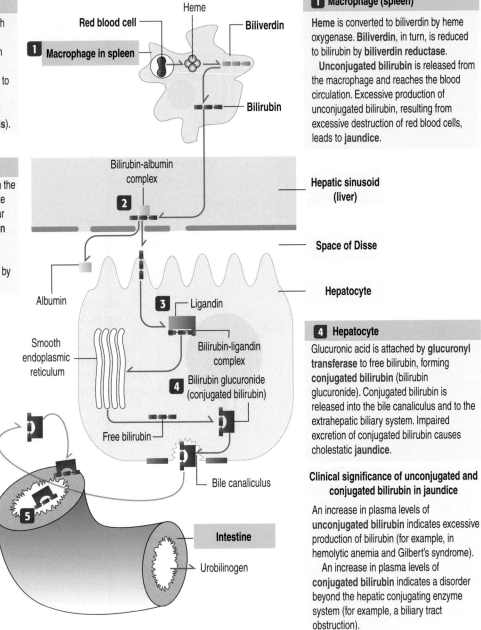

2 Blood

In blood, bilirubin forms a complex with albumin. The **bilirubin-albumin complex** is too large to be excreted in urine. This form of bilirubin is water-soluble and can enter the brain to cause severe neurologic disorders (**kernicterus**) in hemolytic disease of the newborn (**erythroblastosis fetalis**).

1 Macrophage (spleen)

Heme is converted to biliverdin by heme oxygenase. **Biliverdin**, in turn, is reduced to bilirubin by **biliverdin reductase**.

Unconjugated bilirubin is released from the macrophage and reaches the blood circulation. Excessive production of unconjugated bilirubin, resulting from excessive destruction of red blood cells, leads to **jaundice**.

3 Hepatocyte

Lipid-soluble bilirubin, detached from the albumin carrier, enters the hepatocyte and binds to **ligandin**, an intracellular carrier protein. The **bilirubin-ligandin complex** reaches the smooth endoplasmic reticulum and **free bilirubin** is released into the cytosol by enzymatic action.

4 Hepatocyte

Glucuronic acid is attached by **glucuronyl transferase** to free bilirubin, forming **conjugated bilirubin** (bilirubin glucuronide). Conjugated bilirubin is released into the bile canaliculus and to the extrahepatic biliary system. Impaired excretion of conjugated bilirubin causes cholestatic **jaundice**.

Clinical significance of unconjugated and conjugated bilirubin in jaundice

An increase in plasma levels of **unconjugated bilirubin** indicates excessive production of bilirubin (for example, in hemolytic anemia and Gilbert's syndrome).

An increase in plasma levels of **conjugated bilirubin** indicates a disorder beyond the hepatic conjugating enzyme system (for example, a biliary tract obstruction).

5 Intestine

In the intestine, glucuronides are split and bacteria convert bilirubin into **urobilinogens**, which are then excreted in the urine (as **urobilin**), eliminated with feces, or returned to the liver. About 20% of the urobilinogens are reabsorbed in the ileum and colon.

---

gradient necessary for osmotic water flow into the bile canaliculus. In addition, an **ion exchanger** enables the passage of HCO_3^- and Cl^- ions. Finally, hydrolytic enzymes associated with the plasma membrane (**ectoenzymes**) of the bile canaliculus and bile duct produce nucleoside and amino acid breakdown products, which are reabsorbed by ductular epithelial cells.

A genetic defect in MDR2 causes focal hepatocyte necrosis, proliferation of bile ductules, and an inflammatory reaction in the portal space. Very low levels of phospholipids are detected in the bile of MDR2 mutants.

Metabolism of bilirubin

Bilirubin is the end product of heme catabolism and about 85% originates from senescent red blood cells destroyed mainly in the spleen by macrophages (Figure 17-21).

Bilirubin is released into the circulation, where it is bound to albumin and transported to the liver. **Unlike albumin-bound bilirubin, free bilirubin is toxic to the brain.** Recall from our discussion of **erythroblastosis fetalis** (see Chapter 6, Blood and Hematopoiesis) that an antibody-induced hemolytic disease in the newborn is caused by blood group incompatibility between the mother and fetus. The hemolytic process results in hyperbilirubinemia caused by elevated amounts of **free bilirubin**, which causes irreversible damage to the central nervous system (**kernicterus**).

When albumin-conjugated bilirubin reaches the hepatic sinusoids, the **albumin-bilirubin complex** dissociates, and bilirubin is transported across the plasma membrane of hepatocytes after binding to a plasma membrane receptor. Inside the hepatocyte, bilirubin binds to **ligandin**, a protein that prevents bilirubin reflux into the circulation. The **bilirubin-ligandin complex** is transported to the smooth endoplasmic reticulum, where **bilirubin is conjugated to glucuronic acid** by the uridine diphosphate (UDP)–glucuronyl transferase system. This reaction results in the formation of a **water-soluble bilirubin diglucuronide**, which diffuses through the cytosol into the bile canaliculus, where it is secreted into the bile.

In the small intestine, conjugated bilirubin in bile remains intact until it reaches the distal portion of the small intestine and colon, where **free bilirubin is generated by the intestinal bacterial flora**.

Unconjugated bilirubin is then reduced to **urobilinogen**. Most urobilinogen is excreted in the feces. A small portion returns to the liver following absorption by a process known as **enterohepatic bile circulation**. Another small fraction is excreted in the urine.

Composition of the bile

The human liver produces about 600 mL of bile per day. The bile consists of **organic components** (such as **bile acids**, the major component; **phospholipids**, mainly lecithins; **cholesterol**; and **bile pigments, bilirubin**) and **inorganic components** (predominantly Na^+ and Cl^- **ions**).

Bile acids (cholic acid, chenodeoxycholic acid, deoxycholic acid, and lithocholic acid) are synthesized by the hepatocytes. Cholic and chenodeoxycholic acids are synthesized from cholesterol as a precursor and are called **primary bile acids**. Deoxycholic and lithocholic acids are called **secondary bile acids** because they are produced in the intestinal lumen by the action of intestinal bacteria on the primary bile acids.

The synthetic bile acid pathway is the major mechanism of elimination of cholesterol from the body. **Micelles** are formed by the aggregation of bile acid molecules conjugated to taurine or glycine. Cholesterol is located inside the micelles. Bile pigments are not components of the micelles.

Bile secreted by the liver is stored in the gallbladder and released into the duodenum during a meal to facilitate the breakdown and absorption of fats (see Figure 16-9 in Chapter 16, Lower Digestive Segment). About 90% of both primary and secondary bile acids is absorbed from the intestinal lumen by

enterocytes and transported back to the liver through the portal vein. This process is known as the **enterohepatic circulation**.

The absorption of bile acids by the enterocyte is mediated at the apical plasma membrane by an Na^+-dependent transporter protein and released through the basolateral plasma membrane by an Na^+-independent anion exchanger.

Bilirubin is not absorbed in the intestine. Bilirubin is reduced to **urobilinogen** by bacteria in the distal small intestine and colon (see Figure 17-21). Urobilinogen is partially secreted in the feces, part returns to the liver through the portal vein, and some is excreted in urine as **urobilin**, the oxidized form of urobilinogen.

Bile acids establish an osmotic gradient that mobilizes water and electrolytes into the bile canaliculus. HCO_3^- ions, secreted by epithelial cells lining the bile ducts, are added to the bile, which becomes alkaline as Na^+ and Cl^- ions and water are absorbed. **Secretin** increases the active transport of HCO_3^- into the bile.

The flow of bile into the duodenum depends on:

1. The secretory pressure generated by the actively bile-secreting hepatocytes.

2. The flow resistance in the bile duct and **sphincter of Oddi**.

The sphincter of Oddi is a thickening of the circular muscle layer of the bile duct at the duodenal junction. During fasting, the sphincter of Oddi is closed and bile flows into the gallbladder. The gallbladder's ability to concentrate bile 5 to 20 times compensates for the limited storage capacity of the gallbladder (20 to 50 mL of fluid) and the continuous production of bile by the liver.

Bile secretion during meal digestion is initiated by the **cholecystokinin**-induced contraction of the muscularis of the gallbladder in response to lipids in the intestinal lumen, assisted by the muscular activities of the common bile duct, the sphincter of Oddi, and the duodenum.

Cholecystokinin stimulates the relaxation of the sphincter of Oddi, enabling bile to enter the duodenum. Note that **cholecystokinin has opposite effects**: it stimulates **muscle contraction** of the **gallbladder** and induces **muscle relaxation** of the **sphincter of Oddi**.

Pathology: Conditions affecting bile secretion

Because bile secretion involves the hepatocytes, bile ducts, gallbladder, and intestine, any perturbation along this pathway can result in a pathologic condition. For example, destruction of hepatocytes by viral infection (**viral hepatitis**) and toxins can lead to a decrease in bile production as well as an increase in bilirubin in blood (**jaundice**).

Obstruction of the passages by **gallstones, biliary**

Figure 17-22. **The gallbladder**

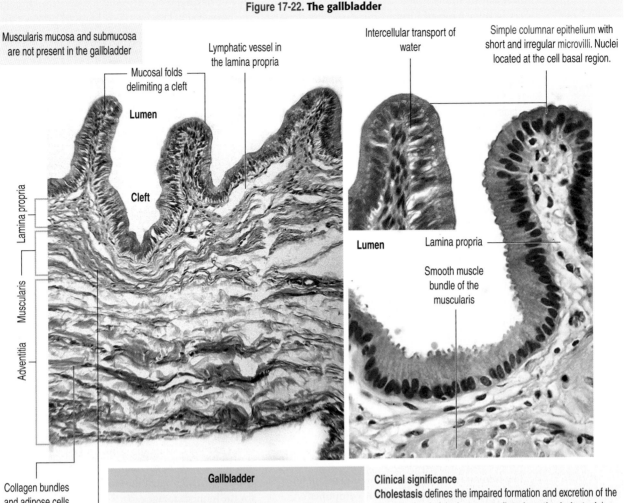

Muscularis mucosa and submucosa are not present in the gallbladder

Mucosal folds delimiting a cleft

Lumen

Lymphatic vessel in the lamina propria

Cleft

Lamina propria

Muscularis

Adventitia

Collagen bundles and adipose cells

Smooth muscle fibers

Intercellular transport of water

Simple columnar epithelium with short and irregular microvilli. Nuclei located at the cell basal region.

Lumen

Lamina propria

Smooth muscle bundle of the muscularis

Gallbladder

The major functions of the gallbladder are:
1. Concentration (up to 10-fold) and storage of bile between meals.
2. Release of bile by contraction of the muscularis in response to **cholecystokinin** stimulation (produced by enteroendocrine cells in the duodenum) and **neural stimuli**, together with **relaxation of the sphincter of Oddi** (a muscular ring surrounding the opening of the bile duct in the wall of the duodenum).
3. Regulation of hydrostatic pressure within the biliary tract.

Clinical significance
Cholestasis defines the impaired formation and excretion of the bile at the level of the hepatocyte (**intrahepatic cholestasis**) or a structural (tumor of the pancreas or biliary tract, cholangiocarcinoma) or mechanical (**cholelithiasis**, produced by gallstones) perturbation in the excretion of bile (**extrahepatic cholestasis**).

Clinically, cholestasis is detected by (1) the presence in blood of **bilirubin** and bile acids, secreted into bile under normal conditions; (2) elevation in serum of **alkaline phosphatase** (an enzyme associated with the plasma membrane of the bile canaliculus); and (3) **radiologic examination** (many gallstones are radiopaque and can be detected on a plain radiograph).

tract diseases (such as **primary sclerosing cholangitis**), or **tumors** (for example, **cholangiocarcinoma**) can block the flow of bile, with bile reflux to the liver and then to the systemic circulation.

Clinical significance: Hyperbilirubinemia
Several diseases occur when one or more of the metabolic steps of bilirubin formation are disrupted. A characteristic feature is **hyperbilirubinemia**, an increase in the concentration of bilirubin in the blood (more than 0.1 mg/mL).

Gilbert's syndrome is the most common inborn error of metabolism causing moderate hyperbilirubinemia. Elevated levels of unconjugated bilirubin,

with no serious health consequences, are detected in the bloodstream. The cause is the reduced activity of the enzyme **glucuronyl transferase**, which conjugates bilirubin (see Figure 17-21).

An inherited defect in the **UDP–glucuronyl transferase system**, known as **Crigler-Najjar disease**, results in failure to conjugate bilirubin in hepatocytes and the absence of conjugated bilirubin diglucuronide in bile. Infants with this disease develop **bilirubin encephalopathy**.

The **Dubin-Johnson syndrome** is a familial disease caused by a **defect in the transport of conjugated bilirubin to the bile canaliculus**. In addition to the transport of conjugated bilirubin, there is a general defect in the transport and excretion of organic anions in these patients.

Gallbladder

The main functions of the gallbladder are **storage**, **concentration**, and **release of bile**. Dilute bile from the hepatic ducts is transported through the cystic duct into the gallbladder. After concentration, bile is discharged into the common bile duct.

The wall of the gallbladder consists of a **mucosa**, a **muscularis**, and an **adventitia** (Figure 17-22). The portion of the gallbladder that does not face the liver is covered by the peritoneum.

The mucosa displays multiple **folds** lined by a **simple columnar epithelium** and is supported by a lamina propria that contains a **vascular lymphatic plexus**. The mucosa creates with time deep clefts known as **Rokitansky-Aschoff sinuses**. In the **neck region** of the gallbladder, the lamina propria contains **tubuloacinar glands**.

There is no muscularis mucosa and submucosa in the gallbladder. The **muscularis** is represented by smooth muscle bundles associated with collagen and elastic fibers.

Essential concepts | **Digestive Glands**

• The three major digestive glands are:
(1) The salivary glands: the parotid, submandibular, and sublingual glands.
(2) The exocrine pancreas.
(3) The liver.

• Salivary glands consist of branched ducts and secretory portions, acini, producing a mucous, serous, or mucous-serous product. They are classified as branched (compound) tubuloalveolar glands.

Each acinus is drained sequentially by:
(1) An intercalated duct, lined by low squamous-to-cuboidal simple epithelium. An intercalated duct links an acinus to a striated duct.
(2) A striated duct, lined by a cuboidal-to-columnar simple epithelium with abundant basal mitochondria. The striated duct is well developed in the submandibular gland.
Intercalated and striated ducts are seen within a lobule. They are intralobular ducts.
Striated ducts converge toward interlobular ducts found between lobules in the interlobular septa. They are lined by a pseudostratified columnar epithelium.
Interlobular ducts merge with lobar ducts located in interlobar septa. They are lined by a stratified columnar epithelium.
Lobar ducts join the main duct, which displays a stratified squamous epithelium near its opening in the oral cavity.
Connective tissue septa provide support to the branching duct system. Blood vessels, lymphatics, and nerves are found in the septa along the ducts.

Saliva is the major product of salivary glands. Saliva contains protein, glycoproteins, ions, water, and immunoglobulin A. Submandibular glands produce 70% of the saliva; the parotid glands contribute 25%. Proteins in saliva form pellicles, a protective film on the teeth.
The main products in saliva are:
(1) Lysozyme, which attacks the walls of bacteria.
(2) Lactoferrin, which chelates iron necessary for bacterial growth.

(3) SIgA, which neutralizes bacteria and viruses.
The digestive function of saliva relies on:
(1) Amylase (ptyalin), which initiates the digestion of carbohydrates (starch) in the oral cavity.
(2) Lingual lipase, which participates in the hydrolysis of dietary lipids.

The **parotid gland** consists of serous acini surrounded by myoepithelial cells. The parotid gland has the longest intercalated ducts.
The **submandibular gland** contains mixed seromucous and serous acini, also surrounded by myoepithelial cells. Serous cells form demilunes capping the mucous cells of the serous-mucous acinus. Secretion of the serous cells is transported to the acinar lumen along intercellular secretory canaliculi.
The **sublingual gland** has predominant mucous acini; a few seromucous acini can be found. Myoepithelial cells are present. The intercalated and striated ducts are poorly developed.

• The two most frequent benign tumors of the parotid gland are:
(1) The slow-growing salivary gland **mixed tumor** (pleomorphic adenoma). This tumor consists of myxochondroid zones with ductal epithelial and mesenchyme-like myoepithelial cells. Its surgical removal is complicated by the need to protect the facial nerve running through the parotid gland. Enucleation of mixed tumors results in a multifocal high recurrence rate.
(2) **Warthin tumor** (papilloma cystoadenoma lymphomatosum). This tumor occurs in the parotid gland with a high risk incidence in smokers. The tumor stroma consist of a papillary arrangement of lymphoid tissue centers surrounded by squamous, mucous, and sebaceous epithelial cells. This tumor may develop from intraparotid or periparotid lymph nodes.

• **Exocrine pancreas.** The pancreas is a combined exocrine branched tubuloacinar gland and endocrine gland (islet of Langerhans).

The pancreas is surrounded by a connective tissue but does not have a capsule proper. Lobules are separated by connective tissue partitions.
The pancreatic acinus contains serous-secreting cells and centroacinar cells, unique to the pancreas. Intercalated ducts, lined by a low cuboidal epithelium, drain the acinus.
Neither striated ducts nor myoepithelial cells are present in the exocrine pancreas.
Intercalated ducts converge to form interlobular ducts lined by a simple columnar epithelium.
Secretin and cholecystokinin regulate the function of the pancreatic acinus and intercalated duct. Cholecystokinin and acetylcholine trigger the release of inactive forms of trypsin, chymotrypsin, and carboxylpeptidases produced by the pancreatic acinar cells. Lipase, amylase, cholesterol esterase, and phospholipase are also secreted. Secretin stimulates the secretion of water, sodium, and bicarbonate ions by centroacinar cells and epithelial cells of the intercalated duct.

Acute pancreatitis is the result of pancreatic tissue autodigestion by the premature activation of pancreatic enzymes, in particular trypsin.
This condition usually follows trauma, heavy meals or excessive alcohol ingestion or biliary tract disease. The clinical features of acute pancreatitis are severe abdominal pain, nausea, and vomiting.
A rapid elevation of amylase and lipase in serum (within 24 to 72 hours) are typical diagnostic features. Acute pancreatitis can give rise to complications, such as abscess formation and cysts.

Chronic pancreatitis is characterized by fibrosis and partial or total destruction of the pancreatic tissue. Alcoholism is the major cause of chronic pancreatitis, leading to a permanent loss of pancreatic endocrine and exocrine functions.

Cystic fibrosis is an inherited disease affecting mucus-secreting tissues of the respiratory,

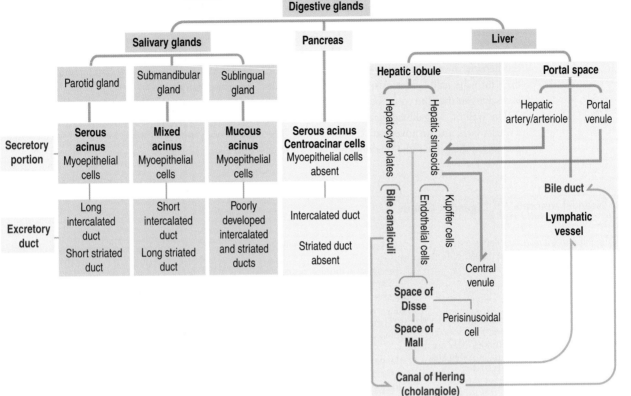

digestive, reproductive, and integumentary systems. Chronic pancreatitis in cystic fibrosis is characterized by a loss of acini, dilation of the pancreatic excretory ducts, and extensive fibrosis (increase in connective tissue). A genetic defect in the cystic fibrosis transmembrane conductance regulator (CFTR) protein prevents the transport of chloride ions. Mucus becomes thick and prone to bacterial infections.

• **Carcinoma of the pancreas**. The pancreatic duct–bile duct anatomic relationship is of clinical significance in carcinoma of the pancreas localized in the head region, because compression of the bile duct causes obstructive jaundice.

Ductal adenocarcinoma is the most common primary malignant tumor of the pancreas. Tumoral masses obstruct and dilate the distal common bile and pancreatic ducts. Hyperplasia and carcinoma in situ of the duct epithelial lining are the precursor changes of the infiltrating ductal adenocarcinoma.

Activation of the oncogene K-*ras* and inactivation of tumor suppressor genes, including *p53*, are molecular characteristics of the tumor.

The close association of the pancreas with large blood vessels, the extensive and diffuse abdominal drainage to lymph nodes, and the frequent spread of carcinoma cells to the liver via the portal vein are factors contributing to the ineffectiveness of surgical removal of pancreatic tumors.

Cystic tumors of the pancreas. This category includes serous cystoadenomas (with cysts containing a clear fluid) and mucinous cystoadenomas (with cysts filled with a mucoid product). Untreated mucinous cystoadenomas evolve into an infiltrating tumor (mucinous cystoadenocarcinoma).

Endocrine tumors of the pancreas can be detected as isolated pancreatic masses or a component of the multiple endocrine neoplasia syndrome, type 1 (MEN1). MEN1 is an autosomal dominant hereditary endocrine cancer syndrome characterized primarily by tumors of the parathyroid glands, gastroenteroendocrine cells, and adenohypophysis.

This tumor type does not show activation of the K-ras gene or p53 gene inactivation. Mutations in the *MEN1* (producing the tumor suppressor menin), *RET* (Ret protoncogene producing receptor tyrosine kinase), and *CDKN1B* (for cyclin-dependent kinase inhibitor 1B, encoding the tumor suppressor p27) genes can cause MENs.

Gastrinomas, insulinomas, and glucagonomas are examples of endocrine tumors showing cytoplasmic secretory granules. This tumors belong to the category of syndromic functioning tumors (associated with a syndrome). For example, as we have already seen, gastrinomas produce the Zollinger-Ellison syndrome characterized by multiple peptic ulcers caused by gastrin continuous stimulation of HCl production by parietal cells in stomach.

• **Liver**. The liver consists of poorly defined lobes surrounded by a collagen–elastic fiber capsule (of Glisson).

Blood is supplied by two vessels:

(1) The portal vein supplies 75% to 80% of the afferent deoxygenated blood volume from the digestive tract, spleen, and pancreas.

(2) The hepatic artery supplies 20% to 25% of oxygenated blood.

Blood from the portal vein and hepatic artery mixes in the hepatic sinusoid of the liver lobules. Sinusoidal blood converges to the central venule (or vein), and is drained sequentially by the sublobular vein, collecting vein, and hepatic vein into the inferior vena cava.

Bile, the exocrine product of the liver, is collected by the intrahepatic bile duct, and drained by the right and left hepatic ducts. Bile is stored in the gallbladder and released in the descending second part of the duodenum through the common bile duct.

The **hepatic lobule** is the structural and functional unit of the liver. The hepatic lobule consists of anastomosing plates of hepatocytes limiting blood sinusoidal spaces lined by endothelial cells and Kupffer cells. The space of Disse is interposed between the sinusoidal space and the hepatocytes. Perisinusoidal cells of Ito (the storage site of retinoids) are present in the space of Disse. A central venule (or vein) collects the sinusoidal blood.

Branches of the portal vein and hepatic artery, together with a bile duct, form the portal triad found in the connective tissue surrounding the hepatic lobule.

A **limiting plate** of hepatocytes is the boundary between the hepatocyte parenchyma and the connective tissue stroma.

Bile, produced by hepatocytes, flows in opposite direction to the blood. Bile is transported through bile canaliculi into the canal of Hering (or cholangiole), and then into the bile duct in the portal triad space.

• The liver lobule can be conceptualized as:
(1) The **classic hepatic lobule** (described above).
(2) The **portal lobule**, based on the bile drainage pathway; the portal triad is the center of the portal lobule.
(3) The **liver acinus**, based on the zone gradient distribution of deoxygenated–oxygenated blood along the sinusoidal spaces).

• The hepatocyte is the functional endocrine and exocrine cell of the liver. The hepatocyte has a **basolateral domain** with abundant microvilli extending into the space of Disse. Excess of fluid in the space of Disse, not absorbed by the hepatocytes, is drained into the lymphatic circulation through the space of Mall located adjacent to the limiting plate.

The basolateral domain participates in the absorption of blood-borne substances (for example, bilirubin, peptide and steroid hormones, vitamin B_{12}, and substances to be detoxified), and the secretion of plasma proteins (for example, albumin, fibrinogen, prothrombin, coagulation factors, and complement proteins).

The **apical domain** borders the bile canaliculus, a trenchlike depression lined by microvilli and sealed by tight junctions.

Hepatocytes contain smooth endoplasmic reticulum (SER) associated with glycogen inclusions. The functions of the SER include:
(1) Synthesis of cholesterol and bile salts.
(2) Glucuronide conjugation of bilirubin, steroids, and drugs.
(3) The breakdown of glycogen into glucose.
(4) The detoxification of lipid-soluble drugs (for example, phenobarbital).

The rough endoplasmic reticulum (RER) and Golgi apparatus participate in the synthesis and glycosylation of the secretory proteins indicated above. Peroxisomes are prominent in hepatocytes.

Severe liver diseases can result from the excessive storage of iron and copper.

Hereditary hemochromatosis is an example of a disease characterized by increased iron absorption and accumulation in lysosomal hepatocytes. Cirrhosis and cancer of the liver are complications of hemochromatosis.

Wilson's disease (hepatolenticular degeneration) is a hereditary disorder of copper metabolism in which excessive deposits of copper in liver and brain lysosomes produce chronic hepatitis and cirrhosis.

• Alcoholism and fatty liver. Hepatocytes participate in the metabolism of ethanol. Long-term consumption of ethanol results in fatty liver, a reversible process if alcohol ingestion is discontinued. If alcohol consumption continues, hepatocyte injury can lead to cirrhosis (collagen proliferation of fibrosis of the liver) and hepatocellular carcinoma (malignant transformation of hepatocytes).

Ethanol can be metabolized by the alcohol dehydrogenase (ADH) pathway, and the microsomal ethanol-oxidizing system (MEOS).

In the ADH pathway, ethanol is oxidized to acetaldehyde in the cytoplasm and acetaldehyde is converted to acetate in mitochondria. Excess of acetaldehyde and protons can cause hepatocyte injury.

In the MEOS pathway, ethanol metabolized in the SER produces acetaldehyde and excess of oxygen radicals (instead of protons). Both produce hepatocyte injury.

• The perisinusoidal cell (of Ito) is found in the space of Disse, in the proximity of hepatic sinusoids.

These cells:
(1) Store and release retinoids.
(2) Produce and turn over extracellular matrix components.
(3) Regulate blood flow in the sinusoids.

Perisinusoidal cells remain in a quiescent, nonproliferative state, but can proliferate when activated by Kupffer cells and hepatocytes. Activation occurs after partial hepatectomy, focal hepatic lesions, and in different conditions that lead to fibrosis.

In pathologic conditions, perisinusoidal cells change into myofibroblasts and contribute to fibrogenesis during chronic liver disease by producing type I and type II collagens and extracellular matrix proteins.

Once activated, myofibroblasts secrete transforming growth factor-β (TGF-β) to stimulate, by an autocrine mechanism, their own activity and promote type 2 epithelial-mesenchymal transition (EMT) of hepatocytes.

Let us review the highlights of EMT:
(1) Type 1 EMT occurs during embryonic development.
(2) Type 2 EMT takes place during the repair of tissue injury and inflammation. Liver fibrogenesis is an example of type 2 EMT. It requires fibroblasts and mesenchymal cells to repair acute and chronic hepatitis.
(3) Type 3 EMT occurs in cancer and metastasis. A possible progression of cirrhosis into hepatocellular cancer occurs when hepatitis Bx (HBx) antigen, a regulatory protein of the hepatitis B virus, stimulates cancer stem cells into hepatocellular cancer pathogenesis.

• **Chronic hepatitis and cirrhosis**. Hepatitis is an inflammatory condition of the liver determined predominantly by viruses but also by bacteria (of intestinal origin or hema-togenous) and parasites (amebiasis and schistosomiasis).

Viral hepatitis can be caused by hepatotropic viruses, in particular hepatitis virus A (HAV), B (HBV), and C (HCV), the most common.

(1) HAV causes acute hepatitis that rarely becomes chronic. HAV infections are caused by spread through the ingestion of contaminated food or water.

(2) HBV infection can be determined by sexual contact and the transfer of blood or serum through shared needles in drug abusers. About 10% of the infected individuals develop chronic hepatitis.

(3) HCV is caused in about 90% of the cases by blood transfusion and about 50-70% of the affected individuals develop chronic hepatitis. Therapy of HCV infection is based in the oral administration of combined direct-acting antiviral agents.

Other types of viral hepatitis includes virus types D, E, and G. Immunity determined by one type of virus does not protect against infection caused by other viruses.

Typical clinical manifestations of acute hepatitis are loss of appetite, nausea, vomiting, and jaundice.

Biochemical abnormalities include:
(1) An elevation in serum of liver aminotransferases (aspartate aminotransferase, AST, and alanine aminotrasferase, ALT), resulting from the enzyme leakage of injured hepatocytes into blood.
(2) Viral antibodies detected in blood within weeks of infection.

The histopathologic features of **acute hepatitis** are hepatocyte injury (necrosis) and apoptosis and accumulation of bile within hepatocytes. Inflammatory cells, including neutrophils, lymphocytes, and macrophages, are seen in the sinusoids around the central venule (zone III of the liver acinus) and portal spaces.

Chronic hepatitis is defined by the presence of fibrosis, together with hepatocyte necrosis and inflammatory lymphocytic activity. Disruption of the limiting plate (zone I of liver acinus), progression of fibrosis into the portal spaces, nodular regeneration of hepatocytes, and proliferation of bile ductules (cholangiolar proliferation) are indications of a possible progression to cirrhosis.

• Bile is a mixture of organic and inorganic substances produced by the hepatocyte. Bile participates in the excretion of cholesterol, phospholipids, bile salts, conjugated bilirubin, and electrolytes. Fat absorption in the intestinal lumen depends on the fat-emulsifying function of bile salts. Bile transports IgA to the intestinal mucosa (enterohepatic circulation), and inhibits bacterial growth in the small intestine.

The secretion of bile into the bile canaliculus is an adenosine triphosphate (ATP)-mediated process involving multidrug resistance 1 and 2 transporters (MDR1 and MDR2), multispecific organ anionic transporter (MOAT), and biliary acid transporter (BAT).

- Metabolism of bilirubin. Bilirubin is the end product of heme catabolism:

(1) About 85% of bilirubin originates from senescent red blood cells destroyed in the spleen by macrophages.

(2) Macrophages convert heme into biliverdin, which is transformed into unconjugated bilirubin released into the blood circulation.

(3) In the blood circulation, bilirubin forms a complex with albumin.

(4) When the bilirubin-albumin complex reaches the hepatic sinusoids, albumin detaches and bilirubin is internalized by the hepatocyte.

(5) Bilirubin binds to ligandin in the hepatocyte cytosol and is transported to the SER, which releases free bilirubin that becomes conjugated with glucuronic acid.

(6) Bilirubin glucuronide is released into the bile canaliculus and transported to the small intestine. Glucuronide separates from bilirubin in the small intestine and bilirubin is converted by intestinal bacteria into urobilinogen, which is excreted. Urobilin is eliminated by urine.

Hyperbilirubinemia, an increase in the concentration of bilirubin circulating in blood, can occur when bilirubin cannot be conjugated in the hepatocyte (**Crigler-Najjar disease**). Infants with this disease develop bilirubin encephalopathy.

A defect in the transport of conjugated bilirubin to the bile canaliculus is the cause of the **Dubin-Johnson syndrome**. **Gilbert's syndrome** is a common inborn error of metabolism causing moderate hyperbilirubinemia without significant clinical manifestations.

- The **gallbladder** is the storage, concentration, and release site of bile. The wall of the gallbladder consists of a mucosa with folds and deep clefts, lined by a simple columnar epithelium. There are no muscularis mucosa and submucosa. A muscularis (smooth muscle) and adventitia can be seen. Blood vessels predominate in the adventitia.

18. Neuroendocrine System

The neuroendocrine system combines functions of the nervous system and the endocrine system aimed at the regulation of several physiologic processes. A key component of the neuroendocrine system is the hypothalamus, a site where neurons, acting as neurosecretory cells, release their neuropeptides into blood vessels to reach the adjacent hypophysis so they can collectively communicate with their target organs and tissues and receive information through feedback loops. Furthermore, the hypothalamus regulates the activities of the parasympathetic and sympathetic nervous system, including cardiovascular responses and glucose metabolism. This chapter addresses the structure and function of the hypophysis and the pineal gland. Both are endocrine glands located behind the blood-brain barrier, but their secretory products are released outside the blood-brain barrier in a cyclic, rhythmic, or pulsatile manner.

Hypophysis

The hypophysis (Greek *hypo*, under; *physis*, growth), (also known as the **pituitary gland**), consists of two embryologically distinct tissues (Figure 18-1):

1. The **adenohypophysis**, the **glandular epithelial** portion.

2. The **neurohypophysis**, the **neural** portion.

The **adenohypophysis** is formed by three subdivisions or parts:

1. The **pars distalis**, or **anterior lobe**, is the main part of the gland.

2. The **pars tuberalis** envelops, like a partial or total collar, the infundibular stem or stalk, a neural component. Together they make up the pituitary stalk.

3. The **pars intermedia**, or intermediate lobe, is rudimentary in the adult. It is a thin wedge separating the pars distalis from the neurohypophysis.

The **neurohypophysis** is formed by two subdivisions:

1. The **pars nervosa**, or neural lobe.

2. The **infundibulum**. The infundibulum, in turn, consists of two components: the **infundibular process**

Figure 18-1. Regions of the hypophysis (pituitary gland)

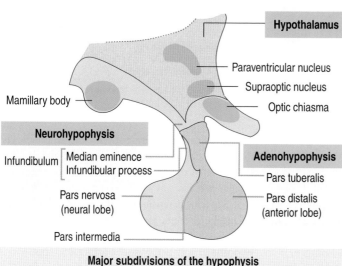

Hypothalamus
Paraventricular nucleus
Supraoptic nucleus
Optic chiasma
Mamillary body
Neurohypophysis
Infundibulum — Median eminence / Infundibular process
Adenohypophysis
Pars nervosa (neural lobe)
Pars tuberalis
Pars distalis (anterior lobe)
Pars intermedia

Major subdivisions of the hypophysis

The **adenohypophysis** is formed by three major subdivisions: (1) the **pars distalis**, or **anterior lobe**, the main glandular epithelial component; (2) the **pars tuberalis**, a collar-like nonsecretory tissue enveloping the infundibulum of the neurohypophysis; and (3) the **pars intermedia**, a narrow wedge forming a cap around the pars nervosa (neural lobe).

The **neurohypophysis** consists of two parts: the **pars nervosa**, or neural lobe, and the **infundibulum**. The infundibulum is formed by two structures: (1) the **median eminence**, a funnel-shaped extension of the hypothalamus; and (2) the **infundibular process**.

The **hypothalamus** is divided into two symmetric halves by the third ventricle. It is limited rostrally by the **optic chiasma**, caudally by the **mamillary bodies**, laterally by the **optic tracts**, and dorsolaterally by the **thalamus**.

The **pars intermedia**, a rudiment of the Ratke's pouch, consists of small colloid–containing folicles and scattered epithelial cells.

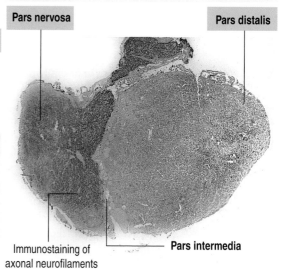

Pars nervosa
Pars distalis
Immunostaining of axonal neurofilaments
Pars intermedia

Immunohistochemistry panel from Martín-Lacave I, García-Caballero T: Atlas of Immunohistochemistry. Madrid, Spain. Ed. Díaz de Santos, 2012.

Figure 18-2. **Development of the hypophysis**

Infundibulum

Diencephalon

1

Infundibulum

Stomodeum

Notochord

2

3 Rathke's pouch elongates toward the infundibulum.

4

3

4 The infundibular process descends along the dorsal side of the elongating Rathke's pouch.

1 A diverticulum, called the **infundibulum**, develops in the floor of the diencephalon and grows toward the stomodeum.

2 Simultaneously, an ectodermal region in the roof of the stomodeum invaginates to form a diverticulum called **Rathke's pouch**.

Infundibulum recess

Posterior lobe

Anterior lobe

The inner layer of Rathke's pouch becomes the pars intermedia.

Two **signaling molecules** from the diencephalon control the development of Rathke's pouch: (1) **bone morphogenetic protein-4** induces formation of the pouch rudiment; (2) **fibroblast growth factor-8** activates the key regulator genes *Lhx3* and *Lhx4*, and subsequent development of the pouch rudiment into a definitive pouch. *Lhx3* belongs to the family of **Lim-type homeobox-containing genes**.

5 The regressing stalk of Rathke's pouch can leave residual tissue, which may become a tumor called a **craniopharyngioma**.

5

Developing sphenoid bone

Roof of the pharynx

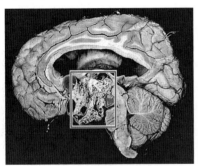

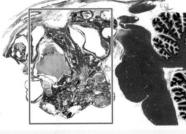

Craniopharyngiomas are epithelial tumors derived from remnants of the stalk of Rathke's pouch. They have some histologic similarities to odontogenic tumors.
There are two subtypes of craniopharyngiomas: (1) **Adamantinomatous craniopharyngioma**, common in children, and (2) **papillary craniopharyngioma**, frequent in adults.

Adamantinomatous craniopharyngioma in a 11-year old boy. It consists of cysts lined by squamous epithelial cells and necrotic areas.

Photographs from Burger PC, Scheithauer BW, Vogel FS: Surgical Pathology of the Nervous System and its Coverings, 4th ed. Philadelphia, Churchill Livingstone, 2002.

and the **median eminence**, a funnel-like extension of the hypothalamus.

Embryologic origin of the hypophysis

The anterior hypophysis and neurohypophysis have different embryologic origins (Figure 18-2). The anterior hypophysis derives from an evagination (**Rathke's pouch**) of the ectodermal lining of the future oral cavity extending upward toward the developing neurohypophysis.

The neurohypophysis develops from an **infundibular downgrowth from the floor of the diencephalon**. The connecting stem attached to Rathke's pouch disappears. However, the connecting stem of the neurohypophysis remains as the core of the infundibular stem, or stalk.

Rathke's pouch develops into three different regions:

1. Cells of the anterior surface of the pouch give rise to the pars distalis (the bulk of the gland).

2. Cells of the posterior surface invade the infundibular process.

3. Superior extensions of the pouch surround the infundibular stem, forming the pars tuberalis.

Hypothalamohypophyseal portal circulation

The hypothalamus and the hypophysis form an integrated neuroendocrine network known as the **hypothalamohypophyseal system**.

The hypothalamohypophyseal system consists of two components:

1. The **hypothalamic adenohypophyseal system**, connecting the hypothalamus to the anterior hypophysis.

2. The **hypothalamic neurohypophyseal system**, linking the hypothalamus to the posterior hypophysis.

Figure 18-3. Blood supply to the hypophysis

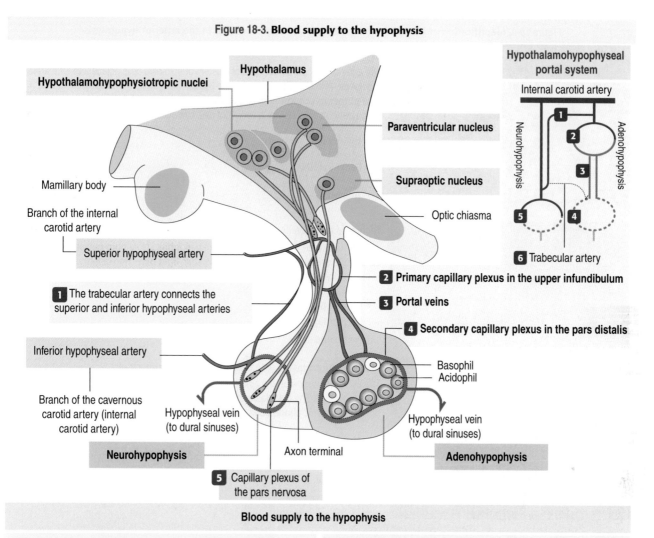

The **superior hypophyseal artery** forms a **primary capillary plexus** in the infundibulum (formed by the median eminence and infundibular stem). The primary capillary plexus receives releasing and inhibitory hormones from the neuroendocrine **hypothalamohypophysiotropic nuclei**.
The primary capillary plexus is drained by **portal veins**.

Portal veins supply blood to the **secondary capillary plexus**, with which basophils and acidophils are associated.

By this mechanism, hypothalamic releasing and inhibitory peptides act directly on cells of the pars distalis (anterior hypophysis) to regulate their endocrine function.

The primary and secondary capillary plexuses linked by the portal veins form the **hypothalamohypophyseal portal system**.

The **inferior hypophyseal artery** supplies the pars nervosa, forming a capillary plexus, which collects vasopressin (antidiuretic hormone) and oxytocin produced by neuroendocrine cells of the supraoptic and paraventricular nuclei, respectively.

The superior and inferior hypophyseal arteries are connected by the **trabecular artery**, whose capillaries bypass the portal circulation of the adenohypophysis (see **6**).

The **hypothalamus**, corresponding to the floor of the diencephalon and forming part of the walls of the third ventricle, consists of at least twelve clusters of neurons, called **nuclei**, some of which secrete hormones.

The neurosecretory cells of the hypothalamus exert **positive** and **negative** effects on the hypophysis through neuropeptides (called **releasing** and **inhibitory hormones** or **factors**), have a **very short response time** to neurotransmitters (fractions of a second), and send **axons** into the neurohypophysis. In contrast, the effects of hormones derived from the epithelial cells of the anterior hypophysis have a longer response time (minutes or hours) and can persist for as long as a day or even a month.

A pair of **superior hypophyseal arteries** (derived from the internal carotid arteries) (Figure 18-3) enter the median eminence and upper part of the infundibular stem and form the **first sinusoidal capillary plexus (primary capillary plexus)**, which receives the secretion of the neurosecretory cells grouped in the **hypothalamic hypophysiotropic nuclei** of the hypothalamus.

Capillaries arising from the primary capillary plexus project down the infundibulum and pars tuberalis to form the **portal veins**. Capillaries arising from the

Figure 18-4. Identification of basophil, acidophil, and chromophobe cells in the anterior hypophysis

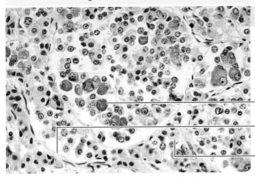

Hematoxylin-eosin staining (H&E)

The anterior hypophysis consists of clusters of epithelial cells adjacent to fenestrated capillaries. With hematoxylin and eosin (H&E), the cytoplasm of **basophils** stains **blue-purple (glycoproteins)** and **acidophils** stain **light pink (proteins)**. Chromophobe cells display a very light pink cytoplasm.

— **Basophil**

— **Fenestrated capillary**

— **Acidophil**

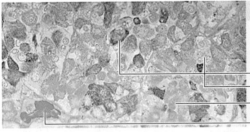

Trichrome stain (aniline blue, orange G, and azocarmine)

With the trichrome stain, the cytoplasm of **basophils** stains **blue-purple** and **acidophils orange. Chromophobe cells** stain **light blue**. Red blood cells in the lumen of the capillaries stain **deep orange**.

— **Basophil**
— **Chromophobe**
— **Acidophil**
— **Red blood cells**

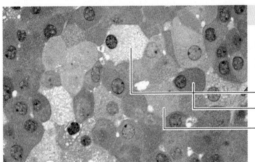

Plastic section stained with basic fuchsin and hematoxylin

The polygonal shape of the epithelial cells of the anterior hypophysis is well defined in this preparation. The cytoplasm of **basophils** stains **dark pink, acidophils** stain **light pink**, and **chromophobe cells** are **unstained**.

— **Chromophobe**

— **Basophil**

— **Acidophil**

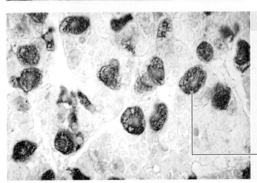

Immunohistochemistry (immunoperoxidase)

An antibody against the β chain of follicle-stimulating hormone (FSH) has been used to identify gonadotrophs within the anterior hypophysis in this illustration.

The use of specific antibodies against hormones produced in the anterior hypophysis has enabled (1) the precise identification of all hormone-producing cells of the anterior hypophysis; (2) the identification of hormone-producing **adenomas**; and (3) the elucidation of the negative and positive feedback pathways regulating the secretion of hypophyseal hormones.

— **FSH-secreting cell (classified as basophil by H&E staining)**

portal veins form a **secondary capillary plexus** that supplies the anterior hypophysis and receives secretions from endocrine cells of the anterior hypophysis. **There is no direct arterial blood supply to the anterior hypophysis.**

The hypothalamohypophyseal portal system enables:

1. The transport of hypothalamic releasing and inhibitory neuropeptides from the primary capillary plexus to the hormone-producing epithelial cells of the anterior hypophysis.

2. The secretion of hormones from the anterior hypophysis into the secondary capillary plexus and to the general circulation.

3. The functional integration of the hypothalamus with the anterior hypophysis, provided by the **portal veins**.

A **third capillary plexus**, derived from the inferior hypophyseal artery, supplies the neurohypophysis. This third capillary plexus collects secretions from neurosecretory cells present in the hypothalamus. The secretory products (vasopressin [antidiuretic hormone] and oxytocin) are transported along the axons into the neurohypophysis.

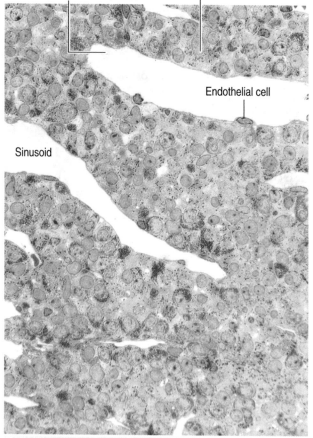

Cell with hormone-containing cytoplasmic granules

Sinusoid (fenestrated capillary)

Endothelial cell

Sinusoid

Light microscopy (plastic section)
Cells of the pars distalis are surrounded by sinusoids (fenestrated capillaries) that receive the secreted hormones. Hormones are then transported in the bloodstream to regulate the function of target cells.

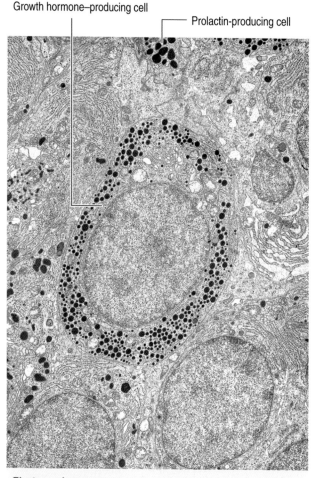

Growth hormone–producing cell

Prolactin-producing cell

Electron microscopy
Electron microscopy has provided a powerful tool for examining the **size**, **distribution**, **content**, and **mode of synthesis** and **secretion** of the various hormones stored in secretory granules in the cytoplasm of endocrine cells of the anterior hypophysis.

Histology of the pars distalis (anterior lobe)

The pars distalis is formed by three components:

1. Cords of **epithelial cells** (Figure 18-4).

2. Minimal supporting **connective tissue stroma**.

3. **Fenestrated capillaries** (or **sinusoids**) (Figure 18-5), which are parts of the secondary capillary plexus.

There is no blood-brain barrier in the anterior hypophysis.

The epithelial cells are arranged in cords surrounding fenestrated capillaries carrying blood from the hypothalamus. Secretory hormones diffuse into a network of capillaries, which drain into the hypophyseal veins and from there into the dural venous sinuses.

There are three distinct types of endocrine cell in the anterior hypophysis (see Figure 18-4):

1. **Acidophils** (cells that stain with an acidic dye), which are prevalent at the sides of the gland.

2. **Basophils** (cells that stain with a basic dye and are periodic acid–Schiff [PAS]-positive), which are predominant in the middle of the gland.

3. **Chromophobes** (cells lacking cytoplasmic staining).

Acidophils secrete two major **peptide hormones**: **growth hormone** and **prolactin**.

Basophils secrete **glycoprotein hormones**: the **gonadotropin follicle-stimulating hormone (FSH)**, **luteinizing hormone (LH)**, **thyroid-stimulating hormone (TSH)**, and **adrenocorticotropic hormone (ACTH)**, or corticotropin. Chromophobes include cells that have depleted their hormone content and lost the staining affinity typical of acidophils and basophils.

The precise identification of the endocrine cells of the anterior hypophysis is by **immunohistochemistry**, which demonstrates their hormone content using specific antibodies (see Figure 18-4).

Figure 18-6. **Growth hormone**

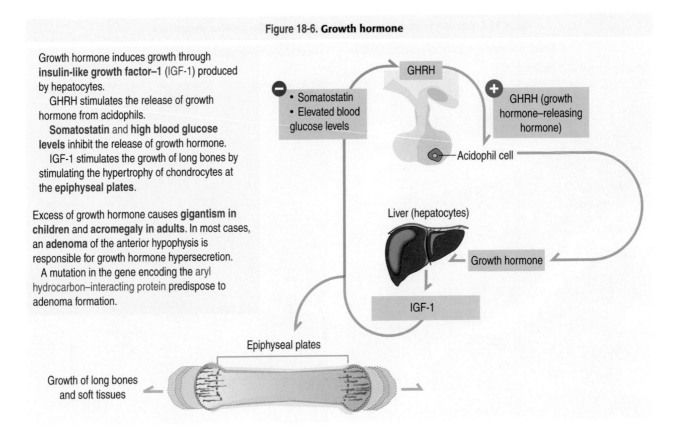

Growth hormone induces growth through **insulin-like growth factor–1** (IGF-1) produced by hepatocytes.

GHRH stimulates the release of growth hormone from acidophils.

Somatostatin and **high blood glucose levels** inhibit the release of growth hormone.

IGF-1 stimulates the growth of long bones by stimulating the hypertrophy of chondrocytes at the **epiphyseal plates**.

Excess of growth hormone causes **gigantism in children** and **acromegaly in adults**. In most cases, an **adenoma** of the anterior hypophysis is responsible for growth hormone hypersecretion.

A mutation in the gene encoding the aryl hydrocarbon–interacting protein predispose to adenoma formation.

Hormones secreted by acidophils: Growth hormone and prolactin

Acidophils secrete **growth hormone**, also called **somatotropin**. These acidophilic cells, called **somatotrophs**, represent a large proportion (40% to 50%) of the cell population of the anterior hypophysis. Prolactin-secreting cells, or **lactotrophs**, represent 15% to 20% of the cell population of the anterior hypophysis.

Growth hormone

Growth hormone is a peptide of 191 amino acids in length (22 kd). It has the following characteristics (Figure 18-6):

1. Growth hormone has structural homology similar to prolactin and human placental lactogen. There is some overlap in the activity of these three hormones.

2. It is released into the blood circulation in the form of **pulses** throughout a 24-hour sleep-wake period, with **peak secretion occurring during the first two hours of sleep**.

3. Despite its name, growth hormone does not directly induce growth; rather, it acts by stimulating in hepatocytes the production of **insulin-like growth factor-1** (IGF-1), also known as **somatomedin C**. The cell receptor for IGF-1 is similar to that for insulin (formed by dimers of two glycoproteins with integral cytoplasmic protein tyrosine kinase domains).

4. The release of growth hormone is regulated by two neuropeptides.

A **stimulatory** effect is determined by **growth hormone–releasing hormone** (GHRH), a peptide of 44 amino acids. An **inhibitory** effect is produced by **somatostatin** (a peptide of 14 amino acids) and by **elevated blood glucose levels**. Both GHRH and somatostatin derive from the hypothalamus. Somatostatin is also produced in the islet of Langerhans (pancreas).

IGF-1 (7.5 kd) stimulates the overall growth of bone and soft tissues. In children, IGF-1 stimulates the growth of long bones at the epiphyseal plates. Clinicians measure IGF-1 in blood to determine growth hormone function. **A drop in IGF-1 serum levels stimulates the release of growth hormone.**

IGF target cells secrete several **IGF-binding proteins** and **proteases**. The latter can regulate the delivery and action of IGF on target cells by reducing available IGF-binding proteins.

Clinical significance: Gigantism (in children) and acromegaly (in adults)

Excessive secretion of growth hormone can occur in the presence of a benign tumor called an **adenoma**.

When the growth hormone–secreting tumor occurs during childhood and puberty, at a time when the epiphyseal plates are still active, **gigantism** (Greek *gigas*, giant; extremely tall stature) is observed. If excessive growth hormone secretion occurs in the adult, when the epiphyseal plates are inactive, **acromegaly** (Greek *akron*, end or extremity; *megas*, large)

Figure 18-7. Prolactin

Prolactin stimulates lactation postpartum.

The secretion of prolactin by **acidophils** is regulated primarily by inhibition rather than by stimulation.

Dopamine is the main inhibitor of prolactin secretion.

Suckling during lactation is the major stimulus of prolactin secretion.

A prolactin-secreting adenoma of the anterior hypophysis causes **hyperprolactinemia**, which in turn accounts for **galactorrhea** (nonpuerperal milk secretion).

Hyperprolactinemia leads to reversible **infertility** in both females and males.

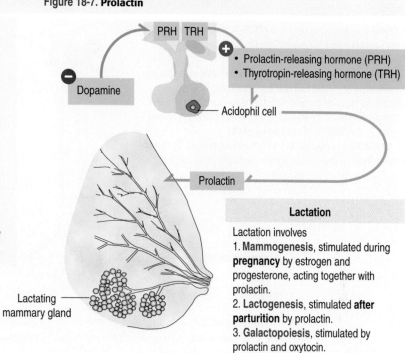

Prolactin
- **Prolactin-releasing hormone (PRH)**
- **Thyrotropin-releasing hormone (TRH)**

Lactation

Lactation involves
1. **Mammogenesis**, stimulated during **pregnancy** by estrogen and progesterone, acting together with prolactin.
2. **Lactogenesis**, stimulated **after parturition** by prolactin.
3. **Galactopoiesis**, stimulated by prolactin and oxytocin.

develops. In acromegaly, the hands, feet, jaw, and soft tissues become enlarged. Long bones do not grow in length, but cartilage (nose, ears) and membranous bones (mandible and calvarium) continue to grow, leading to gross deformities.

A growth hormone–secreting adenoma does not show the typical pulsatile secretory pattern of the hormone. A **decrease** in the secretion of growth hormone in children results in short stature (**dwarfism**).

Prolactin

Prolactin is a 199-amino-acid single-chain protein (22 kd). Prolactin, growth hormone, and human placental lactogen share some amino acid homology and overlapping activity,

The predominant action of prolactin is to stimulate the initiation and maintenance of **lactation** post partum (Figure 18-7). Lactation involves the following:

1. **Mammogenesis**, the growth and development

Figure 18-8. Gonadotropins (FSH and LH)

Neurons in the **arcuate nucleus** of the hypothalamus secrete **GnRH** (gonadotropin-releasing hormone). GnRH is secreted in pulses at 60- to 90-minute intervals and stimulates the pulsatile secretion of **gonadotropins** by the basophilic gonadotrophs.

In the female, FSH stimulates **granulosa cells** of the ovarian follicle to proliferate and secrete **estradiol**, **inhibin**, and **activin**. LH stimulates progesterone secretion by the **corpus luteum**.

In the male, FSH stimulates **Sertoli cell** function in the seminiferous epithelium (synthesis of **inhibin**, **activin**, and **androgen-binding protein**). LH stimulates the production of **testosterone** by **Leydig cells**. A lack of FSH and LH in females and males leads to **infertility**.

Kallmann's syndrome is characterized by **delayed** or **absent puberty** and **anosmia** (impaired sense of smell). It is clinically defined as **hypogonadotropic hypogonadism (HH)**. Mutations in genes prevent the migration of GnRH–secreting neurons to the hypothalamic arcuate nucleus and olfactory neurons to the olfactory bulb.

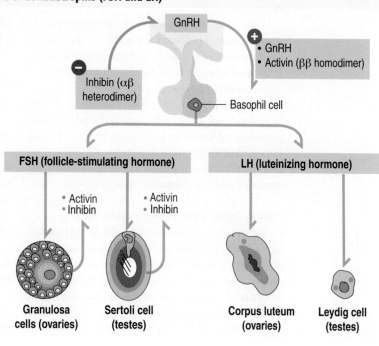

GnRH
- GnRH
- Activin (ββ homodimer)

Inhibin (αβ heterodimer)

Basophil cell

FSH (follicle-stimulating hormone)
- Activin
- Inhibin

LH (luteinizing hormone)
- Activin
- Inhibin

Granulosa cells (ovaries) **Sertoli cell (testes)** **Corpus luteum (ovaries)** **Leydig cell (testes)**

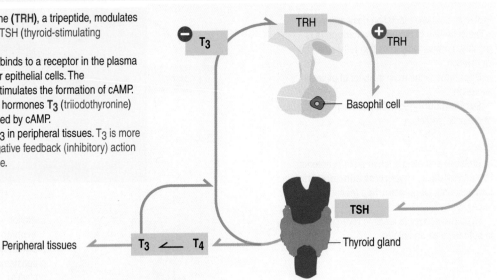

Figure 18-9. Thyroid-stimulating hormone (TSH)

Thyrotropin-releasing hormone (**TRH**), a tripeptide, modulates the synthesis and release of TSH (thyroid-stimulating hormone) from basophils.

TSH is a glycoprotein that binds to a receptor in the plasma membrane of thyroid follicular epithelial cells. The hormone-receptor complex stimulates the formation of cAMP. The production of the thyroid hormones T$_3$ (triiodothyronine) and T$_4$ (thyroxine) is stimulated by cAMP.

Some T$_4$ is converted to T$_3$ in peripheral tissues. T$_3$ is more active than T$_4$ and has a negative feedback (inhibitory) action on TSH synthesis and release.

Labels in figure: TRH; TRH; T$_3$; Basophil cell; TSH; Thyroid gland; Peripheral tissues; T$_3$; T$_4$

---

of the mammary gland, is stimulated primarily by estrogen and progesterone in coordination with prolactin and human placental lactogen.

2. **Lactogenesis**, the initiation of lactation, is triggered by prolactin acting on the developed mammary gland by the actions of estrogens and progesterone. Lactation is inhibited during pregnancy by high levels of estrogen and progesterone, which decline at delivery. Either estradiol or prolactin antagonists are used clinically to stop lactation.

3. **Galactopoiesis**, the maintenance of milk production, requires both prolactin and oxytocin.

The effects of prolactin, placental lactogen, and steroids on the development of the lactating mammary gland are discussed in Chapter 23, Fertilization, Placentation, and Lactation.

Unlike other hormones of the anterior hypophysis, **the secretion of prolactin is regulated primarily by inhibition rather than by stimulation.** The main inhibitor is **dopamine**. Dopamine secretion is stimulated by prolactin to inhibit its own secretion.

A **stimulatory** effect on prolactin release is exerted by **prolactin-releasing hormone** (PRH) and **thyrotropin-releasing hormone** (TRH). Prolactin is released from **acidophils** in a pulsatile fashion, coinciding with and following each period of suckling. **Intermittent surges of prolactin stimulate milk synthesis.**

Clinical significance: Hyperprolactinemia

Prolactin-secreting tumors alter the hypothalamo-hypophysial-gonadal axis, leading to gonadotropin deficiency. Hypersecretion of prolactin in women can be associated with **infertility,** caused by the lack of **ovulation** and **oligomenorrhea** or **amenorrhea** (dysfunctional uterine bleeding).

A decrease in fertility and libido is found in males. These antifertility effects are found in both genders and are usually reversible. **Galactorrhea** (nonpuerperal milk secretion) is a common problem in **hyperprolactinemia** and can also occur in males.

Hormones secreted by basophils: Gonadotropins, TSH, and ACTH

Gonadotropins (FSH and LH) and TSH have common features:

1. They are glycoproteins (hence the PAS-positive staining of basophils).

2. They consist of **two chains**. The α chain is a glycoprotein common to FSH, LH, and TSH, but the β chain is specific for each hormone. Therefore, **the β chain confers specificity to the hormone.**

Gonadotropins: Follicle-stimulating hormone and luteinizing hormone

Gonadotrophs (gonadotropin-secreting cells) (Figure 18-8) secrete **both FSH and LH.** Gonadotrophs constitute about 10% of the total cell population of the anterior hypophysis.

The release of gonadotropins is stimulated by **gonadotropin-releasing hormone (GnRH; also called luteinizing hormone–releasing hormone [LHRH]),** a decapeptide produced in the **arcuate nucleus** of the hypothalamus. GnRH is secreted in pulses at 60- to 90-minute intervals into the portal vasculature. **A single basophil can synthesize and release both FSH and LH** in a pulsatile fashion.

In the female, **FSH** stimulates the development of the ovarian follicles by a process called **folliculogenesis.** In the male, FSH acts on **Sertoli cells** in the testes to stimulate the aromatization of estrogens from androgens and the production of **androgen-binding protein**, with binding affinity to testosterone.

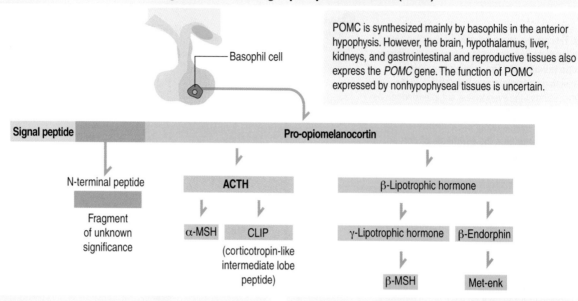

Figure 18-10. Processing of pro-opiomelanocortin (POMC)

POMC is synthesized mainly by basophils in the anterior hypophysis. However, the brain, hypothalamus, liver, kidneys, and gastrointestinal and reproductive tissues also express the *POMC* gene. The function of POMC expressed by nonhypophyseal tissues is uncertain.

N-terminal peptide, adrenocorticotropic hormone (ACTH), and β-lipotrophic hormone (β-LPH) are produced in the anterior hypophysis.

The cleavage products of β-LPH (γ-LPH and β-endorphin) are released into the circulation and may have a functional role in humans.

β-LPH and γ-LPH are lipolytic hormones and their role in fat mobilization in humans is not known.

γ-LPH gives rise to β-melanocyte–stimulating hormone (β-MSH).

β-Endorphin contains the sequences of met-enkephalin (met-enk). There is no evidence that β-endorphin is cleaved in the hypophysis to form met-enk. β-MSH is not secreted in humans.

ACTH is cleaved to α-melanocyte–stimulating hormone (α-MSH) and CLIP only in species with a prominent pars intermedia. α-MSH and β-MSH determine the dispersion of melanin granules in melanophores of fish, reptiles, and amphibians to darken the skin. The human hypophysis lacks a prominent pars intermedia (except during fetal development), and the processing of ACTH to α-MSH and CLIP (unknown function) does not occur.

In the female, **LH** stimulates **steroidogenesis** in the ovarian follicle and corpus luteum. In the male, LH controls the rate of **testosterone** synthesis by **Leydig cells** in the testis. The function of FSH and LH in the male is analyzed in Chapter 20, Spermatogenesis.

The release of FSH and GnRH is **inhibited** by:

1. **Inhibin**, a **heterodimer** protein formed by α- and β-peptide chains, secreted by the male and female target cells (Sertoli cells and granulosa cells and cells of the anterior hypophysis).

2. **Estradiol**.

The release of FSH in both females and males is **enhanced** by a homodimer protein, called **activin**, secreted by Sertoli cells and granulosa cells. It consists of two β chains. Little is known about what controls αβ (inhibin) and ββ (activin) dimerization.

Kallmann's syndrome is characterized by **delayed** or **absent puberty** and **anosmia** (impaired sense of smell). It is determined by mutations in genes whose encoded proteins are responsible for the migration and survival of GnRH–secreting neurons to the hypothalamic arcuate nucleus and olfactory neurons to the olfactory bulb.

This condition affects the production of FSH and LH, two gonadotropins that regulate male and female sexual development at puberty. It is clinically defined as **hypogonadotropic hypogonadism (HH)**.

We discuss in Chapter 20, Spermatogenesis, and Chapter 22, Follicle Development and The Menstrual Cycle, the functions of FSH and LH in spermatogenesis, Leydig cell function, folliculogenesis, and luteogenesis. Additional molecular aspects of Kallmann's syndrome are discussed in Chapter 22.

Clinical significance: Infertility

The secretion of FSH and LH can decrease when there is a deficient secretion of GnRH, caused by anorexia or a tumor of the hypophysis, which can destroy the gonadotrops, thereby decreasing FSH and LH secretion.

A decrease in fertility and reproductive functions can be observed in females and males. Females can have menstrual disorders. Small testes and infertility can be seen in males (a condition known as **hypogonadotropic hypogonadism**) when GnRH secretion is deficient.

Castration (**ovariectomy** in the female and **orchidectomy** in the male) causes a significant **increase** in the synthesis of FSH and LH as a result of a **loss of feedback inhibition**. Hyperfunctional gonadotropic cells are large and vacuolated and are called **castration cells**.

Figure 18-11. Adrenocorticotropic hormone (ACTH)

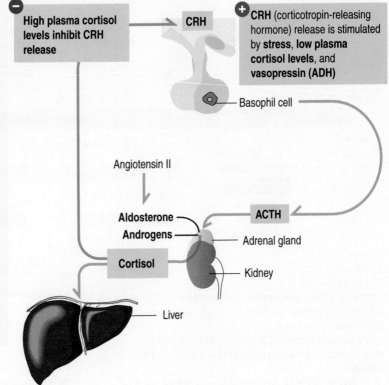

ACTH controls predominantly the function of two zones of the adrenal cortex (**zona fasciculata** and **zona reticularis**). The zona glomerulosa is regulated by **angiotensin II** derived from the processing of the liver protein angiotensinogen by the proteolytic action of renin (kidneys) and converting enzyme (lungs).

ACTH stimulates the synthesis of cortisol (a glucocorticoid) and androgens. Cortisol and other steroids are metabolized in liver.

Low levels of cortisol in blood, stress, and vasopressin (antidiuretic hormone [ADH]) stimulate ACTH secretion from basophils by stimulation of CRH release (positive feedback). **Cortisol is the dominating regulatory factor.**

ACTH increases the pigmentation of skin. Skin darkening in **Addison's disease** and **Cushing's disease** is not determined by melanocyte-stimulating hormone (MSH), which is not normally present in human serum.

High plasma cortisol levels inhibit CRH release

CRH

CRH (corticotropin-releasing hormone) release is stimulated by **stress**, **low plasma cortisol levels**, and **vasopressin (ADH)**

Basophil cell

Angiotensin II

Aldosterone
Androgens

ACTH

Adrenal gland

Cortisol

Kidney

Liver

Thyroid-stimulating hormone (thyrotropin)

Thyrotropic cells represent about 5% of the total population of the anterior hypophysis.

TSH is the regulatory hormone of **thyroid function** (Figure 18-9) and **growth**. The mechanism of action of TSH on thyroid cell function is discussed in the thyroid gland section of Chapter 19, Endocrine System.

Thyrotropin-releasing hormone (TRH), a 3-amino-acid-peptide produced in the hypothalamus, **stimulates** the synthesis and release of TSH from **basophils**. TRH also stimulates the release of prolactin. The release of TSH is **inhibited** by increased concentrations of the thyroid hormones triiodothyronine (T_3) and thyroxine (T_4).

Clinical significance: Hypothyroidism

A deficiency in the secretion of TSH (observed in rare cases of congenital hypoplasia of the hypophysis) produces **hypothyroidism**, characterized by reduced cell metabolism and temperature and basal metabolic rate and mental lethargy. Hypothyroidism is also observed in the autoimmune disorder **Hashimoto's disease**. Hypothyroidism can also result from a disease of the thyroid gland or a deficiency in dietary iodine. We discuss **hyperthyroidism** in the thyroid gland section of Chapter 19, Endocrine System when describing **Graves' disease**.

Adrenocorticotropic hormone

ACTH, or **corticotropin**, is a **single-chain** protein, 39 amino acids in length (4.5 kd), with a short circulating time (7 to 12 minutes). Its primary action is **to stimulate growth** and **steroid synthesis** in the zonae fasciculata and reticularis of the **adrenal cortex**. The zona glomerulosa of the adrenal cortex is under the control of angiotensin II (see the adrenal gland section of Chapter 19, Endocrine System).

The effects of ACTH on the adrenal cortex are mediated by cyclic adenosine monophosphate (cAMP). ACTH also acts beyond the adrenal gland by increasing skin pigmentation and lipolysis.

ACTH derives from a large glycosylated precursor of 31 kd called **pro-opiomelanocortin** (POMC), processed in the anterior hypophysis. The products of POMC are the following (Figure 18-10):

1. An **N-terminal peptide** of unknown function, **ACTH**, and β-**lipotrophic hormone** (β-LPH). These three POMC derivatives are secreted by the anterior hypophysis.

2. The cleavage products of β-**LPH**, γ-**LPH**, and β-**endorphin** are released into circulation. β-LPH and γ-lipotrophic hormone (γ-LPH) have **lipolytic action**, but their precise role in fat mobilization in humans is unknown.

3. γ-LPH contains the amino acid sequence of β-**melanocyte–stimulating hormone** (β-MSH; not

Figure 18-12. Neurohypophysis

The hormones **antidiuretic hormone (or arginine vasopressin)** and **oxytocin** are synthesized in the neurons of the **supraoptic** and **paraventricular nuclei**, respectively.

The hormones are transported along the axons forming the **hypothalamic hypophyseal tract**, together with the carrier protein **neurophysin**, and are released at the axon terminals. The hormones enter **fenestrated capillaries** derived from the inferior hypophyseal artery.

Paraventricular nucleus (primarily **oxytocin**)
Hypothalamic area
Mamillary body
Infundibulum — **Median eminence** / **Infundibular process**
Pars nervosa (neural lobe)
Neurohypophysis — Axon terminal
Inferior hypophyseal artery
Supraoptic nucleus (primarily **antidiuretic hormone**)
Optic chiasma
Hypothalamic hypophyseal tract
Anterior hypophysis

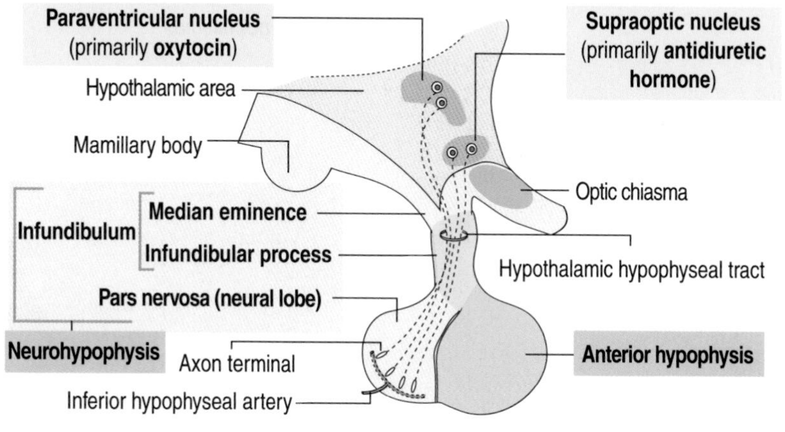

The neurohypophysis is formed by supporting neuroglial cells, the **pituicytes**, whose cytoplasmic processes surround the **unmyelinated nerve fibers** arising from neurons of the paraventricular and supraoptic nuclei. Abundant capillaries are visualized.

Antidiuretic hormone and oxytocin accumulate temporarily in axon dilations, forming the **Herring bodies** (not seen in these micrographs).

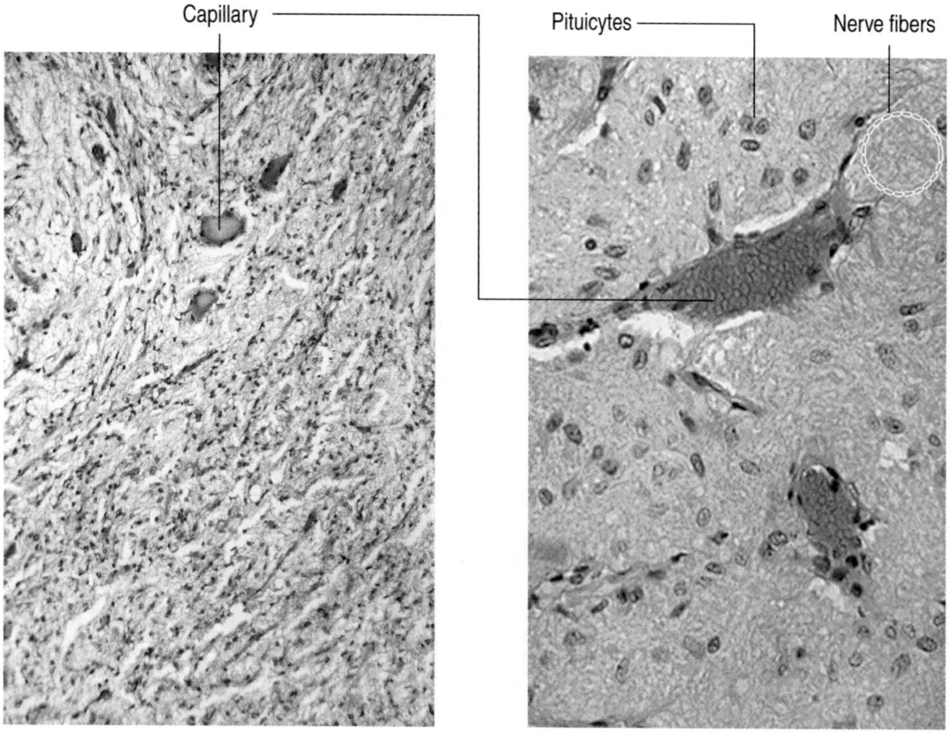

Capillary

Pituicytes — Nerve fibers

secreted in humans). β-Endorphin contains the sequences of **met-enkephalin** (met-enk). There is no evidence that β-endorphin is cleaved in the hypophysis to form met-enk.

4. ACTH is cleaved to α-melanocyte–stimulating hormone (α-MSH) and **corticotropin-like intermediate peptide** (CLIP). α-MSH and CLIP hormones, found in species with a hypophysis with a prominent pars intermedia, cause dispersion of melanin granules in melanophores and darkening of the skin of many fish, amphibians, and reptiles.

The release of ACTH is controlled by the following (Figure 18-11):

1. A stimulatory effect determined by **corticotropin-releasing hormone** (CRH) from the hypothalamus. CRH co-localizes with **antidiuretic hormone** (ADH; see later section, Neurohypophysis) in the

paraventricular nuclei. Both ADH and angiotensin II potentiate the effect of CRH on the release of ACTH.

2. An **inhibitory** effect caused by high levels of **cortisol** in blood either by preventing the release of CRH or by blocking the release of ACTH by basophil **corticotropic cells** (ACTH-secreting cells).

ACTH is secreted in a circadian manner (morning peaks followed by a slow decline afterward).

Clinical significance: Cushing's disease

An ACTH-secreting adenoma of the hypophysis causes **Cushing's disease**. This disease is characterized by an increase in the production of cortisol by the zona fasciculata of the adrenal cortex (see the adrenal gland section in Chapter 19, Endocrine System), obesity, osteoporosis, and muscle wasting. A **reduction** in the secretion of ACTH results in diminished

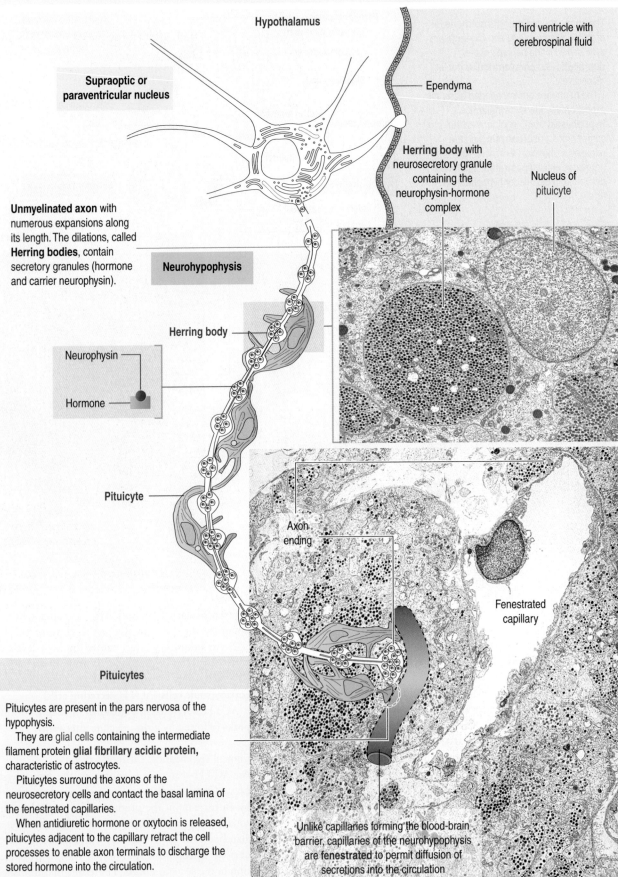

Figure 18-13. Structure and function of the neuroendocrine cell

Hypothalamus

Third ventricle with cerebrospinal fluid

Supraoptic or paraventricular nucleus

Ependyma

Herring body with neurosecretory granule containing the neurophysin-hormone complex

Nucleus of pituicyte

Unmyelinated axon with numerous expansions along its length. The dilations, called **Herring bodies**, contain secretory granules (hormone and carrier neurophysin).

Neurohypophysis

Herring body

Neurophysin

Hormone

Pituicyte

Axon ending

Fenestrated capillary

Pituicytes

Pituicytes are present in the pars nervosa of the hypophysis.

They are glial cells containing the intermediate filament protein **glial fibrillary acidic protein,** characteristic of astrocytes.

Pituicytes surround the axons of the neurosecretory cells and contact the basal lamina of the fenestrated capillaries.

When antidiuretic hormone or oxytocin is released, pituicytes adjacent to the capillary retract the cell processes to enable axon terminals to discharge the stored hormone into the circulation.

Unlike capillaries forming the blood-brain barrier, capillaries of the neurohypophysis are **fenestrated** to permit diffusion of secretions into the circulation

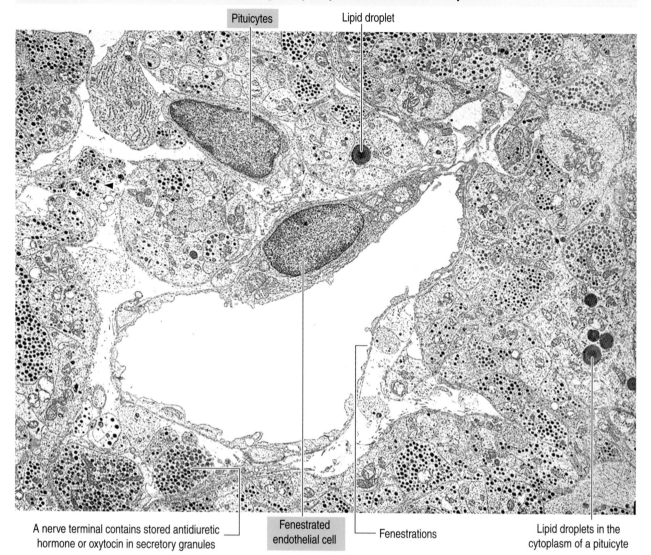

Pituicytes

Lipid droplet

A nerve terminal contains stored antidiuretic hormone or oxytocin in secretory granules

Fenestrated endothelial cell

Fenestrations

Lipid droplets in the cytoplasm of a pituicyte

secretion of cortisol and in hypoglycemia.

A loss of ACTH decreases adrenal androgen secretion. In females, androgen deficiency causes loss of pubic and axillary hair. This effect is not observed in males because it is compensated for by the testicular secretion of androgens.

Neurohypophysis

The neurohypophysis consists of three histologic components (Figures 18-12 and 18-13):

1. **Pituicytes**, resembling astrocytes, provide support to the axons.

2. **Unmyelinated axons**, derived from neuroendocrine cells called **magnicellular neurons** (because their cell bodies are large). Axons have **Herring bodies,** bulging intermittent segments and terminals containing secretory products, the **neurophysin-hormone complex.**

Neurophysin is a protein of 10 kd containing 90 to 97 amino acids derived by cleavage from **pre-prooxiphysin.** It is transported, stored, and secreted bound to the hormone. Neurophysin does not have an apparent biologic action other than serving as a hormone carrier during axonal transport.

3. **Fenestrated capillaries** are derived from the inferior hypophyseal artery.

Pituicytes are astrocyte-like glial cells with abundant **glial fibrillary acidic proteins**, an intermediate filament protein, and a few **lipid droplets** in their cytoplasm. The cytoplasmic processes of pituicytes (Figure 18-14):

1. Embrace the axons derived from the neuroendocrine cells.

2. Extend between the axon terminals and the basal lamina surrounding fenestrated capillaries.

3. Retract the cytoplasmic processes to enable the release into the blood of secretory granules stored in the axon terminals (see Figure 18-14).

Axons in the neurohypophysis derive from the **supraoptic nuclei** and the **paraventricular nuclei.**

Figure 18-15. **Antidiuretic hormone (vasopressin) and oxytocin**

Arginine vasopressin and oxytocin have similar molecular structures. Each consists of nine amino acids arranged as a ring formed by the linkage of two molecules of cysteine (a disulfide linkage) and a short side chain. The structure of the two hormones differs only at amino acids 3 and 8. There are two forms of vasopressin: **arginine vasopressin** has arginine at position 8; **lysine vasopressin** has lysine at position 8.

Antidiuretic hormone increases the **permeability of the collecting tubule to water** and also has an **arteriolar vasoconstrictive** action (hence the alternative name **vasopressin**). The action of antidiuretic hormone is mediated by **cAMP**, which stimulates membrane channels to increase the diffusion of water. Consequently, urine flow decreases.

Oxytocin acts on **uterine contraction** and **milk release during suckling**.

Estrogens increase the response of the myometrium to oxytocin; progesterone decreases the response.

During lactation, oxytocin release is mediated by a neurohumoral reflex triggered by suckling. Suckling activates sensory receptors in the nipple and areola. Sensory fibers are linked to the hypothalamic neurons producing oxytocin. When the stimulus arrives, an action potential transmitted along the axons of the paraventricular neurons extending into the pars nervosa causes the release of oxytocin into the blood.

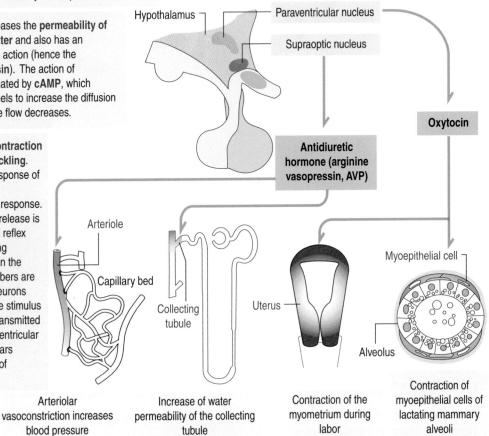

Some neurons of the paraventricular nuclei are small and their axons project to the median eminence rather than to the pars nervosa. These neurons, called **parvicellular neurons** (Latin *parvus*, small), secrete arginine vasopressin (ADH) and oxytocin entering the hypophyseal portal blood at the median eminence.

Large neurons of the supraoptic and paraventricular nuclei, called **magnicellular neurons** (Latin *magnus*, large), give rise to axons forming the **hypothalamic hypophyseal tract**. The terminals of these neurons are located in the pars nervosa.

In general, neurons of the supraoptic and paraventricular nuclei synthesize vasopressin and oxytocin. However, **neurons of the supraoptic nuclei produce primarily vasopressin and neurons of the paraventricular nuclei synthesize primarily oxytocin**. Neurophysin I is a carrier for oxytocin; neurophysin II is a carrier for vasopressin.

Vasopressin and oxytocin are transported down the axons and stored in nerve terminals within secretory granules, packaged together with neurophysin. The released hormones circulate in blood in an unbound form and have a half-life of 5 minutes.

In addition to these two nuclei, the hypothalamus has additional nuclei, **the hypothalamic hypophysiotropic nuclei**, with neurons producing releasing and inhibitory hormones to be discharged at the fenestrated capillaries of the primary plexus (see earlier, Blood supply of the hypophysis).

Although the neuroendocrine cells of the supraoptic and paraventricular nuclei are located **behind the blood-brain barrier**, their products are transported to nerve terminals and released **outside the blood-brain barrier** into fenestrated capillaries.

Clinical significance: Diabetes insipidus
Oxytocin participates in the **contraction of smooth muscle**, in particular the **uterus during labor**, and **myoepithelial cells** lining the secretory acini and lactiferous ducts of the mammary gland to facilitate

Figure 18-16. **Development of the pineal gland**

1 A dorsal diverticulum, an outpocketing of the diencephalon, initiates the formation of the pineal gland during the 10th week of development.

2 The wall of the vesicular evagination thickens. The lumen is occluded, except at the base of the outpocketing, where the **pineal recess** persists and communicates with the third ventricle in the adult.

3 The pineal gland becomes a compact structure containing two cell types derived from the primordial neuroepithelial cells: (1) **pinealocytes**; and (2) **glial-like interstitial cells**. Meninges envelop and invade the developing pineal gland, forming **connective tissue septa**.

1 Diverticulum

Diencephalon

Infundibulum (the site of origin of the neurohypophysis)

2 Pineal recess

3 Connective tissue septum

Meninges

Blood vessel

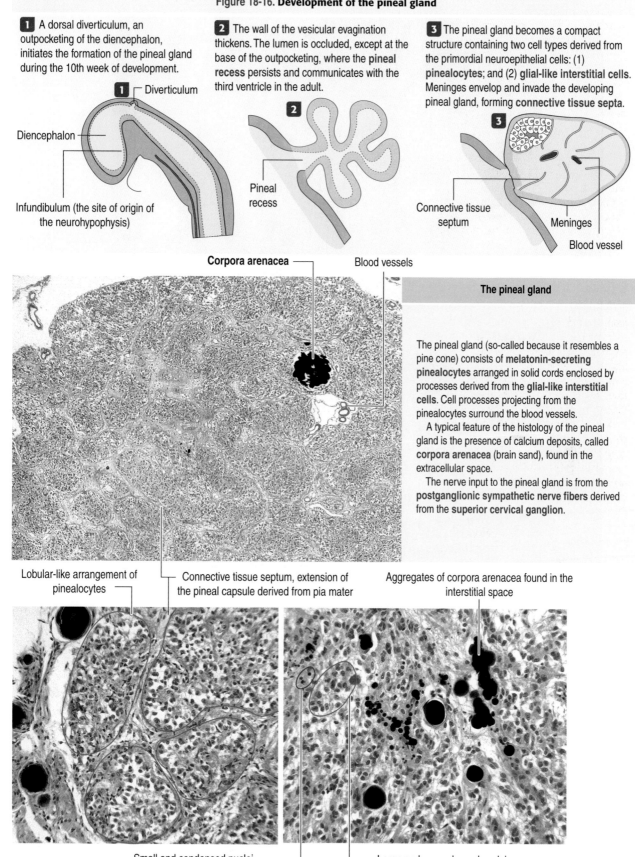

Corpora arenacea — Blood vessels

The pineal gland

The pineal gland (so-called because it resembles a pine cone) consists of **melatonin-secreting pinealocytes** arranged in solid cords enclosed by processes derived from the **glial-like interstitial cells**. Cell processes projecting from the pinealocytes surround the blood vessels.

A typical feature of the histology of the pineal gland is the presence of calcium deposits, called **corpora arenacea** (brain sand), found in the extracellular space.

The nerve input to the pineal gland is from the **postganglionic sympathetic nerve fibers** derived from the **superior cervical ganglion**.

Lobular-like arrangement of pinealocytes

Connective tissue septum, extension of the pineal capsule derived from pia mater

Aggregates of corpora arenacea found in the interstitial space

Small and condensed nuclei correspond to **glia-like intestitial cells**

Large and uncondensed nuclei correspond to **pinealocytes**

Figure 18-17. **Structure of the pinealocyte**

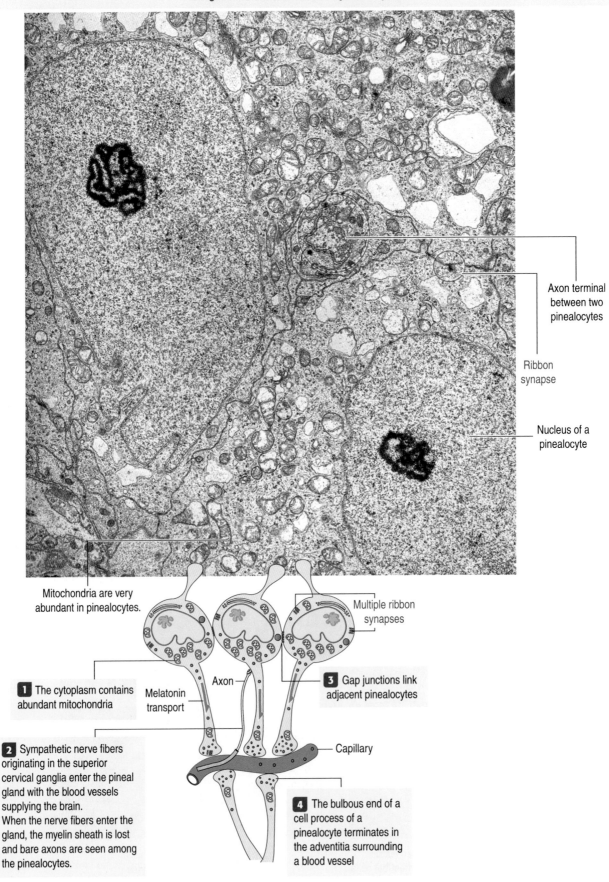

Axon terminal
between two
pinealocytes

Ribbon
synapse

Nucleus of a
pinealocyte

Mitochondria are very
abundant in pinealocytes.

Multiple ribbon
synapses

1 The cytoplasm contains
abundant mitochondria

Melatonin
transport

Axon

3 Gap junctions link
adjacent pinealocytes

2 Sympathetic nerve fibers
originating in the superior
cervical ganglia enter the pineal
gland with the blood vessels
supplying the brain.
When the nerve fibers enter the
gland, the myelin sheath is lost
and bare axons are seen among
the pinealocytes.

Capillary

4 The bulbous end of a
cell process of a
pinealocyte terminates in
the adventitia surrounding
a blood vessel

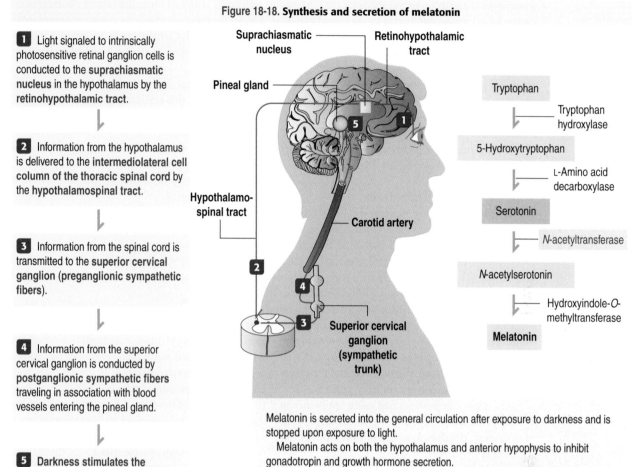

Figure 18-18. Synthesis and secretion of melatonin

1 Light signaled to intrinsically photosensitive retinal ganglion cells is conducted to the **suprachiasmatic nucleus** in the hypothalamus by the **retinohypothalamic tract**.

2 Information from the hypothalamus is delivered to the **intermediolateral cell column of the thoracic spinal cord** by the **hypothalamospinal tract**.

3 Information from the spinal cord is transmitted to the **superior cervical ganglion (preganglionic sympathetic fibers)**.

4 Information from the superior cervical ganglion is conducted by **postganglionic sympathetic fibers** traveling in association with blood vessels entering the pineal gland.

5 **Darkness stimulates the production of melatonin**. Light rapidly suppresses production of melatonin.

Suprachiasmatic nucleus

Retinohypothalamic tract

Pineal gland

Hypothalamo-spinal tract

Carotid artery

Superior cervical ganglion (sympathetic trunk)

Tryptophan → Tryptophan hydroxylase → 5-Hydroxytryptophan → L-Amino acid decarboxylase → Serotonin → N-acetyltransferase → N-acetylserotonin → Hydroxyindole-O-methyltransferase → **Melatonin**

Melatonin is secreted into the general circulation after exposure to darkness and is stopped upon exposure to light.

Melatonin acts on both the hypothalamus and anterior hypophysis to inhibit gonadotropin and growth hormone secretion.

Tumors of the pineal gland are associated with **precocious puberty**.

milk ejection (or **letdown of milk**) during lactation (Figure 18-15).

Antidiuretic hormone regulates water excretion in the kidneys and is also a **potent vasoconstrictor at high doses** (see Figure 18-15). This is the basis for its alternative name, vasopressin (arginine vasopressin [AVP]).

An increase in osmotic pressure in circulating blood or reduced blood volume triggers the release of ADH. Retention of water reduces plasma osmolality, which acts on hypothalamic osmoreceptors to suppress the secretion of ADH.

Neurogenic diabetes insipidus occurs when the secretion of ADH is reduced or absent. **Polyuria** is a common clinical finding. Patients with diabetes insipidus can excrete up to 20 L of urine in 24 hours.

Neurogenic diabetes insipidus is caused by a head injury, an invasive tumor damaging the hypothalamic hypophyseal system, or autoimmune destruction of vasopressin-secreting neurons.

Nephrogenic diabetes insipidus occurs in certain chronic renal diseases that are **nonresponsive** to vasopressin or as a result of genetic defects in renal receptors for vasopressin.

Pineal gland

The pineal gland, or **epiphysis**, is an endocrine organ formed by cells with a neurosecretory function. It lies in the center of the brain, behind the third ventricle and is connected to the brain by a stalk.

There are no direct nerve connections of the pineal gland with the brain. Instead, **postganglionic sympathetic nerve fibers derived from the superior cervical ganglia** supply the pineal gland.

Preganglionic fibers to the superior cervical ganglia derive from the lateral column of the spinal cord. The function of the pineal gland is regulated by **sympathetic nerves**.

In brief,, the mammalian pineal gland is a **neuroendocrine transducer** handling photic information sent from the retina.

Development of the pineal gland

The pineal gland develops from a saccular outpocketing of the posterior diencephalic roof in the midline of the third ventricle (Figure 18-16).

Continued diverticulation and infolding result in a solid parenchymal mass of **cords** and **clusters of pinealocytes** and **glial-like interstitial cells** supported by a meninges-derived connective tissue (pia mater) that carries blood vessels and nerves to the pineal gland.

Histology of the pineal gland

In fishes and amphibians, the pineal gland is a neurosensory **photoreceptor** organ. In reptiles and birds, the photosensory function has been replaced by a secretory function. In mammals, the pineal gland has a neurotransmitter secretory function.

The pineal gland is a highly vascular gland consisting of two cell types (see Figure 18-16):

1. The **pinealocytes**.
2. The **glial-like interstitial cells**.

The **pinealocytes** are neuroepithelial secretory cells organized into cords and clusters resting on a basal lamina and surrounded by connective tissue, blood vessels lined by fenestrated endothelial cells, and nerves. The pinealocyte lacks an axon; it has two or more cell processes ending in bulbous expansions. One of the processes ends near a capillary. The cytoplasm contains **abundant mitochondria and randomly distributed multiple synaptic ribbons** (Figure 18-17). In contrast, **single ribbon synapses** can be seen at the **synaptic end** of sensory cells of the **retina** (see Figure 9-18) and **inner ear** (see Figure 9-28).

Pinealocytes can be identified using antibodies to **synaptophysin**, a cell membrane glycoprotein marker of neurosecretory cells, as well as tumors arising from these cells.

Interstitial cells are found among pinealocytes. The glial-like interstitial cells, identified by the presence of **glial fibrillary acidic protein (GFAP)** in the cytoplasm, and the connective tissue provide stromal support to the functional pinealocytes.

The neural input to the pineal gland is **norepinephrine**, and the output is **melatonin**. The function of pinealocytes is regulated by β-**adrenergic receptors**. The metabolic activity of pinealocytes is inhibited by β-adrenergic antagonists.

An important feature of the pineal gland is the presence of defined **areas of calcification**, called **corpora arenacea** (brain sand). Pinealocytes secrete an extracellular matrix in which hydroxyl or carbonate apatite crystals deposit (see Figure 18-16). They develop from early infancy, increase with age and are radiologically visible after the second decade of life.

Calcification has no known effect on the function of the pineal gland. **A calcified pineal gland is an important radiographic marker of the midline of the brain.**

Pinealocytes secrete melatonin

Melatonin is the major biologically active substance secreted by the pineal gland. The synthesis and release of melatonin are stimulated by darkness and inhibited by light.

During daylight hours, the retinal photoreceptor cells are hyperpolarized and the release of norepinephrine is inhibited. Consequently, the retinohypothalamic–pineal system is resting and little melatonin is secreted.

When darkness starts, the photoreceptors release norepinephrine, that activates α1- and β1-adrenergic receptors in the pinealocytes to increase their melatonin synthetic activity.

Melatonin is rapidly metabolized, mainly in the liver, by hydroxylation to 6-hydroxymelatonin and, after conjugation with sulfuric or glucuronic acid, is excreted in the urine.

In summary, light has two effects on melatonin:

1. Day–night light cycles modify the rhythm of melatonin secretion.

2. Brief pulses of light of sufficient intensity and duration can rapidly suppress the production of melatonin.

Melatonin is synthesized from **tryptophan** and immediately secreted (Figure 18-18). **Serotonin**, a neurotransmitter, is a precursor of melatonin. Serotonin is acetylated and then methylated to produce melatonin. Serotonin *N*-acetyltransferase is the rate-limiting enzyme in melatonin synthesis. In fact, exposure to light or administration of β-adrenergic blocking agents causes a rapid decrease in *N*-acetyltransferase and a consequent decline in melatonin synthesis.

During night, with complete darkness, the melatonin content of the pineal gland is highest.

Melatonin is released by passive diffusion into the general circulation:

1. **To act on the hypothalamus and hypophysis, and, in many species, to inhibit gonadotropin and growth hormone secretion.**

2. To induce **sleepiness**. Melatonin integrates photoperiods and modulate circadian rhythms. An unproved hypothesis is that melatonin contributes to drowsiness when lights are turned down.

Two melatonin G protein-coupled cell surface receptors, designated **Mel1A** and **Mel1B**, are differentially expressed in different tissues and account for the varying biologic effects of melatonin.

Light is a regulator of circadian rhythms

The circadian rhythm of melatonin secretion is of endogenous origin; signals originate in the suprachiasmatic nucleus. A 24-hour biologic circadian (Latin *circa*, about; *dies*, day) clock regulates sleep and alert patterns and is linked to the periodic light-dark cycle or sleep-wake cycle.

We previously indicated that the mammalian pineal gland is a neuroendocrine transducer handling information sent from the retina.

The retina has two functions:

1. The **detection of light for the formation of images**

by transforming photon energy into an electrical signal, as we discuss in Chapter 9, Sensory Organs.

2. **Non-image forming (NIF)** visual functions required for adjusting the internal circadian clock to light and sleep. NIF visual functions involve a subset of retinal ganglion cells

The **retinohypothalamic tract** conducts light signals to the hypothalamic suprachiasmatic nucleus (the central circadian pacemaker) as the initial step in the regulation of melatonin synthesis and secretion by the way of a polysynaptic pathway (see Figure 18-18).

The **suprachiasmatic nucleus (SCN)** is located adjacent to the optic chiasm and contains a network of neurons operating as **an endogenous pacemaker regulating circadian rhythmicity**. Neurons that contain melatonin Mel1A and Mel1B receptors are **circadian oscillators** connected to specialized **melanopsin-producing ganglion cells** of the retina.

Cells with **NIF** visual functions are called **intrinsically photosensitive retinal ganglion cells (ipRGCs)**.

The ipRGCs function as **luminance detectors** resetting the circadian oscillators. There is some evidence that the SCN sends signals to the circadian pacemakers of the rest of the body through the proteins **transforming growth factor-α and prokineticin 2**.

When a SCN is transplanted to a recipient with a damaged suprachiasmatic nucleus, it displays the circadian pacemaker properties of the donor rather than those of the host. This indicates that ipRGCs and the SCN, in addition to its circadian pacemaker function, project to several regions of the brain to drive rhythms involved in inducing sleep or influence mood.

Patients with depression report sleep alteration weeks before the reappearance of depression symptoms. **Seasonal affective disorder (SAD)** is a type of depression related to the shorter day length of the winter months. SAD has been observed in patients with bipolar disorders, characterized by a significant switch in mood between periods of mania and depression.

Jet lag, a condition associated with fatigue, insomnia, and disorientation experienced by many travelers flying across time zones, is caused by a temporary disruption of the circadian rhythm by shifting or dissociation of the light-dark/sleep-wake cycles.

Resetting of the circadian clock, caused by a tempo-rary lack of alignment between the circadian rhythm and local time, involves appropriate timed exposure to light and/or the administration of melatonin.

Together, these observations indicate that the synchronization of the circadian system impacts on mental health issues.

Pathology: Pineocytomas

A tumor of the pineal gland, called **pineocytoma**, causes compression symptoms, invades local structures or disseminates beyond the tumor site.

About 10 percent of lesions of the pineal gland are essentially benign, including **pineal cysts**. Another 10 percent of tumors are relatively benign, including **low-grade gliomas**. The remaining 80 percent of pineal region neoplasms are highly malignant lesions. These include **germ cell tumors** (pineal germinoma), **embryonal carcinoma** and **malignant pineoblastoma**.

Germinomas derive from primordial germ cells (PGCs) that originate from yolk-sac endoderm and migrate to the gonadal ridges of the embryo. A lack of normal involution of PGCs at any migratory site (see Chapter 21, Sperm Transport and Maturation) can develop into a germinoma.

Magnetic resonance imaging (MRI) provides tumor and anatomic details (cystic, calcified, extension into the lateral ventricles or the suprasellar region).

The extent and nature of the tumor can be assessed by cytologic examination of the cerebrospinal fluid (to determine the presence of malignant cells) and determination of α-fetoprotein (AFP), a marker of a germ cell tumor. Ophthalmologic examination is required to determine the regional extent of the tumor.

Precocious puberty or **delayed onset of sexual maturation** is seen in about 10 percent of male patients with pineal tumors. Precocious puberty is characterized by the onset of androgen secretion and spermatogenesis in boys before the age of 9 or 10 years and the initiation of estrogen secretion and cyclic ovarian activity in girls before age 8.

Precocious puberty is probably caused by the effect of the tumor on the function of the hypothalamus rather than by a direct effect of pineal tumors on sexual function.

Pineocytomas cause a neurologic disorder known as **Parinaud's syndrome** (paralysis of upward gaze, looking steadily in one direction, pupillary areflexia to light, paralysis of convergence, and wide-based gait).

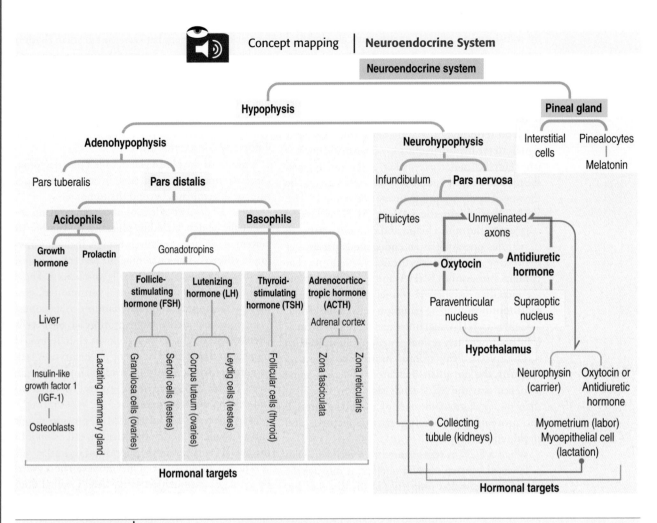

Concept mapping | Neuroendocrine System

Essential concepts | Neuroendocrine System

• General organization of the neuroendocrine system. The hypothalamus and the hypophysis (pituitary gland) form an integrated system known as the hypothalamohypophyseal system consisting of two components:

(1) The hypothalamic adenohypophyseal system (linking the hypothalamus to the anterior hypophysis).

(2) The hypothalamic neurohypophyseal system (connecting the hypothalamus to the neurohypophysis).

• Functional aspects of the neuroendocrine system. The hypothalamus contains clusters of neurons called nuclei. Some of the neurons are neuroendocrine cells exerting positive and negative effects on the two components of the hypophysis. These effects are mediated by releasing and inhibitory hormones or factors.

The transport of signaling molecules is mediated by the hypothalamohypophyseal portal circulation consisting of:

(1) A primary capillary plexus in the lower hypothalamus.

(2) The primary capillary plexus is connected by portal veins to a secondary capillary plexus in the anterior lobe of the hypophysis.

(3) A third capillary plexus supplies the neurohypophysis.

The primary capillary plexus is supplied by the superior hypophyseal artery; the third capillary plexus is supplied by the inferior hypophyseal artery. The two arteries are connected by the trabecular artery. There is no connection between the secondary and third capillary plexuses. The hypophyseal vein drains the second and third capillary plexuses to the dural sinuses.

• The hypophysis consists of two embryologically distinct portions:

(1) The adenohypophysis or glandular component, derived from Rathke's pouch, an invagination of the roof of the future oral cavity.

(2) The neurohypophysis or neural component, an infundibular downgrowth from the floor of the diencephalon.

The adenohypophysis consists of three subdivisions:

(1) The pars distalis (anterior lobe).

(2) The pars tuberalis, surrounding the neural infundibular stem or stalk.

(3) The pars intermedia (the rudimentary intermediate lobe).

The neurohypophysis consists of two subdivisions:

(1) The pars nervosa.

(2) The median eminence.

The anterior lobe contains three components:

(1) Epithelial cell cords.

(2) A connective tissue stroma.

(3) Fenestrated capillaries (sinusoids) of the secondary capillary plexus.

There are three distinct cell populations:

(1) Acidophil cells, stain with an acidic dye.

(2) Basophil cells, stain with a basic dye.

(3) Chromophobe cells, lacking cytoplasmic staining).

Acidophil cells secrete peptide hormones (growth hormone and prolactin); basophils secrete glycoprotein hormones (gonadotropins FSH and LH, TSH, and ACTH). Chromophobe cells are cells that have depleted their cytoplasmic hormonal content.

• Growth hormone (also called somatotropin). It is secreted in a pulsatile pattern with peak secretion occurring during the first 2 hours of sleep. Growth hormone exerts its actions through insulin-like growth factor-1 (IGF-1) produced in hepatocytes after stimulation by growth hormone.

The release of growth hormone is stimulated by growth hormone–releasing hormone produced in the hypothalamus and by high blood levels of IGF-1. Inhibition of growth hormone release is mediated by somatostatin (also produced in the hypothalamus and in the islets of Langerhans in the pancreas) and high blood levels of glucose.

Gigantism during childhood and puberty is caused by excessive secretion of growth hormone (usually produced by a benign tumor of the hypophysis called adenoma). **Acromegaly** (enlargement of hands, feet, jaw, and soft tissues) is seen in adults when growth hormone production is high.

• **Prolactin** has a main function: to stimulate the initiation and maintenance of lactation postpartum. Lactation involves:

(1) Mammogenesis, the growth and development of the mammary glands.

(2) Lactogenesis, the initiation of lactation.

(3) Galactopoiesis, the maintenance of milk production.

A secondary function is to facilitate the steroidogenic action of LH in Leydig cells by up-regulating the expression of the luteinizing hormone (LH) receptor. The pulsatile secretion of prolactin is regulated primarily by an inhibitory mechanism rather than by stimulation. The main inhibitor is dopamine.

Prolactin-releasing hormone and thyrotropin-releasing hormone, both originating in the hypothalamus, stimulate prolactin release.

Excessive secretion of prolactin (hyperprolactinemia) by a benign tumor of the hypophysis in both genders causes gonadotropin deficiency. In women, hyperprolactinemia is associated with infertility, anovulation, and oligomenorrhea or amenorrhea (dysfunctional uterine bleeding). A decrease in fertility and libido is seen in males. Galactorrhea (nonpuerperal milk secretion) caused by hyperprolactinemia is common in both genders.

• **Gonadotropins: FSH and LH.** The release of gonadotropins is stimulated by gonadotropin-releasing hormone (GnRH; also called luteinizing hormone–releasing hormone or LHRH). GnRH is secreted in pulses at 60- to 90-minute intervals. A single basophil cell can produce both FSH and LH.

In the female, FSH stimulates folliculogenesis (the development of the ovarian follicle).

In the male, FSH targets Sertoli cells in the testes to convert testosterone into estrogen (by aromatization) and produce androgen-binding protein (ABP).

In the female, LH stimulates steroidogenesis in the ovarian follicle and corpus luteum. In the male, LH controls the production of testosterone by Leydig cells.

The release of FSH and GnRH is inhibited by inhibin (an $\alpha\beta$ heterodimer) produced by the target cells (follicular cells and Sertoli cells), and estradiol. The release of FSH is enhanced by activin (a $\beta\beta$ homodimer).

A drop in the secretion of GnRH, caused by anorexia nervosa, a tumor of the hypophysis, or a condition known as **hypogonadotropic hypogonadism (HH)**, can abolish the secretion of FSH and LH. Castration (ovariectomy or orchidectomy) causes a significant increase in the synthesis of FSH and LH and the vacuolization of gonadotropin-secreting cells (castration cells).

Kallmann's syndrome consists in delayed or absent puberty and anosmia (impaired sense of smell). It is determined by mutations in genes whose encoded proteins are responsible for the migration of GnRH–secreting neurons to the hypothalamic arcuate nucleus and olfactory neurons to the olfactory bulb.

• **Thyroid-stimulating hormone (TSH**; or thyrotropin) regulates thyroid function. Thyrotropin-releasing hormone stimulates the release of TSH (and prolactin). Thyroid hormones triiodothyronine (T_3) and thyroxine (T_4) inhibit the release of TSH.

Hypothyroidism, characterized by reduced cell metabolism and temperature, is caused by deficient secretion of TSH and by the autoimmune disorder **Hashimoto's disease.** **Hyperthyroidism** is usually determined by an autoantibody directed against the TSH receptor in thyroid follicular cells (Graves' disease).

• **Adrenocorticotropic hormone (ACTH**; or corticotropin) stimulates growth and steroid synthesis in the zona fasciculata and zona reticularis of the adrenal cortex.

ACTH derives from the large precursor pro-opiomelanocortin (POMC) processed in the anterior hypophysis.

Corticotropin-releasing hormone (CRH) derived from neuroendocrine neurons of the paraventricular nuclei, which also produce antidiuretic hormone (ADH), stimulates the release of ACTH. This CRH stimulatory effect is potentiated by ADH and angiotensin II (ANGII). High levels of cortisol prevent the release of CRH or ACTH.

Cushing's disease, caused by an ACTH-producing adenoma of the hypophysis, results in the overproduction of cortisol by cells of the zona fasciculata of the adrenal cortex, obesity, osteoporosis, and muscle wasting.

• **Neurohypophysis.** Three histologic components form the neurohypophysis:

(1) Pituicytes, astrocyte-like cells containing the intermediate filament protein glial fibrillary acidic protein and providing support to axons.

(2) Unmyelinated axons derived from neuroendocrine cells of the hypothalamic supraoptic and paraventricular nuclei forming the hypothalamic hypophyseal tract.

(3) Fenestrated capillaries.

Axons display intermittent bulging segments called Herring bodies containing neuroendocrine secretory granules.

Each secretory granule consists of two components: the carrier protein neurophysin and the associated hormone ADH (also called arginine vasopressin) or oxytocin.

Oxytocin participates in the contraction of uterine smooth muscle during labor, and of myoepithelial cells in the lactating mammary alveoli to facilitate milk ejection. ADH regulates water excretion in the kidneys and, at a higher concentration, is also a potent vasoconstrictor.

Neurogenic diabetes insipidus occurs when the secretion of ADH is reduced. It is caused by severe head injury, an invasive tumor disrupting the hypothalamic hypophysial tract, or the autoimmune destruction of ADH-

producing neurons. Polyuria is a common clinical finding.

Nephrogenic diabetes insipidus occurs in certain chronic renal diseases that are not responsive to ADH.

• **Pineal gland.** The pineal gland is an endocrine organ consisting of cells with a neurosecretory function and without direct nerve connection with the brain.

The pineal gland is supplied by postganglionic sympathetic nerve fibers derived from the superior cervical ganglia (SCG). Preganglionic fibers to the SCG derive from the lateral column of the spinal cord.

The pineal gland develops from a saccular outpocketing of the posterior diencephalic roof in the midline of the third ventricle. It contains cells called pinealocytes, arranged in cords and clusters, and supporting glial-like interstitial cells.

The pinealocyte displays cytoplasmic extensions with bulbar endings. These cell processes end close to a capillary. Pinealocytes contain abundant mitochondria and characteristic multiple ribbon synapses.

Remember that ribbon synapses are also seen in photoreceptor cells of the retina and in hair cells of the inner ear.

An important landmark of the pineal gland are calcified deposits called corpora arenacea ("brain sand").

Functional aspects of the pineal gland. The pineal gland can be regarded as a neuroendocrine transducer collecting information sent from the retina.

During daylight hours, the retinal photoreceptor cells are hyperpolarized and the release of norepinephrine is inhibited. Consequently, the retinohypothalamic–pineal system is resting and little melatonin is secreted.

When darkness starts, the photoreceptors release norepinephrine, that activates $\alpha 1$- and $\beta 1$-adrenergic receptors in the pinealocytes to increase their melatonin synthetic activity.

The neural input to the pineal gland is norepinephrine, and the output is melatonin. The function of pinealocytes is regulated by β-adrenergic receptors. The metabolic activity of pinealocytes is inhibited by β-adrenergic antagonists.

Melatonin is synthesized from tryptophan and immediately secreted into the bloodstream. Serotonin, a neurotransmitter, is a precursor of melatonin. Serotonin is acetylated and then methylated to produce melatonin.

Serotonin N-acetyltransferase is the rate-limiting enzyme in melatonin synthesis. In fact, exposure to light or administration of β-adrenergic blocking agents causes a rapid decrease in N-acetyltransferase and a consequent decline in melatonin synthesis.

The retinohypothalamic tract conducts light signals from the retina, in particular from melanopsin-producing ganglion cells that function as luminance detectors, to the hypothalamic suprachiasmatic nucleus (SCN), regarded as the circadian clock. Neurons of the SCN that contain melatonin Mel1A and

Mel1B receptors, are circadian oscillators connected to specialized melanopsin-producing ganglion cells of the retina.

The following signaling steps are involved:

(1) Signals from the SCN are delivered to the intermediolateral cell column of the thoracic spinal cord by the hypothalamospinal tract.

(2) Signals from the spinal cord are transmitted to the superior cervical ganglion by preganglionic sympathetic fibers.

(3) Signals from the superior cervical ganglion are conducted by postganglionic sympathetic fibers traveling in association with blood vessels entering the pineal gland.

As noted earlier, the neural input to the pineal gland is norepinephrine, and the output is melatonin.

Remember that retinal photoreceptors are the starting point of the neuronal input to pinealocytes.

The retina has two functions:

(1) The detection of light for the formation of images by transforming photon energy into an electrical signal, as we discuss in Chapter 9, Sensory Organs: Vision and Hearing.

(2) Non-image forming (NIF) visual functions required for adjusting the internal circadian clock to light and sleep. NIF visual functions involve a subset of melanopsin-producing retinal ganglion cells as indicated above. These cells, with NIF visual functions, are called intrinsically photosensitive retinal ganglion cells (ipRGCs). The ipRGCs function as luminance detectors resetting the circadian oscillators.

Two clinical conditions related to the function of the pineal gland are significant:

(1) Seasonal affective disorder (SAD) is a type of depression related to the shorter day length of the winter months. SAD has been observed in patients with bipolar disorders, characterized by a significant switch in mood between periods of mania and depression.

This indicates that ipRGCs and the SCN, in addition to its circadian pacemaker function, project to several regions of the brain to drive rhythms involved in inducing sleep or influence mood.

(2) Jet lag, a sleep disorder associated with fatigue, insomnia, diminished physical performance, and disorientation experienced by many travelers, is caused by a temporary lack of alignment between the circadian rhythm and local time.

Appropriately timed exposure to light and/or the administration of melatonin are strategies for jet lag treatment.

Pineocytomas are tumors of the pineal gland. About 10 percent of lesions of the pineal gland are essentially benign, including pineal cysts. Another 10 percent of tumors are relatively benign, including low-grade gliomas.

The remaining 80 percent of pineal region neoplasms are highly malignant lesions. These include germ cell tumors (pineal germinoma), embryonal carcinoma, and malignant pineoblastoma.

Pineocytomas are associated with **precocious puberty** and with a neurologic disorder known as **Parinaud's syndrome** (paralysis of upward gaze, looking steadily in one direction, pupillary areflexia to light, paralysis of convergence, and wide-based gait).

These findings provide support for the hypothesis that melatonin participates in the timing of puberty.

19. Endocrine System

The endocrine system is represented by a group of single cells and glands that produce and secrete peptide and steroid hormones in the bloodstream to modulate many functions of the body. Several endocrine glands, like the thyroid gland and the adrenal glands, are regulated by the hypothalamic–hypophyseal system. Others, like the parathyroid glands, responds to variations in the blood levels of calcium; and the main function of the pancreatic islet of Langerhans is under the control sugar levels in blood. In addition, there is a massive population of single endocrine cells distributed in several tissue of the body that are independent of the hypothalamic–hypophyseal system and have a significant functional and pathologic role. One of these cells is the C cell, housed in the thyroid gland and whose secretory product, calcitonin, balances the calcium regulatory function of the parathyroid glands. The cell target of the parathyroid glands is the osteoblast, whereas C cell targets the osteoclast. This chapter covers the structure and function of the thyroid gland, the adrenal glands, the parathyroid glands, the C cells, and the islets of Langerhans and provides insights concerning clinical and pathologic conditions.

Thyroid gland

Development of the thyroid gland

The thyroid gland (Greek *thyreos,* shield; *eidos,* form) develops as a median **endodermal** downgrowth at the base of the tongue. A transient structure, the **thyroglossal duct**, connects the developing gland to its point of origin, the **foramen cecum**, at the back of the tongue.

The thyroglossal duct disappears completely, leaving the thyroid to develop as a ductless gland. Persistent thyroglossal duct tissue remnants may generally give rise to a **cysts** in the front area of the neck that looks like a lump. Surgical removal of an enlarging thyroglossal cyst in children may be necessary to alleviate breathing and swallowing problems and the prevention of infections and even malignant transformation during adulthood.

Maternal thyroid hormone is transferred to the fetus across the placenta throughout the first trimester of pregnancy. High levels of thyroid hormone are found in the fetal cerebral cortex between weeks 12 and 20.

At about week 22, the fetal thyroid gland responds to **thyroid-stimulating hormone (TSH)** by producing **endogenous thyroid hormone** to enable perinatal brain development.

The congenital absence of the thyroid gland causes irreversible neurologic damage in the infant (**cretinism**). In adults, thyroid dysfunction correlates with neurologic and behavioral disorders.

Histologic organization of the thyroid gland

The thyroid gland consists of two lobes connected by a narrow band of thyroid tissue called the **isthmus.**

The thyroid gland is located below the larynx and the lobes rest on the sides of the trachea. The larynx provides a convenient landmark for locating the thyroid gland. Remember that the **recurrent laryngeal nerves** are closely related to the thyroid gland, an anatomic relationship of importance when a thyroidectomy procedure is required.

The thyroid gland is surrounded by a connective tissue capsule. Two pairs of parathyroid glands, designated as superior and inferior parathyroid glands, are located on the lateral lobes of the thyroid gland.

Each lobe of the thyroid gland consists of numerous **follicles**. The **thyroid follicle**, or acinus, is the structural and functional unit of the gland.

A thyroid follicle consists of a single layer of cuboidal epithelial cells, the **follicular epithelium** (Figures 19-1 and 19-2), enclosing a central lumen containing a **colloid** substance, The colloid is rich in **thyroglobulin**, an iodinated glycoprotein, yielding a periodic acid–Schiff (PAS)–positive reaction.

The follicular epithelium also contains about 10% of scattered **parafollicular cells**, also called **C cells**. C cells, derived from the **neural crest**, contain small cytoplasmic **granules** representing the stored hormone **calcitonin** (hence the designation C cells).

When the thyroid gland is **hypoactive**, as in **dietary iodide deficiency**, the follicle is enlarged with colloid. Because no **triiodothyronine** (T_3) or **thyroxine** (T_4) is made to exert a negative feedback, TSH synthesis and secretion increase. TSH stimulates growth and vascularization of the thyroid gland. Consequently, the gland enlarges.

When the thyroid gland is **active**, the follicular epithelium is columnar, and **colloid droplets** may be seen within the cells as well as large apical pseudopodia and microvilli (see Figure 19-2).

The thyroid epithelium is surrounded by a basal lamina and reticular fibers. A network of vasomotor and sympathetic nerve fibers and blood vessels, including fenestrated capillaries, can be observed in the connective tissue among thyroid follicles.

Function of the thyroid gland

In contrast to other endocrine organs, which have a

Figure 19-1. **Histology of the thyroid gland**

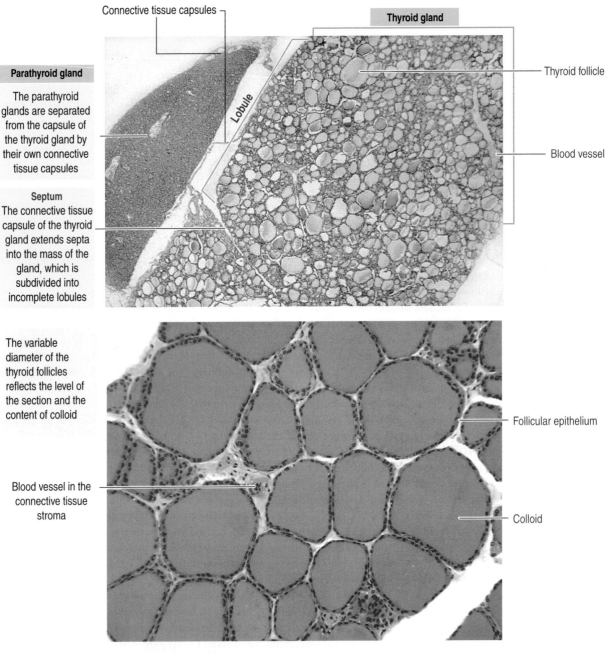

Connective tissue capsules

Thyroid gland

Parathyroid gland

The parathyroid glands are separated from the capsule of the thyroid gland by their own connective tissue capsules

Thyroid follicle

Lobule

Blood vessel

Septum
The connective tissue capsule of the thyroid gland extends septa into the mass of the gland, which is subdivided into incomplete lobules

The variable diameter of the thyroid follicles reflects the level of the section and the content of colloid

Follicular epithelium

Blood vessel in the connective tissue stroma

Colloid

Area of colloid resorption

A **C cell** can be distinguished from surrounding follicular cells by its pale cytoplasm.

Follicular epithelium
In the resting follicle, the follicular epithelium is simple low cuboidal, or squamous. During their active secretory phase, the cells become columnar

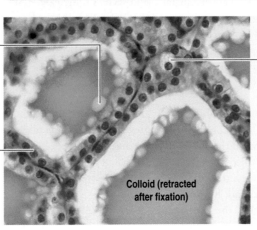

Two more effective identification approaches are:
1. Immunocytochemistry, using an antibody to calcitonin.

2. Electron microscopy, to visualize calcitonin-containing cytoplasmic granules.

Colloid (retracted after fixation)

Figure 19-2. **Structure of the thyroid follicular cells**

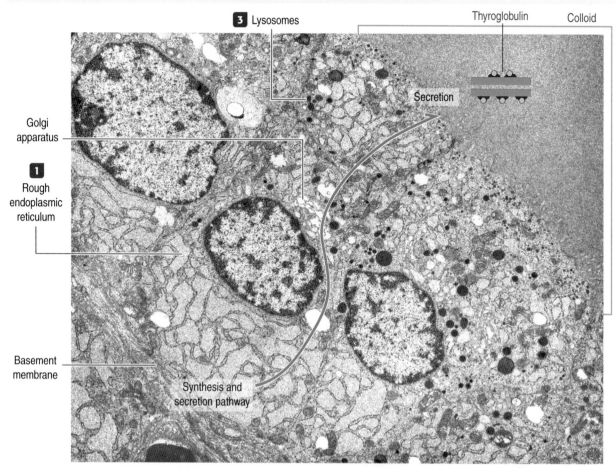

Lysosomes

Thyroglobulin   Colloid

Secretion

Golgi apparatus

1

Rough endoplasmic reticulum

Basement membrane

Synthesis and secretion pathway

1 The synthesis of thyroglobulin, the precursor of triiodothyronine (T_3) and thyroxine (T_4), starts in the rough endoplasmic reticulum (RER). The cisternae of the RER are distended by the newly synthesized precursor and the cytoplasmic regions are reduced to very narrow areas. Thyroglobulin molecules are glycosylated in the Golgi apparatus.

2 Under the light microscope, thyroglobulin synthetic activity can be visualized in the cytoplasm of the follicular cells as optically clear vesicular spaces.

3 The apical domain of the follicular cells displays abundant lysosomes involved in the processing of the prohormone thyroglobulin into thyroid hormones.

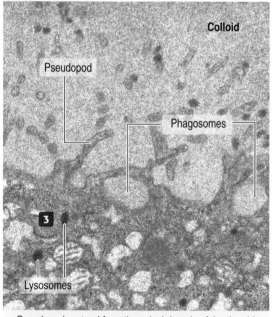

Colloid

Pseudopod

Phagosomes

3

Lysosomes

Pseudopods extend from the apical domain of the thyroid follicular cells and, after surrounding a portion of the colloid (thyroglobulin), organize an intracellular phagosome. Lysosomes fuse with the phagosome and initiate the proteolytic breakdown of thyroglobulin while moving toward the basal domain of the follicular cell.

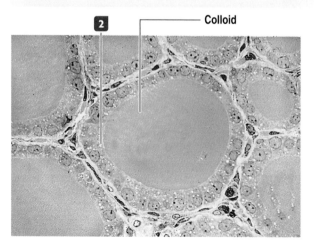

2   Colloid

Figure 19-3. Synthesis and secretion of thyroid hormones T₃ and T₄

4 At the **apical plasma membrane**, **thyroid peroxidase** is activated and converts **iodide** into **iodine**. Two iodine atoms are linked to each tyrosyl residue. Iodination occurs within the lumen of the thyroid follicle.

After proteolytic processing, one monoiodotyrosine peptide combines with diiodotyrosine to form **T₃ (triiodothyronine)**. Two diiodotyrosines combine to form **T₄ (thyroxine)**. One iodinated thyroglobulin molecule yields four molecules of T₃ and T₄.

Clinical significance: Propylthiouracil and **methyl mercaptoimidazole (MMI)** inhibit thyroid peroxidase–mediated iodination of tyrosine in thyroglobulin.

5 A droplet in the colloid of the thyroid follicle, containing iodinated thyroglobulin, is endocytosed by a pseudopod extension of the apical domain of a follicular epithelial cell. The **intracellular colloid droplet**, guided by cytoskeletal components, fuses with a **lysosome**. T₃ and T₄ molecules are released by the proteolytic action of lysosomal enzymes.

Clinical significance: Propylthiouracil can block the conversion of T₄ to T₃ in peripheral tissues (liver).

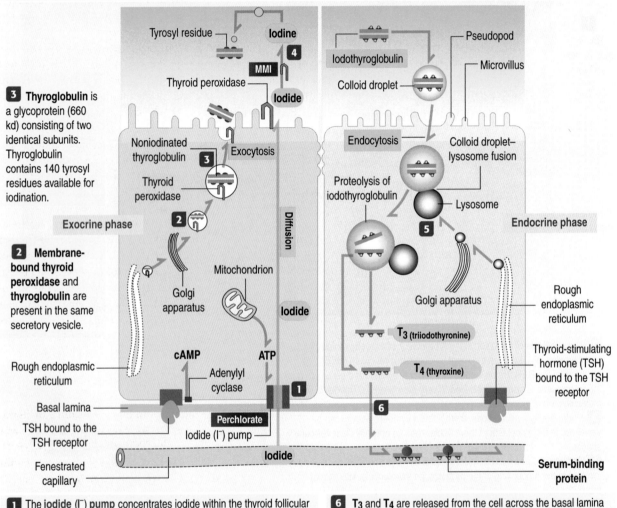

3 **Thyroglobulin** is a glycoprotein (660 kd) consisting of two identical subunits. Thyroglobulin contains 140 tyrosyl residues available for iodination.

2 **Membrane-bound thyroid peroxidase** and **thyroglobulin** are present in the same secretory vesicle.

1 The **iodide (I⁻) pump** concentrates iodide within the thyroid follicular cell 20- to 100-fold above serum levels. An Na⁺, K⁺-dependent ATPase and adenosine triphosphate (ATP) provide the energy for iodide transport.

Clinical significance: Thyroid follicular cell activity can be determined by measuring **radioactive iodine uptake (RAIU)**. Radiation thyroidectomy can be implemented by using larger amounts of radioactive iodine in cases of thyroid hyperfunction. Also, the iodide pump can be inhibited by **perchlorate**, a competitive anion.

6 T₃ and T₄ are released from the cell across the basal lamina of the thyroid follicle into a **fenestrated capillary** and bind to **serum-binding proteins**. Tissue-specific **deiodinases** expressed in peripheral tissues can increase local concentrations of T₃ from circulating T₄. T₃ has a shorter half-life (18 hours) than T₄ (5 to 7 days). T₃ is 2 to 10 times more active than T₄. Thyroid hormone action is predominantly mediated by **thyroid hormone receptors** (THRs), which are encoded by the thyroid hormone receptor α *(THRA)* and thyroid hormone receptor β *(THRB)* genes.

limited storage capacity, the production of thyroid hormones depends on the follicular storage of the prohormone thyroglobulin in the colloid.

A characteristic feature of the thyroid follicular epithelium is its ability to concentrate iodide from the blood and synthesize the hormones T₃ and T₄.

The synthesis and secretion of thyroid hormones involve two phases (Figure 19-3):

1. An **exocrine phase**.
2. An **endocrine phase**.

Both phases are regulated by TSH by a mechanism that includes receptor binding and cyclic adenosine monophosphate (cAMP) production, as discussed in Chapter 3, Cell Signaling.

The **exocrine phase** (see Figure 19-3) consists of:

1. The uptake of inorganic **iodide** from the blood, stimulated by TSH.

2. The synthesis of **thyroglobulin**.

3. The incorporation of **iodine** into tyrosyl residues of thyroglobulin by **thyroid peroxidase**.

The uptake of iodide requires an adenosine triphosphate (ATP)–driven iodide pump present in the basal plasma membrane of the follicular cells. This active transport system is referred to as the **iodide trap**. Intracellular iodide rapidly diffuses against concentration and electrical gradients to end up in the colloid. Anions, such as **perchlorate** (ClO_4^-), are used clinically as a **competitive inhibitor of the iodide pump** to block iodide uptake by the thyroid follicular cell.

The rough endoplasmic reticulum and Golgi apparatus are sites involved in the synthesis and glycosylation of **thyroglobulin**, a 660-kd glycoprotein composed of two identical subunits. Thyroglobulin is packed in secretory vesicles and released by exocytosis into the colloidal lumen. Thyroglobulin contains about 140 tyrosine residues available for iodination.

Thyroid peroxidase, the enzyme responsible for the iodination of thyroglobulin, is a heme-containing glycoprotein anchored in the membrane of the same secretory vesicle that contains thyroglobulin. After exocytosis, thyroid peroxidase is exposed at the luminal surface of the thyroid follicular epithelium.

Thyroid peroxidase, activated during exocytosis, **oxidizes iodide to iodine within the colloid**; the iodine is then transferred to acceptor tyrosyl residues of thyroglobulin.

Thyroid peroxidase activity and the iodination process can be inhibited by **propylthiouracil** and **methyl mercaptoimidazole (MMI)**. These antithyroid drugs primarily interfere with the synthesis of thyroid hormones in hyperactive glands.

The **endocrine phase** starts with the TSH-stimulated endocytosis of iodinated thyroglobulin into the follicular cell (see Figure 19-3):

1. **Colloid droplets** are enveloped by apical **pseudopods** and internalized to become colloid-containing vesicles.

2. Cytoskeletal components guide the colloid droplets to lysosomes, which fuse with the colloid droplets.

3. **Lysosomal enzymes degrade iodothyroglobulin to release T$_3$, the active form of the hormone, T$_4$,** and other intermediate products. Iodotyrosines, amino acids, and sugars are recycled within the cell.

4. Thyroid hormones are then released across the basal lamina of the thyroid follicular epithelium and gain access to **serum carrier proteins** within the fenestrated capillaries.

T$_3$ has a shorter half-life (18 hours), is **more potent**, and **less abundant than T$_4$**. The half-life of T$_4$ is 5 to 7 days and represents about 90% of the secreted thyroid hormones.

Tissue-specific **deiodinases** increase the local concentrations of T$_3$ from circulating T$_4$. There are three deiodinases:

1. **Deiodinase 1** is found primarily in the liver.

2. **Deiodinase 2** is only expressed in astrocytes and tanycytes, glial cell-derived located in the hypothalamus.

3. **Deiodinase 3** is selectively expressed in neurons. Deiodinase 3 can also inactivate T$_4$ and T$_3$ to T$_3$ and T$_2$ by inner ring deiodination. Inactivation serves to down-regulate local concentrations of thyroid hormone and protect the neurons from excessive levels of thyroid hormone.

In the central nervous system, thyroid hormones cross the blood-brain barrier utilizing transporters of the choroid plexus cells and through gaps between the end feet of astrocytes that fail to complete cover the brain capillaries.

The primary site of action of T$_3$, and to a lesser extent T$_4$, is the **cell nucleus**. T$_3$ binds to thyroid hormone receptor bound to a specific DNA region, called **thyroid hormone–responsive element (TRE)**, to induce or repress specific gene transcription. In cardiocytes, thyroid hormone regulates the expression of genes encoding **phospholamban** in the sarcoplasmic reticulum, β-adrenergic receptors, Ca^{2+}-ATPase, and others.

Clinical significance: Graves' disease and hypothyroidism

Graves' disease, an **autoimmune disorder predominant in women, is caused by an antibody that acts as an agonist on the TSH receptor.** (Figure 19-4). Binding of autoantibodies to TSH receptors results in the unregulated synthesis of thyroid hormone.

Toxic adenoma and **multinodular goiter** (see Box 19-A) also cause unregulated synthesis of thyroid hormone but this effect is triggered by a **mutation in the *TSH receptor* gene**, which results in constitutive activation. Spontaneous remission occurs in approximately 30% of patients with Graves' disease but not in patients with toxic adenoma and multinodular goiter. A non-toxic adenoma is not associated with high thyroid hormone production.

Thyroid follicular cells in Graves' disease show hypertrophy and hyperplasia and secrete large amounts of thyroid hormones in the blood circulation in an unregulated fashion. Serum TSH level is suppressed and levels of serum T$_4$ and T$_3$ are elevated.

Enlargement of the thyroid gland (**goiter**), bulging

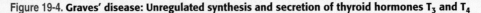

Graves' disease: Pathogenesis

Excessive production of thyroid hormone is caused by the activation of thyroid stimulating hormone receptors (TSHRs) by an autoimmune response (antibodies produced against the TSHR).

Inflammatory cells in the stroma of the thyroid gland produce cytokines (interleukin-1, tumor necrosis factor–α, and interferon-γ), that stimulate thyroid cells to produce cytokines, thus reinforcing the thyroidal autoimmune process. Antithyroid drugs reduce the production of cytokines (immunosuppressive effect), leading to remission in some patients.

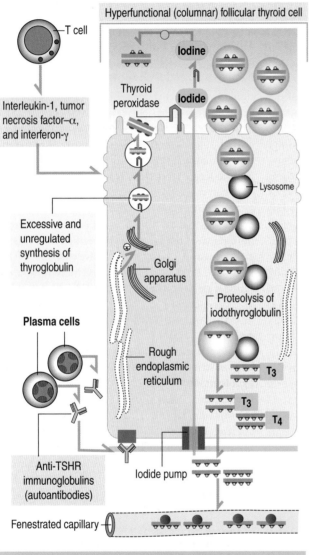

Exophthalmos

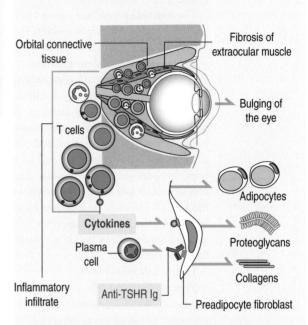

Graves' ophthalmopathy is characterized by inflammation of the extraocular muscles and an increase in orbital adipose and connective tissue. Circulating anti-TSHR Igs bind to the specific receptor expressed by fibroblasts in the retrobulbar tissue.

Cytokines produced by T cells in the inflammatory infiltrate stimulate adipogenesis from preadipocyte fibroblasts.

Fibroblasts produce proteoglycans and collagen fibers leading to retrobulbar edema and fibrosis of the extraocular muscles.

Myocardial contractility

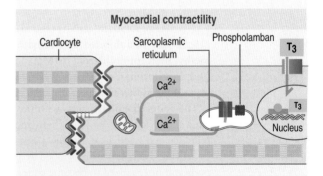

Triiodothyronine (T₃) enters the nucleus of a cardiocyte, binds to its nuclear receptors, and then binds to thyroid hormone response element in target genes.

T₃ stimulates phospholamban, a protein involved in the release and uptake of Ca^{2+} into the sarcoplasmic reticulum. This step is critical for systolic contraction and diastolic relaxation. The activity of phospholamban is regulated by its phosphorylation. Increased diastolic function in patients with hyperthyroidism is related to the role of phospholamban in thyroid hormone–mediated changes in the contractility of cardiac muscle.

Graves' disease: Clinical characteristics

Two characteristics of Graves' disease are exophthalmos and cardiac manifestations (palpitations and tachycardia).

Exophthalmos consists in the presence of an inflammatory infiltrate (T cells, macrophages, and neutrophils) in the extraocular muscles and orbital tissue. Cytokines (produced by T cells) and anti-TSHR immunoglobulins (Igs) (produced by extraocular plasma cells) stimulate the function of orbital fibroblasts and their differentiation into adipocytes.

Overproduction of fat and the hygroscopic nature of proteoglycans contribute to the development of exophthalmos.

of the eyes (**exophthalmos**; see Figure 19-4), **tachycardia**, **warm skin**, and **fine finger tremors** are typical clinical features. Toxic adenoma and multinodular goiter are not associated with exophthalmos.

From a functional perspective, an **excess of thyroid hormones increases the basal metabolic and cardiac rate** and **the consumption of oxygen and nutrients**.

1. A **high metabolic condition** increases appetite.

2. **Increased body heat production**, determined by high oxygen consumption, makes patients feel hot.

3. Tachycardia is one of the consequences of thyroid hormone actions in heart. **Increased cardiac rate** is caused by the up-regulation of **β1 adrenergic receptors** in cardiocytes in the sinoatrial node stimulated by thyroid hormones. **Increase in cardiac muscle contractibility and cardiac output** is triggered by the up-regulation of β1 adrenergic receptors in the ventricular cardiac muscle. The active transport of Ca^{2+} into the lumen of the sarcoplasmic reticulum of cardiocytes is controlled by **phospholamban**, whose activity is regulated by thyroid hormones (see Figure 19-4).

In summary, the classical symptoms of **thyrotoxicosis** are found in patients with Graves' disease. Thyrotoxicosis means an excess of thyroid hormone in the body.

How are patients with Graves' disease treated?

The objective is to neutralize the effects of thyroid hormones by decreasing their synthesis and actions.

1. Thyroid hormone synthesis can be inhibited with drugs (see Figure 19-3).

2. Radioiodine can be given orally as a single dose of ¹³¹I-labeled sodium iodide ($Na^{131}I$) in liquid or capsule form. Beta ray emissions of the radionuclide causes tissue necrosis, resulting in the functional reduction or inactivation of follicular thyroid cells over the course of 6 to 18 weeks, when thyroid function normalizes (**euthyroidism**: characterized by normal serum levels of thyroid hormone).

3. Use of **propranolol**, a β-adrenergic antagonist, to block β1 adrenergic receptors to manage tachycardia. This treatment also offsets increases in cardiac output and arterial blood pressure as well as the elevated thermogenesis caused by the hyperadrenergic state.

Surgery is required in patients with toxic adenoma and toxic multinodular goiter.

In the **adult**, hypothyroidism is generally caused by a thyroid disease. A **decrease** in the **basal metabolic rate**, **hypothermia**, and **cold intolerance** are observed. Decreased sweating and cutaneous vasoconstriction make the skin dry and cool. Afflicted individuals tend to feel cold in a warm room.

Hypothyroidism in the adult is manifested by coarse skin with a puffy appearance due to the accumulation of proteoglycans and retention of fluid in the dermis of the skin (**myxedema**) and muscle. Cardiac output is reduced, and the pulse rate slows down. Except for developmental disturbances, most symptoms are reversed when the thyroid disorder is corrected.

As previously mentioned, the requirement of thyroid hormone for development is most apparent in the **central nervous system**, where severe thyroid hormone deficiency in fetal and neonatal periods results in **cretinism**, a disorder characterized by **mental retardation**, **deafness**, and **ataxia**. These conditions are irreversible if not treated soon after birth.

Hashimoto's thyroiditis, also called **chronic lymphocytic thyroiditis** or **autoimmune thyroiditis** (see Box 19-A), is a **disease** associated with **hypothyroidism** and **accumulation of lymphocytes in the stroma of the thyroid gland**.

Hashimoto's thyroiditis is caused by autoantibodies targeting **thyroid peroxidase** and **thyroglobulin** (anti–thyroid peroxidase [anti–TPO] and anti-thyroglobulin [anti–TG] antibodies). Progressive destruction of the thyroid follicles leads to a decrease in the function of the thyroid gland. The level of T_4 in blood is lower than normal, whereas the level of TSH are above normal. The size of the thyroid gland is enlarged (goiter). Patients are treated with synthetic T_4 (Synthroid).

Additional inflammatory conditions of the thyroid gland includes de **Quervain's thyroiditis** and **Riedel's thyroiditis**.

Finally, **papillary carcinoma** is the most frequent malignant tumor of the thyroid gland. This tumor is locally invasive and spreads to cervical lymph nodes. **Follicular carcinoma**, is the second most frequent tumor of the thyroid gland (see Box 19-A). It is a slow growing tumor that usually spreads to bone by the hematogenous route.

Box 19-A | Concept mapping: Pathology of the thyroid gland

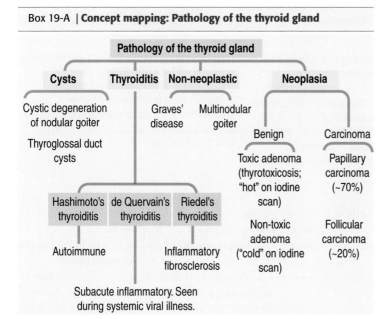

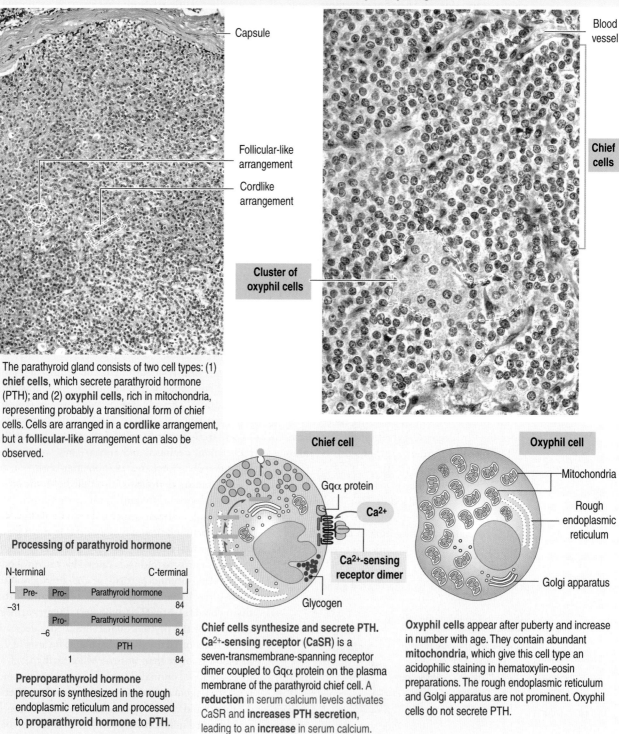

Figure 19-5. **Structure and function of the parathyroid gland**

Capsule

Follicular-like
arrangement

Cordlike
arrangement

Cluster of
oxyphil cells

Blood
vessel

Chief
cells

The parathyroid gland consists of two cell types: (1) **chief cells**, which secrete parathyroid hormone (PTH); and (2) **oxyphil cells**, rich in mitochondria, representing probably a transitional form of chief cells. Cells are arranged in a **cordlike** arrangement, but a **follicular-like** arrangement can also be observed.

Processing of parathyroid hormone

N-terminal   C-terminal

| Pre- | Pro- | Parathyroid hormone |
−31   84

| Pro- | Parathyroid hormone |
−6   84

| PTH |
1   84

Preproparathyroid hormone precursor is synthesized in the rough endoplasmic reticulum and processed to **proparathyroid hormone** to PTH.

Chief cell

Gqα protein

Ca²⁺

Ca²⁺-sensing
receptor dimer

Glycogen

Chief cells synthesize and secrete PTH. Ca²⁺-sensing receptor (CaSR) is a seven-transmembrane-spanning receptor dimer coupled to Gqα protein on the plasma membrane of the parathyroid chief cell. A **reduction** in serum calcium levels activates CaSR and **increases PTH secretion**, leading to an **increase** in serum calcium.

Oxyphil cell

Mitochondria

Rough
endoplasmic
reticulum

Golgi apparatus

Oxyphil cells appear after puberty and increase in number with age. They contain abundant **mitochondria**, which give this cell type an acidophilic staining in hematoxylin-eosin preparations. The rough endoplasmic reticulum and Golgi apparatus are not prominent. Oxyphil cells do not secrete PTH.

Calcium regulation

Ca^{2+} is found inside and outside cells, is a major component of the skeleton, is required for muscle contraction, blood clotting, nerve impulse transmission, and enzymatic activities. Ca^{2+} is an essential mediator in cell signaling (for example, through **calcium-binding calmodulin**).

Ca^{2+} homeostasis is regulated by:

1. **Parathyroid hormone (PTH)**, secreted from the parathyroid glands. PTH acts on **bone** and the **kidneys** to **raise Ca^{2+} levels in blood**.

2. **Calcitonin**, produced by C cells lodged in the thyroid gland, **lowers Ca^{2+} levels in blood**.

3. **Vitamin D** (calcitriol, or 1,25-dihydroxychole-calciferol) enhances the uptake of Ca^{2+} by the small intestine by stimulating the synthesis of Ca^{2+}-

binding protein **calbindin** by intestinal epithelial cells (enterocytes). These two last aspects will be discussed later in this chapter.

The key element in monitoring extracellular Ca^{2+} levels is the extracellular **Ca^{2+}-sensing receptor** (**CaSR**) of the parathyroid chief or principal cells.

Parathyroid glands
Development of the parathyroid glands

The four parathyroid glands derive from the third and fourth branchial pouches. The third branchial pouch differentiates into the inferior parathyroid glands and the thymus. The fourth branchial pouch develops into the superior parathyroid glands and the ultimobranchial body.

The parathyroid glands are on the posterolateral regions of the thyroid gland, located between the thyroid capsule and the surrounding cervical connective tissue. The yellow color of the adipose tissue-containing parathyroid glands may be confused with surrounding fat. The accidental surgical removal of the normal parathyroid glands during thyroid surgery (thyroidectomy) causes **tetany**, characterized by spasms of the thoracic and laryngeal muscles, leading to asphyxia and death.

Histologic organization of the parathyroid glands

The parenchyma of the parathyroid glands consists of two cell populations supplied by sinusoidal capillaries (Figure 19-5):

1. The more numerous **chief** or **principal cell**.

2. The **oxyphil** or **acidophilic cell**.

Cells are arranged in cordlike or follicular-like clusters. **Chief** or **principal cells** contain cytoplasmic granules with PTH, an 84-amino-acid peptide derived from a large precursor of 115 amino acids (**preproPTH**). This precursor gives rise to **proPTH** (90 amino acids), which is processed by a proteolytic enzyme in the Golgi apparatus into **PTH**. PTH is stored in **secretory granules**. Magnesium is essential for PTH secretion. PTH is secreted into the blood and has a half-life of about 5 minutes. Serum Ca^{2+} levels normally average **9.5 mg/dL**.

Oxyphil or **acidophilic cells** contain abundant mitochondria, which give this cell its typical pink-reddish stain. Oxyphils may represent transitional chief cells.

Signal transduction mediated by CaSR

A **CaSR dimer** is present in the plasma membrane of chief cells. CaSR activates **Gqα**, a subunit of heterotrimeric **G proteins**.

The G protein–linked cascade stimulates the action of **phospholipase C**. Phospholipase C hydrolyzes phosphatidylinositol 4,5-bisphosphate (PIP2) to release intracellular IP3 (inositol trisphosphate) and diacylglycerol (DAG). IP3 and DAG trigger the release of Ca^{2+} from intracellular storage sites followed by a flux of extracellular Ca^{2+} into the cytosol of the chief cells.

The increase of intracellular Ca^{2+} levels prevents PTH, contained in the secretory granules, to be released. An **increase** in serum Ca^{2+} levels (**hypercalcemia**) triggers intracellular signaling **suppressing** the secretion of PTH, with the consequent decrease in the serum Ca^{2+} concentration. When the serum Ca^{2+} concentration decreases (**hypocalcemia**), the secretion of PTH is **stimulated**, resulting in an increase in serum Ca^{2+}. Magnesium, like calcium, can activate CaSR and suppress PTH release.

In most cells, Ca^{2+} enters a cell through a membrane-associated channel. Chief cells are rather unusual because Ca^{2+} is a ligand for the CaSR resulting in the activation of Gqα protein subunit.

Functions of the parathyroid hormone

PTH regulates the Ca^{2+} and PO_4^{3-} balance in blood by acting on two main sites:

1. In **bone tissue**, PTH stimulates the **resorption of mineralized bone by osteoclasts** and the release of Ca^{2+} into the blood.

2. In the **uriniferous tubules**, PTH activates the **production of active vitamin D (calcitriol)** by stimulating the activity of **1α-hydroxylase**. Vitamin D, in turn, **stimulates the intestinal resorption of Ca^{2+}**. As you can see, PTH regulates **indirectly** Ca^{2+} levels by inducing the synthesis of an enzyme involved in the production of the active vitamin D metabolite in the kidneys.

When Ca^{2+} levels are low, PTH reestablishes homeostasis by acting on **osteoblasts** to induce osteoclastogenesis. As already discussed, PTH binds to a cell surface receptor of the osteoblast to regulate the synthesis of three proteins essential for the differentiation and function of osteoclasts (review the discussion of osteoclastogenesis in Chapter 4, Connective Tissue).

Clinical significance: Hyperparathyroidism and hypoparathyroidism

Hyperparathyroidism is caused by a functional benign tumor of the gland (**adenoma**). An abnormal increase in the secretion of PTH causes:

1. **Hypercalcemia** and **phosphaturia** (increased urinary excretion of PO_4^{3-} anions).

2. **Hypercalciuria** (increased urinary excretion of Ca^{2+}) leading to the formation of **renal stones** in the calyces of the kidneys. When stones descend to the ureter, there is severe pain, caused by spasmodic contraction of the smooth muscle, **hematuria** (blood in the urine), and infections of the renal tract (**pyelonephritis**).

Figure 19-6. **Synthesis and mechanism of action of calcitonin**

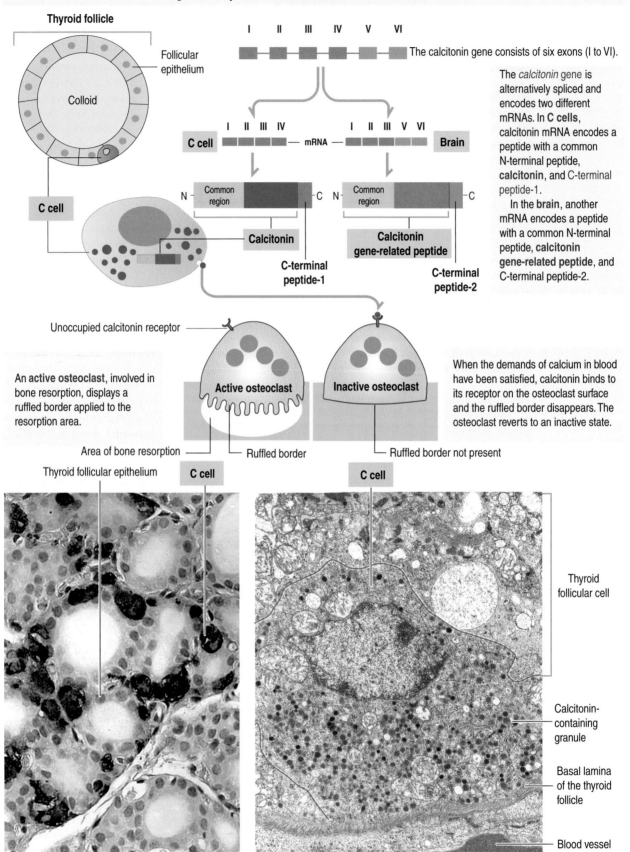

Thyroid follicle

Follicular epithelium

Colloid

C cell

The calcitonin gene consists of six exons (I to VI).

C cell I II III IV — mRNA — I II III V VI Brain

N – Common region – C

N – Common region – C

Calcitonin

C-terminal peptide-1

Calcitonin gene-related peptide

C-terminal peptide-2

The *calcitonin* gene is alternatively spliced and encodes two different mRNAs. In **C cells**, calcitonin mRNA encodes a peptide with a common N-terminal peptide, **calcitonin**, and C-terminal peptide-1.

In the **brain**, another mRNA encodes a peptide with a common N-terminal peptide, **calcitonin gene-related peptide**, and C-terminal peptide-2.

Unoccupied calcitonin receptor

An **active osteoclast**, involved in bone resorption, displays a ruffled border applied to the resorption area.

Active osteoclast

Inactive osteoclast

When the demands of calcium in blood have been satisfied, calcitonin binds to its receptor on the osteoclast surface and the ruffled border disappears. The osteoclast reverts to an inactive state.

Area of bone resorption — Ruffled border

Ruffled border not present

Thyroid follicular epithelium

C cell

C cell

Thyroid follicular cell

Calcitonin-containing granule

Basal lamina of the thyroid follicle

Blood vessel

Immunohistochemistry panel from Martín-Lacave I, García-Caballero T: Atlas of Immunohistochemistry. Madrid, Spain:Ed. Díaz de Santos, 2012.

3. **Hypercalcemia, the result of bone demineralization.** Extensive bone resorption results in the development of **cysts.**

Hypoparathyroidism is seen during the **inadvertent removal or irreversible damage (disrupted blood supply) to the parathyroid glands during surgery of the thyroid gland.**

The occurrence of hypoparathyroidism depends on the surgeon's experience and extent of thyroid resection determined by an underlying thyroid disease.

Within 24 to 48 hours of surgical removal of the parathyroid glands, hypocalcemia determines increased excitability of nervous tissue, including **paresthesia** (sensation of pins and needles), muscle cramping, twitching, and spasms. Attacks of **laryngospasm, bronchospasm, tetany,** and **seizures** occur. These severe symptoms require intravenous calcium therapy followed by continuous infusions to achieve safe ionized Ca^{2+} blood levels.

Neuromuscular symptoms caused by acute low blood Ca^{2+} concentration can be clinically tested:

1. A positive **Chvostek sign** is the twitching of facial muscles when the facial nerve is tapped.

2. **Trousseau sign** results in carpopedal spasm (contraction of the muscles and hands and feet) when a blood pressure cuff is applied.

Administration of vitamin D and calcium and magnesium supplements or synthetic PTH 1-34, given twice daily, correct these alterations.

Clinical significance: CaSR mutations

Inactivating mutations of the **CaSR are responsible for familial hypocalciuric hypercalcemia (FHH)** and **neonatal severe hyperparathyroidism (NSHPT).**

Heterozygous individuals with FHH have one defective copy of the *CaSR* gene. Because of the dimeric arrangement of the CaSR, the intact copy can rescue the function of the mutated copy.

Two defective copies (homozygous condition) detected in the newborn causes NSHPT, associated with severe hypercalcemia, bone demineralization and multiple fractures. NSHPT requires immediate parathyroidectomy early in life to prevent a fatal outcome.

An activating mutation of the CaSR, **autosomal dominant hypocalcemia,** leads the parathyroid gland into assuming that the Ca^{2+} serum level is elevated when it is not.

This condition determines a reduction in serum Ca^{2+} and PTH levels. In addition, CaSR can also be a target of autoimmunity determined by autoantibodies against the receptor that can either activate the CaSR or inactivate the CaSR (causing a syndrome similar to FHH).

Calcimimetic synthetic drugs, which activate CaSR, reduce pathologic elevations of PTH. CaSR-blocking drugs, called **calcilytics,** may be useful for the treatment of osteoporosis.

C cells (thyroid follicle)

C cells derive from **neural crest cells** and are associated with thyroid follicles. C cells:

1. Represent about 0.1% of the mass of thyroid tissue.

2. May be present within (or outside) the thyroid follicle but are not in contact with the colloid.

3. Produce **calcitonin,** encoded by a gene located on the short arm of chromosome 11 (Figure 19-6).

Calcitonin is a 32-amino-acid peptide derived from a 136-amino-acid precursor. It is stored in secretory granules. The calcitonin gene is also expressed in other tissues (hypothalamus and hypophysis), giving rise to a **calcitonin gene–related peptide (CGRP)** consisting of 37 amino acids. CGRP has neurotransmitter and vasodilator properties.

The main function of calcitonin is **to antagonize the effects of PTH. Calcitonin suppresses the mobilization of calcium from bone by osteoclasts** triggered by an increase in cAMP. Calcitonin secretion is stimulated by an **increase** in blood levels of calcium (hypercalcemia).

Vitamin D

Vitamin D_2 is formed in the **skin** by the conversion of 7-dehydrocholesterol to **cholecalciferol** following exposure to ultraviolet light (Figure 19-7). Cholecalciferol is then absorbed into the blood circulation and transported to the **liver** where it is converted to **25-hydroxycholecalciferol** by the addition of a hydroxyl group to the side chain.

In the **nephron,** two events can occur:

1. **Low calcium levels** and hypophosphatemia can determine PTH to stimulate the enzymatic activity of mitochondrial **1α-hydroxylase** to add another hydroxyl group to 25-hydroxycholecalciferol to form **1,25-dihydroxycholecalciferol (calcitriol),** the active form of vitamin D.

2. **High Ca^{2+} levels** can stimulate the enzymatic activity of **24-hydroxylase** to convert 25-hydroxycholecalciferol to biologically inactive 24,25-hydroxycholecalciferol.

Calcitriol (active form) and 24,25-hydroxycholecalciferol (inactive form) circulate in blood bound to a **vitamin D–binding protein.**

The main function of vitamin D is to stimulate the absorption of Ca^{2+} by the intestinal mucosa. Ca^{2+} is absorbed by:

1. **Transcellular absorption (active mechanism)** in the duodenum, an active process that involves the import of Ca^{2+} by enterocytes through **voltage-insensitive channels,** its transport across the cell, assisted by the carrier protein **calbindin,** and its release from

Figure 19-7. Metabolism of vitamin D and calcium absorption

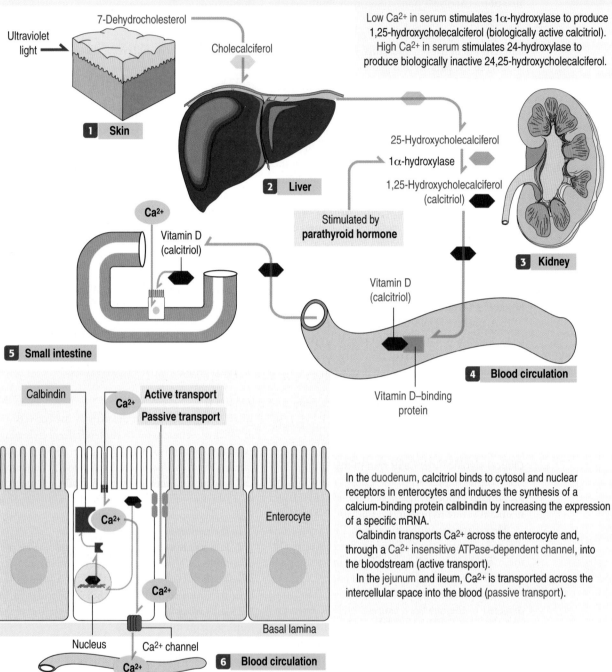

Low Ca^{2+} in serum stimulates 1α-hydroxylase to produce 1,25-hydroxycholecalciferol (biologically active calcitriol). High Ca^{2+} in serum stimulates 24-hydroxylase to produce biologically inactive 24,25-hydroxycholecalciferol.

7-Dehydrocholesterol

Ultraviolet light

Cholecalciferol

1 **Skin**

2 **Liver**

25-Hydroxycholecalciferol

1α-hydroxylase

1,25-Hydroxycholecalciferol (calcitriol)

Stimulated by **parathyroid hormone**

3 **Kidney**

Ca^{2+}

Vitamin D (calcitriol)

5 **Small intestine**

Vitamin D (calcitriol)

4 **Blood circulation**

Vitamin D–binding protein

Calbindin

Ca^{2+}

Active transport

Passive transport

Ca^{2+}

Enterocyte

Ca^{2+}

Ca^{2+}

Nucleus

Ca^{2+} channel

Basal lamina

6 **Blood circulation**

Ca^{2+}

In the duodenum, calcitriol binds to cytosol and nuclear receptors in enterocytes and induces the synthesis of a calcium-binding protein **calbindin** by increasing the expression of a specific mRNA.

Calbindin transports Ca^{2+} across the enterocyte and, through a Ca^{2+} insensitive ATPase-dependent channel, into the bloodstream (active transport).

In the jejunum and ileum, Ca^{2+} is transported across the intercellular space into the blood (passive transport).

---

the cell by a Ca^{2+}-ATPase–mediated mechanism.

2. **Paracellular absorption (passive mechanism)** in the jejunum and ileum, through tight junctions into the intercellular spaces, and into blood. A small fraction (about 10%) of Ca^{2+} absorption takes place in the large intestine by active and passive mechanisms.

Vitamin D, like all steroids, is transported to the **nucleus** of the intestinal cell to induce the synthesis of a calcium-binding protein, calbindin.

Clinical significance: Rickets and osteomalacia
In children, a deficiency of vitamin D causes **rickets**.

In adults, the corresponding clinical condition is **osteomalacia**. The calcification of the bone matrix osteoid is deficient in both conditions.

In **rickets**, bone remodeling is defective. The ends of the bones bulge (rachitic rosary at the costochondral junctions), and poor calcification of the long bones causes bending (bowlegs or knock-knees).

In **osteomalacia**, pain, partial bone fractures, and muscular weaknesses are typical in the adult.

Chronic renal failure or a congenital disorder, resulting in the lack of 1α-hydroxylase, can also cause rickets or osteomalacia.

Adrenal (suprarenal) glands

Development of the adrenal gland

The adrenal (or suprarenal) glands develop from two separate embryologic tissues:

1. The **neural crest ectoderm.**
2. The **mesoderm.**

During the sixth to seventh week of embryonic development:

1. Cells from the celomic epithelium aggregate on each side, between the developing gonads and the dorsal mesentery, to form the **fetal cortex.**

2. The medulla originates from neural crest cells migrating from the adjacent sympathetic ganglia into the medial region of the fetal cortex.

3. A layer of mesodermic cells surrounds the fetal cortex to form the **precursor of the adult adrenal cortex.**

4. Mesenchymal cells surround each developing adrenal gland and differentiate into fibroblasts that form the perirenal fascia and capsule. At this time, blood vessels and nerves of each adrenal gland develop.

At birth, the adrenal glands are 20 times relatively larger than they are in the adult. The zonae glomerulosa and fasciculata are present. They produce corticosteroids as well as androgen and estrogen precursors under the control of adrenocorticotropic hormone (ACTH) secreted by the fetal pituitary gland. The zona reticularis is not apparent. Modest amounts of epinephrine are produced by the adrenal medulla.

By the third month after birth, the celomic-derive fetal cortex regresses and disappears within the first year of life. The mesoderm-derived adrenal cortex precursor, consisting of the zona glomerulosa and the zona fasciculata, remains as the definitive cortex. The zona reticularis develops by the end of the third year.

Ectopic adrenocortical or medullary tissue may be found retroperitoneally, inferior to the kidneys, along the aorta, and in the pelvis. Aggregates of ectopic chromaffin cells, called **paraganglia,** can be a site of tumor growth (**pheochromocytoma**).

Functions of the fetal adrenal cortex

During the early stage of gestation, the adrenal cortex synthesizes **dehydroepiandrosterone,** a precursor of the synthesis of estrogen by the placenta. A lack of 3β-hydroxysteroid dehydrogenase activity prevents the synthesis of progesterone, glucocorticoids, and androstenedione.

The interaction between the fetal adrenal cortex and the placenta constitutes the **fetoplacental unit** (see Chapter 23, Fertilization, Placentation, and Lactation).

Glucocorticoids, either of maternal origin or synthesized from placental progesterone by the fetus, are essential for three main developmental events:

1. The production of surfactant by type II alveolar cells after the eighth month of fetal life.

2. The development of a functional hypothalamo-pituitary axis.

3. The induction of thymic involution.

Histologic organization of the adrenal cortex

The adrenal glands (Latin *ad*, near; *ren*, kidney) are associated with the superior poles of each kidney. Each gland consists of a yellowish outer cortex (80% to 90% of the gland) and a reddish inner medulla (10% to 20%).

Each adrenal gland is surrounded by perinephritic fat and enclosed by the renal fascia. A thin connective tissue capsule separates each gland from its associated kidney. An **arterial plexus,** derived from three adrenal arteries, is located in the adrenal gland capsule. We discuss later the functional significance of the adrenal vasculature.

Each adrenal gland has a **cortex** and a **medulla.**

The **adrenal cortex** consists of three concentric zones (Figures 19-8):

1. The **outermost layer of the cortex is the zona glomerulosa,** just under the capsule (see Figure 19-8).

2. The **middle layer of the cortex is the zona fasciculata** (Figure 19-9).

3. The **innermost** layer of the cortex, **adjacent to the adrenal medulla,** is the **zona reticularis** (Figure 19-10).

Zona glomerulosa

The **zona glomerulosa** (Latin *glomus,* ball) has the following characteristics (see Figure 19-8):

1. It lies under the capsule.

2. It represents 10% to 15% of the cortex.

3. Its cells aggregate into a glomerulus-like arrangement and have a **moderate amount of lipid droplets** in the cytoplasm.

4. It lacks the enzyme 17α-**hydroxylase (CYP17)** and, therefore, cannot produce cortisol or sex steroids (Figure 19-11).

The zona glomerulosa is primarily **angiotensin II (ANG II)–dependent;** it is not ACTH–dependent. ANG II stimulates the growth of the zona glomerulosa and the synthesis of the mineralocorticoid **aldosterone** (see Figure 19-11, Figure 19-12).

ANG II is an octapeptide derived from the conversion of the **angiotensin I (ANG I) decapeptide** in the pulmonary circulation by **angiotensin-converting enzyme (ACE,** see Chapter 14, Urinary System).

Aldosterone has a half-life of 20 to 30 minutes and acts directly on the distal convoluted tubule and collecting tubule, where it increases Na^+ reabsorption and water (as a consequence of Na^+ reabsorption) and excretion of K^+ and H^+.

During aldosterone action, aldosterone binds to **intracellular receptor proteins** to activate transcription

Figure 19-8. Histologic organization of the adrenal gland

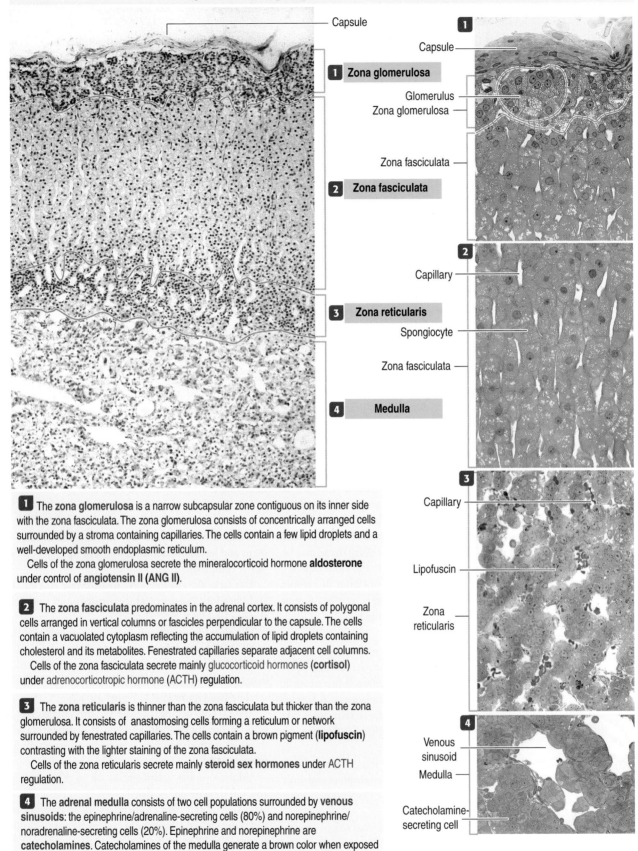

Capsule

1 Zona glomerulosa

2 Zona fasciculata

3 Zona reticularis

4 Medulla

Capsule

Glomerulus
Zona glomerulosa

Zona fasciculata

Capillary

Spongiocyte

Zona fasciculata

Capillary

Lipofuscin

Zona reticularis

Venous sinusoid
Medulla

Catecholamine-secreting cell

1 The **zona glomerulosa** is a narrow subcapsular zone contiguous on its inner side with the zona fasciculata. The zona glomerulosa consists of concentrically arranged cells surrounded by a stroma containing capillaries. The cells contain a few lipid droplets and a well-developed smooth endoplasmic reticulum.

Cells of the zona glomerulosa secrete the mineralocorticoid hormone **aldosterone** under control of **angiotensin II (ANG II)**.

2 The **zona fasciculata** predominates in the adrenal cortex. It consists of polygonal cells arranged in vertical columns or fascicles perpendicular to the capsule. The cells contain a vacuolated cytoplasm reflecting the accumulation of lipid droplets containing cholesterol and its metabolites. Fenestrated capillaries separate adjacent cell columns.

Cells of the zona fasciculata secrete mainly glucocorticoid hormones (**cortisol**) under adrenocorticotropic hormone (ACTH) regulation.

3 The **zona reticularis** is thinner than the zona fasciculata but thicker than the zona glomerulosa. It consists of anastomosing cells forming a reticulum or network surrounded by fenestrated capillaries. The cells contain a brown pigment (**lipofuscin**) contrasting with the lighter staining of the zona fasciculata.

Cells of the zona reticularis secrete mainly **steroid sex hormones** under ACTH regulation.

4 The **adrenal medulla** consists of two cell populations surrounded by **venous sinusoids**: the epinephrine/adrenaline-secreting cells (80%) and norepinephrine/noradrenaline-secreting cells (20%). Epinephrine and norepinephrine are **catecholamines**. Catecholamines of the medulla generate a brown color when exposed to air or the oxidizing agent potassium dichromate (**chromaffin reaction**).

factors that enhance the expression of specific genes.

Aldosterone-responsive cells do not respond to the glucocorticoid cortisol because cortisol is converted in the liver to **cortisone** by the enzyme 11β-hydroxysteroid dehydrogenase. Cortisone does not bind to the aldosterone receptor.

Zona fasciculata

The **zona fasciculata** (Latin *fascis,* bundle) makes up 75% of the cortex. It consists of cuboid cells, with the structural features of steroid-producing cells, arranged in longitudinal cords separated by cortical **fenestrated capillaries**, or **sinusoids**.

The cytoplasm of zona fasciculata cells shows three components that characterize their steroidogenic function (see Figures 19-8 and 19-9):

1. The steroid hormone precursor cholesterol is stored in abundant **lipid droplets**. When lipids are extracted during histologic preparation or are unstained by the standard hematoxylin-eosin (H&E) procedures, the cells of the zona fasciculata display a foamy appearance and are called **spongiocytes**.

2. **Mitochondria with tubular cristae** containing steroidogenic enzymes.

3. Well-developed **smooth endoplasmic reticulum**, also with enzymes involved in the synthesis of steroid hormones.

Cells of the zona fasciculata are stimulated by ACTH. In the presence of 17α-**hydroxylase** (**CYP17**), cells of the zona fasciculata produce glucocorticoids, mainly **cortisol** (see Figures 19-11 and 19-12). Cortisol is not stored in the cells and new synthesis, stimulated by ACTH, is required for achieving a cortisol increase in blood circulation. Cortisol is converted in hepatocytes to cortisone.

Cortisol has two major effects:

1. **A metabolic effect:** The effects of cortisol are opposite to those of insulin. In the liver, cortisol stimulates gluconeogenesis to increase the concentration of glucose in blood. Remember this concept. It becomes useful to understand fluctuations in blood glucose levels in the diabetic patient.

2. **An anti-inflammatory effect:** Cortisol suppresses tissue responses to injury and decreases cellular and humoral immunity.

Zona reticularis

The **zona reticularis** (Latin *rete,* net) makes up 5% to 10% of the cortex. Cells of the zona reticularis form an anastomosing network of short cellular cords separated by fenestrated capillaries.

The cells of this zone are acidophilic, due to abundant **lysosomes**, large **lipofuscin granules**, and **fewer lipid droplets** (see Figures 19-8 and 19-10).

Cells of the zona fasciculata are stimulated by corticotropin (ACTH) and produce sex hormones.

Dehydroepiandrosterone (DHEA) and **androstenedione** are the predominant androgens produced by the cortex of the adrenal gland (see Figures 19-11 and 19-12).

Although DHEA and androstenedione are weak androgens, they can be converted to testosterone and even to estrogen in peripheral tissues. It is interesting to note that the female hormone estradiol derives from the male hormone testosterone, and that testosterone has the female hormone progesterone as a precursor.

The adrenal gland is the major source of androgens in women; these androgens stimulate the growth of pubic and axillary hair during puberty.

Adrenal medulla

The adrenal medulla contains **chromaffin cells**, so named because of their ability to acquire a **brown coloration** when exposed to an aqueous solution of **potassium dichromate**. This reaction is due to the **oxidation of catecholamines** by chrome salts to produce a brown pigment.

Chromaffin cells (see Figure 19-8) are **modified sympathetic postganglionic** neurons, without postganglionic processes, derived from the **neural crest** and forming epithelioid cords surrounded by **fenestrated capillaries**.

In addition, small numbers of **sympathetic ganglion cells** are commonly observed in the medulla (Figure 19-13).

The cytoplasm of chromaffin cells contains membrane-bound **dense granules** consisting in part of matrix proteins, called **chromogranins**, and one class of **catecholamine**, either **epinephrine** or **norepinephrine** (adrenaline or noradrenaline). Some granules contain both epinephrine and norepinephrine. Minimal secretion of **dopamine** also occurs, but the role of adrenal dopamine is not known.

Catecholamines are secreted into the blood instead of being secreted into a synapse, as in postganglionic terminals. The adrenal medulla is innervated by **sympathetic preganglionic fibers** that release **acetylcholine**.

Two different chromaffin cell types are present. About **80% of the cells produce epinephrine** and **20% synthesize norepinephrine**. These two cell populations can be distinguished at the electron microscope level by the morphology of the membrane-bound granules:

1. Norepinephrine is stored in granules with an **eccentric core** (not shown).

2. Epinephrine-containing granules are smaller and occupy a **central core** (see Figure 19-13).

Note an important difference with cells of the adrenal cortex: **cells from the adrenal cortex do not store their steroid hormones in granules.**

Figure 19-9. Fine structure of steroid-producing cells of the adrenal cortex (zona fasciculata)

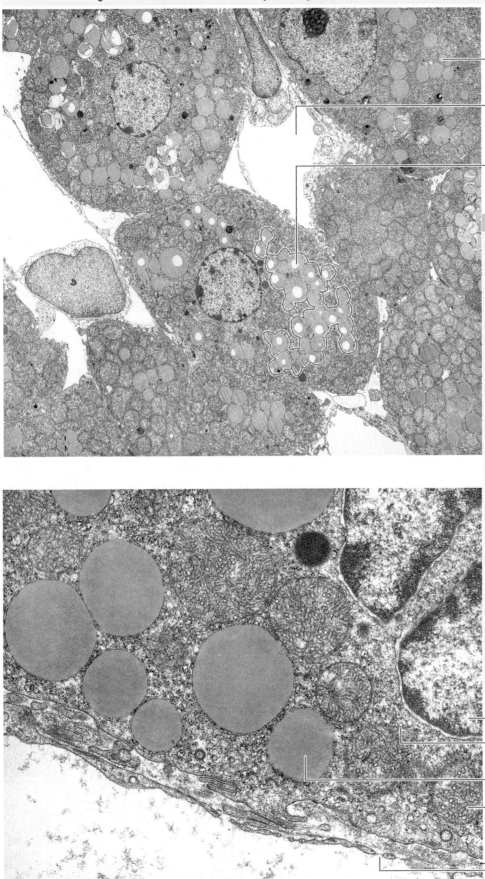

Spongiocyte of the zona fasciculata

Fenestrated capillary

Cluster of lipid droplets

Spongiocytes

The ultrastructure of cells of the zona fasciculata and their close relationship with capillaries lined by **fenestrated endothelial cells** demonstrate their participation in the synthesis of steroid hormones released into the blood vascular system. Like steroid-producing cells of the theca interna and corpus luteum of the ovaries and Leydig cells of the testes, cells of the zona fasciculata display three characteristic structural features representative of steroidogenesis: (1) **lipid droplets** containing cholesterol; (2) **mitochondria with tubular cristae** housing the enzymes involved in steroidogenesis; and (3) **smooth endoplasmic reticulum**, also containing membrane-associated enzymes involved in the production of steroids.

Nucleus

Smooth endoplasmic reticulum

Lipid droplet

Mitochondria with tubular cristae

Basal lamina

Fenestrated endothelial cell

Figure 19-10. **Fine structure of steroid-producing cells of the adrenal cortex (zona reticularis)**

Lipid droplet   Mitochondria with tubular cristae   Lysosome   Lipofuscin

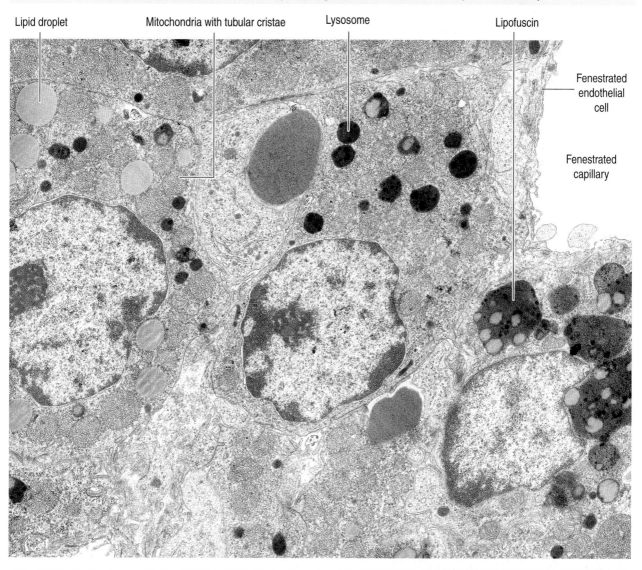

Fenestrated endothelial cell

Fenestrated capillary

Cells of the **zona reticularis** are smaller than the cells of the zonae glomerulosa and fasciculata and contain fewer lipid droplets and mitochondria. However, mitochondria still display the characteristic tubular cristae. A structural feature not prominent in the cells of the other cortical zones is the presence of **lysosomes** and deposits of **lipofuscin**.

Lipofuscin is a remnant of lipid oxidative metabolism reflecting degradation within the adrenal cortex.

There are other relevant characteristics of the zona reticularis. (1) It receives steroid-enriched blood from the zonae glomerulosa (mineralocorticoids) and fasciculata (mainly cortisol). (2) It is in close proximity to the catecholamine-producing cells of the adrenal medulla. (3) In response to adrenocorticoptropic hormone (ACTH) stimulation, cells of **the zonae reticularis and fasciculata produce androgens** (dehydroepiandrosterone and androstenedione). **Cells of the zona reticularis synthesize dehydroepiandrosterone sulfate.**

Clinical significance: Adrenogenital syndrome

Although dehydroepiandrosterone, androstenedione, and dehydroepiandrosterone sulfate are weak androgens, they can be converted outside the adrenal cortex into more potent androgens and also estrogens.

This androgen conversion property has clinical significance in pathologic conditions such as the **adrenogenital syndrome**.

An excessive production of androgens in the adrenogenital syndrome in women leads to masculinization (abnormal sexual hair development, **hirsutism**, and enlargement of the clitoris).

In the male, adrenal androgens do not replace testicular androgens produced by Leydig cells. In women, adrenal androgens are responsible for the growth of axillary and pubic hair.

Catecholamines are synthesized from **tyrosine** to **DOPA** (3,4-dihydroxyphenylalanine) in the presence of **tyrosine hydroxylase** (see Figure 19-13). DOPA is converted to **dopamine** by **DOPA decarboxylase.**

Dopamine is transported into existing granules and converted inside them by **dopamine β-hydroxylase** to **norepinephrine.**

The **membrane of the granules** contains the

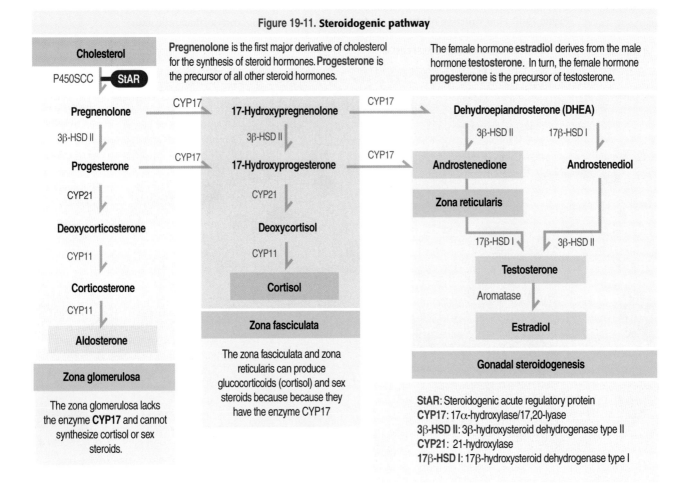

Figure 19-11. Steroidogenic pathway

Pregnenolone is the first major derivative of cholesterol for the synthesis of steroid hormones. **Progesterone** is the precursor of all other steroid hormones.

The female hormone **estradiol** derives from the male hormone **testosterone**. In turn, the female hormone **progesterone** is the precursor of testosterone.

The zona glomerulosa lacks the enzyme **CYP17** and cannot synthesize cortisol or sex steroids.

The zona fasciculata and zona reticularis can produce glucocorticoids (cortisol) and sex steroids because because they have the enzyme CYP17

StAR: Steroidogenic acute regulatory protein
CYP17: 17α-hydroxylase/17,20-lyase
3β-HSD II: 3β-hydroxysteroid dehydrogenase type II
CYP21: 21-hydroxylase
17β-HSD I: 17β-hydroxysteroid dehydrogenase type I

enzymes required for catecholamine synthesis and ATP-driven pumps for the transport of substrates.

Once synthesized, norepinephrine leaves the granule **to enter the cytosol**, where it is converted to epinephrine in a reaction driven by the enzyme **phenylethanolamine *N*-methyltransferase** (**PNMT**). The synthesis of PNMT is induced by **glucocorticoids** transported from the cortex to the medulla by the adrenocortical capillary system. When the conversion step to epinephrine is completed, epinephrine **moves back to the membrane-bound granule** for storage.

The degradation of catecholamines in the presence of the enzymes **monoamine oxidase** (**MAO**) and **catechol *O*-methyltransferase** (**COMT**) yields the main degradation products **vanillylmandelic acid** (**VMA**) and **metanephrine**, which are eliminated in urine. Urinary VMA and metanephrine are used clinically to determine the level of catecholamine production in a patient.

Adrenergic receptors α and β

Catecholamines bind to α- and β-**adrenergic receptors** in target cells. There are α_1-, α_2-, β_1-, and β_2-adrenergic receptors.

Epinephrine has greater binding affinity for β_2-adrenergic receptors than norepinephrine. Both hormones have similar binding affinity for β_1-, α_1-, and α_2-adrenergic receptors.

The stimulation of α-adrenergic receptors of blood vessels by epinephrine causes **vasoconstriction**. In blood vessels of **skeletal muscle**, activation of β_2-adrenergic receptors by epinephrine causes **vasodilation**.

The adrenergic receptors of the cardiac muscle are β_1-adrenergic receptors, and both epinephrine and norepinephrine have comparable effects. Remember the clinical consequences of the up regulation of β_1-adrenergic receptors in Graves' disease.

Blood supply to the adrenal gland

Similar to all endocrine organs, the adrenal glands are highly vascularized. Arterial blood derives from three different sources (Figure 19-14):

1. The **inferior phrenic artery**, which gives rise to the **superior adrenal artery**.

2. The **aorta**, from which the **middle adrenal artery** branches out.

3. The **renal artery**, which gives rise to the **inferior adrenal artery**.

All three adrenal arteries enter the adrenal gland capsule and form an **arterial plexus**. Three sets of branches emerge from the plexus:

Figure 19-12. Synthesis of steroids in the adrenal cortex

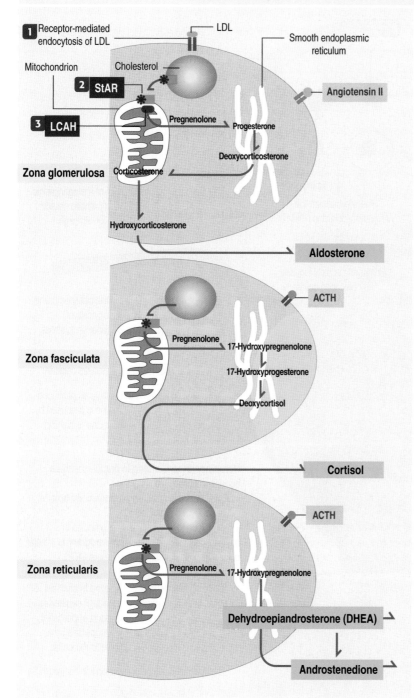

1 Most of the **cholesterol**, the precursor for the biosynthesis of all steroid hormones, derives from circulating **low-density lipoprotein (LDL)**. Cholesterol is esterified by acylCoA cholesterol acyltransferase to be stored in cytoplasmic lipid droplets.

Cholesterol is modified by a series of hydroxylation reactions. Enzymes located in the mitochondria and smooth endoplasmic reticulum participate in the reactions. The substrates shuttle from mitochondria to smooth endoplasmic reticulum to mitochondria during steroidogenesis.

Steroidogenic acute regulatory protein (StAR)

2 The **steroidogenic acute regulatory protein (StAR)** is a cholesterol transfer protein. StAR regulates the synthesis of steroids by **transporting cholesterol across the outer mitochondrial membrane to the inner mitochondrial membrane,** where cytochrome **P450SCC**, the rate-limiting enzyme of steroidogenesis is located.

3 A mutation in the gene encoding StAR or P450SCC is detected in individuals with defective synthesis of adrenal and gonadal steroids (**lipoid congenital adrenal hyperplasia, LCAH**).

Congenital adrenal hyperplasia (CAH)

CAH results from genetic enzymatic defects in the synthesis of cortisol. However, the adrenal cortex is responsive to adrenocorticotropic hormone (ACTH) and, therefore, cortical hyperplasia develops.

In a large number of patients (90%), CAH is caused by an inborn defect in 21-hydroxylase (CYP21), the enzyme that converts 17-hydroxyprogesterone to deoxycorticosterone. The precursor is instead converted to androgens. Aldosterone is lacking and hypoaldosteronism develops (with hypotension and low Na^+ in plasma). Circulating androgens are high and virilization is found in female infants.

1. One set supplies the **capsule**.

2. The second set enters the cortex forming **straight fenestrated capillaries** (also called **sinusoids**), percolating between the zonae glomerulosa and fasciculata, and forming a capillary network in the zona reticularis before entering the medulla.

3. The third set generates **medullary arteries** that travel along the cortex and, **without branching, supply blood only to the medulla.**

This blood vessel distribution results in:

1. **A dual blood supply to the adrenal medulla.**

2. The **transport of cortisol to the medulla**, necessary for the synthesis of PNMT, required for the conversion of norepinephrine to epinephrine.

3. The **direct supply of blood to the adrenal medulla,** involved in rapid responses to stress.

There are no veins or lymphatics in the adrenal cortex.

The adrenal cortex and medulla are drained by the **central vein**, present in the adrenal medulla.

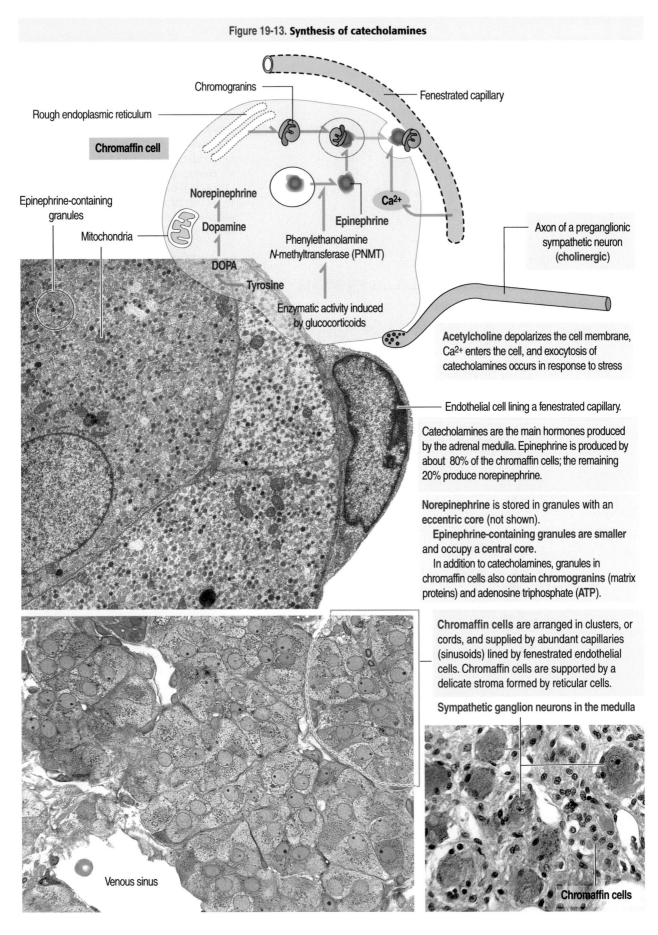

Figure 19-13. **Synthesis of catecholamines**

Chromogranins

Fenestrated capillary

Rough endoplasmic reticulum

Chromaffin cell

Norepinephrine

Epinephrine-containing granules

Dopamine

Mitochondria

Epinephrine

DOPA

Phenylethanolamine N-methyltransferase (PNMT)

Ca^{2+}

Tyrosine

Enzymatic activity induced by glucocorticoids

Axon of a preganglionic sympathetic neuron **(cholinergic)**

Acetylcholine depolarizes the cell membrane, Ca^{2+} enters the cell, and exocytosis of catecholamines occurs in response to stress

Endothelial cell lining a fenestrated capillary.

Catecholamines are the main hormones produced by the adrenal medulla. Epinephrine is produced by about 80% of the chromaffin cells; the remaining 20% produce norepinephrine.

Norepinephrine is stored in granules with an **eccentric core** (not shown).
   Epinephrine-containing granules are smaller and occupy a **central core**.
   In addition to catecholamines, granules in chromaffin cells also contain **chromogranins** (matrix proteins) and adenosine triphosphate (**ATP**).

Chromaffin cells are arranged in clusters, or cords, and supplied by abundant capillaries (sinusoids) lined by fenestrated endothelial cells. Chromaffin cells are supported by a delicate stroma formed by reticular cells.

Sympathetic ganglion neurons in the medulla

Venous sinus

Chromaffin cells

Figure 19-14. **Blood supply to the adrenal gland**

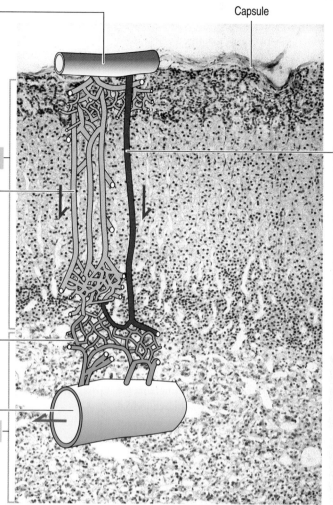

Blood vessels derived from the **capsular plexus**, formed by the **superior** and **middle adrenal arteries**, supply the three zones of the cortex. **Fenestrated cortical capillaries** derive from these blood vessels.

Cortex

Fenestrated cortical capillaries (also called sinusoids) percolate through the zonae glomerulosa and fasciculata and form a network within the zona reticularis before entering the medulla.

Medullary venous sinuses Mineralocorticoids, cortisol, and sexual steroids enter the medullary venous sinuses.

Central vein

Medulla

Capsule

The medullary artery, derived from the **inferior adrenal artery**, enters the cortex within a connective tissue trabecula and supplies blood directly to the adrenal medulla.

Medullary artery

The medullary artery **bypasses the cortex without branching**. In the medulla, the artery joins with branches from the cortical capillaries to form **medullary venous sinuses**. Thus, **the medulla has two blood supplies:** one from cortical capillaries and the other from the medullary artery.

The conversion of norepinephrine to epinephrine by chromaffin cells is dependent on **phenylethanolamine *N*-methyltransferase (PNMT)**, an enzyme activated by cortisol transported by the cortical capillaries to the medullary venous sinuses.

Pathology: The adrenal cortex

Zona glomerulosa: A tumor localized in the zona glomerulosa can cause excessive secretion of aldosterone. This rare condition is known as **primary hyperaldosteronism**, or **Conn's syndrome**. A more common cause of hyperaldosteronism is an increase in renin secretion (**secondary hyperaldosteronism**).

Zona fasciculata: An increase in aldosterone, cortisol, and adrenal androgen production, secondary to ACTH production, occurs in **Cushing's** *disease*. Cushing's disease is caused by an **ACTH-producing tumor of the anterior hypophysis**.

Adrenocortical adenoma, a functional tumor of the adrenal cortex can also result in overproduction of cortisol, as well as of aldosterone and adrenal androgens.

This clinical condition is described as **Cushing's** *syndrome* (as opposed to Cushing's *disease*). The symptoms of Cushing's syndrome reflect the multiple actions of an excess of glucocorticoids, in particular, on the carbohydrate metabolism. The effects of cortisol are opposite to those of insulin.

Zona reticularis: When compared with the gonads, the zona reticularis secretes insignificant amounts of sex hormones. However, sex hormone hypersecretion becomes significant when an adrenalcortical adenoma is associated with virilization or feminization.

An **acute destruction** of the adrenal gland by meningococcal septicemia in infants is the cause of **Waterhouse-Friderichsen syndrome** (or **hemorrhagic adrenalitis**) producing adrenocortical insufficiency.

A **chronic destruction** of the adrenal cortex by an autoimmune process or tuberculosis results in the classic **Addison's disease**.

In Addison's disease, ACTH secretion increases because of the cortisol deficiency. ACTH can cause an increase in skin pigmentation, in particular in the skin folds and gums. The loss of mineralocorticoids leads to hypotension and circulatory shock.

A loss of cortisol decreases vasopressive responses to catecholamines and leads to an eventual drop in peripheral resistance, thereby contributing to hypotension. A deficiency in cortisol causes muscle weakness (asthenia).

Pathology: Pheochromocytoma

Adrenal **pheochromocytoma** (or adrenal **medullary paraganglioma**) is a rare neoplasm that arises from the chromaffin cells.

Pheochromocytoma causes sustained or episodic **hypertension, tachycardia,** and **tremor**. The gross appearance of a pheochromocytoma is a hemorrhagic mass. Microscopically, the tumor displays a cellular cluster and/or a trabecular pattern surrounded by an abundant sinusoidal-capillary network. Chromogranins are markers for pheochromocytoma.

When pheochromocytomas are associated with other endocrine tumors, they are a component of the **multiple endocrine neoplasia (MEN) syndrome**. The presence of large amounts of VMA in urine has diagnostic relevance.

Clinical significance: Congenital adrenal hyperplasia

Lipoid congenital adrenal hyperplasia is a familial inherited condition in which a mutation in the gene encoding **steroidogenic acute regulatory protein (StAR)** or **cytochrome P450SCC**, causes a deficiency in adrenocortical and gonadal steroidogenesis. StAR regulates the synthesis of steroids **by transporting cholesterol across the outer mitochondrial membrane** to the inner mitochondrial membrane. Cytochrome P450SCC is the rate-limiting enzyme of steroidogenesis located in the inner mitochondrial membrane. **A steroidogenic deficiency increases ACTH secretion, leading to adrenal hyperplasia.**

Adrenal hyperplasia is seen in individuals with a deficiency of the enzyme **21-hydroxylase** who cannot produce cortisol or mineralocorticoids. These individuals are hypotensive because of a difficulty in retaining salt and maintaining extracellular volume. A deficiency in the enzyme **11-hydroxylase** (CYP11) results in the synthesis and accumulation of the mineralocorticoid deoxycorticosterone (DOC). Patients with this deficiency retain salt and water and become hypertensive.

See Figure 19-11 for the roles of 21-hydroxylase (CYP21) and 11-hydroxylase (CYP11) in the synthesis of cortisol and mineralocorticoids.

Endocrine pancreas

Development of the pancreas

By week 4, two outpocketings from the endodermal lining of the duodenum develop as the ventral and dorsal pancreas, each with its own duct. The ventral pancreas forms the head of the pancreas and associates with the common bile duct. The dorsal pancreas forms part of the head, body, and tail of the pancreas. By week 12, pancreatic acini develop from the ducts. The endocrine pancreas develops at the same time as the exocrine pancreas. Endocrine cells are first observed along the base of the differentiating exocrine acini by weeks 12 to 16.

Islets of Langerhans

The pancreas has two portions:

1. The **exocrine pancreas**, consisting of acini involved in the synthesis and secretion of several digestive enzymes transported by a duct system into the duodenum (see Chapter 17, Digestive Glands).

2. The **endocrine pancreas** (2% of the pancreatic mass), formed by the **islets of Langerhans** scattered throughout the pancreas.

Each islet of Langerhans is formed by two components:

1. A **vascular component**, the **insuloacinar portal system** (see Figure 19-15), which consists of an afferent arteriole giving rise to a capillary network lined by fenestrated endothelial cells. Venules leaving the islets of Langerhans supply blood to adjacent pancreatic acini. This portal system enables the local action of insular hormones on the exocrine pancreas.

An independent vascular system, the **acinar vascular system**, supplies blood directly to the exocrine pancreatic acini.

2. **Anastomosing cords** of endocrine cells, A (α cells), B (β cells), D (δ cells), and F cells, each secreting a single hormone (Figure 19-16).

A cells (α cells) produce **glucagon**, beta cells synthesize **insulin, delta cells** secrete **gastrin** and **somatostatin**, and **F cells** produce **pancreatic polypeptide**.

Glucagon, a 29-amino-acid peptide, is stored in granules that are released by exocytosis when there is a **decrease** in the plasma levels of **glucose**. Glucagon increases glucose blood levels by increasing **hepatic glycogenolysis**. Glucagon binds to a specific membrane-bound receptor and this binding results in the synthesis of cAMP.

B cells (β cells) **produce** insulin, a 6-kd polypeptide consisting of two chains (Figure 19-17):

1. **Chain A**, with 21 amino acids,
2. **Chain B**, with 30 amino acids.

Chains A and B are linked by disulfide bonds.

Insulin derives from a large single-chain precursor, **preproinsulin**, encoded by a gene located on the short arm of chromosome 11. Preproinsulin is synthesized in the rough endoplasmic reticulum and is processed in the Golgi apparatus.

The large precursor gives rise to **proinsulin** (9 kd; 86 amino acids) in which **C peptide** connects A and B chains. Removal of C peptide by specific proteases results in:

1. The separation of chains A and B.

2. The organization of a crystalline core consisting of a hexamer and zinc atoms. C peptide surrounds the crystalline core.

An **increase in blood glucose stimulates the release of both insulin and C peptide stored in secretory granules.**

Glucose is taken up by B cells by an **insulin-independent, glucose transporter protein-2 (GLUT-2),**

Figure 19-15. Blood supply to the islets of Langerhans

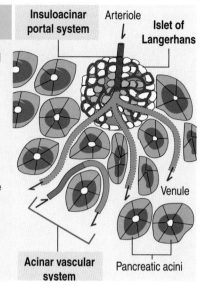

Dual blood supply: Acinar and insuloacinar vascular systems

Each islet of Langerhans is supplied by afferent arterioles, forming a network of capillaries lined by fenestrated endothelial cells. This network is called the **insuloacinar portal system**.

Venules leaving the islet supply blood to the pancreatic acini surrounding the islet. This vascular system enables a local action on the exocrine pancreas of hormones produced in the islet.

An independent arterial system, the **acinar vascular system**, supplies the pancreatic acini.

Labels in figure: Insuloacinar portal system — Arteriole — Islet of Langerhans — Venule — Acinar vascular system — Pancreatic acini

and stored insulin is released in a Ca^{2+}–dependent manner.

If glucose levels remain high, new synthesis of insulin occurs. GLUT-2 is also present in hepatocytes.

Insulin is required for increasing the transport of glucose in cells (predominantly in hepatocytes, skeletal and cardiac muscle, fibroblasts, and adipocytes). This is accomplished by:

1. The transmembrane transport of glucose and amino acids.

2. The formation of glycogen in hepatocytes and skeletal and cardiac muscle cells.

3. The conversion of glucose to triglycerides in adipose cells (Figure 19-18).

Insulin initiates its effect by binding to the α subunit of its receptor. The **insulin receptor** consists of two subunits, α and β. The intracellular domain of the β **subunit** has **tyrosine kinase activity**, which autophosphorylates and triggers a number of intracellular responses.

One of these responses is the translocation of **glucose transporter protein-4 (GLUT-4)** from the Golgi apparatus to the plasma membrane to facilitate the uptake of glucose. **GLUT-4 is insulin-dependent** and is present in adipocytes and skeletal and cardiac muscle.

Note the functional difference between GLUT-2 and GLUT-4:

1. **GLUT-2 is insulin-independent and serves to transport glucose to insular B cells and hepatocytes.**

2. **GLUT-4 is insulin-dependent and serves to remove glucose from blood.**

A (α) **cells** produce **glucagon**, a 29-amino-acid peptide (3.5 kd) derived from a large precursor, **pre-proglucagon**, encoded by a gene present on chromosome 2. In addition to the pancreas, glucagon can be found in the gastrointestinal tract (enteroglucagon) and brain. About 30% to 40% of glucagon in blood derives from the pancreas; the remainder comes from the gastrointestinal tract. Circulating glucagon, of pancreatic and gastrointestinal origin, is transported to the liver and about 80% is degraded before reaching the systemic circulation. The liver is the primary target site of glucagon. Glucagon induces hyperglycemia by its glycogenolytic activity in hepatocytes.

Neither C peptide nor zinc is present in glucagon-containing secretory granules.

The actions of glucagon are antagonistic to those of insulin. The secretion of glucagon is stimulated by:

1. A fall in the concentration of glucose in blood.

2. An increase of arginine and alanine in serum.

3. Stimulation of the sympathetic nervous system.

D (δ) cells produce **gastrin** (see discussion of enteroendocrine cells in Chapter 15, Upper Digestive Segment) and **somatostatin**. **Somatostatin** is a 14 amino-acid peptide identical to somatostatin produced in the hypothalamus. Somatostatin **inhibits the release of insulin and glucagon** in a paracrine manner.

Somatostatin also **inhibits the** secretion of HCl by parietal cells of the fundic stomach, the release of gastrin from enteroendocrine cells, the secretion of pancreatic bicarbonate and enzymes, and the contraction of the gallbladder. Somatostatin is also produced in the hypothalamus and inhibits the secretion of growth hormone from the anterior hypophysis.

Pancreatic polypeptide is a 36-amino-acid peptide that **inhibits the secretion of somatostatin**. Pancreatic polypeptide also inhibits the secretion of pancreatic enzymes and blocks the secretion of bile by inhibiting contraction of the gallbladder. Its function is to conserve digestive enzymes and bile between meals.

Cholecystokinin stimulates the release of pancreatic polypeptide.

Cell types in the islets of Langerhans can be identified by:

1. **Immunocytochemistry**, using antibodies specific for each cell product.

2. **Electron microscopy**, to distinguish the size and structure of the secretory granules.

3. The **cell distribution** in the islet. B cells are centrally located (core distribution) and surrounded by the other cell types (mantle distribution; see Figure 19-16).

Clinical significance: ATP-sensitive K+ channel and insulin secretion

The **ATP-sensitive potassium (K_{ATP}) channel**, a complex of the **sulfonylurea receptor 1 (SUR1)** and the **inward-rectifying K+ channel (Kir6.2) subunits**, are the key regulators of insulin release.

SUR1 is encoded by the *KCNJ11* (potassium channel J member 11) gene. Kir6.2 is encoded by

Figure 19-16. **Islet of Langerhans**

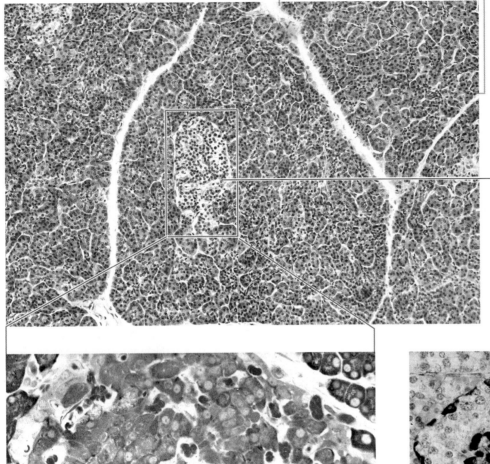

Exocrine pancreas

Formed by protein secretory acini with apically located zymogen granules

Islet of Langerhans

Each islet consists of 2000 to 3000 cells surrounded by a network of fenestrated capillaries and supported by reticular fibers. About one million islets of Langerhans are scattered throughout the pancreas.

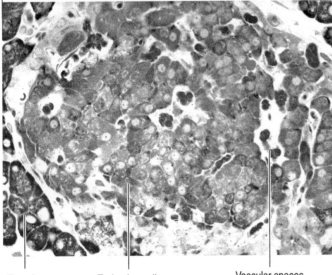

Exocrine pancreas

Endocrine cells forming cords

Vascular spaces (sinusoids)

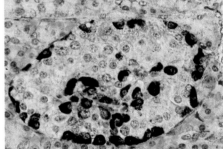

A (α) cells secrete **glucagon** and are located at the periphery of the islet

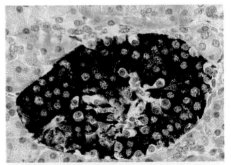

B (β) cells, the predominant cell type, secrete **insulin** and are found in the core of the islet

Immunocytochemistry (immunoperoxidase shown in the four panels) and electron microscopy (to identify secretory granules of varying diameters, densities and internal structures; see Figure 19-17), are valuable approaches to the recognition of specific cell types

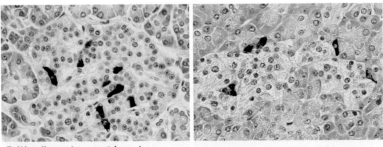

D (δ) cells produce **gastrin** and **somatostatin** (shown)

F cells secrete **pancreatic polypeptide**

Immunohistochemistry panels from Martín-Lacave I, García-Caballero T: Atlas of Immunohistochemistry. Madrid, Spain:Ed. Díaz de Santos, 2012.

Figure 19-17. Fine structure and synthesis and secretion of insulin by B cells of an islet of Langerhans

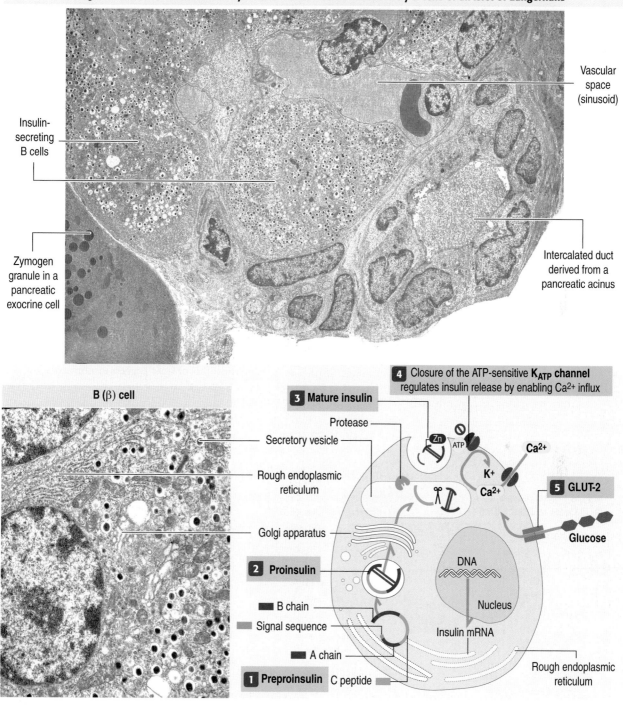

Vascular space (sinusoid)

Insulin-secreting B cells

Zymogen granule in a pancreatic exocrine cell

Intercalated duct derived from a pancreatic acinus

B (β) cell

4 Closure of the ATP-sensitive **K_ATP channel** regulates insulin release by enabling Ca^{2+} influx

3 **Mature insulin**

Protease

Secretory vesicle

Rough endoplasmic reticulum

Golgi apparatus

2 **Proinsulin**

B chain

Signal sequence

A chain

1 **Preproinsulin** C peptide

Zn

ATP

Ca^{2+}

K^+

Ca^{2+}

5 GLUT-2

Glucose

DNA

Nucleus

Insulin mRNA

Rough endoplasmic reticulum

1 **Preproinsulin** is synthesized in the rough endoplasmic reticulum and the signal sequence is removed. Proinsulin is produced.

Proinsulin is transferred to the Golgi apparatus. Proinsulin consists of a connecting (C) peptide bound to A and B chains, held together by disulfide bonds.

2 **Proinsulin** is enclosed in a secretory vesicle that contains a specific **protease**.

Within the secretory vesicle, the **protease** releases the C peptide from the linked A and B chains.

3 **Mature insulin molecules, in the presence of zinc**, yield a dense crystalloid surrounded by C peptides.

4 Closing of the adenosine triphosphate (ATP)–sensitive potassium channel (**K_ATP**) enables Ca^{2+} influx by depolarization of the plasma membrane following accumulation of K^+ in the cytosol. Ca^{2+} influx causes exocytosis of the secretory vesicle and the release of insulin into the bloodstream.

5 Glucose enters the B cell through **insulin-independent glucose transporter protein-2 (GLUT-2)** and triggers the immediate release of insulin.

Adenosine triphosphate (ATP) from glucose metabolism closes the K_{ATP} channel, causing accumulation of intracellular K^+.

Figure 19-18. Adipose cell, lipid storage, and insulin

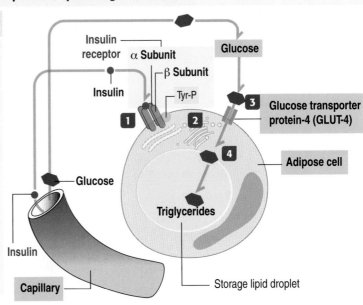

Mechanism of action of insulin in an adipose cell

1 Insulin binds to the α subunit of the insulin receptor and activates the autophosphorylation (**Tyr-P**) of the adjacent β subunit (a tyrosine kinase).

2 An activated insulin receptor stimulates DNA synthesis, protein synthesis, and the translocation of insulin-dependent **glucose transporter protein-4 (GLUT-4)** from the Golgi apparatus to the plasma membrane.

3 GLUT-4 translocation facilitates the cellular uptake of glucose.

4 This mechanism demonstrates that, in diabetic individuals, a lack of insulin decreases the **utilization of glucose** in target cells.

---

the *ABCC8* (ATP-binding cassette, subfamily C, member 8) gene.

K_{ATP} channel modulates the influx of Ca^{2+} through voltage-gated Ca^{2+} channels. In the normal resting state, the K_{ATP} channel is open and the voltage-gated Ca^{2+} channel remains closed. No insulin is secreted.

When glucose is taken up by B cells by GLUT-2,

the K_{ATP} channel closes utilizing ATP derived from glucose metabolism. K^+ accumulates in the cell, the Ca^{2+} channel opens by membrane depolarization, and the influx of Ca^{2+} triggers insulin exocytosis (see Figure 19-17).

The clinical significance of this mechanism is highlighted by mutations in *SUR1* and *Kir6.2* genes.

Gain-of-function mutations of *SUR1* and *Kir6.2*

Figure 19-19. Diabetes mellitus: Clinical forms

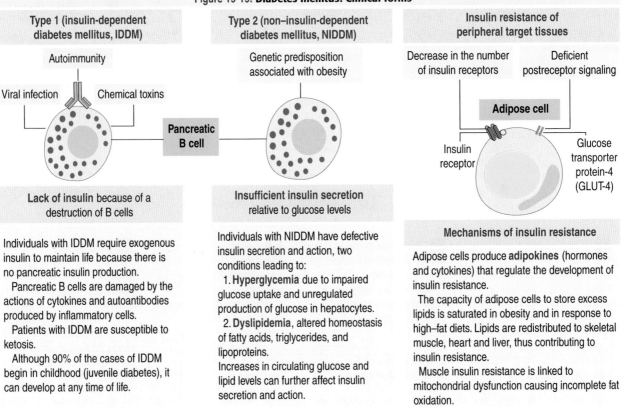

Type 1 (insulin-dependent diabetes mellitus, IDDM)

Autoimmunity

Viral infection — Chemical toxins

Pancreatic B cell

Lack of insulin because of a destruction of B cells

Individuals with IDDM require exogenous insulin to maintain life because there is no pancreatic insulin production.

Pancreatic B cells are damaged by the actions of cytokines and autoantibodies produced by inflammatory cells.

Patients with IDDM are susceptible to ketosis.

Although 90% of the cases of IDDM begin in childhood (juvenile diabetes), it can develop at any time of life.

Type 2 (non–insulin-dependent diabetes mellitus, NIDDM)

Genetic predisposition associated with obesity

Insufficient insulin secretion relative to glucose levels

Individuals with NIDDM have defective insulin secretion and action, two conditions leading to:

1. **Hyperglycemia** due to impaired glucose uptake and unregulated production of glucose in hepatocytes.

2. **Dyslipidemia**, altered homeostasis of fatty acids, triglycerides, and lipoproteins.

Increases in circulating glucose and lipid levels can further affect insulin secretion and action.

Insulin resistance of peripheral target tissues

Decrease in the number of insulin receptors

Deficient postreceptor signaling

Adipose cell

Insulin receptor

Glucose transporter protein-4 (GLUT-4)

Mechanisms of insulin resistance

Adipose cells produce **adipokines** (hormones and cytokines) that regulate the development of insulin resistance.

The capacity of adipose cells to store excess lipids is saturated in obesity and in response to high–fat diets. Lipids are redistributed to skeletal muscle, heart and liver, thus contributing to insulin resistance.

Muscle insulin resistance is linked to mitochondrial dysfunction causing incomplete fat oxidation.

Figure 19-20. Clinical aspects of types 1 and 2 diabetes: Late complications

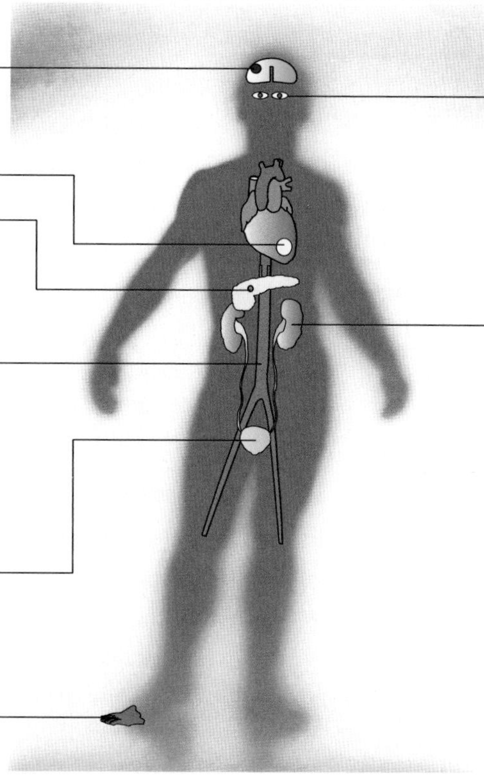

Cerebral infarcts and hemorrhage

Myocardial infarct

Loss of B cells (islets of Langerhans)

A major target of diabetes is the **vascular system**. **Atherosclerosis** of the aorta and large and medium-sized blood vessels leads to myocardial and brain infarctions and gangrene of the lower extremities. **Arteriolosclerosis** (thickening of the wall of the arterioles) is associated with hypertension.

Urinary bladder neuropathy (alteration in the autonomic nervous system)

Gangrene caused by blood vessel obstruction as a consequence of vascular arteriosclerosis

Eye complications of diabetes can cause total blindness. Damage of the retina (**retinopathy**), opacity of the lens (**cataract**), or **glaucoma** (impaired drainage of the aqueous humor) is frequently observed.

Glomerulosclerosis, arteriosclerosis, and **pyelonephritis** are frequently seen kidney diseases in diabetic patients. The most significant damage to the kidneys is the **diffuse thickening of the basal lamina of the glomerular capillaries and proliferation of mesangial cells.**

This glomerular change is known as the **Kimmelstiel-Wilson lesion.**

cause K_{ATP} channels to remain **open**, thereby decreasing insulin secretion and leading to **neonatal diabetes mellitus. Loss-of-function mutations** of *SUR1* and *Kir6.2* genes cause K_{ATP} channels to remain **closed**, thereby causing unregulated secretion of insulin leading to **neonatal hyperinsulinemic hypoglycemia.**

Clinical significance: Insulin and diabetes

When blood glucose levels rise in a normal person, the immediate release of insulin ensures a return to normal levels within 1 hour. In a diabetic individual, increased blood glucose levels (**hyperglycemia**) remain high for a prolonged period of time.

The **glycated hemoglobin test**, also called hemoglobin A1c (**HbA1c**) test, provides an average of blood glucose measurements over a 6 to 12 week period. When blood glucose levels are high, the sugar combines with hemoglobin that becomes glycated (coated). The HbA1c test range in normal individuals is between 4% and 5.6%. Individuals with diabetes should have a HbA1c level less of 6.5%.

Hyperglycemia can be the result of the following (see Figure 19-18):

1. A **lack of insulin**, caused by autoimmune, toxic, or viral damage to B cells (**type 1 diabetes mellitus; insulin-dependent diabetes mellitus [IDDM]**). Insulinitis with an infiltration of lymphocytes is characteristic of the early stages of IDDM. This type of diabetes, also known as **juvenile diabetes**, accounts

for about 90% of cases and often occurs before the age of 25 years (between 10 and 14). However, IDDM can occur at any age.

2. **Insufficient insulin secretion** relative to glucose levels and **resistance of peripheral target tissues to insulin (type 2 diabetes mellitus; non–insulin-dependent diabetes mellitus [NIDDM]**).

3. **The association between excess lipid storage in the form of obesity and insulin resistance.** Following carbohydrate ingestion, glucose is deposited in muscle and the liver as glycogen. Defective insulin responsiveness in these organs result in fasting hyperglycemia

The lack of responsiveness to insulin by target cells can be caused by a decrease in the number of available insulin receptors in the target cells and deficiency in postreceptor signaling (for example, the translocation of GLUT-4 from the Golgi apparatus to the plasma membrane to facilitate glucose uptake). This latter type of defect is most frequent (80%) and is observed in the adult.

The symptoms and consequences of type 1 and type 2 diabetes are generally similar. **Hyperglycemia, polyuria** (increased frequency of micturition and urine volume), and **polydipsia** (sensation of thirst and increased fluid intake) are the three characteristic symptoms.

The clinical forms of diabetes mellitus are presented in Figure 19-19. The late complications of diabetes mellitus are summarized in Figure 19-20.

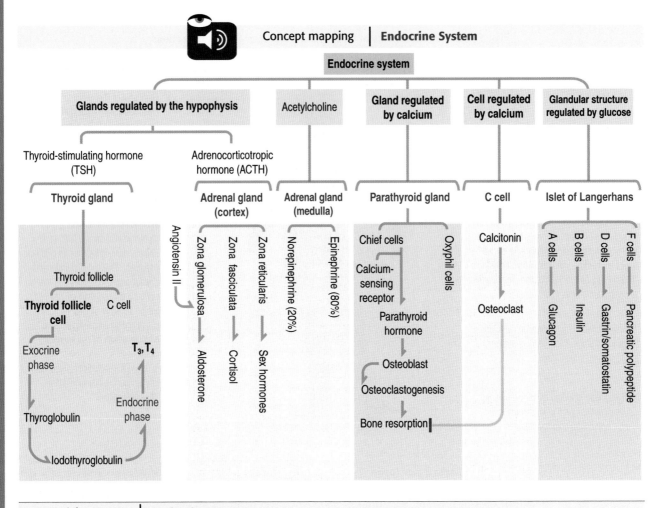

Endocrine system

- Glands regulated by the hypophysis
  - Thyroid-stimulating hormone (TSH)
    - Thyroid gland
      - Thyroid follicle
      - **Thyroid follicle cell** — C cell
        - Exocrine phase
        - Thyroglobulin
        - Iodothyroglobulin
        - Endocrine phase
        - T_3, T_4
  - Adrenocorticotropic hormone (ACTH)
    - Adrenal gland (cortex)
      - Angiotensin II
      - Zona glomerulosa → Aldosterone
      - Zona fasciculata → Cortisol
      - Zona reticularis → Sex hormones
- Acetylcholine
  - Adrenal gland (medulla)
    - Norepinephrine (20%)
    - Epinephrine (80%)
- Gland regulated by calcium
  - Parathyroid gland
    - Chief cells
      - Calcium-sensing receptor
      - Parathyroid hormone
        - Osteoblast
        - Osteoclastogenesis
        - Bone resorption
    - Oxyphil cells
- Cell regulated by calcium
  - C cell
    - Calcitonin
    - Osteoclast
- Glandular structure regulated by glucose
  - Islet of Langerhans
    - A cells → Glucagon
    - B cells → Insulin
    - D cells → Gastrin/somatostatin
    - F cells → Pancreatic polypeptide

Essential concepts | Endocrine System

- **Thyroid gland.** The thyroid gland develops from an endodermal downgrowth at the base of the tongue, connected by the thyroglossal duct. C cells, derived from the neural crest, are present in the thyroid gland.

The thyroid gland consists of thyroid follicles lined by a simple cuboidal epithelium, whose height varies with functional activity. The lumen contains a colloid substance rich in thyroglobulin, the precursor of the thyroid hormones triiodothyronine (T_3) and thyroxine (T_4). The main function of thyroid hormones is the regulation of the body's basal metabolism.

The synthesis and secretion of thyroid hormones involve two phases:
(1) An excretory phase.
(2) An endocrine phase.
Both phases can occur in the same thyroid cell and are regulated by thyroid stimulating hormone (TSH), produced by basophil cells in the anterior hypophysis.

The exocrine phase consists of the synthesis and secretion of thyroglobulin into the colloid-containing lumen and the uptake of inorganic iodide from blood through an ATP-dependent iodide pump. The enzyme thyroid peroxidase, present in the membrane of the secretory vesicle, which also contains thyroglobulin, converts iodide into iodine. Iodine atoms are attached to tyrosil residues on thyroglobulin, which become iodothyroglobulin.

The endocrine phase consists of the reuptake and processing of iodothyroglobulin. Colloid droplets, containing iodothyroglobulin, are enveloped by pseudopods and internalized to become colloid-containing vesicles. Lysosomes fuse with the internalized vesicles and iodothyroglobulin is processed to release T_3 and T_4 across the basal domain of the thyroid cell into the bloodstream. T_3 and T_4 are transported in the blood by serum carrier proteins. Thyroid hormones enter the cell nucleus of a target cell, and bind to the thyroid hormone–responsive element to activate specific gene expression.

- **Graves' disease** is an autoimmune disease that causes hyperfunction of the thyroid gland (hyperthyroidism). Autoantibodies against the TSH receptor stimulate the unregulated function of the thyroid gland. Patients have an enlargement of the thyroid gland (goiter), bulging eyes (exophthalmos), and accelerated heart rate (tachycardia).

Hashimoto's thyroiditis is an autoimmune disease associated with hypofunction of the thyroid gland (hypothyroidism). It is caused by autoantibodies to thyroid peroxidase (anti-TPO) and thyroglobulin (anti-TG).

Additional inflammatory conditions of the thyroid gland includes de Quervain's thyroiditis (a subacute inflammatory process seen during systemic viral illness) and Riedel's thyroiditis (inflammatory fibrosclerosis).

Papillary carcinoma is the most frequent malignant tumor of the thyroid gland. This tumor is locally invasive and spreads to cervical lymph nodes. Follicular carcinoma, is the second most frequent tumor of the thyroid gland. It is a slow growing tumor that usually spreads to bone by the hematogenous route

- **Ca^{2+} regulation.** The maintenance of Ca^{2+} levels in blood is regulated by
(1) Parathyroid hormone.
(2) Calcitonin.
(3) Vitamin D.
Parathyroid gland. The four parathyroid glands derive from the third and fourth branchial pouches. The parathyroid gland consists of two cell populations arranged in cords or clusters:
(1) Chief or principal cells, producing parathyroid hormone.
(2) Oxyphil cells, presumably a transitional chief cell. Chief cells secrete parathyroid hormone.
A Ca^{2+}-sensing receptor (CaSR) in the plasma membrane of chief cells detects Ca^{2+}

concentration in serum. When Ca^{2+} levels go down, the secretion of parathyroid hormone is stimulated. Parathyroid hormone regulates the Ca^{2+} and PO_4^{3-} balance by acting on:

(1) The bone tissue, stimulating the function of osteoclasts.

(2) The uriniferous tubule, by stimulating the resorption of Ca^{2+} by osteoclasts and activating the production of vitamin D.

Parathyroid hormone induces the production of proteins in osteoblasts, which stimulate osteoclastogenesis. Proteins produced by osteoblasts and involved in osteoclastogenesis are macrophage-colony stimulating factor, RANKL, and osteoprotegerin.

• **Hyperparathyroidism** is caused by an adenoma (benign tumor) of the parathyroid gland. Excessive secretion of parathyroid hormone causes hypercalcemia, phosphaturia, and hypercalciuria. Complications include the formation of renal stones and bone cysts caused by excessive removal of mineralized bone. Inactivating mutations of CaSR cause **familial benign hypercalcemia.** Activating mutations of CaSR result in **idiopathic hypoparathyroidism.**

C cells, present in the lining of the thyroid follicle, produce calcitonin, which antagonizes the effects of parathyroid hormone.

Vitamin D. Cholecalciferol is formed in the skin from 7-dehydrocholesterol. Before reaching its active form, cholecalciferol undergoes two hydroxylation steps, first in the liver (25-hydroxycholecalciferol) and the second in the kidneys.

Low Ca^{2+} levels stimulate 1α-hydroxylase to convert 25-hydroxycholecalciferol into calcitriol, the active form of vitamin D. The main function of vitamin D (calcitriol) is to stimulate the absorption of calcium by the intestinal mucosa.

Calcitriol is transported to the small intestine through the bloodstream, bound to vitamin D–binding protein. In the duodenum, calcitriol is taken up by enterocytes, which are stimulated by vitamin D to produce calbindin, a calcium-binding protein.

Calcium is absorbed in the duodenum by transcellular absorption, an active process that requires calbindin (for transcellular transport), and a voltage-insensitive channel controlled by calcium-ATPase (for export to the bloodstream). Calcium is absorbed in the jejunum and ileum by a passive paracellular absorption mechanism.

In children, a deficiency of vitamin D causes **rickets.** In adults, it causes **osteomalacia.**

• **Adrenal (suprarenal) gland.** The adrenal glands develop from two separate embryologic tissues:

(1) The neural crest ectoderm.

(2) The mesoderm.

Cells from the celomic epithelium aggregate on each side, between the developing gonads and the dorsal mesentery, to form the fetal cortex.

The medulla originates from neural crest cells migrating from the adjacent sympathetic ganglia into the medial region of the fetal cortex.

A layer of mesodermic cells surrounds the fetal cortex to form the precursor of the adult adrenal cortex.

Mesenchymal cells surround each developing adrenal gland and differentiate into fibroblasts that form the perirenal fascia and capsule.

At birth, the adrenal glands are 20 times relatively larger than they are in the adult. The zonae glomerulosa and fasciculata are present. The zona reticularis is not apparent.

By the third month after birth, the celomic-derive fetal cortex regresses and disappears within the first year of life. The mesoderm-derived adrenal cortex precursor, consisting of the zona glomerulosa and the zona fasciculata, remains as the definitive cortex. The zona reticularis develops by the end of the third year.

During the early stage of gestation, the fetal adrenal cortex synthesizes dehydroepiandrosterone, a precursor of the synthesis of estrogen by the placenta. A lack of 3β-hydroxysteroid dehydrogenase activity prevents the synthesis of progesterone, glucocorticoids, and androstenedione.

The interaction between the fetal adrenal cortex and the placenta constitutes the **fetoplacental unit.**

Glucocorticoids, either of maternal origin or synthesized from placental progesterone by the fetus, are essential for:

(1) The production of surfactant by type II alveolar cells after the eighth month of fetal life.

(2) The development of a functional hypothalamopituitary axis.

(3) The induction of thymic involution.

The adrenal gland consists of two components:

(1) The adrenal cortex, derived from the mesoderm.

(2) The adrenal medulla, derived from neural crest cells.

The fetal adrenal cortex plays an important role during early gestation: it synthesizes dehydroepiandrosterone (DHEA), a precursor for the synthesis of estrogen by the placenta. This interaction is known as the fetoplacental unit. After the eighth month of gestation, glucocorticoids are essential for the production of surfactant by type II alveolar cells.

The adrenal cortex consists of three zones:

(1) The outermost, subcapsular zona glomerulosa, which produces the mineralocorticoid aldosterone.

(2) The middle layer of the zona fasciculata, which produces glucocorticoids, mainly cortisol.

(3) The inner layer of the zona reticularis, which synthesizes the androgens DHEA and androstenedione. The function of the zona glomerulosa is controlled by angiotensin II (ANG II), and the functions of the zona fasciculata and zona reticularis are regulated by adrenocorticotropic hormone (ACTH).

The significant structural characteristics of steroid-producing cells are lipid droplets (containing cholesterol), mitochondria with

tubular cristae (housing the enzymes involved in steroidogenesis), and smooth endoplasmic reticulum cisternae (also containing membrane-associated enzymes involved in the production of steroids).

• **Congenital adrenal hyperplasia** results from a genetic enzymatic defect in the synthesis of cortisol. The adrenal cortex is responsive to ACTH and the adrenal cortex enlarges (adrenal hyperplasia).

Lipoid congenital adrenal hyperplasia is caused by a mutation in the gene encoding steroidogenic acute regulatory protein (StAR), a protein that transports cholesterol across the outer mitochondrial membrane. The synthesis of adrenal and gonadal steroids is affected.

Primary hyperaldosteronism or **Conn's syndrome** is caused by a tumor in the zona glomerulosa that produces excessive aldosterone.

Cushing's *disease* is caused by an ACTH-producing tumor of the anterior hypophysis, resulting in an increased production of cortical steroids. **Cushing's** *syndrome* is caused by a functional tumor of the adrenal cortex, resulting in the overproduction of aldosterone, glucocorticoids, and androgens.

Waterhouse-Friderichsen syndrome, seen in infants, is the acute destruction of the adrenal gland by meningococcal septicemia.

Addison's disease is the chronic destruction of the adrenal cortex by an autoimmune process or tuberculosis.

• The **adrenal medulla** consists of two cell populations of chromaffin, catecholamine-producing cells or modified sympathetic postganglionic neurons:

(1) Epinephrine-producing cells (80%).

(2) Norepinephrine-producing cells (20%).

Epinephrine is stored in granules with a dense eccentric core; norepinephrine-containing granules are smaller and occupy a less dense central core than epinephrine-containing granules.

The synthesis of catecholamines includes the following steps:

(1) Tyrosine is converted to DOPA,

(2) DOPA is converted to dopamine, which changes into norepinephrine stored in a vesicle in the form of an eccentric granule.

(3) Norepinephrine leaves the granule, enters the cytosol, and becomes epinephrine under the influence of phenylethanolamine *N*-methyltransferase (PNMT).

(4) The synthesis of PNMT is stimulated by glucocorticoids arriving in the adrenal medulla from the zona fasciculata.

(5) Epinephrine enters a vesicle and forms a complex with chromogranins, and is released into fenestrated capillaries following stimulation by a cholinergic axon from a preganglionic sympathetic neuron in the presence of calcium.

In contrast to the adrenal medulla, cells of the adrenal cortex do not store steroid hormones in granules. Vanillylmandelic acid and metanephrine are metabolic products of catecholamines. They are used clinically to determine the production level of catecholamines.

Adrenal pheochromocytoma (or adrenal medullary paraganglioma) is a rare neoplasm that arises from the chromaffin cells. Pheochromocytoma causes sustained or episodic hypertension, tachycardia, and tremor. The gross appearance of a pheochromocytoma is a hemorrhagic mass. Microscopically, the tumor displays a cluster and/or a trabecular pattern surrounded by an abundant sinusoidal-capillary network. Chromogranins are markers for pheochromocytoma.

• The adrenal medulla has a **dual blood supply**:
(1) Blood vessels from the capsular plexus supply the three zones of the cortex. Fenestrated capillaries (called sinusoids) percolate between cells of the zona glomerulosa and zona fasciculata, and form a capillary network in the zona reticularis before entering the medulla. Medullary sinuses collect aldosterone, cortisol, and sexual steroids, which are drained by the central vein of the medulla.
(2) The medullary artery (derived from the inferior adrenal artery) enters the cortex and supplies blood only to the medulla without branching in the adrenal cortex.
There are no veins or lymphatics in the adrenal cortex.

• **Endocrine pancreas**. The pancreas has two portions:

(1) The exocrine pancreas, consisting of acini involved in the production of enzymes transported to the duodenum.
(2) The endocrine pancreas or islets of Langerhans.
The islets of Langerhans are formed by two components:
(1) The endocrine cells A (α cells), B (β cells), D (δ cells), and F cells, each secreting a single hormone.
(2) A vascular component, the insuloacinar portal system, which enables a local action of insular hormone on the exocrine pancreas.
A cells secrete glucagon (which increases glucose blood levels).
B cells secrete insulin (which increases the transport of glucose into cells; such as hepatocytes and skeletal and cardiac muscle cells).
D cells secrete gastrin (which stimulates production of HCl by parietal cells in the stomach) and somatostatin (which inhibits the release of insulin and glucagon, and the secretion of HCl by parietal cells).
F cells produce pancreatic polypeptide (which inhibits the secretion of somatostatin and the secretion of pancreatic enzymes).

The secretion of insulin is stimulated by an influx of Ca^{2+} into B cells through voltage-gated Ca^{2+} channels. Ca^{2+} influx occurs when the adenosine triphosphate (ATP)-sensitive K^+ channel (K_{ATP}) closes and K^+ accumulates in the cytosol.
Mutations in the *sulfonyurea receptor* (*Sur1*) gene and the *inward rectifying K+ channel* (*Kir6.2*) gene, components of the K_{ATP}

channel, are seen in patients with **neonatal diabetes mellitus**.

• **Diabetes** is characterized by hyperglycemia, polyuria, and polydipsia.
The glycated hemoglobin test, also called hemoglobin A1c (HbA1c) test, provides an average of blood glucose measurements over a 6 to 12 week period. When blood glucose levels are high, the sugar combines with hemoglobin that becomes glycated (coated).
The HbA1c test range in normal individuals is between 4% and 5.6%. Individuals with diabetes should have HbA1c less of 6.5%.
Type 1 diabetes (also known as juvenile diabetes) is determined by autoimmunity, viral infection, and chemical toxins affecting insulin-producing B cells. There is a lack of insulin in type I diabetes.
Type 2 diabetes is caused by a genetic predisposition. The levels of insulin are insufficient relative to glucose levels. In addition, tissues decrease responsiveness to insulin (insulin resistance).
Chronic diabetes affects the vascular system. Atherosclerosis of the aorta and large and medium-sized blood vessels leads to myocardial and brain infarctions and gangrene of the lower extremities. Capillaries are also affected. Retinopathy, cataract, and glaucoma can cause total blindness.
Glomerulopathy (**Kimmelstiel-Wilson lesion**), consists of thickening of the glomerular basal lamina of glomerular capillaries, and proliferation of mesangial cells that affects glomerular filtration of the kidneys.

20. Spermatogenesis

The male reproductive system is responsible for (1) the continuous production, nourishment, and temporary storage of the haploid male gamete (spermatozoa [sing. spermatozoon], or sperm); and (2) the synthesis and secretion of male sex hormones (androgens). The male reproductive system consists of (1) the testes, which produce sperm and synthesize and secrete androgens; (2) the epididymis, vas deferens, ejaculatory duct, and a segment of the male urethra, which form the excurrent duct system responsible for the transport of spermatozoa to the exterior; (3) accessory glands, the seminal vesicle, the prostate gland, and the bulbourethral glands of Cowper, whose secretions form the bulk of the semen and provide nutrients to ejaculated spermatozoa; and (4) the penis, the copulatory organ, formed of erectile tissue. The testes, epididymis, and the initial part of the vas deferens are located in the scrotal sac, a skin-covered pouch enclosing a mesothelium-lined cavity—the tunica vaginalis. This chapter is focused on structural and functional aspects of sperm development, pathologic conditions related to male infertility, genomic imprinting, and testicular tumors.

The testes

The testes are paired organs located in the scrotum, outside the abdominal cavity. This location enables maintenance of the testes at a temperature 2°C to 3°C below body temperature. A temperature of 34°C to 35°C is essential for normal **spermatogenesis**.

The posterior surface of the mature testes is associated with the epididymis. Both testes and epididymis are suspended in the scrotal sac by the **spermatic cord**, which contains the **vas deferens**, the **spermatic artery**, and the **venous** and **lymphatic plexuses**.

Each testis is enclosed by the **tunica albuginea**, which is thickened to form the **mediastinum** where the **rete testis** is located (Figure 20-1). Fibrous septa from the mediastinum project into the testicular mass, dividing the tissue into 250 to 300 **lobules**. Each lobule contains one to four **seminiferous tubules**.

Each seminiferous tubule is about 150 μm in diameter and 80 cm long; it is U-shaped with the two ends opening in the **rete testis**. The rete testis is a

Figure 20-1. Testes, epididymis, and vas deferens

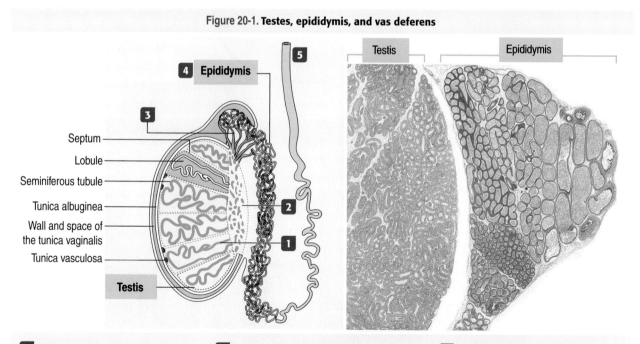

1 **Tubulus rectus**, links the seminiferous tubule to the rete testis.

2 **Rete testis**, a network of spaces contained within the connective tissue of the mediastinum.

3 **Ductuli efferentes**. About 12 to 20 spiral winding ductuli efferentes arise from the rete testis.

4 **Epididymis**. Ductuli efferentes become confluent with a single epididymal highly coiled duct. Note the variation in diameter of the coiled duct containing sperm in the lumen.

5 **Vas deferens**, a muscular tube, continuous with the epididymal duct. Peristaltic contractions of the smooth muscle wall move sperm along the vas.

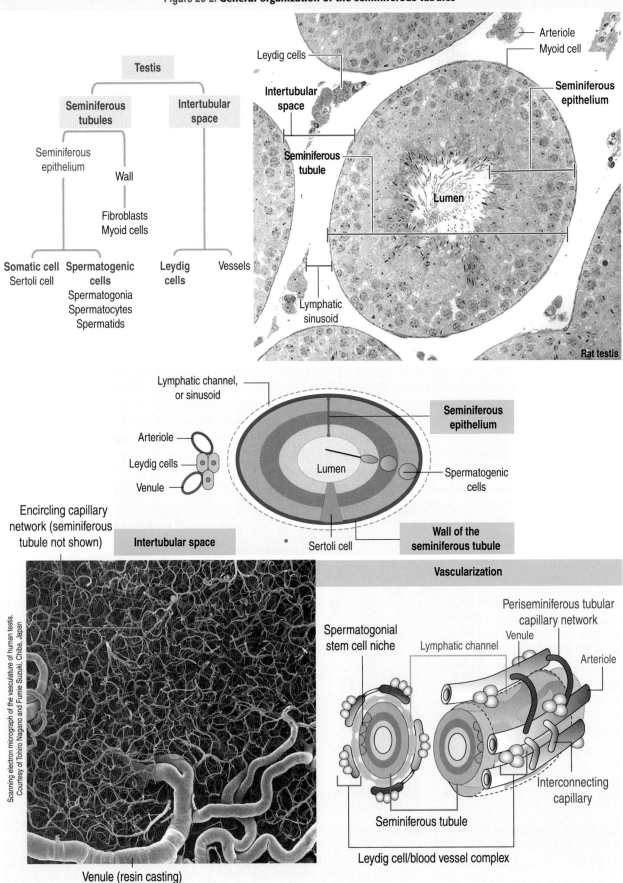

Figure 20-2. General organization of the seminiferous tubules

Testis

Seminiferous tubules

Seminiferous epithelium

Wall

Fibroblasts
Myoid cells

Somatic cell
Sertoli cell

Spermatogenic cells
Spermatogonia
Spermatocytes
Spermatids

Intertubular space

Leydig cells

Vessels

Leydig cells

Intertubular space

Seminiferous tubule

Arteriole
Myoid cell

Seminiferous epithelium

Lumen

Lymphatic sinusoid

Rat testis

Lymphatic channel, or sinusoid

Arteriole

Leydig cells

Venule

Seminiferous epithelium

Lumen

Spermatogenic cells

Intertubular space

Sertoli cell

Wall of the seminiferous tubule

Encircling capillary network (seminiferous tubule not shown)

Scanning electron micrograph of the vasculature of human testis.
Courtesy of Tohiro Nagano and Fumie Suzuki, Chiba, Japan

Venule (resin casting)

Vascularization

Spermatogonial stem cell niche

Lymphatic channel

Periseminiferous tubular capillary network

Venule

Arteriole

Interconnecting capillary

Seminiferous tubule

Leydig cell/blood vessel complex

Figure 20-3. **General histologic structure of the testes**

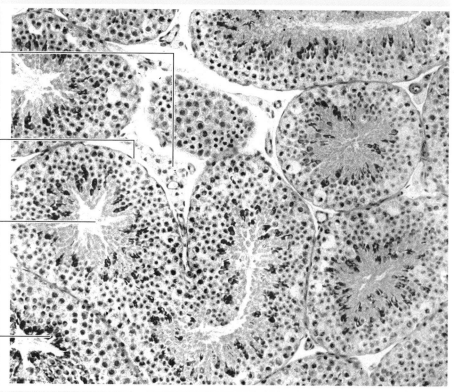

Clusters of **Leydig cells** are present in the intertubular space. Leydig cells are in close contact with blood vessels and lymphatic channels. The major product of Leydig cells is testosterone.

The **wall of the seminiferous tubule** consists of **peritubular myoid cells** separated from the seminiferous epithelium by a basement membrane.

The **lumen of a seminiferous tubule** displays the free ends of the tails of developing spermatids. Fluid and secretory proteins from Sertoli cells are also found in the lumen.

Periodic acid–Schiff staining detects glycoproteins in the developing acrosome of spermatids adjacent to the lumen of the seminiferous tubule.

Although variations are observed in the cellular composition of the seminiferous epithelium, reflecting both synchrony and overlap of spermatogenic cell progenies during their development, Sertoli cells are the permanent somatic components of the epithelium.

Sertoli cells:
1. Maintain a close relationship with spermatogonia, primary and secondary spermatocytes, and spermatids.
2. Are postmitotic in the adult testis.

network of channels that collects the products of the **seminiferous epithelium** (testicular sperm, secretory proteins, fluid, and ions).

The seminiferous tubule (Figure 20-2) consists of a central lumen lined by a specialized seminiferous epithelium containing **two distinct cell populations:**
1. The **somatic Sertoli cells.**
2. The **spermatogenic cells** (spermatogonia, spermatocytes, and spermatids).

The seminiferous epithelium is encircled by a **basement membrane** and a wall formed by **collagenous fibers, fibroblasts,** and **contractile myoid cells.** Myoid cells are responsible for the **rhythmic contractile activity** that propels the **nonmotile sperm** to the rete testis. Sperm acquire forward motility after they have passed through the epididymal duct.

The space in between the seminiferous tubules is occupied by abundant blood vessels (arterioles, capillaries, and venules) and aggregates of the androgen-producing **Leydig cells.** Lymphatic channels, in close proximity to Leydig cells, encircle each seminiferous tubule (see Figure 20-2).

We initiate this chapter by describing the histology of the testes seen with light microscopy (Figures 20-3 and 20-4) and electron microscopy (Figure 20-5).

Seminiferous epithelium

The seminiferous epithelium can be classified as a stratified epithelium with rather unusual characteristics not found in any stratified epithelium of the body.

In this stratified epithelium, somatic columnar Sertoli cells interact with mitotically dividing spermatogonia, meiotically dividing spermatocytes, and a haploid population of spermatids undergoing a differentiation process called **spermiogenesis.**

Figure 20-3 illustrates several cross sections of seminiferous tubules. Note that irregular arrangement of seminiferous tubules generates different profiles in the sections.

A more detailed view of the seminiferous epithelium is seen in Figure 20-4. Different structural types of nuclei can be appreciated:

1. The nuclei of spermatogonia and Sertoli cells are closely associated to the seminiferous tubular wall.

2. Overlying the spermatogonial cell population are the primary spermatocytes. Their nuclei are larger and clumps of chromatin represent the meiotic chromosomes.

3. Close to the lumen are the early spermatids with a round light nucleus and the late spermatids with a cylindrical-shaped condensed nuclei.

Figure 20-4. **Identification of seminiferous epithelial cells**

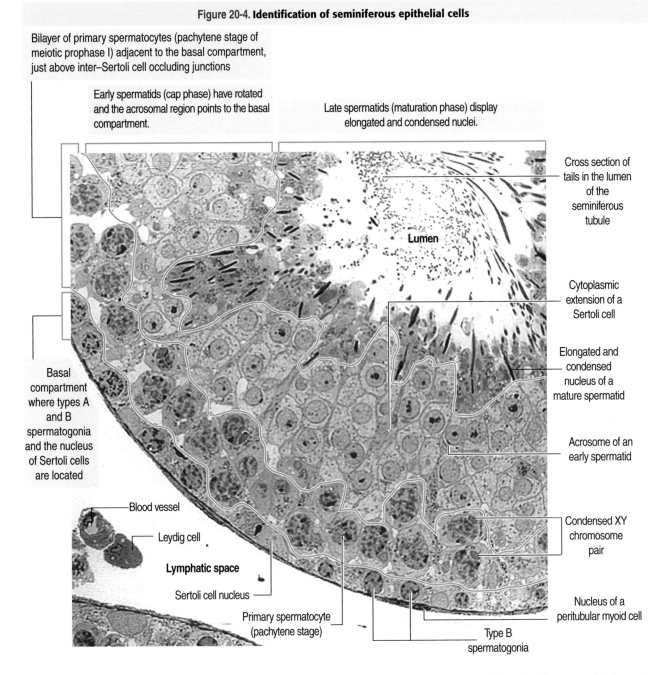

Bilayer of primary spermatocytes (pachytene stage of meiotic prophase I) adjacent to the basal compartment, just above inter–Sertoli cell occluding junctions

Early spermatids (cap phase) have rotated and the acrosomal region points to the basal compartment.

Late spermatids (maturation phase) display elongated and condensed nuclei.

Cross section of tails in the lumen of the seminiferous tubule

Lumen

Cytoplasmic extension of a Sertoli cell

Basal compartment where types A and B spermatogonia and the nucleus of Sertoli cells are located

Elongated and condensed nucleus of a mature spermatid

Acrosome of an early spermatid

Blood vessel

Leydig cell

Lymphatic space

Sertoli cell nucleus

Primary spermatocyte (pachytene stage)

Condensed XY chromosome pair

Nucleus of a peritubular myoid cell

Type B spermatogonia

Figure 20-5 illustrates in an electron micrograph the basal lamina and fibrillar components of the seminiferous tubular wall and the nuclear characteristics of two Sertoli cells, spermatogonia, and primary spermatocytes. Note how Sertoli cell processes extend between the spermatogenic cells.

The next step is to provide additional information to help understand why each cell progeny occupies a specific space in the seminiferous epithelium

The basal and adluminal compartments of the seminiferous epithelium

Sertoli cells are columnar cells extending from the basal lamina to the lumen of the seminiferous tubule

(see Figures 20-2 and 20-5). They act as **bridge cells** between the intertubular space and the lumen of the seminiferous tubule and as **nurse cells**, supporting spermatogenic cell survival.

The apical and lateral plasma membranes of Sertoli cells have an irregular outline because they provide **niches** and **crypts** to house the developing spermatogenic cells (Figure 20-6).

At their **basolateral** domain, Sertoli cells form **tight junctions** with adjoining Sertoli cells. Most epithelia have tight junctions at the apical domain. Therefore, tight junctions at the basolateral domain of Sertoli cells represents an exception to the rule.

If you consider that molecules and fluids in a stan-

Figure 20-5. **Human seminiferous epithelium**

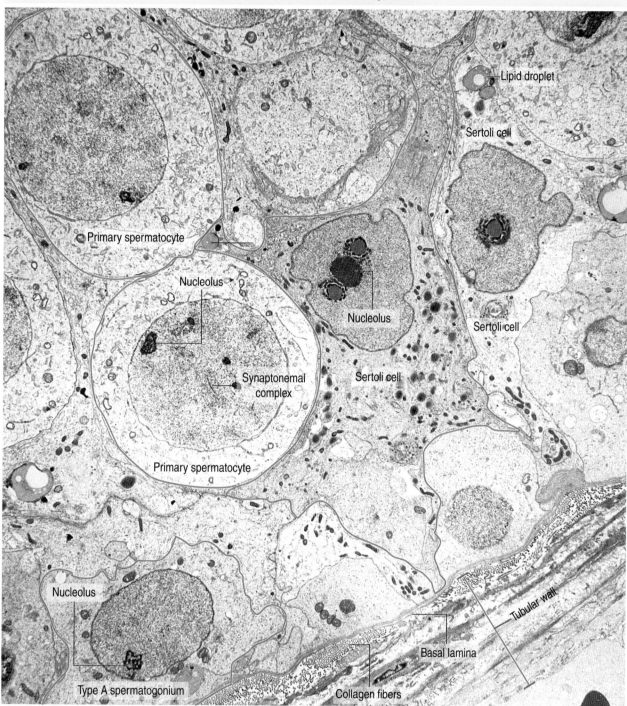

Sertoli cells display a columnar shape, with the cytoplasm extending like a bridge from the lumen to the basal lamina of the seminiferous epithelium and cytoplasmic processes enveloping adjacent spermatogenic cells, forming **niches**. The **irregularly shaped nucleus**, with a prominent nucleolus and associated heterochromatin masses, is observed in the **basal portion of the cell**. **Lipid droplets** are present.

Spermatogonia are in contact with the basal lamina. In human testes, spermatogonia A include two subtypes based on the nuclear appearance (not shown): (1) **spermatogonium A pale** (A$_{pale}$) and (2) **spermatogonium A dark** (A$_{dark}$).

Spermatocytes are located above the blood-testis barrier, represented by inter–Sertoli cell tight junctions. Most spermatocytes are **primary spermatocytes**. They are recognized by three specific features, depending on the stage of meiotic prophase I: (1) a condensed chromatin mass adjacent to the nuclear envelope, corresponding to the XY chromosome pair (see Figure 20-4); (2) nucleolar masses originated in several autosomal bivalents, and (3) sections of the synaptonemal complex, connecting homologous chromosomes in preparation for crossing-over events.

The **tubular wall** is thick. It consists of three to five layers of myoid cells, fibroblasts and adjacent collagen and elastic fibers.

Figure 20-6. **Two compartments of the seminiferous epithelium**

The **Sertoli cell** spans from the seminiferous tubular wall to the lumen and has cell-cell contacts with all proliferating and differentiating spermatogenic cells.

The cytoplasm of Sertoli cells encloses (1) spermatogonial **niches** in the basal compartment, between themselves and the basal lamina; (2) spermatocytes and early spermatids, in adluminal **niches** between adjacent Sertoli cells; and (3) late spermatids, in **crypts** at the luminal surfaces of Sertoli cells.

Basal tight junctions between adjacent Sertoli cells form the **blood-testis barrier.** The barrier prevents proteins, including antibodies, from reaching developing spermatogenic cells.

In an opposite direction, the barrier prevents proteins in developing spermatogenic cells from leaking and triggering an immune response.

Tight junctions divide the seminiferous epithelium into a **basal compartment**, below the junctions, and an **adluminal compartment**, above the junctions. Spermatogonia are located in the basal compartment and spermatocytes and spermatids occupy the adluminal compartment.

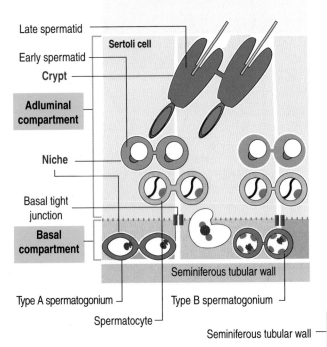

Seminiferous tubular lumen

Late spermatid — Sertoli cell

Early spermatid

Crypt

Adluminal compartment

Niche

Basal tight junction

Basal compartment

Seminiferous tubular wall

Type A spermatogonium — Type B spermatogonium

Spermatocyte

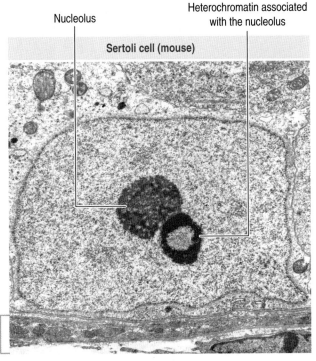

Nucleolus — Heterochromatin associated with the nucleolus

Sertoli cell (mouse)

Seminiferous tubular wall

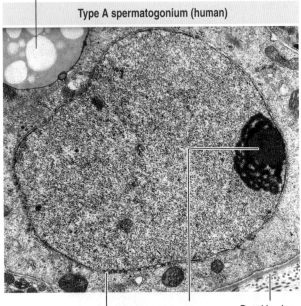

Lipid droplet (Sertoli cell)

Type A spermatogonium (human)

Nuclear envelope   Nucleolus   Basal lamina

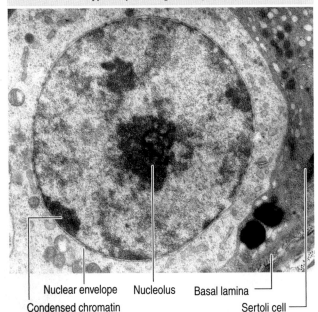

Type B spermatogonium (human)

Nuclear envelope   Nucleolus   Basal lamina

Condensed chromatin   Sertoli cell

dard epithelium follow the apical-to-basal transport direction across tight junctions, in the seminiferous tubules the transporting direction is reversed: basal-to-apical. In fact, the source of fluid and nutrients is not in the luminal space but rather in the inter-seminiferous tubular space.

Basolateral tight junctions subdivide the seminiferous epithelium into:

1. A **basal compartment**.
2. An **adluminal compartment** (see Figure 20-4). Note that:

• The spermatogonial cell population is housed in **niches** within the basal compartment. This location has ample access to nutrients and signaling molecules derived from vessels in the inter-seminiferous tubular space.

• Inter-Sertoli tight junctions are components of the so-called **blood-testes barrier**. This barrier protects developing spermatocytes and spermatids, located within the adluminal compartment, from autoimmune reactions.

The spermatogenic cell sequence
The basic concepts to remember are:

• Somatic Sertoli cells represent the **stable** members of the seminiferous tubule cell population.

• The spermatogenic cell progenies are **transient**.

Figure 20-7 illustrates relevant aspects of a mammalian spermatogenic cell sequence.

1. At puberty, a **spermatogonial stem cell (SSC)**, derived from a primordial germinal cell in the fetal testes, divides by mitosis to generate two daughter cells. **One daughter cell initiates a spermatogenic cell sequence. The other cell becomes a SSC with self-renewal capacity and able to soon initiate another spermatogenic cell sequence.** We have seen in Chapter 3, Cell Signaling, that stem cells can self-renew and give rise to another stem cell and a cell entering a terminal differentiation pathway. The same rule applies to SSCs.

2. After cell division, all **spermatogenic cells remain interconnected by intercellular bridges** because cytokinesis is incomplete.

3. Spermatogonia, spermatocytes, and spermatids complete their proliferation and differentiation sequence in a timely manner.

Each spermatogenic cell cohort proliferates and differentiates synchronously.

4. SSCs periodically initiate spermatogenic cell series to ensure the continuous production of sperm. We will study later how spermatogenic cell cycles overlap in a segment of a seminiferous tubule and generate distinct combinations of spermatogenic cell cohorts called **cellular associations**.

Now that you have been exposed to the basic aspects of the organization of a mammalian testis, the next step is to understand how the different spermatogenic cells types are distributed in the seminiferous epithelium with respect to the Sertoli cell.

Sertoli cells
Sertoli cells are the predominant cell type of the seminiferous epithelium until **puberty**. After puberty, they represent about 10% of the cells lining the seminiferous tubules. Sertoli cells are **postmitotic after puberty**. No mitotic cell division is observed in the adult testes. In elderly men, when the population of spermatogenic cells decreases, Sertoli cells again become the major component of the epithelium.

The **cytoskeleton of Sertoli cells** (microtubules, actin microfilaments, and the intermediate filament vimentin) facilitates the displacement of differentiating spermatogenic cells farther away from the periphery of the seminiferous tubule and closer to the lumen.

Members of the spermatogonia progeny, interconnected by intercellular bridges, complete the mitotic amplification cycle, translocate from the basal compartment to the adluminal compartment, and initiate the meiotic cycle as primary spermatocytes. Inter-Sertoli tight junctions unzip and re-zip to enable the massive migration of interconnected cells.

How can Sertoli cells be identified in a histology preparation?

The most useful parameter is the Sertoli **cell nucleus**. The cytoplasmic processes of a Sertoli cell are tortuous and difficult to resolve with the light microscope.

The Sertoli cell **nucleus** is located at the base of the cell, near the basal lamina. It displays **indentations** and a **large nucleolus** with associated **heterochromatin masses** (see Figures 20-5 and 20-6).

The cytoplasm contains smooth and rough endoplasmic reticulum, mitochondria, lysosomes, lipid droplets, an extensive Golgi apparatus, and a rich cytoskeleton.

The **functions** of Sertoli cells are:

1. To support, protect, and nourish developing spermatogenic cells.

2. To eliminate by **phagocytosis** excess cell portions, called **residual bodies**, discarded by spermatids at the end of **spermiogenesis**.

3. To facilitate the release of mature spermatids into the lumen of the seminiferous tubule by actin-mediated contraction, a process called **spermiation**.

4. To secrete a fluid rich in proteins, lactate, and ions into the seminiferous tubular lumen.

Sertoli cells respond to **follicle-stimulating hormone (FSH)** stimulation and express **androgen receptors**. Androgens acting through Sertoli cells stimulate spermatogenesis by a still undefined mechanism (see Box 20-A). FSH regulates the synthesis

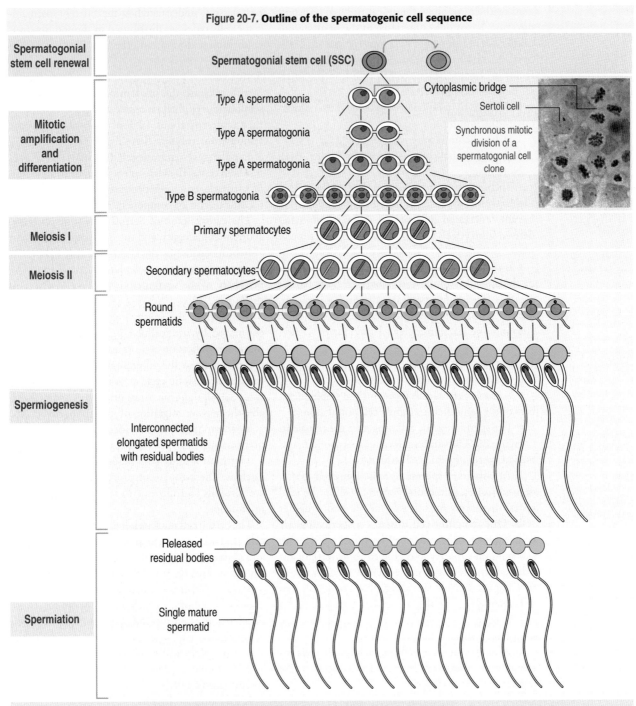

Figure 20-7. **Outline of the spermatogenic cell sequence**

Spermatogonial stem cell renewal — Spermatogonial stem cell (SSC)

Mitotic amplification and differentiation — Type A spermatogonia · Type A spermatogonia · Type A spermatogonia · Type B spermatogonia — Cytoplasmic bridge · Sertoli cell · Synchronous mitotic division of a spermatogonial cell clone

Meiosis I — Primary spermatocytes

Meiosis II — Secondary spermatocytes

Spermiogenesis — Round spermatids · Interconnected elongated spermatids with residual bodies

Spermiation — Released residual bodies · Single mature spermatid

The spermatogenic cell sequence: Highlights to remember

Spermatogenesis starts at puberty when **spermatogonial stem cells (SSC) derived from primordial germinal cells (PGCs)** undergo mitotic cell division to produce two daughter cells. One daughter cell remains as a SSC; the other initiates a mitotic amplification and differentiation sequence giving rise to morphologically distinct spermatogonia type A and type B.

Type B spermatogonia complete the S phase (DNA synthesis) of their cell cycle and advance to G_2. Instead of undergoing mitotic cell division, they translocate to the adluminal compartment and initiate meiosis I.

A characteristic feature of spermatogenesis is **incomplete**

cytokinesis. Cells are conjoined to each other by **cytoplasmic bridges**, a condition that persists until the completion of spermatogenesis.

Another typical aspect of spermatogenesis is **cell cycle synchrony** (see image inset). All the cells initiate, progress, and complete a differentiation sequence in a coordinated manner.

The conjoined condition terminates when mature spermatids are released at the end of spermiogenesis by the process of **spermiation. Residual bodies**, linked by cytoplasmic bridges, separate from the spermatids and are phagocytosed by Sertoli cells. Mature spermatids become single cells transported to the rete testis.

• Testosterone, produced in the testes by Leydig cells in response to luteinizing homone (LH) stimulation, is released into peripheral blood and lymphatic channels encircling seminiferous tubules and diffuses into the seminiferous epithelium. Testosterone levels in the testes are about 25–125-fold higher than in serum. Only one-third of testosterone is bound to androgen binding protein (ABP), a secretory product of Sertoli cells.

• Testosterone effects are mediated by the **androgen receptor** (**AR**) localized in the cytosol and nucleus of Sertoli cells. AR is also present in the contractile peritubular myoid cells and vascular smooth muscle cells. No functional AR has been found in spermatogenic cells.

• In humans, AR in Sertoli cells is detected at the age of 5 months and AR gene expression in Sertoli cells is cyclical (dependent on the stages of the spermatogenic cycle; described later in this chapter).

• Testosterone is required for: (1) the maintenance of the blood-testis barrier; (2) the progression and completion of meiosis; (3) the adhesion of spermatids to Sertoli cells; and (4) release of mature spermatids (spermiation). Details of the molecular and cellular of some of these events regulated by testosterone remain to be characterized.

and secretion of **androgen-binding protein** (**ABP**).

ABP is a secretory protein with high binding affinity for the androgens **testosterone** and **dihydrotestosterone**. The androgen-ABP complex, whose function is unknown at present, is transported to the proximal segments of the epididymis.

We come back to this aspect later in this chapter and in Chapter 21, Sperm Transport and Maturation.

Note that although both ABP and the androgen receptor have binding affinity for androgens, they are distinct proteins. ABP is a secretory protein, whereas the androgen receptor is a cytoplasmic and nuclear protein with DNA binding activity.

Sertoli cells secrete **inhibin** and **activin** subunits (α and β subunits):

1. Inhibin (an αβ **heterodimer**) exerts a **negative feedback** on gonadotropin-releasing factor and FSH release by the hypothalamus and anterior hypophysis.

2. **Activin** (an αα or ββ **homodimer**) exerts a **positive feedback** on the release of FSH (see Chapter 18, Neuroendocrine System).

Sertoli cells also secrete regulatory proteins required

for spermatogonial cell differentiation (discussed later).

Clinical significance: Sertoli cell–only syndrome
Sertoli cell–only syndrome (SCOS) is a clinical condition defined by **germinal aplasia**, the absence of spermatogenic cells in seminiferous tubules. Seminiferous tubules are lined only by Sertoli cells. SCOS can be determined by congenital (including Y chromosome abnormalities) or acquired factors (see Box 20-B).

Spermatogonia
Spermatogonia are diploid spermatogenic cells residing in a unique environment, or **niche, directly in contact with the basal lamina** in the basal compartment in association with Sertoli cells (see Figure 20-6). They are located below the inter–Sertoli cell occluding junctions and therefore **outside** the blood-testes barrier.

Two major morphologic spermatogonial cell types can be observed:

1. **Type A spermatogonia** display an oval euchromatic nucleus and a nucleolus attached to the nuclear envelope (see Figure 20-6). Subclasses of type A spermatogonia (with a dark nucleus, called **A dark spermatogonium,** and with a lighter nucleus, called **A pale spermatogonium**) are observed in human testes.

2. **Type B spermatogonia** have a round nucleus, masses of heterochromatin attached to the nuclear envelope, and a central nucleolus (see Figures 20-4 and 20-6).

Stimulated by follicle-stimulating hormone, FSH, Sertoli cells secrete **GDNF** (for glial cell line-derived neurotrophic factor) that stimulates SSC renewal and differentiation by binding to the GDNF family receptor α1 (GFRα1) (Figure 20-8).

There is a balance between SSC renewal and spermatogonial differentiation. Maintenance of this balance determines an input-output equilibrium between the number of SCCs being produced (input)

• **Sertoli cell–only syndrome** (SCOS) is also known as germinal cell aplasia or Del Castillo syndrome. SCOS is characterized by the presence of Sertoli cells only. Spermatogenic cells are absent. Leydig cells display crystals of Reinke in the cytoplasm.

• SCOS is associated with permanent and irreversible **azoospermia** (no sperm are produced). The diagnosis is based on testicular biopsy findings.

• SCOS can be congenital or acquired. **Congenital factors** include a failure of primordial germinal cells (PGCs) to migrate to the gonadal ridges during embryonic development, cryptorchidism, Y chromosome abnormalities (microdeletions in the Yq11 region of the Y chromosome, encoding the **AZF, azoospermia factor**), and deficiency in gonadotropins (follicle-stimulating hormone and luteinizing hormone). **Acquired factors** responsible for the loss of spermatogenic cells include radiation therapy, chemotherapy, and severe trauma.

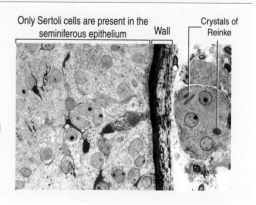

Only Sertoli cells are present in the seminiferous epithelium — Wall — Crystals of Reinke

Figure 20-8. Outline of the spermatogenic cycle

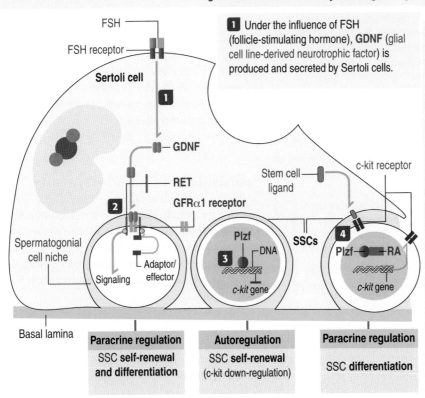

1 Under the influence of FSH (follicle-stimulating hormone), **GDNF** (glial cell line-derived neurotrophic factor) is produced and secreted by Sertoli cells.

2 Sertoli cell-derived GDNF binds to the GFRα1 receptor on SSCs forming a binary complex that binds to the adjacent tyrosine kinase receptor, **RET**. GDNF binding induces tyrosine phosphorylation of the RET intracellular domains to enable binding of adaptor/effector proteins. This **paracrine regulatory event** initiated by Sertoli cells triggers a downstream cascade leading to spermatogonial stem cell (SSC) **self-renewal** and **differentiation**.

3 In contrast, an **autoregulatory** event takes place in SSCs. It is mediated by the transcription factor **Plzf** (promyelocyte leukemia zinc finger) to maintain stable the pool of SSCs. Plzf represses the *c-kit* tyrosine kinase receptor gene to prevent the differentiation of SSCs.

4 Retinoic acid (RA) down-regulates the transcription factor Plzf to enable the expression of *c-kit* receptor gene. Then, Sertoli cell-derived stem cell ligand binds to c-kit receptor to trigger SSC differentiation.

Paracrine regulation
SSC **self-renewal and differentiation**

Autoregulation
SSC **self-renewal** (c-kit down-regulation)

Paracrine regulation
SSC **differentiation**

and the number of sperm released (output).

The transcription factor **Plzf** (for promyelocytic leukemia zinc finger) deters SSC self-renewal by blocking the gene expressing the **c-kit tyrosine kinase receptor**.

When SSCs are ready to start their self-renewal process, retinoic acid down-regulates the transcription factor Plzf, thereby **unblocking** the expression of the c-kit receptor that becomes available for binding to the **stem cell ligand**. The ligand is bound to the plasma membrane of Sertoli cells (see Figure 20-8).

There are two regulatory mechanisms of SSCs:

1. A **paracrine regulatory mechanism** exerted by the **GDNF-GFRα1-RET complex** and the **c-kit receptor-stem cell ligand complex**. By this mechanism Sertoli cells regulate SSC self-renewal and differentiation.

2. An **autoregulatory mechanism**, mediated by the **retinoic acid–Plzf interplay** that modulates the expression of the *c-kit* gene. This mechanism determines whether SCCs undergo self-renewal.

SSCs have important implications for male fertility. SSCs are relatively quiescent and therefore resistant to radiation and cancer chemotherapy. Mitotically dividing spermatogonia, meiotically dividing spermatocytes, and differentiating spermatids are sensitive to radiation and cancer chemotherapy. After cessation of radiotherapy or anticancer chemotherapy, SSCs can reestablish the spermatogenic

developmental sequence. Postmitotic Sertoli cells are highly resistant to these therapies.

Failure of spermatogonia to undergo differentiation in humans results in a neoplastic transformation into carcinoma in situ leading to a **testicular germ cell carcinoma** in the adult.

Spermatocytes

Type B spermatogonia enter meiotic prophase **immediately after completing the last S phase (DNA synthesis)**. This last round of major DNA synthetic activity in the lifetime of spermatogenic cells determines that a primary spermatocyte starting meiotic prophase I will have **two times the amount of DNA of a spermatogonium**. The primary spermatocyte has a 4C DNA value, where 1C equals about 1.5 pg of DNA per cell.

Spermatocytes divide by **two successive meiotic cell divisions** (Figure 20-9) and are located in the **adluminal compartment** of the seminiferous epithelium, just above the inter–Sertoli cell occluding junctions. Therefore, meiosis occurs **inside** the blood-testes barrier.

A **primary spermatocyte** undergoes the first meiotic division (or **reductional division**) without significant DNA synthesis (only repair DNA synthesis occurs) to produce two **secondary spermatocytes**.

The secondary spermatocytes rapidly undergo the second meiotic division (or **equational division**).

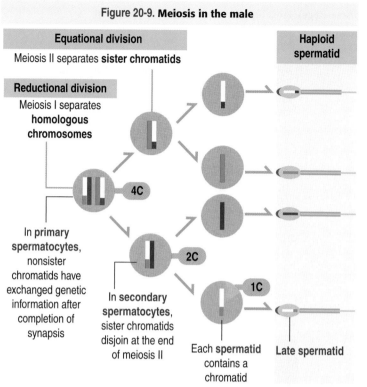

Figure 20-9. Meiosis in the male

Equational division
Meiosis II separates **sister chromatids**

Haploid spermatid

Reductional division
Meiosis I separates **homologous chromosomes**

4C

In **primary spermatocytes**, nonsister chromatids have exchanged genetic information after completion of synapsis

In **secondary spermatocytes**, sister chromatids disjoin at the end of meiosis II

2C

1C

Each **spermatid** contains a chromatid

Late spermatid

Each secondary spermatocyte forms two spermatids that mature without further cell division into sperm.

By the end of the first meiotic division, the original 4C DNA content of a primary spermatocyte is reduced to 2C in a secondary spermatocyte. By the end of the second meiotic division, the 2C DNA content is reduced to 1C. The resulting spermatids

are the haploid spermatids and initiate a complex differentiation process called **spermiogenesis**.

Because the first meiotic division is a long process (days) and the second meiotic division is very short (minutes), primary spermatocytes are the most abundant cells observed in the seminiferous epithelium.

Figure 20-10 illustrates for comparison the meiotic process of the female gamete that is initiated in the ovary during fetal development (see Chapter 23, Fertilization, Placentation, and Lactation).

Meiosis

As already indicated, soon after the last mitotic division of type B spermatogonia, the resulting daughter cells synthesize DNA (S phase), advance into the G_2 phase, and start the first meiotic division with a 4C DNA content. The first meiotic division is characterized by a **long prophase**, lasting about 10 days.

The **prophase substages** of the **first meiotic division** are (Figures 20-11 and 20-12):

1. **Leptotene** (threadlike chromosomes).
2. **Zygotene** (pairing of chromosomes).
3. **Pachytene** (thickening of chromosomes).
4. **Diplotene** (chromosomes appearing double).
5. **Diakinesis** (chromosomes moving apart).

These substages are characterized by four major events:

1. The formation of a **synaptonemal complex** (see Box 20-C) during zygotene-pachytene to facilitate the pairing or **synapsis** of homologous chromosomes (autosomes and sex chromosomes X and Y).

2. The pairing of homologous chromosomes

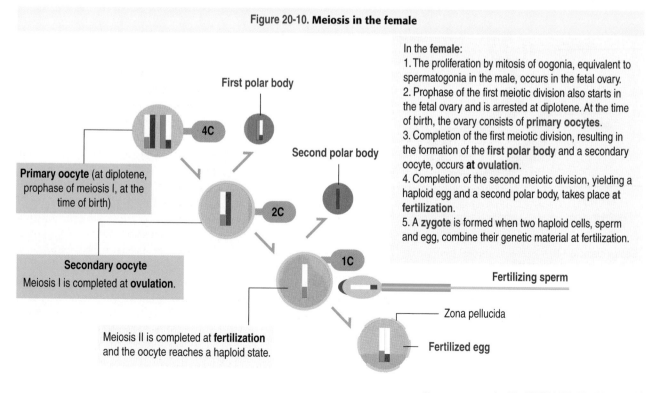

Figure 20-10. Meiosis in the female

First polar body

4C

Second polar body

Primary oocyte (at diplotene, prophase of meiosis I, at the time of birth)

2C

Secondary oocyte
Meiosis I is completed at **ovulation**.

1C

Meiosis II is completed at **fertilization** and the oocyte reaches a haploid state.

Fertilizing sperm

Zona pellucida

Fertilized egg

In the female:
1. The proliferation by mitosis of oogonia, equivalent to spermatogonia in the male, occurs in the fetal ovary.
2. Prophase of the first meiotic division also starts in the fetal ovary and is arrested at diplotene. At the time of birth, the ovary consists of **primary oocytes**.
3. Completion of the first meiotic division, resulting in the formation of the **first polar body** and a secondary oocyte, occurs **at ovulation**.
4. Completion of the second meiotic division, yielding a haploid egg and a second polar body, takes place **at fertilization**.
5. A **zygote** is formed when two haploid cells, sperm and egg, combine their genetic material at fertilization.

Figure 20-11. First meiotic division (prophase stage): From leptotene to zygotene to pachytene

A Leptotene

Each homologous chromosome consists of two **sister** chromatids. Chromosomes attach to the inner membrane of the nuclear envelope.

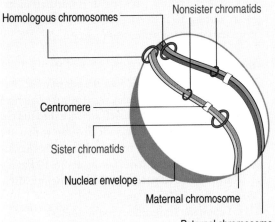

Homologous chromosomes
Nonsister chromatids
Centromere
Sister chromatids
Nuclear envelope
Maternal chromosome
Paternal chromosome

B Zygotene

Synapsis of homologous chromosomes starts.
 Starting from nuclear envelope attachment points, a synaptonemal complex develops between the homologous chromosomes.

1 Initiation of the assembly of the synaptonemal complex

2 Initiation of synapsis of homologous chromosomes

Synapsis

Centrioles

Synaptonemal complex of an autosome

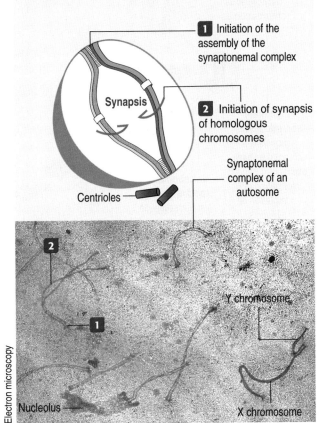

Electron microscopy

2

1

Y chromosome

X chromosome

Nucleolus

C Pachytene

When each homologous chromosome becomes entirely linked by a synaptonemal complex, synapsis is complete. **Cohesin** stabilizes the association between sister chromatids.
 Homologous stretches of paternal and maternal DNA are in register with each other and crossing over between nonsister chromatids starts.

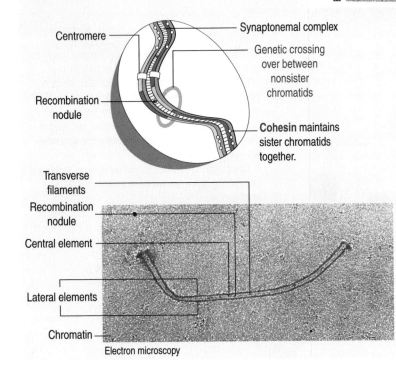

Centromere
Synaptonemal complex
Genetic crossing over between nonsister chromatids
Recombination nodule
Cohesin maintains sister chromatids together.

Transverse filaments
Recombination nodule
Central element
Lateral elements
Chromatin

Electron microscopy

XY chromosomal pair

Autosomal bivalent

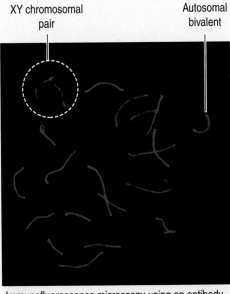

Immunofluorescence microscopy using an antibody to detect synaptonemal complex protein 3 (**SCP3**) in the synaptonemal complex.

(**synapsis**) so recombination sites are co-aligned and bridged.

3. **Crossing over** is the exchange of genetic information between **non-sister chromatids** of homologous chromosomes. Crossovers foster genetic diversity and establish physical links between homologues to ensure precise segregation.

Meiotic recombination starts by DNA **double-strand breaks** (**DSBs**), which take place at precise sites as the synaptonemal complex develops.

Crossovers along any given chromosome pair are evenly spaced over distances from 300 nm to 30 μm. This regularly spaced distribution, known as **crossover interference**, involves the catalytic activity of **topoisomerase II** (**TopoII**), an enzyme that breaks and rejoins double-stranded DNA. Crossover interference means that crossover at a given chromosomal site prevents another crossover to occur too close to it.

4. **Disjunction** (the separation of paired homologous chromosomes) after completion of crossover.

After this prolonged prophase, **pairs of sister chromatids** pass through metaphase, anaphase, and telophase and are separated into daughter cells, the **secondary spermatocytes**.

During the second meiotic division, prophase, metaphase, anaphase, and telophase separate **sister chromatids** into daughter cells, the **spermatids**.

In the female (see Figure 20-10), **a primary oocyte** (with a 4C DNA content) completes the first meiotic division **at ovulation** to produce a **secondary oocyte** (2C DNA content) and the **first polar body. When fertilization occurs,** the secondary oocyte completes the second meiotic division to reach the haploid state (1C DNA content), and a **second polar body** is generated.

The three most important **events of meiosis** are:

1. Sperm and oocytes contain only one representative of each homologous pair of chromosomes.

2. Maternal and paternal chromosomes are randomly assorted.

3. Crossing over increases genetic variation.

Spermatids

Haploid spermatids are located in the **adluminal compartment**, in proximity to the seminiferous tubular lumen. There are two main types of spermatids:

1. **Round** or **early spermatids,** housed in **niches** in the cytoplasm of Sertoli cells.

2. **Elongated** or **late spermatids,** housed in **crypts,** deep invaginations in Sertoli cell apical cytoplasm.

Spermatids are engaged in a highly differentiated cell process designated **spermiogenesis. Spermiogenesis is the last step of spermatogenesis.**

Mature spermatids are released into the seminiferous tubular lumen by a process called **spermiation**. Spermiation involves contractile forces generated by F-actin–containing hoops at the apical ectoplasmic region of Sertoli cells, embracing the head of a mature spermatid.

Spermatids are highly polarized cells. Their polarity is determined by the opposite position of the Golgi-acrosome-acroplaxome complex and the **head-tail coupling apparatus** (HTCA) with respect to the nucleus.

Four major events characterize spermiogenesis (Figures 20-13 and 20-14):

1. The development of the **acrosome**.
2. The development of the **manchette**.
3. The development of the **tail**.
4. The shaping and condensation of the spermatid **nucleus**.

We emphasize details of these four events because of their important contribution to male fertility and to an understanding of causes of male infertility.

1. **Development of the acrosome**. The acrosome contains **hydrolytic enzymes** released at fertilization by a mechanism called **acrosome reaction** (discussed in detail in Chapter 23, Fertilization, Placentation, and Lactation).

The development of the acrosome consists of four sequential phases:

1. The **Golgi phase**.
2. The **cap phase**.
3. The **acrosomal phase**.
4. The **maturation phase** (see Figures 20-13 and 20-14).

• During the **Golgi phase,** proacrosomal vesicles containing **hyaluronidase, proacrosin,** and other hydrolytic enzymes, are transported from the Golgi to the **acroplaxome** along microtubules and actin microfilaments using motor proteins (kinesins and myosin Va, respectively). The acroplaxome (Greek *akros,* topmost; *platys,* flat; *sōma,* body) **is** an actin-

---

Box 20-C | Synaptonemal complex

• The function of the synaptonemal complex is to facilitate the **synapsis** of homologous chromosomes by stabilizing their axial alignment and association.
• Sister chromatids are maintained in close contact by the **cohesin protein complex**.
• The separation between synapsed homologous chromosomes is 100 nm.
• A synaptonemal complex consists of **two lateral elements** (closely associated to chromosomal chromatin loops) and a **central element**.
• The **lateral elements** are formed by the **cohesin protein complex** (Rec8, SCM1, and SCM3 proteins), SCP2, and SCP3 (**SCP** stands for synaptonemal complex protein).
• The lateral elements are bridged by transverse fibrous **SCP1 dimers**, whose terminal globular regions overlap in the center of the synaptonemal complex to form the **central element**.
• **Recombination nodules** are present along the synaptonemal complex during pachytene. They represent sites where genetic recombination between nonsister chromatids (called **reciprocal exchange**) will occur.

D Diplotene

Disjunction of homologous chromosomes takes place when crossing over terminates. Chromosomes remain connected by one or more **chiasmata**, or crossing points.

Centrioles duplicate in preparation for metaphase.

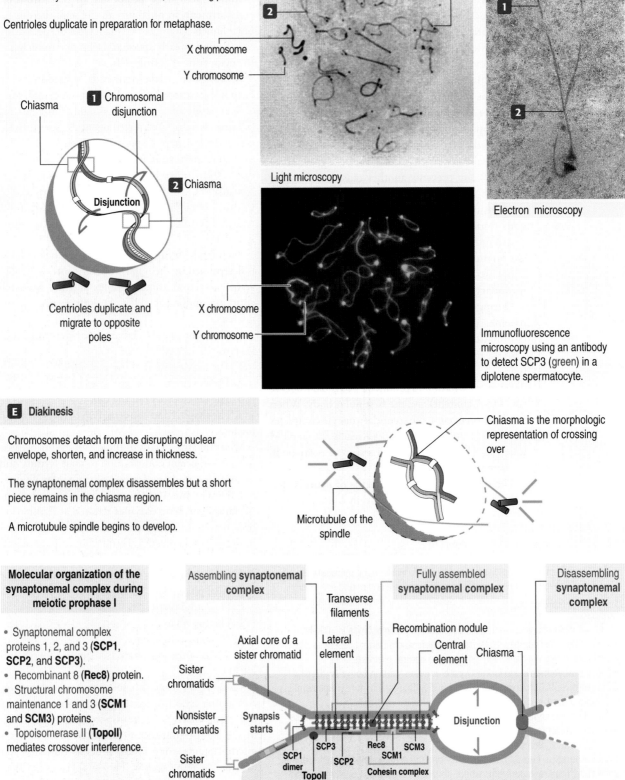

Chiasma

1 Chromosomal disjunction

2 Chiasma

Disjunction

Centrioles duplicate and migrate to opposite poles

X chromosome
Y chromosome

Light microscopy

X chromosome
Y chromosome

Electron microscopy

Immunofluorescence microscopy using an antibody to detect SCP3 (green) in a diplotene spermatocyte.

E Diakinesis

Chromosomes detach from the disrupting nuclear envelope, shorten, and increase in thickness.

The synaptonemal complex disassembles but a short piece remains in the chiasma region.

A microtubule spindle begins to develop.

Chiasma is the morphologic representation of crossing over

Microtubule of the spindle

Molecular organization of the synaptonemal complex during meiotic prophase I

- Synaptonemal complex proteins 1, 2, and 3 (**SCP1**, **SCP2**, and **SCP3**).
- Recombinant 8 (**Rec8**) protein.
- Structural chromosome maintenance 1 and 3 (**SCM1** and **SCM3**) proteins.
- Topoisomerase II (**TopoII**) mediates crossover interference.

Assembling **synaptonemal complex**

Fully assembled **synaptonemal complex**

Disassembling **synaptonemal complex**

Transverse filaments

Axial core of a sister chromatid

Recombination nodule

Lateral element

Central element

Chiasma

Sister chromatids

Nonsister chromatids

Synapsis starts

Sister chromatids

SCP1 dimer

TopoII

SCP3

SCP2

Rec8

SCM1

SCM3

Cohesin complex

Disjunction

Leptotene | Zygotene | Pachytene | Diplotene | Diakinesis

cytokeratin–containing plate anchored to the nuclear envelope.

Proacrosomal vesicles tether and dock to the acroplaxome and fuse to form first the **acrosome vesicle** and then the **acrosomal sac**.

• During the **cap phase**, Golgi-derived proacrosomal vesicles continue to merge into the progressively enlarging acrosomal sac that initiates its caudal descent in parallel to the elongation of the spermatid nucleus.

The acrosome acquires a cap-like shape and its narrow descending recess is anchored to the nuclear envelope by the desmosome-like, keratin intermediate filament protein–containing **marginal ring** of the acroplaxome. The acroplaxome plate anchors the acrosome to the nuclear envelope by a spermiogenesis-specific **LINC** (for **linker of nucleoskeleton and cytoskeleton**) protein complex. LINC connects the dense nuclear lamina to F-actin in the acroplaxome (Figure 20-15).

• During the **acrosomal and maturation phases**, the shape of the acrosome-acroplaxome complex adjusts to the profile of the elongating spermatid head. Mutations in the genes encoding two proacrosomal vesicle fusion proteins, **Hrb** and **GOPC** (for Golgi-associated PDZ and coiled-coil motif-containing protein), disrupts acrosome development. **A lack of an acrosome results in round-headed sperm** (called **globozoospermia**) **and male infertility**.

2. **Development of the manchette.** Soon after the development of the acrosome starts, a transient and predominant microtubule-containing manchette develops at the caudal site of the acrosome-acroplaxome complex.

The manchette consists of a **perinuclear ring** assembled just beneath the desmosome-like marginal ring of the acroplaxome. Microtubules are inserted into the perinuclear ring (see Figures 20-13 and 20-15, and Box 20-D). Therefore, two juxtaposed rings embrace the caudal region of the elongating spermatid nucleus. The acroplaxome and manchette reduce the diameter of their circumvallate rings to comply with an equivalent reduction of the elongating nucleus.

The opposite nuclear region is encircled by **F-actin hoops** of the adjacent Sertoli cells (see Figure 20-15).

From a mechanical perspective, the exogenous clutching forces exerted by the Sertoli cell F-actin hoops, combined with the endogenous force modulation of the acrosome–acroplaxome–manchette (AAM) complex, contribute to the shaping of the gradually elongating spermatid nucleus. Abnormal assembly and function of the AAM complex cause a variety of sperm head shape aberrations leading to infertility.

The manchette is involved in the trafficking of proteins between the nucleus and the cytoplasm and in the transport of proteins involved in the development of the HTCA and the tail.

Intramanchette transport of various cargos engage motor proteins (kinesins, dyneins, and myosin Va) and proteins of the **intraflagellar transport system** (**IFT proteins**; see Figure 1-6 in Chapter 1, Epithelium). Disruption of the intramanchette transport machinery by a defective IFT protein (IFT88) results in abortive spermatid tail development

The manchette disassembles once the elongation and condensation of the spermatid nucleus is near completion.

3. The centriolar pair migrates from the Golgi-region to the opposite pole of the spermatid nucleus to initiate the development of the future sperm tail (see Figure 20-13). The **axoneme** of the sperm tail develops from the **distal centriole**. The **proximal centriole and pericentriolar matrix** give rise to the HTCA, connecting the sperm head to the tail.

The HTCA withstands the mechanical stress of the strong wave-like motion of the sperm tail during sperm motility. Sperm decapitation, a cause of male infertility, takes place when the position and assembly of the HTCA are aberrant.

Additional structural aspects of the sperm head and tail are discussed below (see Figure 20-15).

4. **Nuclear condensation.** Nuclear condensation occurs when somatic histones are replaced by **arginine- and lysine-rich protamines**. This replacement stabilizes and protects sperm DNA.

After the somatic histone-to-protamine shift occurs, nucleosomes disappear and smooth chromatin fibers associate side-by-side to condense the nuclear material (see Figure 20-13). There is no significant RNA transcription after the spermatid maturation phase, when the spermatid nucleus is fully condensed.

Box 20-D | Intramanchette transport

• The manchette is a transient microtubular structure that occupies a perinuclear position during the elongation and condensation of the spermatid nucleus.
• Microtubules are the major component of the manchette. They are formed by the polymerization of tubulin dimers with post-translational modifications (such as acetylation). F-actin microfilaments, aligned along microtubules, are present to a lesser extent.
• Molecules involved in **nucleocytoplasmatic transport** (such as Ran GTPase; see Chapter 1, Epithelium, Figure 1-39), 26S proteasome, and microtubule- and F-actin–based molecular motors are present in the manchette.
• Molecules targeted to construct the spermatid centriolar region and derived developing tail are mobilized along microtubules of the manchette. Intramanchette transport appears essential for cargo delivery during spermiogenesis.
• Intramanchette transport has structural and functional similarities with the intraflagellar transport pathway, with which it interfaces during spermiogenesis.
• **Tg737 mutant mice** have a defect in the gene expressing **Polaris/IFT88**, a component of the protein raft mobilized by a molecular motor along microtubules. This protein is present in the manchette of normal mice but abnormal in Tg737 mutants, which have defective bronchial cilia and abortive sperm tails.

Figure 20-13. **Spermiogenesis**

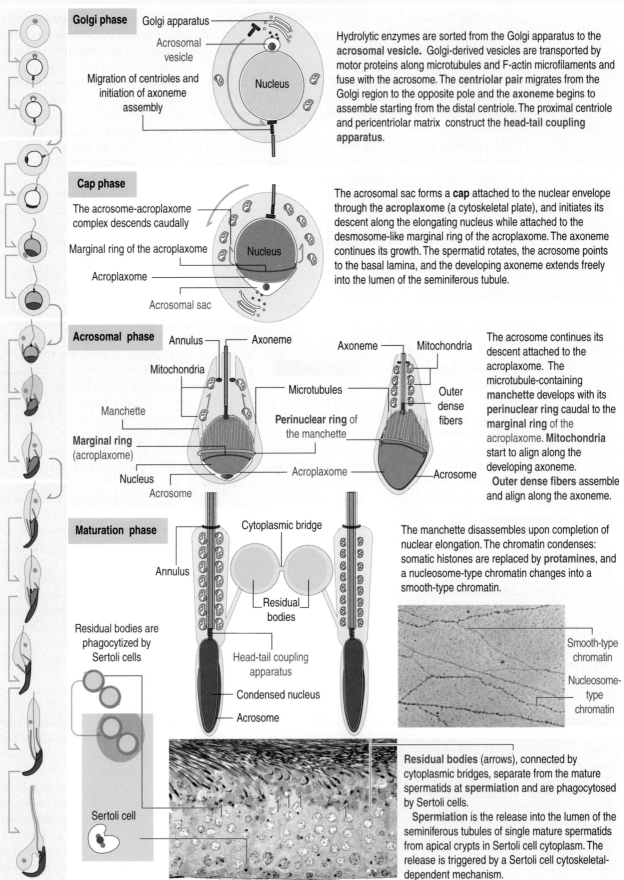

Golgi phase

Golgi apparatus

Acrosomal vesicle

Migration of centrioles and initiation of axoneme assembly

Nucleus

Hydrolytic enzymes are sorted from the Golgi apparatus to the **acrosomal vesicle.** Golgi-derived vesicles are transported by motor proteins along microtubules and F-actin microfilaments and fuse with the acrosome. The **centriolar pair** migrates from the Golgi region to the opposite pole and the **axoneme** begins to assemble starting from the distal centriole. The proximal centriole and pericentriolar matrix construct the **head-tail coupling apparatus.**

Cap phase

The acrosome-acroplaxome complex descends caudally

Marginal ring of the acroplaxome

Nucleus

Acroplaxome

Acrosomal sac

The acrosomal sac forms a **cap** attached to the nuclear envelope through the **acroplaxome** (a cytoskeletal plate), and initiates its descent along the elongating nucleus while attached to the desmosome-like marginal ring of the acroplaxome. The axoneme continues its growth. The spermatid rotates, the acrosome points to the basal lamina, and the developing axoneme extends freely into the lumen of the seminiferous tubule.

Acrosomal phase

Annulus — Axoneme

Mitochondria

Manchette

Marginal ring (acroplaxome)

Nucleus

Acrosome

Microtubules

Perinuclear ring of the manchette

Acroplaxome

Axoneme — Mitochondria

Outer dense fibers

Acrosome

The acrosome continues its descent attached to the acroplaxome. The microtubule-containing **manchette** develops with its **perinuclear ring** caudal to the **marginal ring** of the acroplaxome. **Mitochondria** start to align along the developing axoneme.

Outer dense fibers assemble and align along the axoneme.

Maturation phase

Annulus

Cytoplasmic bridge

Residual bodies

Residual bodies are phagocytized by Sertoli cells

Head-tail coupling apparatus

Condensed nucleus

Acrosome

Sertoli cell

The manchette disassembles upon completion of nuclear elongation. The chromatin condenses: somatic histones are replaced by **protamines**, and a nucleosome-type chromatin changes into a smooth-type chromatin.

Smooth-type chromatin

Nucleosome-type chromatin

Residual bodies (arrows), connected by cytoplasmic bridges, separate from the mature spermatids at **spermiation** and are phagocytosed by Sertoli cells.

Spermiation is the release into the lumen of the seminiferous tubules of single mature spermatids from apical crypts in Sertoli cell cytoplasm. The release is triggered by a Sertoli cell cytoskeletal-dependent mechanism.

Figure 20-14. Spermiogenesis

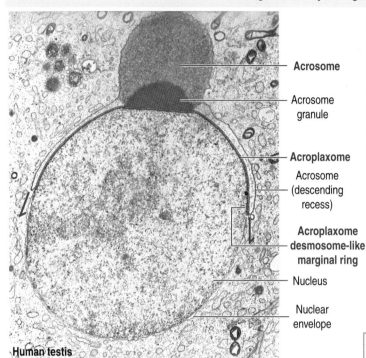

Human testis

The arrows indicate the descending recess of the acrosome, attached to the desmosome-like marginal ring of the acroplaxome

Labels: Acrosome; Acrosome granule; **Acroplaxome**; Acrosome (descending recess); **Acroplaxome desmosome-like marginal ring**; Nucleus; Nuclear envelope

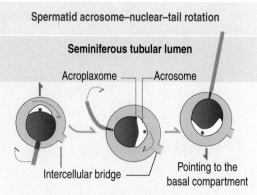

Spermatid acrosome–nuclear–tail rotation

Seminiferous tubular lumen

Labels: Acroplaxome; Acrosome; Intercellular bridge; Pointing to the basal compartment

During the cap phase of spermiogenesis, the acrosome-nucleus-tail complex rotates. At the end of the rotation, the acrosome points toward the basal compartment and the developing tail extends freely into the seminiferous tubular lumen.

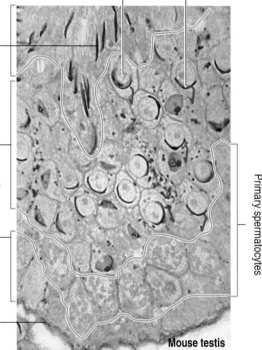

Mouse testis

Labels: Nucleus of the spermatid; PAS-positive cap-shaped acrosome; Primary spermatocytes

Mature spermatids have extended and condensed nuclei, each associated with an **elongated periodic acid–Schiff (PAS)-positive acrosome** (all of them pointing downward).

During the cap phase, early spermatids have round-to-elongating nuclei associated with **PAS-positive cap acrosomes.** Note that some of the acrosomes are pointing to the tubular wall (arrows); others are undergoing rotation.

Spermatogonia and the nuclear region of Sertoli cells are located along the tubular wall (in the basal compartment, below inter–Sertoli cell tight junctions).

PAS-positive reaction of the components of the seminiferous tubular wall

Completion of spermiogenesis and spermiation

During the final spermatid maturation phase:

1. **Mitochondria** complete their alignment along the proximal segment of the developing axoneme, surrounded by outer dense fibers.

2. The **nucleus** achieves complete elongation and chromatin packaging.

3. The **manchette** migrates caudally and disassembles.

4. The **residual body**, an excess of cytoplasm from the mature spermatid, that contains the no longer needed Golgi apparatus, is released and phagocytosed by Sertoli cells just before **spermiation**.

Spermiation is the release over several days of mature spermatids from the apical edge of Sertoli cells into the lumen of the seminiferous tubule; see Figure 20-13. The intercellular bridges, linking members of a spermatid progeny, become part of the residual body. As a result the conjoined mature spermatids become separated from each other.

Spermiation is preceded by:

1. The complete remodelling of the spermatid

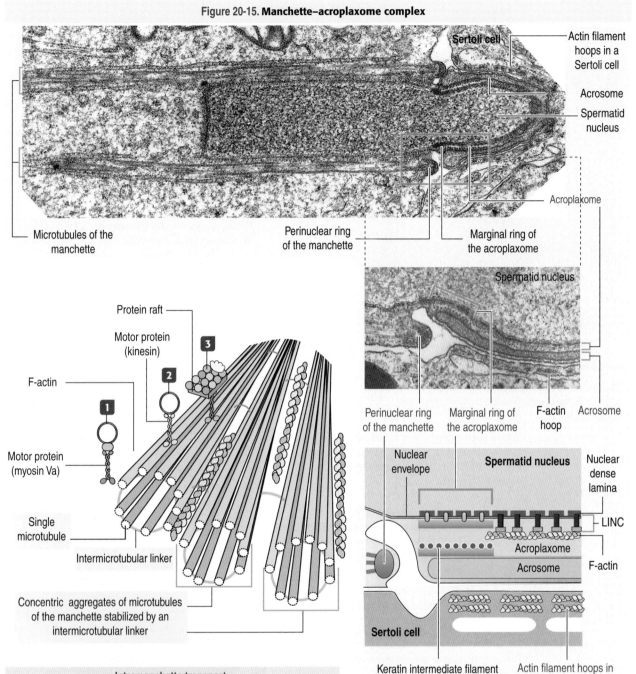

Figure 20-15. **Manchette–acroplaxome complex**

Sertoli cell

Actin filament hoops in a Sertoli cell

Acrosome

Spermatid nucleus

Microtubules of the manchette

Perinuclear ring of the manchette

Marginal ring of the acroplaxome

Acroplaxome

Spermatid nucleus

Perinuclear ring of the manchette

Marginal ring of the acroplaxome

F-actin hoop

Acrosome

Protein raft

Motor protein (kinesin)

F-actin

Motor protein (myosin Va)

Single microtubule

Intermicrotubular linker

Concentric aggregates of microtubules of the manchette stabilized by an intermicrotubular linker

Nuclear envelope

Spermatid nucleus

Nuclear dense lamina

LINC

Acroplaxome

Acrosome

F-actin

Sertoli cell

Keratin intermediate filament bundles in the desmosome-like marginal ring

Actin filament hoops in a Sertoli cell

Intramanchette transport

Intramanchette transport consists of the mobilization of cargos (vesicles or protein rafts) along F-actin filaments **1** (present in the manchette) and microtubules **2** mediated by motor proteins (myosin Va, cytoplasmic dynein, and kinesins).

Molecular motors transport proteins associated with a protein raft **3** along microtubules.

We discuss in Chapter 1, Epithelium, that microtubules participate in the intracellular traffic of vesicles and nonvesicle cargos. Examples are **axonemal transport** (including **ciliary transport** and **intraflagellar transport**), **axonal transport,** and **intramanchette transport**. Intraflagellar transport was first described in the biflagellated green alga *Chlamydomonas*.

Defective intramanchette and axonemal transport results in abnormal sperm tail development.

The acroplaxome

The acroplaxome is an F-actin-keratin–containing cytoskeletal plate with a desmosome-like **marginal ring** containing keratin intermediate filaments. The ring fastens the descending recess of the acrosome to the spermatid nuclear envelope.

During acrosome development, Golgi-derived proacrosomal vesicles are transported to the acroplaxome where they dock and fuse to form the acrosome. A **LINC** complex (for linker of nucleoskeleton and cytoskeleton) anchors the spermatid nuclear dense lamina to F-actin in the acroplaxome.

Sertoli cell **F-actin hoops** embrace the acrosome-acroplaxome portion of the elongating spermatid head.

head, capture of residual bodies by the phagocytic Sertoli cell, and separation of mature spermatids from each other.

2. The uncoupling of spermatid finger-like anchoring structures, the **tubulobulbar complexes**, inserted in the neighboring Sertoli cells.

3. The release of mature spermatids from the Sertoli cell deep apical **crypts**. A cytoskeletal-dependent mechanism and the breakdown of cell adhesion molecules (including $\alpha_6\beta_1$ integrins, the afadin–nectin–F-actin complex, and junctional adhesion molecules C, JAM-C) assist in the disengagement of mature spermatids from the crypts.

Mature spermatids become nonmotile sperm upon release into the seminiferous tubular lumen and are propelled to the epididymal duct, where they undergo a **maturation** process resulting in the **acquisition of forward motility** leading to fertilization capability.

Structure of the sperm

The mature sperm consists of two components (Figure 20-16): the **head** and the **tail**. The **HTCA** links the head to the tail. A plasma membrane surrounds the head and tail regions of the sperm.

The **head** is composed of a flattened, condensed, and elongated **nucleus** partially capped by the **acrosome**. The acrosome covers the anterior one half of the nucleus and contains **hydrolytic enzymes** (proteases, acid phosphatase, hyaluronidase, and neuraminidase, among others), usually found in lysosomes.

The acroplaxome anchors the acrosome to the nuclear envelope.

The **tail** is subdivided into three segments:

1. The **middle piece**.
2. The **principal piece**.
3. The **end piece**.

The **HTCA**, linking the head to the tail, consists of a **pair of centrioles and associated proteins**. The **distal centriole** gives rise to the **axoneme**, whereas the proximal centriole participates in the anchoring of the HTCA to the nuclear envelope.

The **middle piece** of the tail consists of:

1. A helically arranged **mitochondrial sheath**.
2. The **axoneme**.
3. **Nine longitudinal columns**, called **outer dense fibers**, surrounding the axoneme and projecting down the tail from the HTCA.

The lower limit of the middle piece is marked by the termination of the mitochondrial helical sheath at the **annulus**, a cortical ring that contains the protein **septin 4**.

Septin 4 is a member of the septin family of cytoskeletal proteins distinct from microfilaments, microtubules, and intermediate filaments. Septins are GTPases that form cortical corset-like structures. Septin 4 mutant male mice are sterile due to sperm immotility (a condition known as **asthenospermia**, see Box 20-E). Sperm lack the cortical ring at the annulus region and the kinesin-mediated intraflagellar transport of cargo proteins, required for sperm tail development, stalls beneath the annulus.

The **principal piece** is the longest segment of the tail. It consists of the central axoneme surrounded by **seven outer dense fibers** (instead of nine, as in the middle piece) and a **fibrous sheath**. Outer dense fibers are not seen in cilia.

The fibrous sheath is formed by **concentric ribs** projecting from equidistant **longitudinal columns**. Outer dense fibers and the fibrous sheath provide a rigid scaffold during microtubular sliding and bending of the tail during sperm **forward motility**.

The **end piece** is a very short segment of the tail in which only the axoneme is present because of an early termination of the outer dense fibers and fibrous sheath.

Pathology: Conditions affecting male fertility
Temperature

A temperature of 35ºC is critical for spermatogenesis. This temperature is achieved in the scrotum by the **pampiniform plexus** of veins surrounding the spermatic artery and functions as a **countercurrent heat exchanger** to dissipate heat.

When the temperature is below 35ºC, contraction of the **cremaster muscle** in the spermatic cord and of

---

Box 20-E | Semen analysis

The microscopic screening of **semen** samples explores three main sperm characteristics: **concentration**, **morphology**, and **motility**.

   Sperm normal concentration is about 20-40 million sperm/mL of semen. Normal sperm should display a regular oval head connected to a long straight tail. Abnormal sperm have atypical shaped heads (round heads, pin heads, large heads, or double heads) and short or absent tails. Morphology is a valuable predictor for in vitro fertilization (IVF) procedures.

• The frequent cause of male infertility is a low sperm concentration (less than 15 million sperm/mL of semen). This condition is called **oligospermia** (or oligozoospermia). A reduced volume of semen (lower than 2.0 mL-1.5 mL) is called **hypospermia** (or hypozoospermia). Semen volumes between 2.0 mL and 6.5 mL are normal.

• Low sperm motility is called **asthenospermia** (or asthenozoospermia) (Greek *astheneia*, weakness).

• Low sperm concentration and poor sperm motility often coexist. This condition is called **oligoasthenospermia** (or oligoasthenozoospermia).

• The presence in semen of sperm with abnormal morphology is called **teratospermia** (or teratozoospermia) (Greek *teras*, monster).

• The absence of sperm in semen is called **aspermia** (or azoospermia).

• The presence of dead sperm in semen is called **necrospermia** (or necrozoospermia)

• According to the World Health Organization (WHO) criteria described in 2010, sperm motility is graded as: **Grade a**: sperm have fast forward motility in a straight line. **Grade b**: sperm have slow forward or slow nonlinear motility (curved or crooked line). **Grade c**: sperm lack forward motility; sperm move their tails but do not advance forward. **Grade d**: sperm are immotile. Sperm classified Grade c and d are regarded as poor and associated with male infertility.

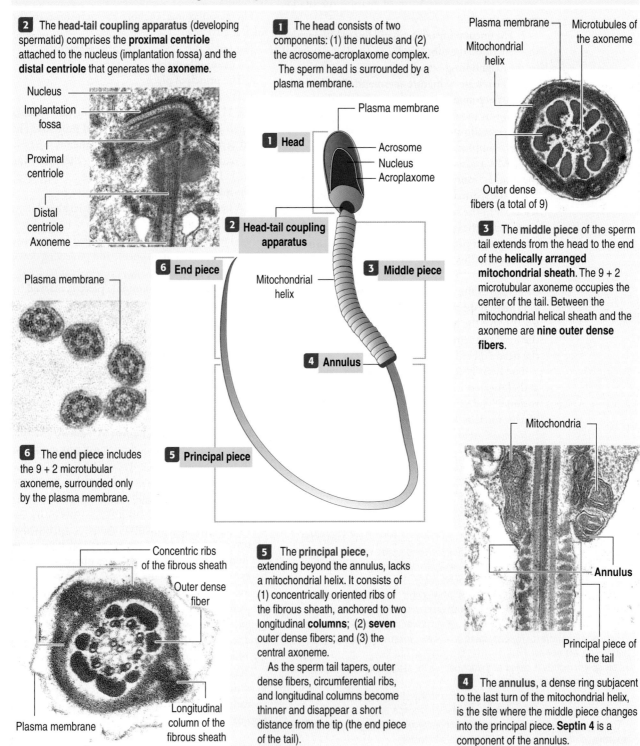

Figure 20-16. Sperm structure: Head and tail components

2 The **head-tail coupling apparatus** (developing spermatid) comprises the **proximal centriole** attached to the nucleus (implantation fossa) and the **distal centriole** that generates the **axoneme**.

Nucleus
Implantation fossa
Proximal centriole
Distal centriole
Axoneme

Plasma membrane

6 The **end piece** includes the 9 + 2 microtubular axoneme, surrounded only by the plasma membrane.

1 The **head** consists of two components: (1) the nucleus and (2) the acrosome-acroplaxome complex. The sperm head is surrounded by a plasma membrane.

Plasma membrane

1 Head

Acrosome
Nucleus
Acroplaxome

2 Head-tail coupling apparatus

6 End piece

Mitochondrial helix

3 Middle piece

4 Annulus

5 Principal piece

Plasma membrane
Mitochondrial helix

Microtubules of the axoneme

Outer dense fibers (a total of 9)

3 The **middle piece** of the sperm tail extends from the head to the end of the **helically arranged mitochondrial sheath**. The 9 + 2 microtubular axoneme occupies the center of the tail. Between the mitochondrial helical sheath and the axoneme are **nine outer dense fibers**.

Mitochondria

Annulus

Principal piece of the tail

4 The **annulus**, a dense ring subjacent to the last turn of the mitochondrial helix, is the site where the middle piece changes into the principal piece. **Septin 4** is a component of the annulus.

Concentric ribs of the fibrous sheath
Outer dense fiber
Plasma membrane
Longitudinal column of the fibrous sheath

5 The **principal piece**, extending beyond the annulus, lacks a mitochondrial helix. It consists of (1) concentrically oriented ribs of the fibrous sheath, anchored to two longitudinal **columns**; (2) **seven** outer dense fibers; and (3) the central axoneme.

As the sperm tail tapers, outer dense fibers, circumferential ribs, and longitudinal columns become thinner and disappear a short distance from the tip (the end piece of the tail).

the **dartos muscle** in the scrotal sac brings the testes close to the body wall to increase the temperature.

Cryptorchidism

In cryptorchidism (or **undescended testes**), the testes fails to reach the scrotal sac during development and remains in the abdominal cavity or inguinal canal.

Under these conditions, the normal body temperature (37°C to 38°C) inhibits spermatogenesis and sterility occurs if the condition is bilateral and not corrected.

Fetal and neonatal testicular descent is controlled by the testes-produced hormones **insulin-like 3 (INSL3)** and **androgens** that regulate the development of the **gubernaculum**, a ligament connecting each testis-epididymis complex to the future scrotal sac.

The gubernaculum consists of a core of mesenchymal cells surrounded by striated muscle innervated by the genitofemoral nerve. INSL3 binds to the relaxin/insulin-like peptide family receptor 2 (**RXFP2**) in the gubernaculum skeletal muscle cells. INSL3 appears to trigger a neuromuscular downstream pathway leading to the production of muscle-derived neurotrophic proteins required for the completion of testes descent.

A high incidence of **testicular tumors** is associated with the untreated cryptorchid testes. Cryptorchidism is an asymptomatic condition that is detected by physical examination of the scrotal sac after birth and before puberty.

Hormonal treatment (administration of human chorionic gonadotropin) may induce testicular descent. If that is unsuccessful, **surgery** is the next step, in which the testes is attached to the wall of the scrotal sac (a process called **orchiopexy**).

Inguinal hernia, cysts and hydrocele

You may remember from Embryology that the descent of the testes to the scrotal sac involves:

1. The **gubernaculum**, a ligament that originates at the testis-epidydymal complex and inserts in the genital swelling, the future scrotal sac.

2. An evagination of the peritoneum, the **vaginal process**, that facilitates the sliding of the descending testes through the inguinal canal.

Between week 7 and 12, the gubernaculum shortens and drags the testes, the deferent duct and blood vessels toward the scrotal sac by a mechanism described above.

During the first year of life, the upper section of the vaginal process closes leaving behind the **peritoneal-vaginal ligament**. The lower section becomes the **tunica vaginalis**, consisting of a parietal and a visceral layer.

A **congenital inguinal hernia** will occur if the vaginal process is wide enough and does not close.

If the unclosed space above the testis is narrow, fluid, instead of an intestinal loop, can accumulate forming a **cyst of the spermatic cord**.

If fluid collects between the parietal and visceral layers of the tunica vaginalis, a **testicular hydrocele** is formed.

Cancer chemotherapy

Young male patients treated with antitumoral drugs may become transiently aspermatogenic because spermatogonial mitosis and spermatocyte meiosis can be affected. However, dormant **spermatogonial stem cells**, not involved in DNA synthesis and cell division, can repopulate the seminiferous epithelium once anticancer chemotherapy is discontinued.

We discuss later the timing and dynamics of spermatogenesis, concepts that enable the physician to determine the recovery time frame of spermatogenesis upon completion of cancer chemotherapy.

Viral orchitis

Mumps is a systemic viral infection with a 20% to 30% incidence of unilateral or bilateral **acute orchitis** (sudden edema and infiltration of lymphocytes of the seminiferous intertubular space) in postpubertal males. In general, no alterations in spermatogenic function can be expected following mumps-caused orchitis. **Coxsackie B virus** is another pathogen for viral orchitis.

Spermatic cord torsion

Twisting of the spermatic cord may disrupt the arterial blood supply to, and venous drainage from, the testes. This condition, that can appear up to adolescence, is generally caused by physical trauma or an abnormally mobile testes within the tunica vaginalis.

If torsion is not treated immediately (within the first 6 hours), hemorrhagic infarction and necrosis of the whole testes occur.

Varicocele

This condition is caused by the abnormal dilation of the veins of the spermatic cord (varicosities of the pampiniform plexus) caused by prolonged stagnation of blood. A consequence of varicocele is a decrease in sperm production (**oligospermia**). Recall that veins in the spermatic cord play a significant role in maintaining testicular temperature at 35°C by a countercurrent exchange mechanism with the spermatic artery.

Leydig cells

Aggregates of Leydig cells are present in the intertubular space in proximity to blood vessels and lymphatic channels or sinusoids (Figure 20-17). Like most steroid-producing cells, Leydig cells contain **lipid droplets, mitochondria with characteristic tubular cristae**, and a well-developed **smooth endoplasmic reticulum**.

After puberty and upon stimulation with **luteinizing hormone** (LH) by a cyclic adenosine monophosphate (cAMP)–mediated mechanism, Leydig cells produce **testosterone**, which can be converted to **dihydrotestosterone** by the enzyme 5α-reductase. About 95% of the testosterone found in serum (bound to **sex hormone–binding globulin** [SHBG] and other proteins) is synthesized by Leydig cells; the remaining testosterone is produced by the adrenal cortex.

Testosterone can also be aromatized to estrogens

Figure 20-17. Leydig cell: The androgen-producing cell of the testes

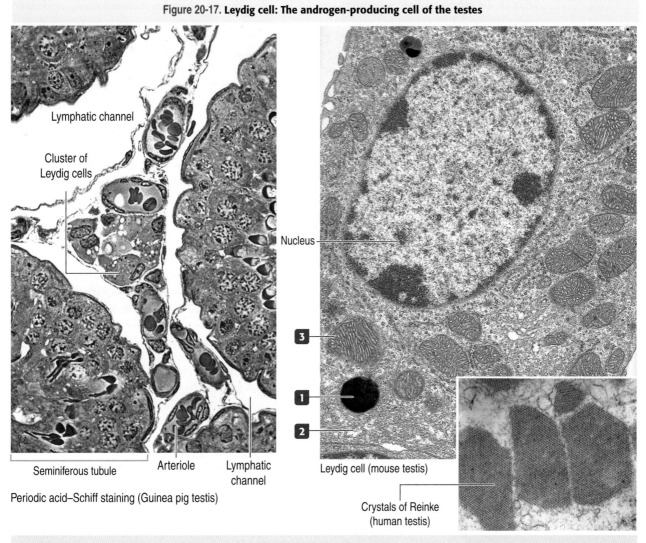

Lymphatic channel

Cluster of Leydig cells

Seminiferous tubule

Arteriole

Lymphatic channel

Periodic acid–Schiff staining (Guinea pig testis)

Nucleus

3

1

2

Leydig cell (mouse testis)

Crystals of Reinke (human testis)

Leydig cell: Androgen production

Aggregates of Leydig cells are found in the intertubular space, in close contact with blood vessels and lymphatic channels surrounding the seminiferous tubules.

Like all steroid-producing cells, Leydig cells have abundant lipid droplets containing esterified cholesterol, smooth endoplasmic reticulum (with enzymes involved in steroidogenesis), and mitochondria with tubular cristae (processing cholesterol transported by StAR).

Leydig cell function is regulated by two hormones of the anterior hypophysis:

1 Luteinizing hormone (LH), which stimulates testosterone production.

2 Prolactin, which induces the expression of LH receptor.

3 Testosterone, which binds to the androgen receptor in Sertoli cells and maintains spermatogenesis, male libido, and the function of the male accessory glands (prostate and seminal vesicle). Crystals of Reinke are inclusions of proteins in the cytoplasm of human Leydig cells.

4 StAR (steroidogenic acute regulatory protein) regulates the synthesis of steroids by transporting cholesterol across the outer mitochondrial membrane. A mutation in the gene encoding StAR is detected in individuals with defective synthesis of adrenal and gonadal steroids (lipoid congenital adrenal hyperplasia).

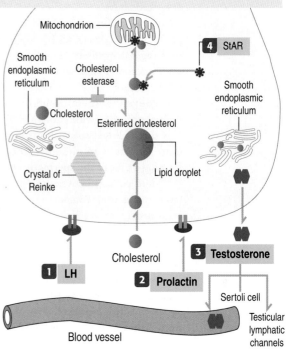

Mitochondrion

4 StAR

Smooth endoplasmic reticulum

Cholesterol esterase

Cholesterol

Esterified cholesterol

Smooth endoplasmic reticulum

Crystal of Reinke

Lipid droplet

Cholesterol

1 LH

2 Prolactin

3 Testosterone

Sertoli cell

Testicular lymphatic channels

Blood vessel

in many tissues, in particular adipose tissue. ABP produced by Sertoli cells after stimulation by FSH, maintains a high concentration of testosterone in the proximity of developing spermatogenic cells.

Clinical significance: Steroidogenic acute regulatory protein (StAR)

Fetal Leydig cells are steroidogenically active between 8 and 18 weeks of gestation. By week 18 of gestation, the Leydig cell population predominates in the testes. The androgens produced by fetal Leydig cells at this time are critical for the development of the male reproductive tract (see the development of the testes in Chapter 21, Sperm Transport and Maturation). In the neonate, testicular steroidogenesis reaches high levels at 2 to 3 months post partum and then decreases. Androgen levels remain low until puberty, when an increase in LH activates androgen synthesis.

LH and prolactin regulate the function of Leydig cells (Figure 20-17; see also Figure 20-18). Prolactin regulates the gene expression of the LH receptor. LH is responsible for the production of testosterone. **Hyperprolactinemia** inhibits male reproductive function by decreasing gonadotropin secretion and action on the testes. Excessive prolactin can decrease the production of androgens by Leydig cells, diminish spermatogenesis, and lead to erectile dysfunction and infertility.

During the synthesis of testosterone, plasma **cholesterol** enters the cell, is esterified by **acetyl coenzyme A** (acetyl CoA) and is stored in the cytoplasm as lipid droplets. **Fatty acids** are processed to cholesterol in the smooth endoplasmic reticulum.

Cholesterol is transported from the lipid droplet to mitochondria by **steroidogenic acute regulatory protein (StAR)** (synthesized in the cytosol by polyribosomes), and pregnenolone is produced.

Enzymes in the smooth endoplasmic reticulum convert pregnenolone to progesterone to testosterone. Two other less potent androgens produced by Leydig cells are **dehydroepiandrosterone (DHEA)** and **androstenedione**.

In the human testes, the cytoplasm of Leydig cells contains **crystals of Reinke**, inclusions of proteins in a geometric array, which become more apparent with age.

Hormonal control of the male reproductive tract

FSH and LH regulate the function of Sertoli and Leydig cells, respectively (see Figure 20-18). **FSH stimulates the production of inhibin and activin by Sertoli cells.** Inhibin exerts a **negative feedback** on the hypothalamic gonadotropin–releasing hormone (**GnRH**) and hypophyseal release of FSH. Activin has an opposite effect.

FSH and LH are mandatory regulators of the spermatogenic process, as demonstrated by the arrest of spermatogenesis following experimental removal of the hypophysis (**hypophysectomy**).

The synthesis and secretion of **ABP** by Sertoli cells are stimulated by FSH. ABP binds androgens (testosterone or dihydrotestosterone) and the ABP-androgen complex maintains high levels of androgens in the proximity of developing spermatogenic cells. In addition, the complex, released into the lumen of the seminiferous tubule, is transported to the epididymis, where it keeps high concentration of androgens.

Sertoli cells in the **adult testes** produce three major secretory proteins:
1. **Inhibin.**
2. **Activin.**
3. **ABP.**

Fetal Sertoli cells synthesize and secrete **anti-müllerian hormone (AMH)**.

As we have already discussed, LH stimulates the synthesis of testosterone by Leydig cells (see Box 20-F). Testosterone and dihydrotestosterone, the latter a metabolite of testosterone after reduction by **steroid 5α-reductase (SRD5A)**, bind to the same **androgen receptor** (unrelated to ABP).

The **androgen receptor (AR)** is a member of the **steroid–thyroid–retinoic acid superfamily** of receptors and as such it has three domains:
1. A **DNA binding domain** that recognizes the **androgen-responsive element**.
2. A **transcription factors–binding domain**
3. An **androgen-binding domain**.

Recall that a defective AR, encoded by a gene in the X chromosome, determines the **androgen insensitivity syndrome (AIS)** also known as **testicular feminization**. The magnitude of symptoms in individuals with this genetic defect is variable depending on the partial to complete inability of the AR to bind to androgens.

Testosterone has a **negative feedback** effect on the release of LH. An excess of testosterone in circulating blood prevents the release of LH from the anterior hypophysis. Testosterone stimulates the function of the **seminal vesicles**, whereas dihydrotestosterone acts on the **prostate gland**.

The spermatogenic cell sequence

When you examine a number of seminiferous tubules under the light microscope, you will see a variable combination of spermatogenic cells. Spermatogenic cells are not arranged at random but are organized into well-defined combinations called **cellular associations** (Figures 20-19 to 20-20).

For example, in a particular region of the seminiferous epithelium, spermatids, completing their differentiation, can be seen only in specific combination with early spermatids, spermatocytes, and spermatogonia at their respective developmental stages.

Figure 20-18. Hormonal regulation of testicular function

1 Gonadotropin–releasing hormone (GnRH) in the hypothalamus stimulates the secretion of FSH and LH by basophils located in the **2** adenohypophysis. Prolactin is secreted by acidophils.

3 FSH binds to its receptor in Sertoli cells and stimulates the synthesis and secretion of **4** androgen binding protein (ABP). After binding to testosterone, the ABP-testosterone complex is transported to the epididymis.

5 Prolactin (PL) stimulates Leydig cells to express LH receptors. **6** LH binds to its receptor to trigger the production of testosterone.

Testosterone follows three secretory routes: **7** the blood circulation, **8** the lymphatic channels surrounding the seminiferous tubules, and to **9** Sertoli cells, where it binds to the androgen receptor.

There are two feedback loops that regulate spermatogenesis:
(1) Following FSH stimulation, Sertoli cells produce **10** inhibin to down-regulate FSH secretion. When the levels of FSH decrease, Sertoli cells secrete **11** activin to up-regulate FSH secretion.
(2) When **12** testosterone levels are high, the secretion of LH decreases. When the testosterone levels decrease, LH is released. GnRH in the hypothalamus modulates the FSH-inhibin-activin feedback loop and the LH-testosterone feedback loop.

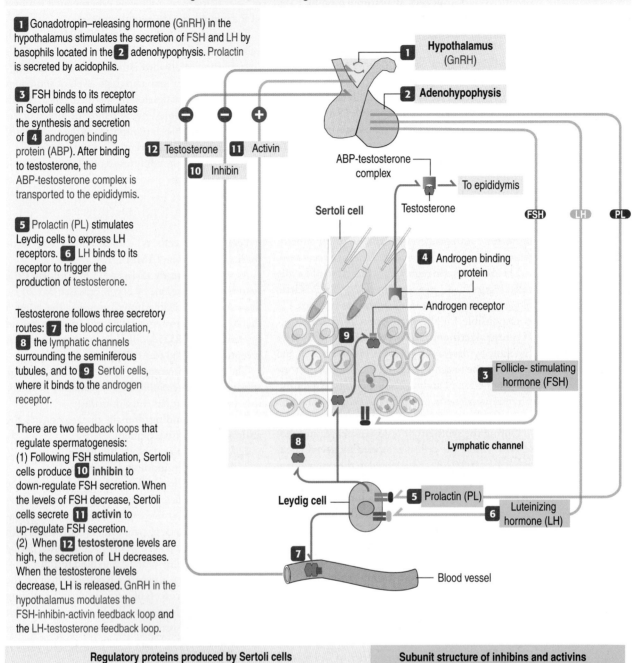

1 Hypothalamus (GnRH)

2 Adenohypophysis

12 Testosterone   **11** Activin   **10** Inhibin

ABP-testosterone complex

To epididymis

Sertoli cell   Testosterone

FSH   LH   PL

4 Androgen binding protein

Androgen receptor

3 Follicle- stimulating hormone (FSH)

Lymphatic channel

8

9

Leydig cell   **5** Prolactin (PL)   **6** Luteinizing hormone (LH)

7   Blood vessel

Regulatory proteins produced by Sertoli cells

Inhibins are dimers containing the α subunit and one of the two β subunits (βA or βB).

Activins lack the α subunit but are composed of two β subunits. They can be homodimers (βAβA or βBβB) or heterodimers (βAβB).

Inhibins and activins are synthesized in the ovaries, testes, hypophysis, and probably in other tissues.

Inhibins and activins are members of the family of polypeptides that include transforming growth factor-β and anti-müllerian hormone (AMH).

Subunit structure of inhibins and activins

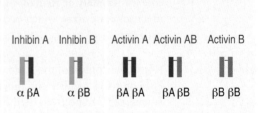

Inhibin A	Inhibin B	Activin A	Activin AB	Activin B
α βA	α βB	βA βA	βA βB	βB βB

These cellular associations (designated by Roman numerals) succeed one another at a given site of the seminiferous tubule and this sequence repeats itself regularly.

You should realize that it takes several cycles, each consisting of precise cellular associations that repeat themselves (at least four times as illustrated in Figure 20-20), to produce mature spermatids released into

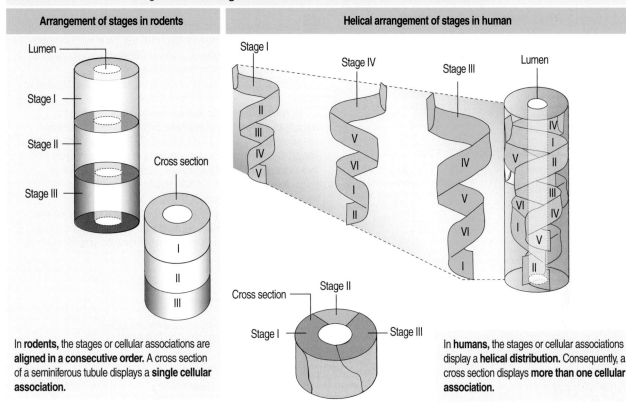

Figure 20-19. Arrangement of cellular associations in seminiferous tubules

Arrangement of stages in rodents

Lumen

Stage I

Stage II

Stage III

Cross section

I

II

III

In **rodents,** the stages or cellular associations are **aligned in a consecutive order.** A cross section of a seminiferous tubule displays a **single cellular association.**

Helical arrangement of stages in human

Stage I

Stage IV

Stage III

Lumen

Cross section

Stage II

Stage I

Stage III

In **humans,** the stages or cellular associations display a **helical distribution.** Consequently, a cross section displays **more than one cellular association.**

the tubular lumen by the process of spermiation.

How do these combinations of spermatogenic cells occur?

Let us examine Figure 20-20 that presents a **hypothetical example**. Note that all generations of spermatogenic cells (spermatogonia, spermatocytes, and spermatids) coexist. The difference rests on their step of differentiation in a given segment of a seminiferous epithelium. The development of any single generation takes place concomitantly with the development of the earlier and later generations.

Each defined cell association or combination represents a **stage** in the sequential process of spermatogenesis initiated by a SSC.

Because several spermatogonial stem cells give rise to a spermatogenic cell progeny at regular intervals along the seminiferous tubule and the progenies overlap, it is possible to understand that cellular associations derive from overlapping progenies at a given point in the seminiferous tubule.

Now, we need to discuss the difference between **spermatogenic cycle** and **spermatogenic wave** (see Figure 20-21). You realize that at a given point in the seminiferous tubule, the cohorts of spermatogenic cells will change with time as early and late progenies continue their development. It is just a question of time (hours and days) for the stages of the cycle (represented by cellular associations) to change.

A **spermatogenic cycle is defined by the time it takes for a sequence of cellular associations (or stages of the cycle) at a particular point of the seminiferous tubule to change.**

We now want to determine the alignment of cell associations **along the length of the seminiferous tubule.** You realize that we have changed our parameter from time to distance.

We isolate a seminiferous tubule, prepare serial histologic sections along its length, and use already available tables to verify whether cellular associations are present.

After examining a number of serial sections covering a distance of a few millimeters or centimeters, we realize **the presence of successive cellular associa-**

Box 20-F | Androgen actions: Highlights to remember

In the male fetus
• Regulation of the differentiation of the male internal and external genitalia.
• Stimulation of the growth, development, and function of male internal and external genitalia.
In the adult male
• Stimulation of sexual hair development.
• Stimulation of the secretion of sebaceous glands of the skin.
• Binding to androgen receptor in Sertoli cells, peritubular myoid cells and Leydig cells and to androgen-binding protein produced by Sertoli cells after FSH stimulation.
• Initiation and maintenance of spermatogenesis.
• Maintenance of the secretory function of accessory sex glands (seminal vesicle and prostate).

Figure 20-20. Spermatogenic cell sequence

The spermatogenic cell sequence

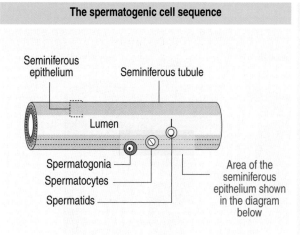

Seminiferous epithelium

Seminiferous tubule

Lumen

Spermatogonia
Spermatocytes
Spermatids

Area of the seminiferous epithelium shown in the diagram below

2 Because the development of each spermatogenic cell progeny (starting from a spermatogonial stem cell, SSC) is in synchrony with preceding and later progenies, a series of different cell associations can be seen along the seminiferous tubule.

A series of consecutive cell associations constitute the stages of a cycle.

The number of cycles is species-dependent. Note that in the diagram of a **hypothetical example**, **cycle 1** consists of sucessive cell associations labeled **I to VI**. Then **cycle 2** appears starting with **stage I**. **Cycle 3** and **cycle 4** are repeats of cycle 1 and cycle 2. **In this example, a total of four cycles** must be completed before sperm derived from the initial SSC can be released into the seminiferous tubular lumen.

In the human, each cycle lasts 16 days, and the progeny initiated from a spermatogonial stem cell must pass through 4 cycles (or 64 days) before release of mature spermatids from the seminiferous epithelium (spermiation).

1 Distinct spermatogenic cells in the seminiferous epithelium are only found in association with other specific spermatogenic cells. This constant cell combination is known as **cell association** and is designated by a Roman numeral.

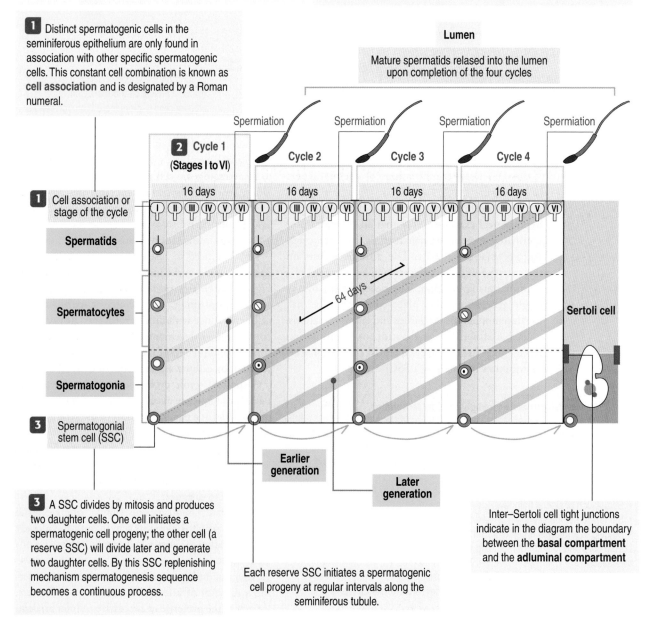

Lumen

Mature spermatids relased into the lumen upon completion of the four cycles

Spermiation · Spermiation · Spermiation · Spermiation

2 Cycle 1 (Stages I to VI) · Cycle 2 · Cycle 3 · Cycle 4

16 days · 16 days · 16 days · 16 days

1 Cell association or stage of the cycle

Spermatids

Spermatocytes

64 days

Sertoli cell

Spermatogonia

3 Spermatogonial stem cell (SSC)

Earlier generation

Later generation

3 A SSC divides by mitosis and produces two daughter cells. One cell initiates a spermatogenic cell progeny; the other cell (a reserve SSC) will divide later and generate two daughter cells. By this SSC replenishing mechanism spermatogenesis sequence becomes a continuous process.

Each reserve SSC initiates a spermatogenic cell progeny at regular intervals along the seminiferous tubule.

Inter–Sertoli cell tight junctions indicate in the diagram the boundary between the **basal compartment** and the **adluminal compartment**

Figure 20-21. **Spermatogenic cycle: Waves and cycles**

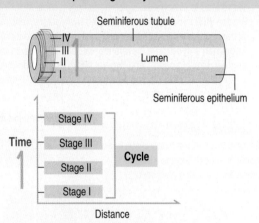

Spermatogenic cycle

A **spermatogenic cycle** involves cellular association changes **with time** at one particular point of the seminiferous tubule. These changes occur as overlapping spermatogenic cell progenies advance in their development.

Imagine that you can monitor changes in the cellular associations or stages of a cycle using a time-lapse camera placed at that given point of the seminiferous tubule.

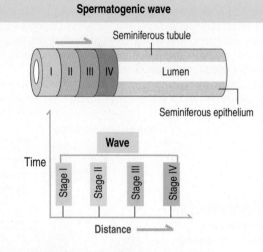

Spermatogenic wave

A **spermatogenic wave** involves changes **along a seminiferous tubule (distance)**.

Imagine that you can visualize a wave by "traveling" along the length of a seminiferous tubule.

A wave is not distinct in the human testis because of the **helical progression** of spermatogenic cell progenies.

tions (or stages of a cycle) along the length of the seminiferous tubule.

We realize that **all 6 cellular associations or stages (equivalent to one cycle) occur in a wavelike succession along a stretch of a seminiferous tubule** (as illustrated in Figure 20-20).

The series of cycles, each formed by 6 consecutive stages, repeat themselves again and again. We measure the distance between two consecutive cycles (each represented by 6 consecutive cellular associations or stages of a cycle) and define what a **spermatogenic wave** is.

The number of cellular associations or stages in a cycle is constant for any given species (14 stages in the rat, **6 stages in man**, 12 in the monkey). Things are not that simple in human testis.

In human testes, spermatogenic cell generations are organized in a **helical fashion** instead of a longitudinal and consecutive sequence as in rodents (see Figure 20-19). Consequently, a cross section of a seminiferous tubule will display three or four cellular associations instead of the single one observed in the rat testes. In man, the **duration of one cycle is 16 days**. It takes **four cycles** (64 days) to develop spermatogonia into testicular sperm.

Clinical significance: Epigenetics reprogramming
We have seen that somatic histones are removed from spermatids and replaced by arginine-, lysine-rich protamines.

This histone-protamine shift results in:

1. RNA transcriptional inactivation (called **gene silencing**).

2. Changes in chromatin structure from a nucleosomal-type to a smooth-type of chromatin in late spermatids (see Figure 20-13). This structural modification enables the condensation of chromatin and protects DNA from degradation.

Changes in DNA and histones can modify gene activity without changing DNA sequence. Such modifications are called **epigenetic (getting around conventional genetics): epigenetic modifications affect gene expression without modifying DNA sequence.** As we will see, **DNA methylation**, consisting in methyl groups added to DNA, can initiate a cascade of events silencing RNA transcription.

There are important concepts to remember:

1. During **gametogenesis** (spermatogenesis and oogenesis), **genetic imprints are differentially erased to allow epigenetic reprogramming** to be transmitted to embryos by the gametes.

DNA of mature spermatids is highly methylated (Figure 20-22), in comparison with a more modest methylation pattern during oogenesis.

2. Immediately after **fertilization**, there is significant sperm DNA demethylation, followed by an extensive loss of DNA methylation from most of the genomic DNA in human embryos.

3. After **implantation**, DNA methylation increases rapidly when embryonic cells acquire the characteristics of cell and tissue differentiation.

In summary, reprogramming during gameto-

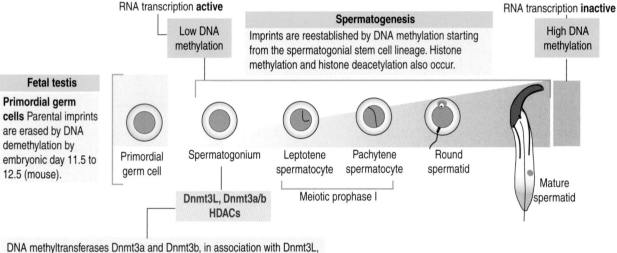

Figure 20-22. Epigenetics reprogramming

Gametogenesis (spermatogenesis and oogenesis) in mammals is under the control of genetic and epigenetic mechanisms. Epigenetics consists in the reprogramming of specific gene expression by two major mechanisms: **DNA methylation** and **histone modifications** (acetylation, phosphorylation, methylation, and ubiquitylation).

The major objectives are to erase and reprogram methylation patterns to reset imprints and/or eliminate acquired epigenetic modifications.

A disruption of DNA methylation and histone modifications of alleles lead to abnormal developmental processes, including **Prader-Willi syndrome** (characterized by hypotony, respiratory distress, obesity, short stature, and mild mental retardation) and **Angelman's syndrome** (severe mental retardation, excessive laughter, lack of speech, and hyperactivity). Both syndromes have an epigenetic defect caused by a lack of methylation of several paternally derived alleles.

RNA transcription **active**

Low DNA methylation

Spermatogenesis

Imprints are reestablished by DNA methylation starting from the spermatogonial stem cell lineage. Histone methylation and histone deacetylation also occur.

RNA transcription **inactive**

High DNA methylation

Fetal testis

Primordial germ cells Parental imprints are erased by DNA demethylation by embryonic day 11.5 to 12.5 (mouse).

Primordial germ cell

Spermatogonium

Leptotene spermatocyte

Pachytene spermatocyte

Round spermatid

Mature spermatid

Meiotic prophase I

Dnmt3L, Dnmt3a/b HDACs

DNA methyltransferases Dnmt3a and Dnmt3b, in association with Dnmt3L, establish a paternal DNA methylation pattern from spermatogonia on.

In addition, histone hypoacetylation-deacetylation is controlled by histone deacetylases (HDACs) and histone methyltransferases.

genesis is required for the resetting of imprints or eliminating acquired epigenetic modifications. The pluripotent inner cell mass of the blastocyst erases the epigenetic memory before implantation. The epigenetic memory is back so embryo cells can achieve tissue-specific patterns.

There is a close relationship between gene imprinting, chromatin structure, and DNA methylation. During gametogenesis, the differential expression of **alleles** (Greek *allos,* another) can be inhibited in paternal and maternal gametes. As you remember from previous discussions, genes come in pairs, one copy or allele inherited from each parent. During spermatogenesis and oogenesis one copy of the imprinted gene is selectively silenced. Imprinting disorders are seen when the alternative maternal or paternal copy (allele) does not appear.

Defects in parental imprinting include (see Figure 20-22):

1. **Prader-Willi syndrome**.

2. **Angelman's syndrome**.

Prader-Willi syndrome is characterized by hypotony, respiratory distress, obesity, short stature, and mild mental retardation. It is caused by the deletion of a paternal allele or the retention of two maternal copies.

Angelman syndrome includes severe mental retardation, excessive inappropriate laughter, lack of speech, and hyperactivity. In contrast to Prader-Willi syndrome, the maternal allele has been lost or two paternal copies are retained. Although two alleles are available (one inherited from each parent), the affected individuals have mutations in the DNA regions controlling gene imprinting of the two alleles.

We now address with this background the molecular aspects of epigenetics reprogramming (Figure 20-23).

Epigenetics is focused on the following basic premises:

1. **Differences in gene expression patterns are not determined by heritable changes in DNA sequence.**

2. **DNA methylation occurs on cytosine bases in the dinucleotide sequence cytosine-guanine: CpG, where p denotes the DNA phosphate backbone.**

Because C pairs with G on complementary DNA strands, islands of CpG dinucleotides align in both strands and are methylated in the same site. This means that methylation patterns can be passed to daughter cells when cells divide so they can maintain their epigenetic identity. A large number of CpG islands are present in transcription initiation sites and in promoters of active genes.

2. **Histone modifications** take place, in particular **histone deacetylation**.

Figure 20-23. **DNA methylation and histone deacetylation**

1 Transcriptionally active chromatin consists of transcription factors and RNA polymerase bound to the gene promoter region. Histones in the nucleosomal core are acetylated.

2 Transcriptional silencing starts when DNA methyltransferases methylate CpG islands on DNA. Methylated DNA binding proteins (MBD), including histone deacetylase, are recruited to the methylated CpG islands. Histone deacetylase relocates to the histone core and removes acetyl groups from histones.

3 Histone deacetylation enables histone methyltransferase to attach methyl groups to histones and heterochromatin protein-1 (HP1) is recruited to histone methylated sites.
    Chromatin is condensed and transcription stops.

A mutation on the *Dnmt3b* gene is observed in patients with the rare disease called **ICF** (immunodeficiency, centromeric instability, and facial anomalies syndrome).
    A mutation in the *MeCP2* gene, encoding one of the MBD proteins, is the cause of the **Rett syndrome** in young girls (mental retardation).

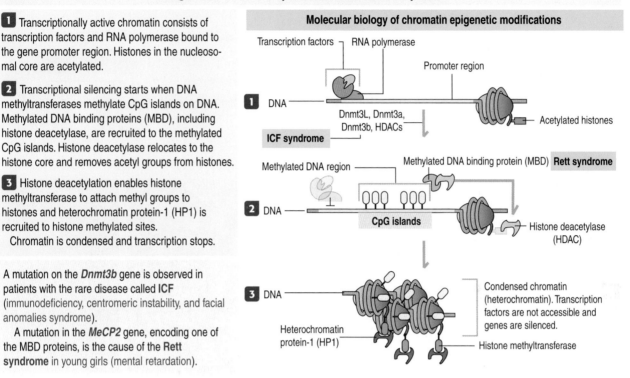

Chromatin of an actively transcribing gene (euchromatin) has acetylated histones and the CpG islands are unmethylated. This "open" chromatin organization enables transcription factors and RNA polymerase to transcribe a gene. Chromatin can be condensed (heterochromatin) to become transcriptionally inactive.

Two events take place to accomplish this task:
1. DNA methyltransferases methylate CpG islands.
2. Histone deacetylases remove acetyl groups from the N-terminal tail of the nucleosomal histones.

Methylation consists of the attachment of a methyl group to a biological molecule by methyltransferases. **DNA methyltransferases** (Dnmt1, Dnmt3a, and Dnmt3b, with the participation of Dnmt3L) attach methyl groups to CpG dinucleotides. **Histone methyltransferases** attach methyl groups to histones after they have become deacetylated by **histone deacetylases**.

How do histone deacetylases know when to remove acetyl groups from histones? **Methylated DNA-binding protein** (MBD) and **histone deacetylase** (which removes acetyl groups) are recruited to the CpG island when they become methylated. Histone deacetylation is a prerequisite for histone methylation, which involves **histone methyltransferase** targeting histone 3 (H3). H3 methylation results in the recruitment of the effector **heterochromatin protein-1** (HP1). Chromatin condenses and transcription is inactivated ("closed" chromatin).

The clinical significance of DNA and histone methylation, coupled with histone deacetylation, points to the therapeutic reactivation of abnormally silenced tumor-suppressor genes. DNA methylation inhibitors and histone deacetylase inhibitors are promising agents in cancer treatment.

Pathology: Testicular tumors

Testicular tumors are detected in 30- to 40-year old individuals. Two significant risk factors are cryptorchidism and gonadal dysgenesis (for example, Klinefelter's syndrome or the testicular feminization syndrome). An increase in X-chromosome number is a common feature of testicular germ cell tumors.

Serum tumor markers are α-**fetoprotein** (**AFP**), the β subunit of human chorionic gonadotropin (β-**hCG**) and lactate dehydrogenase isoenzyme 1.

Testicular tumors are classified into three major groups (Figure 20-24):
1. **Seminomas.**
2. **Testicular germ cell tumors** (**TGCTs**).
3. **Sex cord cell tumors**.

Seminoma occurs in younger patients and is the most common testicular tumor. Seminomas are well delimited lobulated yellowish tumoral masses confined to the testis. It consists of nodules surrounded by connective tissue cells. Tumor cells are large and uniform with large nuclei and prominent nucleoli. Sincytiotrophoblasts may be present in testicular seminomas. Serum levels of β-hCG are moderately

Figure 20-24. **Testicular tumors**

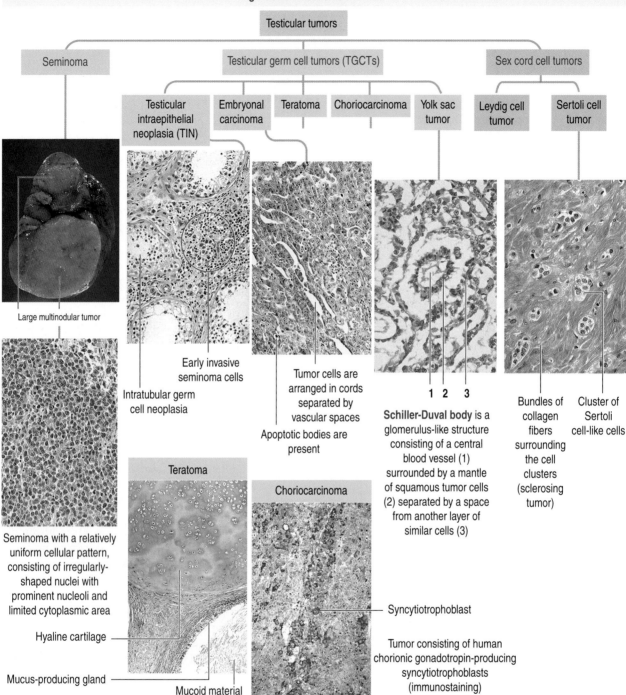

Large multinodular tumor

Seminoma with a relatively uniform cellular pattern, consisting of irregularly-shaped nuclei with prominent nucleoli and limited cytoplasmic area

Intratubular germ cell neoplasia

Early invasive seminoma cells

Teratoma

Hyaline cartilage

Mucus-producing gland

Mucoid material

Tumor cells are arranged in cords separated by vascular spaces

Apoptotic bodies are present

Choriocarcinoma

Syncytiotrophoblast

Tumor consisting of human chorionic gonadotropin-producing syncytiotrophoblasts (immunostaining)

1 2 3

Schiller-Duval body is a glomerulus-like structure consisting of a central blood vessel (1) surrounded by a mantle of squamous tumor cells (2) separated by a space from another layer of similar cells (3)

Bundles of collagen fibers surrounding the cell clusters (sclerosing tumor)

Cluster of Sertoli cell-like cells

Images from Weidner N, Cote RJ, Suster S, Weiss LM: Modern Surgical Pathology, St. Louis, Saunders, 2003.

elevated. **Spermatocytic seminoma** is regarded as a variant of seminoma. It is seen in older patients. Histologically, it mimics meiotic cells (spermatocytes).

TGCTs include **testicular intraepithelial neoplasia (TIN)**, **embryonal carcinoma**, **teratoma**, **choriocarcinoma** and **yolk sac tumor**.

TIN (also called **intratubular germ cell neoplasia**) is the initial phase of invasive TGCTs that develops in 70% of the cases after an average of 7 years. Malignant cells resembling seminoma cells are confined within seminiferous tubules. Tumor cells stain positive for membrane-associated **placental-like alkaline phosphatase (PLAP)** and **c-kit receptor**. As you remember, c-kit receptor is expressed in primordial germ cells and differentiating spermatogonia.

TGCTs, as indicated above, correlate with all kinds of X chromosome gains. In fact, the gene *TGCT1* located to the long arm (Xq27) appears associated with a risk of bilateral TGCTs, presumably mediated by the increased expression of two X chromosome-linked oncogenes (ARAF1, encoding a serine/threonine kinase, and ELK1, a transcription factor).

Male infertility is associated with TIN, a clinical observation to be taken into account during the differential diagnostic process in all young men. Radical orchiectomy is generally performed through an inguinal incision. Organ-preserving surgery is an alternative to orchiectomy in patients who want to father children and the TIN has a reduced size.

In a few patients, germ cell tumors may have an **extragonadal localization** (in the retroperitoneum or mediastinum) in addition to TIN. Remember that primordial germinal cells that do not reach the gonadal ridges during gonadogenesis and are not destroyed by apoptosis can give rise to germ cell tumors. Elevated AFP or β-hCG correlate with a extragonadal germ cell tumor that is generally confirmed by biopsy.

Embryonal carcinoma consists of epithelial cells arranged in cords. The tumor cells show large nuclei with an irregular outline and noticeable nucleoli. Tumor cells are PLAP- and cytokeratin-positive.

Teratoma is a benign germ cell tumor derived from a combination of the tissues from all three embryonic layers (ectoderm, mesoderm, and endoderm). Teratomas are seen in prepubertal and postpubertal patients. The tumor consists of cysts (containing mucoid material and nodules of cartilage), solid tissue (immature form) and malignant transformed teratomas.

Choriocarcinoma is a malignant tumor with trophoblastic cells found in teenagers. In contrast to germ cell tumors, it presents metastasis before a testicular mass is found. Serum levels of β-HCG are significantly elevated and gynecomastia is frequent.

Yolk sac tumor is the most common testicular tumor of childhood. The tumor consists of blood vessels surrounded by squamous tumor cells organizing glomerular-like structures known as **Schiller-Duval bodies**.

Sex cord cell tumors include **Leydig cell tumor** and **Sertoli cell tumor**.

Leydig cell tumor, the most frequent sex cord cell tumor, is seen at any age. Tumor cells display a vacuolated cytoplasm, representing the presence of abundant lipid droplets, and occasional crystals of Reinke (a typical feature of human Leydig cells as we have seen). Tumor cells stain positively for inhibin.

Sertoli cell tumor are generally benign and small. Tumor cells are vimentin- and cytokeratin-positive.

Typical seminoma may mimic a Sertoli cell tumor because of the microlobular organization and presence of cells with clear nuclei and conspicuous nucleolus like Sertoli cells.

Essential concepts | **Spermatogenesis**

- Components of the male reproductive system. It consists of:
  (1) The testes (the site of production of sperm and androgens).
  (2) The epididymis (the site of sperm maturation).
  (3) The excurrent duct system (vas deferens, ejaculatory ducts, and urethra).
  (4) The accessory glands (seminal vesicles, prostate gland, and bulbourethral glands of Cowper).
  (5) The penis (the copulatory organ).

- The testes are located in the scrotal sac. Each testes is surrounded by the tunica albuginea (dense connective tissue) concentrated in the mediastinum, where the rete testis is located. The network of blood vessels under the tunica albuginea is called tunica vasculosa. Septa or partitions derived from the mediastinum divide the testes into 250 to 300 lobules. Each lobule contains 1 to 4 seminiferous tubules.

- The seminiferous tubule consists of:
  (1) The seminiferous tubular wall.
  (2) The seminiferous epithelium surrounding a central lumen.
  The wall consists of collagen-producing fibroblasts and contractile myoid cells. A basement membrane, consisting of a basal lamina and reticular lamina, separates the wall from the seminiferous epithelium.

The two ends of the tubule open into the rete testis, a network of channels collecting testicular sperm, secretory proteins, and fluid produced by the seminiferous epithelium.

The space between seminiferous tubules is called the intertubular space. It contains blood vessels, lymphatic channels, and clusters of the androgen-producing Leydig cells.

- The seminiferous epithelium consists of:
  (1) Somatic Sertoli cells.
  (2) Spermatogenic cells.
  The stratified cellular arrangement of spermatogenic cells (spermatogonia, primary and secondary spermatocytes, and spermatids) enables the classification of the seminiferous epithelium as stratified with structural and functional characteristics not found in other stratified epithelia.
  For example, a postmitotic cell population of somatic Sertoli cells interacts with mitotically dividing spermatogonia, meiotically dividing spermatocytes, and differentiating haploid spermatids. The only permanent member of the epithelium is the Sertoli cell.

- The mammalian spermatogenic sequence starts at puberty from a spermatogonial stem cell (SSC) derived from the primordial germ cells (PGCs) colonizing the gonadal ridges.
  SSC divide by mitosis to produce two daughter cells. One daughter cell initiates a spermatogenic cycle. The other daughter cell,

a reserve SCC, retains self-renewal capacity and initiate a separate spermatogenic series at a later time. Reserve SCC are resistant to radiation and cancer chemotherapy. This is an important consideration regarding the fertility of young patients undergoing one or both treatments.

There are two significant characteristics to remember:
  (1) All spermatogenic cells remain connected by cytoplasmic bridges after cell division.
  (2) Spermatogenic cell cohorts proliferate and differentiate synchronously.

- Sertoli cells. It is the predominant mitotically dividing cell type in the postnatal testes. After puberty, Sertoli cells become postmitotic.
  Sertoli cells are columnar cells extending from the tubular wall to the lumen. They are linked to each other by basally located tight junctions. Tight junctions, the basis for the blood-testes barrier, divide the seminiferous epithelium into a basal compartment (housing spermatogonia) and an adluminal compartment (where spermatocytes and spermatids are located).
  The nucleus of the Sertoli cells is usually found close to the seminiferous wall. It has an irregular outline with euchromatin and a large nucleolus flanked by two masses of heterochromatin.
  After puberty, Sertoli cell function is regulated by follicle-stimulating hormone (FSH).

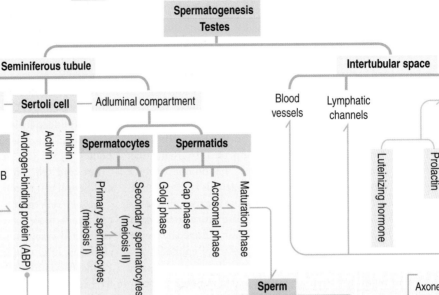

Sertoli cells secrete the αβ heterodimer **inhibin**, which exerts a negative feedback on the mechanism of release of FSH, and the αα or ββ homodimer **activin**, which has positive feedback action on FSH release.

FSH stimulates the production of androgen-binding protein (ABP), a Sertoli cell secretory protein.

In the fetal testes, Sertoli cells secrete anti-müllerian hormone (AMH), a glycoprotein that prevents the development of the müllerian duct. Sertoli cells take up by phagocytosis residual bodies left behind by mature spermatids upon their release from Sertoli cell crypts at spermiation.

• **Spermatogonia**. Spermatogonial cells are diploid cells. They derive from the SCC progenitor and divide by mitosis several times while retaining cytoplasmic bridges. They are in direct contact with the tubular wall.

There are two major types:

(1) Type A spermatogonia, with an oval euchromatic nucleus and eccentric nucleolus.

(2) Type B spermatogonia, with round nuclei displaying clumps of chromatin near the nuclear envelope and a central nucleolus.

In the human testes, type A spermatogonia can be subdivided into type A pale and type A dark based on the nuclear characteristics.

• **Spermatocytes**. There are:

(1) Primary spermatocytes, derived from type B spermatogonia committed to meiosis

(instead of mitosis) after duplicating their DNA content.

(2) Secondary spermatocytes, derived from the first meiotic division of primary spermatocytes.

Meiosis has two major objectives:

(1) The exchange of genetic information between nonsister chromatids (called reciprocal exchange) of paired homologous chromosomes.

(2) To achieve a haploid status at the end of meiosis II.

It is important to remember that oogenesis in the female starts in the fetal ovary, in contrast to the male, which starts spermatogenesis after puberty.

In the fetal ovary, oogonia, the spermatogonia-equivalent in the male, divide by mitosis a number of times, enter meiosis I as primary oocytes and do not advance beyond the last phase of meiotic prophase I until after puberty. Primary oocytes, but not oogonia, are present in the ovary at the time of birth.

It is also relevant that the completion of meiosis I of a primary oocyte (which occurs at ovulation) yields a secondary oocyte and a cell rudiment called a first polar body.

If the secondary oocyte is fertilized, meiosis II is completed and a second polar body is produced. The objective here is to have the secondary oocyte pronucleus reach a haploid state at the time when the haploid male pronucleus penetrates the egg.

• **Meiosis** consists of two steps:

(1) **Meiosis I, reductional division**, when homologous chromosomes, each consisting of two sister chromatids, separate.

(2) **Meiosis II, equational division**, when sister chromatids separate.

Meiosis I is prolonged (days) because it has a long prophase; meiosis II is shorter (minutes) and is not preceded by DNA synthesis.

Meiotic prophase I consists of well-defined substages:

(1) Leptotene, in which each chromosome consists of two sister chromatids.

(2) Zygotene, when homologous chromosomes (autosomes and sex chromosomes) start to pair (a process called synapsis) at the time when the synaptonemal complex starts to assemble.

(3) Pachytene, the longest substage of meiotic prophase I in which a synaptonemal complex is fully assembled and crossing over between nonsister chromatids of the paired chromosomes begins.

(4) Diplotene, a substage when disjunction (separation) of paired chromosomes occurs.

(5) Diakinesis, represented by chiasmata (crossing points) and the disassembly of the synaptonemal complex.

The synaptonemal complex is a protein-containing ribbon. It consists of two lateral elements and a central element. Each lateral element, representing the remnant of the axial chromosomal core of each paired chromosome, contains a cohesin protein complex and proteins SCP3 and SCP2 (SCP stands for synaptonemal complex protein).

- **Spermatids**. There are two major morphologic types of spermatid:
  (1) Round or early spermatids.
  (2) Elongated or late spermatids.
  Spermatids are haploid cells derived from the division of secondary spermatocytes. They are involved in a process called spermiogenesis, the last phase of spermatogenesis, consisting of the development of the acrosome and the tail, and the elongation and condensation of the nucleus.

  Spermiogenesis consists of four phases:
  (1) Golgi phase: Golgi-derived proacrosomal vesicles are transported by motor proteins (kinesins and myosin Va) along microtubules and F-actin to the acroplaxome, where they tether, dock, and fuse to form the acrosomal vesicle. The Golgi-associated centrosome initiates its migration to the opposite nuclear pole to develop the spermatid tail.
  (2) Cap phase: Gradual fusion of Golgi-derived proacrosomal vesicles change the acrosomal vesicle into the acrosomal sac. The acrsosomal sac forms a cap to the elongating spermatid nucleus and initiates, together with the acroplaxome, its caudal descent.
  A desmosome-like structure, the marginal ring of the acroplaxome, fastens the descending acrosomal sac recess to the spermatid nuclear envelope. The manchette initiates its development just below the marginal ring of the acroplaxome by assembling a perinuclear ring, the insertion site of manchette microtubules.
  (3) Acrosomal phase. Spermatid nuclear condensation and elongation take place as somatic-type of nucleosome-containing chromatin is replaced by smooth chromatin fibers as somatic histones are replaced by protamine. RNA transcription becomes gradually silent.
  (4) Maturation phase. The manchette disassembles as mitochondria migrate and surround the proximal segment of the developing spermatid tail.
  These four phases describe the morphogenesis of the acrosome and the spermatid nucleus. Yet, there are significant changes in gene expression during spermiogenesis. Defective gene expression result in abnormal sperm development, a condition known as teratozoospermia, that affects male fertility.
  Spermiogenesis includes the development of the tail, a structure that contains the axoneme surrounded by outer dense fibers and a fibrous sheath.
  The **acrosome** is a sac consisting of an outer acrosomal membrane and an inner acrosomal membrane and contains hydrolytic enzymes to be released following the acrosome reaction during fertilization.
  The inner acrosomal membrane is attached to the spermatid nuclear envelope and subjacent nuclear lamina by a cytoskeletal plate called the acroplaxome. The acroplaxome consists of F-actin, actin-polymerizing proteins, and keratin 5.
  The **manchette** is a transient microtubular structure positioned caudally with respect

to the acrosome-acroplaxome complex. The manchette participates in:
  (1) Nucleocytoplasmic transport, an important event during the somatic histone-protamine shift during nuclear condensation.
  (2) Intramanchette transport of cargos required for tail development.
  (3) Together with the acrosome-acroplaxome complex, the manchette has a role in spermatid head shaping. Round-shaped sperm, unable to fertilize, develop when there are deficiencies in the structure and function of the acrosome-acroplaxome-manchette complex.

- **Sperm**. Nonmotile mature spermatids are released into the seminiferous tubular lumen and transported to the rete testis. Transport depends on fluid flowing along the lumen of the seminiferous tubules and the contractile activity of myoid cells present in the seminiferous peritubular wall.
  The sperm consists of a head and a tail connected to each other at the neck region by the head-tail coupling apparatus derived from the centrosome. The head contains the acrosome and the condensed nucleus. The acroplaxome, a cytoskeletal plate, links the acrosome to the nuclear envelope.
  The tail consists of three segments:
  (1) The middle piece contains the axoneme, outer dense fibers, and a mitochondrial sheath. Mitochondria provide adenosine triphosphate (ATP) as a source of energy for the sliding of axonemal microtubules during tail beating.
  (2) The principal piece consists of the axoneme, outer dense fibers, a pair of concentric ribs, and the fibrous sheath.
  (3) The end piece is a short segment containing the terminal portion of the axoneme. An annulus, containing the protein septin 4, represents the limiting ring between the middle piece and the principal piece.

- **Conditions affecting male fertility**
  A **temperature** of 35°C is essential for spermatogenesis. This temperature is achieved in the scrotum by the pampiniform plexus and spermatid artery participating in countercurrent heat exchange.
  Varicocele (dilation of the veins of the pampiniform plexus) hampers heat exchange and may lead to a decrease in sperm production.
  Spermatic cord torsion is caused by the twisting of the spermatic cord that disrupts the arterial blood supply to, and venous drainage from, the testes. This condition, that can appear up to adolescence, is generally caused by physical trauma or an abnormally mobile testes within the tunica vaginalis.

  Cryptorchidism (or undescended testes) is the failure of one or both testes to reach the scrotal sac. Fetal and neonatal testicular descent is controlled by the testis-produced hormones insulin-like 3 (INSL3) and androgens that regulate the development of the gubernaculum, a ligament attached cpnnecting

the testis-epidymis complex to the scrotal sac. INSL3 binds to the relaxin/insulin-like peptide family receptor 2 (RXFP2) in the gubernaculum skeletal muscle. Mutations in the *INSL3* gene have been associated with bilateral cryptorchidism.
  Viral orchitis. Mumps is a systemic viral infection with a 20% to 30% incidence of unilateral or bilateral acute orchitis (sudden edema and infiltration of lymphocytes of the seminiferous intertubular space) in postpubertal males. Coxsackie B virus is another pathogen for viral orchitis.

- **Leydig cells**. Clusters of Leydig cells are observed in the intertubular space associated with blood vessels and lymphatic channels. Leydig cells produce testosterone when stimulated by luteinizing hormone (LH) and prolactin. As in all steroid-producing cells (for example, in the adrenal cortex and the corpus luteum of the ovary), cholesterol is esterified by acetyl coenzyme A and stored as cytoplasmic lipid droplets. Cholesterol is transported to mitochondria by steroidogenic acute regulatory protein (StAR) to produce pregnenolone. Enzymes of the smooth endoplasmic reticulum convert pregnenolone to progesterone to testosterone.

- **Hormonal regulation of spermatogenesis**. Sertoli cell activities are dependent on the FSH-activin-inhibin complex. The production of testosterone by Leydig cells is under control of LH. Therefore, FSH and LH are mandatory regulators of spermatogenesis as demonstrated by the collapse of spermatogenesis following hypophysectomy (surgical removal of the hypophysis). Testosterone binds to ABP, produced by Sertoli cells following FSH stimulation. The ABP-testosterone complex is transported to the epididymis together with mature spermatids. Recall the importance of cytosol and nuclear androgen receptor in mediating androgen effects. As we have seen, the gene encoding androgen receptor is located in the X chromosome and patients with androgen insensitivity syndrome (testicular feminization) have a defective androgen receptor gene.

- **The spermatogenic developmental sequence**. A few concepts need to be reviewed.
  (1) A SSC gives rise by mitosis to a daughter cell that initiates a spermatogenic cell progeny, and another daughter cell that becomes a reserve SSC. The reserve SSC will divide again and continue the same self-renewal cycle of its progenitor. This event starts at puberty.
  (2) At a given developmental time, several progenies will coexist: early and late progenies. A section of a seminiferous tubule represents the coexistence of two or more spermatogenic cell progenies started by different SSCs.
  (3)The progression of spermatogenesis is a precise timely process coordinated by the existence of cytoplasmic bridges within a spermatogonial, spermatocyte, and spermatid cohort. As a result, it is possible to determine

with great precision a series of cellular combinations in sections of seminiferous tubules (except in man). Each cellular combination is called a **cellular association**.

(4) It was noted that the cellular association sequence repeats a number of times. Each repeat of cellular associations is known as a **cycle**. Therefore, a cycle consists of cellular associations, each representing a stage of the cycle.

(5) If you can trace a progeny starting from a radiolabeled spermatogonial stem cell, you will realize that no radiolabeled mature spermatids are ready for release at the end of the first cycle. It takes three additional cycles to accomplish this goal.

By following day-by-day the radiolabeled progeny, it is possible to determine the duration of a cycle.

If the completion of one cycle occurs within 16 days and four cycles are needed for mature spermatids to be ready for release, we can say that it takes 64 days to produce mature spermatids from a starting spermatogonial stem cell.

(6) You should be able to distinguish the difference between a spermatogenic cycle and a spermatogenic wave.

A **spermatogenic cycle** is defined by changes in cellular associations that occur with **time**.

A **spermatogenic wave** is defined by the sequence of cellular associations that occurs along the **length** of a seminiferous tubule.

(7) Although the concept of a spermatogenic cycle applies to human spermatogenesis, the concept of a spermatogenic wave is not as precise as in rodents. It will take 16 days for each of the four cycles (each consisting of 6 cellular associations) to result in the release, after 64 days, of mature spermatids from the human seminiferous epithelium.

There is, however, a complication concerning the spermatogenic wave: the progression of the spermatogenic cell progenies, started by a spermatogonial stem cell, is helicoidal (instead of linear as in rodents). The turns of at least three helices, each with a different cellular association, can be visualized in a cross section of a human seminiferous tubule.

- **Epigenetics**. During spermatogenesis and oogenesis, genetic imprints are erased to allow epigenetic reprogramming to be transmitted to embryos by the gametes.

Reprogramming determines the differential expression of a number of alleles in the paternal and maternal gametes. One copy of an imprinted gene is silenced during gametogenesis. A defect in parental imprinting can give rise to **Prader-Willi syndrome** and **Angelman's syndrome.**

Important concepts to remember:
(1) During gametogenesis (spermatogenesis and oogenesis), genetic imprints are differentially erased to allow epigenetic reprogramming to be transmitted to embryos by the gametes.
(2) Immediately after fertilization, there is significant sperm DNA demethylation, followed by an extensive loss of DNA methylation from most of the genomic DNA in human embryos.

(3) After implantation, DNA methylation increases rapidly when embryonic cells acquire the characteristics of cell and tissue differentiation.

Epigenetics is the study of differences in gene expression patterns that are not determined by heritable changes in DNA sequence.

The basis of epigenetics is the methylation of cytosine-phospho-guanosine (CpG) islands seen predominantly in actively transcribing genes.

When DNA methylation occurs, with the participation of DNA methyl-transferases, transcription factors and RNA polymerase fail to transcribe a gene "silenced" by methylation. Methylated CpG islands recruit methylated DNA-binding proteins. One of them is histone deacetylase.

For transcription to occur, the N-terminal tail of histones must be acetylated. Histone deacetylation enables histone methyltransferases to methylate histone 3 and recruit heterochromatin protein-1 to trigger chromatin condensation. As you already know, heterochromatin (condensed chromatin) is transcriptionally inactive.

There are important concepts to remember:
(1) During gametogenesis (spermatogenesis and oogenesis), genetic imprints are differentially erased to allow epigenetic reprogramming to be transmitted to embryos by the gametes. DNA of mature spermatids is highly methylated (Figure 20-22), in comparison with a more modest methylation pattern during oogenesis.
(2) Immediately after fertilization, there is significant sperm DNA demethylation, followed by an extensive loss of DNA methylation from most of the genomic DNA in human embryos.
(3) After implantation, DNA methylation increases rapidly when embryonic cells acquire the characteristics of cell and tissue differentiation.

Remember that reprogramming during gametogenesis is required for the resetting of imprints or eliminating acquired epigenetic modifications. The pluripotent inner cell mass of the blastocyst erases the epigenetic memory before implantation. The epigenetic memory is back so embryo cells can achieve tissue-specific patterns.

- **Testicular tumors**
Testicular tumors are detected in 30- to 40-year old individuals. Two significant risk factors are cryptorchidism and gonadal dysgenesis (for example, Klinefelter's syndrome or the testicular feminization syndrome). An increase in X-chromosome number is a common feature of testicular germ cell tumors. Serum tumor markers are α-fetoprotein (AFP), the β subunit of human chorionic gonadotropin (β-hCG) and lactate dehydrogenase isoenzyme 1.
Testicular tumors are classified into three major groups:
(1) **Seminomas**.
(2) **Testicular germ cell tumors (TGCTs)**.

(3) **Sex cord cell tumors**.
Seminoma occurs in younger patients and is the most common testicular tumor. Serum levels of β-hCG are moderately elevated.
Spermatocytic seminoma is regarded as a variant of seminoma. It is seen in older patients.
TGCTs include testicular intraepithelial neoplasia (TIN), embryonal carcinoma, teratoma, choriocarcinoma, and yolk sac tumor.
TIN (also called intratubular germ cell neoplasia) is the initial phase of invasive TGCTs that develops in 70% of the cases after an average of 7 years. Tumor cells stain positive for membrane-associated placental-like alkaline phosphatase (PLAP) and c-kit receptor. As you remember, c-kit receptor is expressed in PGCs and differentiating spermatogonia.

Male infertility is associated with TIN, a clinical observation to be taken into account during the differential diagnostic process in all young men. Radical orchiectomy is generally performed through an inguinal incision. Organ-preserving surgery is an alternative to orchiectomy in patients who want to father children and the TIN has a reduced size.

TGCTs correlate with all kinds of X chromosome gains. In fact, the gene TGCT1 located to the long arm (Xq27) appears associated with a risk of bilateral TGCTs, presumably mediated by the increased expression of two X chromosome-linked oncogenes (ARAF1, encoding a serine/threonine kinase, and ELK1, a transcription factor). In a few patients, germ cell tumors may have an extragonadal localization (in the retroperitoneum or mediastinum) in addition to TIN. Remember that primordial germinal cells that do not reach the gonadal ridges during gonadogenesis and are not destroyed by apoptosis can give rise to germ cell tumors.
Embryonal carcinoma consists of epithelial cells arranged in cords. The tumor cells show large nuclei with an irregular outline and noticeable nucleoli. Tumor cells are PLAP- and cytokeratin-positive.
Teratoma is a benign germ cell tumor derived from a combination of the tissues from all three embryonic layers (ectoderm, mesoderm, and endoderm). Teratomas are seen in prepubertal and postpubertal patients.
Choriocarcinoma is a malignant tumor with trophoblastic cells found in teenagers. In contrast to germ cell tumors, it presents metastasis before a testicular mass is found. Serum levels of β-HCG are significantly elevated and gynecomastia is frequent.
Yolk sac tumor is the most common testicular tumor of childhood. The tumor consists of blood vessels surrounded by squamous tumor cells organizing glomerular-like structures known as Schiller-Duval bodies.
Sex cord cell tumors include Leydig cell tumor and Sertoli cell tumor.
Leydig cell tumor, the most frequent sex cord cell tumor, is seen at any age. Sertoli cell tumor are generally benign and small. Tumor cells are vimentin- and cytokeratin-positive.

21. Sperm Transport and Maturation

Mature spermatids released from the seminiferous tubules complete, as sperm, a maturation process in the epididymal duct consisting in the acquisition of forward motility, essential for eventual fertilization. Secretions from the epididymal duct, combined mainly with additional products of the prostate and seminal vesicles, contribute to the maturation and viability of the male gamete. This chapter starts by reviewing the major developmental steps of the gonads and excurrent (efferent) ducts. This review will lead us to an understanding of the histology, function, and clinical significance of the pathway followed by male and female gametes in the pursuit of fertilization.

Development of the gonads

An important aspect of gonadogenesis is that the cell precursors of the male and female gametes migrate from the primary ectoderm into the wall of the yolk sac to become **extra-embryonic. Bone morphogenetic protein**, together with signals from the extraembryonic mesoderm and visceral endoderm specify pluripotent **epiblast cells** to become **primordial germinal cells (PGCs)**. PGCs appear first in the primitive streak and endoderm in the 4-week embryo (Figure 21-1).

The induction of epiblast cells to PGCs is at the level of transcription regulation mediated by **BLIMP1** (B lymphocyte-induced maturation protein 1). BLIMP1 stimulates the expression of the PGC–specific gene *Stella*. *Stella* maintains the pluripotent state of the migrating PGCs by repressing transcription of genes specific to somatic cells. A lack of BLIMP1 prevents the appropriate differentiation and migration of PGCs.

Between 4 and 6 weeks, about 10 to 100 PGCs migrate by **ameboid movements** from the yolk sac back to the embryo into the wall of the rectum tube and from there to the right and left sides of the gonadal ridges through the dorsal mesentery. The initiation of PGC migration is regulated by the cell surface protein **IFITM1** (interferon-induced transmembrane protein 1). A lack of IFITM1 protein prevents PGCs to migrate into the endoderm. On migration of the PGCs to the genital ridge, the expression of *Stella* persists.

How do PGCs find their way to the gonadal ridges along the complex journey? There is a chemoattractant system that guides PGCs to the gonadal ridges:

1. **SDF1** (stromal-derived factor 1) is expressed at the gonadal ridges and in the surrounding mesenchyme.

2. The **chemokine CXCR4**, expressed by PGCs, is the receptor for SDF1.

A lack of SDF1 or CXCR4 causes very few PGCs to reach the gonadal ridges. If there is an ectopic expression of SDF1, PGCs migrate to ectopic sites.

PGCs that do not reach the gonadal ridges undergo apoptosis. Bax, a member of the Bcl2 protein family, initiates the apoptotic cascade. Yet, some PGCs avoid apoptosis and can later give rise to **extragonadal germ cell tumors**.

As PGCs migrate, they proliferate by mitotic division. PGCs reach the gonadal ridges by the 6th week and continue their proliferation as they interact with somatic cells to develop the indifferent gonads.

There are at least three additional factors that participate in the migration of PGCs:

1. The rate of migration and proliferation of PGCs are dependent on the interaction of the **c-kit receptor**, a **tyrosine kinase**, with its corresponding cell membrane ligand, **stem cell factor** (or **c-kit ligand**). The c-kit receptor is produced by PGCs; stem cell factor is produced by somatic cells along the migration route.

A lack of the c-kit receptor or stem cell factor results in gonads deficient in PGCs because they migrate at a significant reduced rate. As we have already seen, hematopoiesis and the development of melanocytes and mast cells depend on the c-kit receptor and its stem cell ligand.

2. **E-cadherin** expressed by PGCs is required as PGCs migrate to the hindgut.

3. PGCs express β**1 integrin**, also required for entry to the gonadal ridges.

About 2500 to 5000 PGCs lodge in the mesenchyme and induce cells of the mesonephros and lining coelomic epithelium to proliferate, forming a pair of **gonadal ridges**. Coelomic epithelial cords grow into the mesenchyme of the gonadal ridge to form an **outer cortex** and **inner medulla** of the indifferent gonad.

Testis-determining factor controls the development of the testes

Until the seventh week of fetal development, there is one type of gonad common to both genders. This is the "**indifferent**" stage of gonadal development.

Thereafter, **in the female, the cortex develops into**

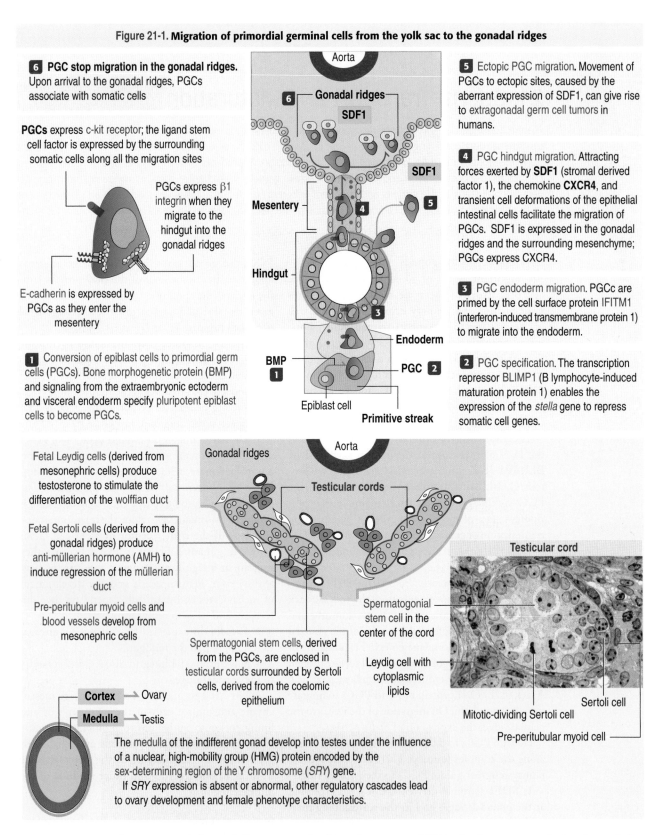

Figure 21-1. Migration of primordial germinal cells from the yolk sac to the gonadal ridges

6 PGC stop migration in the gonadal ridges. Upon arrival to the gonadal ridges, PGCs associate with somatic cells

PGCs express c-kit receptor; the ligand stem cell factor is expressed by the surrounding somatic cells along all the migration sites

PGCs express β1 integrin when they migrate to the hindgut into the gonadal ridges

E-cadherin is expressed by PGCs as they enter the mesentery

1 Conversion of epiblast cells to primordial germ cells (PGCs). Bone morphogenetic protein (BMP) and signaling from the extraembryonic ectoderm and visceral endoderm specify pluripotent epiblast cells to become PGCs.

Aorta
Gonadal ridges
SDF1
SDF1
Mesentery
Hindgut
BMP 1
Endoderm
PGC 2
Epiblast cell
Primitive streak

5 Ectopic PGC migration. Movement of PGCs to ectopic sites, caused by the aberrant expression of SDF1, can give rise to extragonadal germ cell tumors in humans.

4 PGC hindgut migration. Attracting forces exerted by **SDF1** (stromal derived factor 1), the chemokine **CXCR4**, and transient cell deformations of the epithelial intestinal cells facilitate the migration of PGCs. SDF1 is expressed in the gonadal ridges and the surrounding mesenchyme; PGCs express CXCR4.

3 PGC endoderm migration. PGCc are primed by the cell surface protein IFITM1 (interferon-induced transmembrane protein 1) to migrate into the endoderm.

2 PGC specification. The transcription repressor BLIMP1 (B lymphocyte-induced maturation protein 1) enables the expression of the *stella* gene to repress somatic cell genes.

Fetal Leydig cells (derived from mesonephric cells) produce testosterone to stimulate the differentiation of the wolffian duct

Fetal Sertoli cells (derived from the gonadal ridges) produce anti-müllerian hormone (AMH) to induce regression of the müllerian duct

Pre-peritubular myoid cells and blood vessels develop from mesonephric cells

Spermatogonial stem cells, derived from the PGCs, are enclosed in testicular cords surrounded by Sertoli cells, derived from the coelomic epithelium

Gonadal ridges
Aorta
Testicular cords

Testicular cord

Spermatogonial stem cell in the center of the cord

Leydig cell with cytoplasmic lipids

Sertoli cell

Mitotic-dividing Sertoli cell

Pre-peritubular myoid cell

Cortex → Ovary
Medulla → Testis

The medulla of the indifferent gonad develop into testes under the influence of a nuclear, high-mobility group (HMG) protein encoded by the sex-determining region of the Y chromosome (*SRY*) gene.
If *SRY* expression is absent or abnormal, other regulatory cascades lead to ovary development and female phenotype characteristics.

the ovary, and the medulla regresses. In the male, the cortex regresses and the medulla forms the testis.

The development of each medulla into a testis is controlled by a transcription factor encoded by the **sex-determining region of the Y chromosome (*SRY*)** gene. SRY is also known as **testicular-determining factor.**

SRY upregulates **Sox9** (for sex determining region Y-box 9), another transcription factor, whose expression, together with fibroblast growth factor 9, causes

Figure 21-2. Development of the male genitalia

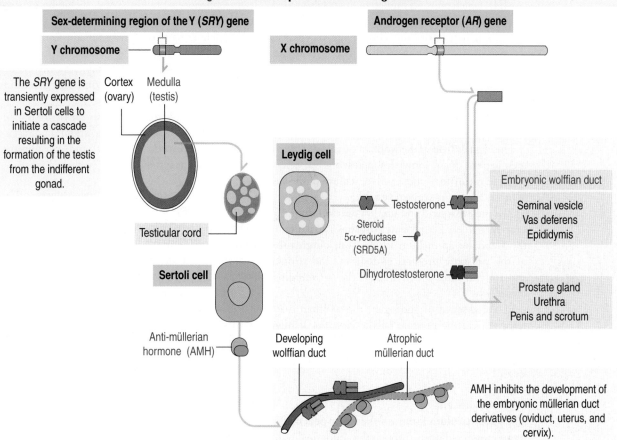

The development of **testicular cords**, the precursors of the seminiferous tubules. We have learned in Chapter 4, Connective Tissue, that Sox9 participates in chondrogenesis, by enabling cells in the perichondrium to differentiate into chondrocytes. Therefore, Sox9 is important for the development of the male reproductive system and the skeleton.

The initial step of testicular development is the differentiation of the Sertoli cell population regulated by the Y chromosome. Fetal Sertoli cells, in turn, regulate the differentiation of the mesenchymal–derived Leydig cells, that initially proliferate under the influence of insulin-like growth factor I (IGF-I).

Fetal precursors of peritubular myoid cells and the vasculature develop around the testicular cords.

Fetal Leydig cells produce testosterone stimulated by luteinizing hormone produced by the fetal adenohypophysis. Testosterone production ceases postnatally, reassumes at puberty and continues throughout adulthood.

Spermatogonial stem cells (SSCs), derived from PGCs, are mitotically quiescent and located in the center of the testicular cords surrounded by mitotically dividing Sertoli cells (see Figure 21-1). Close to puberty, SSCs migrate to the future seminiferous tubular wall and initiate their mitotic amplification cycle, the starting point of spermatogenesis.

A loss of Sox9 function results in **XY gonadal dysgenesis** in which patients have undeveloped gonadal structures (streak gonads) and absence of virilization (persistence of müllerian-derived structures). Mutations of the *Sox9* gene cause **campomelic dysplasia** involving skeletal abnormalities.

Development of male and female internal genitalia
The fetal testis is formed by testicular cords connected to the rete testis by tubuli recti. The cords are formed by **Sertoli cells**, derived from the coelomic epithelium, and SSCs. **Leydig cells**, derived from the mesonephric mesenchyme, are present between the testicular cords.

Box 21-A | Development of internal genitalia: Highlights to remember

- When Sertoli cell–derived AMH is not present, the müllerian ducts become the fallopian tubes (oviducts), uterus, cervix, and upper one third of the vagina.
- When Leydig cell–derived testosterone is present, the wolffian ducts become the epididymis, vas deferens, seminal vesicles, and ejaculatory ducts.
- When steroid 5-α reductase (SRD5A) is present, testosterone is converted into dihydrotestosterone (DHT). DHT induces the genital tubercle, genital fold, genital swelling, and urogenital sinus to become the penis, scrotum, and prostate.
- When DHT is not present, the genital tubercle, genital fold, genital swelling, and urogenital sinus become the labia majora, labia minora, clitoris, and lower two thirds of the vagina.

Fetal Sertoli cells secrete **anti-müllerian hormone (AMH)**, which prevents müllerian ducts (also called paramesonephric ducts) from developing into the uterovaginal primordium (Figure 21-2). In the absence of AMH, the müllerian ducts persist and become the female internal genitalia.

By 8 weeks of gestation, fetal Leydig cells produce testosterone, which is regulated by placental human chorionic gonadotropin (hCG), because the fetal hypophysis is not secreting luteinizing hormone (LH).

The cephalic end of the wolffian ducts (also called mesonephric ducts) forms the epididymis, vas deferens, and ejaculatory duct. A diverticulum of the vas deferens forms the seminal vesicles.

The prostate gland and urethra develop from the urogenital sinus. The prostate gland has a dual origin: the glandular epithelium forms from outgrowths of the prostatic urethral endoderm; the stroma and smooth muscle derive from the surrounding mesoderm.

In the absence of androgen, the wolffian duct regresses and the prostate fails to develop. If high levels of androgen are present in the **female fetus**, both müllerian and wolffian ducts can persist (see Box 21-A).

Testicular descent

The **gubernaculum** forms on the lower pole of the testis, crosses obliquely through the abdominal wall, and attaches the testis to the genital swelling, the future scrotal sac.

Between month 3 and 7 of pregnancy, the testis remains near the inguinal canal. In month 9 of pregnancy or immediately after birth, the testes reach the scrotal sac after moving across the inguinal canal. The gubernaculum shortens, the vaginal process lengthens and each testis is drawn into the scrotum. As the vaginal process lengthens, it traps muscle fibers of the oblique internal muscle and the transverse muscle to form the cremaster muscle.

For additional details, see Cryptorchidism (or undescended testis) in Chapter 20, Spermatogenesis.

Clinical significance: Klinefelter's syndrome

Klinefelter's syndrome is observed in males with an **extra X chromosome (47,XXY)** as a result of chromosomal non-disjunction during male or female meiosis.

Individuals with this syndrome:

1. Are phenotypically males (presence of the Y chromosome).

2. Have small testes and few spermatogenic cells are present.

3. Have high follicle-stimulating hormone (FSH) levels because the function of Sertoli cells is abnormal (failure to produce inhibin).

4. Have low testosterone levels (hypogonadism), but **high estradiol levels**. The excess of estradiol can lead to phenotypic feminization, including **gynecomastia (breast enlargement)**.

Klinefelter's syndrome may remain undiagnosed until the patient consults because of infertility. Chromosome analysis (karyotyping), testosterone and estrogen determination and sperm count determine the nature of the syndrome.

Klinefelter's syndrome increases the risk of testicular germ cell tumor, breast cancer, attention deficient hyperactivity disorder (ADHD) and autoimmune diseases (such as systemic lupus erythematosus).

Clinical significance: Androgen insensitivity syndrome (AIS)

Androgen insensitivity syndrome (**AIS**), or testicular feminization (Tfm) syndrome, results from a defect in the gene controlling the expression of the **androgen receptor**. This gene is located on the X chromosome.

Three phenotypes are observed:

1. **Complete a**ndrogen insensitivity syndrome (**CAIS**) with female external genitalia.

2. **Partial a**ndrogen insensitivity syndrome (**PAIS**, Reifenstein syndrome) with predominantly female, predominantly male, or ambiguous genitalia.

3. **Mild a**ndrogen insensitivity syndrome (**MAIS**) with male external genitalia. Spermatogenesis and/or pubertal virilization may be impaired.

Although the karyotype is 46,XY, a deficiency in the action of androgen results in the lack of development of the wolffian duct and regression of the müllerian duct because testes development takes place and Sertoli cell–derived AMH is available.

No functional **internal genitalia** are present in patients with CAIS: the testes remain in the abdomen (recall that androgens stimulate testicular descent). Inguinal hernia with testes can be detected during a physical examination. The testes may be removed after puberty (until feminization is complete) because of the risk of testicular cancer, just like in the undescended testis condition.

The **external genitalia** develop as female but no uterus is present. Individuals with complete AIS have labia, a clitoris, and a short vagina (these structures are not müllerian duct derivatives). Pubic and axillary hair is absent (sexual hair development is androgen-dependent). Individuals with PAIS may have male and female physical characteristics (ambiguous genitalia).

At puberty, the production of both androgen and estradiol increases (the latter from peripheral aromatization of androgens). Androgens cannot inhibit LH secretion (because a defective androgen receptor prevents LH feedback inhibition), and plasma levels of androgens remain high.

AIS can be diagnosed by pelvic ultrasound, hormonal determinations and chromosome analysis.

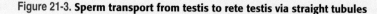

Figure 21-3. Sperm transport from testis to rete testis via straight tubules

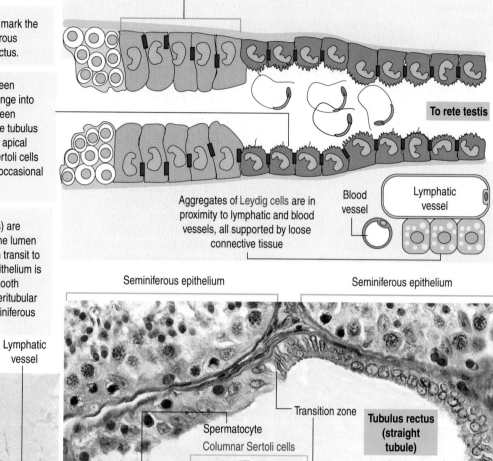

Columnar Sertoli cells only mark the transition from the seminiferous epithelium to the tubulus rectus.

Basal tight junctions between columnar Sertoli cells change into apical tight junctions between cuboidal Sertoli cells at the tubulus rectus and rete testis. The apical domain of the cuboidal Sertoli cells displays microvilli and an occasional primary cilium.

Tubuli recti (straight tubules) are shown in a cross section. The lumen contains immature sperm in transit to the rete testis. The lining epithelium is cuboidal and peritubular smooth muscle cells continue the peritubular myoid cells layer of the seminiferous tubules.

To rete testis

Aggregates of Leydig cells are in proximity to lymphatic and blood vessels, all supported by loose connective tissue

Blood vessel

Lymphatic vessel

Leydig cells   Blood vessel   Lymphatic vessel

Straight tubules

Seminiferous epithelium   Seminiferous epithelium

Spermatocyte
Columnar Sertoli cells

Transition zone

Tubulus rectus (straight tubule)

Cuboidal Sertoli cells

Lymphatic vessel

Clinical significance: Steroid 5α-reductase 2 deficiency

There are three isoenzymes of **steroid 5α-reductase (SRD5A)**: **SRD5A1**, **SRD5A2**, and **SRD5A3**. A defect in the activity of **SRD5A2** results in decreased conversion of testosterone to the more potent androgen, dihydrotestosterone (DHT) in individuals with SRD5A deficiency.

Individuals with mutations of the *SRD5A2* gene, located on the short arm of chromosome 2, are genetically males. Affected individuals have normal internal genitalia (whose development from the wolffian duct is androgen-dependent) but nonmasculinized external genitalia (whose development is DHT-dependent). They are often mistaken for females at birth.

Although the external genitalia may be female, the vagina consists of only the lower two-thirds of a normal vagina, creating a blind-ending vaginal pouch (see Box 21-A). Because Sertoli cell–derived AMH is present and determines the regression of the müllerian duct, individuals with SRD5A2 deficiency lack a uterus and oviducts.

Individuals with SRD5A2 deficiency can produce sperm but fertility is compromised by a lack of development of seminal vesicles and prostate. In addition, SRD5A2 deficiency is associated with an increased risk of cryptorchidism and testicular cancer.

The discovery of congenital SRD5A2 deficiency made possible a better understanding of two androgen hormones: testosterone and DHT, in the drug therapy of benign prostatic hyperplasia and prostate cancer as

Figure 21-4. Sperm transport and fluid reabsorption in the efferent ductule and proximal epididymis

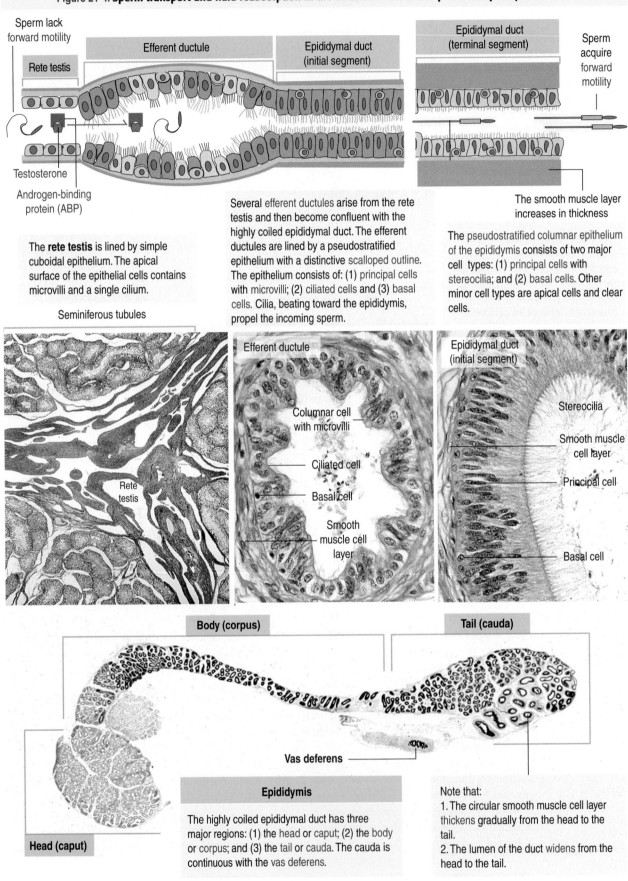

Sperm lack forward motility

Rete testis

Efferent ductule

Epididymal duct (initial segment)

Epididymal duct (terminal segment)

Sperm acquire forward motility

Testosterone

Androgen-binding protein (ABP)

The **rete testis** is lined by simple cuboidal epithelium. The apical surface of the epithelial cells contains microvilli and a single cilium.

Several efferent ductules arise from the rete testis and then become confluent with the highly coiled epididymal duct. The efferent ductules are lined by a pseudostratified epithelium with a distinctive scalloped outline. The epithelium consists of: (1) principal cells with microvilli; (2) ciliated cells and (3) basal cells. Cilia, beating toward the epididymis, propel the incoming sperm.

The smooth muscle layer increases in thickness

The pseudostratified columnar epithelium of the epididymis consists of two major cell types: (1) principal cells with stereocilia; and (2) basal cells. Other minor cell types are apical cells and clear cells.

Seminiferous tubules

Rete testis

Efferent ductule

Columnar cell with microvilli

Ciliated cell

Basal cell

Smooth muscle cell layer

Epididymal duct (initial segment)

Stereocilia

Smooth muscle cell layer

Principal cell

Basal cell

Body (corpus)

Tail (cauda)

Vas deferens

Head (caput)

Epididymis

The highly coiled epididymal duct has three major regions: (1) the head or caput; (2) the body or corpus; and (3) the tail or cauda. The cauda is continuous with the vas deferens.

Note that:
1. The circular smooth muscle cell layer thickens gradually from the head to the tail.
2. The lumen of the duct widens from the head to the tail.

Figure 21-5. Epididymis

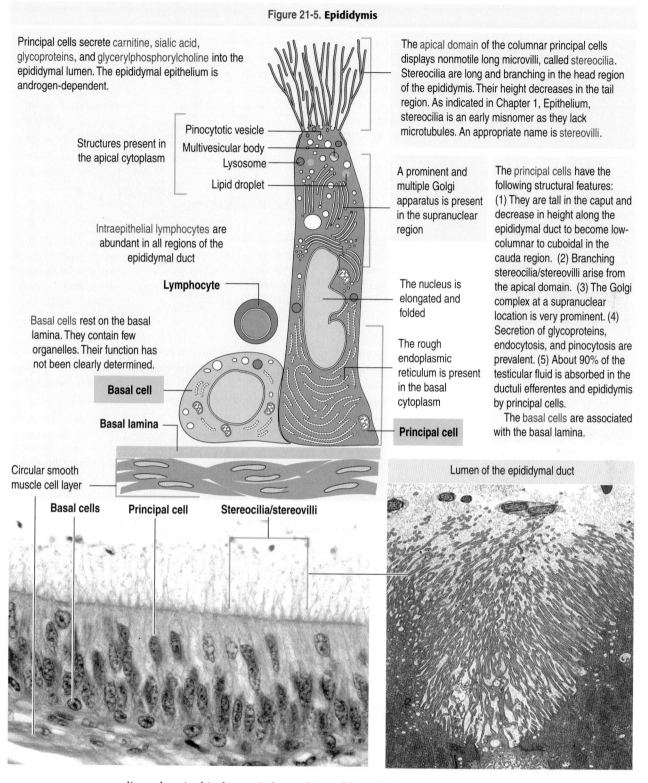

Principal cells secrete carnitine, sialic acid, glycoproteins, and glycerylphosphorylcholine into the epididymal lumen. The epididymal epithelium is androgen-dependent.

Structures present in the apical cytoplasm

- Pinocytotic vesicle
- Multivesicular body
- Lysosome
- Lipid droplet

Intraepithelial lymphocytes are abundant in all regions of the epididymal duct

Lymphocyte

Basal cells rest on the basal lamina. They contain few organelles. Their function has not been clearly determined.

Basal cell

Basal lamina

Circular smooth muscle cell layer

The apical domain of the columnar principal cells displays nonmotile long microvilli, called stereocilia. Stereocilia are long and branching in the head region of the epididymis. Their height decreases in the tail region. As indicated in Chapter 1, Epithelium, stereocilia is an early misnomer as they lack microtubules. An appropriate name is stereovilli.

A prominent and multiple Golgi apparatus is present in the supranuclear region

The nucleus is elongated and folded

The rough endoplasmic reticulum is present in the basal cytoplasm

Principal cell

The principal cells have the following structural features: (1) They are tall in the caput and decrease in height along the epididymal duct to become low-columnar to cuboidal in the cauda region. (2) Branching stereocilia/stereovilli arise from the apical domain. (3) The Golgi complex at a supranuclear location is very prominent. (4) Secretion of glycoproteins, endocytosis, and pinocytosis are prevalent. (5) About 90% of the testicular fluid is absorbed in the ductuli efferentes and epididymis by principal cells.

The basal cells are associated with the basal lamina.

Basal cells   Principal cell   Stereocilia/stereovilli

Lumen of the epididymal duct

we discuss later in this chapter. Polymorphism of the *SRD5A2* gene (by single amino acid substitutions) may be associated with the risk of developing prostate cancer or having an aggressive form of the tumor.

Sperm maturation pathway

After transport to the **rete testis** through a connecting **tubulus rectus** (Figure 21-3), mature spermatids

(or immature sperm) enter the **ductuli efferentes**.

Ductuli efferentes link the rete testis to the initial segment of the epididymal duct, an irregularly coiled duct extending to the **ductus**, or **vas deferens**. Remember that the epididymal duct and ductus or vas deferens differentiate from the mesonephric duct (wolffian duct).

Tubuli recti (**straight tubules**) are located in the

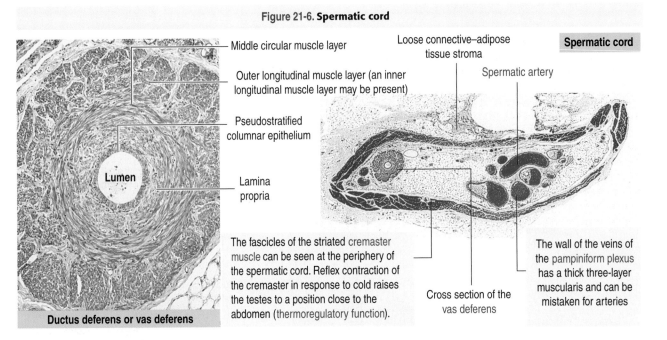

Figure 21-6. Spermatic cord

Middle circular muscle layer

Outer longitudinal muscle layer (an inner longitudinal muscle layer may be present)

Pseudostratified columnar epithelium

Lumen

Lamina propria

Ductus deferens or vas deferens

The fascicles of the striated cremaster muscle can be seen at the periphery of the spermatic cord. Reflex contraction of the cremaster in response to cold raises the testes to a position close to the abdomen (thermoregulatory function).

Loose connective–adipose tissue stroma

Spermatic artery

Spermatic cord

Cross section of the vas deferens

The wall of the veins of the pampiniform plexus has a thick three-layer muscularis and can be mistaken for arteries

---

mediastinum of the testis. They are lined by a **simple cuboidal epithelium** with structural features similar to those of Sertoli cells except that occluding junctions are now at the **apical domain**, instead of at the basal domain. Spermatogenic cells are not present.

The **rete testis** consists of irregularly anastomosing channels within the mediastinum of the testis (Figure 21-4). These channels are lined by a **simple cuboidal epithelium**. The wall, formed by fibroblasts and smooth muscle cells, is surrounded by large lymphatic channels and blood vessels associated with large clusters of Leydig cells (see Figure 21-3).

About 12 to 20 **ductuli efferentes (efferent ductules)** link the rete testis to the epididymis after piercing the testicular tunica albuginea. Each ductule is lined by:

1. **Columnar cells with microvilli/stereocilia**, with a role in the reabsorption of fluid from the lumen.

2. **Ciliated cells,** which contribute to the transport of **nonmotile sperm** toward the epididymis.

3. **Basal cells,** the cell precursor of the ciliated and nonciliated epithelial cells.

The pseudostratified epithelium has a characteristic scalloped outline that enables identification of the ductuli efferentes (see Figure 21-4). A thin inner circular layer of **smooth muscle cells** underlies the epithelium and its basal lamina.

Androgen-binding protein, produced by Sertoli cells, binds androgens. The protein-steroid complex is present in the lumen of the rete testis and the initial segments of the epididymis. Consequently, the rete testis contains a larger concentration of androgens than arterial blood. Intraluminal androgens appear to favor the normal function of the head of the epididymis.

The epididymal ducts

The **epididymides** (Greek *epi*, following; *didymos*, pair) (Pl **epididymides**) are a highly elongated and coiled tubules (about 6 meters in length in the adult human) where sperm mature.

Sperm maturation consists in the acquisition of **forward motility**, essential to sperm **fertilizing ability**. Mature sperm are stored in the terminal portion of the epididymal duct before ejaculation.

The epididymal duct is classically subdivided into three major segments:

1. The **head** or **caput**.

2. The **body** or **corpus**.

3. The **tail** or **cauda** (see Figure 21-4).

The epithelium is **pseudostratified columnar** with

Box 21-B | Epididymal duct: Highlights to remember

The epididymis has three main functions:
• Sperm transport by peristalsis to the storage region, the tail of the epididymis. The time of sperm epididymal maturation is from 2 to 12 days.
• Sperm storage until ejaculation.
• Sperm maturation. Sperm collected from the head region of the epididymis are unable to fertilize. The fertilizing ability is acquired from the body to the tail of the epididymis.
  Sperm maturation includes:
  1. Stabilization of condensed chromatin.
  2. Changes in plasma membrane surface charge.
  3. Acquisition by sperm of new surface proteins.
  4. Acquisition of sperm forward motility.
• The development of the epididymal ducts, derived from the wolffian ducts, requires normal expression of *Homeobox A10 (Hoxa10)* and *Hoxa11* genes. Mutations in the genes encoding bone morphogenetic protein (Bmp) 4, Bmp7, and Bmp8 result in the defective differentiation of specific segments of the epididymal duct.

Figure 21-7. Ejaculatory ducts

The ducts of the seminal vesicles pierce the capsule of the prostate gland and join the vas deferens of the same side to form the ejaculatory duct.

The ejaculatory duct opens onto the posterior wall of the prostatic urethra. The wall of the ejaculatory ducts is folded and lined by simple columnar epithelium surrounded by connective tissue and bundles of smooth muscle.

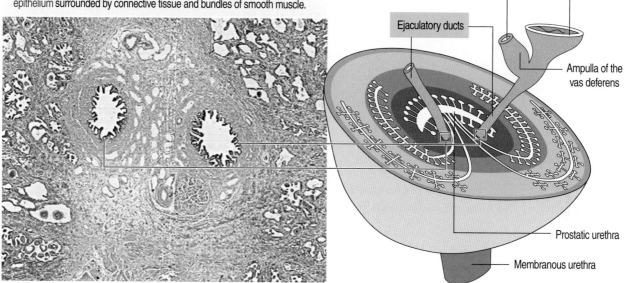

long and branched **stereocilia**. The epithelium consists of **two major cell types** (Figure 21-5):

1. Columnar **principal cells**, extending from the lumen to the basal lamina. The apical domain of principal cells displays **branched stereocilia/stereovilli** and a well-developed Golgi apparatus, lysosomes, and vesicles.

2. **Basal cells** associated with the basal lamina. Basal cells are regarded as the undifferentiated precursors of principal cells.

Other cell types are the **apical cells**, rich in mitochondria and predominant in the head of the epididymis, and the **clear cells**, predominant in the tail of the epididymis. **Intraepithelial lymphocytes** are distributed throughout the epididymis. They may be an important component of the epididymal immunologic barrier.

The **height of the epithelium** varies with respect to the segment of the epididymal duct. The epithe-lium is **taller in the head region** and **shorter in the tail region**. In an opposite fashion, the lumen of the epididymal duct is narrow in the head region and wider in the tail region.

Regional differences exist in the organization of the **smooth muscle cell layer**, responsible for the rhythmic peristaltic contractions moving sperm along the epididymal duct (see Box 21-B). The initial portions of the epididymal duct are surrounded by a circular smooth muscle cell layer. The terminal portions (body and tail) display an increase in the thickness of the inner circular smooth muscle layer and the development of an outer longitudinal smooth muscle cell layer.

The **vas deferens** (ductus deferens) is a 45-cm-long muscular tube with the following features:

1. The lining epithelium is **pseudostratified columnar with stereocilia/stereovilli** similar to that of the epididymis, and is supported by a connective tissue lamina propria with elastic fibers.

2. The muscular wall consists of **inner** and **outer** layers of longitudinally oriented muscle separated by a **middle circular layer**.

3. The external layer consists of loose connective tissue and adipose cells.

In addition to the vas deferens, the **spermatic cord** contains the following components (Figure 21-6):

1. The **cremaster muscle**.

2. **Arteries** (spermatic artery, cremasteric artery, and artery to the vas deferens).

3. **Veins of the pampiniform plexus**.

4. **Nerves** (genital branch of the genitofemoral

Box 21-C | Seminal plasma (semen)

• The seminal plasma or semen consists of the combination of alkaline secretions of epididymal epithelium and the accessory glands (predominantly the prostate and seminal vesicles). The fresh ejaculate coagulates within one minute in the vaginal cavity and neutralizes the acidic contents of the vagina. Proteases (fibrinolysin and fibrinogenase) present in the prostate secretions change the coagulated ejaculate to a fluid state after 15 to 20 minutes.
• Proteins of the seminal plasma coat the sperm plasma membrane and supply nutrients, including fructose, and activator of sperm forward motility.
• Seminal vesicles contribute about 75% of the volume of the seminal plasma; about 20-25% of the volume derives from the prostate gland.

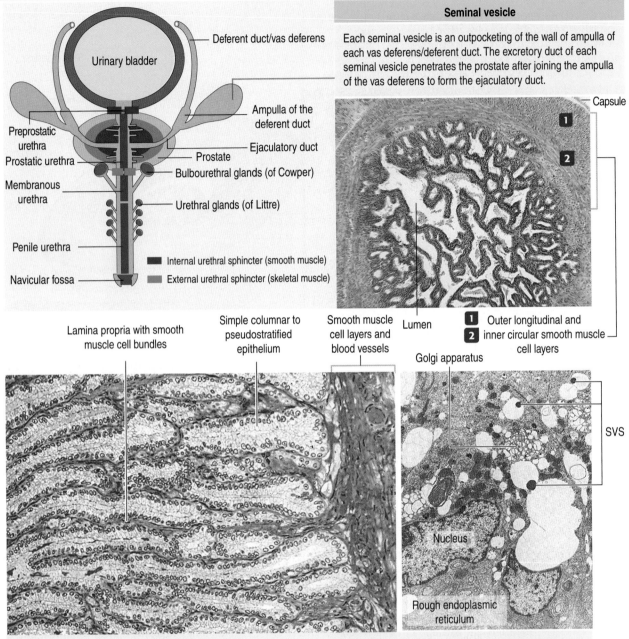

Figure 21-8. Seminal vesicle

Seminal vesicle

Each seminal vesicle is an outpocketing of the wall of ampulla of each vas deferens/deferent duct. The excretory duct of each seminal vesicle penetrates the prostate after joining the ampulla of the vas deferens to form the ejaculatory duct.

Deferent duct/vas deferens

Urinary bladder

Ampulla of the deferent duct

Preprostatic urethra

Ejaculatory duct

Prostatic urethra

Prostate

Bulbourethral glands (of Cowper)

Membranous urethra

Urethral glands (of Littre)

Penile urethra

Navicular fossa

■ Internal urethral sphincter (smooth muscle)
■ External urethral sphincter (skeletal muscle)

Capsule

1

2

1 Outer longitudinal and
2 inner circular smooth muscle cell layers

Lumen

Lamina propria with smooth muscle cell bundles

Simple columnar to pseudostratified epithelium

Smooth muscle cell layers and blood vessels

Golgi apparatus

SVS

Nucleus

Rough endoplasmic reticulum

Each seminal vesicle has a highly folded mucosa with primary epithelial folds branching into secondary and tertiary folds. Epithelial folds are supported by loose connective tissue (lamina propria of the mucosa).

At high magnification, the epithelium is simple columnar to pseudostratified. The apical cytoplasm is vacuolated. It contains

seminal vesicle secretory (SVS) proteins (coagulating proteins) seen as dense secretory granules eccentrically located in large and clear vesicles. The seminal vesicles contribute about 75% of the volume of the semen. Sperm are not stored in the seminal vesicles. The secretion also consists of fructose and prostaglandins.

nerve, cremasteric nerve, and sympathetic branches of the testicular plexus).

All these structures are surrounded by **loose connective tissue**.

An **ampulla**, the dilated portion of the vas deferens, leads directly into the prostate gland (Figure 21-7). The distal end receives the ducts of the seminal vesicle, forming the **ejaculatory ducts,** which pass

through the prostate gland to empty secretion into the prostatic urethra at the seminal colliculus.

Clinical significance: Causes of male infertility

We have seen that the *SRY* gene, located on the Y chromosome, encodes a transcription factor called sex-determining region Y protein responsible, together with Sox9, for the development of the testes.

A fetus with a mutation in the SRY gene develops as a female despite having a Y chromosome.

The Y chromosome also harbors the *azoospermia factor (AZF)* region gene, a determinant of spermatogenesis. Deletions in the *AZF* region, located in the long arm of human Y chromosome, are implicated in male infertility.

There are three AZF regions: *AZFa, AZFb,* and *AZFc.* Each AZF region contains several genes with a role in spermatogenesis.

Deletions of the AZFa region are less frequent and account for the Sertoli cell–only syndrome (SCOS; see Chapter 20, Spermatogenesis).

AZFb deletions are associated with meiotic arrest (spermatocytes).

Deletions of the AZFc region result in a reduction in sperm production (oligozoospermia) and can be transmitted to the offspring. Males with Y chromosome infertility have small testes and short stature.

Y chromosome infertility is characterized by **azoospermia** (absence of sperm) and **oligozoospermia** (less than 15 million sperm/mL of semen). Normal sperm count is 20-40 million sperm/mL of semen.

In addition to deletions in the AZF region of the Y chromosome, other causes of male infertility include:

1. Obstruction of the ejaculatory duct.

2. Cystic fibrosis transmembrane conductance regulator (CFTR)–related disorders, including cystic fibrosis and congenital bilateral absence of the vas deferens (because of the atrophy, fibrosis and absence of wolffian–derived structures). Affected men have azoospermia.

3. Bilateral viral orchitis (mumps), epididymitis and urethritis.

4. Chemotherapy or exposure to radiation.

5. Klinefelter's syndrome (XXY).

6. Sertoli cell–only syndrome (SCOS).

Accessory genital glands

The accessory glands of the male reproductive tract include two **seminal vesicles**, the **prostate gland,** two **bulbourethral glands** of Cowper and urethral glands of Littré (the latter also present in the female urethra).

The seminal vesicles and the prostate produce most of the seminal fluid, and their function is regulated by androgens (testosterone and DHT).

Seminal vesicles

The seminal vesicles are androgen-dependent organs. Each seminal vesicle is an outpocketing of the wall of ampulla of each vas deferens. It consists of three components (Figure 21-8):

1. An **external connective tissue capsule.**

2. A **middle smooth muscle layer** (inner circular and outer longitudinal layers).

3. An **internal highly folded mucosa** lined by a **simple cuboidal-to-pseudostratified columnar epithelium**.

The epithelial cells display a large Golgi apparatus with vesicles containing **seminal vesicle secretory (SVS) granules** (coagulating proteins). Seminal vesicles secrete an alkaline viscous fluid rich in **fructose** and **prostaglandins.** The fluid contributes about 75% of the human ejaculate.

Fructose is the major source of energy of the ejaculated sperm. Seminal vesicles do not store sperm. They contract during ejaculation and their secretion contributes to the semen.

The excretory duct of each seminal vesicle penetrates the prostate after joining the ampulla of the vas deferens/deferent duct to form the ejaculatory duct (see Figures 21-7 and 21-8; see Box 21-C).

Prostate gland

The prostate is the largest accessory genital gland surrounded by a capsule. It consists of 30 to 50 branched **tubuloalveolar glands** that empty their contents into the **prostate urethra** via long excretory ducts.

The male urethra consists of four segments (see Figure 21-8):

1. **Preprostatic urethra,** a short segment (1 cm) surrounded by the internal urethral sphincter (smooth muscle cells) that, when contracted, prevents the retrograde flow of semen into the urinary bladder during ejaculation.

2. **Prostatic urethra,** a 3 to 4 cm long segment embedded in the prostate gland, is the end site of prostatic ducts transporting glandular secretions, and the ejaculatory ducts, carrying semen and secretions of the seminal vesicles during ejaculation.

3. **Membranous urethra** is a segment that crosses through the deep perineal pouch and is surrounded by skeletal muscle of the external urethral sphincter.

4. **Penile urethra** (spongy urethra), surrounded by erectile tissue (the corpus spongiosum) of the penis.

Remember the segmental distribution of the male urethra because it will become useful when performing **urethral catheterization** to drain urine from patients unable to micturate.

The prostate glands are arranged in three zones (Figure 21-9):

1. A **central zone** with **periurethral mucosal glands**.

2. A **transition zone** with **periurethral submucosal glands**.

3. A **peripheral zone** consisting of **branched (compound) glands.** About 70% to 80% of prostate cancer originates in the peripheral zone.

The prostate glands are lined by **simple** or **pseudostratified columnar epithelium** (Figure 21-10). The lumen contains **concretions (corpora amylacea)** rich in glycoproteins and, sometimes, a site of **calcium**

Figure 21-9. **Prostate gland**

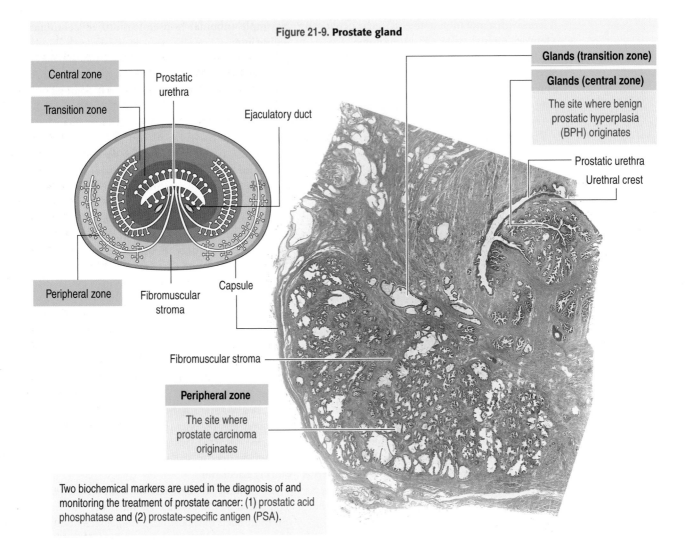

Central zone

Transition zone

Prostatic urethra

Ejaculatory duct

Peripheral zone

Fibromuscular stroma

Capsule

Glands (transition zone)

Glands (central zone)

The site where benign prostatic hyperplasia (BPH) originates

Prostatic urethra

Urethral crest

Fibromuscular stroma

Peripheral zone

The site where prostate carcinoma originates

Two biochemical markers are used in the diagnosis of and monitoring the treatment of prostate cancer: (1) prostatic acid phosphatase and (2) prostate-specific antigen (PSA).

Benign prostatic hyperplasia

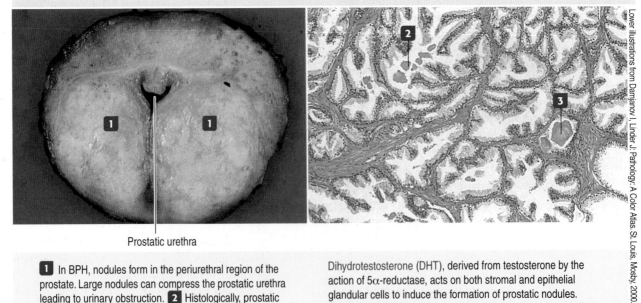

Prostatic urethra

1 In BPH, nodules form in the periurethral region of the prostate. Large nodules can compress the prostatic urethra leading to urinary obstruction. **2** Histologically, prostatic glands are enlarged and the epithelial lining is folded. **3** Corpora amylacea are seen in the glandular lumen.

Dihydrotestosterone (DHT), derived from testosterone by the action of 5α-reductase, acts on both stromal and epithelial glandular cells to induce the formation of prostatic nodules. Because the enzyme 5α-reductase is present in stromal cells, stromal cells have a pivotal role in generating DHT and BPH.

Figure 21-10. Prostate tubuloalveolar glands

Prostate gland

The prostate is a muscular and glandular organ. It consists of three groups of glands: (1) periurethral mucosal glands (in the central zone); (2) periurethral submucosal glands, linked to the urethra by short ducts (in the transition zone); and (3) main prostatic glands (in the peripheral zone). About 30 to 50 tubuloalveolar glands open directly into the prostatic urethra through 15 to 30 long ducts ending at the sides of the urethral crest.

The epithelium of the main prostatic glands is simple columnar or pseudostratified and arranged into folds supported by a lamina propria. The lumen may contain corpora amylacea, a condensed structure rich in glycoproteins and cell fragments, with a tendency to calcify in older men.

The secretion of the prostate contains fibrinolysin, with a role in the liquefaction of semen. Citric acid, zinc, amylase, prostate-specific antigen, and acid phosphatase are present in high concentrations in prostate fluid secreted in the semen.

Prostate-specific antigen screening

Although the digital rectal examination (DRE) has been the primary screening test for prostate cancer, a large number of cancers detected by this method are at an advanced stage. Prostate-specific antigen blood testing (PSA) was introduced in the late 1980s to increase early-stage cancer detection of prostate cancer as compared to DRE. Values above 4 ng/ml, considered to be abnormal, are associated with benign prostatic hyperplasia (BPH), prostatitis or cystitis (false-positive). A normal PSA value does not rule out prostate cancer (false-negative). At present, patients are informed about inconsistent evidence of PSA screening.

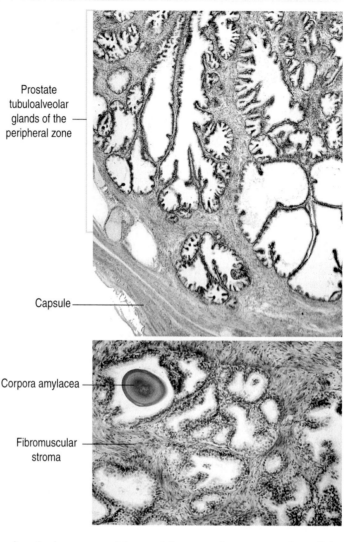

Prostate tubuloalveolar glands of the peripheral zone

Capsule

Corpora amylacea

Fibromuscular stroma

deposition. Cells contain abundant rough endoplasmic reticulum and Golgi apparatus.

The prostate produces a zinc-rich alkaline fluid that neutralizes the acidic vaginal content, provides nutrients and transports sperm, and liquefies semen.

Protein products include **prostate-specific acid phosphatase**, **prostate-specific antigen** (**PSA**, a marker for early detection of prostate cancer), **amylase**, and **fibrinolysin**.

Pathology: Benign prostate hyperplasia

Benign prostate hyperplasia (**BPH**), a condition that occurs with aging, is a noncancerous enlargement of the prostate gland that can restrict the flow of urine through the prostatic urethra.

The periurethral mucosal (central zone) and submucosal (transition zone) prostate glands and cells of the stroma undergo **nodular hyperplasia** (see Figure 21-9) in older men.

Periurethral nodular hyperplasia produces:

1. Difficulty in urination and urinary obstruction caused by partial or complete compression of the prostatic urethra by the nodular growth.

2. Retention of urine in the bladder or inability to empty the urinary bladder completely. The possibility of infection leads to inflammation of the urinary bladder (**cystitis**) and urinary tract infection (**pyelonephritis**). Acute and persistent urinary retention requires emergency urethral catheterization.

BPH is attributed to **DHT**, a metabolite of testosterone. (Figure 21-11). DHT is converted in the prostate from circulating testosterone by the action of the enzyme SRD5A2 (steroid 5α-reductase type 2). This enzyme is localized predominantly in the stromal cells, the predominant androgen conversion site. The participation of DHT in determining periurethral nodular hyperplasia is supported by the clinical use of **finasteride**, an inhibitor of SRD5A that lowers DHT levels of the prostate, reduces prostate size and alleviates to a large extent BPH symptoms.

There are two Federal Drug Administration (FDA)-approved SRD5A inhibitors: **finasteride** in-

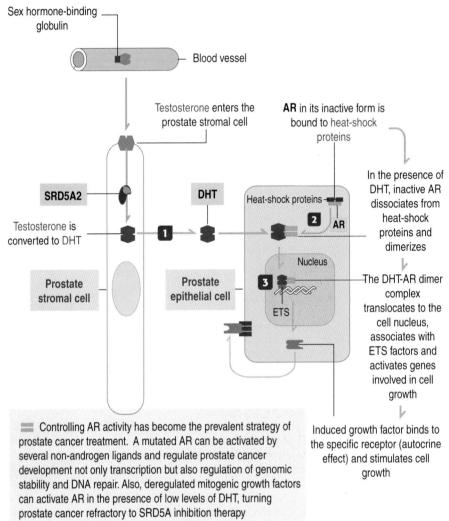

Figure 21-11. Stromal-prostate epithelial cell interaction

1 Because prostate stromal cells, but not prostate epithelial cells, contain steroid 5α-reductase 2 (SRD5A2), they are the main source of dihydrotestosterone (DHT) for neighboring prostate epithelial cells. DHT acts in a paracrine fashion on prostate epithelial cells. Prostate epithelial cells contain SRD5A3 that can also convert testosterone to DHT (not shown in the diagram).

Like prostate epithelial cells, prostate stromal cells can also produce growth factors with paracrine and autocrine effects (not shown).

2 Inactive androgen receptor (AR) in prostate epithelial cells is bound to heat-shock proteins (mainly HSP90). DHT binds to AR, that dimerizes after dissociation from HSPs.

3 The DHT-AR dimer complex translocates to the nucleus of the prostate epithelial cell, associates with other transcription factors, including ETS factors, binds to androgen-response elements on DNA and induces the production of mitogenic growth factors to stimulate cell survival and growth.

Therapy with inhibitors of SRD5A reduces the production of DHT, the synthesis of mitogenic growth factors, and decreases the size of the nodular hyperplasia and urinary obstruction.

Sex hormone-binding globulin

Blood vessel

Testosterone enters the prostate stromal cell

AR in its inactive form is bound to heat-shock proteins

SRD5A2

DHT

Heat-shock proteins

In the presence of DHT, inactive AR dissociates from heat-shock proteins and dimerizes

2 AR

Testosterone is converted to DHT

1

Nucleus

Prostate stromal cell

Prostate epithelial cell

3

ETS

The DHT-AR dimer complex translocates to the cell nucleus, associates with ETS factors and activates genes involved in cell growth

Controlling AR activity has become the prevalent strategy of prostate cancer treatment. A mutated AR can be activated by several non-androgen ligands and regulate prostate cancer development not only transcription but also regulation of genomic stability and DNA repair. Also, deregulated mitogenic growth factors can activate AR in the presence of low levels of DHT, turning prostate cancer refractory to SRD5A inhibition therapy (castration-resistant prostate cancer, CRPC).

Induced growth factor binds to the specific receptor (autocrine effect) and stimulates cell growth

hibits the SRD5A2 isoenzyme, leading to decreases in serum dihydrotestosterone levels by 70 to 90%, whereas **dutasteride** blocks SRD5A1 and SRD5A2 isoenzymes, reducing dihydrotestosterone to levels close to zero.

Rectal examination (palpation of the prostate through the rectum) may reveal a markedly enlarged prostate. **Transrectal ultrasonography** and determination of blood levels of **prostate specific antigen** (**PSA**) are indicated to rule out prostate cancer.

Pathology: Prostate cancer

The enzyme **SRD5A2**, present mainly in prostate **stromal cells**, converts testosterone to DHT. As discussed earlier in this chapter, a congenital lack of SRD5A2 results in a vestigial prostate gland. Castration in a man leads to atrophy of the prostate gland.

Testosterone and DHT bind to **androgen receptors**

(**ARs**). We have seen from AIS (androgen insensitivity syndrome) that the AR has an important role in the development of the prostate gland. In addition, AR activity plays an important role at different stages of prostate cancer.

In its inactive state, AR forms in the cytoplasm a complex with **heat shock proteins** (**HSPs**), including HSP90, when testosterone or DHT are not present (see Figure 21-11).

Upon binding of androgens, transported to the prostate gland by the bloodstream bound to **sex hormone-binding globulin** (**SHBG**), the AR detaches from HSPs, forms dimers that bind to the androgen and the androgen-AR dimer complex translocates to the nucleus.

In the nucleus, AR, regarded as a transcription factor, binds to DNA and to transcription factors, including ETS (for E26), to induce the expression of autocrine and paracrine survival and growth factors to prostate epithelial cells and prostate stromal cells.

Note that androgen binding triggers dimerization of AR and translocation to the nucleus. Therefore, **the major therapeutic objective is to prevent androgen binding to AR to block dimerization, nuclear translocation and eventual transcription of genes that depend on AR during prostate cancer development.**

In addition to the classical AR activation following androgen binding, additional changes take place during prostate cancer progression:

1. **Overexpression of AR** is able to increase the activity of cell cycle regulators that can turn cell proliferation refractory to androgen deprivation therapy (a clinical condition called **castration-resistant prostate cancer, CRPC**).

2. **Expression of AR splice variants** can lack an androgen-binding domain without affecting the recruitment of AR to DNA. This event can induce genomic reprogramming leading to the down regulation of repressors or maximizing the expression of AR co-regulators, including ETS transcription factors.

3. **Mutations that uphold AR activity** by conversion of antagonistic drug responses to agonist responses.

Prostate cancer originates from the main prostate glands of the peripheral zone, farthest from the urethra. Urinary symptoms are not present at the early stage and tumor growth is often detected by digital palpation of the prostate, by elevated serum levels of **PSA**, or by back pain caused by vertebral **metastasis**. Transperineal or transrectal **biopsy**, if required, confirm a clinical diagnosis.

Surgery (radical prostatectomy by retropubic or perineal surgery) and radiotherapy (external beam radiation therapy or radioactive seed implants in the prostate) are appropriate when the tumor is localized as determined by computer imaging techniques.

Male and female urethra

The urethra in the **male** is 20 cm long and, as already described, it has four segments: preprostatic urethra, prostatic urethra, membranous urethra and penile or spongy urethra (see Figure 21-8).

The penile urethra receives the excretory ducts of the bulbourethral gland (of Cowper; Figure 21-12) and the urethral glands (of Littré).

Urethral glands produce a glycosaminoglycan-containing secretion that protects and lubricates the surface of the urethral epithelium.

The epithelium of the prostate urethra is **transitional (urothelium)**. It changes to a pseudostratified-to-stratified columnar epithelium in the membranous and penile urethra. The **muscle layer** in the membranous urethra consists of a smooth muscle sphincter (involuntary) and a striated muscle sphincter (voluntary). It controls the passage of urine or semen.

The urethra in the **female** is 4 cm long and is lined by **transitional epithelium** changing to pseudostratified columnar and stratified squamous nonkeratinized epithelium near the urethral meatus.

The mucosa contains mucus-secreting glands (see Figure 21-12). An inner layer of smooth muscle is surrounded by a circular layer of striated muscle that closes the urethra when contracted.

Bulbourethral glands

The bulbourethral glands consist of several lobules containing tubuloalveolar secretory units and a main excretory duct lined by a stratified columnar epithelium.

The lining epithelium of the secretory units is columnar and secretes a mucus product. The secretion, containing abundant **galactose** and a moderate amount of **sialic acid**, is discharged into the **penile urethra**. This secretion has a **lubrication function** and precedes the emission of semen along the penile urethra (see Figure 21-8).

Penis

The penis consists of three cylindrical columnar masses of **erectile tissue** (see Figure 21-12): the right and left **corpora cavernosa**, and the ventral **corpus spongiosum**, transversed by the penile urethra. The three columns converge to form the shaft of the penis. The distal tip of the corpus spongiosum is the **glans penis**.

The corpora cavernosa and corpus spongiosum contain irregular and communicating blood spaces, or sinusoids, supplied by an artery and drained by venous channels. During erection, arterial blood fills the sinusoids, which enlarge and compress the draining venous channels (Figure 21-13).

Two chemicals control erection:

1. **Nitric oxide.**

2. **Phosphodiesterase** (see Figure 21-13).

Sexual stimulation, via the cerebral cortex and hypothalamus and transported down the spinal cord to autonomic nerves in the penis, causes the branches of the **dorsal nerve**, the end point of the pudendal nerve, to produce **nitric oxide**.

Nitric oxide molecules spread rapidly across **gap junctions** of **smooth muscle cells** surrounding the blood sinusoids.

Within smooth muscle cells, nitric oxide molecules activate **guanylyl cyclase** to produce **cyclic guanosine monophosphate (cGMP)** from **guanosine triphosphate (GTP)**.

cGMP **relaxes the smooth muscle cell wall** surrounding the sinusoids by inducing the **sequestration of Ca^{2+}** within intracellular storage sites. The lowered concentrations of Ca^{2+} determine the relaxation of

Figure 21-12. **Female and male urethra**

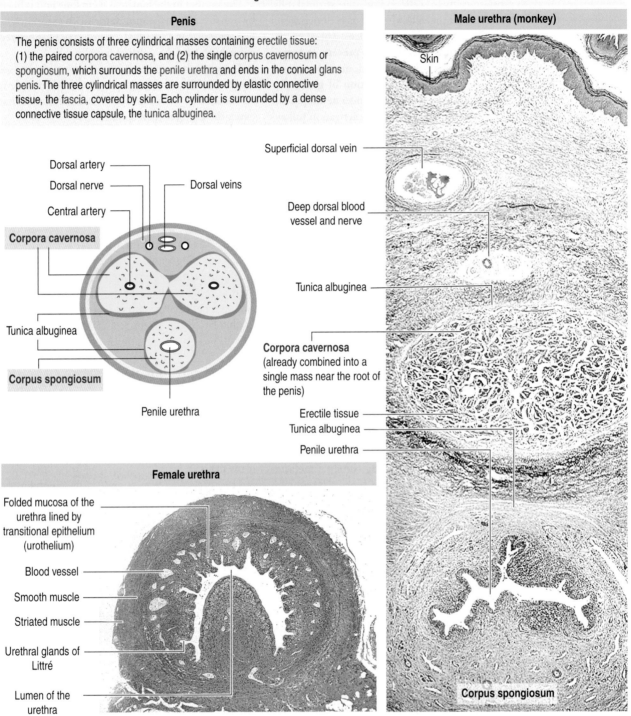

Penis

The penis consists of three cylindrical masses containing erectile tissue: (1) the paired corpora cavernosa, and (2) the single corpus cavernosum or spongiosum, which surrounds the penile urethra and ends in the conical glans penis. The three cylindrical masses are surrounded by elastic connective tissue, the fascia, covered by skin. Each cylinder is surrounded by a dense connective tissue capsule, the tunica albuginea.

Dorsal artery
Dorsal nerve
Central artery
Dorsal veins
Corpora cavernosa
Tunica albuginea
Corpus spongiosum
Penile urethra

Male urethra (monkey)

Skin
Superficial dorsal vein
Deep dorsal blood vessel and nerve
Tunica albuginea
Corpora cavernosa (already combined into a single mass near the root of the penis)
Erectile tissue
Tunica albuginea
Penile urethra
Corpus spongiosum

Female urethra

Folded mucosa of the urethra lined by transitional epithelium (urothelium)
Blood vessel
Smooth muscle
Striated muscle
Urethral glands of Littré
Lumen of the urethra

smooth muscle cells, which leads to the accumulation of blood in the sinusoids by the rapid flow of arterial blood from the dorsal and cavernous arteries (see Figure 21-13). Sinusoids engorged with blood compress the small veins that drain blood from the penis and the penis becomes erect.

The enzyme **phosphodiesterase** (PDE) is produced to destroy cGMP and terminate erection. By blocking PDE activity, cGMP levels remain elevated and the penis remains erect.

Clinical significance: Erectile dysfunction
Factors that affect the cerebral cortex–hypothalamus–spinal cord–autonomic nerve pathway and vascular diseases can cause erectile dysfunction. Traumatic head and spinal cord injuries, stroke, Parkinson's disease, and systemic diseases, such as diabetes and multiple sclerosis, reduce nerve function and lead to erectile dysfunction. In addition, anxiety disorders can be a primary cause of erectile dysfunction.

Sildenafil (Viagra) was originally tested as a treat-

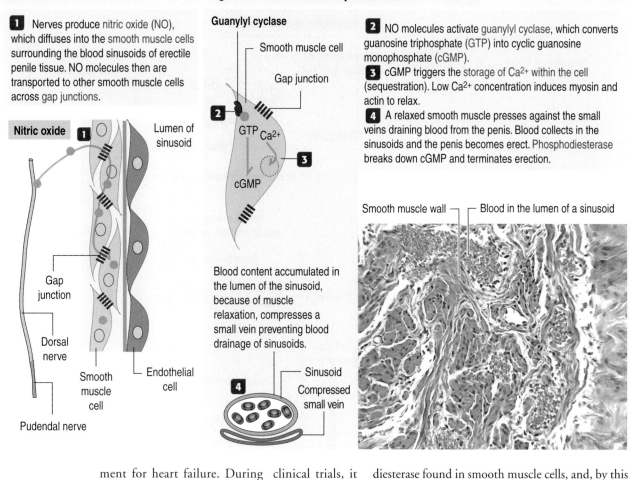

Figure 21-13. Mechanism of penile erection

1 Nerves produce nitric oxide (NO), which diffuses into the smooth muscle cells surrounding the blood sinusoids of erectile penile tissue. NO molecules then are transported to other smooth muscle cells across gap junctions.

Nitric oxide **1**

Lumen of sinusoid

Gap junction

Dorsal nerve

Smooth muscle cell

Endothelial cell

Pudendal nerve

Guanylyl cyclase

Smooth muscle cell

Gap junction

2

GTP Ca^{2+}

cGMP

3

Blood content accumulated in the lumen of the sinusoid, because of muscle relaxation, compresses a small vein preventing blood drainage of sinusoids.

4

Sinusoid

Compressed small vein

2 NO molecules activate guanylyl cyclase, which converts guanosine triphosphate (GTP) into cyclic guanosine monophosphate (cGMP).

3 cGMP triggers the storage of Ca^{2+} within the cell (sequestration). Low Ca^{2+} concentration induces myosin and actin to relax.

4 A relaxed smooth muscle presses against the small veins draining blood from the penis. Blood collects in the sinusoids and the penis becomes erect. Phosphodiesterase breaks down cGMP and terminates erection.

Smooth muscle wall — Blood in the lumen of a sinusoid

ment for heart failure. During clinical trials, it was noticed that a significant number of patients were getting erections after taking the drug. This observation initiated an independent clinical study to evaluate the effect of sildenafil in the treatment of erectile dysfunction.

In the penis, sildenafil blocks a specific phospho-diesterase found in smooth muscle cells, and, by this mechanism, inhibits the degradation of cGMP. High levels of cGMP induce Ca^{2+} to enter storage areas in the cell and induce the perisinusoidal smooth muscle cells to relax. Sildenafil can cause dose-dependent side effects such as facial flushing, gastrointestinal distress, headaches, and a blue tinge to vision.

Essential concepts | **Sperm Transport and Maturation**

• Primordial germinal cells (PGCs) have an extra-embryonic origin.

Precursors of the male and female gametes migrate from the primary ectoderm into the wall of the yolk sac and become extra-embryonic. They appear first in the wall of the yolk sac in the 4-week embryo.

Bone morphogenetic protein and signals from the extraembryonic mesoderm and visceral endoderm specify pluripotent epiblast cells to become PGCs.

BLIMP1 (B lymphocyte-induced maturation protein 1) stimulates the expression of the PGC–specific gene *Stella*. Stella represses transcription of genes specific to somatic cells.

Between 4 and 6 weeks, PGCs migrate to the gonadal ridges by translocation from the yolk sac to the hindgut.

The initiation of PGC migration is regulated by the cell surface protein IFITM1 (interferon-induced transmembrane protein 1).

Migration from the hindgut to the gonadal ridges across the mesentery is guided by:

(1) SDF1 (stromal-derived factor 1), expressed at the gonadal ridges and in the surrounding mesenchyme.

(2) The chemokine CXCR4, expressed by PGCs.

There are at least three additional factors that participate in the migration of PGCs:

(1) The rate of migration and proliferation of PGCs are dependent on the interaction of the c-kit receptor, a tyrosine kinase, with its corresponding cell membrane ligand, stem cell factor (or c-kit ligand).

(2) E-cadherin, expressed by PGCs.

(3) PGCs express β$_1$ integrin, required for entry to the gonadal ridges.

PGCs that do not reach the gonadal ridges undergo apoptosis. PGCs that avoid apoptosis can later give rise to extragonadal germ cell tumors.

PGCs reach the gonadal ridges by the 6th week and continue their proliferation as they interact with somatic cells to develop the indifferent gonads.

In the gonadal ridges, XX chromosome-containing PGCs occupy the cortex, and XY chromosome-containing PGCs localize in the medulla, the central portion of the gonadal ridges.

After 7 weeks, the indifferent gonad contains a cortex, which develops into an ovary, and a

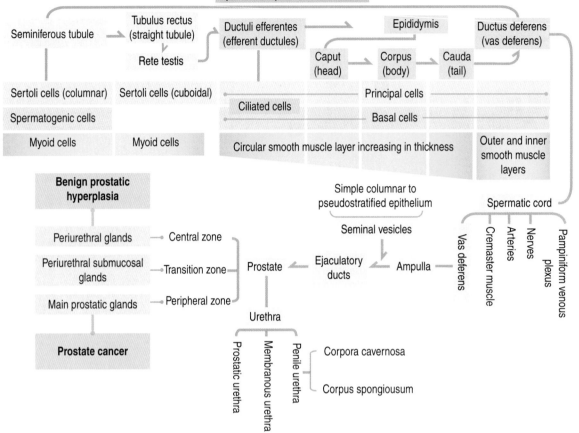

Sperm transport and maturation

Seminiferous tubule → Tubulus rectus (straight tubule) → Ductuli efferentes (efferent ductules) → Epididymis → Ductus deferens (vas deferens)

Rete testis

Caput (head) → Corpus (body) → Cauda (tail)

Sertoli cells (columnar) — Sertoli cells (cuboidal) — Principal cells

Ciliated cells — Basal cells

Spermatogenic cells

Myoid cells — Myoid cells — Circular smooth muscle layer increasing in thickness — Outer and inner smooth muscle layers

Benign prostatic hyperplasia

Periurethral glands → Central zone

Simple columnar to pseudostratified epithelium

Seminal vesicles

Spermatic cord

Periurethral submucosal glands → Transition zone → Prostate ← Ejaculatory ducts ← Ampulla ← Vas deferens / Cremaster muscle / Arteries / Nerves / Pampiniform venous plexus

Main prostatic glands → Peripheral zone

Prostate cancer

Urethra — Prostatic urethra / Membranous urethra / Penile urethra — Corpora cavernosa / Corpus spongiousum

---

medulla, which develops into a testis.

The development of the testis is controlled by testis-determining factor, a product of a gene on the sex-determining region of the Y chromosome (*SRY*).

The initial components of the fetal testis are the testicular cords. A testicular cord contains Sertoli cells and spermatogonial stem cells (SSCs) derived from PGCs. Leydig cells are present between the testicular cords.

Fetal Sertoli cells secrete anti-müllerian hormone (AMH), which induces regression by apoptosis of the müllerian duct (paramesonephric duct).

Leydig cells, stimulated by human chorionic gonadotropin, secrete testosterone. Testosterone is converted to dihydrotestosterone (DHT) by the enzyme steroid 5α-reductase 2 (SRD5A2).

Testosterone stimulates the wolffian duct (mesonephric duct) to develop the epididymis, vas deferens, and seminal vesicle.

DHT stimulates the development of the prostate gland and urethra from the urogenital sinus. Testosterone and DHT bind to androgen receptor, encoded by a gene on the X chromosome.

Klinefelter's syndrome (47,XXY) is observed in males with an extra X chromosome. Individuals are phenotypically males, have atrophic testes, and the blood levels of testosterone are low but the levels of estradiol are high. Excess of estradiol causes gynecomastia.

Androgen insensitivity syndrome (AIS, also called testicular feminization) is determined by a complete or partial defect in the expression of androgen receptor. A lack of development of the wolffian duct and regression of the müllerian duct are observed. Testes remain in the abdomen, and external genitalia develop as female. Blood levels of androgens and estradiol are high.

Three phenotypes are observed:

(1) Complete androgen insensitivity syndrome (CAIS) with female external genitalia. The testes remain in the abdomen. They may be removed after puberty (until feminization is complete) because of the risk of testicular cancer.

(2) Partial androgen insensitivity syndrome (PAIS, Reifenstein syndrome) with predominantly female or male, or ambiguous genitalia.

(3) Mild androgen insensitivity syndrome (MAIS) with male external genitalia. Spermatogenesis and/or pubertal virilization may be impaired.

Steroid SRD5A2 deficiency determines a decrease in the conversion of testosterone to DHT. Individuals with mutations of the *SRD5A2* gene are genetically males.

Affected individuals have normal internal genitalia (whose development from the wolffian duct is androgen-dependent) but nonmasculin-ized external genitalia (whose development is DHT-dependent).

• **Sperm maturation pathway.** After leaving the seminiferous tubule, immature sperm follow this sequential pathway:

(1) Tubuli recti (straight tubules): Narrow tubular structures lined by a simple cuboidal epithelium with microvilli and a single cilium. Tight junctions occupy an apical position, in contrast to the basally located inter–Sertoli cell tight junctions.

(2) Rete testis: A network of anastomosing channels lined by simple cuboidal epithelium. The wall consists of myoid cells and fibroblasts.

(3) Ductuli efferentes (efferent ductules): They connect the rete testis to the initial region of the epididymal duct. The epithelial lining consists of principal cells with microvilli (instead of stereocilia) and ciliated cells, involved in the transport of nonmotile sperm toward the epididymis. Clusters of these two cell types, differing in height, give the epithelium a characteristic scalloped outline.

(4) Epididymis: A highly coiled duct (about 6 meters long) with three typical anatomic regions: Head or caput, body or corpus, and tail or cauda. The lining epithelium is pseudostratified columnar with stereocilia/stereovilli. The wall contains smooth muscle cells. The two major epithelial cell types are

the columnar principal cells with apical stereo-cilia/stereovilli, and basal cells, associated with the basal lamina. Intraepithelial lymphocytes are frequently seen. The height of the principal cells decreases towards the tail region. Consequently, the lumen becomes progressively wider. The thickness of the muscle wall increases toward the epididymal tail region.

(5) Vas deferens (ductus deferens): A muscular tube with a length of 45 cm. It can be seen in the spermatic cord. The vas deferens is lined by pseudostratified columnar epithelium with stereocilia/stereovilli. The smooth muscle cell layer consists of a middle circular layer surrounded by inner and outer longitudinal layers.

Additional components of the spermatic cord include the cremaster muscle, arteries (spermatic, cremasteric, and vas deferens arteries), veins of the pampiniform plexus (important for spermatic artery—pampiniform plexus heat transfer to maintain testicular temperature 2°C to 3°C below body temperature for normal spermatogenesis), and nerves.

The vas deferens ends in a dilated ampulla receiving the duct of the seminal vesicle to form the ejaculatory duct passing through the prostate gland.

• **Accessory genital glands.** The accessory glands of the male reproductive system are the seminal vesicles, the prostate gland, and the bulbourethral glands of Cowper.

Each seminal vesicle has three components:
(1) An external connective tissue capsule.
(2) A middle smooth muscle layer.
(3) An internal highly folded mucosa lined by a simple cuboidal-to-pseudostratified columnar epithelium supported by a lamina propria.

Under the influence of androgens, the seminal vesicle epithelium contributes 70% to 85% of an alkaline fluid to the human ejaculate. The fluid contains seminal coagulating proteins, fructose, and prostaglandins.

The **prostate gland** is a branched (compound) tubuloalveolar gland. It consists of three zones:
(1) **Central zone**, with periurethral mucosal glands.
(2) **Transition zone**, with periurethral submucosal glands.

(3) **Peripheral zone**, with branched tubuloalveolar glands, called main glands. Glands are lined by simple or pseudostratified columnar epithelium. The lumen contains corpora amylacea, rich in glycoproteins.

The alkaline fluid produced by the prostate gland contains acid phosphatase and prostate-specific antigen (PSA).

A combined enlargement of the periurethral mucosal and submucosal glands and surrounding stroma accounts for **benign prostate hyperplasia (BPH)**. BPH is determined by growth factors with mitogenic action produced by both stromal and glandular epithelial cells stimulated by DHT. Testosterone is converted to DHT by the enzyme SRD5A2, present mainly in prostate stromal cells.

Periurethral nodular hyperplasia produces:
(1) Difficulty in urination and urinary obstruction caused by partial or complete compression of the prostatic urethra by the nodular growth.
(2) Retention of urine in the bladder or inability to empty the urinary bladder completely. The possibility of infection leads to inflammation of the urinary bladder (cystitis) and urinary tract infection (pyelonephritis).

Blocking agents of SRD5A2 activity and antiandrogens are used in the nonsurgical treatment of BPH.

Cancer of the prostate is the result of the malignant transformation of the prostate glands of the peripheral zone. Blood levels of PSA are elevated in patients with prostate cancer.

Let us review how androgens work in the prostate:
(1) Testosterone and DHT bind to androgen receptors (ARs).
(2) In its inactive state, AR forms in the cytoplasm a complex with heat shock proteins (HSPs) when testosterone or DHT are not present.
(3) Upon binding of androgens, transported by the bloodstream bound to sex hormone-binding globulin (SHBG), the AR detaches from HSPs, forms dimers that bind to androgen, and the androgen-AR dimer complex translocates to the nucleus.
(4) In the nucleus, AR, regarded as a transcription factor, binds to DNA and to transcription factors to induce the expression of auto-

crine and paracrine growth factors to prostate epithelial cells and prostate stromal cells.

Bulbourethral glands secrete a lubricating mucus product into the penile urethra.

• **Male and female urethra.** The male urethra has a length of 20 cm and consists of three segments:
(1) The prostatic urethra, whose lumen receives fluid transported by the ejaculatory ducts and products from the prostatic glands.
(2) The membranous urethra.
(3) The penile urethra, which receives a lubricating fluid from the bulbourethral glands.

The epithelium of the prostatic urethra is transitional (urothelium) with regional variations. Smooth muscle and striated muscle sphincters are present in the membranous urethra.

The female urethra is shorter (4 cm long) and is lined by transitional epithelium, also with regional variations. The mucosa contains mucus-secreting glands. Inner smooth and outer striated muscle cell layers are observed.

• **Penis.** The penis consists of three cylindrical structures of erectile tissue: a pair of corpora cavernosa and a single corpus spongiosum. The three cylindrical structures converge to form the shaft of the penis. The tip of the corpus spongiosum is the glans penis. The erectile tissue contains vascular spaces, called sinusoids, supplied by arterial blood and drained by venous channels. During erection, arterial blood fills the sinusoids, which compress the adjacent venous channels preventing draining. Nitric oxide, produced by branches of the dorsal nerve, spreads across gap junctions between smooth muscle cells surrounding the sinusoids. Within smooth muscle cells, nitric oxide activates guanylyl cyclase to produce cyclic guanosine monophosphate (cGMP) from guanosine triphosphate (GTP). cGMP relaxes the smooth muscle by sequestering calcium into intracellular storage sites, and arterial blood accumulates in the distended sinusoids and the penis becomes erect. The enzyme phosphodiesterase degrades cGMP, thus terminating erection. Sildenafil, a phosphodiesterase inhibitor, is used to prevent rapid cGMP degradation in cases of **erectile dysfunction.**

22. Follicle Development and The Menstrual Cycle

The menstrual cycle represents the reproductive status of a female. It starts with menarche at puberty and ends with menopause about 40 years later. There are two coexisting events during the menstrual cycle: the ovarian cycle and the uterine cycle. During the ovarian cycle, several ovarian follicles, each housing a primary oocyte, undergo a growing process (folliculogenesis) in preparation for ovulation into the oviducts or fallopian tubes. During the concurrent uterine cycle, the endometrium, the lining of the uterus, is preparing for embryo implantation. If fertilization of the ovulated egg does not take place, the endometrium is shed, menstruation occurs and a new menstrual cycle starts. This chapter is focused on structural and functional aspects of the ovarian and uterine cycle, including specific hormonal disorders and pathologic conditions of the uterine cervix.

Development of the female reproductive tract

The reproductive tract develops through the differentiation of wolffian ducts (male reproductive tract anlage) and müllerian ducts (female reproductive tract anlage). The female reproductive system consists of the **ovaries**, the **ducts** (**oviduct, uterus,** and **vagina**), and the **external genitalia** (**labia majora, labia minora,** and **clitoris**).

Knowledge of the developmental sequence from the **indifferent stage** to the fully developed stage is helpful in understanding the structural anomalies that can be clinically observed. The molecular aspects of the development of the ovary, female genital ducts, and external genitalia are summarized in the next sections.

Development of the ovary

The differentiation of a testis or an ovary from the indifferent gonad is a complex developmental process involving various genes and hormones.

Wnt4 is a major player in the ovarian-determination pathway and sexual differentiation. Wnt4 is a member of the **Wingless** (**Wnt**) family of proteins (see Chapter 3, Cell Signaling).

The **testis-determining factor** (**TDF**), encoded by the gene *SRY*, on the sex-determining region of the Y chromosome, and the *Sox9* (for sex determining region Y-box 9) gene are responsible for the development of the indifferent gonads into testes. As previously indicated, Sox9 participates in the development of the skeleton (see Chondrogenesis in Chapter 4, Connective Tissue).

As discussed in Chapter 21, Sperm Transport and Maturation, the **cortical region** of the primitive gonad develops into an ovary. The cortical region of the **indifferent gonad** initially contains the **primary sex cords** (fifth week of development).

One week later, cells of the primary cell cords degenerate and are replaced by **secondary sex cords** that surround individual **oogonia** (Figure 22-1).

Oogonia result from the mitotic division of mi-

grating **primordial germinal cells** derived from the yolk sac. Primordial germinal cells contain two X chromosomes.

In the fetal ovary, oogonia enter meiotic prophase I to become **primary oocytes.** Primary oocytes are arrested after completion of crossing over (exchange of genetic information between nonsister chromatids of homologous chromosomes). **Meiotic prophase arrest continues until puberty,** when one or more ovarian follicles are recruited to initiate their development.

Development of the female genital ducts

During development, the **cranial ends of the müllerian ducts** (paramesonephric ducts) remain separated to form the **oviducts.** The oviducts open into the coelomic cavity (the future peritoneal cavity). The **caudal segments of the müllerian ducts** (mesonephric ducts) fuse to develop into the **uterovaginal primordium** that becomes the **uterus** and **upper part of the vagina.** The **broad ligaments** of the uterus, derived from two peritoneal folds, approach each other when the müllerian ducts fuse.

The **primitive cloaca** is divided by the **urorectal septum** into two regions:

1. The **ventral urogenital sinus.**
2. The **dorsal anorectal canal.**

The urorectal septum fuses with the cloacal membrane (the future site of the perineal body), which is divided into the **dorsal anal membrane** and the larger **ventral urogenital membrane.** By week 7, the membranes rupture.

The contact of the uterovaginal primordium with the urogenital sinus results in the formation of the **vaginal plate.** The **canalization of the vaginal plate** results in the development of the middle and lower portions of the vagina:

1. The solid mass of cells of the vaginal plate extends from the urogenital sinus into the uterovaginal primordium.

2. The central cells of the vaginal plate disappear, forming the lumen of the vagina.

Figure 22-1. From the indifferent gonad to the ovary and testis

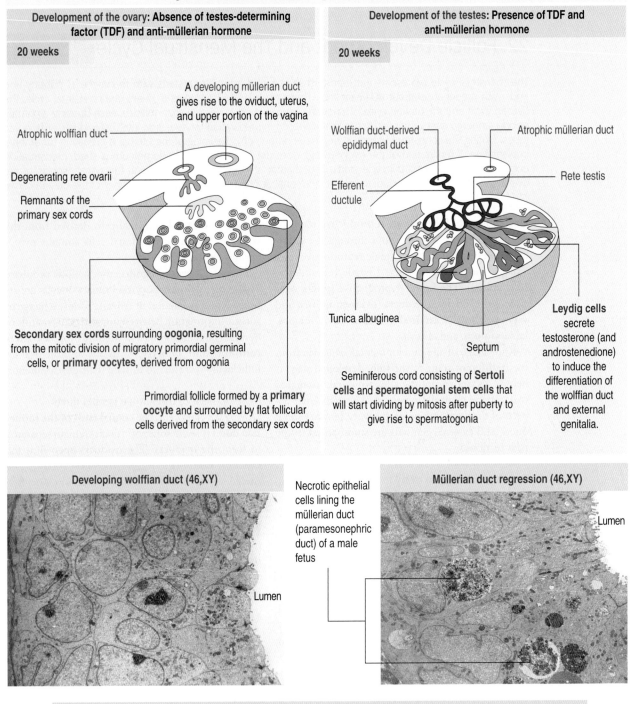

Development of the ovary: Absence of testes-determining factor (TDF) and anti-müllerian hormone

20 weeks

Atrophic wolffian duct

A developing müllerian duct gives rise to the oviduct, uterus, and upper portion of the vagina

Degenerating rete ovarii

Remnants of the primary sex cords

Secondary sex cords surrounding **oogonia**, resulting from the mitotic division of migratory primordial germinal cells, or **primary oocytes**, derived from oogonia

Primordial follicle formed by a **primary oocyte** and surrounded by flat follicular cells derived from the secondary sex cords

Development of the testes: Presence of TDF and anti-müllerian hormone

20 weeks

Wolffian duct-derived epididymal duct

Atrophic müllerian duct

Efferent ductule

Rete testis

Tunica albuginea

Septum

Seminiferous cord consisting of **Sertoli cells** and **spermatogonial stem cells** that will start dividing by mitosis after puberty to give rise to spermatogonia

Leydig cells secrete testosterone (and androstenedione) to induce the differentiation of the wolffian duct and external genitalia.

Developing wolffian duct (46,XY)

Lumen

Necrotic epithelial cells lining the müllerian duct (paramesonephric duct) of a male fetus

Müllerian duct regression (46,XY)

Lumen

Persistent müllerian duct syndrome

In the **female**, the müllerian ducts (paramesonephric ducts) develop into the oviducts, uterus and cervix and the upper two-third of the vagina. The wolffian ducts (mesonephric ducts) degenerate in the absence of androgens.

In the **male**, the müllerian ducts undergo regression in presence of **anti-müllerian hormone (AMH)**, a member of the **transforming growth factor-β family** produced by Sertoli cells in the testes. AMH regressive actions on the epithelial lining of the müllerian duct are indirect; they are mediated by binding of AMH to AMH receptor 2 (AMHR2) on the surrounding mesenchymal cells.

Persistent müllerian duct syndrome (PMDS) in human males is associated with **cryptorchidism** (undescended testis) or **ectopic testis** accompanied by **inguinal hernia**. Gene mutations of AMH and AMHR2 are found in individuals with PDMS (displaying oviducts, uterus and cervix in addition to male external genitalia).

3. The peripheral cells persist and form the vaginal epithelium.

The urogenital sinus also gives rise to the urinary bladder, urethra, vestibular glands, and hymen.

Development of the external genitalia

By week 4, the **genital tubercle**, or **phallus**, develops at the cranial end of the **cloacal membrane**. Then, **labioscrotal swellings** and **urogenital folds** develop at either side of the cloacal membrane.

The genital tubercle enlarges in both the female and male. In the absence of androgens, the external genitalia are feminized: the **phallus** develops into the **clitoris**. The **urogenital folds** form the **labia minora**, and the **labioscrotal swellings** develop into the **labia majora**.

Clinical significance: Developmental anomalies of the müllerian duct

Failure of müllerian development occurs in 46,XX female patients with **müllerian agenesis (Mayer–Rokitansky–Küster–Hauser syndrome)**. Müllerian agenesis is characterized by the absence of the uterus, cervix, and upper vagina. Kidney abnormalities, including a pelvic kidney or the more severe unilateral agenesis of the kidney, are observed.

Inactivation of the *Wnt4* gene has been implicated in this disorder. Wnt4 is secreted by the müllerian-duct epithelium. WNT4 suppresses the synthesis of gonadal androgen in females by antagonizing the **nuclear-receptor steroid factor 1 (SF-1)**, thereby inhibiting steroidogenic enzymes.

Persistent müllerian duct syndrome (PMDS) occurs in 46,XY males as a rare form of male pseudohermaphroditism. It is caused by a defect in either the *AMH* gene or its receptor (AMHR2). Patients with this syndrome retain müllerian ducts and have unilateral or bilateral undescended testes. See Figure 22-1 concerning the **PMDS** in human males.

Clinical significance: Turner's syndrome

The central genetic defect recognized in prepubertal and pubertal girls with **Turner's syndrome** is the absence of all or part of a second X chromosome **(45,X)** and **a lack of Barr bodies**.

The prenatal diagnosis of Turner's syndrome is based on the finding of fetal edema on ultrasonography, abnormal levels of human chorionic gonadotropin, and α-fetoprotein during the screening of maternal serum. A 45,X fetus often aborts spontaneously.

Physical findings include **congenital lymphedema**, **short stature**, and **gonadal dysgenesis**. The ovaries are represented by **streaks**. **Puffy hands** and **feet** or **redundant nuchal skin** are characteristic clinical findings.

Gonadal dysgenesis is a typical feature of Turner's syndrome. Ovarian failure is characterized by decreased or absent production of estrogens in association with elevated levels of gonadotropins, resulting in a failure to establish secondary sexual development (because of a lack of estrogens).

Patients require hormone-replacement therapy to initiate puberty and complete growth. Recombinant growth hormone administration is recommended when there is evidence of growth failure. Hormone replacement therapy (estrogen and progesterone) compensates for ovarian atrophy.

The ovaries

Each ovary is lined by a **simple squamous-to-low cuboidal epithelium** (called **ovarian surface epithelium**, see Box 22-A) and a subjacent connective tissue layer, the **tunica albuginea**.

A **cortex** and a **medulla** without distinct demarcation can be visualized in a cross section. The broad cortex contains connective tissue and **primordial follicles** housing **primary oocytes** (at the end of meiotic prophase I). The **medulla** consists of connective tissue, interstitial cells, nerves, lymphatics, and blood vessels reaching the ovary through the **hilum** (Figure 22-2).

The functions of the ovary are:
1. The production of the female gamete.
2. The secretion of estrogens and progesterone.
3. The regulation of postnatal growth of reproductive organs.
4. The development of secondary sexual characteristics.

The ovarian cycle

The three phases of the ovarian cycle are:
1. The **follicular phase (folliculogenesis)**.
2. The **ovulatory phase**.
3. The **luteal phase**.

The **follicular phase** consists of the sequential development of several primordial follicles (Figures 22-3 and 22-4):
1. Primary **(unilayered) follicle**.
2. Secondary **(multilayered) follicle**.
3. **Preantral follicle**.
4. **Antral follicle**.

Box 22-A | Lgr5⁺ stem cells in the ovarian surface epithelium

- The **ovarian surface epithelium (OSE)** has **Lgr5⁺** (for leucine-rich repeat-containing G-protein coupled receptor 5) stem cells that repair the damage caused to the ovarian surface cell lining after each ovulation. Lgr5 is a marker of stem cells in many organs, including the crypts of Lieberkühn as we discuss in Chapter 16, Lower Digestive Segment.
- In the fetal ovary, cells of the **OSE are the progenitor cells of granulosa cells** and **stromal cells** that constitute the growing ovarian follicles after birth. This function persists in the OSE and hilum of the adult ovary and fimbria of the oviduct.
- The observation of Lgr5⁺ cells on the OSE, ovarian hilum, and fimbria of the oviduct has been associated to the development of serous ovarian carcinomas that spread to the entire ovary and metastasize extensively.

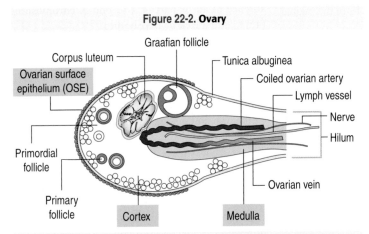

Figure 22-2. Ovary

Graafian follicle

Corpus luteum

Ovarian surface epithelium (OSE)

Tunica albuginea

Coiled ovarian artery

Lymph vessel

Nerve

Hilum

Primordial follicle

Primary follicle

Ovarian vein

Cortex

Medulla

The ovary is covered by the **ovarian surface epithelium** (simple cuboidal-to-squamous epithelium) and consists of an outer **cortex** and a central **medulla**. The medulla contains connective tissue supporting large blood vessels (a **coiled and tortuous ovarian artery** and vein), lymph vessels, and nerves. The cortex displays clusters of **primordial follicles**. The **tunica albuginea**, a thin layer of connective tissue, is observed at the periphery of the cortex.

5. Preovulatory follicle (Graffian follicle).

The following structural changes occur during the development of the ovarian follicles:

• **Primordial follicles.** Several primordial follicles, about 25 μm in diameter, each surrounded by **simple squamous layer** of granulosa cells (see Figure 22-3) are recruited to initiate the process of folliculogenesis.

• **Primary (unilayered) follicles.** Primordial follicles become primary follicles when the single layer of squamous granulosa cells changes into **simple cuboidal layer** of granulosa cells. A basal lamina separates the granulosa cells from the stroma of the ovary. At the same time, the **zona pellucida** initiates its assembly, separating gradually the primary oocyte from the granulosa cells.

• **Secondary (multilayered) follicles.** Granulosa cells proliferate into a **stratified cuboidal epithelium**. A cellular shell or **theca** (*theca folliculi*; Greek *theke*, box) surrounds the follicle. The theca begins to organize two distinct layers:

1. The **theca interna**, a vascularized cell layer adjacent to the basal lamina supporting the granulosa cells of the follicle.

2. The **theca externa**, a fibrous cellular layer continuous with the ovarian stroma.

• **Preantral follicles.** Small intercellular spaces, named **Call-Exner bodies**, develop between the granulosa cells. These spaces contain **follicular fluid** (liquor folliculi). Follicular fluid derives from the blood vessels of the theca interna, reaching the antrum by an osmotic gradient.

• **Antral follicle.** The Call-Exner bodies coalesce into a single space called **antrum** (see Figure 22-4). At this stage, granulosa cells, stimulated by FSH, actively synthesize and secrete estrogen.

• **Preovulatory follicle (Graffian follicle).** The antrum reaches its maximum size. The fluid of the antrum segregates the granulosa cells into three specific regions:

1. The **cumulus oophorous**, a cluster of granulosa cells anchoring the primary oocyte to the wall of the follicle (see Figure 22-4). The cumulus prevents the primary oocyte-from floating freely in the antrum fluid. It is also the nutrient delivery channel to the primary oocyte.

2. The **mural granulosa cells**, lining the wall of the follicle (see Figure 22-4).

3. The **corona radiata**, the layer of granulosa cells firmly anchored to the zona pellucida by zona–penetrating cellular processes (see Figure 22-4).

A preovulatory or graafian follicle reaches about **20 mm** in diameter, as compared to the **25 μm** in diameter of a primordial follicle.

The **theca externa** forms a connective tissue capsule-like layer, continuous with the ovarian stroma. In contrast, the **theca interna** is a well-vascularized cell layer adjacent to the basal lamina of the follicle. It consists of elongated cells with small lipid droplets in the cytoplasm acquiring the characteristics of steroid-secreting cells.

In summary, folliculogenesis occurs around a centrally located primary oocyte arrested at the end of meiotic prophase.

It involves a progressive increase in the population of estrogen-producing granulosa cells, the assembly of a thick glycoprotein-containing zona pellucida coat, and the development of the vascularized steroid-producing theca interna.

A basal lamina separates theca cells from granulosa cells. The zona pellucida separates the primary oocyte from the granulosa cells.

Upon the formation of the antrum, granulosa cells become segregated into two cell populations:

1. The clustered granulosa cells, surrounding the zona pellucida–encased primary oocyte. The clustered granulosa cells secrete a hyaluronic acid–rich product that enables the capture of the ovulated ovum in the fallopian tube.

2. The mural granulosa cells, lining the outer perimeter of the follicle. The mural cells are in close proximity to cells of the theca interna. As discussed later, this relationship is largely responsible for the production of steroid hormones.

Paracrine signaling and cell-cell communication during folliculogenesis

Two forms of paracrine cell-cell interaction take place during folliculogenesis (Figure 22-5):

1. **Granulosa cell–primary oocyte bidirectional signaling.**

2. **Theca interna–granulosa cell synergistic communication.**

Figure 22-3. From primordial to primary follicle

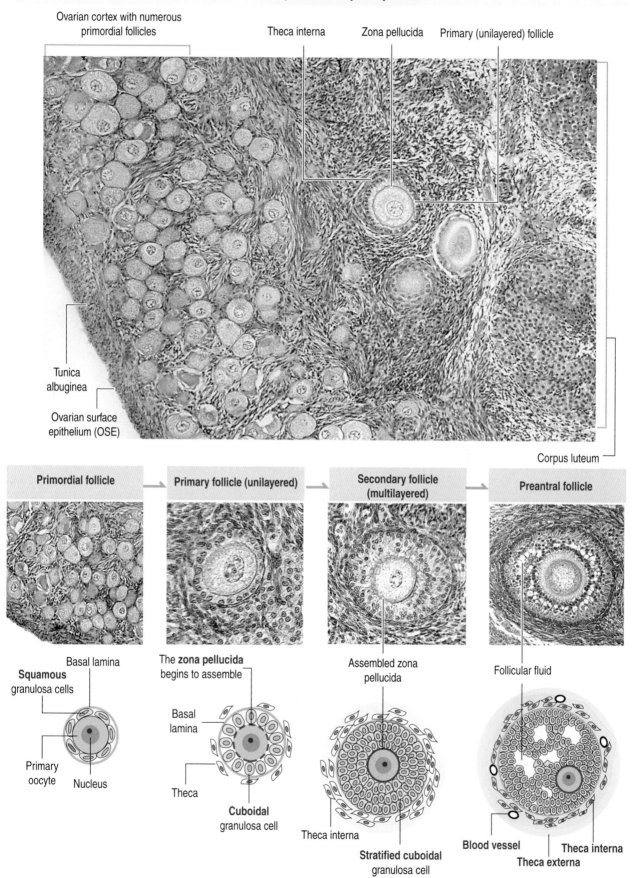

Ovarian cortex with numerous primordial follicles

Theca interna

Zona pellucida

Primary (unilayered) follicle

Tunica albuginea

Ovarian surface epithelium (OSE)

Corpus luteum

| Primordial follicle | Primary follicle (unilayered) | Secondary follicle (multilayered) | Preantral follicle |

Primordial follicle

Basal lamina

Squamous granulosa cells

Primary oocyte

Nucleus

Primary follicle (unilayered)

The **zona pellucida** begins to assemble

Basal lamina

Theca

Cuboidal granulosa cell

Secondary follicle (multilayered)

Assembled zona pellucida

Theca interna

Stratified cuboidal granulosa cell

Preantral follicle

Follicular fluid

Blood vessel

Theca interna

Theca externa

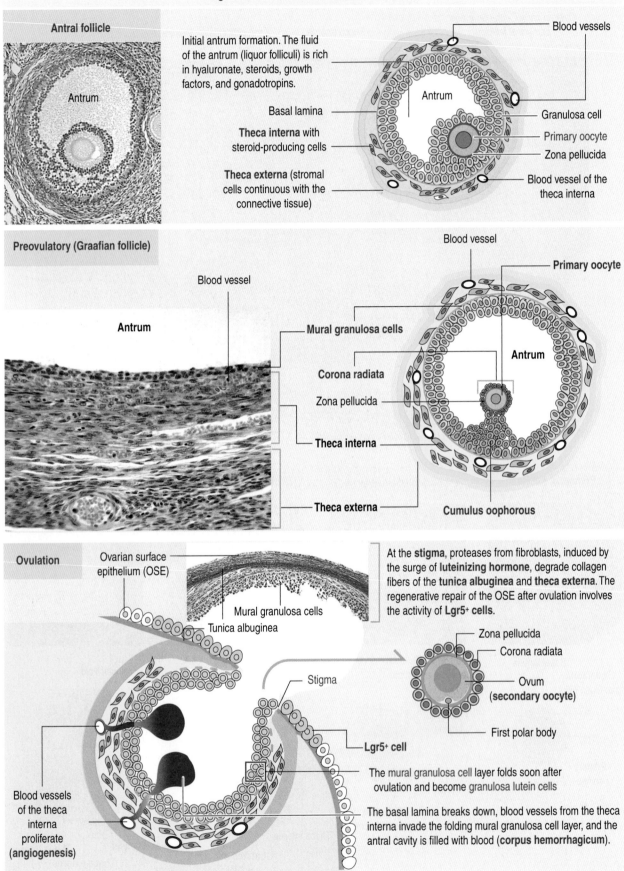

Figure 22-4. **From antral follicle to ovulation**

Antral follicle

Antrum

Initial antrum formation. The fluid of the antrum (liquor folliculi) is rich in hyaluronate, steroids, growth factors, and gonadotropins.

Blood vessels

Basal lamina

Theca interna with steroid-producing cells

Theca externa (stromal cells continuous with the connective tissue)

Antrum

Granulosa cell

Primary oocyte

Zona pellucida

Blood vessel of the theca interna

Preovulatory (Graafian follicle)

Antrum

Blood vessel

Blood vessel

Primary oocyte

Mural granulosa cells

Corona radiata

Zona pellucida

Theca interna

Theca externa

Antrum

Cumulus oophorous

Ovulation

Ovarian surface epithelium (OSE)

Mural granulosa cells

Tunica albuginea

At the **stigma**, proteases from fibroblasts, induced by the surge of **luteinizing hormone**, degrade collagen fibers of the **tunica albuginea** and **theca externa**. The regenerative repair of the OSE after ovulation involves the activity of **Lgr5+ cells**.

Zona pellucida

Corona radiata

Ovum (**secondary oocyte**)

First polar body

Stigma

Lgr5+ cell

Blood vessels of the theca interna proliferate (angiogenesis)

The mural granulosa cell layer folds soon after ovulation and become granulosa lutein cells

The basal lamina breaks down, blood vessels from the theca interna invade the folding mural granulosa cell layer, and the antral cavity is filled with blood (**corpus hemorrhagicum**).

Granulosa cell–primary oocyte bidirectional signaling

Zona pellucida is a glycoprotein coat that separates a corona radiata layer of granulosa cells from the primary oocyte. It consists of three zonula pellucida (**ZP**) glycoproteins: **ZP-1**, **ZP-2**, and **ZP-3**.

The zona pellucida is penetrated by thin cytoplasmic processes originated in granulosa cells of the corona radiata that contact the microvilli of the oocyte plasma membrane. This cell-cell communication mechanism coordinates the growth of the primary oocyte as well as its cell cycle progression (see Figure 22-5).

Granulosa cell-primary oocyte bidirectional signaling involves:

1. **Gap junctions** and **adherent junctions** at the granulosa cell-oocyte contact sites.

2. The intercellular transfer of specific members of the **transforming growth factor-β** (**TGF-β**) family.

Gap junctions enable metabolic cooperation between oocytes and granulosa cells mediated by the transfer of nutrients and substrates to the growing oocyte. Gap junctions are also seen between granulosa cells.

Connexin 37 is present in gap junctions connecting granulosa cells to the primary oocyte. **Connexin 43** is found in gap junctions interlinking granulosa cells. A lack of connexin 37, encoded by the *Gja4* gene, stops follicle development and interferes with the capacity of the primary oocyte to resume meiosis and epigenetic modifications essential for fetal development. A lack of connexin 43 disrupts folliculogenesis during the preantral phase.

Two **oocyte-derived** members of the **TGF-β family** transferred to granulosa cells are (see Figure 22-5):

1. **Growth and differentiation factor-9 (GDF-9)**.

2. **Bone morphogenetic protein-15 (BMP-15)**.

GDF-9 and BMP-15 function in a cooperative manner to regulate the energy metabolism and cholesterol biosynthesis of granulosa cells, thus enhancing female fertility by supporting the metabolic needs of the primary oocyte. GDF-9 is also required for the formation by granulosa cells of cell processes that penetrate and cross the zona pellucida.

Granulosa cell-derived members of the TGF-β superfamily, **AMH**, **inhibin**, and **activin**, are also involved in the regulation of granulosa cell function during folliculogenesis.

AMH appears to control the rate at which follicles become available for preovulatory development. As you are aware, AMH is secreted in the male fetus by Sertoli cells, the male somatic cell equivalent to granulosa cells. AMH triggers the regression of the müllerian duct.

FSH stimulates the proliferation and estrogen secretion by granulosa cells. Activin enhances granulosa cell responsiveness to FSH. Inhibin down-regulates the release of FSH and promotes luteinizing hormone (LH)–stimulated androgen synthesis. As we discuss below, an androgen precursor is required for estrogen production by granulosa cells.

As you can see, members of the TGF-β superfamily participate not only in the bidirectional signaling between granulosa cells and the primary oocyte but also in FSH regulation of folliculogenesis.

What prevents the primary oocyte from completing meiotic prophase I during folliculogenesis? **Granulosa cell-derived proteins** include (see Figure 22-5):

1. **Oocyte maturation inhibitor (OMI)**.

2. **Stem cell factor**.

OMI prevents the resumption of meiosis by primary oocytes prior to the surge of FSH and LH at ovulation.

Stem cell factor binds to the oocyte **c-kit receptor** and stimulates oocyte growth and survival. As you remember, c-kit receptor and its ligand play significant roles in the migration of mast cells (see Chapter 4, Connective Tissue) and primordial germinal cells to the gonadal ridges (see Chapter 21, Sperm Transport and Maturation).

Polycystic ovary syndrome (PCOS) is a clinical condition resulting from disrupted folliculogenesis caused by a defective paracrine oocyte-granulosa cell signaling mechanism. PCOS is associated with infrequent or prolonged menstrual periods, excess hair growth (**hirsutism**), acne, and obesity. Blood levels of androgens are elevated. Infrequent or absent menstruation in adolescents may raise suspicion for PCOS (see Box 22-B).

Then, how does the primary oocyte complete meiosis I before ovulation?

Just before ovulation, the oocyte activates itself by inducing completion of meiotic prophase. The **cyclin B–Cdc2 complex** constitutes the **maturation promoting factor** (**MPF**) that triggers the **breakdown of the oocyte nuclear envelope**, an event called **germinal vesicle breakdown (GVBD)**.

MPF action leads to the formation of the **secondary oocyte** and release of the **first polar body**.

Box 22-B | Polycystic ovary syndrome

- A breakdown in the bidirectional oocyte-granulosa cell signaling mechanism takes place in **polycystic ovary syndrome (PCOS)**, characterized by a disruption in folliculogenesis associated with **ovarian hyperandrogenism** (excess androgen), **insulin resistance** (resulting in high blood sugar), and **infertility**.
- The ovaries are enlarged and contain numerous cysts that can be detected by ultrasound.
- Infrequent or prolonged menstrual periods, excess hair growth (hirsutism), acne, and obesity are the clinical aspects of PCOS.
- A combination of endocrine and paracrine abnormalities affecting granulosa cell-oocyte communication are regarded as a possible cause of PCOS.

Figure 22-5. Granulosa cell–primary oocyte interaction

Granulosa cell–primary oocyte bidirectional signaling

1 Defect in primary oocyte meiotic progression is seen in the absence of **connexin 37** (encoded by the *Gja4* gene) in granulosa cell-oocyte gap junctions.

2 Granulosa cell–drived **stem cell factor (c-kit ligand)** bind to **c-kit receptor** on the oocyte surface. A lack of c-kit ligand and GDF-9 blocks follicular development before formation of secondary follicles.

3 Knockout mice lacking oocyte-derived **zona pellucida protein 3 (ZP-3)** or **ZP-2** have defects in the development of preantral and antral follicles, formation of the cumulus oophorous, and ovulation.

4 Oocyte-derived **GDF-9** and **BMP-15** cooperate with granulosa cells to maintain the metabolic needs of the primary oocyte and maximize female fertility. Granulosa cell processes crossing zona pellucida are lacking in the absence of GDF9 and FSH. GDF-9 and BMP-15 are members of the transforming growth factor-β superfamily.

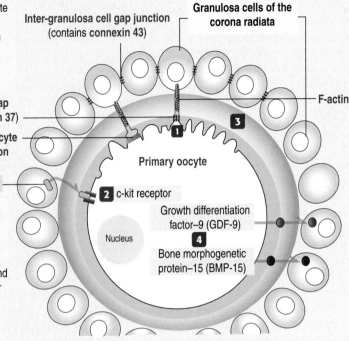

Inter-granulosa cell gap junction (contains **connexin 43**)

Granulosa cells of the corona radiata

Granulosa cell-oocyte gap junction (contains **connexin 37**)

Granulosa cell-oocyte adherens junction

Stem cell factor

F-actin

Primary oocyte

2 c-kit receptor

Nucleus

Growth differentiation factor–9 (GDF-9)

4

Bone morphogenetic protein–15 (BMP-15)

Meiotic prophase arrest and progression of a primary oocyte

5 OMI is a **granulosa cell** protein with a small molecular mass (1 to 2 kd) that reaches the oocyte through a gap junction. OMI prevents the **premature completion of meiotic prophase of the primary oocyte.**

Cortical granule containing **ovastacin**, a protease that proteolytically cleaves ZP2 after gamete fusion

Cortical polarity is a cap-like cortical region of the oocyte lacking microvilli but rich in F-actin and myosin II

6 Just before ovulation, the oocyte activates itself to induce completion of meiotic prophase. The cyclin B–Cdc2 complex constitutes the maturation promoting factor (MPF). MPF induces the breakdown of the nuclear envelope (**germinal vesicle breakdown, GVBD**) before metaphase I. MPF action results in formation of the secondary oocyte and release of the **first polar body**, that is retained in the perivitelline space.

Zona pellucida

GVBD

5 Oocyte maturation inhibitor (OMI)

6

Maturation promoting factor (MPF)

Cdc2

Cyclin B

Primary oocyte

Perivitelline space

The primary oocyte overcomes meiotic arrest and continues meiosis I in response to the LH surge. This process results in GVBD, completion of meiotic prophase I, and the assembly of the meiotic spindle. As a result, the **first polar body** is formed and released into the **perivitelline space**. The secondary oocyte retains most of the cytoplasm and the first polar body degenerates within hours of formation.

Meiosis II reaches metaphase and awaits **fertilization** for completion and extrusion of the **second polar body**. A haploid state is reached.

Figure 22-6. Theca interna–granulosa cell interaction

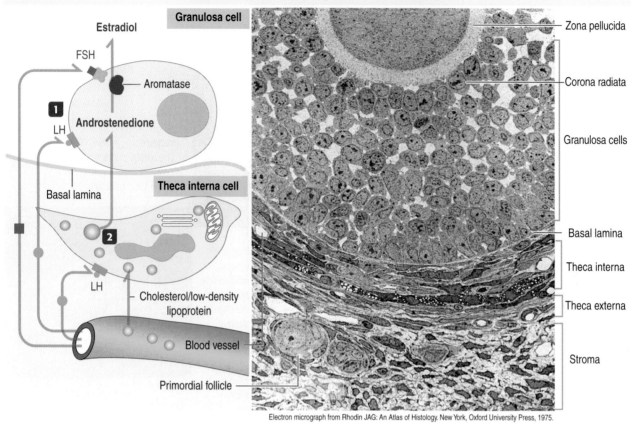

Electron micrograph from Rhodin JAG: An Atlas of Histology. New York, Oxford University Press, 1975.

Functional synergism between granulosa cells and theca interna cells during early folliculogenesis

1 In the primary and secondary follicle, granulosa cells have follicle-stimulating hormone (FSH) receptors. In the graafian follicle, luteinizing hormone (LH) receptors appear and coexist with FSH receptors. **The acquisition of LH receptors is essential for the luteinization of the ruptured follicle following ovulation.**

2 Estradiol is the major steroid produced by granulosa cells under stimulation by FSH. However, **granulosa cells depend on the supply of androstenedione by theca interna cells, regulated by LH, to produce estradiol** (by aromatization of the androgen) since granulosa cells lack the required enzymes for producing the precursor of estradiol.

Theca interna–granulosa cell synergistic communication

A basal lamina separates granulosa cells from theca interna cells. Yet, significant molecular flow initiated in the theca interna cells ensures the production of estrogens by granulosa cells (Figure 22-6).

Cells of the theca interna secrete **androstenedione**, an androgen precursor that is **transferred across the basal lamina to the granulosa cells** for the production of estradiol (see Figure 22-6; see Box 22-C). The androgen is then converted to **estradiol** by aromatase. Granulosa cells lack enzymes required for the direct production of estrogens. As a result, **granulosa cells cannot produce steroid precursors during folliculogenesis.**

Follicular atresia or degeneration

Several primary follicles initiate the maturation process, but generally only one follicle completes its development; the remainder degenerate by an apoptotic process called **atresia.**

Atresia refers to the failure of a follicle to ovulate. Atresia is also observed in the fetal ovary and after

---

Box 22-C | Ovarian hormones

• **Estradiol** (estradiol-17β) is the most abundant and most potent ovarian estrogen, produced mainly by granulosa and granulosa lutein cells. Significant amounts of **estriol**, a less potent estrogen, is produced from estrone in the **liver** during **pregnancy**. Most **estrone**, the least potent of the three estrogens, is predominant in the **postmenopausal woman** and is formed in **peripheral tissues** by the conversion of estradiol or androstenedione.

• **Progesterone**, a precursor of androgens and estrogens, is synthesized by follicular and luteal cells.

• Weak **androgens** (**dehydroepiandrosterone** and **androstenedione**) are produced by theca interna cells.

• Other ovarian hormones are **inhibin, activin,** and **relaxin. Relaxin,** produced by both the ovary and the placenta, induces **relaxation of the pelvic ligaments** and **softens the cervix to facilitate childbirth.**

Figure 22-7. **Atretic follicle**

A woman ovulates about 400 oocytes during her reproductive years. During a reproductive cycle, a group of follicles starts the maturation process.

However, only one or two follicles complete folliculogenesis and are eventually ovulated. The others undergo, at any time of their development, a degenerative process called **follicular atresia**.

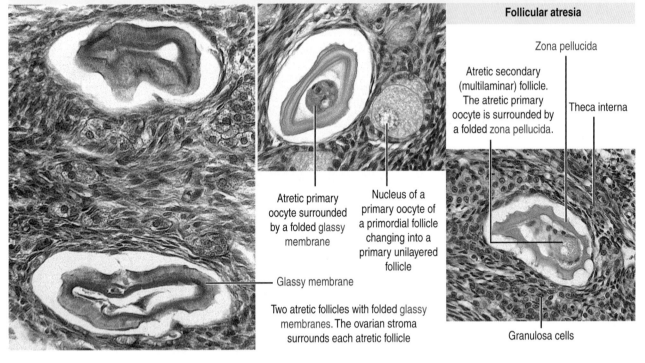

Follicular atresia

Zona pellucida

Atretic secondary (multilaminar) follicle. The atretic primary oocyte is surrounded by a folded zona pellucida.

Theca interna

Atretic primary oocyte surrounded by a folded glassy membrane

Nucleus of a primary oocyte of a primordial follicle changing into a primary unilayered follicle

Glassy membrane

Two atretic follicles with folded glassy membranes. The ovarian stroma surrounds each atretic follicle

Granulosa cells

birth. Follicles can become atretic at any stage of their development but the proportion of follicles that become atretic increases with follicle size (see Box 22-D).

Apoptosis is the mechanism of follicular atresia. Apoptosis ensures regression of the follicle without eliciting an inflammatory response.

Atretic follicles display thick folded basement membrane material, called **glassy membrane** (Figure 22-7). Folded zona pellucida and apoptotic fragmented oocyte can be seen.

Why so many follicles enter the folliculogenesis process when generally only one ovulates? Atresia ensures that only viable follicles, containing oocytes of optimal quality for fertilization, are available throughout the reproductive period. Furthermore, a large number of atretic follicles retain steroidogenic activity, thereby contributing to the endocrine function of the ovary that prepares the endometrium for implantation.

From a clinical perspective, follicular atresia correlates with the menopause-like **premature ovarian failure** (**POF**) and **PCOS** (see Box 22-B), two pathological conditions leading to infertility.

Ovulatory phase
At the time of ovulation, the mature follicle protrudes from the ovarian surface, forming the **stigma** (see Figure 22-4). Proteolytic activity within the theca externa and tunica albuginea, induced by a surge of LH, facilitates the rupture of the now mature preovulatory graafian follicle.

The released gamete enters the closely apposed uterine tube or oviduct as it completes meiosis I and becomes a secondary oocyte that still needs to finish meiosis II to become a haploid cell. A few hours before ovulation, changes occur in the **mural granulosa cell layer** and the **theca interna in preparation for luteinization.** Lgr5+ cells of the OSE repair the damage of the site following the rupture of the follicle.

Luteal phase: Luteinization and luteolysis
Following ovulation, the residual mural granulosa cell layer folds and becomes part of the **corpus luteum**, a major hormone-secreting gland (Figure 22-8).

Box 22-D | **Folliculogenesis and follicular atresia**

• The development of the ovarian follicle and steroidogenesis are controlled by gonadotropin-releasing hormones (GnRH), in part by ovarian steroids and autocrine and paracrine secretions of the granulosa cells.
• About 7 million primary oocytes are present in the fetal ovary by midgestation. There is a gradual loss of oocytes and, at birth, approximately 400,000 oocytes remain. Only 400 follicles ovulate after puberty. The remaining follicles degenerate and are called **atretic follicles**.
• The follicular phase begins with the development of 6 to 12 primary follicles. This development is FSH-dependent. By the sixth day of the cycle, one follicle predominates and the others become atretic.

Figure 22-8. Development, function, and involution of the corpus luteum

Formation of the corpus luteum (luteinization)

Following ovulation, the **follicular membrane** (also called granulosa cell mural layer) of the preovulatory follicle becomes folded and is transformed into part of the **corpus luteum**. A surge in luteinizing hormone (LH) correlates with luteinization.

Luteinization includes the following:

(1) The lumen, previously occupied by the follicular antrum, is filled with fibrin, which is then replaced by connective tissue and new blood vessels piercing the basement membrane.

(2) Granulosa cells enlarge and lipid droplets accumulate in the cytoplasm. They become **granulosa lutein cells**.

(3) The spaces between the folds of the granulosa cell layer are penetrated by theca interna cells, blood vessels, and connective tissue. Theca interna cells also enlarge and store lipids. They are now **theca lutein cells**.

1 Folded granulosa cell mural containing **granulosa lutein cells** store lipids.

The spaces between the folds are occupied by theca lutein cells, connective tissue, and blood vessels.

Fibroblast in connective tissue

Blood vessels

Theca externa

2 The former antrum filled with fibrin is replaced by connective tissue and blood vessels.

3 A breakdown of the basement membrane enables blood vessels of the theca interna to invade the ruptured follicle.

Function of the corpus luteum

The function of the corpus luteum is regulated by two gonadotropins: FSH and LH.

Follicle-stimulating hormone (FSH) stimulates the production of **progesterone** and **estradiol** by granulosa lutein cells.

LH stimulates the production of progesterone and androstenedione by theca lutein cells. Androstenedione is translocated into granulosa lutein cells for aromatization into **estradiol**.

During pregnancy, **prolactin** and **placental lactogens** up-regulate the effects of estradiol produced by granulosa lutein cells by enhancing the production of estrogen receptors.

Estradiol stimulates granulosa lutein cells to take up cholesterol from blood, which is then stored in lipid droplets and transported to mitochondria for progesterone synthesis.

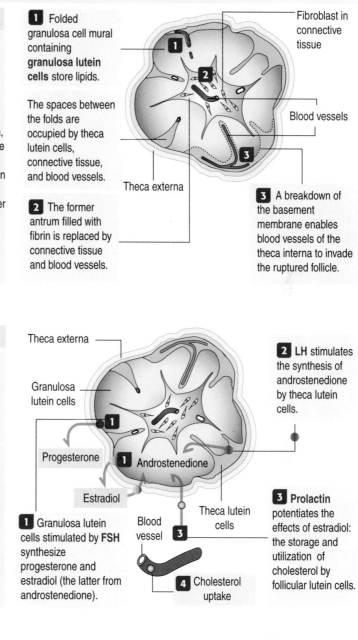

Theca externa

Granulosa lutein cells

Progesterone

Estradiol

1 Androstenedione

2 LH stimulates the synthesis of androstenedione by theca lutein cells.

Theca lutein cells

Blood vessel

3

4 Cholesterol uptake

1 Granulosa lutein cells stimulated by **FSH** synthesize progesterone and estradiol (the latter from androstenedione).

3 Prolactin potentiates the effects of estradiol: the storage and utilization of cholesterol by follicular lutein cells.

Regression of the corpus luteum (luteolysis)

If fertilization does not occur, the corpus luteum undergoes a process of regression called **luteolysis**.

Luteolysis involves a programmed cell death (apoptosis) sequence. It is triggered by endometrial **prostaglandin F2a**. The following events take place:

(1) A **reduction in the blood flow** within the corpus luteum causes a decline in oxygen (hypoxia).

(2) **T cells** reach the corpus luteum and produce **interferon-γ**, which, in turn, acts on the endothelium to enable the arrival of macrophages.

(3) **Macrophages** produce **tumor necrosis factor ligand** and the apoptotic cascade starts.

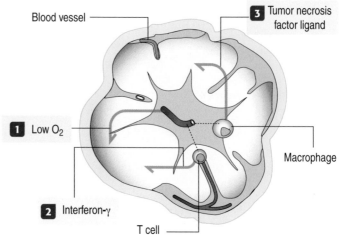

Blood vessel

3 Tumor necrosis factor ligand

1 Low O_2

Macrophage

2 Interferon-γ

T cell

Figure 22-9. **Lutein cell**

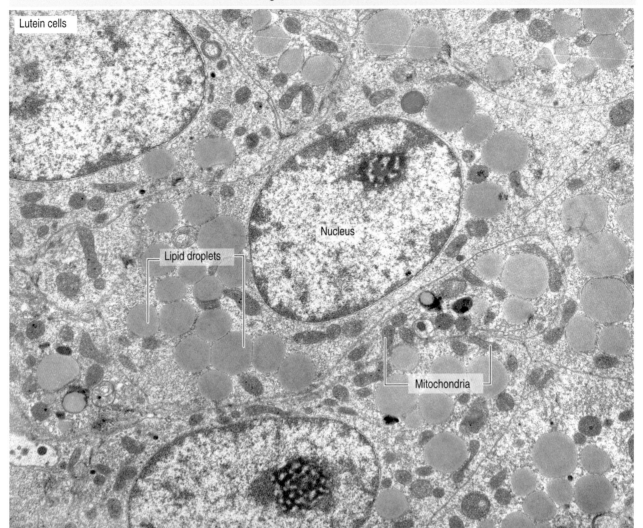

Lutein cells

Lipid droplets

Nucleus

Mitochondria

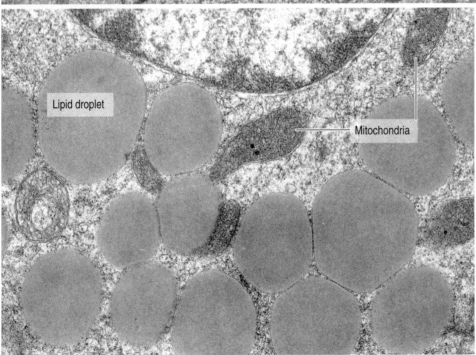

Lipid droplet

Mitochondria

Corpus luteum

Steroid-producing cells of the corpus luteum display the three characteristic features already seen in the adrenal cortex: (1) **lipid droplets**; (2) **mitochondria with tubular cristae**; (3) **abundant smooth endoplasmic reticulum**. The participation of these three elements in steroidogenesis has been stressed in discussions of the adrenal cortex (Chapter 19) and Leydig cells (Chapter 20).

When comparing mitochondria in cells of the corpus luteum and adrenal cortex, the number of tubular cristae in the latter is considerably higher.

Figure 22-10. Granulosa lutein–theca lutein cell cooperation

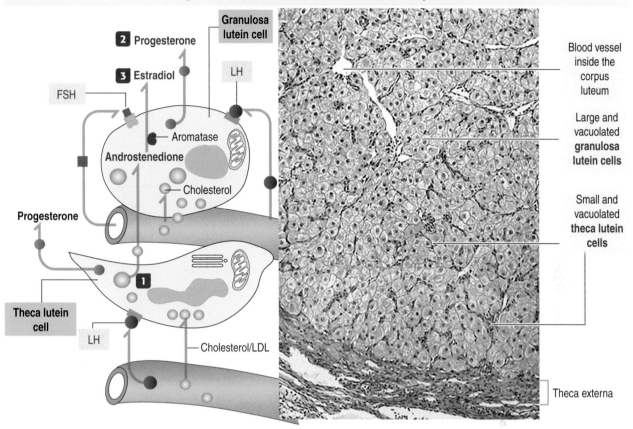

Granulosa lutein cell

2 Progesterone

3 Estradiol

FSH

LH

Aromatase

Androstenedione

Cholesterol

Progesterone

1

Theca lutein cell

LH

Cholesterol/LDL

Blood vessel inside the corpus luteum

Large and vacuolated **granulosa lutein cells**

Small and vacuolated **theca lutein cells**

Theca externa

Functional cooperation between theca lutein cells and granulosa lutein cells

1 Theca lutein cells, stimulated by luteinizing hormone (LH), take up cholesterol or low-density lipoprotein (LDL), or both, from blood. Cholesterol is used for steroidogenesis. The steroid product, androstenedione, is transported to granulosa lutein cells.

2 Granulosa lutein cells are under control of both follicle-stimulating hormone (FSH) and LH. These cells can store cholesterol taken up from blood and use it for the synthesis of progesterone.

3 In addition, granulosa lutein cells utilize androstenedione, delivered by theca lutein cells, to produce estradiol.

Figure 22-11. Corpus albicans

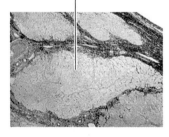

Corpus albicans (low magnification)

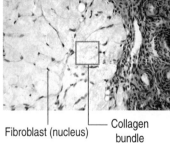

Corpus albicans (detail)

Stroma of the ovary with blood vessels

Fibroblast (nucleus)

Collagen bundle

In the absence of fertilization, the corpus luteum undergoes involution and regression (luteolysis), luteal cells are phagocytized by macrophages and the former corpus luteum becomes the corpus albicans, a scar of white fibrous tissue containing type I collagen produced by fibroblast.

Luteinization involves:

1. A **breakdown of the basal lamina of the follicle**.
2. **Invasion of blood vessels** into the wall of the now empty antrum.

Blood flows into the former antral space and coagulates, forming a transient **corpus hemorrhagicum**. The fibrin clot is then penetrated by newly formed blood vessels (**angiogenesis**), fibroblasts, and collagen fibers. Note that angiogenesis is a normal physiologic process that takes place during each menstrual cycle.

3. A **transformation of mural granulosa cells and theca interna cells**. Mural granulosa cells change into **granulosa lutein cells**. They display the typical features of steroid-secreting cells (lipid droplets, a well-developed smooth endoplasmic reticulum, and mitochondria with tubular cristae, Figure 22-9).

Granulosa lutein cells secrete **progesterone** and **estrogen in response to both FSH and LH stimula-**

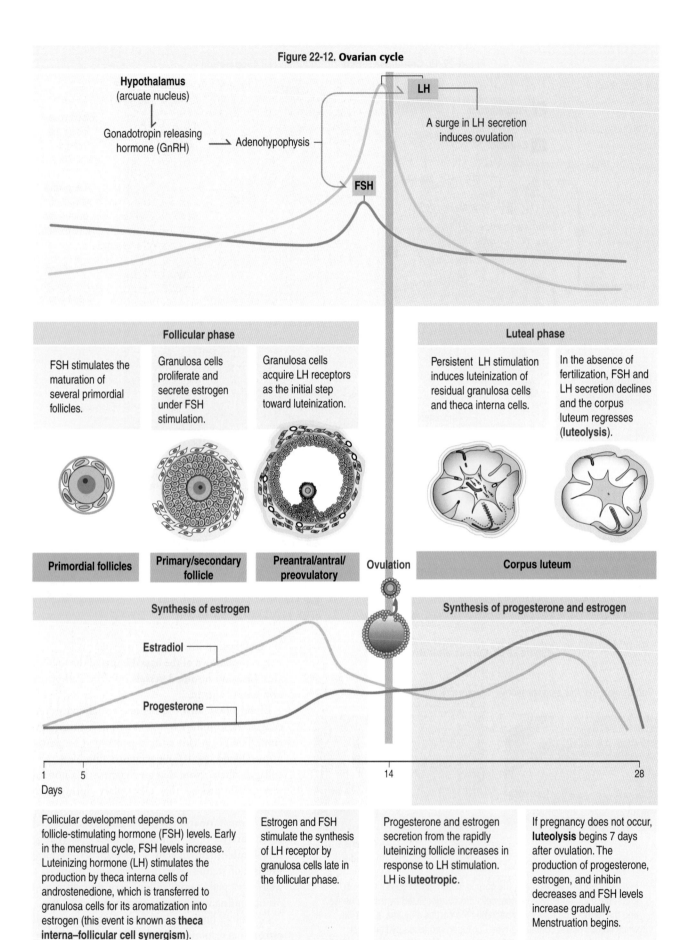

Figure 22-12. **Ovarian cycle**

Hypothalamus
(arcuate nucleus)

Gonadotropin releasing
hormone (GnRH) → Adenohypophysis

LH

A surge in LH secretion
induces ovulation

FSH

Follicular phase

FSH stimulates the maturation of several primordial follicles.

Granulosa cells proliferate and secrete estrogen under FSH stimulation.

Granulosa cells acquire LH receptors as the initial step toward luteinization.

Luteal phase

Persistent LH stimulation induces luteinization of residual granulosa cells and theca interna cells.

In the absence of fertilization, FSH and LH secretion declines and the corpus luteum regresses (**luteolysis**).

Primordial follicles

Primary/secondary follicle

Preantral/antral/ preovulatory

Ovulation

Corpus luteum

Synthesis of estrogen

Synthesis of progesterone and estrogen

Estradiol

Progesterone

1   5   14   28
Days

Follicular development depends on follicle-stimulating hormone (FSH) levels. Early in the menstrual cycle, FSH levels increase. Luteinizing hormone (LH) stimulates the production by theca interna cells of androstenedione, which is transferred to granulosa cells for its aromatization into estrogen (this event is known as **theca interna–follicular cell synergism**).

Estrogen and FSH stimulate the synthesis of LH receptor by granulosa cells late in the follicular phase.

Progesterone and estrogen secretion from the rapidly luteinizing follicle increases in response to LH stimulation. LH is **luteotropic**.

If pregnancy does not occur, **luteolysis** begins 7 days after ovulation. The production of progesterone, estrogen, and inhibin decreases and FSH levels increase gradually. Menstruation begins.

Figure 22-13. **Oviduct**

3 In the **isthmus**, the muscle layer is thick and capable of rhythmic contractions toward the uterus. Contractions help the displacement of sperm toward the egg and the fertilized egg toward the uterus.

2 The lumen of the ampulla is occupied by folds of the mucosa forming convoluted channels. The displacement of the ovum through the ampulla is slow. This is the site where fertilization occurs. A fertilized egg may implant in the mucosa of the oviduct (**ectopic pregnancy**). The progression of pregnancy is disrupted by the rupture of the oviduct and is accompanied by internal bleeding.

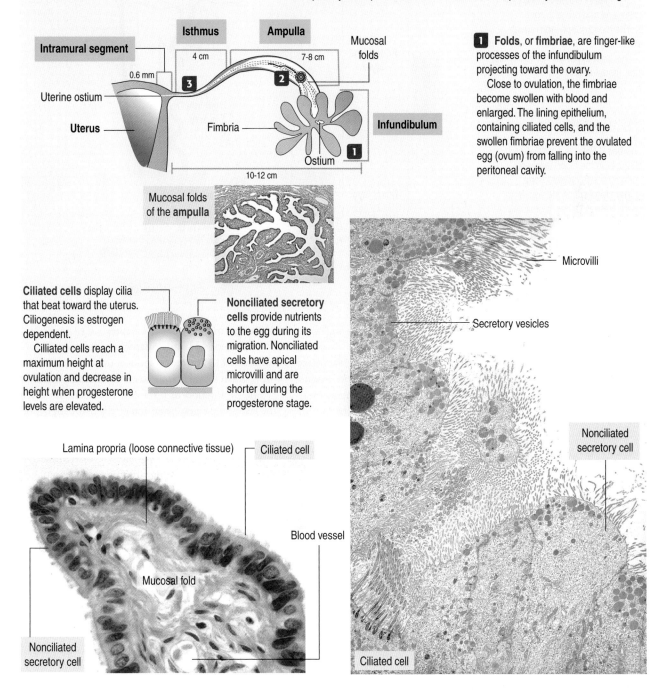

1 **Folds**, or **fimbriae**, are finger-like processes of the infundibulum projecting toward the ovary.

Close to ovulation, the fimbriae become swollen with blood and enlarged. The lining epithelium, containing ciliated cells, and the swollen fimbriae prevent the ovulated egg (ovum) from falling into the peritoneal cavity.

Mucosal folds of the **ampulla**

Ciliated cells display cilia that beat toward the uterus. Ciliogenesis is estrogen dependent.

Cilliated cells reach a maximum height at ovulation and decrease in height when progesterone levels are elevated.

Nonciliated secretory cells provide nutrients to the egg during its migration. Nonciliated cells have apical microvilli and are shorter during the progesterone stage.

tion. The expression of LH receptors by granulosa cells is an essential step in the luteinization process.

The theca interna cells change into **theca lutein cells**, which produce **androstenedione** and **progesterone in response to LH stimulation** (Figure 22-10).

Granulosa lutein cells still lack the steroido- **genic enzyme required for the complete synthesis of estradiol** (see Box 22-C). Yet, they can synthesize progesterone.

Theca lutein cells cooperate with granulosa lutein cells by providing androstenedione, which is then converted into estradiol by aromatase within follicular lutein cells (see Figure 22-10).

Figure 22-14. Endometrial glands

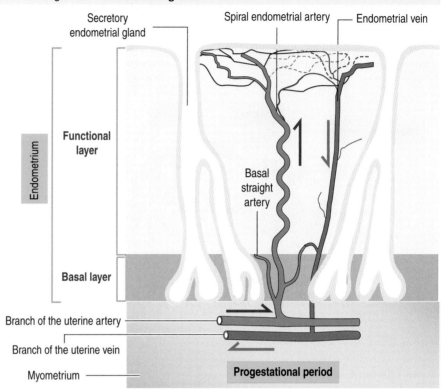

Figure 22-14. Endometrial glands

Functional layer

The **functional layer** of the endometrium is most affected by:
1. Changes in the blood levels of estrogens and progesterone.
2. The blood supply from spiral arteries.

This layer is partially or totally lost after menstruation.

Basal layer

The **basal layer** is not affected by changes in the blood levels of estrogens and progesterone.

The blood supply derives from basal arteries rather than spiral arteries.

This layer is not lost after menstruation. The functional layer regenerates after menstruation from the basal-functional layer boundary.

The corpus luteum continues to enlarge and enters an involution stage about 14 days after ovulation unless fertilization occurs. If fertilization takes place, the corpus luteum continues to enlarge and produce **progesterone** and **estrogen** under the stimulatory action of **human chorionic gonadotropin (hCG)** synthesized by the **trophoblast** of the implanted embryo.

Regression of the corpus luteum, **luteolysis**, leads to the formation of the **corpus albicans**, resulting from the stromal connective tissue replacing the mass of degenerating luteal cells of the corpus luteum (Figure 22-11).

The corpus albicans remains in the ovary; it decreases in size but seldom disappears.

Hormonal regulation of ovulation and the corpus luteum

Let us review the hormonal regulation of the menstrual cycle.

Two hormones of the anterior hypophysis, controlled by **gonadotropin-releasing hormone (GnRH)** produced by neurons of the **arcuate nucleus** in the hypothalamus, regulate follicular growth (Figure 22-12):

1. **Follicle-stimulating hormone** stimulates folliculogenesis and ovulation as well as the production of estrogen.

2. **Luteinizing hormone** stimulates the secretion of progesterone by the corpus luteum.

FSH and LH effects are mediated by a cAMP-

dependent mechanism (see Chapter 3, Cell Signaling).

A surge of LH immediately precedes ovulation. Continued LH secretion induces the **luteinization** of the residual mural granulosa cell layer after ovulation.

The production of FSH and LH decreases when the levels of progesterone and estrogen are high, and then the corpus luteum enters involution (luteolysis).

Keep in mind that activin and inhibin originated in the ovarian follicles regulate hypothalamic and hypophysis gonadotropic responses by a feedback mechanism.

At the initiation of menstruation, estrogen and progesterone levels are low and increase gradually during the preovulatory period. Estrogen reaches maximum levels just before the LH peak precedes ovulation.

Coinciding with the FSH and LH secretory pattern, the FSH-dependent synthesis of estrogen by granulosa cells stimulates the **proliferation of the endometrial glands**. LH-dependent synthesis of progesterone by the corpus luteum **initiates and maintains the secretory activity of the endometrial glands**.

Oviduct, fallopian or uterine tube

The oviduct is the site of fertilization and early cleavage of the **zygote** (fertilized ovum). Each tube is divided into **four anatomic regions** (Figure 22-13):
1. The proximal fimbriated **infundibulum**.
2. A long and thin-walled **ampulla**.
3. A short and thick-walled **isthmus**.

Figure 22-15. **Endometrial cycle**

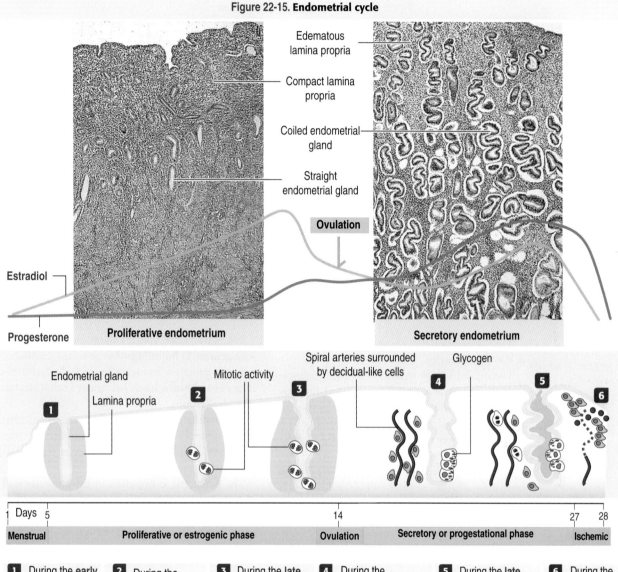

Edematous lamina propria

Compact lamina propria

Coiled endometrial gland

Straight endometrial gland

Ovulation

Estradiol

Progesterone

Proliferative endometrium

Secretory endometrium

Spiral arteries surrounded by decidual-like cells

Glycogen

Endometrial gland

Lamina propria

Mitotic activity

1 **2** **3** **4** **5** **6**

Days 5 14 27 28

Menstrual **Proliferative or estrogenic phase** **Ovulation** **Secretory or progestational phase** **Ischemic**

1 During the **early proliferative period**, the glands are short, straight, and narrow. The lamina propria is compacted.

2 During the **midproliferative period**, the glands are longer and straight. The epithelium is mitotically active. The lamina propria is slightly edematous.

3 During the **late proliferative period**, mitotic activity is intense, the glands grow rapidly and become tortuous.

The lamina propria is more edematous.

4 During the **midsecretory period**, glycogen accumulates in the **basal portion** of the glandular epithelial cells.

The glands have a **saw-toothed appearance**.

The cells of the stroma surrounding the spiral arteries enlarge and become **decidual-like**.

5 During the **late secretory period**, glycogen shifts to the **apical portion** of the glandular epithelium.

The glands have secretion in the lumen.

The stromal cells surrounding the spiral arteries are mitotically active, an indication of a decidual change.

6 During the **ischemic period**, the upper region of the endometrial stroma contains numerous decidual cells.

The spiral arteries contract and ischemia starts.

Lamina propria

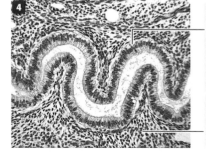

The basal region of columnar epithelial cells lining the endometrial gland contains glycogen deposits (not visible with hematoxylin-eosin [H & E] stain), and the nucleus is displaced to the center or apical portion of the cell.

The surrounding stroma will undergo a decidual transformation as the secretory phase progresses.

Figure 22-16. Premenstrual endometrium

Premenstrual or ischemic stage

1 Periodic contractions of the spiral artery, triggered by a reduction in progesterone, deprive the supply of oxygen (hypoxia) to the functional layer.

2 A breakdown of the spiral artery floods the lamina propria with blood.

3 The functional layer, consisting of glands and decidual-like cells, detaches and sheds into the uterine cavity (**menses**).

4 The basal layer is not affected because basal straight arteries provide independent blood supply to this layer.

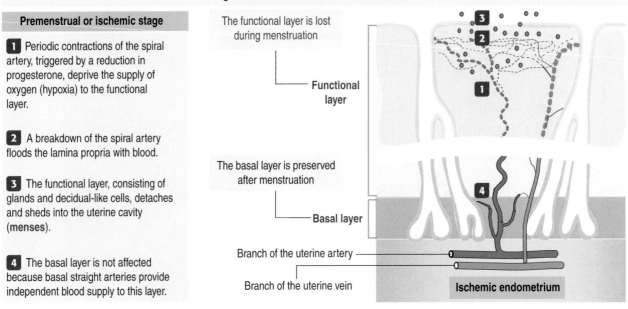

The functional layer is lost during menstruation

— Functional layer

The basal layer is preserved after menstruation

— Basal layer

Branch of the uterine artery —

Branch of the uterine vein —

Ischemic endometrium

4. An **intramural** portion opening into the lumen of the uterine cavity.

The infundibulum consists of numerous finger-like projections of mucosal tissue called **fimbriae**. The ampulla and the isthmus are lined by **mucosal folds** projecting into the lumen of the tube. The isthmus has fewer mucosal folds than the ampulla.

The wall of the oviduct consists of three layers:

1. A **mucosa** layer supported by a **lamina propria**, consisting of loose connective tissue and a few scattered smooth muscle cells.

2. A smooth **muscle layer**.

3. A **serosa layer**.

The mucosa lining consists of a **simple columnar epithelium** with two cell populations (see Figure 22-13) under **hormonal control**:

1. **Ciliated cells**, which enlarge and produce cilia (**ciliogenesis**) as folliculogenesis and estrogen production is in progress. Estrogens increase the rate of the ciliary beat. During luteolysis, ciliated cells lose their cilia (**deciliation**).

2. **Nonciliated secretory cells** (called **peg cells**), whose secretory activity is also stimulated by estrogens. Nonciliated cells in some species have apical microvilli.

The **peristaltic contraction** of the muscular wall, with an **inner circular-spiral layer** and an **outer longitudinal layer**, as well as the ciliary activity of the lining epithelial cells, propel the oocyte or fertilized egg/embryo toward the uterus.

The surface of the oviduct is covered by the peritoneal **mesothelium**. Large blood vessels are observed under the serosa.

Uterus

The uterus consists of two anatomic segments:

1. The **corpus** or **body**.

2. The **cervix**.

The wall of the body of the uterus consists of three layers:

1. The **endometrium** (Figures 22-14 and 22-15).

2. The **myometrium**.

3. The **adventitia** or **serosa**.

The major component of the wall is the myometrium, lined by a mucosa, the endometrium.

The myometrium has three poorly defined smooth muscle layers. The central layer is thick with circularly arranged muscle fibers and abundant blood vessels, which give the name **stratum vasculare** to this particular layer. The outer and inner layers contain longitudinally or obliquely arranged muscle fibers.

Figure 22-17. Decidual cells

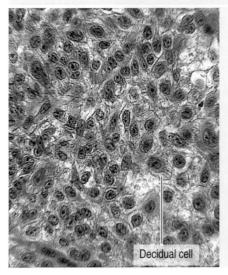

Decidual cell

The **decidual reaction** consists in the hypertrophy of endometrial stromal cells. Implantation of the fertilized egg depends on a hormonally primed endometrium (see Chapter 23, Fertilization, Placentation, and Lactation) consisting of secretory endometrial glands surrounded by decidual cells. In addition, high progesterone levels keep the myometrium relatively quiescent.

Figure 22-18. **Decidual cell**

Decidual cells

Decidual cells derive from the epithelial-like transformation of endometrial **stroma cells** (**decidual reaction** in preparation for embryo implantation).

- Decidual cells **modulate trophoblast cell invasion**.
- Decidual cells **provide nutrients to the developing embryo**.
- Together with trophoblast cells, decidual cells **prevent the immunologic rejection** of genetically different embryonic and fetal tissues.
- Decidual cells have an **endocrine role**: the production of **decidual prolactin**, related to pituitary prolactin, with a trophic effect on the **corpus luteum**.

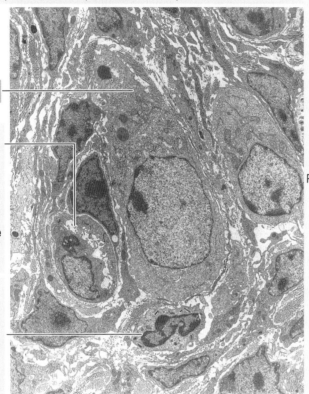

Decidual cell

Vascular changes
An increase in the permeability of endometrial blood vessels and angiogenesis occurs in response to embryo implantation.

Recruitment of inflammatory cells
Lymphocytes, macrophages, and eosinophils are attracted to the implantation site.

Electron micrograph courtesy of Patricia C. Cross, Stanford, California.

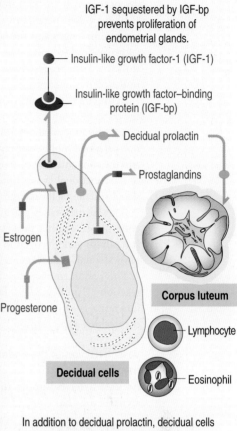

IGF-1 sequestered by IGF-bp prevents proliferation of endometrial glands.

— Insulin-like growth factor-1 (IGF-1)

Insulin-like growth factor–binding protein (IGF-bp)

Decidual prolactin

Prostaglandins

Estrogen

Progesterone

Corpus luteum

Lymphocyte

Decidual cells

Eosinophil

In addition to decidual prolactin, decidual cells produce **prostaglandins** and **relaxin**.

- Decidual cells have receptors for **estrogens** and **progesterone**.
- Decidual cells secrete **IGF-binding proteins** which bind IGFs to prevent their proliferative action on endometrial cells.

During pregnancy, myometrial smooth muscle enlarges (**hypertrophy**) and the fibers increase in number (**hyperplasia**).

Inhibition of myometrial contraction during pregnancy is controlled by **relaxin**, a peptide hormone produced in the ovary and placenta. **Myometrial contraction during parturition** is under the control of **oxytocin**, a peptide hormone secreted from the neurohypophysis.

The **endometrium** consists of a **simple columnar epithelial lining**, associated with simple tubular endometrial glands, and the **lamina propria**, called the **endometrial stroma**.

Functionally, the endometrium consists of two layers (see Figure 22-14):

1. A superficial **functional layer**, lost during menstruation.

2. A **basal layer**, retained as the source of regenera-tion of a new functional layer following menstruation.

A menstrual cycle consists of four consecutive phases: **menstrual**, **proliferative**, **secretory**, and **ischemic phases** (see Figure 22-15).

The **menstrual phase** (4 to 5 days) is the initial phase of the cycle.

The **proliferative phase** (also called the estrogenic or follicular phase) is of about 9 days duration. During the proliferative phase, the thickness of the endometrium (0.5 to 1 mm) increases as a result of the stimulatory activity of **estrogen** produced by maturing ovarian follicles. Mitotic activity is detected in both the lamina propria and the epithelium.

After day 14, when ovulation occurs, the endometrium begins its **secretory** or **progestational phase**, which lasts approximately 13 days. During this phase, the endometrium has a thickness of 5 to 7 mm and endometrial glands initiate their secretory activity.

The outline of the tubular glands becomes irregular and coiled, the lining epithelium accumulates **glycogen**, and secretions rich in glycogen and glycoproteins are present in the glandular lumen.

Blood vessels parallel to the endometrial glands increase in length and the lamina propria contains excessive fluid (edema). The secretory phase is controlled by both **progesterone** and **estrogen** produced in the corpus luteum.

At the end of the menstrual cycle, the regression of the corpus luteum leads to an endometrial **ischemic phase** (duration of about 1 day). A reduction in the normal blood supply, causing intermittent **ischemia** and the consequent hypoxia, determine the necrosis of the **functional layer** of the endometrium, which sloughs off during the menstrual phase (Figure 22-16).

If pregnancy takes place, **decidual cells** in the endometrial lamina propria increase in size and store lipids and glycogen in response to increasing progesterone levels (Figures 22-17 and 22-18).

This endometrial change is known as a **decidual reaction** (Latin *deciduus*, falling off) because the functional layer of the endometrium will be shed as the **decidua** at parturition.

Vascularization of the endometrium and menstruation

Arcuate arteries supply the endometrium. An arcuate artery has two segments (see Figure 22-14):

1. A **straight segment**, supplying the **basal layer** of the endometrium.

2. A **coiled segment,** supplying the **functional layer** of the endometrium.

The coiled segment stretches as the endometrium grows in thickness. Before menstruation, **contraction of the artery at the straight-coiled interface reduces the blood flow resulting in the destruction of the functional layer of the endometrium.**

Clinical significance: Delayed puberty and hypothalamic amenorrhea

The onset of puberty requires a functional hypothalamic–hypophysis–gonadal axis represented by an increase in the pulsatile secretion of GnRH to trigger sexual maturation leading to reproductive function.

Two clinical conditions, **delayed puberty** and **functional hypothalamic amenorrhea** (absence of menses), illustrate the importance of GnRH in reproductive function:

1. **Delayed puberty** is the delayed or absence of testicular development in boys or breast development in girls at the pubertal timing of the age of 14 years in boys and 13 years in girls.

The designation **hypogonadotropic hypogonadism (HH)** indicates the unavailability of GnRH responsible for a delayed or absent gonadal develop-

ment. This condition can be permanent or transient.

Permanent HH is characterized by low levels of LH and FSH determined by hypothalamic or pituitary congenital disorders. **Transient HH** can be functional.

Kallmann's syndrome is permanent HH associated with **anosmia** (loss of the sense of smell). Males with permanent HH are often born with a small penis (micropenis) and undescended testes (cryptorchidism). Puberty is incomplete or delayed. Affected females usually do not begin menstruating at puberty and breast development is absent.

Kallmann's types 1 to 4 syndromes are caused by a congenital defect in the secretion of GnRH determined by defects in the *KAL1* (Kallmann syndrome 1 sequence), *PROKR2* (prokineticin receptor 2), and *PROK2* (prokinecitin 2) genes responsible for the migration of GnRH–secreting hormones to the hypothalamus.

The X chromosome–located *KAL1* gene encodes the protein **anosmin-1**, that controls the migration of olfactory neurons to the olfactory bulb, and GnRH–producing neurons to the hypothalamus.

In addition, the *FGFR1* (fibroblast growth factor receptor 1) gene controls the fate specification, migration, and survival of GnRH-secreting neurons. Proteins encoded by *KAL1*, *PROKR2*, *PROK2,* and *FGFR1* are expressed not only during development but also in the adult hypothalamus.

Thus, the secretion of FSH and LH is compromised by the absence of GnRH. Exogenous therapy with pulsatile GnRH or gonadotropin therapy usually restores normal pubertal development and fertility.

2. **Functional hypothalamic amenorrhea** can be determined by stress conditions (weight loss, excessive exercise, eating disorders, and psychologic distress) inhibiting the hypothalamic pulsatile secretion of GnRH. Elimination of stressors and administration of exogenous pulsatile GnRH can restore functionality of the hypothalamic–pituitary–gonadal axis.

However, a decrease in the function of the above indicated genes can predispose individuals to abnormal GnRH secretion leading to functional hypothalamic amenorrhea.

Clinical significance: Endometriosis

Endometriosis is a relatively common and painful disorder in which clusters of endometrium become implanted outside the uterus (predominantly in the oviduct, ovaries, and the peritoneal lining of the pelvis). During the menstrual cycle, the implanted endometrial tissue (called **endometrioma**) continues to proliferate, secrete, and bleed in relation to the hormonal levels as the endometrium does. Trapped

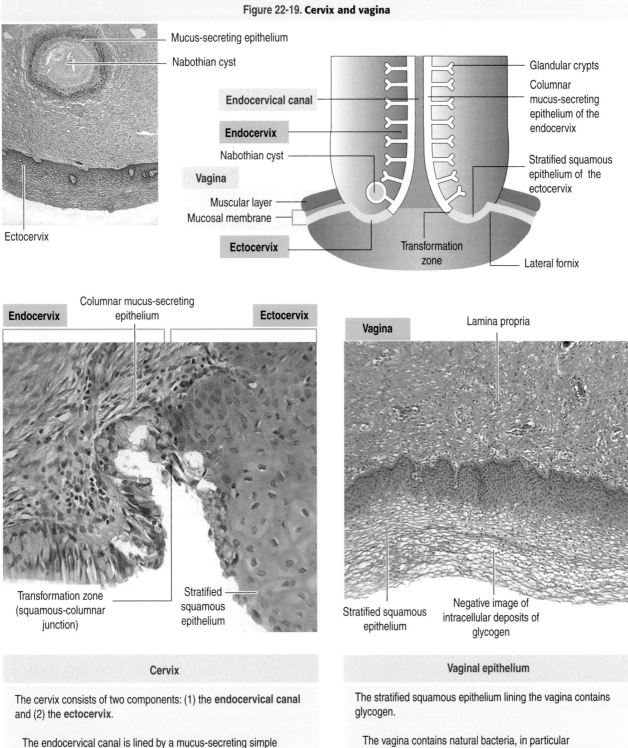

Figure 22-19. Cervix and vagina

Mucus-secreting epithelium

Nabothian cyst

Ectocervix

Endocervical canal

Endocervix

Nabothian cyst

Vagina

Muscular layer

Mucosal membrane

Ectocervix

Glandular crypts

Columnar mucus-secreting epithelium of the endocervix

Stratified squamous epithelium of the ectocervix

Transformation zone

Lateral fornix

Endocervix

Columnar mucus-secreting epithelium

Ectocervix

Transformation zone (squamous-columnar junction)

Stratified squamous epithelium

Vagina

Lamina propria

Stratified squamous epithelium

Negative image of intracellular deposits of glycogen

Cervix

The cervix consists of two components: (1) the **endocervical canal** and (2) the **ectocervix**.

The endocervical canal is lined by a mucus-secreting simple columnar epithelium extending into the lamina propria in the form of glandular crypts. The ectocervix is lined by a stratified squamous epithelium continuous with the vaginal epithelial lining.

Before puberty, the endocervical epithelium extends over the convexity of the ectocervix and becomes exposed to the vaginal environment. The area between the "old" and "new" squamous-columnar epithelial junction is called the **transformation zone**. About 95% of **cervical intraepithelial neoplasias** originates within the transformation zone.

Vaginal epithelium

The stratified squamous epithelium lining the vagina contains glycogen.

The vagina contains natural bacteria, in particular *Lactobacillus acidophilus,* which produces **lactic acid** by the breakdown of **glycogen**. Lactic acid creates an acidic coat (pH 3.0) on the vaginal surface that prevents the proliferation of bacteria. The acidic environment does not protect from **trichomoniasis**, a sexually transmitted infection caused by the flagellated protozoan parasite *Trichomonas vaginalis*.

Antibiotics can destroy the vaginal flora, and *Candida albicans*, a natural fungal component of the vagina, develops on the mucosal surface.

bleeding can give rise to cysts, scar tissue, and peritoneal adhesions.

Chronic pelvic pain occurs during menstruation (**dysmenorrhea**). Excessive bleeding during the menstrual period (**menorrhagia**) or bleeding between periods (**menometrorrhagia**) can be seen. Endometriosis is commonly first diagnosed in patients seeking treatment for **infertility**.

The cause of endometriosis remains elusive. Possible causes include a flow back of endometrial tissue through the oviduct to the implanting site and the dissemination of endometrial cells through the bloodstream.

Diagnosis is established by ultrasound and laparoscopy. The treatment includes pain medications, hormone therapy (oral contraceptives and gonadotropin-releasing hormone agonists and antagonists to block the production of ovarian hormones by creating an induced menopause), and laparoscopy to remove implanted endometriomas. Management of infertility of women with endometriosis consists in gonadotropin-induced superovulation with intrauterine insemination as well as in vitro fertilization.

Cervix

The cervix is the lower extension of the uterus. It communicates with the uterine cavity and the vagina through the **endocervix**.

The endocervix is lined by a folded mucosa consisting of **deep crypts** arranged in different orientations mimicking a system of mucus-secreting tubular glands. This glandular-like arrangement increases the surface area of mucus-producing cells consisting of **simple columnar cells** (Figure 22-19) whose height varies with the time of the menstrual cycle and their secretory activity. Occasionally, some of the crypts become occluded and dilated by the accumulated mucus secretion. These formations are called **cysts of Naboth** or **nabothian cysts**.

The stroma consists predominantly of collagen bundles (dense irregular connective tissue), some smooth muscle cells and abundant blood vessels.

The secretory activity of the **endocervical epithelium** is regulated by **estrogens** and is **maximal at the time of ovulation**. The secreted mucus lubricates the vagina during sexual intercourse and acts as a bacterial protective barrier blocking access to the uterine cavity.

During ovulation, the mucus is **less viscous**, is hydrated, and has an **alkaline pH**, conditions favorable for the migration of sperm. The high content of ions (Na^+, K^+, and Cl^-) is responsible for the **crystallization of the mucus** into a fernlike pattern in the ovulatory phase. This feature of cervical mucus is used clinically to assess the optimal time for fertilization to occur.

After ovulation, the mucus is **highly viscous** with an **acidic pH**, detrimental conditions for sperm penetration and viability.

Pathology: Cervical intraepithelial neoplasia and human papillomavirus infection

The external segment of the cervix, the **ectocervix**, is lined by **stratified squamous epithelium**. There is an abrupt epithelial transition between the endocervix and the ectocervix, called the **transformation zone**.

At the transformation zone, **dysplasia**, an abnormal but reversible condition, may occur. Dysplasia is characterized by disorganized epithelial cells that slough off before reaching full stratified maturity.

However, dysplasia can progress into **carcinoma in situ**, a condition in which proliferation of epithelial cells is very active but within the limits of the basal lamina (**cervical intraepithelial neoplasia or CIN**). This condition can be reversible or can progress (if undetected) into an **invasive carcinoma** that breaks the continuity of the basal lamina and invades the underlying connective tissue. Dysplasia and carcinoma in situ can be detected by the routine **Papanicolaou smear** (Pap smear).

Various strains of the **human papillomavirus (HPV)**, a sexually transmitted infection, have been associated with the majority of cervical cancer cases. Like the Pap smear, cells collected from the cervix can be used to determine by an HPV test whether a patient is infected with any of the 13 types of HPV. This test can detect high-risk HPV strains (for example, HPV-16 and HPV-18) in cell DNA before the development of CIN.

Vagina

The vagina is a fibromuscular tube consisting of three layers:

1. An inner **mucosal layer** (stratified squamous epithelium with a **lamina propria** usually infiltrated by neutrophils and lymphocytes; see Figure 22-19).

2. A middle **muscularis layer** (circular and longitudinal smooth muscle).

3. An outer **adventitial layer** (dense connective tissue).

The surface of the mucosa is kept moist by mucus secreted by uterine and endocervical glands and the **glands of Bartholin** in the vestibule. The wall of the vagina lacks glands.

The vaginal epithelium undergoes cyclic changes during the menstrual cycle. The **differentiation of vaginal epithelium** is stimulated by **estrogens**. At ovulation, the stratified epithelium is fully differentiated, and abundant acidophilic squamous cells can be seen in the Pap smear.

After ovulation, when **progesterone** predominates, the number of squamous cells declines and

Figure 22-20. Diagnostic cytopathology

Physiologic cytohormonal patterns

Menstruation phase

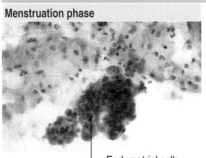

Endometrial cells

Estrogen phase

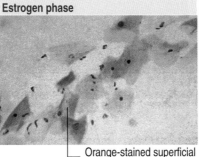

Orange-stained superficial cell of exocervix or vagina

Progesterone phase

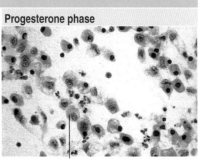

Light green-stained intermediate cell of exocervix or vagina

Human papillomavirus (HPV) infection

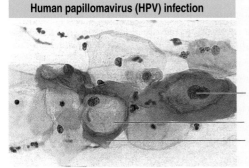

Binucleated koilocyte

Perinuclear halo

Cytoplasmic rim

The presence of koilocytic (Greek *koilos*, hollow; *kytos*, cell) cells in cervicovaginal smear is regarded as a reliable evidence of HPV infection. Koilocytes are squamous cells with a large light perinuclear halo surrounded by a densely stained cytoplasmic rim. The nucleus is enlarged. Cells are often binucleated and multinucleated.

Cervical intraepithelial neoplasia

Dyskaryotic cell

Carcinoma cells extend into the stroma

Carcinoma cells extend into a cervical gland

Inflammatory cells

Cluster of dyskaryotic cells from an early invasive squamous cell carcinoma

Light green-stained nonkeratinized cell

Orange-stained keratinized cell

CIN 3

Severe dyskaryosis of an invasive squamous cell carcinoma

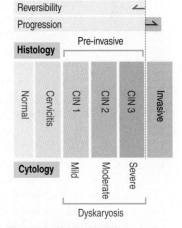

		Pre-invasive			
Reversibility ↰					
Progression →					
Histology					
Normal	Cervicitis	CIN 1	CIN 2	CIN 3	Invasive
Cytology		Mild	Moderate	Severe	
			Dyskaryosis		

The cervical intraepithelial neoplasia (CIN) classification defines cytologic and histologic changes that precede an invasive squamous carcinoma of the cervix. CIN 3 stage can regress or progress into an invasive phase (breakdown of the basement membrane, extension of tumor cells into the stroma, and invasion of blood and lymphatic vessels).

The term dyskaryosis (Greek *dys*, difficult; *karyon*, nucleus; *osis*, condition) designates abnormalities in the structure of the nucleus.

Photographs from Gray W, McKee G: Diagnostic Cytopathology, 2nd edition, Churchill Livingstone, Oxford, UK, 2003.

Figure 22-21. Female urethra

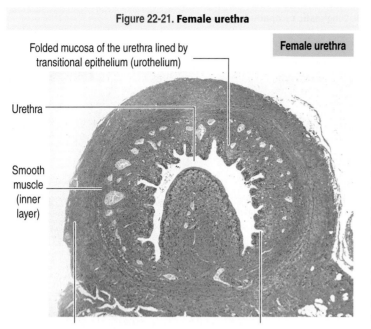

Female urethra

Folded mucosa of the urethra lined by transitional epithelium (urothelium)

Urethra

Smooth muscle (inner layer)

Striated muscle (outer layer)

Mucus-secreting glands

more basophilic polygonal cells appear, together with neurophils and lymphocytes. The vaginal smear provides rapid information on estrogen and progesterone levels during the menstrual cycle and is also useful for monitoring the hormonal status during pregnancy.

Pathology: Diagnostic cytopathology

Diagnostic cytopathology is based on observations of normal and abnormal cells, either exfoliated, or in imprints and scrapes, in correlation with tissue analysis.

The sample collection and staining procedures were introduced in 1941 by George N. Papanicolaou (1883–1962), an anatomist, and Herbert E. Traut (1894-1963), a gynecologist. The diagnostic potential of cytohormonal evaluation using vaginal smears was reported in 1925 by Papanicolaou.

The **Pap smear** is a standard procedure for the early detection of cervicovaginal malignancies. Two components of the Papanicolaou stain are alcohol-based cytoplasmic stains: **eosin**, which stains superficial squamous cells pink or orange, and **light green**, which stains the cytoplasm of less differentiated cells close to the basal lamina. The nuclei are stained with **hematoxylin**.

Estrogens stimulate the differentiation of the superficial layers of the stratified squamous epithelium of the vagina. Once the epithelium has differentiated under the influence of estrogens, progesterone causes rapid desquamation of the topmost pink-orange stained squamous cells and light green-stained polygonal cells of the intermediate layers are seen in the smears (Figure 22-20).

Cervical smears provides evidence of **HPV infection**. The presence of **koilocytes**, squamous cells with a large and well-demarcated clear perinuclear zone surrounded by a dense peripheral cytoplasmic rim are characteristic (see Figure 22-20).

Microinvasive carcinoma of the cervix, preceded by **cervical intraepithelial neoplasia (CIN)** stages 1 and 2 (CIN 1 and CIN 2), is shown in Figure 22-20 (stage CIN 3). The carcinoma extends into a endocervical gland and deep into the stroma in the form of tongues and islands of tumoral cells surrounded by inflammatory cells. The Pap smear detects severe dyskaryosis, inflammatory cells, and keratinized superficial cells, features that alert the cytologist to the possibility of early tumor invasion.

Mons pubis, labia majora, and labia minora

The mons pubis, labia majora, and labia minora are modified skin structures. The **mons pubis** (mons veneris) is skin lined by **keratinized stratified squamous epithelium** with hair follicles covering subcutaneous fat overlying the symphysis pubis.

The **labia majora** are extensions of the mons pubis at each side of the vaginal introitus. In addition to skin with hair follicles and glands (**apocrine sweat glands** and **sebaceous glands**) covering the fat pad, smooth muscle fibers are detected in the subcutaneous fat. Hair follicles and fat accumulation are regulated by sex hormones at the onset of sexual maturity (by the age of 10 to 13 years old).

The **labia minora** are skin folds without adipose tissue and hair follicles but with abundant blood vessels, elastic fibers, and sebaceous glands opening directly onto the surface of the melanin-pigmented epidermis. Pigmentation of the epidermis of both labia majora and minora appears at the initiation of puberty.

The **hymen** is the limit between the internal and external genitalia. It consists of a thin fibrous membrane lining the lower vagina, covered on its external surface by a **keratinized stratified squamous epithelium** and on the internal surface by **nonkeratinizing stratified squamous epithelium** with glycogen (like the vaginal epithelium).

The **clitoris**, located below the mons pubis, is the female equivalent of the penis. Like the penis, it consists of two side-by-side corpora cavernosa (erectile vascular tissue) separated by a septum, surrounded by a fibrous collagenous sheath. The clitoris is partially covered by skin containing rich sensory nerves and receptors but lacking hair follicles and glands.

Urethral meatus and glands (paraurethral glands and Bartholin's glands)

The urethral meatus communicates with the exterior close to the clitoris. **Para-urethral glands of Skene** are distributed around the meatus and are lined by **pseudostratified columnar epithelium**.

Bartholin's vulvovaginal glands are found around the lower vagina and consist of acini with mucus-secreting cells. A duct covered by a transitional epithelium connects these glands to the posterolateral side of the vagina.

The **female urethra** is covered by a **folded mucosa** lined by a pseudostratified columnar epithelium changing to **transitional epithelium** and, near the urethral meatus, to a nonkeratinizing stratified squamous epithelium. **Mucus-secreting glands** are observed in the **mucosa** (Figure 22-21). The **muscular wall** consists of a **single longitudinal layer of smooth muscle (involuntary sphincter)**. A **circular striated muscle (voluntary sphincter)** is observed outside the smooth muscle layer. A connective tissue rich in elastic fibers provides support to the muscle layers.

Essential concepts	Follicle Development and The Menstrual Cycle

• Development of the ovary. The cortical region of the indifferent gonad develops into an ovary.

Primary sex cords, derived from the coelomic epithelium, are replaced by secondary sex cords surrounding oogonia. Oogonia are mitotically dividing cells derived from primordial germ cells with two X chromosomes. Oogonia complete mitosis and enter meiotic prophase I to become primary oocytes. Meiosis is arrested following crossing over, a stage that persists until puberty. Therefore, at the time of birth, primary oocytes at the diplotene stage of Meiosis I are surrounded by granulosa cells.

• Development of the female genital ducts. The cranial ends of the müllerian ducts remain separated to form the oviduct. The caudal segments fuse to develop into the uterovaginal primordium, which becomes the uterus and upper part of the vagina. The canalization of the vaginal plate (the contact point of the uterovaginal primordium with the urogenital sinus) results in the middle and lower parts of the vagina. The genital tubercle (phallus) develops at the cranial end of the cloacal membrane. The labioscrotal swellings (that will give rise to the labia majora) and urogenital folds (that will give rise to the labia minora) develop at either side of the cloacal

membrane. In the absence of androgens, the phallus develops into the clitoris.

• Failure of müllerian development occurs in 46,XX female patients with müllerian agenesis (Mayer–Rokitansky–Küster–Hauser syndrome). Müllerian agenesis is characterized by the absence of the uterus, cervix, and upper vagina. Kidney abnormalities, including a pelvic kidney or the more severe unilateral agenesis of the kidney, are observed. Inactivation of the *Wnt4* gene has been implicated in this disorder.

Persistent müllerian duct syndrome (PMDS) occurs in 46,XY males as a rare form of male

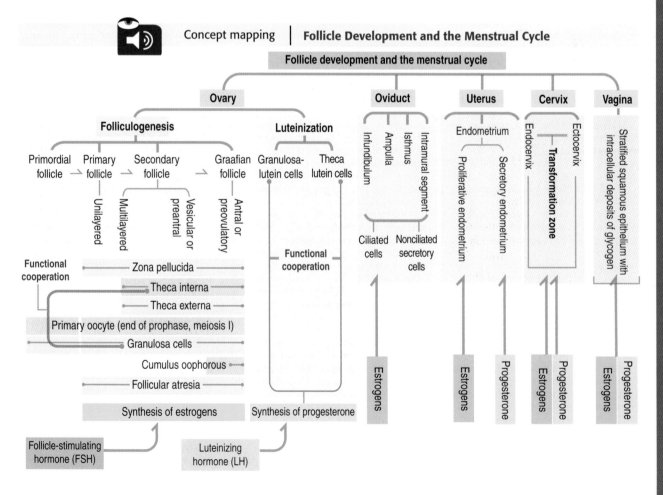

Concept mapping | **Follicle Development and the Menstrual Cycle**

pseudohermaphroditism. It is caused by a defect in either the *AMH* gene or its receptor (AMHR2).

Turner's syndrome is determined by the absence of all or part of a second X chromosome (45,X) and a lack of Barr bodies. The prenatal diagnosis of Turner's syndrome is based on the finding of fetal edema on ultrasonography, abnormal levels of human chorionic gonadotropin, and α-fetoprotein during the screening of maternal serum. A 45,X fetus often aborts spontaneously.

Physical findings recognized in prepubertal and pubertal girls include congenital lymphedema, short stature, and gonadal dysgenesis. The atrophic ovaries are represented by streaks. Puffy hands and feet or redundant nuchal skin are characteristic clinical findings.

• The ovary is lined by an ovarian surface epithelium (OSE; simple squamous-to-low cuboidal epithelium) with Lgr5-positive (Lgr5+). OSE cells are capable of regenerative repair after ovulation. The OSE is supported by a layer of connective tissue, the tunica albuginea. The ovary has a cortex and a medulla. The cortex houses the primordial follicles; the medulla is connected to the hilum consisting of blood vessels (ovarian artery and vein), nerves, and lymphatic vessels. Lgr5+ cells are present in the ovarian hilum.

The **ovarian cycle** comprises three phases:
(1) Follicular phase, consisting of the development of a primordial follicle into a preovulatory, antral or graafian follicle.
(2) Ovulatory phase, characterized by the rupture of the graafian follicle, completion of meiosis I (resulting in the formation of the first polar body), and release of the now secondary oocyte from the ovary.
(3) Luteal phase, the transformation of the residual mural granulosa cell layer and theca interna cells into a vascularized, steroid-producing corpus luteum.

The **follicular phase** (or folliculogenesis) results in the following sequence:
(1) Primordial follicle: a primary oocyte is surrounded by a single layer of flattened squamous granulosa cells supported by a basal lamina.
(2) Primary (unilayered) follicle: a primary oocyte surrounded by a single layer of cuboidal granulosa cells.
(3) Secondary (multilayered) follicle: the primary oocyte becomes gradually separated from multilayered proliferating granulosa cells by the developing zona pellucida.
Cell processes of the granulosa cells adjacent to the zona pellucida (the future corona radiata) penetrate the thickened zona pellucida and establish contact with the plasma membrane of the primary oocyte.
Reciprocal molecular cooperation occurs between the primary oocyte and granulosa cells. Gap junctions are present at the contact points and between adjacent granulosa cells.
(4) Preantral follicle: enlarging intercellular

spaces separate granulosa cells from each other. In addition, spaces containing fluid (liquor folliculi; also named Call-Exner bodies) appear between the multilayered granulosa cells. These spaces will coalesce to form the antrum in the mature follicle.

Stromal cells surrounding the developing follicle differentiate into two layers:
The highly vascularized theca interna, producing androstenedione that is transferred to granulosa cells across the basal lamina so they can produce estrogen.
The theca externa, a connective tissue continuous with the ovarian stroma.
(5) Antral follicle: consists of a primary oocyte surrounded by the zona pellucida. A single large space containing fluid, the antrum, is seen.
(6) Preovulatory follicle (Graffian follicle): the granulosa cells become displaced by the fluid in the antrum and segregate the granulosa cells into two distinct regions:
The cumulus granulosa cell region, represented by granulosa cells surrounding the zona pellucida-primary oocyte complex.
The mural granulosa cell region, lining the wall of the follicle. The cumulus prevents the primary oocyte-zona pellucida-corona radiata complex from floating freely in the antrum fluid.
Follicular atresia is a physiologic apoptotic process consisting of a failure of ovarian follicles to complete folliculogenesis at any point in development.

• Two forms of paracrine signaling take place during folliculogenesis:
(1) Granulosa cell–primary oocyte bidirectional signaling.
(2) Theca interna–granulosa cell synergistic communication.
Zona pellucida, a glycoprotein coat that separates a corona radiata from the primary oocyte, is penetrated by thin cytoplasmic processes of granulosa cells of the corona radiata and contact the microvilli of the oocyte.
These contact sites:
(1) Are mediated by gap junctions and adherent junctions.
(2) Enable specific members of the transforming growth factor-β (TGF-β) family to prevents the untimely completion of meiotic prophase of the primary oocyte. Gap junctions are also seen between granulosa cells.
Connexin 37 is present in gap junctions linking granulosa cells of the corona radiata and the primary oocyte. Connexin 43 is found in gap junctions connecting granulosa cells.
A lack of connexin 37, encoded by the *Gja4* gene, stops follicle development and interferes with the capacity of the primary oocyte to resume meiosis. A lack of connexin 43 disrupts folliculogenesis during the preantral phase.
Two oocyte-derived members of the TGF-β family facilitate the growth and maturation of the primary oocyte:
(1) Growth and differentiation factor-9 (GDF-9).
(2) Bone morphogenetic protein-15 (BMP-15).

GDF-9 and BMP-15 regulate the energy metabolism and cholesterol biosynthesis of granulosa cells. GDF-9 is also required for the formation by granulosa cells of cell processes that penetrate and cross the zona pellucida.

Granulosa cell-derived members of the TGF-β superfamily, AMH, inhibin, and activin, are also involved in the regulation of granulosa cell function during folliculogenesis.

How does the meiotic prophase stage of the primary oocyte remain frozen during folliculogenesis and is not completed before ovulation?
Granulosa cell-derived proteins include:
(1) Oocyte maturation inhibitor (OMI).
(2) Stem cell factor.
OMI prevents the resumption of meiosis by primary oocytes of antral follicles prior to the surge of FSH and LH at ovulation.
Stem cell factor binds to the oocyte c-kit receptor and stimulates oocyte growth and survival.

Polycystic ovary syndrome (PCOS) result from disrupted folliculogenesis caused by a defect in the paracrine oocyte-granulosa cell signaling mechanism. PCOS refers to a clinical condition associated with infrequent or prolonged menstrual periods, excess hair growth (hirsutism), acne, and obesity. Blood levels of androgens are elevated. Infrequent or absent menstruation in adolescents may raise suspicion for PCOS.

How does the primary oocyte complete meiosis I before ovulation?
Just before ovulation, the oocyte activates itself by inducing completion of meiotic prophase. The cyclin B–Cdc2 complex constitutes the maturation promoting factor (MPF) that induces the breakdown of the oocyte nuclear envelope (an event called germinal vesicle breakdown, GVBD). MPF action results in formation of the secondary oocyte and release of the first polar body, that is retained in the perivitelline space.

• Two hormones of the anterior hypophysis regulate follicular growth and the menstrual cycle:
(1) Follicle-stimulating hormone (FSH) stimulates folliculogenesis and ovulation as well as the production of estrogen.
(2) Luteinizing hormone (LH) stimulates the secretion of progesterone by the corpus luteum.
Remember the following key steps of hormonal regulation:
(1) A surge of LH immediately precedes ovulation.
(2) Continued LH secretion induces the luteinization of the residual mural granulosa cell layer after ovulation.
(3) The production of FSH and LH decreases when the levels of progesterone and estrogen are high, and then the corpus luteum enters involution (if no pregnancy occurs).
(4) Note that the events originated in the ovaries are the ones that determine hypothalamic and hypophysis responses.

(5) At the initiation of menstruation, estrogen and progesterone levels are low and increase gradually during the preovulatory period.

(6) Estrogen reaches maximum levels just before the LH peak precedes ovulation.

(7) The FSH-dependent synthesis of estrogen by granulosa cells stimulates the proliferation of the endometrial glands.

(8) LH-dependent synthesis of progesterone by the corpus luteum triggers and maintains the secretory activity of the endometrial glands.

• The following endometrial changes take place during the **menstrual cycle**:

(1) During the early proliferative period, the endometrial glands are short, straight, and narrow.

(2) During the midproliferative period, the endometrial glands are longer and straight. The epithelium is mitotically active.

(3) During the late proliferative period, the mitotic activity is intense and the endometrial glands grow rapidly and become tortuous. The cells of the stroma surrounding the spiral arteries enlarge and become decidual-like.

(4) During the midsecretory period, glycogen accumulates in the basal portion of the glandular epithelial cells. The endometrial glands have a saw- toothed appearance.

(5) During the late secretory period, glycogen translocates from the basal to the apical portion of the glandular epithelial cells and secretion accumulates in the lumen. The stromal cells surrounding the spiral arteries are mitotically active, an indication of a decidual change.

(6) During the ischemic period, the upper region of the endometrial stroma contains numerous decidual cells. The spiral arteries contract and ischemia starts.

• A mechanism prevents primary oocytes from completing meiosis I while they remain inside the developing follicle.

Granulosa cells produce oocyte maturation inhibitor, which is transferred from granulosa cells to the oocyte through cytoplasmic processes crossing the zona pellucida and connected to the oocyte by gap junctions.

Just before ovulation, the oocyte produces maturation promoting factor (Cdc2-cyclin B complex), which induces completion of meiosis I and formation of the first polar body.

The luteal phase occurs soon after ovulation and consists of the formation of the corpus luteum (a process called luteinization).

Luteinization consists of:

(1) The breakdown of the basal lamina of the follicle.

(2) The invasion of blood vessels from the theca interna.

(3) The transformation of the remnant mural granulosa cells into granulosa lutein cells and of the theca interna cells into theca lutein cells.

The secretion of estrogen and progesterone takes place in response to FSH and LH stimulation. Theca lutein cells cooperate with follicular lutein cells to produce estradiol; both cell types can independently synthesize progesterone.

When fertilization occurs, the secondary oocyte completes meiosis II, produces the second polar body, and becomes a haploid pronucleus that fuses with the haploid sperm pronucleus to form a zygote.

The trophoblastic cells of the implanted embryo produce chorionic gonadotropin, which will take over the control of corpus luteum estrogen and progesterone secretory function.

If fertilization does not occur, the corpus luteum undergoes degeneration (a process called luteolysis) and changes into a connective tissue scar called corpus albicans.

• **Oviduct** (fallopian tube or uterine tube). The oviduct is a muscular tube with four anatomic regions:

(1) Infundibulum has finger-like folds called fimbriae, responsible for capturing the ovulated complex from the ovary.

(2) Ampulla is the site where fertilization takes place.

(3) Isthmus is the site where:

• The muscle layer of the tube thickens.

• Muscle contraction helps the displacement of sperm toward the ovulated egg or ovum.

• Muscle contraction propels the fertilized embryo to the uterus.

(4) Intramural segment at the oviduct-uterine junction.

The wall of the oviduct consists of three layers:

(1) The mucosa, consisting of a simple columnar epithelium with ciliated and nonciliated cells supported by a lamina propria.

(2) A smooth muscular cell layer.

(3) A serosa layer.

• Mons pubis, labia majora, and labia minora are modified skin structures. The mons pubis is skin lined by keratinized stratified squamous epithelium. The labia majora have, in addition to skin, apocrine sweat glands and sebaceous glands. Labia minora are melanin-pigmented epidermal skin folds with abundant blood vessels, elastic fibers, and sebaceous glands.

• Female urethra. The female urethra has a folded mucosa lined by columnar pseudostratified epithelium changing into transitional epithelium with mucosa glands. Near the urethral meatus, the epithelium changes into a nonkeratinizing stratified squamous epithelium.

The muscle wall consists of an inner smooth muscle layer (involuntary sphincter) and an outer striated muscle layer (voluntary sphincter).

Note that the presence of Lgr5+ cells in the OSE, hilum of the ovary and fimbriae of the oviduct indicates a potential for neoplastic transformation in these three sites.

• **Uterus**. The uterus consists of two anatomic segments: the corpus or body, and the cervix.

The body of the uterus consists of three layers: the endometrium, the myometrium, and the serosa/adventitia.

The myometrium has three poorly defined smooth muscle layers. During pregnancy, the myometrial smooth muscle enlarges (hypertrophy) and the fibers increase in number (hyperplasia).

Inhibition of myometrial contraction during pregnancy is controlled by relaxin, a peptide hormone produced in the ovary and placenta.

Myometrial contraction during parturition is under the control of oxytocin, a peptide hormone secreted from the neurohypophysis.

The endometrium consists of a simple columnar epithelial cell lining that invaginates to form simple tubular endometrial glands surrounded by a lamina propria, the endometrial stroma.

The endometrium has:

(1) A superficial functional layer, lost during menstruation.

(2) A basal layer, retained during menstruation as a reserve for tissue regeneration.

The superficial functional layer is supplied by a spiral endometrial artery; the basal layer is supplied by a basal straight artery, an independent blood supply.

Four consecutive phases characterize the menstrual cycle:

(1) The menstrual phase (days 1 to 5).

(2) The proliferative or estrogenic phase (days 5 to 14).

(3) The secretory or progestational phase (days 15 to 27).

(4) The ischemic phase (days 27 to 28).

Contraction of the spiral endometrial artery during the ischemic phase reduces blood flow and triggers the destruction of the functional endometrial layer.

Ovulation marks the end of the proliferative phase and the beginning of the secretory phase.

If pregnancy takes place, cells of the endometrial stroma change into an epithelial-like shape and become decidual cells. This change is called the decidual reaction.

Decidual cells modulate trophoblast-driven embryo implantation, provide nutrients to the developing embryo, and, together with the trophoblast, prevent immunologic rejection of genetically different embryonic and fetal tissues.

• **Endometriosis** is a disorder characterized by the implantation and growth of endometrial tissue (called endometrioma) in the oviduct, ovaries, and pelvic peritoneal surface.

The ectopic endometrial tissue responds to hormonal stimulation, like the endometrium.

Pelvic pain during menstruation (dysmenorrhea), excessive bleeding during menstruation (menorrhagia), or bleeding between periods (menometrorrhagia) are characteristic clinical findings.

Infertility is associated with endometriosis.

• Cervix. The cervix consists of two components:
   (1) The endocervical canal.
   (2) The ectocervix.
   The endocervical canal is lined by a mucus-secreting simple columnar epithelium extending into the lamina propria forming glandular crypts.
   During ovulation, the mucus is less viscous and alkaline, two conditions favoring sperm penetration. After ovulation, the mucus becomes viscous and acidic, two unfavorable conditions for sperm penetration.
   Occlusion of the glandular crypts gives rise to cysts, called cysts of Naboth or nabothian cysts.
   The ectocervix is lined by a stratified squamous epithelium. The simple columnar-stratified squamous epithelial junction is called the transformation zone, the site of origin of most cervical intraepithelial neoplasias (CINs).

• Human papillomavirus (HPV), a sexually transmitted infection, has been associated with the development of CINs. CIN can be reversible or can progress (if undetected) into a microinvasive cervical carcinoma.
   About 13 strains of the HPV exist. The high-risk HPV strains are HPV-16 and HPV-18.

   The Papanicolaou test (Pap smear) has played a significant role in the early detection of cervical cancer.
   Cervical smears provides evidence of HPV infection by detecting koilocytes, squamous cells with a large and well-demarcated clear perinuclear zone surrounded by a dense peripheral cytoplasmic rim.
   Microinvasive carcinoma of the cervix CIN stage 3 (CIN 3) is preceded by CIN stages 1 and 2 (CIN 1 and CIN 2).
   In CIN 3, the carcinoma extends deep into the stroma in the form of tongues and islands of tumoral cells surrounded by inflammatory cells.
   At this stage, the Pap smear detects severe dyskaryosis, inflammatory cells, and keratinized superficial cells, features that alert the cytologist to the possibility of early tumor invasion.

• Vagina. A fibromuscular tube consisting of three layers: an inner mucosa layer (stratified squamous epithelium, rich in glycogen, supported by a lamina propria), a middle smooth muscle layer, and an outer connective tissue adventitial layer. The differentiation of the vaginal epithelium is hormone-dependent and undergoes cyclic changes during the

menstrual cycle. The breakdown of glycogen by *Lactobacillus acidophilus* into lactic acid creates an acidic vaginal coat preventing proliferation of bacteria but not sexually transmitted pathogens.

• Mons pubis, labia majora, and labia minora are modified skin structures. The mons pubis is skin lined by keratinized stratified squamous epithelium with hair follicles covering subcutaneous fat overlying the symphysis pubis.
   The labia majora have, in addition to skin, apocrine sweat glands and sebaceous glands. The labia minora are melanin-pigmented epidermal skin folds with abundant blood vessels, elastic fibers, and sebaceous glands.

• Female urethra. The female urethra has a folded mucosa lined by a pseudostratified columnar epithelium changing into transitional epithelium with mucus-secreting glands in the mucosa. Near the urethral meatus, the epithelium changes into a nonkeratinizing stratified squamous epithelium.
   The muscular wall consists of an inner smooth muscle layer (involuntary sphincter) and an outer striated muscle layer (voluntary sphincter).

23. Fertilization, Placentation, and Lactation

During fertilization, a haploid sperm and a haploid egg fuse to form a diploid zygote. The resulting zygote forms soon after capacitated sperm are guided by chemoattractants to the egg. After crossing a layer of granulosa cells and binding to the sperm receptor on the zona pellucida, the first sperm completing the journey achieves sperm-egg fusion. The embryo travels along the oviduct, finds its way to the uterus, implants in a receptive endometrium, and secures fetal development by constructing a placenta. The mother provides nourishment to the newborn by milk produced in the mammary glands prepared for lactation during pregnancy.

Fertilization

Fertilizing sperm must complete **maturation** and **capacitation** before sperm-egg fusion can take place.

Sperm released from the testis and entering the epididymal duct display **circular motion**. After a 2-week **maturation** process during epididymal transit, sperm acquire **forward motility**, a requirement for fertilization.

After ejaculation, a number of sperm undergo a **capacitation process** in a storage site in the isthmus of the oviduct. Capacitated sperm are then guided by a combination of chemotaxis and thermotaxis from the storage site to the ovum or egg in the ampulla of the oviduct where fertilization takes place.

Capacitation is a biochemical event that can be induced in vitro to enable in vitro fertilization. During capacitation:

1. Non-covalently bound epididymal and seminal glycoproteins are diluted from the sperm plasma membrane by fluids of the female reproductive tract .

2. The sperm influx of external **bicarbonate ions** stimulates the activity of a specific adenylyl cyclase (ADCY10) to maximize intracellular cyclic adenosine monophosphate (cAMP) levels, contributing to the **start** of capacitation.

3. Sperm membrane permeability to Ca^{2+} increases. An influx of Ca^{2+}, enabled through a flagellar pH-sensitive **CatSper** (for Cation Sperm) Ca^{2+} channel (Figure 23-1), starts in the principal piece of the sperm tail, reaching the sperm head in a few seconds.

Figure 23-1. Acrosome reaction

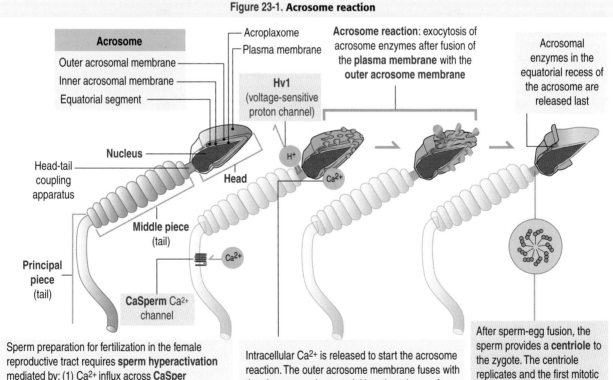

Acrosome
Outer acrosomal membrane
Inner acrosomal membrane
Equatorial segment

Acroplaxome
Plasma membrane

Acrosome reaction: exocytosis of acrosome enzymes after fusion of the **plasma membrane** with the **outer acrosome membrane**

Acrosomal enzymes in the equatorial recess of the acrosome are released last

Hv1
(voltage-sensitive proton channel)

H^+

Ca^{2+}

Nucleus
Head-tail coupling apparatus

Head

Middle piece
(tail)

Principal piece (tail)

Ca^{2+}

CaSperm Ca^{2+} channel

Sperm preparation for fertilization in the female reproductive tract requires **sperm hyperactivation** mediated by: (1) Ca^{2+} influx across **CaSper channels** and (2) sperm intracellular alkalinization and regulation of sperm intracellular Ca^{2+} levels through **Hv1**, the voltage-gated proton channel.

Intracellular Ca^{2+} is released to start the acrosome reaction. The outer acrosome membrane fuses with the plasma membrane to initiate the release of acrosomal enzymes. Membrane fusion is a calcium-dependent process.

After sperm-egg fusion, the sperm provides a **centriole** to the zygote. The centriole replicates and the first mitotic spindle is assembled in the zygote. **The unfertilized egg lacks centrioles.**

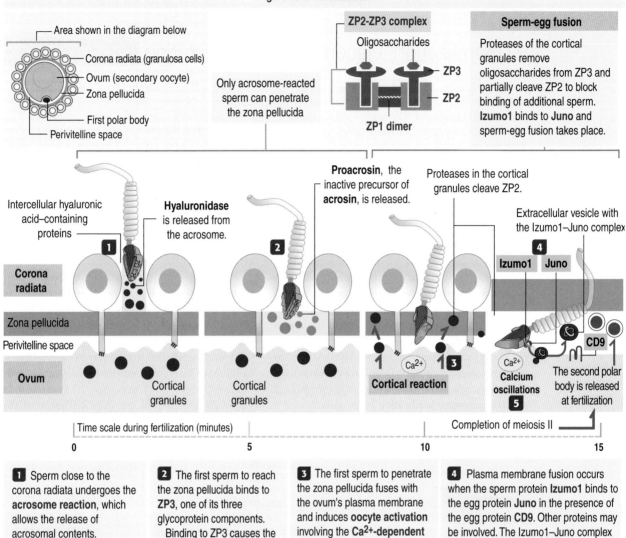

Figure 23-2. Fertilization

Area shown in the diagram below
- Corona radiata (granulosa cells)
- Ovum (secondary oocyte)
- Zona pellucida
- First polar body
- Perivitelline space

Only acrosome-reacted sperm can penetrate the zona pellucida

ZP2-ZP3 complex
Oligosaccharides
ZP3
ZP2
ZP1 dimer

Sperm-egg fusion
Proteases of the cortical granules remove oligosaccharides from ZP3 and partially cleave ZP2 to block binding of additional sperm. **Izumo1** binds to **Juno** and sperm-egg fusion takes place.

Intercellular hyaluronic acid–containing proteins

Hyaluronidase is released from the acrosome.

Proacrosin, the inactive precursor of **acrosin**, is released.

Proteases in the cortical granules cleave ZP2.

Extracellular vesicle with the Izumo1–Juno complex

Izumo1   Juno

Corona radiata

Zona pellucida

Perivitelline space

Ovum

Cortical granules

Cortical granules

Cortical reaction

Ca²⁺

CD9

Ca²⁺

Calcium oscillations

The second polar body is released at fertilization

Time scale during fertilization (minutes)   Completion of meiosis II

0   5   10   15

1 Sperm close to the corona radiata undergoes the **acrosome reaction**, which allows the release of acrosomal contents.
   Hyaluronidase released from the acrosome dissolves the intercellular material between granulosa cells of the corona radiata.

2 The first sperm to reach the zona pellucida binds to **ZP3**, one of its three glycoprotein components.
   Binding to ZP3 causes the release of **acrosin** from the inner acrosomal membrane.
   Acrosin facilitates penetration of the zona by the sperm head.

3 The first sperm to penetrate the zona pellucida fuses with the ovum's plasma membrane and induces **oocyte activation** involving the **Ca²⁺-dependent exocytosis of protease–containing cortical granules** located just beneath the oocyte plasma membrane. This process, called **cortical reaction**, prevents polyspermy.

4 Plasma membrane fusion occurs when the sperm protein **Izumo1** binds to the egg protein **Juno** in the presence of the egg protein **CD9**. Other proteins may be involved. The Izumo1–Juno complex is released to prevent polyspermy.
5 Sperm fusion causes oocyte intracellular **calcium oscillations** in response to a sperm-specific phospholipase C. Calcium oscillations lead the oocyte to complete meiosis II.

4. Sperm cytoplasmic acidic pH (lower than pH 6.5) changes to an alkaline intracellular pH (pH 7.4) through the extrusion of H⁺ through **Hv1**, a **voltage-sensitive proton channel**. An increase in sperm intracellular pH **completes** capacitation.

Why is Ca²⁺ and alkalinization so important to achieve sperm capacitation?

Increases in Ca²⁺ concentration induce the exocytotic **acrosome reaction** in the sperm head and alkalinization triggers sperm **hyperactivation** (intensification of the beating of the sperm tail).

What is **acrosome reaction**?

We have seen in Chapter 20, Spermatogenesis, that the **sperm head** consists of three components:

1. The **condensed elongated nucleus.**

2. The **acrosome,** bound to the **acroplaxome,** a cytoskeletal plate anchoring the acrosome to the nuclear envelope.

Box 23-A | Tetraspanins

- **Tetraspanins,** first discovered on the human leukocyte surface, have four transmembrane domains, two extracellular loops (small and large), and short intracytoplasmic N- and C-terminal tails.
- The transmembrane domains enable the association of additional tetraspanins to assemble the tetraspanin web in which integrins are included.
- The large extracellular loop is involved in protein-protein interaction with laterally positioned proteins.
- The intracellular short tails are linked to intracellular cytoskeletal and signaling molecules.

3. The **plasma membrane**.

The **acrosome**, in turn, consists of:

- The **outer acrosomal membrane**.
- The **inner acrosomal membrane**.
- A content of **hydrolytic enzymes** (mainly **hyaluronidase** and **acrosin,** the latter derived from the precursor **proacrosin**).

The thin portion of the acrosomal sac, extending toward the tail, is the **equatorial segment** (see Figure 23-1). The equatorial region of the acrosome does not participate in the acrosome reaction. Three sequential events take place during fertilization:

1. The **acrosome reaction**.
2. **Sperm binding to a receptor on ZP3,** a glycoprotein of the zona pellucida (ZP).
3. **Sperm-egg fusion** (Figure 23-2).

In the proximity of the ovum, and in the presence of free Ca^{2+}, **the sperm plasma membrane fuses with the outer acrosomal membrane,** an event known as **acrosome reaction.**

Small openings created by membrane fusion permit

the leakage of hydrolytic enzymes (see Figures 23-1 and 23-2). **Hyaluronidase** breaks down proteins present in the intercellular space of granulosa cells of the corona radiata. Proacrosin changes into **acrosin** and enables the fertilizing sperm to cross the zona pellucida.

Male infertility may occur when the acrosome reaction fails to occur or takes place before the sperm reaches the oocyte, also called **egg**.

After crossing the zona pellucida, the plasma membrane of the sperm (the post-acrosomal equatorial region) and plasma membrane of the egg fuse to enable the sperm nucleus to reach the cytoplasm of the oocyte. The insertion of the sperm nucleus into the cytoplasm of the egg is called **impregnation**.

How does sperm-egg fusion take place?

Two membrane proteins are regarded essential for sperm-egg fusion:

1. **Izumo1,** a protein of the immunoglobulin superfamily, is inserted in the sperm plasma membrane.
2. **Juno,** present in the egg plasma membrane.

In the presence of CD9, Izumo1 binds to Juno to achieve sperm–egg fusion. Then, the Izumo1-Juno complex is sequestered within a membrane-bound vesicle and ejected into the perivitelline space (see Figure 23-2).

This event, together with a conformation change in the molecular organization of the zona pellucida, block the binding and fusion of additional sperm, thus preventing polyspermy.

CD9 is a member of the tetraspanin superfamily of transmembrane proteins (see Box 23-A). Other proteins, such as ADAMs (a disintegrin and metalloprotease), may participate in this reaction.

We discussed in Chapter 1, Epithelium, how the disintegrin domain of ADAMS participates in the shedding of the ectoplasmic portion of transmembrane proteins.

Sperm-egg fusion causes a local mild depolarization of the egg plasma membrane that generates within 5 to 20 seconds **calcium oscillations** across the cytoplasm of the fertilized egg. Calcium oscillations result in **oocyte activation** involving two fundamental steps in the process of fertilization (see Box 23-B):

1. The **exocytosis of the protease ovastacin from cortical granules.** During this event, a vesicle is formed to dispose the Izumo1–Juno complex into the perivitelline space.

2. To trigger the secondary oocyte to **complete meiosis II**. The second polar body is released into the perivitelline space and the secondary oocyte achieves a haploid state. Completion of meiosis II starts the early embryogenesis developmental program as a zygote.

Remember that the sperm contributes the **centrosome** responsible for assembling the first mitotic spindle of the new embryo and that **mitochondria** derive from the fertilized egg.

Figure 23-3. Implantation of the blastocyst

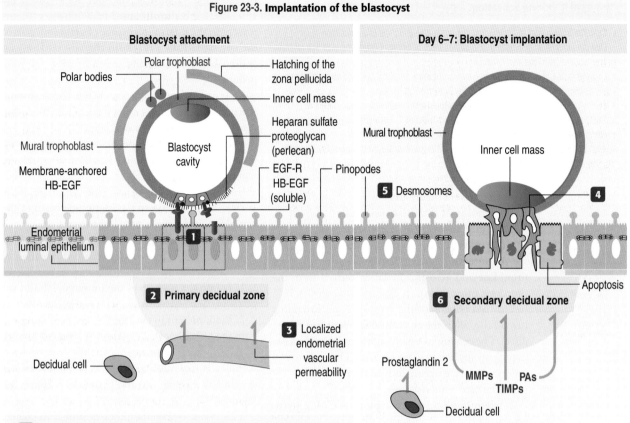

Blastocyst attachment

- Polar bodies
- Polar trophoblast
- Hatching of the zona pellucida
- Inner cell mass
- Mural trophoblast
- Blastocyst cavity
- Heparan sulfate proteoglycan (perlecan)
- Membrane-anchored HB-EGF
- EGF-R HB-EGF (soluble)
- Pinopodes
- Endometrial luminal epithelium

Day 6–7: Blastocyst implantation

- Mural trophoblast
- Inner cell mass
- **5** Desmosomes
- **4**
- Apoptosis

2 Primary decidual zone

- Decidual cell
- **3** Localized endometrial vascular permeability

6 Secondary decidual zone

- Prostaglandin 2
- MMPs
- PAs
- TIMPs
- Decidual cell

1 At the site of blastocyst apposition, uterine endometrial cells express **heparin-bound epidermal growth factor–like factor** (HB-EGF) with binding affinity to **heparan sulfate proteoglycans** and **EGF receptor** (EGF-R) on the surface of the trophoectoderm.

Binding of membrane-anchored or soluble HB-EGF to EGF-R induces receptor autophosphorylation. The apical domain of uterine epithelial cells contains microprocesses, the **pinopodes**, interacting with microvilli on the apical surface of polar trophoblast cells.

2 Decidual cells become epithelial-like and proliferate and the **primary decidual zone** develops. Fibronectin, laminin, entactin, and types I, III, IV, and V collagen are components of the primary decidual zone. Bone morphogenetic protein-2 and -7, fibroblast growth factor-2, Wnt-4, and proteins of the Hedgehog family are expressed.

3 **Localized vascular permeability** is observed at the implantation site.

4 Processes of the polar trophoblast cells penetrate between uterine luminal cells that undergo apoptosis.

5 A reduction in the number of desmosomes facilitates embryo penetration.

6 A **secondary decidual zone** replaces the primary decidual zone. Matrix metalloproteinases (**MMPs**), tissue inhibitors of MMPs (**TIMPs**), plasminogen activators (**PAs**), and inhibitors regulate the **remodeling of the decidual zone** in the presence of **prostaglandin 2**.

The normal site of implantation is the endometrium of the posterior wall of the uterus, nearer to the fudus than to the cervix

Zona pellucida during fertilization

We have discussed in Chapter 22, Follicle Development and The Menstrual Cycle, aspects of the development of the zona pellucida.

The plasma membrane of mammalian eggs is surrounded by a 6- to 7-μm-thick zona pellucida (plural zonae pellucidae), a glycoprotein coat produced mainly by the primary oocyte during folliculogenesis, as early as during the primary follicle stage.

The zona pellucida has important roles in fertilization and implantation of the embryo in the endometrium. In vitro fertilization procedures overcome the inability of some sperm of penetrating the zona pellucida, a form of infertility (see Box 23-C).

The zona pellucida is composed of three glycoproteins (see Figure 23-2):

1. **ZP1**, a dimer of 200 kd.
2. **ZP2**, 120 kd.
3. **ZP3**, 83 kd.

ZP2 and ZP3 interact to form a long filament interconnected by ZP1 dimers at regular intervals.

There are four functional aspects related to ZP3 to keep in mind:

1. ZP3 is responsible for sperm binding, mediated

by *O*-oligosaccharides linked to ZP3 with binding affinity to sperm receptors.

2. **Only acrosome-reacted sperm can interact with ZP3.**

3. **ZP3 is essential for species specific sperm binding.** It prevents sperm from a different species to fertilize the egg.

4. After the first sperm fertilizes the egg, the protease ovastacin, released from the cortical granules of the egg, removes oligosaccharides from ZP3 and partially cleaves ZP2. This process, called **cortical reaction**, together with the disposal of the Izumo1-Juno complex, prevent polyspermy. Polyspermy results in nonviable zygotes. Ovastacin is an oocyte-specific member of the astacin family of metalloendoproteases.

Putting things together, **sperm maturation** in the epididymis, **sperm capacitation** in the female reproductive tract, and **acrosome reaction** in the proximity of the ovulated secondary oocyte are sequential steps leading to fertilization.

Sperm reach a **storage site** in the isthmus region of the oviduct and a fraction of them undergoes capacitation. Sperm reach the oviduct assisted by **sperm motility** as well as on a passive drag by **waves of muscular contractile activity** of the vagina, cervix, and uterus.

Fertilization takes place in the ampulla of the oviduct.

Sperm are guided to the egg by:

1. A **chemoattractant gradient** present in the oviductal fluid and originated in the egg and granulosa cells anchored to the zona pellucida.

2. A **temperature gradient** between the storage site (34.7°C) and the fertilization site (36.3°C).

3. Contractions of the oviduct wall.

Two barriers that the fertilizing sperm confront during fertilization are the **corona radiata** and the **zona pellucida**. Enzymes released following the acrosome reaction enable the sperm to cross these barriers. The final step of fertilization is the **fusion of the plasma membranes** of the sperm and the secondary oocyte. Two plasma membrane proteins, **Izumo1** in sperm and **Juno** in the oocyte, achieve sperm-egg fusion.

Recall from our discussion in Chapter 20, Spermatogenesis, that sperm condensed chromatin lacks nucleosomes. Somatic histones have been replaced by a protamine complex during spermiogenesis. Therefore, the zygote needs to resolve differences in the chromatin state of the egg and sperm pronuclei to make sure that:

1. The first mitotic division can take place.

2. The embryo can take full control of gene expression for embryonic development by a process termed **zygotic genome activation**.

The **calcium oscillations** across the cytoplasm of the fertilized egg that we mentioned before, responsible for the completion of meiosis II, trigger the rapid removal of the protamine complex of the sperm pronucleus and DNA is re-wrapped by somatic histones donated by the egg.

One final point: remember that the embryo undergoes extensive epigenetic reprogramming, which involves **DNA demethylation** (see Chapter 20, Spermatogenesis). This change is required for the zygote to acquire **totipotency**. The expression of cell lineage specific transcription factors starts in the blastocyst, when the outer **trophoblast** and the pluripotent **inner cell mass** acquire cellular identity.

Preimplantation of the fertilized egg or zygote

You have learned in the Embryology course that the first rounds of cell divisions of the zygote, the fertilized egg, are designated **cleavage**. The daughter cells are named **blastomeres**. The embryo consists of a compact or ball structure, called **morula**, once it has attained an 8-cell number of blastomeres.

Two different cell populations appear in the **blastocyst**: the **inner cell mass**, that produces the embryo, and the **trophoblast**, which gives rise to the extraembryonic tissue to support embryonic development. In direct contact with the inner cell mass is the **polar trophoblast layer**. Surrounding the **blastocyst cavity** is the **mural trophoblast layer**.

The embryo and the maternal endometrium begin to cooperate to form the placenta as soon as the blastocyst implants in the endometrium. Box 23-D provides the time-course of events preceding egg implantation soon after fertilization.

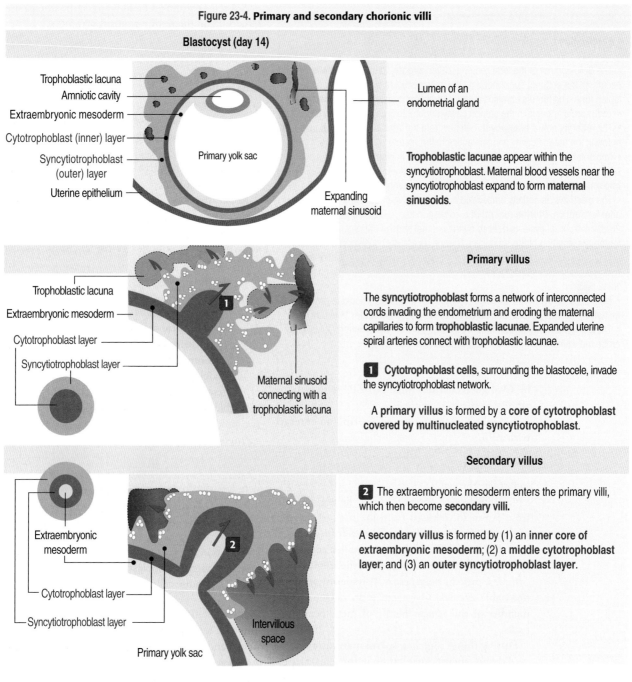

Figure 23-4. Primary and secondary chorionic villi

Blastocyst (day 14)

Trophoblastic lacuna
Amniotic cavity
Extraembryonic mesoderm
Cytotrophoblast (inner) layer
Syncytiotrophoblast (outer) layer
Uterine epithelium

Primary yolk sac

Lumen of an endometrial gland

Expanding maternal sinusoid

Trophoblastic lacunae appear within the syncytiotrophoblast. Maternal blood vessels near the syncytiotrophoblast expand to form **maternal sinusoids**.

Primary villus

Trophoblastic lacuna
Extraembryonic mesoderm
Cytotrophoblast layer
Syncytiotrophoblast layer

Maternal sinusoid connecting with a trophoblastic lacuna

The **syncytiotrophoblast** forms a network of interconnected cords invading the endometrium and eroding the maternal capillaries to form **trophoblastic lacunae**. Expanded uterine spiral arteries connect with trophoblastic lacunae.

1 **Cytotrophoblast cells**, surrounding the blastocele, invade the syncytiotrophoblast network.

A **primary villus** is formed by a **core of cytotrophoblast covered by multinucleated syncytiotrophoblast**.

Secondary villus

Extraembryonic mesoderm
Cytotrophoblast layer
Syncytiotrophoblast layer

Intervillous space

Primary yolk sac

2 The extraembryonic mesoderm enters the primary villi, which then become **secondary villi**.

A **secondary villus** is formed by (1) an **inner core of extraembryonic mesoderm**; (2) a **middle cytotrophoblast layer**; and (3) an **outer syncytiotrophoblast layer**.

Implantation of the blastocyst

On day 4 of pregnancy, the blastocyst is within the uterine cavity. The coordinated effect of ovarian estrogens and progesterone has already conditioned **uterine receptivity** for implantation, including an increase in endometrial vascular permeability at the implantation site (see Box 23-D).

On day 5, the **blastocyst hatches from the zona pellucida** and exposes the **polar trophoblast** to the endometrium. If zona pellucida hatching fails to occur, the embryo will not implant.

The **receptive time** of the endometrium for the incoming embryo, called the **implantation window**, lasts 4 days (20-23 days of the menstrual cycle).

The implantation of the blastocyst involves:

1. An initial **unstable** adhesion of the blastocyst to the endometrial surface, called **apposition**, followed by a more **stable adhesion** phase.

2. The **decidualization** of the endometrial stroma (Figure 23-3). Failure of the uterine stroma to undergo decidualization can lead to spontaneous abortion.

Implantation of the embryo requires the interaction of the trophoblast cells and the endometrium:

1. The apical surface of the endometrial epithelial cell is coated with bound and soluble forms of **heparin-bound epidermal growth factor-like factor (HB-EGF)**, a member of the transforming growth factor-α family.

Figure 23-5. Tertiary chorionic villi (3rd week, late)

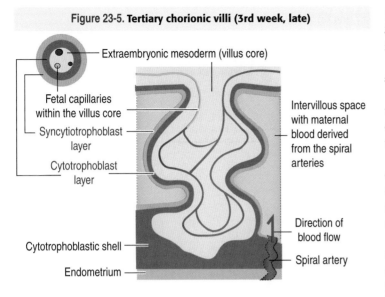

- Extraembryonic mesoderm (villus core)
- Fetal capillaries within the villus core
- Syncytiotrophoblast layer
- Cytotrophoblast layer
- Cytotrophoblastic shell
- Endometrium
- Intervillous space with maternal blood derived from the spiral arteries
- Direction of blood flow
- Spiral artery

2. **Epidermal growth factor receptor (EGF-R)**, on the surface of the trophoblast cells, autophosphorylates and **heparan sulfate proteoglycan** (also called perlecan) binds strongly to HB-EGF.

Then, cytoplasmic processes of trophoblast cells interact with small processes on the apical surface of the endometrial epithelial cells, called **pinopodes**, and penetrate the intercellular spaces between endometrial cells. Penetration is facilitated by a decrease in the number of desmosomes linking the endometrial cells that undergo **apoptosis**.

As you recall, the lamina propria of the endometrium undergoes a **decidual transformation** during the secretory phase of the menstrual cycle. This **primary decidual zone** is remodeled by the action of metalloproteinases into a **secondary decidual zone** that houses the implanting embryo (see Figure 23-3).

Box 23-E | Trophoblast cells: Highlights to remember

- The blastocyst has two distinct cell populations: (1) **trophoblast cells**, derived from the trophoectoderm and surrounding the blastocyst; and (2) the **inner cell mass**, which gives rise to the embryo.
- Trophoblast cells (the collective designation of cytotrophoblast cells and syncytiotrophoblast cells) are always the outermost layer of fetal cells covering the mesenchyme and fetal capillaries of the chorionic villi.
- The wall of maternal blood vessels is infiltrated and ruptured by trophoblast cells. Maternal blood is released into the intervillous space, and the outer layer of the chorionic villi (syncytiotrophoblast cells) is immersed in maternal blood like a sponge in a container of blood.
- The uterine spiral arteries are converted to **uteroplacental arteries**. Trophoblast cells replace the endothelium and tunica media of the uteroplacental arteries, which deliver blood, at low pressure, to the intervillous space. Basal straight arteries are not involved in these changes.
- When trophoblast cell replacement of spiral arteries is incomplete, the development of uteroplacental arteries is deficient and blood flow is reduced.
- **Preeclampsia** occurs when there is a reduced development of the branches of the chorionic villus tree and limited fetal growth.

Differentiation of the trophoblast

Soon after implantation, the trophoblast differentiates into two layers:

1. An inner layer of mitotically active **mononucleated cytotrophoblast cells**.

2. An outer layer of **multinucleated syncytiotrophoblast cells** at the embryonic pole, facing the endometrium. **Syncytiotrophoblast cells arise from the fusion of cytotrophoblast cells.**

The syncytiotrophoblast produces **proteolytic enzymes**, penetrates the primary decidua, and the entire blastocyst is rapidly surrounded by the endometrium. Invasion of the endometrium at the edge of the myometrium is called **interstitial invasion**.

The blastocyst has a cavity containing fluid and the eccentric **inner cell mass**, which gives rise to the embryo and some extraembryonic tissues. The mural trophoblast cells, proximal to the inner cell mass, begin to develop the **chorionic sac**. The chorionic sac consists of two components: the **trophoblast** and the underlying **extraembryonic mesoderm**.

Proteases released by the syncytiotrophoblast erode the branches of the spiral uterine arteries to form spaces or **lacunae** of maternal blood within the syncytiotrophoblast mass.

This endometrial eroding event, called **endovascular invasion**, marks the initiation of the **primitive uteroplacental circulation**.

Decidualization allows an orderly access of trophoblastic cells to the maternal nutrients by modulating their invasion of uterine spiral arteries.

The **syncytiotrophoblast** begins the secretion of **human chorionic gonadotropin (hCG)** into the maternal lacunae.

The secretion of estrogens and progesterone by the corpus luteum is now under the control of hCG, an LH-equivalent.

Immunoprotective decidua during implantation

On the maternal side, decidual cells, close to the mass of invading syncytiotrophoblast cells, degenerate and release glycogen and lipids, thus providing, together with products of the endometrial glands and maternal blood in the lacunae, the initial nutrients for embryonic development.

The **decidual reaction** provides an immune-protective environment for the development of the embryo. The decidual reaction involves:

1. The production of immunosuppressive substances (mainly **prostaglandins**) by decidual cells to inhibit the activation of **natural killer cells** at the implantation site.

2. Infiltrating leukocytes in the endometrial stroma that secrete **interleukin-2** to prevent maternal tissue rejection of the implanting embryo.

Syncytiotrophoblast cells do not express **major**

Figure 23-6. **Anatomy and histology of the placenta**

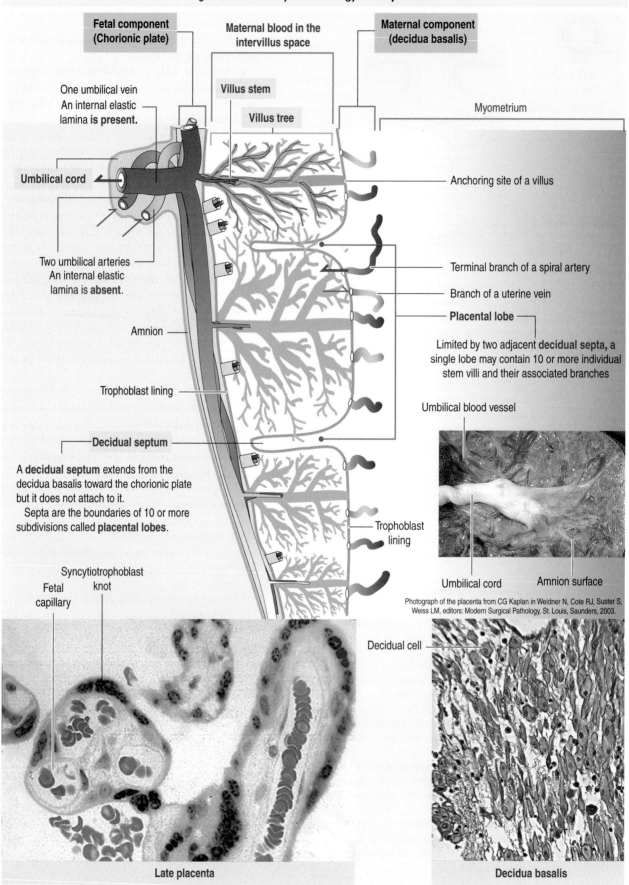

Fetal component (Chorionic plate)

Maternal blood in the intervillus space

Maternal component (decidua basalis)

One umbilical vein
An internal elastic lamina **is present.**

Villus stem

Villus tree

Myometrium

Umbilical cord

Anchoring site of a villus

Two umbilical arteries
An internal elastic lamina is **absent**.

Terminal branch of a spiral artery

Branch of a uterine vein

Placental lobe

Amnion

Limited by two adjacent **decidual septa**, a single lobe may contain 10 or more individual stem villi and their associated branches

Trophoblast lining

Umbilical blood vessel

Decidual septum

A **decidual septum** extends from the decidua basalis toward the chorionic plate but it does not attach to it.
  Septa are the boundaries of 10 or more subdivisions called **placental lobes**.

Trophoblast lining

Umbilical cord   Amnion surface

Photograph of the placenta from CG Kaplan in Weidner N, Cote RJ, Suster S, Weiss LM, editors: Modern Surgical Pathology, St. Louis, Saunders, 2003.

Syncytiotrophoblast knot

Fetal capillary

Decidual cell

Late placenta

Decidua basalis

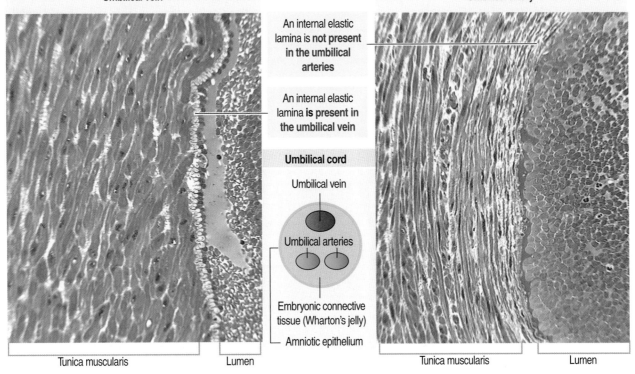

Figure 23-7. Differences between umbilical vein and umbilical artery

Umbilical vein

Umbilical artery

An internal elastic lamina is **not present** in the umbilical arteries

An internal elastic lamina **is present** in the umbilical vein

Umbilical cord

Umbilical vein

Umbilical arteries

Embryonic connective tissue (Wharton's jelly)

Amniotic epithelium

Tunica muscularis

Lumen

Tunica muscularis

Lumen

histocompatibility complex class II. Therefore, the syncytiotrophoblast cannot present antigens to maternal CD4$^+$ T cells.

Primary, secondary, and tertiary villi

At the end of the second week, cytotrophoblast cells proliferate under the influence of the extraembryonic mesoderm, and extend into the syncytiotrophoblast mass, forming the **villi.**

There are three different types of chorionic or placental villi:

1. **Primary villi** (Figure 23-4).
2. **Secondary villi** (see Figure 23-4).
3. **Tertiary villi** (Figure 23-5).

Primary villi represent the first step in the development of the chorionic villi of the placenta. A primary villus is formed by a core of cytotrophoblast cells covered by syncytiotrophoblast.

Early in the third week, the **extraembryonic mesoderm** extends into the primary villi, forming the secondary villi.

A secondary villus consists of a core of extraembryonic mesoderm surrounded by a middle cytotrophoblast layer and an outer layer of syncytiotrophoblast layer (see Figure 23-4).

Soon after, cells of the extraembryonic mesoderm differentiate into capillary and blood cells and **tertiary villi** are developed (Figure 23-5). A tertiary villus is formed by a core of extraembryonic mesoderm with

capillaries, surrounded by a middle cytotrophoblast layer and an outer layer of syncytiotrophoblast. The difference between the secondary and tertiary villi is the presence of capillaries in the latter. The capillaries in the tertiary villi interconnect to form **arteriocapillary networks** leading to the embryonic heart.

Histology of the placenta

The placenta and embryonic-fetal membranes (amnion, chorion, allantois, and yolk sac) protect the embryo-fetus and provide for nutrition, respiration, excretion, and hormone production during development. The membranes are formed by the embryo.

The mature placenta is 3 cm thick, has a diameter of 20 cm, and weighs about 500 g.

The **fetal side** of the placenta is smooth and associated with the amniotic membrane (Figure 23-6).

The **maternal side** of the placenta is partially subdivided into 10 or more **lobes** by **decidual septa** derived from the decidua basalis and extending toward the chorionic plate. The decidual septa do not fuse with the chorionic plate.

Each lobe contains 10 or more stem villi and its branches.

The 50- to 60-cm-long and 12-mm-thick and twisted **umbilical cord** is attached to the chorionic plate and contains **two umbilical arteries** (transporting **deoxygenated** blood) and **one umbilical vein** (transporting **oxygen-rich** blood).

Figure 23-8. Uterine and fetal membranes

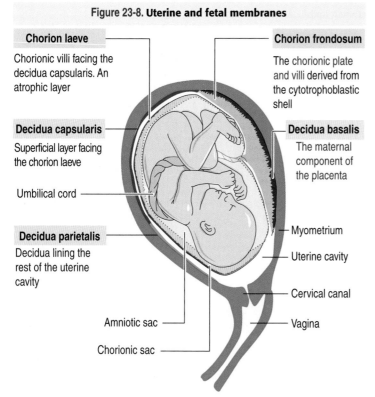

Chorion laeve
Chorionic villi facing the decidua capsularis. An atrophic layer

Chorion frondosum
The chorionic plate and villi derived from the cytotrophoblastic shell

Decidua capsularis
Superficial layer facing the chorion laeve

Decidua basalis
The maternal component of the placenta

Umbilical cord

Myometrium

Uterine cavity

Decidua parietalis
Decidua lining the rest of the uterine cavity

Cervical canal

Amniotic sac

Vagina

Chorionic sac

The **umbilical vessels** (Figure 23-7) are embedded in **embryonic connective tissue**, called **Wharton's jelly** (see Chapter 4, Connective Tissue).

Embryonic connective tissue cushions the umbili-

cal cord blood vessels to ensure steady blood flow by preventing twisting and compression. The cord is lined by amniotic epithelium.

Blood collected from the vein of the severed umbilical cord from a newborn baby (following detachment from the newborn) contains **stem cells**, including hematopoietic stem cells, useful for transplantation to patients with leukemia, lymphoma, and anemia.

Placenta: Decidua basalis and villus corion

In **summary**, the placenta consists of a maternal component, the **decidua basalis**, and a fetal component, the **villus corion** (Figure 23-8).

The **maternal component** is represented by the **decidua**. The decidua (Latin *deciduus*, falling off; a tissue shed at birth) is the endometrium of the gravid uterus.

There are **three regions of the decidua**, named according to their relation to the developing fetus:

1. The **decidua basalis** is the maternal component of the placenta. Chorionic villi facing the decidua basalis are highly developed and form the **chorion frondosum** (bushy chorion).

2. The **decidua capsularis** is the superficial layer covering the developing fetus and its chorionic sac.

3. The **decidua parietalis** is the rest of the decidua lining the cavity of the uterus not occupied by the fetus.

The **fetal component** is the **villus corion**, represented by the **chorion frondosum**: the **chorionic plate** and derived **chorionic villi**.

Chorionic villi facing the decidua capsularis un-

Figure 23-9. Structure of the chorionic villus

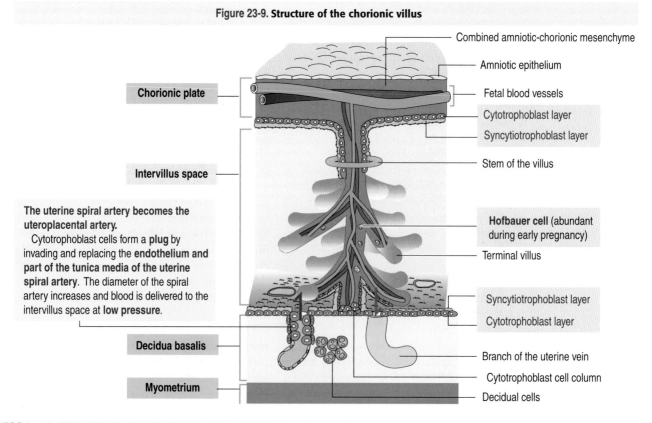

Combined amniotic-chorionic mesenchyme

Amniotic epithelium

Chorionic plate

Fetal blood vessels

Cytotrophoblast layer

Syncytiotrophoblast layer

Stem of the villus

Intervillus space

The uterine spiral artery becomes the uteroplacental artery.
Cytotrophoblast cells form a **plug** by invading and replacing the **endothelium and part of the tunica media of the uterine spiral artery**. The diameter of the spiral artery increases and blood is delivered to the intervillus space at **low pressure**.

Hofbauer cell (abundant during early pregnancy)

Terminal villus

Syncytiotrophoblast layer

Cytotrophoblast layer

Decidua basalis

Branch of the uterine vein

Cytotrophoblast cell column

Myometrium

Decidual cells

Figure 23-10. The blood-placental barrier

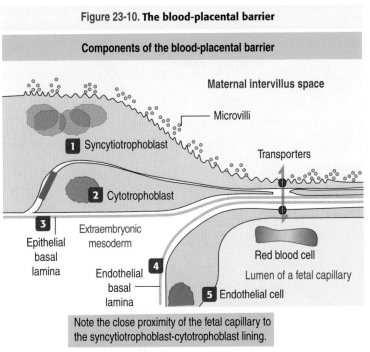

Components of the blood-placental barrier

Maternal intervillus space

Microvilli

1 Syncytiotrophoblast

Transporters

2 Cytotrophoblast

3

Epithelial basal lamina

Extraembryonic mesoderm

4

Endothelial basal lamina

Red blood cell

Lumen of a fetal capillary

5 Endothelial cell

Note the close proximity of the fetal capillary to the syncytiotrophoblast-cytotrophoblast lining.

The blood-placental barrier has a significant role in placental function and fetal development. The presence of a brush border-like domain at the apical domain of the syncytiotrophoblast, facing maternal blood, points to an absorption function. A number of transporters in the syncytiotrophoblast and endothelial cells of fetal capillaries provide pathways for exogenous and endogenous substances.

dergo atrophy, resulting in the formation of the **chorion laeve** (smooth chorion).

The **intervillous space** between the maternal and fetal components contains circulating maternal blood (see Figures 23-6).

Arterial blood, derived from the open ends of the spiral arteries, flows into the intervillous space and moves blood into the uterine veins. **A plug of cytotrophoblast cells** and the **contraction of the smooth muscle wall** of the artery **control the flow of blood** (Figure 23-9).

Placental blood circulation

Placental blood circulation has two relevant characteristics:

1. The **fetal blood circulation** is **closed** (within blood vessels).

2. The **maternal blood circulation** is **open** (not bound by blood vessels).

Maternal blood enters the intervillous space under reduced pressure, regulated by the cytotrophoblast cell plugs, and leaves through the uterine veins after exchanges occur with the fetal blood in the terminal branched villi.

The **umbilical vein** has a **subendothelial elastic lamina**; the **two umbilical arteries lack an elastic lamina** (see Figure 23-6).

The **umbilical vein carries 80% oxygenated fetal blood**. Although the partial pressure of oxygen in fetal blood is low (20 to 25 mm Hg), the higher cardiac output in organ blood flow, higher hemoglobin concentration in fetal red blood cells, and higher oxygen saturation provide adequate oxygenation to the fetus.

The **umbilical arteries return deoxygenated fetal blood to the placenta**.

Recall that **fetal circulation** involves three circulatory shunts:

1. The **ductus venosus**, which allows blood from the placenta to bypass the liver.

2. The **ductus arteriosus** and **foramen ovale**, which allow blood to bypass the developing lungs.

Structure of the chorionic villus

The chorionic villus is involved in maternal-fetal exchanges. It originates from the chorionic plate and derives from a **stem villus** giving rise to villous branches (see Figure 23-9).

When you examine a histologic preparation of placenta, you are visualizing cross sections of villi corresponding to the villous branches. You may also be able to see a longitudinal section of a stem villus.

Fetal vessels are separated from maternal blood in the intervillous space by the **placental barrier** (Figure 23-10), which is formed by:

1. The **cytotrophoblast** and **syncytiotrophoblast** cells and supporting **basal lamina**.

2. **Endothelial cells** and **basal lamina of the fetal blood capillaries**.

Each villus has a core of **mesenchymal connective tissue** and **fetal blood vessels** (arterioles, capillaries and venules).

The mesenchymal core contains two major cell types:

1. **Mesenchymal cells**, which differentiate into fibroblasts, involved in the synthesis of various types of collagens (types I, III, V, and VI) and extracellular matrix components (Figure 23-11).

2. **Hofbauer cells**, phagocytic cells predominant in **early pregnancy**.

The mesenchymal core is covered by two cell types:

1. **Syncytiotrophoblast cells**, in contact with the maternal blood in the intervillous space. The apical surface of the syncytiotrophoblast contains numerous **microvilli** extending into the intervillous space.

2. **Cytotrophoblast cells**, subjacent to the syncytiotrophoblast and supported by a basal lamina. Cytotrophoblast cells are linked to each other and to the overlying syncytiotrophoblast by **desmosomes**.

Deposits of fibrin are frequently seen on the villus surface on areas lacking syncytiotrophoblast cells.

After the fourth month of pregnancy, the fetal blood vessels become dilated and are in direct contact with the subepithelial basal lamina. Cytotrophoblast cells

Figure 23-11. **Fine structure of the chorionic villus**

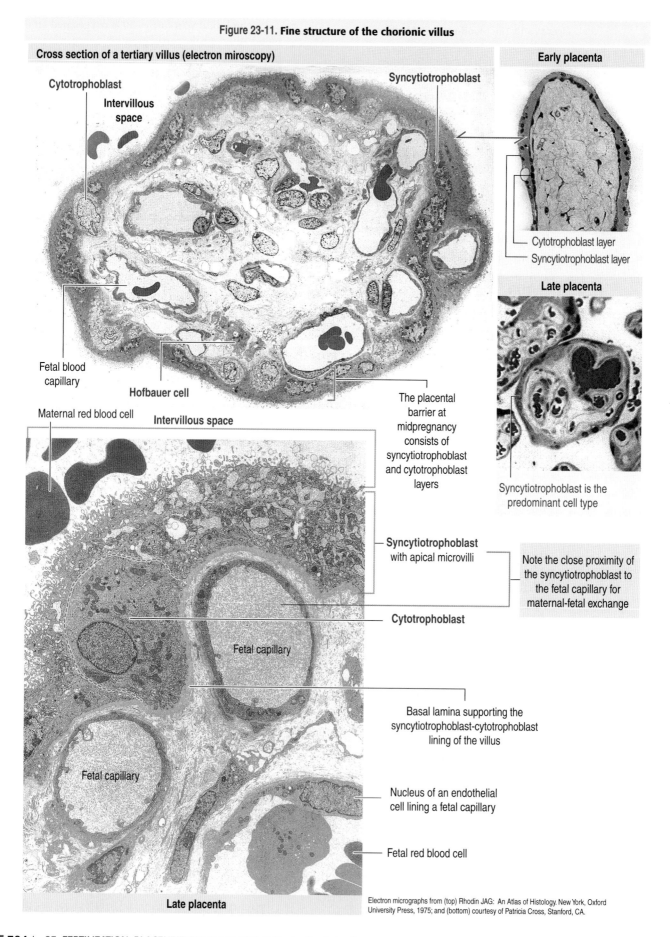

Cross section of a tertiary villus (electron miroscopy)

Cytotrophoblast

Intervillous space

Syncytiotrophoblast

Early placenta

Cytotrophoblast layer

Syncytiotrophoblast layer

Fetal blood capillary

Hofbauer cell

Maternal red blood cell

Intervillous space

The placental barrier at midpregnancy consists of syncytiotrophoblast and cytotrophoblast layers

Late placenta

Syncytiotrophoblast is the predominant cell type

Syncytiotrophoblast with apical microvilli

Note the close proximity of the syncytiotrophoblast to the fetal capillary for maternal-fetal exchange

Cytotrophoblast

Fetal capillary

Basal lamina supporting the syncytiotrophoblast-cytotrophoblast lining of the villus

Fetal capillary

Nucleus of an endothelial cell lining a fetal capillary

Fetal red blood cell

Late placenta

Electron micrographs from (top) Rhodin JAG: An Atlas of Histology. New York, Oxford University Press, 1975; and (bottom) courtesy of Patricia Cross, Stanford, CA.

Figure 23-12. **Functions of the placenta**

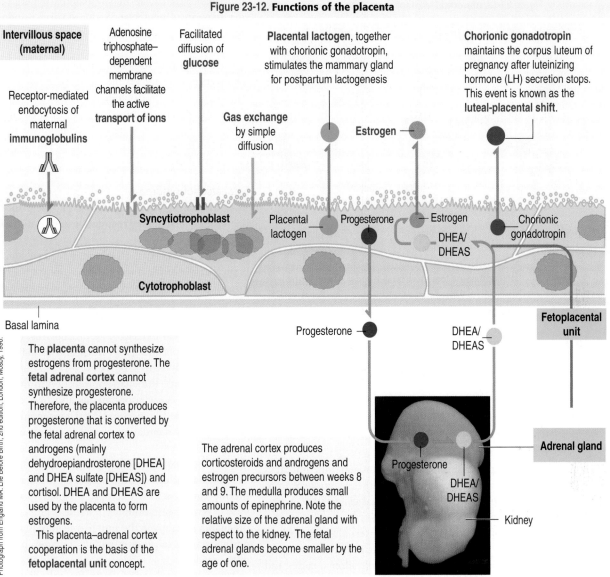

Intervillous space (maternal)

Receptor-mediated endocytosis of maternal **immunoglobulins**

Adenosine triphosphate–dependent membrane channels facilitate the active **transport of ions**

Facilitated diffusion of **glucose**

Gas exchange by simple diffusion

Placental lactogen, together with chorionic gonadotropin, stimulates the mammary gland for postpartum lactogenesis

Estrogen

Chorionic gonadotropin maintains the corpus luteum of pregnancy after luteinizing hormone (LH) secretion stops. This event is known as the **luteal-placental shift**.

Syncytiotrophoblast

Placental lactogen

Progesterone

Estrogen

DHEA/ DHEAS

Chorionic gonadotropin

Cytotrophoblast

Basal lamina

Progesterone

DHEA/ DHEAS

Fetoplacental unit

The **placenta** cannot synthesize estrogens from progesterone. The **fetal adrenal cortex** cannot synthesize progesterone. Therefore, the placenta produces progesterone that is converted by the fetal adrenal cortex to androgens (mainly dehydroepiandrosterone [DHEA] and DHEA sulfate [DHEAS]) and cortisol. DHEA and DHEAS are used by the placenta to form estrogens.

This placenta–adrenal cortex cooperation is the basis of the **fetoplacental unit** concept.

The adrenal cortex produces corticosteroids and androgens and estrogen precursors between weeks 8 and 9. The medulla produces small amounts of epinephrine. Note the relative size of the adrenal gland with respect to the kidney. The fetal adrenal glands become smaller by the age of one.

Progesterone

DHEA/ DHEAS

Adrenal gland

Kidney

Photograph from England MA: Life Before Birth, 2nd edition, London, Mosby, 1996.

decrease in number and syncytiotrophoblast cells predominate. This arrangement facilitates maternal-fetal exchange activities.

In **summary**, chorionic villi of an **early placenta** consist of two distinct cytotrophoblast and syncytiotrophoblast layers (see Figure 23-11). Hofbauer cells predominate in the mesenchyme. In a **late placenta**, syncytiotrophoblast cells form distinct clusters, called **syncytiotrophoblast knots** (see Figure 23-6).

Functions of the placenta

The main function of the placenta is the regulation of the fetal-maternal exchange of molecules, ions, and gases.

This function is accomplished at specialized areas of the syncytiotrophoblast adjacent to fetal capillaries. The transfer of molecules across the placental barrier can follow **intercellular** and **transcellular** pathways.

Figure 23-12 illustrates the main functional aspects

of the placenta that are of clinical and physiologic relevance.

Exchange of gases

Oxygen, carbon dioxide, and carbon monoxide exchange through the placenta is by **simple diffusion**. Nitrous oxide anesthesia (used in the treatment of dental disease) should be avoided during pregnancy.

Transfer of maternal immunoglobulins

Maternal antibodies, mainly **immunoglobulin G (IgG)**, are taken up by the syncytiotrophoblast and then transported to fetal capillaries for **passive immunity**.

The larger **immunoglobulin M (IgM)** molecules do not cross the placental barrier.

Rh (D antigen) isoimmunization

Maternal antibodies against D antigen (present in the

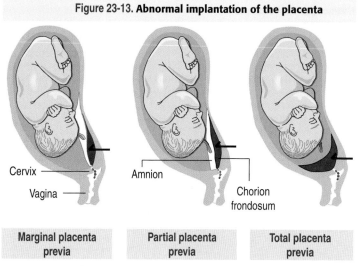

Figure 23-13. Abnormal implantation of the placenta

Cervix

Vagina

Amnion

Chorion frondosum

Marginal placenta previa

Partial placenta previa

Total placenta previa

Rh system of fetal red blood cells) cause hemolytic disease (**erythroblastosis fetalis**). The fetus is Rh-positive (Rh D antigen received from the father), but the mother lacks the D antigen (she is Rh-negative). **Isoimmunization** refers to maternal exposure and sensitization to fetal Rh$^+$ red blood cells, mainly during delivery. In a subsequent pregnancy, antibodies to D antigen (IgG) cross the placenta and cause hemolysis of fetal red blood cells (see Chapter 6, Blood and Hematopoiesis).

The fetoplacental unit

The placenta can synthesize progesterone but lacks 17-hydroxylase activity to synthesize estrogens from progesterone. The fetal adrenal cortex cannot synthesize progesterone.

Consequently, a fetal-maternal cooperation, known as the **fetoplacental unit**, enables the transport of **placental progesterone** to the adrenal cortex and its conversion to dehydroepiandrosterone (DHEA), which can be sulfated to form DHEA sulfate (DHEAS) (see Figure 23-12).

When DHEA and DHEAS are transported to the syncytiotrophoblast, the conversion to estrone (E_1) and estradiol (E_2) occurs. DHEA can be hydroxylated in the liver and serves as a substrate for the synthesis of estriol (E_3) by the syncytiotrophoblast.

The luteal-placental shift

Chorionic gonadotropin, instead of **maternal luteinizing hormone**, maintains the **corpus luteum** during pregnancy. This switch, from the corpus luteum to the placenta, is called the **luteal-placental shift**.

Placental lactogen (also called chorionic somatomammotropin) stimulates fetal growth and conditions the mammary gland for lactation. Placental lactogen has a **diabetogenic effect**: It increases the resistance of peripheral tissues and liver to the effects of **insulin**.

Pregnancy is characterized by maternal **hyperglycemia**, **hyperinsulinemia**, and **reduced tissue response to insulin**.

Active transport of ions and glucose

The transport of ions is mediated by an adenosine triphosphate (ATP)–dependent mechanism.

Glucose enters the placenta by facilitated diffusion using a glucose transporter. Fetal glucose levels depend on maternal levels. The fetus does not depend on maternal insulin.

Fetal alcohol syndrome

The excessive ingestion of alcohol during pregnancy is the cause of **fetal mental retardation** and **craniofacial abnormalities**.

Alcohol can cross the placenta and fetal blood-brain barrier causing direct toxicity. Indirect toxicity is mediated by the alcohol metabolite **acetaldehyde**.

Infectious agents

Rubella (German measles), cytomegalovirus, herpes simplex, toxoplasmosis, syphilis, and human immunodeficiency virus type 1 (HIV-1) are potential infectious agents. **Rubella** viral infection in the first trimester can cause spontaneous abortion or the **congenital rubella syndrome** (fetal congenital heart disease, mental retardation, deafness, and cataracts).

Clinical significance: Ectopic pregnancy

The **implantation of the blastocyst outside the uterine cavity** is called **ectopic pregnancy**. About 95% of ectopic gestations occur in the oviduct (**tubal pregnancy**), mainly in the ampullar region. A predisposing factor is **salpingitis**, an inflammatory process of the oviduct.

A major complication is profuse bleeding and rupture of the wall of the oviduct caused by the trophoblastic erosion of blood vessels and tissue layers. **Abdominal pain, amenorrhea**, and **vaginal bleeding** in a sexually active woman of reproductive age are symptoms of a suspected tubal pregnancy. A rapid and precise diagnosis of ectopic pregnancy is essential to reduce the risk of complications or death.

Pathology: Placenta previa

The **abnormal extension of the placenta over or close to the internal opening of the cervical canal** is called **placenta previa**. A possible cause is **abnormal vascularization of the placenta**.

There are three types of placenta previa (Figure 23-13):

1. **Marginal placenta previa**, when the margin of the placenta lies close to the internal cervical os (low implantation of the placenta).

2. **Partial placenta previa**, when the edge of the

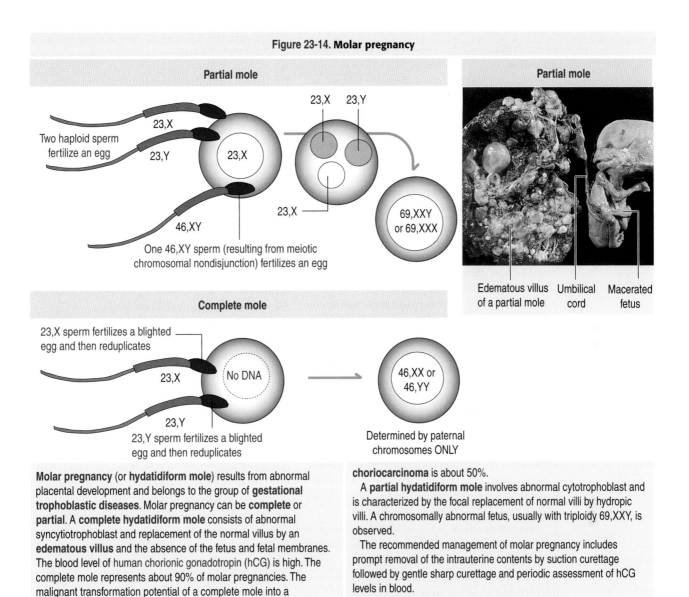

Figure 23-14. Molar pregnancy

Partial mole

23,X

Two haploid sperm fertilize an egg

23,Y

23,X

46,XY

One 46,XY sperm (resulting from meiotic chromosomal nondisjunction) fertilizes an egg

23,X   23,Y

23,X

69,XXY or 69,XXX

Partial mole

Edematous villus of a partial mole   Umbilical cord   Macerated fetus

Complete mole

23,X sperm fertilizes a blighted egg and then reduplicates

23,X

No DNA

23,Y

23,Y sperm fertilizes a blighted egg and then reduplicates

46,XX or 46,YY

Determined by paternal chromosomes ONLY

Molar pregnancy (or **hydatidiform mole**) results from abnormal placental development and belongs to the group of **gestational trophoblastic diseases**. Molar pregnancy can be **complete** or **partial**. A **complete hydatidiform mole** consists of abnormal syncytiotrophoblast and replacement of the normal villus by an **edematous villus** and the absence of the fetus and fetal membranes. The blood level of human chorionic gonadotropin (hCG) is high. The complete mole represents about 90% of molar pregnancies. The malignant transformation potential of a complete mole into a

choriocarcinoma is about 50%.

A **partial hydatidiform mole** involves abnormal cytotrophoblast and is characterized by the focal replacement of normal villi by hydropic villi. A chromosomally abnormal fetus, usually with triploidy 69,XXY, is observed.

The recommended management of molar pregnancy includes prompt removal of the intrauterine contents by suction curettage followed by gentle sharp curettage and periodic assessment of hCG levels in blood.

Photograph from Damjanov I, Linder J: Pathology: A Color Atlas. St. Louis, Mosby, 2000.

Box 23-F | Hydramnios

• The functions of the amniotic fluid during pregnancy is to cushion the fetus inside the uterus, provide space for fetal movements, and regulates fetal body temperature.

• Initially, the amniotic fluid is produced by dialysis through placental maternal and fetal blood vessels. Later, amniotic fluid is essentially **fetal urine**; it is absorbed by fetal swallowing. The maximum amount of amniotic fluid is reached by the 36th week of pregnancy and then decreases gradually.

• Severe **hydramnios** (excessive amniotic fluid) may indicate a genetic defect, a fetal defect in the central nervous system or blockage of the gastrointestinal tube. Clinical signs include abdominal pain, significant swelling or bloating and breathlessness. Hydramnios can be confirmed by ultrasound. Amniocentesis is recommended to determine a possible chromosomal problem. A mild form of hydramnios may be detected during the second trimester of pregnancy and return spontaneously to a normal condition.

• **Oligohydramnios** is a condition opposite to hydramnios in which there is no sufficient amniotic fluid (less than 400 ml). It may indicate a problem with fetal development (such as **renal agenesis**) or the placenta or the consequence of high blood pressure of the mother. A decrease in amniotic fluid does not provide cushion protection to the fetus and the umbilical cord.

placenta extends across part of the internal ostium.

3. **Total placenta previa**, when the placenta covers the internal cervical ostium.

Spontaneous painless bleeding, caused by partial separation of the placenta from the lower portion of the uterus and cervix due to mild uterine contractions, is commonly observed.

Pathology: Abnormal separation and implantation of the placenta

The normal separation of the placenta from the uterus during labor is determined by a cleavage at the decidua basalis region.

After separation, the placenta is ejected by strong uterine contractions, which also constrict the spiral arteries of the vascular decidual bed to prevent excessive bleeding.

A placenta may be retained in the uterine cavity when the process of cleavage or ejection is incomplete.

After expulsion, every placenta must be inspected **to detect missing lobes**, which may remain inside the uterus.

When some placental tissue remains in the uterus, uterine contractions are deficient and excessive bleeding is observed. Curettage with a suction apparatus may remove the retained tissue.

The following pathologic conditions can be seen during pregnancy and labor:

1. **Uterine atony** occurs when **the contractions of the uterine muscles are not strong enough and postpartum bleeding occurs.**

Predisposing factors of uterine atony include **abnormal labor**, **substantial enlargement of the uterus** (because of hydramnios; excessive amniotic fluid, see Box 23-F), or **uterine leiomyomas** (benign tumors of the myometrium).

Intravenous infusion of **oxytocin** stimulates uterine contractions and decreases the possibility of uterine atony.

2. **Placental abruption** is the **premature separation** of the normally implanted placenta from the inner uterine wall. Hemorrhage into the decidua basalis leads to premature placental separation and bleeding. Separation of the placenta from the uterus impairs oxygenation of the fetus.

Possible causes include **trauma**, **maternal hypertension** (preeclampsia or eclampsia), **blood clotting abnormalities**, and **cocaine use** by the mother. Spontaneous painful bleeding and uterine contractions are typical symptoms.

3. **Placenta accreta** (Latin *accretus,* overgrown) is an **abnormally strong and deep attachment of part or the entire placenta to the uterine wall.** Abnormalities in the uterine wall, usually due to previous uterine surgery (such as cesarean section or scar tissue following uterine curettage [Asherman syndrome]), increase the possibilities of placenta accreta.

The incidence of placenta accreta has increased in parallel to the increasing repeated cesarean delivery rate and the incidence of placenta previa overlying an uterine scar.

Ultrasonography and magnetic resonance imaging enable diagnosis of placenta accreta before delivery to reduce possible maternal hemorrhagic morbidity or neonatal morbidity and mortality.

There are three forms of placenta accreta, based on how deeply the placenta penetrates the myometrium.

• **Placenta accreta**: The placenta invades the uterine wall but does not penetrate the myometrium. This condition, accounts for 75 percent of all cases.

• **Placenta increta**: The invading placenta penetrates through the myometrium. Placenta increta is seen in 15 percent of cases.

• **Placenta percreta**: The placenta extends into the uterine wall and its muscles, pierces the uterine serosa, and may attach to other adjacent organs (urinary bladder or rectum). Placenta percreta occurs in 10 percent of the cases.

Pathology: Gestational trophoblastic diseases

Gestational trophoblastic diseases are classified into three distinct types:

1. **Hydatidiform mole.**
2. **Invasive mole.**
3. **Choriocarcinoma.**

Hydatidiform mole designates the **partial** or **complete** replacement of normal villi by dilated or hydropic (edematous) translucent vesicles. A fetus or embryo is often found in partial hydatidiform mole but no fetus is recognizable in complete hydatidiform mole.

The villi are avascular with no blood present in remnant vessels of complete hydatidiform mole. In contrast, capillaries containing blood can be seen in the villi of partial hydatidiform mole.

Complete hydatidiform moles are of **paternal origin** and result from the fertilization of a blighted (empty) ovum by a haploid sperm that reduplicates within the egg (Figure 23-14). The frequent karyotype of a complete hydatidiform mole is 46,XX or 46,YY, and no fetus is observed.

The fetus of a **partial hydatidiform mole** is usually 69,XXY (triploid): one haploid set of maternal chromosomes (23,X) and two haploid sets of paternal chromosomes (46,XY; arising from meiotic nondisjunction or from two haploid fertilizing sperm).

Extremely high levels of hCG are characteristic in patients with hydatidiform mole. Failure of high levels of hCG to regress after initial removal of intrauterine contents suggests a need for further treatment.

Invasive mole is the most frequent form of trophoblastic disease generally diagnosed by persistent high blood levels of hCG. It invades the uterine wall and cannot be detected on evacuated specimens. This condition responds to chemotherapy.

Choriocarcinoma is a malignant neoplasm observed in about 50% of patients with molar pregnancies. Choriocarcinoma is a hemorrhagic tumor in primary and metastatic sites. Treatment with combined chemotherapy agents is usually curative.

Lactation
The mammary glands

The breasts, or mammary glands, develop as a downgrowth of the epidermis. The **nipple** is surrounded by the **areola**, a modified skin with abundant sebaceous glands. The nipple contains connective tissue and smooth muscle cells, forming a **circular sphincter**.

About 15 to 20 **lactiferous ducts** open at the tip of the nipple through individual **lactiferous sinuses**.

In the lactating mammary gland, each lactiferous duct drains one lobe. Like most branched (compound) glands, the mammary glands contain a **duct system**, **lobes**, and **lobules** (Figure 23-15).

Figure 23-15. Structure of the mature female mammary gland

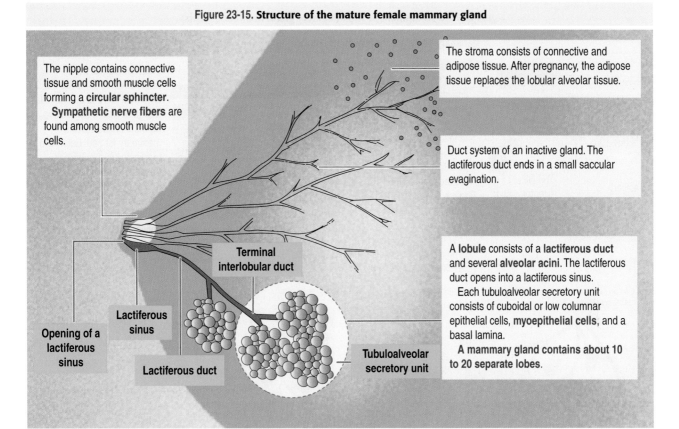

The nipple contains connective tissue and smooth muscle cells forming a **circular sphincter**. **Sympathetic nerve fibers** are found among smooth muscle cells.

The stroma consists of connective and adipose tissue. After pregnancy, the adipose tissue replaces the lobular alveolar tissue.

Duct system of an inactive gland. The lactiferous duct ends in a small saccular evagination.

A **lobule** consists of a **lactiferous duct** and several **alveolar acini**. The lactiferous duct opens into a lactiferous sinus.

Each tubuloalveolar secretory unit consists of cuboidal or low columnar epithelial cells, **myoepithelial cells**, and a basal lamina.

A mammary gland contains about 10 to 20 separate lobes.

Opening of a lactiferous sinus

Lactiferous sinus

Lactiferous duct

Terminal interlobular duct

Tubuloalveolar secretory unit

Each lobe consists of a branching **lactiferous duct** that extends into the **fibroadipose tissue** of the breast.

A **lobe** consists of a group of lobules drained by a **lactiferous duct. Lobules and lobes are not seen in the resting mammary gland**.

Each lactiferous duct is lined by a **simple columnar** or **cuboidal epithelium** and a discontinuous outer layer of **myoepithelial cells**. Each duct is surrounded by loose connective tissue and a capillary network.

In the **resting, nonlactating state**, the mammary glands consist of lactiferous ducts, each ending in a group of blind, saccular evaginations or buds (see Figure 23-15).

During **pregnancy**, the ducts branch and end in clusters of saccules (alveoli or acini), forming a **lobule**. Each lobule consists of various **secretory tubuloacinar units**.

Morphogenesis of the mammary glands

Placental lactogen, progesterone, growth hormone and **estrogen** stimulate the development of the mammary gland through a number of paracrine mechanisms.

Paracrine mechanisms include parathyroid hormone-related protein, amphiregulin, receptor of activated nuclear factor κβ ligand (RANKL), fibroblast growth factor-10, bone morphogenic protein-4, Wnt ligands, the hedgehog signaling pathway and transforming growth factor-β.

Amphiregulin is an epidermal growth factor-like protein that binds to the epidermal growth factor receptor on stromal cells.

Modulated by estrogen, amphiregulin, synthesized by mammary epithelial cells, binds to epidermal growth factor receptor on the surrounding stromal cells, which secrete regulatory factors of mammary development during puberty.

Amphiregulin absence leads to a failure of the elongation of lactiferous ducts and a lack of duct and alveolar epithelial cell proliferation in response to estrogen.

Unlike amphiregulin, RANKL is required for postpubertal ductal side branching and alveolar development rather than pubertal mammary gland development.

In addition, the extracellular matrix and remodeling matrix metalloproteinases and their inhibitors participate in mammary gland branching by controlling the surrounding stroma.

The basic concepts to grasp are:

1. Ovarian hormones, estrogen, and progesterone, and pituitary hormones, prolactin, and growth hormone, drive mammary gland development and differentiation.

2. Paracrine and autocrine signaling link mammary gland epithelial cells and the surrounding stromal cells during mammary gland development, puberty, and pregnancy.

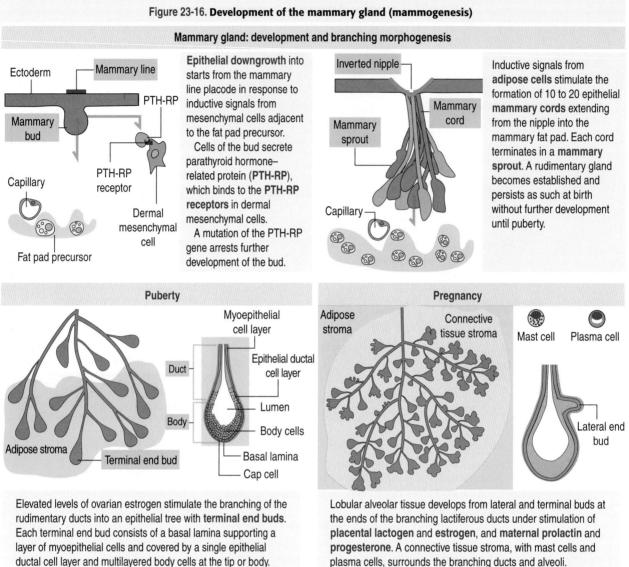

Figure 23-16. Development of the mammary gland (mammogenesis)

Mammary gland: development and branching morphogenesis

Epithelial downgrowth into starts from the mammary line placode in response to inductive signals from mesenchymal cells adjacent to the fat pad precursor.

Cells of the bud secrete parathyroid hormone–related protein (**PTH-RP**), which binds to the **PTH-RP receptors** in dermal mesenchymal cells.

A mutation of the PTH-RP gene arrests further development of the bud.

Inductive signals from **adipose cells** stimulate the formation of 10 to 20 epithelial **mammary cords** extending from the nipple into the mammary fat pad. Each cord terminates in a **mammary sprout**. A rudimentary gland becomes established and persists as such at birth without further development until puberty.

Puberty

Elevated levels of ovarian estrogen stimulate the branching of the rudimentary ducts into an epithelial tree with **terminal end buds**. Each terminal end bud consists of a basal lamina supporting a layer of myoepithelial cells and covered by a single epithelial ductal cell layer and multilayered body cells at the tip or body. Terminal end buds develop under the influence of **progesterone**. Old buds regress and disappear.

Pregnancy

Lobular alveolar tissue develops from lateral and terminal buds at the ends of the branching lactiferous ducts under stimulation of **placental lactogen** and **estrogen**, and **maternal prolactin** and **progesterone**. A connective tissue stroma, with mast cells and plasma cells, surrounds the branching ducts and alveoli.

Lactogenesis is the developmental process by which the mammary gland can produce and maintain the secretion of milk.

Remodeling during mammary gland development
The development of the mammary glands comprise two phases (Figure 23-16):

1. The formation of the **nipple**.
2. The remodeling of the mammary gland.

The nipple is visible by week 6 as an accumulation of ectodermic epithelial cells along the **mammary line placode**, forming a depression, the **inverted nipple**. After birth, the nipple region protrudes and the areola becomes elevated as **areolar sebaceous and sweat glands** develop around the nipple.

Mammary gland development starts when an ectodermic epithelial cell bud, the **mammary bud**, penetrates the underlying mesoderm adjacent to the **fat pad precursor** and capillaries.

During the first trimester, each of 10 to 20 solid epithelial **mammary cords** gives rise to a **mammary sprout** (see Figure 23-16). During the second trimester, the mammary cords become hollow and **terminal end buds** develop by the end of the third trimester. The mammary ducts become lactiferous ducts and the terminal end buds will change into alveolar buds at puberty.

Estrogen, progesterone and prolactin receptors are expressed by a population of luminal duct cells (called **sensor cells**). Under the influence of these hormones, sensor cells secrete paracrine and autocrine signaling molecules to trigger the proliferation of the adjacent luminal glandular epithelial and myoepithelial cells.

The mesoderm differentiates into a connective and adipose stroma as well as into the smooth muscle of the nipple.

Bipotent stem cells give rise to luminal glandular epithelial cells of ducts and alveoli and to myoepi-

Figure 23-17. Histology of the inactive and active mammary gland

Nonlactating mammary gland

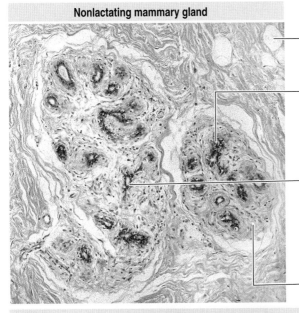

Adipose cell

Secretory units

The progesterone-stimulated acinus contains secretory material in the lumen. Myoepithelial cells are present at the periphery of the acinus.

Lactiferous duct

The lactiferous duct is lined by a two-cell-layered **cuboidal–low columnar epithelium**, sparse **myoepithelial cells**, and a basal lamina.
Myoepithelial cells are vacuolated during the luteal phase (due to glycogen deposits).

Stroma

Dense irregular connective tissue with abundant collagen fibers surrounds the ducts and acini

Active secretory alveoli

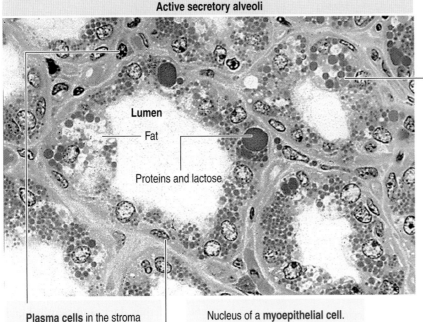

Lumen

Fat

Proteins and lactose

During lactation, alveoli previously formed during pregnancy are lined by a cuboidal epithelium enclosed by the cell processes of myoepithelial cells.
The large and small cytoplasmic masses are proteins and sugars of the milk. The large and small vacuoles are fat deposits.

Lactating mammary gland

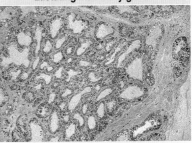

After the brief period of **colostrum** secretion, **transitional milk**, with a lower concentration of IgA and protein, is replaced by **mature milk** (a complex of **protein, milk fat, lactose,** and **water**)

Plasma cells in the stroma secrete immunoglobulin A (IgA) to be transported by transcytosis into the lumen of the alveoli

Nucleus of a **myoepithelial cell**. Myoepithelial cells are 10 to 20 times more sensitive to oxytocin than myometrial smooth muscle cells

thelial cells, which migrate to the basal region of the lining epithelium. Bipotent stem cells are long-lived. They still persist in the adult mammary gland where they participate in homeostasis and morphogenesis (see below).

The epithelium of the lactiferous duct of the mammary glands of newborns of both sexes can respond to maternal hormones and may produce a secretion containing α-lactalbumin, fat, and leukocytes. This secretion is called "witch's milk." In most cases, the simple embryonic-fetal mammary duct system remains unchanged in the infant until the onset of puberty.

In the **male fetus**, the developing duct system undergoes **involution in the presence of testosterone**. The role of the mesoderm and testosterone receptors is well demonstrated in the **androgen insensitivity syndrome** (**testicular feminization syndrome;** see later).

Mammary glands during puberty and pregnancy

At **puberty** (see Figure 23-16), circulating **estrogen**

Figure 23-18. **Function of the mammary alveolar cell**

Lactation and milk composition

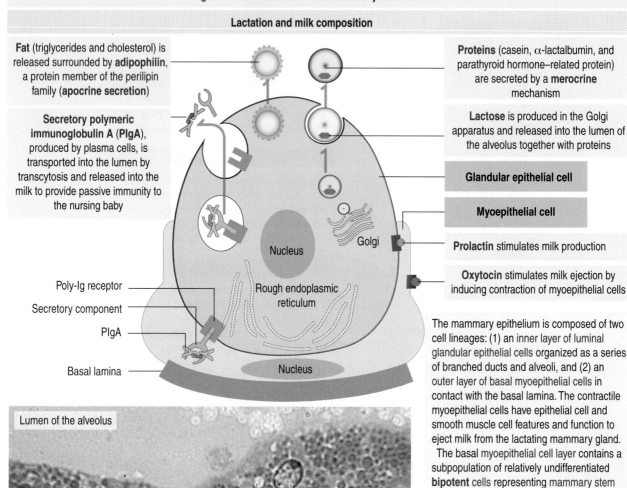

Fat (triglycerides and cholesterol) is released surrounded by **adipophilin**, a protein member of the perilipin family (**apocrine secretion**)

Secretory polymeric immunoglobulin A (PIgA), produced by plasma cells, is transported into the lumen by transcytosis and released into the milk to provide passive immunity to the nursing baby

Poly-Ig receptor

Secretory component

PIgA

Basal lamina

Nucleus

Rough endoplasmic reticulum

Nucleus

Golgi

Proteins (casein, α-lactalbumin, and parathyroid hormone–related protein) are secreted by a **merocrine** mechanism

Lactose is produced in the Golgi apparatus and released into the lumen of the alveolus together with proteins

Glandular epithelial cell

Myoepithelial cell

Prolactin stimulates milk production

Oxytocin stimulates milk ejection by inducing contraction of myoepithelial cells

The mammary epithelium is composed of two cell lineages: (1) an inner layer of luminal glandular epithelial cells organized as a series of branched ducts and alveoli, and (2) an outer layer of basal myoepithelial cells in contact with the basal lamina. The contractile myoepithelial cells have epithelial cell and smooth muscle cell features and function to eject milk from the lactating mammary gland.

The basal myoepithelial cell layer contains a subpopulation of relatively undifferentiated **bipotent** cells representing mammary stem cells forming **mammary repopulating units (MRUs)**. MRUs can generate the basal and luminal components of ductal-alveolar outgrowths in multiple pregnancies. Another population of **unipotent** stem cells regulates homeostasis of the mammary gland ducts by contributing only to the myoepithelial cell layer.

Lumen of the alveolus

Basal lamina

Nucleus of a myoepithelial cell

Fat

Nucleus of an alveolar cell

Proteins and lactose

Box 23-G | Lactation

- Colostrum: early milk (called fore milk) with a lower fat concentration but higher concentration of proteins and minerals. The fat content increases over the next several minutes (mature milk or hind milk).
- Milk: a unique species-specific fluid with nutritive, immunologic, and growth-promoting components.
- Lipids are surrounded by a rim of adiphophilin protein (a member of the perilipin family). Adipophilin becomes a stabilizing interface between fat and the aqueous components of the milk. The cytosol interface allows controlled lipolysis and formation of a micellar aqueous suspension useful for absorption in the small intestine. Lipids include cholesterol, triglycerides, short-chain fatty acids, and long-chain polyunsaturated fatty acids.
- Immunoglobulins: the most abundant immunoglobulin is secretory dimeric immunoglobulin A (IgA). It provides passive acquired defense for several weeks before the baby can produce its own secretory IgA in the small intestine.
- Protective functions of human milk: Milk contains lactoferrin, lysozyme, oligo-saccharides, and mucins. These components enable some intestinal bacteria to become established while others are inhibited.

(in the presence of prolactin) stimulates the development of the **lactiferous ducts and terminal end buds** as well as the enlargement of the surrounding **fat tissue**.

This developmental process is highly regulated by paracrine pathways between duct and terminal bud epithelial cells and cells of the surrounding connective tissue (fibroblasts and adipose cells) and cells of the immune system.

The terminal end buds drive the extension of the mammary gland tissue toward the fat pad. Once the terminal end buds reach the edge of the fat pad, they stop cell proliferation and differentiate into terminal ducts.

The terminal end bud is composed of a **body segment**, consisting of a highly proliferative **cap** and **body bipotent cells** that differentiate into the **luminal**

Figure 23-19. Breast cancer

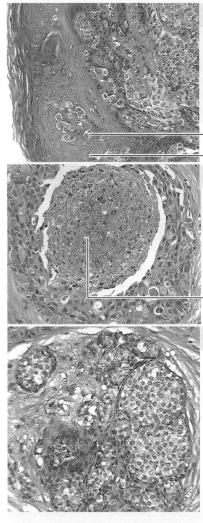

Paget's carcinoma

Paget's carcinoma extends from the lactiferous ducts in the nipple into the adjacent skin of the nipple and areola. Cancerous cells, called **Paget's cells**, invade the epidermis.

— Paget's cells

— Epidermis

Intraductal carcinoma

Intraductal carcinoma consists of cancerous cells proliferating within lactiferous ducts. The tumoral proliferation sites usually have a necrotic center ("comedone-like").

— Central necrosis

Lobular carcinoma

Breast tumors arise in the ductal epithelium (90%) or within the lobular alveolar–ductal epithelium (10%).

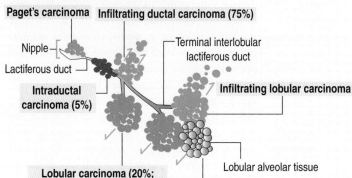

Paget's carcinoma   **Infiltrating ductal carcinoma (75%)**

Nipple —
Lactiferous duct —

Intraductal carcinoma (5%)

Terminal interlobular lactiferous duct

Infiltrating lobular carcinoma

Lobular carcinoma (20%; bilateral multifocal incidence)

Lobular alveolar tissue

glandular epithelial cells and outer **myoepithelial cells** of the duct segment. The **duct segment** displays an inner layer of glandular epithelial cells overlapping the myoepithelial cell layer.

Epithelial cells lining the lactiferous ducts contain cytosolic and nuclear **estrogen receptors**. **Progesterone** stimulates the formation of new terminal end buds, replacing old, regressing buds by apoptosis, which eventually disappear at the end of the ovar-

ian cycle. These cyclic changes are observed in each menstrual cycle.

During **pregnancy** (see Figure 23-16), prolactin and placental lactogen, in the presence of estrogen, progesterone, and growth factors, stimulate the **development of lactiferous ducts** and **secretory alveoli** at the ends of the branched ducts from lateral and terminal end buds.

The induction of the **transcription factor Elf-5 by prolactin** is critical for the differentiation of luminal epithelial cells into the milk producing alveolar cells.

During **lactation**, the lactiferous duct system and the lobular alveolar tissue are fully developed and functional. Myoepithelial cells constrict the alveolar cells to pump milk down the ducts to the nipple.

Histology of the mammary glands

Each mammary gland consists of the following components:

1. A inner layer of **glandular epithelial cells**, organized as a branching system of **lactiferous ducts** ending, when functional, in **secretory alveoli**.

2. **Myoepithelial cells**, surrounding the epithelial lining of the lactiferous ducts and secretory alveoli. A continuous basement membrane encloses the outer layer of myoepithelial cells and the inner layer of glandular epithelial cells (Figure 23-17). The contractile myoepithelial cells have epithelial cell and smooth muscle cell features. They function to eject milk from the lactating mammary gland.

The relevant **regenerative capacity of the mammary glands** evident on successive rounds of pregnancy implies the presence of renewable stem cells. A high proportion of myoepithelial cells are regarded mammary stem cells, giving rise to **bipotent mammary repopulating units (MRUs)**. MRUs produce the basal myoepithelial cells and the luminal glandular epithelial cells of the mammary ducts and alveoli (Figure 23-18). Another population of mammary stem cells of the myoepithelial lineage is **unipotent** and contribute only to the myoepithelial basal cell layer. The definition of bipotent and unipotent stem cells is useful for identifying cells-of-origin and potential biomarkers in breast cancer.

3. A **stroma**, where subcutaneous connective tissue interacts with white adipose tissue.

Each lactiferous duct opens at the tip of the **nipple** in the form of **lactiferous sinuses**.

An epidermic keratinizing stratified squamous epithelium lines the outer surface of the lactiferous ducts. Sebaceous glands discharge their product into the lactiferous ducts.

The **areola** contains melanocytes, sebaceous glands and sweat glands. The stroma of the nipple and areola contains dense irregular connective tissue, bundles of elastic fibers and abundant smooth muscle fibers in a circular and radial distribution.

As previously indicated, a cluster of secretory alveoli drained by a lactiferous duct forms a **lobule**. Figures 23-17 and 23-18 provide a summary of the most relevant histologic and developmental features of the inactive and active mammary gland.

Suckling during lactation

A **neural stimulus** at the nipple resulting from **suckling** determines:

1. The ejection of milk by the release of oxytocin. Oxytocin causes contraction of myoepithelial cells surrounding the alveoli.

2. The inhibition of the release of **luteinizing hormone–releasing factor** by the hypothalamus, resulting in the temporary **arrest of ovulation**.

Milk contains (see Figure 23-18; see Box 23-G):

1. **Proteins** (**casein**, α-**lactalbumin**, and large amounts of **parathyroid hormone–related protein [PTH-RP]**), released by **merocrine secretion** together with lactose.

2. **Lipids** (**triglycerides** and **cholesterol**), released by **apocrine secretion**. Lipid droplets are surrounded by the protein **adipophilin**, a member of the perilipin family.

3. **Sugar** (in particular **lactose,** produced in the Golgi apparatus from glucose and uridine diphosphogalactose). Lactose osmotically draws water into secretory vesicles, a process that accounts for the large volume of milk.

In addition, **plasma cells** present in the stroma surrounding the alveolar tissue secrete **polymeric IgA**. Polymeric IgA is taken up by alveolar cells and transported to the lumen by a mechanism similar to that discussed in Chapter 16, Lower Digestive Segment.

After nursing, prolactin secretion decreases, the mammary alveoli regress, and the lactiferous duct system returns to its normal nonpregnant stage within several months.

Pathology: Benign breast diseases and breast cancer

Each of the structures of the mammary gland (ducts and alveoli) can be the source of a pathologic condition. We have seen how many paracrine pathways and bipotent and unipotent stem cells are involved in the development and differentiation of the mammary glands. Genes participating in these processes may be deregulated during breast carcinogenesis.

Fibrocystic changes are the most common of all benign mammary gland conditions in 20- to 40-year-old patients. Hormonal imbalances are associated with fibrocystic changes. In this condition, a proliferation of the connective tissue stroma and cystic formation of the ducts are observed.

Pain (**mastalgia**) tends to be cyclic as cysts expand rapidly.

Fibroadenoma, the second most common form of benign breast disease, occurs in young women (20 to 30 years old). Fibroadenomas are slow-growing masses of epithelial and connective tissues and are painless.

Gynecomastia, the enlargement of the **male breast**, is caused by a shift in the adrenal cortex estrogen-testis androgen balance. It may be observed during **cirrhosis**, because the liver is responsible for the breakdown of estrogens. Gynecomastia is a typical feature of **Klinefelter's syndrome** (47,XXY).

About 80% of **breast cancers** originate in the epithelial lining of the lactiferous ducts (Figure 23-19). **Epithelial cells lining the lactiferous ducts have estrogen receptors and about 50% to 85% of breast tumors have estrogen receptors.**

There are **two types of estrogen receptors**, α and β. The α receptor has a higher binding affinity for estrogen than the β receptor. The β receptor acts as a physiologic regulator of the α receptor. The expression of the α receptor is higher than the β receptor in invasive tumors than in normal breast tissue. This finding suggests that a balance between the receptors is important in determining the sensitivity of tissue to estrogen and the relative risk of breast tumor development. A large number of estrogen-dependent tumors regress after antiestrogen therapy (treatment with the antiestrogen **tamoxifen**).

The familial inheritance of two autosomal dominant genes, *BRCA1* and *BRCA2*, has been determined in 20% to 30% of patients with breast cancer. *BRCA1* and *BRCA2* encode **tumor suppressor proteins** interacting with other nuclear proteins (see Chapter 3, Cell Signaling, for a discussion on Oncogenes and Tumor Suppressors). Wild-type *BRCA1* can suppress estrogen-dependent transcription pathways related to the proliferation of epithelial cells of the mammary gland. A mutation of *BRCA1* can determine the loss of this ability, facilitating tumorigenesis. Women with *BRCA1* and *BRCA2* mutations have a lifetime risk of invasive breast and ovarian cancer. **Prophylactic bilateral total mastectomy** has been shown to drastically reduce the incidence of breast cancer among women with a *BRCA1* or *BRCA2* mutation.

The mammary gland has a rich blood and lymphatic system, which facilitates metastases. Axillary lymph node metastases are the most important prognostic factor.

Estrogen-replacement therapy in **postmenopausal** women has been implicated as a risk factor for breast cancer. In **premenopausal** women, the ovaries are the predominant source of estrogen. In **postmenopausal** women, estrogen derives predominantly from **aromatization** of adrenal (see Adrenal Gland in Chapter 19, Endocrine System) and ovarian androgens in the liver, muscle, and adipose tissue.

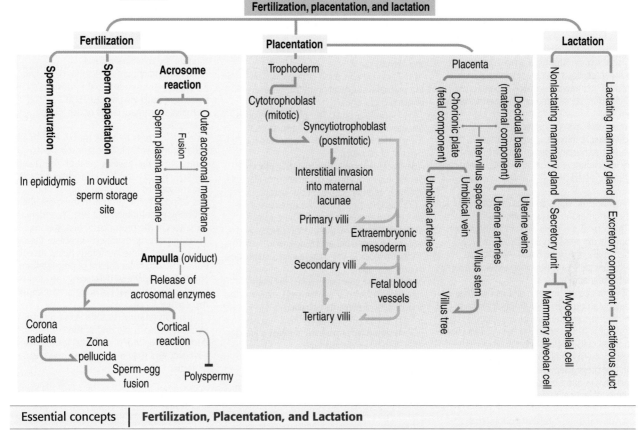

Essential concepts | Fertilization, Placentation, and Lactation

• **Fertilization** encompasses three events:
(1) The acrosome reaction.
(2) Sperm binding to the egg zona pellucida.
(3) Sperm-egg plasma membrane fusion.

As you remember, the acrosome, acroplaxome, and the condensed nucleus are components of the sperm head.

The acrosome contains hydrolytic enzymes (mainly hyaluronidase and proacrosin; the latter gives rise to acrosin during the acrosome reaction).

The acrosome consists of an outer acrosomal membrane facing the plasma membrane, and an inner acrosomal membrane facing the acroplaxome anchored to the nuclear envelope of the condensed sperm nucleus.

The acrosome reaction occurs when the outer acrosomal membrane fuses at different points with the plasma membranes in the presence of Ca^{2+}.

Acrosomal-derived hyaluronidase facilitates sperm penetration across the corona radiata. Acrosin enables sperm penetration of the zona pellucida.

When the first sperm binds to the zona pellucida (consisting of three glycoproteins: ZP1, ZP2, and ZP3), the protease ovastacin is released from the cortical granules located at the periphery of the egg cytoplasm. This event is called cortical reaction.

The following molecules and events are involved in fertilization:

(1) The sperm plasma membrane contains receptors with binding affinity to *O*-oligosaccharides of ZP3.
(2) The first sperm to penetrate the zona pellucida fuses with the eggs plasma membrane. Sperm fusion causes intracellular calcium oscillations in the oocyte in response to a sperm-specific phospholipase C. Ca^{2+}-dependent exocytosis of ovastacin takes place and the conformation of the zona pellucida changes to prevent polyspermy.
(3) Plasma membrane fusion occurs when the sperm protein Izumo1 binds to the egg protein Juno in the presence of the egg plasma membrane protein CD9. Other proteins may be involved.
(4) The Izumo1–Juno complex is sequestered inside a vesicle that is released into the perivitelline space (between the zona pellucida and the plasma membrane of the egg).
(5) Calcium oscillations lead the secondary oocyte to complete meiosis II, release the second polar body, and become haploid.

• **Placentation** starts with the implantation of the blastocyst into the endometrium after the blastocyst hatches from the zona pellucida exposing the trophoblast layer.

Implantation consists in:
(1) The adhesion of the blastocyst to the endometrial surface (a process called apposition).
(2) Apposition is followed by implantation into the decidualized endometrial stroma with

the help of the invasive trophoblast cells. This process is called interstitial invasion.

(3) Uterine receptivity is the optimal state of the endometrium for the implantation of the blastocyst. A primary decidual zone is remodeled into a secondary decidual zone by the action of local matrix metalloproteinases (MMPs) and their tissue inhibitors (TIMPs).

The trophoblast differentiates into:
(1) An inner cell layer, the mitotically dividing cytotrophoblast.
(2) An outer cell layer, the postmitotic syncytiotrophoblast.

Proteolytic enzymes released by the syncytiotrophoblast erode the branches of the spiral uterine arteries, forming lacunae. This event, called endovascular invasion, initiates the uteroplacental circulation. Lacunae represent the starting point of the future intervillous space of the placenta.

Structural differences of the placenta villi:
(1) **Primary villi**, the first step in the development of chorionic villi, are formed at the end of the second week. Primary villi consist of a cytotrophoblast core surrounded by the syncytiotrophoblast layer.
(2) **Secondary villi** are formed early in the third week. Secondary villi consist of a core of extraembryonic mesoderm surrounded by the cytotrophoblast layer in the middle and an outer syncytiotrophoblast layer.
(3) **Tertiary villi** are seen late in the third

week. Tertiary villi have a structure similar to the secondary villus in addition to fetal arteriocapillary networks in the extraembryonic mesoderm.

The **placenta** consists of:
(1) The chorionic plate (fetal component).
(2) The decidua basalis (maternal component). These two components are the boundary of the intervillous space containing maternal blood. The intervillous space is partitioned by decidual septa into compartments, called lobes.

The decidual septa, extending from the decidua basalis into the intervillous space, do not reach the chorionic plate. Therefore, the lobes are incomplete and the intervillous spaces are interconnected.

A **chorionic villus** consists of a stem giving rise to numerous villous branches.

The core of the stem and villous branches contains extraembryonic mesoderm (mesenchymal cells), fetal blood vessels, and Hofbauer cells (a macrophage-like cell seen in early pregnancy).

The surface of the stem and its branches is lined by an outer syncytiotrophoblast layer and an inner cytotrophoblast layer supported by a basal lamina. The apical domain of syncytiotrophoblast cells displays short microvilli extending into the maternal blood space.

In late pregnancy, cytotrophoblast cells decrease in number and disappear and syncytiotrophoblast cells aggregate to form knots.

According to their relation to the fetus, the **decidua** consists of three regions:
(1) Decidua basalis, the maternal component of the placenta.
(2) Decidua capsularis, the superficial layer covering the developing fetus.
(3) Decidua parietalis, covering the uterine cavity not occupied by the fetus.

The **placental barrier** is formed by the syncytiotrophoblast and cytotrophoblast layers supported by a basal lamina and endothelial cells and corresponding basal lamina of the fetal capillaries. Fetal capillaries become closely apposed to the trophoblastic layer. Recall that the population of cytotrophoblast cells decreases with time and syncytiotrophoblast cells aggregate to form knots.

• **Functions of the placenta:**
(1) Exchange of gases by simple diffusion.
(2) Transfer of maternal immunoglobulins.
(3) Production of steroids. Syncytiotrophoblast cells synthesize progesterone, which is transferred to the adrenal cortex for its conversion to weak androgens. Weak androgens are transferred to the syncytiotrophoblast for the conversion to estrogens. The placental–adrenal cortex cooperative mechanism represents the basis for the **fetoplacental unit**.
(4) Synthesis of chorionic gonadotropin (**luteal-placental shift** to maintain the corpus luteum of pregnancy) and placental lactogen (to condition the mammary gland for lactation).
(5) Active transport of ions and glucose.

• **Disorders of the placenta** include:
(1) Ectopic pregnancy, consisting in implantation in the ampulla of the oviduct.
(2) Uterine atony defines weak contractions of the uterine muscle postpartum.
(3) Placenta previa is defined by the abnormal extension of the placenta over or close to the cervical canal.
(4) Placental abruption corresponds to the premature separation of the normally implanted placenta.
(5) Placenta accreta. The placenta invades the uterine wall but does not penetrate the myometrium. This condition, accounts for 75 percent of all cases.
(6) Placenta increta. The invading placenta penetrates through the myometrium. Placenta increta is seen in 15 percent of cases.
(7) Placenta percreta is the extensive invasion of placental villi through the thickness of the myometrium, the uterine serosa, and adjacent organs (urinary bladder and rectum).

Abnormalities in the uterine wall, usually due to previous uterine surgery (such as cesarean section or scar tissue following uterine curettage [Asherman syndrome]), increase the possibilities of placenta accreta.

• **Gestational trophoblastic diseases** are classified into three distinct types:

Hydatidiform mole designates the partial or complete replacement of normal villi by dilated or hydropic (edematous) translucent vesicles. A fetus or embryo is often found in partial hydatidiform mole but no fetus is recognizable in complete hydatidiform mole.

Total moles result from the fertilization of an empty egg (lacking a nucleus) by a haploid sperm that replicates within the egg. High levels of human chorionic gonadotropin (hCG) are characteristic in patients with hydatidiform moles.

Invasive mole is the most frequent form of trophoblastic disease generally diagnosed by persistent high blood levels of hCG. It invades the uterine wall and cannot be detected on evacuated specimens. This condition responds to chemotherapy.

Choriocarcinoma is a malignant neoplasm observed in about 50% of patients with molar pregnancies. Choriocarcinoma is a hemorrhagic tumor in primary and metastatic sites. Treatment with combined chemotherapy agents is usually curative.

• **Lactation** includes the development, structure, and function of the mammary gland. The mammary gland is a branched (compound) organ with lactiferous ducts and tubuloalveolar secretory units forming a lobule in the lactating gland.

A lobe consists of a group of lobules drained by a lactiferous duct. The resting, nonlactating gland is formed by lactiferous ducts, each ending in a group of blind saccular evaginations.

The lactiferous duct is lined by a simple columnar or cuboidal epithelium and a discontinuous layer of myoepithelial cells. Each secretory unit, the alveolus, is lined by the alveolar mammary epithelium and basal myoepithelial cells, both supported by a basal lamina.

• **Development of the mammary gland** (mammogenesis). Placental lactogen, chorionic gonadotropin, and estrogen (produced by syncytiotrophoblast) stimulate the development of the mammary gland.

The mammary bud, an ectodermic epithelial derivative, extends into the mesoderm. Mammary buds give rise to 15 to 25 solid epithelial mammary cords under the influence of estrogens.

Mammary cords become hollow and change into mammary ducts. Bipotent stem cells contribute to the development of alveoli and mammary ducts, the future lactiferous ducts. The mesoderm differentiates into connective and adipose tissue stroma. In the male, the developing mammary duct system undergoes involution in the presence of testosterone.

During **puberty**, estrogens stimulate the development of the lactiferous ducts. Alveolar buds develop under control of progesterone and regress. Epithelial cells lining the lactiferous duct and alveolar buds are precursors of myoepithelial cells.

During **pregnancy** (lactogenesis), lobular alveoli develop at the end of the lactiferous ducts under control of placental lactogen and estrogen, and maternal progesterone and prolactin.

Milk production and ejection. The production of milk in the mammary alveolar cells is controlled by prolactin. The ejection of milk is controlled by oxytocin acting on myoepithelial cells.

Milk contains:
(1) Proteins (casein, α-lactalbumin, parathyroid hormone–related peptide, and others) released by merocrine secretion.
(2) Fat (triglycerides and cholesterol) released by apocrine secretion.
(3) Lactose produced in the Golgi apparatus and released together with proteins.
(4) Secretory polymeric immunoglobulin A (pIgA) produced by plasma cells. PIgA is released into the alveolar lumen by transcytosis.

• **Tumors of the mammary gland.** Benign breast diseases include fibrocystic changes of the lactiferous ducts, and fibroadenoma (masses of epithelial and connective tissue).

Gynecomastia is the enlargement of the male breast.

Breast cancer originates in the epithelial lining of the lactiferous ducts (80%).

Estrogen receptors and the tumor suppressor genes *BRCA1* and *BRCA2* play an important role in breast tumors.

The most frequent breast tumors are the infiltrating duct carcinoma (originating in lactiferous ducts) and lobular carcinoma (derived from the epithelial cells lining the alveolar tissue).

Paget's carcinoma extends from the lactiferous ducts toward the nipple and areola.

Intraductal carcinoma consists of tumor cells growing within the lactiferous duct lumen.